Physical Agents in Rehabilitation

An Evidence-Based Approach to Practice

Physical Agents in Rehabilitation

An Evidence-Based Approach to Practice

Sixth Edition

Michelle H. Cameron, MD, PT, MCR
Professor
Department of Neurology
Oregon Health & Science University
Co-Director
MS Center of Excellence-West
VA Portland Health Care System
Owner
Health Potentials
Portland, Oregon

ELSEVIER

Elsevier

3251 Riverport Lane
St. Louis, Missouri 63043

PHYSICAL AGENTS IN REHABILITATION, SIXTH EDITION   ISBN: 9780323761949

Previous editions copyrighted 2018, 2013, 2009, 2003, and 1999.

Library of Congress Control Number: 2021942177

Senior Content Strategist: Lauren Willis
Senior Content Development Specialists: Melissa Rawe/Laura Klein
Publishing Services Manager: Deepthi Unni
Project Manager: Sindhuraj Thulasingam
Design Direction: Brian Salisbury

Printed in India

Last digit is the print number: 9 8 7 6 5 4 3 2

Working together
to grow libraries in
developing countries

www.elsevier.com • www.bookaid.org

Biography

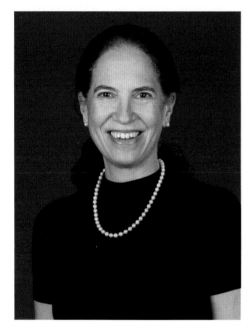

Michelle H. Cameron, MD, PT, MCR, the primary author of *Physical Agents in Rehabilitation: An Evidence-Based Approach to Practice,* is a physical therapist and a physician as well as an educator, researcher, and author. After 10 years working as a clinical physical therapist and teaching rehabilitation providers about physical agents, Michelle furthered her own education through medical training. She now works as a neurologist, focusing on the clinical care of people with multiple sclerosis and on research to optimize mobility in people with multiple sclerosis, while continuing to write, teach about, and do research on the use of physical agents in rehabilitation. Michelle is the co-editor of the texts *Physical Rehabilitation: Evidence-Based Examination, Evaluation, and Intervention* and *Physical Rehabilitation for the Physical Therapist Assistant* and has written and edited many articles on electrical stimulation, ultrasound and phonophoresis, laser light therapy, and wound management. Michelle's discussions of physical agents bring together current research and practice to provide the decision-making and hands-on tools to support optimal care within today's health care environment.

Acknowledgments

First and foremost, I want to thank the instructors who use this book in the classroom and the readers and purchasers of its previous editions. Without you, this book would not exist. In particular, I would like to thank those readers who took the time to contact me with their comments, thoughts, and suggestions about what worked for them and what could be improved.

I would also like to give special thanks to Cassidy Taylor, editorial research assistant, for her help with updating this edition of the book. Her skills and dedication to precision and organization kept me sane and on track and ensured that all the parts and the people came together to make the whole greater than the sum of its parts. I would also like to thank Melissa Rawe and Laura Klein, senior content development specialists at Elsevier, Sindhuraj Thulasingam, project manager at Elsevier, and Lauren Willis, senior content strategist at Elsevier, for their support throughout this project; Diane Allen, Jason Bennett, Tony Rocklin, Bill Rubine, and Gail Widener, contributing authors to this and previous editions, who updated their respective chapters thoroughly and promptly; David Adelson and Erika Hagstrom for their update of Chapter 3 on inflammation and tissue repair; Kimberly Jones who provided insightful updates to Chapter 4 on pain and pain management; Dana Lindberg who contribute to the update of Chapter 5 on tone abnormalities; and particularly Linda Monroe and Michelle Ocelnik, who not only updated their own chapters but also updated and reviewed all the teaching questions and slides that accompany this book.

Thank you all,
Michelle H. Cameron

Contributors

David Adelson, MD, MHCDS
Associate Professor
Department of Dermatology
Oregon Health and Science University
Chief
Dermatology Service
Portland VA Healthcare System
Portland, Oregon

Diane D. Allen, PT, PhD
Professor
Graduate Program in Physical Therapy
University of California San Francisco/San Francisco State
    University
San Francisco, California

Jason E. Bennett, PT, MSPT, PhD, ATC
Board Certified Clinical Specialist in Sports Physical
    Therapy
Assistant Professor
Physical Therapy Department
Carroll University
Waukesha, Wisconsin

Erika Hagstrom, MD
Dermatology
Oregon Health & Science University
Portland, Oregon

Kimberly Dupree Jones, PhD, FNP, FAAN
Dean & Professor
School of Nursing
Linfield University
Portland, Oregon

Dana Lindberg, DPT, CSCS
Doctor of Physical Therapy
Department of Physical Therapy
Samuel Merritt University
Oakland, California

Linda G. Monroe, PT, MPT, OCS
Physical Therapist
John Muir Physical Rehabilitation Services
John Muir Health
Walnut Creek, California;
Adjunct Instructor
Department of Occupational Therapy
Samuel Merritt University
Oakland, California

Michelle Ocelnik, MA, ATC, CSCS
Director of Education and Research
VQ OrthoCare
Irvine, California

Tony Rocklin, PT, DPT, COMT
Therapeutic Associates Downtown Portland Physical
    Therapy
Portland, Oregon

William Rubine, MS, PT
Physical Therapist
Comprehensive Pain Center
Oregon Health and Science University
Portland, Oregon

Ashley L. Shea, MS
Librarian
Albert R. Mann Library
Cornell University
Ithaca, New York

Gail L. Widener, PT, PhD
Professor
Department of Physical Therapy
Samuel Merritt University
Oakland, California

Preface

By writing the first edition of this book, I tried to meet a need that I believed existed—the need for a book on the use of physical agents in rehabilitation that covered the breadth and depth of this material in a readily accessible, systematic, and easily understood manner. I produced a text that leads the reader from the basic scientific and physiological principles underlying the application of physical agents to the research evaluating their clinical use, then to the practical details of selecting and applying each specific physical agent to optimize patient outcomes. The enthusiasm with which the previous editions of this book have been received—including compliments from readers; adoption by many educational programs; translation into multiple languages; and purchase by many clinicians, educators, and students around the world—demonstrates that the need was there and was met.

In all the subsequent editions, I have done my best to keep the most successful aspects from previous editions while bringing the reader new and updated information, further clarifying the presented material, and improving information accessibility. Each edition of this book provides easy-to-follow guidelines for the safe application of all physical agents discussed, as well as the essential scientific rationale and evidence base to select and apply interventions with physical agents safely and effectively. As the quantity of research has increased, along with the quality, this text has become even more important for making clinical decisions. To keep up with the pace of research, new developments in the field of rehabilitation, and technological advances in information delivery, I have added a number of new features to this edition.

The most significant new features in this edition of *Physical Agents in Rehabilitation* are the addition of a chapter on shock wave therapy (Chapter 18); the substantial updating of Chapter 4, on pain; and the reorganization of Chapter 9, on ultrasound, to make it consistent with other chapters, ease access to the information, improve clarity, and maximize comprehension.

In earlier editions, I tried to summarize and reference all the research on the use of each physical agent in rehabilitation. With the exponential growth of research and publication, this became impossible, and with the increased access to information and the growing search skills of clinicians, this has also become unnecessary. This edition focuses on and summarizes only the highest-quality evidence, including the most recent systematic reviews and meta-analyses and subsequent large-scale randomized controlled trials. The case studies then demonstrate how to seek out evidence specific to an individual patient by providing sample MEDLINE search strategies using the Patient, Intervention, Comparison (PICO) framework, followed by summaries of relevant key studies and reviews.

The new chapter on shock wave therapy (Chapter 18) was added in response to consistent feedback and requests from instructors and other readers. Shock wave therapy, which involves the application of brief, high-intensity, focused or radial sound waves, is gaining popularity as a therapeutic agent, particularly in promoting the resolution of chronic tendinopathy and other chronic localized inflammatory conditions. This chapter has the same structure as other chapters in this book and focuses on the use of shock wave therapy for the treatment of chronic musculoskeletal conditions. I am sure you will find it clear and that it meets your needs for a thorough, up-to-date summary of the use of shock wave therapy in rehabilitation.

In addition to the bigger changes, I have also made some smaller but significant changes to this text. I have kept electronic resources for students and practitioners, including PICO charts from the case studies, review questions for each chapter, and the extremely popular *Electrical Stimulation, Ultrasound, and Photobiomodulation (Laser) Handbook*, which has been updated to align with chapter updates and can be printed and used as a clinical quick reference guide. In addition, course instructors have access to PowerPoint slide sets and corresponding Image Collections for each chapter on Evolve (https://evolve.elsevier.com/).

Welcome to the sixth edition of *Physical Agents in Rehabilitation*!

Contents

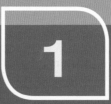

Physical Agents: Essentials

CHAPTER OBJECTIVES

After reading this chapter, the reader will be able to do the following:

- Maximize learning by understanding how to use all of the resources in this book.
- Define *physical agents.*
- List different categories of physical agents.
- Describe the basic effects physical agents have on various indications.
- List general contraindications and precautions for physical agents.
- Evaluate and plan for the use of physical agents.
- Describe attributes to consider when choosing a physical agent.
- Accurately and completely document treatment with physical agents.

How to Use This Book

This book is intended primarily as a course text for those learning to use **physical agents** in **rehabilitation.** It was written to meet the needs of students learning about the theory and practice of applying physical agents and to help practicing rehabilitation professionals review and update their knowledge. This book describes the effects of physical

agents, provides guidelines on when and how physical agents can be most effectively and safely applied and when they should be avoided, and describes the outcomes that can be expected from integrating physical agents within a program of rehabilitation. The book covers the theory underlying the application of each agent and the physiological processes the agent influences, the research concerning its effects, and the rationale for the treatment recommendations. All chapters also include patient case studies with sample online PubMed search strategies used to identify relevant evidence.

After reading this book, the reader should be able to integrate the ideal physical agents and intervention parameters within a complete rehabilitation program to promote optimal patient outcomes. Readers should also feel confident structuring independent search strategies to locate relevant literature in PubMed, a freely accessible, constantly updated search engine that provides access to MEDLINE, a database of biomedical and allied health literature maintained by the U.S. National Library of Medicine.

This book's recommendations regarding the clinical use of physical agents integrate concepts from a variety of sources, including the American Physical Therapy Association's *Guide to Physical Therapist Practice 3.0 (Guide 3.0).*[1] *Guide 3.0* is a normative model of physical therapist professional practice that encompasses the standards for quality assessment; professional conduct, evidence-based practice; and the International Classification of Functioning, Disability and Health (ICF) model of the World Health Organization (WHO). *Guide 3.0* is the most recent edition and is widely used by physical therapists and physical therapist assistants. This book applies the principles of evidence-based practice and the ICF model to guide the selection and application of physical agents. The ICF model (see Fig. 2.1) is used to consider and describe the impact of physical agent interventions on patient outcomes. This model was developed to describe functional abilities and differences and has been adopted globally, particularly among rehabilitation professionals.[2] The specific recommendations presented throughout this book are derived from the best available evidence on the physiological effects and clinical outcomes of physical agents, and the search strategies used to locate the evidence are shared. The book is divided into six parts:

Part I: Introduction to Physical Agents includes this introductory chapter, followed by a chapter introducing the physiological effects of physical agents and their clinical use by various professionals.

Part II: Pathology and Patient Problems starts with a chapter on inflammation and tissue repair, followed by individual chapters on pain, motion restrictions, and tone abnormalities.

Part III: Thermal Agents covers thermal agents, including superficial cold and heat, ultrasound, and diathermy.

Part IV: Electrical Currents starts with a chapter describing the physical properties of electrical currents. This is followed by individual chapters on the use of electrical stimulation for muscle contraction, pain control, and tissue healing and a chapter on electromyographic (EMG) biofeedback.

Part V: Electromagnetic Agents discusses photobiomodulation (previously known as *low-level laser therapy*) and ultraviolet therapy.

Part VI: Mechanical Agents has a new chapter on shock waves, followed by chapters on hydrotherapy, traction, and compression.

The print book includes access to an enhanced eBook with resources for students and practitioners, including PICO charts from the case studies, review questions for each chapter, and the *Electrical Stimulation, Ultrasound, and Photobiomodulation (Laser) Handbook*. In addition, course instructors have access to PowerPoint slide sets and corresponding Image Collections for each chapter on Evolve (https://evolve.elsevier.com/).

What Are Physical Agents?

Physical agents consist of energy and materials applied to patients to assist in their rehabilitation. Physical agents include heat, cold, water, pressure, sound, electromagnetic radiation, and electrical currents. The term *physical agent* can be used to describe the general type of energy, such as electromagnetic radiation or sound; a specific range within the general type, such as **ultraviolet (UV) radiation** or **ultrasound;** and the actual means of applying the energy, such as a UV lamp or an ultrasound transducer. The terms **physical modality,** *biophysical agent, physical agent modality, electrophysical agent,* and **modality** are alternatives for the term *physical agent* and are used interchangeably in this book.

◎ Clinical Pearl

Physical agents are energy and materials applied to patients to assist in their rehabilitation. Physical agents include heat, cold, water, pressure, sound, electromagnetic radiation, and electrical currents.

Categories of Physical Agents

Physical agents can be categorized as thermal, electromagnetic, or mechanical (Table 1.1). **Thermal agents** include superficial-heating agents, deep-heating agents, and superficial-cooling agents. **Electromagnetic agents** include electromagnetic fields and electrical currents. **Mechanical agents** include **sound waves,** water, **traction,** and **compression.** Some physical agents fall into more than one category. Water and ultrasound, for example, can have mechanical and thermal effects.

TABLE 1.1	Categories of Physical Agents	
Category	**Types**	**Clinical Examples**
Thermal	Superficial heating agents	Hot pack, paraffin
	Deep-heating agents	Ultrasound, diathermy
	Cooling agents	Ice pack
Electromagnetic	Electrical currents	TENS
	Electromagnetic fields	Ultraviolet, laser
Mechanical	Sound	Ultrasound, shock waves
	Water	Whirlpool
	Traction	Mechanical traction
	Compression	Elastic bandage, stockings

TENS, Transcutaneous electrical nerve stimulation.

THERMAL AGENTS

Thermal agents transfer energy to a patient to increase or decrease tissue temperature. Examples of thermal agents are hot packs, ice packs, ultrasound, whirlpools, and **diathermy. Cryotherapy** is the therapeutic application of cold. **Thermotherapy** is the therapeutic application of heat. Depending on the thermal agent and the body part to which it is applied, temperature changes may be superficial or deep and may affect one type of tissue more than another. For example, a hot pack produces the greatest temperature increase in superficial tissues with high thermal conductivity in the area directly below it. In contrast, ultrasound produces heat in deeper tissues and produces the most heat in tissues with high **collagen** content and thus high ultrasound absorption coefficients, such as tendon and bone. Diathermy, which involves applying shortwave or microwave electromagnetic energy, heats deep tissues having high electrical conductivity.

Thermotherapy is used to increase circulation, metabolic rate, and soft tissue extensibility or to decrease **pain.** Cryotherapy is applied to decrease circulation, metabolic rate, or pain. A full discussion of the principles underlying the processes of heat transfer; the methods of heat transfer used in rehabilitation; and the effects, **indications,** and **contraindications** for applying superficial heating and cooling agents is provided in Chapter 8. The principles and practice of applying deep-heating agents are discussed in Chapter 9 in the section on thermal applications of ultrasound and in Chapter 10 in the section on diathermy.

Ultrasound is a physical agent that has both thermal and nonthermal effects. *Ultrasound* is defined as sound with a frequency greater than 20,000 cycles/second (i.e., >20,000 hertz [Hz])—too high to be heard by humans. Ultrasound is a mechanical form of energy composed of alternating compression and rarefaction waves. Thermal effects, including increased deep- and superficial-tissue temperature, are produced by continuous ultrasound waves of sufficient intensity, and nonthermal effects are produced by both continuous and **pulsed ultrasound.** Continuous ultrasound is used to heat deep tissues to increase circulation, metabolic rate, and soft tissue extensibility and to decrease pain. Pulsed ultrasound is used to facilitate tissue healing or to promote transdermal drug penetration by nonthermal mechanisms. Further information on the theory and practice of applying ultrasound is provided in Chapter 9.

ELECTROMAGNETIC AGENTS

Electromagnetic agents apply energy in the form of an electrical current or electromagnetic radiation. Agents that use electromagnetic radiation include **infrared (IR) radiation,** light (via **photobiomodulation),** UV radiation, and diathermy.

Electrical currents can be used to induce muscle contractions (motor-level **electrical stimulation [ES]**) and changes in sensation (sensory-level ES), reduce edema, or accelerate tissue healing. The effects and clinical applications of electrical currents vary according to the waveform, intensity, duration, and direction of the current flow and according to the type of tissue to which the current is applied. Electrical currents of sufficient intensity and duration can depolarize nerves, causing sensory or motor responses that may be used to control pain or increase muscle strength and control. Electrical currents with an appropriate direction of flow can attract or repel charged particles and alter cell membrane permeability to control the formation of edema, promote tissue healing, and facilitate transdermal drug delivery. Muscle contractions are associated with changes in ionic activity. This activity can be detected by EMG electrodes placed on the skin and can be fed back to the patient to facilitate or inhibit muscle activity. This is known as *EMG biofeedback.* Further information on the theory and practice of electrical current and EMG biofeedback application is provided in Chapters 11–15.

Electromagnetic radiation can be applied at different frequencies and intensities to produce differing effects at different depths of penetration. For example, IR radiation, which has a frequency of 10^{11} to 10^{14} Hz, produces heat in superficial tissues, whereas UV radiation, which has a frequency of 7.5×10^{14} to 10^{15} Hz, produces erythema and tanning of the skin but does not produce heat. **Lasers** output monochromatic, coherent, directional electromagnetic radiation, and therapeutic laser light is generally in the frequency range of visible light or IR radiation. Continuous shortwave diathermy, which has a frequency of 10^5 to 10^6 Hz, produces heat in superficial and deep tissues. When shortwave diathermy is pulsed (pulsed shortwave diathermy [PSWD]) to provide a low average intensity of energy, it does not produce heat and is known as **nonthermal shortwave therapy (SWT).** SWT is thought to modify cell membrane permeability and cell function by nonthermal mechanisms and thereby control pain and edema. Further information on the theory and practice of photobiomodulation using lasers and other forms of light is provided in Chapter 16. UV radiation and diathermy are discussed in Chapters 17 and 10, respectively.

MECHANICAL AGENTS

Mechanical agents apply force to increase or decrease pressure on the body. Examples of mechanical agents are water, traction and compression, and sound. Water can provide resistance, hydrostatic pressure, and buoyancy for exercise or can apply pressure to clean wounds. Traction decreases the pressure between structures, whereas compression increases the pressure on and between structures. Sound may be applied in the form of ultrasound or shock waves. Both ultrasound and shock waves are compression-rarefaction waves. Ultrasound, as discussed in the section on thermal agents, is high-frequency sound, above 20,000 Hz. In contrast, shock waves are low-frequency sound waves, generally at 1 to 10 Hz, with high, asymmetric compression-rarefaction.

The therapeutic use of water is called **hydrotherapy.** Water can be applied with or without immersion. Immersion in water increases pressure around the immersed area; provides buoyancy; and, if there is a difference in temperature between the immersed area and the water, transfers heat to or from that area. Movement of water produces local pressure that can be used as resistance for exercise when an area is immersed and for cleansing or debriding open wounds with or without immersion. Further information on the theory and practice of hydrotherapy, as well as on negative-pressure wound therapy, is provided in Chapter 19.

Traction is the application of a pulling mechanical force. Traction is most commonly used to alleviate pressure on structures, such as nerves or joints, that produce pain or other sensory changes, or that become inflamed, when compressed. Traction can normalize sensation and prevent or reduce damage or **inflammation** of compressed structures. The pressure-relieving effects of traction may be temporary or permanent, depending on the nature of the underlying **pathology** and the force, duration, and means of applying traction. Further information on the theory and practice of applying traction to the spine and the hips is provided in Chapter 20.

Compression is the application of a compressing mechanical force. Compression is used to counteract fluid pressure and to control or reverse edema. The force, duration, and means of applying compression can be varied to control the magnitude of the effect and to accommodate different patient needs. Further information on the theory and practice of applying compression is provided in Chapter 21.

Because ultrasound is used to heat tissues, it is covered in the discussion of thermal agents. Shock waves, also known as *pressure waves,* are asymmetric compression-rarefaction waves with a frequency of between 1 and 10 Hz produced by pneumatic compression. Shock waves alter cell membrane permeability, thereby modifying inflammation and tissue healing. Shock waves are discussed in detail in Chapter 18.

Effects of Physical Agents

Physical agents primarily reduce tissue inflammation, accelerate tissue healing, relieve pain, modify **muscle tone,** or alter collagen extensibility. A brief review of these processes and tables that summarize the physical agents that modify each of these conditions follow. More complete discussions of the physiological processes affected by physical agents are provided in Chapters 3 through 6, and a full discussion of each of the physical agents is provided in Chapters 7 through 21.

TABLE 1.2	Physical Agents for Promoting Tissue Healing		
Stage of Tissue Healing	**Goals of Treatment**	**Effective Agents**	**Contraindicated Agents**
Initial injury	Prevent further injury or bleeding	Static compression, cryotherapy	Exercise
			Intermittent traction
			Motor-level ES
			Thermotherapy
	Clean open wound	Hydrotherapy (immersion or nonimmersion)	
Chronic inflammation	Prevent/decrease joint stiffness	Thermotherapy	Cryotherapy
		Motor ES	
		Shock waves	
		Whirlpool	
		Fluidotherapy	
	Control pain	Thermotherapy	Cryotherapy
		ES	
		Shock waves	
		Photobiomodulation	
	Increase circulation	Thermotherapy	
		ES	
		Compression	
		Hydrotherapy (immersion or exercise)	
	Progress to proliferation stage	Pulsed ultrasound	
		ES	
		SWT	
		Shock waves	
Remodeling	Regain or maintain strength	Motor ES	Immobilization
		Water exercise	
		EMG biofeedback	
	Regain or maintain flexibility	Thermotherapy	Immobilization
	Control scar tissue formation	Brief ice massage	
		Compression	

EMG, Electromyographic; *ES,* electrical stimulation; *SWT,* nonthermal shortwave therapy.

INFLAMMATION AND TISSUE HEALING

When tissue is damaged, it usually responds predictably. Inflammation is the first phase of recovery, followed by the proliferation and **maturation phases**. Modifying this healing process can accelerate rehabilitation and reduce adverse effects from prolonged inflammation, pain, and disuse. This in turn leads to improved function and more rapid achievement of therapeutic goals. The stages of tissue healing are described in detail in Chapter 3. The selection of physical agents to optimize tissue healing based on the stage of healing is summarized in Table 1.2.

Thermal agents modify inflammation and healing by changing the rates of circulation and chemical reactions. Mechanical agents control motion and alter fluid flow, and electromagnetic agents alter cell function, particularly membrane permeability and transport. Many physical agents affect inflammation and healing, and when appropriately applied, they can accelerate progress, limit adverse consequences of the healing process, and optimize the final patient outcome. However, when poorly selected or misapplied, physical agents may impair or potentially prevent complete healing.

PAIN

Pain is an unpleasant sensory and emotional experience associated with actual or threatened tissue damage. This text follows the recommendations of the International Association for the Study of Pain, considering pain to be a dynamic and multidimensional experience involving an idiosyncratic interaction of biological, physical, psychological, social, and environmental factors.[3] Because pain is complex and multifactorial, the reasoning behind the application of physical agents to pain management can also be somewhat complex. Different physical agents have specific and often beneficial effects on tissues, but they also have nonspecific sensory, cognitive, and emotional effects on patients that should also be accounted for. The selection of physical agents for managing pain at various stages and of various etiologies is summarized in Table 1.3.

Chapter 4 describes the physiology of pain and makes evidence-based recommendations for acute pain management, for reducing the probability of acute pain becoming chronic, for a mechanism-based approach to evaluating and managing common presentations of chronic pain, and for applying physical agents as part of palliative care.

TABLE 1.3	Physical Agents for the Treatment of Pain		
Type of Pain	**Goals of Treatment**	**Effective Agents**	**Contraindicated Agents**
Acute	Control pain	Sensory ES, cryotherapy	
	Control inflammation	Cryotherapy	Thermotherapy
	Prevent aggravation of pain	Immobilization, EMG biofeedback	Local exercise, motor ES
		Low-load static traction	
Referred	Control pain	ES, cryotherapy, thermotherapy	
Spinal radicular	Decrease nerve root compression and inflammation	Traction	
Pain caused by malignancy	Control pain	ES, cryotherapy, superficial thermotherapy	

EMG, Electromyographic; *ES,* electrical stimulation.

MUSCLE TONE

Muscle tone is the underlying tension that serves as the background for the contraction of a muscle. Muscle tone is affected by neural and biomechanical factors and can vary in response to pathology, expected demand, pain, position, and physical agents. Abnormal muscle tone is usually the direct result of nerve pathology or may be a secondary sequela of pain that results from injury to other tissues.

Central nervous system injury, as may occur with head trauma or stroke, can result in increased or decreased muscle tone in the affected area, whereas peripheral motor nerve injury, as may occur with nerve compression, traction, or sectioning, can decrease muscle tone in the affected area. Pain may also increase or decrease muscle tone to protect injured tissue.

Processes underlying changes in muscle tone are discussed fully in Chapter 5.

> **Clinical Pearl**
>
> Physical agents can alter muscle tone directly by altering nerve conduction, nerve sensitivity, or the biomechanical properties of muscle or indirectly by reducing pain or the underlying cause of pain.

Physical agents can alter muscle tone directly by altering nerve conduction, nerve sensitivity, or the biomechanical properties of muscle or indirectly by reducing pain or the underlying cause of pain, as summarized in Table 1.4.

COLLAGEN EXTENSIBILITY AND MOTION RESTRICTIONS

Collagen is the main supportive protein of skin, tendon, bone cartilage, and connective tissue. Tissues that contain collagen can become shortened as a result of being immobilized in a shortened position or being moved through a limited range of motion (ROM). To return soft tissue to its normal functional length and thereby allow full motion without damaging other structures, the collagen must be stretched. Collagen can be stretched most effectively and safely when it is most extensible. Because the extensibility of collagen increases in response to increased temperature, thermal agents are frequently applied before soft tissue stretching to optimize stretching (Fig. 1.1).[4–7] Processes underlying the development and treatment of motion restrictions are discussed in Chapter 6.

Physical agents can be effective adjuncts to the treatment of motion restrictions caused by muscle weakness, pain, soft tissue shortening, or a bony block; however, appropriate interventions for these different sources of motion restriction vary (Table 1.5).

> **Clinical Pearl**
>
> Physical agents can be effective adjuncts to the treatment of motion restrictions caused by muscle weakness, pain, soft tissue shortening, or a bony block.

General Contraindications and Precautions for Physical Agent Use

Restrictions on the use of particular treatment interventions are categorized as contraindications or **precautions.** Contraindications are conditions under which a particular treatment should not be applied, and precautions are conditions under which a particular form of treatment should be applied with special care or limitations. The terms *absolute contraindications* and *relative contraindications*

TABLE 1.4	Physical Agents for the Treatment of Tone Abnormalities		
Tone Abnormality	**Goals of Treatment**	**Effective Agents**	**Contraindicated Agents**
Hypertonicity	Decrease tone	Neutral warmth, prolonged cryotherapy, or EMG biofeedback to hypertonic muscles	Quick ice of agonists
		Motor ES or quick ice of antagonists	
Hypotonicity	Increase tone	Quick ice, motor ES, or EMG biofeedback to agonists	Thermotherapy
Fluctuating tone	Normalize tone	Functional ES	

EMG, Electromyographic; *ES,* electrical stimulation.

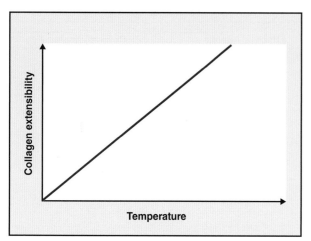

FIGURE 1.1 Changes in collagen extensibility in response to changes in temperature.

can be used in place of *contraindications* and *precautions,* respectively.

Although contraindications and precautions for the application of specific physical agents vary, several conditions are contraindications or precautions for the use of most physical agents. Therefore, caution should be used when applying a physical agent to a patient having any of these conditions. In patients with such conditions, the nature of the restriction, the nature and distribution of the physiological effects of the physical agent, and the distribution of energy produced by the physical agent must be considered.

PREGNANCY

Pregnancy is generally a contraindication or precaution for the application of a physical agent if the energy produced by that agent or its physiological effects may reach the fetus. These restrictions apply because the influences of these types of energy on fetal development usually are unknown and because fetal development is adversely affected by many influences, some of which are subtle.

✳ CONTRAINDICATIONS
for Application of a Physical Agent

- Pregnancy
- Malignancy
- Pacemaker or other implanted electronic device
- Impaired sensation
- Impaired mentation

MALIGNANCY

Malignancy is generally a contraindication or precaution for the application of physical agents if the energy produced by the agent or its physiological effects may reach malignant tissue or alter the circulation to such tissue. Some physical agents are known to accelerate the growth, or metastasis, of malignant tissue. These effects are thought to result from increased circulation or altered cellular function. Care must be taken when considering treatment on any area of the body that currently has or previously had cancer cells because malignant tissue can metastasize and therefore may be present in areas where it has not yet been detected.

PACEMAKER OR OTHER IMPLANTED ELECTRONIC DEVICE

The use of a physical agent is generally contraindicated when the energy of the agent can reach a pacemaker or any other implanted electronic device (e.g., deep brain stimulator, spinal cord stimulator, implanted cardioverter defibrillator) because the energy produced by some of these agents may alter the functioning of the device.

IMPAIRED SENSATION AND MENTATION

Impaired sensation and mentation are contraindications or precautions for the use of many physical agents because the limit for application of these agents is the patient's report of how they feel. For example, for most thermal agents, the patient's report of the sensation of heat as comfortable or painful is used to guide the intensity of treatment. If the patient

---

TABLE 1.5	Physical Agents for the Treatment of Motion Restrictions		
Source of Motion Restriction	**Goals of Treatment**	**Effective Agents**	**Contraindicated Agents**
Muscle weakness	Increase muscle strength	Water exercise, motor ES, EMG biofeedback	Immobilization
Pain			
At rest and with motion	Control pain	ES, cryotherapy, thermotherapy, SWT, spinal traction, EMG biofeedback	Exercise
With motion only	Control pain	ES, cryotherapy, thermotherapy, SWT	Exercise into pain
	Promote tissue healing	Ultrasound, ES, SWT, shock waves	
Soft tissue shortening	Increase tissue extensibility	Thermotherapy	Prolonged cryotherapy
	Increase tissue length	Thermotherapy or brief ice massage and stretch	
Bony block	Remove block	None	Stretching blocked joint
	Compensate	Exercise	
		Thermotherapy or brief ice massage and stretch	

EMG, Electromyographic; *ES,* electrical stimulation; *SWT,* nonthermal shortwave therapy.

cannot feel heat or pain because of impaired sensation or cannot report this sensation accurately and consistently because of impaired mentation or other factors affecting their ability to communicate, applying the treatment is not safe and therefore is contraindicated.

Although these conditions indicate the need for caution with the use of most physical agents, the specific contraindications and precautions for the agent being considered and the patient's situation must be evaluated before an intervention may be used or should be rejected. For example, although applying ultrasound to a pregnant patient is contraindicated in any area where the ultrasound may reach the fetus, this physical agent may be applied to the distal extremities of a pregnant patient because ultrasound penetration is shallow and limited to the area close to the applicator. In contrast, it is recommended that diathermy not be applied to any part of a pregnant patient because the electromagnetic radiation it produces reaches areas distant from the applicator. Specific contraindications and precautions, including questions to ask the patient and features to assess before the application of each physical agent, are provided in Parts III through VI of this book.

Evaluation and Planning for the Use of Physical Agents

Physical agents have direct effects primarily at the level of impairment. These effects can improve activity and participation. For example, for a patient with pain that impairs motion, electrical currents can be used to stimulate sensory nerves to control pain and allow the patient to increase motion and thus increase activity, such as lifting objects, and participation, such as returning to work. Physical agents can also increase the effectiveness of other interventions and should generally be used to facilitate an active treatment program.[8] For example, a hot pack may be applied before stretching to increase the extensibility of superficial soft tissues and promote a safer and more effective increase in soft tissue length when the patient stretches.

When considering the application of a physical agent, one should first check the physician's referral, if one is required, for a medical diagnosis of the patient's condition and any necessary precautions. Precautions are conditions under which a particular treatment should be applied with special care or limitations. The therapist's examination should include, but should not be limited to, the patient's history, which would include information about the history of the current complaint, relevant medical history, and information about current and expected levels of activity and participation; a review of systems; and specific tests and measures. Examination findings and a survey of available evidence in the published literature should be considered in tandem to establish a prognosis and select the interventions and a plan of care, including anticipated goals. This plan may be modified as indicated through ongoing reexamination and reevaluation. The process of staying abreast of the latest clinical evidence is discussed in more detail in Chapter 2, and the sequence of examination, evaluation, and intervention follows in the case studies described in Parts II through VI of this book.

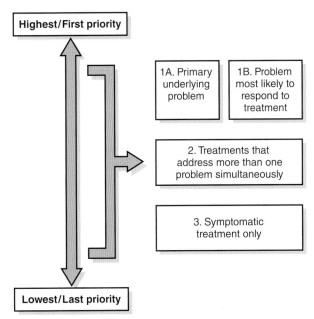

FIGURE 1.2 Prioritizing goals and effects of treatment.

CHOOSING A PHYSICAL AGENT

Physical agents generally assist in rehabilitation by reducing inflammation, pain, and motion restrictions; healing tissue; and improving muscle tone. Guidelines for selecting appropriate interventions based on the direct effects of physical agents are presented here in narrative form and are summarized in Tables 1.2 through 1.5. If the patient presents with more than one problem and so has numerous goals for treatment, only a limited number of goals should be addressed at any one time. It is generally recommended that the primary problems and problems most likely to respond to available interventions should be addressed first; however, the ideal intervention will facilitate progress in a number of areas (Fig. 1.2). For example, if a patient has knee pain caused by acute joint inflammation, treatment should first be directed at resolving the inflammation; however, the ideal intervention would also help to relieve pain. When the primary underlying problem, such as arthritis, cannot benefit directly from intervention with a physical agent, treatment with physical agents may still be used to help alleviate sequelae of these problems, such as pain or swelling.

ATTRIBUTES TO CONSIDER IN THE SELECTION OF PHYSICAL AGENTS

Given the variety of available physical agents and the unique characteristics of each patient, it is helpful to take a systematic approach to selecting the physical agents so that the ideal agent will be applied in each situation (Fig. 1.3).

The first consideration should be the goals of the intervention and the physiological effects required to reach these goals. If the patient has inflammation or delayed tissue healing, pain, problems with muscle tone, or motion restrictions, the use of a physical agent may be appropriate. Looking at the evidence for the effects of a particular physical agent on these conditions is the next step. For example, heat can help during the remodeling phase of healing by promoting increased tissue extensibility and may also temporarily alleviate pain to allow for more activity. Having determined which

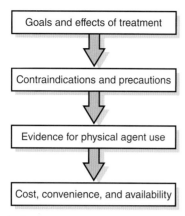

FIGURE 1.3 Attributes to consider when selecting physical agents.

physical agents can promote progress toward determined goals, the clinician should then determine what tissue is affected and then which type of energy is best absorbed by this affected tissue. For example, if a deep tendon is affected, continuous ultrasound would be an appropriate way to provide heat because ultrasound penetrates deeply and is absorbed by tissues with high collagen content. In contrast, if a superficial muscle is affected, a hot pack would be an appropriate way to provide heat because the heat from a hot pack only reaches superficially and is best absorbed by tissues with high water content.

After determining the goals of treatment, physiological effects to achieve these goals, what tissue type is affected, and which type of energy is best absorbed by this type of tissue, the provider should evaluate for contraindications and precautions. Contraindicated interventions should be rejected and all precautions adhered to. If several methods could be effective and applied safely, the ease and cost of application and the availability of resources should also be considered. After selecting physical agents, the clinician should also select the ideal treatment parameters and means of application using the same principles as they used to select the agents. They must then appropriately integrate the chosen agents into a complete rehabilitation program.

USING PHYSICAL AGENTS WITH EACH OTHER AND WITH OTHER INTERVENTIONS

To progress toward the goals of intervention, a number of physical agents may be used simultaneously and/or sequentially. Because physical agents are adjuncts to other therapeutic interventions, they are usually applied in conjunction with or during the same treatment session as other interventions. Interventions are generally combined when they have similar effects or when they address different aspects of a common array of symptoms. For example, splinting, ice, pulsed ultrasound, photobiomodulation, SWT, and phonophoresis or iontophoresis may be used during the acute inflammation phase of healing. Splinting can limit further injury; ice may control pain and limit circulation; pulsed ultrasound, photobiomodulation, and SWT may promote progress toward the proliferation stage of healing; and phonophoresis and iontophoresis may limit the inflammatory response. During the chronic inflammation or proliferation stages of healing, heat, SWT,

shock waves, motor-level ES, and exercise may be used, and ice or other inflammation-controlling interventions may continue to be applied after activity to reduce the risk of recurring inflammation.

Rest, ice, compression, and elevation (RICE) are frequently combined for the treatment of inflammation and edema because these interventions can control inflammation and edema. Rest limits and prevents further injury, ice reduces circulation and inflammation, compression elevates hydrostatic pressure outside the blood vessels, and elevation reduces hydrostatic pressure within the blood vessels of the elevated area to decrease capillary filtration pressure at the arterial end and facilitate venous and lymphatic outflow from the limb. ES may be added to this combination to further control inflammation and the formation of edema by repelling negatively charged blood cells and ions associated with inflammation.

When the goal of intervention is to control pain, a number of physical agents may be used to influence different mechanisms of pain control. For example, cryotherapy or thermotherapy may be used to modulate pain transmission at the spinal cord, whereas motor-level ES may be used to modulate pain by stimulating endorphin release. These physical agents may be combined with other pain-controlling interventions, such as medications, and may be used in conjunction with treatments such as joint mobilization and dynamic stabilization exercise, which are intended to address the underlying impairment causing pain.

When the goal of intervention is to alter muscle tone, various tone-modifying physical agents or other interventions may be applied during or before activity to promote more normal movement and to increase the efficacy of other aspects of treatment. For example, ice may be applied for 30 to 40 minutes to the leg of a patient with hypertonicity of the ankle plantar flexors caused by a stroke to temporarily control the hypertonicity of these muscles, thereby promoting a more normal gait pattern during gait training. Because practicing normal movement is thought to facilitate the recovery of more normal movement patterns, such treatment may promote a superior outcome.

When the goal of intervention is to reverse soft tissue shortening, the application of thermal agents before or during stretching or mobilization is recommended to promote relaxation and increase soft tissue extensibility, thereby increasing the efficacy and safety of treatment. For example, hot packs are often applied in conjunction with mechanical traction to help relax the paraspinal muscles and to increase the extensibility of superficial soft tissues in the area to which traction is being applied.

Physical agents are generally used more extensively during the initial rehabilitation sessions when inflammation and pain control are matters of priority, with progression over time to more active or aggressive interventions, such as exercise or passive mobilization. Progression from one physical agent to another or from the use of a physical agent to another intervention should be based on the course of the patient's problem. For example, hydrotherapy may be applied to cleanse and debride an open wound during initial treatment sessions; however, once the wound is clean, this treatment should be stopped, and ES may be initiated to promote collagen deposition.

Documentation

Documentation involves entering information into a patient's medical record. Documentation communicates examination findings, evaluations, interventions, and plans to other health care professionals; serves as a long-term record for oneself and others; and supports reimbursement for provided services.

> ### ◎ Clinical Pearl
>
> Good documentation effectively, accurately, and completely communicates examination findings, evaluations, interventions, and plans to other health care professionals; serves as a long-term record; and supports reimbursement.

Documentation of a patient encounter may follow any format but is often done in the SOAP note format that includes the four sequential components of subjective (S), objective (O), assessment (A), and plan (P). Alternative documentation schemes may also be used. The SOAP note format is used in this book for consistency and to demonstrate the reasoning used.

Within each component of the SOAP note, details vary depending on the patient's condition and assessment and the interventions applied. When a physical agent is used, documentation should include what agent was used; what area of the body was treated; and all treatment parameters, including intervention duration, outcomes, progress toward goals, and regressions or complications arising from application of the physical agent. This is an example of a SOAP note written after a hot pack was applied to the lower back:

S: Pt reports low back pain and decreased sitting tolerance, which functionally prohibit writing.

O: Pretreatment: Pain level 7/10. Forward and side-bending ROM restricted 50% by pain and muscle spasm. Pt unable to lean forward for writing tasks.

   Intervention: Hot pack to low back, 20 minutes, Pt prone, six layers of towels. Pt performed single knee to chest 2 × 10, double knee to chest 2 × 10.

   Posttreatment: Pain level 4/10. Forward-bending increased, restricted 20%.

   Pt instructed in home program of heating pad on medium for 10 to 20 minutes followed by SKTC and DKTC 3 × 10 daily.

A: Pain decreased, forward bending ROM.

P: Continue use of hot pack as above before stretching. Progress exercise program.

Specific recommendations for SOAP note documentation and examples are given in the text for all physical agents discussed in this book.

Chapter Review

1. Physical agents consist of materials or energy applied to patients to assist in rehabilitation. Physical agents include heat, cold, water, pressure, sound, electromagnetic radiation, and electrical currents. These agents can be categorized as thermal (e.g., hot packs, cold packs), electromagnetic (e.g., lasers, light, ES, UV radiation, EMG biofeedback), or mechanical (e.g., ultrasound, shock waves, water, compression, traction). Some physical agents fall into more than one category. For example, water and ultrasound are both thermal and mechanical agents.

2. Physical agents are components of a complete rehabilitation program. They are rarely the sole intervention.

3. Physical agents are commonly used with each other and with other interventions.

4. The selection of a physical agent is based on integrating findings from the patient examination with evidence of the effects (both positive and negative) of available agents.

5. Physical agents primarily affect inflammation and healing, pain, motion restrictions, and tone abnormalities. Knowledge of normal and abnormal physiology in each area can help in the selection of a physical agent for a patient. These are discussed in Chapters 3 through 6. The specific effects of particular physical agents are discussed in Chapters 7 through 21.

6. Contraindications are circumstances in which a physical agent should not be used. Precautions are circumstances in which a physical agent should be used with caution. General contraindications and precautions, such as pregnancy, malignancy, pacemakers, and impaired sensation and mentation, pertain to the application of all physical agents. Specific contraindications and precautions for each physical agent are discussed in Chapters 7 through 21.

Glossary

Collagen: The protein in the fibers of skin, tendon, bone, cartilage, and all other connective tissue. Collagen is made up of individual polypeptide molecules combined in triplets forming helical tropocollagen molecules that then associate to form collagen fibrils.

Compression: The application of a mechanical force that increases external pressure on a body part to reduce swelling, improve circulation, or modify scar tissue formation.

Contraindications: Conditions in which a particular treatment should not be applied; also called *absolute contraindications*.

Cryotherapy: The therapeutic use of cold.

Diathermy: The application of shortwave or microwave electromagnetic energy to produce heat within tissues, particularly deep tissues.

Electrical stimulation (ES): The use of electrical current to induce muscle contraction (motor level) or changes in sensation (sensory level).

Electromagnetic agents: Physical agents that apply energy to the patient in the form of electromagnetic radiation or electrical current.

Guide to Physical Therapist Practice 3.0 (Guide 3.0): A book used by physical therapists to categorize patients according to preferred practice patterns that include typical findings and descriptive norms of types and ranges of interventions for patients in each pattern.

Hydrotherapy: The therapeutic use of water.

Indications: Conditions under which a particular treatment should be applied.

Inflammation: The body's first response to tissue damage, characterized by heat, redness, swelling, pain, and often loss of function.

Inflammation phase: The first phase of healing after tissue damage.

Infrared (IR) radiation: Electromagnetic radiation in the IR range (wavelength range, approximately 750 to 1300 nm) that can be absorbed by matter and, if of sufficient intensity, can cause an increase in temperature.

Iontophoresis: The delivery of ions through the skin for therapeutic purposes using an electrical current.

Laser: Acronym for *l*ight *a*mplification by *s*timulated *e*mission of *r*adiation. Laser light has the unique properties of being monochromatic, coherent, and directional.

Maturation phase: The final phase of tissue healing, in which scar tissue is modified into its mature form.

Mechanical agents: Physical agents that apply force to increase or decrease pressure on the body.

Modality: Other term for *physical agent*.

Muscle tone: The underlying tension in a muscle that serves as a background for contraction.

Nonthermal shortwave therapy (SWT): The therapeutic use of intermittent shortwave radiation in which heat is not the mechanism of action (previously called *pulsed shortwave diathermy [PSWD]*).

Pain: An unpleasant sensory and emotional experience associated with actual or threatened tissue damage or described in terms of such damage.

Pathology: Alteration of anatomy or physiology as a result of disease or injury.

Phonophoresis: The application of ultrasound with a topical drug to facilitate transdermal drug delivery. Also known as *sonophoresis*.

Photobiomodulation: Light therapy with lasers, light-emitting diodes (LEDs), superluminous diodes (SLDs), or broadband light.

Physical agents: Energy and materials applied to patients to assist in rehabilitation.

Physical modality: Other term for *physical agent*.

Precautions: Conditions in which a particular treatment should be applied with special care or limitations; also called *relative contraindications*.

Pulsed ultrasound: Intermittent delivery of ultrasound during the treatment period.

Rehabilitation: Goal-oriented intervention designed to maximize independence in individuals who have compromised function.

Sound waves: Alternating compression and rarefaction waves that move through a compressible medium.

Thermal agents: Physical agents that increase or decrease tissue temperature.

Thermotherapy: The therapeutic application of heat.

Traction: A mechanical force applied to the body in a way that separates, or attempts to separate, joint surfaces and elongates soft tissues surrounding a joint.

Ultrasound: Sound with a frequency greater than 20,000 cycles per second (Hz) that is used as a physical agent to produce thermal and nonthermal effects.

Ultraviolet (UV) radiation: Electromagnetic radiation with a wavelength from less than 290 to 400 nm, which lies between x-rays and visible light.

References

1. American Physical Therapy Association: *Guide to physical therapist practice 3.0*, Alexandria, VA, 2014, American Physical Therapy Association. http://guidetoptpractice.apta.org/. (Accessed 15 August 2020).
2. World Health Organization (WHO): *Towards a common language for functioning, disability and health: International Classification of Functioning, Disability and Health (ICF)*, Geneva, 2002, WHO.
3. Slater H, Sluka K, Hoeger Bement MK, Sonderlund A: *IASP curriculum outline on pain for physical therapy*, 2018, IASP. https://www.iasp-pain.org/Education/Content.aspx?ItemNumber=1580.
4. Lentell G, Hetherington T, Eagan J, et al: The use of thermal agents to influence the effectiveness of low load prolonged stretch. *J Orthop Sports Phys Ther* 16:200–207, 1992.
5. Warren C, Lehmann J, Koblanski J: Elongation of rat tail tendon: effect of load and temperature. *Arch Phys Med Rehabil* 52:465–474, 1971.
6. Warren C, Lehmann J, Koblanski J: Heat and stretch procedures: an evaluation using rat tail tendon. *Arch Phys Med Rehabil* 57:122–126, 1976.
7. Gersten JW: Effect of ultrasound on tendon extensibility. *Am J Phys Med* 34:362–369, 1955.
8. American Physical Therapy Association: *Choosing wisely: five things physical therapists and patients should question.* November 18, 2015. http://www.choosingwisely.org/societies/american-physical-therapy-association/. (Accessed 5 February 2017).

2

Physical Agents in Clinical Practice

Michelle H. Cameron | Ashley L. Shea

CHAPTER OUTLINE

CHAPTER OBJECTIVES

After reading this chapter, the reader will be able to do the following:

- Describe the history of the use of physical agents in medicine and rehabilitation.
- Explain the role of physical agents as components of rehabilitation intervention.
- Use evidence to guide the integration of physical agents within rehabilitation.
- Use physical agents in rehabilitation within different health care delivery systems.

History of Physical Agents in Medicine and Rehabilitation

Physical agents have been a component of medical and rehabilitative treatment for many centuries and are used across a wide variety of cultures. Ancient Romans and Greeks used heat and water to maintain health and to treat various musculoskeletal and respiratory problems, as evidenced by the remains of ancient bathhouses with steam rooms and pools of hot and cold water still present in many major Roman and Greek cities.[1] The benefits from soaking and exercising in hot water regained popularity in the late 19th century with the advent of health spas in Europe in areas of natural hot springs. Today, the practices of soaking and exercising in water continue to be popular throughout the world because water provides resistance and buoyancy, allowing the development of strength and endurance while reducing weight bearing on compression-sensitive joints.

Other historical applications of physical agents include the use of electrical torpedo fish in approximately 400 BCE to treat headaches and arthritis by applying electrical shocks to the head and feet. Amber was used in the 17th century to generate static electricity to treat skin diseases, inflammation, and hemorrhage.[2] Reports from the 17th century describe the use of charged gold leaf to prevent scarring from smallpox lesions.[3]

Before the widespread availability of antibiotics and effective analgesic and antiinflammatory drugs, physical agents were commonly used to treat infection, pain, and inflammation. Sunlight was used for the treatment of tuberculosis, bone and joint diseases, and dermatological disorders and infections. Warm Epsom salt baths were used to treat sore or swollen limbs.

Although physical agents have been used for their therapeutic benefits throughout history, over time, new uses, applications, and agents have been developed, and certain agents and applications have fallen out of favor. New uses of physical agents have been discovered as a result of increased understanding of the biological processes underlying disease, dysfunction, and recovery and in response to the availability of advanced technology. For example, **transcutaneous electrical nerve stimulation (TENS)** for the treatment of pain was developed on the basis of the **gate control theory of pain modulation,** as proposed by Melzack and Wall.[4] The gate control theory states that nonpainful stimuli can inhibit the transmission of pain at the spinal cord level. Various available modes of TENS application are primarily the result of the development of electrical current generators that allow fine control of the applied electrical current.

A physical agent usually falls out of favor because the intervention is found to be ineffective or because more effective interventions are developed. For example, the superficial heat that infrared (IR) lamps produce was commonly used to dry out open wounds, but IR lamps are no longer used for this application because we now know that wounds heal more rapidly when kept moist.[5,6] During the early years of the 20th century, sunlight was used to treat tuberculosis; however, since the advent of antibiotics to eliminate bacterial infections, physical agents are rarely used to treat tuberculosis or other infectious diseases.

Most recently, the use of a number of physical agents has fallen out of favor. The first of five recommendations in the American Physical Therapy Association (APTA) Choosing Wisely initiative, most recently updated in 2015, is "don't use (superficial or deep) heat to obtain clinically important, long-term outcomes in musculoskeletal conditions."[7] The APTA clarifies this recommendation with the following statement:

There is limited evidence for use of superficial or deep heat to obtain clinically important long-term outcomes for musculoskeletal conditions. While there is some evidence of short-term pain relief for heat, the addition of heat should be supported by evidence and used to facilitate an active treatment program. A carefully designed active treatment plan has a greater impact on pain, mobility, function and quality of life. There is emerging evidence that passive treatment strategies can harm patients by exacerbating fears and anxiety about being physically active when in pain, which can prolong recovery, increase costs and increase the risk of exposure to invasive and costly interventions such as injections or surgery.

Looking at this statement carefully, it does imply that heat can be used to facilitate an active treatment program, as recommended in this book.

In addition, the fifth recommendation of the APTA Choosing Wisely initiative is "don't use whirlpools for wound management." The APTA clarifies this recommendation with the following statement:

Whirlpools are a non-selective form of mechanical debridement. Utilizing whirlpools to treat wounds predisposes the patient to risks of bacterial cross-contamination, damage to fragile tissue from high turbine forces, and complications in extremity edema when arms and legs are treated in a dependent position in warm water. Other more selective forms of hydrotherapy should be utilized, such as directed wound irrigation or a pulsed lavage with suction.

Based on the evidence and this recommendation, the use of whirlpools for wound management was deleted from the fifth and subsequent editions of this book, and details on directed wound irrigation and pulsed lavage with suction are provided.

Furthermore, spinal traction, particularly for the lumbar spine, has come into question in recent years because evidence from randomized controlled trials (RCTs) has failed to prove its benefits and because of concerns that this passive form of treatment may increase the risk of illness behavior and chronicity.[8] Spinal traction is still covered in this book because, as recently as 2015, over 75% of physical therapists reported using lumbar traction[9] for managing low back pain, because there is substantial evidence of traction being associated with effects that may be beneficial in certain patients, and because the evidence for the efficacy of cervical spine traction is more positive.

Physical agents also sometimes wane in popularity because they are cumbersome, have excessive associated risks, interfere with other aspects of treatment, or have just fallen out of fashion. For example, the use of diathermy as a deep-heating agent was very popular over 30 years ago, but because the machines are large and awkward to move around and set up, and because this agent can easily burn patients if not used appropriately and can interfere with the functioning of nearby computer-controlled equipment, diathermy was not commonly used in the United States until more recently. With the development of less cumbersome and safer devices, diathermy is regaining popularity and is presented in this book as a means of deep heating to facilitate an active treatment program and as a nonthermal agent to promote tissue healing.

This book focuses on the physical agents most commonly used in the United States at the present time. Physical agents that are not commonly used in the United States but that were popular in the recent past, as well as agents that are popular abroad or are expected to come back into favor as new delivery systems and applications are developed, are covered briefly. The popularity of particular physical agents is based on their history of clinical use and, in most cases, on evidence to support their efficacy; however, in some cases, their clinical application has continued despite a lack of or limited supporting evidence. More research is needed to clarify which interventions and patient characteristics provide optimal results. Further study is also needed to determine precisely what outcomes should be expected from the application of physical agents in rehabilitation.

Approaches to Rehabilitation

Rehabilitation is a goal-oriented intervention designed to maximize independence in individuals with compromised function. Function is usually compromised because of an underlying pathology and secondary **impairments** and is affected by environmental and personal factors. Compromised function may lead to **disability.** Rehabilitation generally addresses the sequelae of pathology to maximize a patient's function and ability to participate in usual activities, rather than being directed at resolving the pathology itself, and should take into consideration the environmental and personal factors affecting each patient's individual activity and participation limitations and goals.

A number of classification schemes exist to categorize the sequelae of pathology. In 1980, the World Health Organization (WHO) published the first scheme to classify the consequences of diseases, known as the International Classification of Impairments, Disabilities, and Handicaps (ICIDH).[10] This scheme, derived primarily from the work of Wood, is based on a linear model in which the sequelae of pathology or disease are impairments that lead to disabilities and handicaps.[11,12] In this scheme, *impairment* is characterized as an abnormality of structure or function of the body or an organ, including mental function. *Disability* is characterized as a restriction of activities resulting from impairment, and *handicap* is the social level of the consequences of diseases, characterized as the individual's disadvantage resulting from impairment or disability. Shortly after the **ICIDH model** was published, Nagi developed a similar model that classified the sequelae of pathology as impairments, **functional limitations,** and disabilities.[13] He defined *impairments* as alterations in anatomical, physiological, or psychological structures or functions that result from an underlying pathology. In the **Nagi model,** *functional limitations* were defined as restrictions in the ability to perform an activity in an efficient, typically expected, or competent manner, and *disabilities* were defined as the inability to perform activities required for self-care, home, work, and community roles.

The WHO updated the ICIDH model in 2001 to reflect and create changes in perceptions of people with disabilities and to meet the needs of different groups of individuals. The updated version of the ICIDH model is known as the *ICIDH-2* or the *International Classification of Functioning, Disability and Health (ICF)* (Fig. 2.1).[14] The ICF is a classification of health and health-related domains and is the WHO framework for measuring health and disability at both individual and population levels. In contrast to the earlier linear model, the **ICF model** views functioning and disability as a complex,

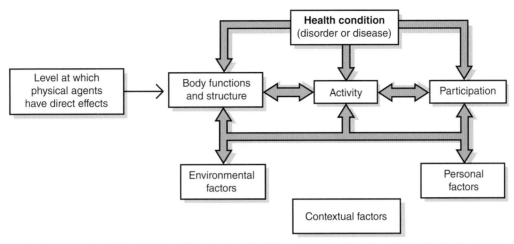

FIGURE 2.1 Model for the International Classification of Functioning, Disability and Health (ICF). (From World Health Organization [WHO]: *ICIDH-2: International Classification of Functioning, Disability and Health,* Geneva, 2001, WHO.)

dynamic interaction between the health condition of the individual and contextual factors of the environment, as well as personal factors. It is applicable to all people, whatever their health condition. The language of the ICF model is neutral to cause, placing the emphasis on function rather than on the condition or disease. It is designed to be relevant across cultures, as well as age groups and genders, making it appropriate for heterogeneous populations. The ICF is operationalized through the WHO Disability Assessment Schedule (WHODAS 2.0).[15]

> ### ◎ Clinical Pearl
> The International Classification of Functioning, Disability and Health (ICF) model views functioning and disability as a complex, dynamic interaction between the health condition of the individual and contextual factors of the environment, as well as personal factors. The ICF model emphasizes function and considers the body, the whole person, and the person in society.

The original ICIDH and Nagi models, developed primarily for use by rehabilitation professionals, were intended to differentiate disease and pathology from the limitations they produced. The new ICF model has a more positive perspective on the changes associated with pathology and disease and is intended for use by a wide range of people, including members of the community, as well as national and global institutions that create policy and allocate resources for persons with disabilities. The ICF model has tried to change the perspective of disability from the negative focus of "consequences of disease" used in the ICIDH model to a more positive focus on "components of health." The ICIDH model used categories of impairments, disabilities, and handicaps to describe sequelae of and limitations associated with pathology, whereas the ICF model uses categories of health conditions, body functions, activities, and participation to focus on abilities rather than limitations.

Consistent with the most recent edition of the APTA's *Guide to Physical Therapist Practice 3.0 (Guide 3.0),*[16] this book uses the terminology and framework of the ICF model to evaluate clinical findings and determine a plan of care for the individuals described in the case studies. The ICF model reflects the interactions between health conditions and contextual factors as they affect disability and functioning. Health conditions include diseases, disorders, and injuries. Contextual factors include environmental factors, such as social attitudes, legal structures, and one's community, and personal factors, such as gender, age, education, experience, and character. The ICF model is intended to be used in conjunction with the International Classification of Diseases (ICD), a classification system used throughout the U.S. health care system to document and code medical diagnoses.

The ICF model is structured around three levels of functioning: (1) the body or a part of the body, (2) the whole person, and (3) the whole person in a social context. Dysfunction at any of these levels is termed a *disability* and results in impairments (at the body level), activity limitations (at the whole-person level), and participation restrictions (at the social level). For example, a person who experienced a stroke may be weak on one side of the body (impairment). This impairment may cause difficulty with activities of daily living (activity limitation). The person may be unable to attend social gatherings that they previously enjoyed (participation restriction).

The ICF model was developed by combining medical and social models of disability. In the medical model, disability is the result of an underlying pathology, and to treat the disability, one must treat the pathology. In the social model, disability is the result of the social environment, and to treat the disability, one must change the social environment to make it more accommodating.

Medical treatment is generally directed at the underlying pathology or disease, whereas rehabilitation focuses primarily on reversing or minimizing impairments, activity limitations, and participation restrictions. Rehabilitation professionals must assess and set goals not only at the levels of impairment, such as pain, decreased range of motion, and **hypertonicity** (increased muscle tone) but also at the levels of activity and participation. These goals should include the patient's goals, such as being able to get out of bed, ride a bicycle, work, or run a marathon.

The Role of Physical Agents in Rehabilitation

Physical agents are tools to be used when appropriate as components of rehabilitation. The position statement of the APTA regarding the *exclusive* use of physical agents, first published in 1995 and reiterated in 2005, stated, "Without documentation which justifies the necessity of the exclusive use of physical agents/modalities, the use of physical agents/modalities, in the absence of other skilled therapeutic or educational interventions, should not be considered physical therapy."[17] In 2015, related to physical agents, as part of its Choosing Wisely initiative, the APTA specifically stated with regard to heat, "don't use (superficial or deep) heat to obtain clinically important long term outcomes in musculoskeletal conditions … the addition of heat should be supported by evidence and used to facilitate an active treatment program."[7] Most recently, in 2018, the APTA updated its position statement on the exclusive use of biophysical agents, stating, "The use of biophysical agents as a standalone intervention, or the use of multiple biophysical agents with a similar physiologic effect, is not considered physical therapy nor is it considered medically necessary without documentation that justifies the use of the biophysical agents for those purposes."[18] In other words, the APTA believes that the use of single or multiple physical agents alone does not constitute physical therapy.

The use of physical agents as a component of rehabilitation involves integration with other appropriate interventions. This integration may include applying a physical agent or educating the patient in its application as part of a complete program to help patients achieve their activity and participation goals. However, because the aim of this book is to give clinicians a better understanding of the theory and appropriate application of physical agents, the emphasis is on the use of physical agents, and other components of the rehabilitation program are described in less detail.

Practitioners Using Physical Agents

Physical therapists, physical therapist assistants, occupational therapists, occupational therapy assistants, athletic trainers, physiatrists, chiropractors, acupuncturists, and patients all apply physical agents. These individuals may have slightly different goals when applying these interventions and slightly different training and educational requirements for their use.

Physical therapists commonly use physical agents and supervise physical therapist assistants in the application of physical agents. The APTA includes physical agents within the interventions that define the practice of physical therapy and notes that when physical agents are used, this should be as a part of a complete rehabilitation program.[19] Training in the use of physical agents is a required part of entry-level education and licensure for physical therapists and physical therapist assistants. The Commission on Accreditation in Physical Therapy Education (CAPTE), the granting agency for the accreditation of physical therapist and physical therapist assistant education programs, requires evidence of "content, learning experiences, and student testing and evaluation" to ensure competent use of biophysical agents.[20] The APTA states that the minimum required skills of a physical therapist graduate at the entry level include competency in the use of physical agents such as cryotherapy, hydrotherapy, ultrasound, and

thermotherapy; mechanical modalities such as compression therapies and traction devices; and electrotherapeutic modalities such as biofeedback, electrotherapeutic delivery of medications (e.g., iontophoresis), and electrical stimulation.[21] When caring for patients, physical therapists are expected to select and use the most appropriate interventions according to the best scientific evidence while considering the patient's perspective and exercising professional judgment.

Occupational therapists and occupational therapy assistants, especially those involved in hand therapy, also commonly use physical agents. In its most recent position paper,[22] published in 2018, the American Occupational Therapy Association (AOTA) referenced a 2014 document supporting that physical agents and mechanical modalities "may be used by occupational therapy practitioners as part of a comprehensive plan of intervention designed to enhance engagement in occupation."[23] The AOTA discourages exclusive or standalone use of physical agents and mechanical modalities and promotes their use as adjunctive to "purposeful and occupation-based intervention activities."[24] Occupational therapists and occupational therapy assistants, under the supervision of occupational therapists, integrate physical agents and mechanical modalities into the intervention plan to prepare clients to complete purposeful and meaningful activities in the areas of activities of daily living, instrumental activities of daily living, rest and sleep, education, work, play, leisure, and social participation, with the overall goal of maximizing functional independence in activities.

The Accreditation Council for Occupational Therapy Education (ACOTE), the body that accredits occupational therapy educational programs in the United States, first introduced physical and mechanical agents into educational standards in 2006 to go into effect in 2008.[25] As of 2018, the ACOTE mandates that entry-level occupational therapy programs include in their curricula coursework that prepares practitioners who can "demonstrate knowledge and use of the safe and effective application of superficial thermal agents, deep thermal agents, electrotherapeutic agents, and mechanical devices as a preparatory measure to improve occupational performance."[26] Similarly, occupational therapy assistant programs must include in their curricula coursework that prepares occupational therapy assistants to understand "the safe and effective application of superficial thermal agents, deep thermal agents, electrotherapeutic agents, and mechanical devices as a preparatory measure to improve occupational performance."[26] Both occupational therapists and occupational therapy assistants must know the indications, contraindications, and precautions for the use of physical agents and mechanical modalities.

As the AOTA notes, it is important for professionals to understand that an association's policies and position do not take precedence over state laws and regulations.[23] Laws and regulations regarding the use of physical agents by occupational therapists vary among states, with many requiring additional training and experience beyond that offered during entry-level education. As of June 2019, only 15 states did not have statutes or regulations regarding the use of physical agents and mechanical modalities by occupational therapy practitioners, whereas the remaining states have, pending or in effect, such statutes or regulations.[26] Occupational therapists and occupational therapy assistants who wish to use physical agents and mechanical modalities in their clinical practice should check the laws and regulations in the state in which they practice and are licensed.

ACOTE requires all accredited occupational therapy programs to address the safe and effective application of superficial thermal and mechanical modalities for pain management and improvement of occupational performance. ACOTE first introduced modalities into educational standards in 2006 to go into effect in 2008. This education must include "foundational knowledge, underlying principles, indications, contraindications, and precautions." Students must also be able to explain the use of deep thermal and electrotherapeutic modalities to improve occupational performance and must know the indications, contraindications, and precautions for the clinical application of these physical agents. ACOTE also requires accredited occupational therapy assistant programs to recognize the use of superficial thermal and mechanical modalities as a preparatory method for other occupational therapy interventions.[25]

The National Athletic Trainers' Association (NATA) states that training in therapeutic modalities is a required part of the curriculum to become a certified athletic trainer for accredited programs.[28,29] Continuing education in modality devices is also a component of required athletic trainer continuing education.[30]

In addition to having physical agents applied by professionals, patients can learn about and apply modalities independently. For example, agents such as heat, cold, compression, and TENS can be safely applied at home after the patient is instructed in and demonstrates proper use of the agent. Patient education has several advantages, including the option for more prolonged and frequent application, decreased cost, and increased convenience for the patient. Most important, education allows patients to be active participants in achieving their own therapeutic goals.

Evidence-Based Practice

If several agents could promote progress toward the goals of treatment, they are not contraindicated, and they can be applied with appropriate precautions, selecting which to use should be based on evidence for or against the intervention. **Evidence-based practice (EBP)** is "the conscientious, explicit, and judicious use of current best evidence in making decisions about the care of individual patients."[31,32] EBP is based on the application of the scientific method to clinical practice. EBP requires that clinical practice decisions be guided by the best available relevant clinical research data in conjunction with the clinician's experience and individual patient's pathology and preferences.

Clinical Pearl

Evidence-based practice (EBP) requires that clinical practice decisions be guided by the best available relevant clinical research data *in conjunction with* the clinician's experience and individual patient's pathology and preferences.

The goal of EBP is to provide the best possible patient care by assessing available research and applying it to each individual patient. When searching for evidence, one may encounter thousands of studies to sift through or very few studies. It is important to understand which studies constitute the

highest level of evidence. To use EBP, the clinician should understand the differences between types of research studies and the advantages and disadvantages of each. Evidence used in EBP can be classified by factors such as study design, types of subjects, the nature of controls, outcome measures, and types of statistical analysis.[33]

Study design: Research studies range in quality from the low-level case report (an individual description of a particular patient that does not necessarily reflect the population as a whole) to the high-level meta-analysis of RCTs (the gold standard of EBP, a quantitative synthesis and summary of the results from previously published high-quality RCTs on the same topic). When directly relevant **meta-analyses** do not exist on a particular therapy or treatment, **systematic reviews** or individual RCTs are preferred to case reports and nonrandomized studies. RCTs minimize bias through blinded, randomized assignment to an intervention or a control group and assessment of outcomes.[34] A general overview of study types is presented in Table 2.1.[35] This table provides the general hierarchy as accepted by

TABLE 2.1	Levels of Evidence From Highest Quality to Lowest[35]
Meta-analyses (highest quality)	The use of statistical methodology to quantify the conclusions of many previously published trials evaluating a particular treatment or intervention. Studies are included in the meta-analysis if they meet predetermined criteria, and the statistical methods used should be well documented.
Systematic reviews	An applied, methodical search of existing literature on a specific treatment and/or pathology. Studies meeting predetermined parameters are included, and a narrative conclusion summarizes the findings. Systematic reviews should include the search strategy used when surveying studies so that the search can be reproduced at a later date.
Randomized controlled trials	A preplanned study that uses random assignment to one of two groups, and blinding of both the investigators to group assignment, in order to minimize bias. One group receives the treatment being evaluated, and the other group does not. In general, the group not receiving the active treatment receives a placebo. The same outcome measures are performed in each group.
Cohort studies	An observational study comparing participants who receive a treatment, or have certain features, to participants who do not receive that treatment, or do not have those features.
Case-control study	An observational study comparing a group of participants with the same diagnosis or pathology with a healthy group without the diagnosis.
Case report	A report of the signs, symptoms, interventions, and outcomes for a single patient.

the clinical community, but there are exceptions. For example, a well-powered observational study run over several decades could provide stronger evidence for a particular treatment than a single RCT with a small sample size. Additionally, not all publications that call themselves "systematic reviews" are equally rigorous. A high-quality systematic review should be exhaustive and reproducible.[36] It should utilize multiple databases so that all relevant literature is found. It should also include the names of the databases searched, the search terms and search strategy used in each database, and the dates the searches were run, and it should provide a **Preferred Reporting Items for Systematic Reviews and Meta-Analyses (PRISMA)** flow diagram giving the number of studies initially found in the search and the final studies selected for inclusion.[37]

Subject type: Studies with demographic variety that include male and female participants of varying ages and from different backgrounds are preferred if the ailment or condition under study affects both sexes across a wide age spectrum. For example, because low back pain commonly affects both men and women of a wide range of ages, with no particular predilection for a specific racial group, studies on the treatment of low back pain should include men and women of various ages and various races to make the results generalizable to the target population. In addition, studies with many participants having homogeneous ailments are preferred over small, heterogeneous groups of participants with varying degrees of ailment, so a study of many people with acute low back pain is better than a study of few people with back pain of varying duration. When an intervention is applied to a group with varying degrees of ailment, the effectiveness of the treatment may be difficult to assess. When the sample size is large and all participants experience the same degree of ailment, the outcomes are more likely to be valid. Subjects with confounding pathologies that may affect the results of treatment should generally be excluded from the study.

Outcome measures: Outcome measures are the assessment strategies used to determine if a treatment is successful. Measures should be reliable—reproducing the same or similar result when repeated, regardless of the test administrator. Measures should also be valid, appropriately assessing the property, unit, or characteristic they intend to measure. Outcome measures can be patient reported,[38] such as self-report on a quality-of-life questionnaire, or clinician measured,[39] such as the speed at which a patient completes a timed walk. Outcome measures can assess functional limitations or the degree of impairment and be sufficiently generic to use across pathologies or specific to pathologies with a specific diagnosis.[40] When considering the quality of outcome measurements, it is important that one consider the reliability and validity of the measure and whether the measurement will provide meaningful data.[41]

Statistical analysis: Once the outcome data have been collected, a study should report the results of preplanned statistical analyses. Results are often considered statistically significant when there is less than a 5% chance that the findings occurred by chance. This is denoted by "$p < 0.05$." Using EBP to guide the selection and application of physical agents as part of rehabilitation is often challenging. It

TABLE 2.2		PICO Table Used by Clinicians When Structuring Questions
P	Patient or Population	The question should apply to a specific person or group (e.g., adults with low back pain; children with lower-extremity spasticity)
I	Intervention	The question should focus on a specific intervention (e.g., specified exercise applied at a specified frequency and duration)
C	Comparison or Control	The question should compare the selected intervention with the gold-standard treatment or no intervention at all
O	Outcome	The question should state clearly the desired outcome from the intervention (e.g., increased walking speed, decrease in self-reported pain)

can be difficult to find published high-quality studies because high-quality studies are difficult to perform. Blinding patients and clinicians to rehabilitation treatments may not be possible, outcomes may be difficult to assess, and it is costly and time consuming to include large numbers of subjects. A good initial approach to evaluating the quality of an individual study is to examine the quality of the question being asked. All well-built questions should have four readily identifiable components: (1) the patients, (2) the intervention, (3) the comparison intervention, and (4) the outcome. These components can be readily remembered by the mnemonic *PICO* (Table 2.2).

When exploring the literature to find applicable evidence, one should use the PICO table to structure well-defined searches. Most databases of the clinical literature rely on the use of **Medical Subject Headings (MeSH)** and other specialized vocabulary when indexing or inputting the literature. Translating PICO terms to the specialized language of the database facilitates a strategic and efficient search. At the end of each subsequent chapter in this book, case studies present various pathologies with structured PICO searches for treatment approaches mapped to MeSH terms that you can apply for yourself in PubMed (Table 2.3). This search will provide citations with abstracts, and often full-text articles, that are continuously updated by the National Library of Medicine.

As noted previously, meta-analyses and systematic reviews typically provide the highest-quality evidence. There are several specialized databases of systematic reviews and meta-analyses of medical and rehabilitation-related research, including the well-respected Cochrane Database of Systematic Reviews and PubMed Health (Box 2.1). For clinical questions not included in these databases, individual studies may be found in other online databases of medical and rehabilitation-oriented publications, such as MEDLINE, which is accessed via PubMed; CINAHL (Cumulative Index of Nursing and Allied Health Literature); and PEDro (Physiotherapy Evidence Database) (Box 2.2). When searching the literature to find and evaluate the latest and most relevant evidence, it is important to understand the strengths and limitations of each database you plan to use. A librarian can suggest the best

TABLE 2.3	Sample Find the Evidence Table With PICO Elements Mapped to MeSH Terms	
PICO Terms	**Natural-Language Example**	**Sample PubMed Search**
P (Population)	Patients with symptoms due to soft tissue shortening	("Contracture*"[MeSH] OR "Contracture"[Text Word] OR "Therapy, Soft Tissue"[MeSH] OR "Tissue Shortening"[Text Word])
I (Intervention)	Ultrasound therapy	AND "Ultrasonic Therapy*"[MeSH] AND English[lang] AND "Humans"[MeSH Terms]
C (Comparison)	No ultrasound therapy	
O (Outcome)	Increased range of motion	

Box 2.1	Databases of Systematic Reviews and Meta-Analyses
The Cochrane Database of Systematic Reviews	A collection of systematic reviews and corresponding editorials that have been carried out by highly trained Cochrane Review Groups
PubMed Health	A resource for systematic reviews provided by the National Library of Medicine including Cochrane's DARE database
Joanna Briggs Institute	A refereed, online library that publishes systematic review protocols and systematic reviews of health care research, as performed by Joanna Briggs Library and international collaboration centers
PROSPERO	An international prospective register of systematic reviews
Epistemonikos	A multilingual database of published research reviews in the clinical, rehabilitation, and public health fields

databases for your study question and demonstrate the various features of the platform so that you can efficiently find relevant literature.

Most databases have advanced search features. For example, when searching MEDLINE through the PubMed interface, you can limit your searches to review articles or randomized trials only. You can also search by keyword at the title level to retrieve only citations that include your selected term or terms in the title. Additionally, in PubMed, articles related to the last selected citation are suggested to you, and references within selected articles are hyperlinked to ease the search and discovery process.

Box 2.2	Sources of Studies Answering Specific Clinical Questions
TRIP Database	A clinical search engine that allows users to structure searches by PICO terms to quickly locate high-quality research evidence
PEDro	An Australian database with citations, abstracts, and full-text articles of more than 23,000 randomized controlled trials, 5200 systematic reviews, and 513 evidence-based clinical practice guides in physiotherapy
MEDLINE (searchable via PubMed)	An online database of over 25 million citations and abstracts from health and medical journals and other news sources
CINAHL	A database of studies and evidence-based care sheets from over 1300 nursing journals
GuidelineCentral	GuidelineCentral is the publisher of American Medical Association guidelines. GuidelineCentral provides a free app and covers a range of rehabilitation topics.

Clinical practice guidelines can also be good sources of evidence. Clinical practice guidelines are systematically developed statements that attempt to interpret current research to provide evidence-based guidelines to guide practitioner and patient decisions about appropriate health care for specific clinical circumstances.[42] Clinical practice guidelines give recommendations for diagnostic and prognostic measures and for preventive and therapeutic interventions. For any of these, the specific types of patients or problems, the nature of the intervention or test, alternatives to the intervention being evaluated, and outcomes of the intervention for which these guidelines apply will be stated. For example, some guidelines for the treatment of acute low back pain and for the treatment of pressure ulcers include evidence-based recommendations for tests and measures, interventions, prevention, and prognosis. Often, such recommendations are classified according to the strength of the evidence supporting them. General clinical practice guidelines used to be available on the Agency for Healthcare Research and Quality (AHRQ) National Guideline Clearinghouse (NGC) website, but funding for this clearinghouse ended, and the clearinghouse closed on July 16, 2018, and has yet to be replaced. Other repositories and libraries with guidelines include the International Guideline Library[44]; the National Institute for Health and Care Excellence (NICE) United Kingdom–based searchable website of evidence-based guidance; and the CPG Infobase, which is the Canadian repository for guidelines.[44] In addition, GuidelineCentral,[45] which provides free access to thousands of current clinical practice guidelines and guideline summaries online and via an app, is currently working with a handful of other organizations to establish a new nonprofit initiative that will aim to fill the gap left by the sudden closure of AHRQ's NGC. This new initiative will include a

Box 2.3	Sources of Clinical Practice Guidelines
International Guideline Library	The International Guideline Library contains around 3000 guidelines, which have mainly been developed or endorsed by organizational members of the Guideline International Network (GIN). The library is free to access.
National Institute for Health and Care Excellence (NICE)	NICE guidelines provide evidence-based recommendations developed by independent committees, including professionals and lay members, and consulted on by stakeholders.
CPG Infobase	This database contains approximately 1200 evidence-based Canadian clinical practice guidelines (CPGs) developed or endorsed by authoritative medical or health organizations in Canada.
Centre for Evidence-Based Medicine (CEBM)	The CEBM website includes information for health care professionals on learning, practicing, and teaching EBM, as well as definitions of terminology and calculators.

database of quick-reference guideline summaries, along with a focus on developing a repository of various guideline-implementation tools (including machine-computable guidelines for electronic health records [EHRs]). This new database will be made available for free to all health care providers in both web and mobile app formats (Box 2.3).

EBP is accepted practice and should be incorporated into every patient's plan of care. However, it is important to remember that every study cannot be applied to every patient, and research-supported interventions should not be applied without considering each patient's situation. EBP requires the careful combination of patient preference, clinical circumstances, clinician expertise, and research findings.

Using Physical Agents Within Different Health Care Delivery Systems

Clinicians may be called on to treat patients within different health care delivery systems in the United States and abroad. These systems may vary in terms of the quantity and nature of available health care resources. Some systems provide high levels of resources in the form of skilled clinicians and costly equipment, and others do not. Over the last several years, the health care delivery system in the United States has tried to contain the growing costs of medical care and focused on the cost-effective use of resources. The emphasis on cost-effectiveness is even greater in socialized medical systems, where there are fewer counterpressures from the for-profit provision of health care.

To help control costs, services that can be self-administered are often not paid for by insurance. For example, since 1997, Medicare has bundled the payment for hot-pack and cold-pack treatments into the payment for all other services, rather than reimbursing separately for these treatments, because hot and cold packs can be administered by patients independently.[46] Nonetheless, this intervention may be indicated, and patients may benefit from education on how and when to apply these agents themselves at home.

Within the context of attending to cost-effectiveness, the goals of health care continue to be, as they always have been, to obtain the best outcome for the patient within the constraints of the health care delivery system. The clinician should find and use the most efficient ways to provide interventions to help patients progress toward the goals of treatment. To use physical agents in this manner, the clinician must be able to assess the presenting problem and know when a physical agent is or is not likely to be an effective component of treatment. The clinician must know when and how to use physical agents most effectively, which ones can be used by patients to treat themselves, and which are not likely to be effective (Box 2.4). To achieve the most cost-effective treatment, the clinician should use evidence-based interventions and optimize the use of practitioners of varying skill levels and of home programs when appropriate. In many cases, the licensed therapist may not need to apply the physical agent but instead may assess and analyze the presenting clinical findings; determine the intervention plan; provide the aspects of care that require the skills of the licensed therapist; and train the patient to apply, or supervise other personnel in applying, interventions that require a lower level of skill. The therapist can then reassess the patient regularly to determine the effectiveness of the interventions provided and the patient's progress toward their goals and can adjust the plan of care accordingly.

Cost-efficiency may also be increased by providing an intervention to groups of patients, such as group water exercise programs for patients recovering from total joint arthroplasty or for patients with osteoarthritis. Such programs may be designed to facilitate the transition to a community-based exercise program when the patient reaches the appropriate level of function and recovery. When used in this manner, physical agents can provide cost-effective care and can involve the patient in promoting recovery and achieving the goals of treatment.

Box 2.4	Requirements for Cost-Effective Use of Physical Agents

- Assess and analyze the presenting problem.
- Know when physical agents can be an effective component of treatment.
- Know when and how to use physical agents most effectively.
- Know the skill level required to apply the different physical agents.
- Optimize the use of different practitioners' skill levels.
- Use home programs when appropriate.
- Treat in groups when appropriate.
- Reassess patients regularly to determine the efficacy of treatments provided.
- Adjust the plan of care according to the findings of reassessments.

Chapter Review

1. The ICF model assesses the impact of a disease or condition on a patient's function. This model considers the effects of a patient's health condition, environment, and personal circumstances on their impairments, activity limitations, and participation restrictions. The ICF model looks at the patient on three levels: body, whole person, and social. Physical agents primarily affect the patient at the body, or impairment, level. A complete rehabilitation program should affect the patient at all levels of functioning, disability, and health.

2. EBP is the incorporation of research-based evidence into a patient's rehabilitation plan. EBP integrates the clinician's experience and judgment with the patient's preferences, the clinical situation, and available evidence. This book attempts to include the current, best-quality evidence available while teaching readers how to conduct independent searches to get the most relevant and up-to-date information when they need it.

3. Physical agents are used in the clinic, at home, and in various health care delivery systems. Depending on the system, the selection and application of physical agents may vary. Reimbursement for applying physical agents is constantly in flux, and the potential for conflict between minimizing cost and maximizing benefit can make intervention selection difficult.

Glossary

Clinical practice guidelines: Systematically developed statements that attempt to interpret current research to provide evidence-based guidelines to guide practitioner and patient decisions about appropriate health care for specific clinical circumstances.

Disability: The inability to perform activities required for self-care, home, work, and community roles.

Evidence-based practice (EBP): The conscientious, explicit, and judicious use of current best evidence in making decisions about the care of individual patients.

Functional limitations: Restrictions in the ability to perform an activity in an efficient, typically expected, or competent manner.

Gate control theory of pain modulation: Theory of pain control and modulation that states that pain is modulated at the spinal cord level by inhibitory effects of nonnoxious afferent input.

Hypertonicity: High muscle tone or increased resistance to stretch compared with normal muscles.

ICF model: International Classification of Functioning, Disability and Health (ICF) model of disability and health created by the World Health Organization (WHO) that views functioning and disability as a complex interaction between the health condition of the individual and contextual factors, including environmental and personal factors. ICF uses categories of health conditions, body functions, activities, and participation to focus on abilities rather than limitations.

ICIDH model: International Classification of Impairments, Disabilities, and Handicaps (ICIDH) model of disability created by the World Health Organization (WHO) that was a precursor to the International Classification of Functioning, Disability, and Health (ICF) model and focused on disability rather than ability.

Impairments: Alterations in anatomical, physiological, or psychological structures or functions as the result of an underlying pathology.

Medical Subject Headings (MeSH): The National Library of Medicine's controlled vocabulary thesaurus.

Meta-analyses: Systematic reviews that use statistical analysis to integrate data from a number of independent studies.

Nagi model: A linear model of disability in which pathology causes impairments, leading to functional limitations that result in disabilities; this was a precursor to the International Classification of Functioning, Disability and Health (ICF) model.

Preferred Reporting Items for Systematic Reviews and Meta-Analyses (PRISMA): An evidence-based minimum set of items for reporting in systematic reviews and meta-analyses. The aim of the PRISMA Statement is to help authors improve the reporting of systematic reviews and meta-analyses.

Systematic reviews: Reviews of studies that answer clearly formulated questions by systematically searching for, assessing, and evaluating literature from multiple sources.

Transcutaneous electrical nerve stimulation (TENS): The application of electrical current through the skin to modulate pain.

References

1. Johnson EW: Back to water (or hydrotherapy). *J Back Musculoskel Med* 4:ix, 1994.
2. Baker LL, McNeal DR, Benton LA, et al: *Neuromuscular electrical stimulation: a practical guide*, ed 3, Downey, CA, 1993, Los Amigos Research & Education Institute.
3. Roberson WS: Digby's receipts. *Ann Med Hist* 7:216–219, 1925.
4. Melzack JD, Wall PD: Pain mechanisms: a new theory. *Science* 150:971–979, 1965.
5. Hyland DB, Kirkland VJ: Infrared therapy for skin ulcers. *Am J Nurs* 80:1800–1801, 1980.
6. Cummings J. Role of light in wound healing. In Kloth L, McCulloch JM, Feedar JA, editors: *Wound healing: alternatives in management*, Philadelphia, 1990, FA Davis.
7. American Physical Therapy Association: *Choosing wisely: five things physical therapists and patients should question*. Released September 15, 2014; recommendation #1 updated November 18, 2015. http://www.choosingwisely.org/societies/american-physical-therapy-association/. (Accessed 17 August 2019).
8. *Evidence-informed primary care management of low back pain. Clinical practice guideline*, ed 3, December 2015, minor revision 2017. http://www.topalbertadoctors.org/download/1885/LBPguideline.pdf?_20160314120252. (Accessed 17 August 2019).
9. Madson TJ, Hollman JH: Lumbar traction for managing low back pain: a survey of physical therapists in the United States. *J Orthop Sports Phys Ther* 45(8):586–595, 2015.
10. World Health Organization (WHO): *International classification of impairments, disabilities and handicaps (ICIDH)*, Geneva, 1980, WHO.
11. Wood PHN: The language of disablement: a glossary relating to disease and its consequences. *Int Rehab Med* 2:86–92, 1980.
12. Wagstaff S: The use of the International Classification of Impairments, Disabilities and Handicaps in rehabilitation. *Physiotherapy* 68:548–553, 1982.
13. Nagi S: Disability concepts revisited. In Pope AM, Tarlov AR, editors: *Disability in America: toward a national agenda for prevention*, Washington, DC, 1991, National Academy Press.
14. World Health Organization (WHO): *ICIDH-2: International classification of functioning, disability and health*, Geneva, 2001, WHO.
15. https://www.who.int/classifications/icf/more_whodas/en/. Updated 14 June 2018. (Accessed 17 August 2019).
16. American Physical Therapy Association: *Guide to physical therapist practice 3.0*, Alexandria, VA, 2014, American Physical Therapy Association. http://guidetoptpractice.apta.org/. (Accessed 23 May 2016).
17. American Physical Therapy Association: *Position on exclusive use of physical agent modalities*, Alexandria, VA, 2005, House of Delegates Reference Committee. P06-95-29-18.

18. https://www.apta.org/uploadedFiles/APTAorg/About_Us/Policies/Practice/ExclusiveUse.pdf. HOD P06-18-17-27. (Accessed 17 August 2019).

19. American Physical Therapy Association: *Guidelines: defining physical therapy in state practice acts.* Last revised December 2009. http://www.apta.org/uploadedFiles/APTAorg/About_Us/Policies/BOD/Practice/DefiningPTinStatePracticeActs.pdf#search=%22physicalagents%22. (Accessed 17 August 2019).

20. Commission on Accreditation in Physical Therapy Education: *Accreditation handbook.* Last revised 7 December 2017. http://www.capteonline.org/AccreditationHandbook/. (Accessed 16 November 2019).

21. American Physical Therapy Association: *Minimum required skills of physical therapist graduates at entry-level.* http://www.apta.org/uploadedFiles/APTAorg/About_Us/Policies/BOD/Education/MinReqSkillsPTGrad.pdf#search=%22physical%20agents%22. (Accessed 9 July 2016).

22. American Occupational Therapy Association: AOTA position paper: physical agents and mechanical modalities. *Am J Occup Ther* 72(Suppl 2): 7212410055p1-7212410055, 2018. doi:10.5014/ajot.2018.72S220.

23. American Occupational Therapy Association: Occupational therapy practice framework: domain and process, ed 3. *Am J Occup Ther* 68(Suppl 1):S2–S48, 2014. doi:10.5014/ajot.2014.68200622.

24. Gillen G, Hunter EG, Lieberman D, Stutzbach M: AOTA's top 5 Choosing Wisely® recommendations. *Am J Occup Ther* 73(2), 2019. doi:10.5014/ajot.2019.732001.

25. Accreditation Council for Occupational Therapy Education (ACOTE): *Standards and interpretive guidelines*, Bethesda, MD, 2011, American Occupational Therapy Association.

26. Accreditation Council for Occupational Therapy Education (ACOTE): *Standards and interpretive guidelines*, Bethesda, MD, 2018, American Occupational Therapy Association.

27. American Occupational Therapy Association, State Affairs Group: *State occupational therapy statutes, regulations and policy statements with specific physical agent modalities provisions.* 2019. https://www.aota.org/~/media/corporate/files/secure/advocacy/licensure/stateregs/otregs/pams-chart-2019.pdf. (Accessed September 30, 2019).

28. Commission on Accreditation of Athletic Training Education: *Standards for accreditation of professional athletic training programs.* 2020. https://caate.net/pp-standards/. (Accessed 18 August 2019).

29. Commission on Accreditation of Athletic Training Education: *Implementation and guide to the CAATE 2020 professional standards.* https://caate.net/wp-content/uploads/2018/09/Guide-to-2020-Standards.pdf. (Accessed 18 August 2019).

30. Rozzie SL, Futrell MG: *Practice analysis*, ed 7, Omaha, NE, 2015, Board of Certification for the Athletic Trainer, Inc.

31. Sackett DL, Rosenberg WMC, Gray JAM, et al: Evidence based medicine: what it is and what it isn't. *BMJ* 312:71–72, 1996.

32. Sackett DL, Straus SE, Richardson WS, et al: *Evidence based medicine: how to practice and teach EBM*, ed 2, Edinburgh, 2000, Churchill Livingstone.

33. https://www.cebm.net/2016/05/ocebm-levels-of-evidence/. (Accessed 21 September 2019).

34. Howick J, Chalmers I, Glasziou P, et al: *The 2011 Oxford CEBM levels of evidence (introductory document).* Oxford Centre for Evidence-Based Medicine. http://www.cebm.net/index.aspx?o=5653.

35. OCEBM Levels of Evidence Working Group: *The Oxford 2011 levels of evidence.* Oxford Centre for Evidence-Based Medicine. https://www.cebm.net/wp-content/uploads/2014/06/CEBM-Levels-of-Evidence-2.1.pdf. (Accessed 21 September 2019).

36. Moher D, Tetzlaff J, Tricco AC, et al: Epidemiology and reporting characteristics of systematic reviews. *PLoS Med* 4:e78, 2007.

37. The *PLoS Medicine* editors: Many reviews are systematic but some are more transparent and completely reported than others. *PLoS Med* 4:e147, 2007.

38. Michener LA, Leggin BG: A review of self-report scales for the assessment of functional limitation and disability of the shoulder. *J Hand Ther* 14:68–76, 2001.

39. Suk M, Hanson BP, Norvell DC, et al: *AO handbook: musculoskeletal outcomes measures and instruments*, Davos, Switzerland, 2005, AO Publishing.

40. Fitzpatrick R, Davey C, Buxton MJ, et al: Review: evaluating patient-based outcome measures for use in clinical trials, *Health Technol Assess* 2:i–iv, 1–74, 1998.

41. Valovich McLeod TC, Snyder AR, Parsons JT, et al. Using disablement models and clinical outcomes assessment to enable evidence-based athletic training practice, part II: clinical outcomes assessment. *J Athl Train* 43:437–445, 2008.

42. Institute of Medicine (US) Committee on Standards for Developing Trustworthy Clinical Practice Guidelines; Graham R, Mancher M, Miller Wolman D, et al: *Clinical practice guidelines we can trust*, Washington, DC, 2011, National Academies Press. https://www.ncbi.nlm.nih.gov/books/NBK209538/.

43. Guidelines International Network: *International Guidelines Laboratory.* https://g-i-n.net/library/international-guidelines-library/. (Accessed 21 September 2019).

44. Joule: *CPG Infobase: clinical practice guidelines.* https://joulecma.ca/cpg/homepage. (Accessed 21 September 2019).

45. Guidelines Central: *Official society guidelines tool.* https://www.guidelinecentral.com. (Accessed 21 September 2019).

46. Department of Health and Human Services: Medicare program; revisions to payment policies under the physician fee schedule for calendar year 1997; proposed rule. *Fed Reg* 61(128), 1997.

Inflammation and Tissue Repair

3

Erika L. Hagstrom | David Adelson

CHAPTER OBJECTIVES

After reading this chapter, the reader will be able to do the following:
- Define *inflammation*.
- Describe the phases of inflammation.
- Explain the tissue healing process.
- List the factors that affect the tissue healing process
- Discuss the healing process of specific musculoskeletal tissues.

Injury to vascularized tissue results in a coordinated, complex, and dynamic series of events collectively referred to as **inflammation** and repair. Although there are variations among the responses of different tissue types, overall, the processes are remarkably similar. The sequelae depend on the source and site of injury, the state of local homeostasis, and whether the injury is acute or chronic. The goal of inflammation and repair is to restore function by eliminating the pathological or physical insult, replacing the damaged or destroyed tissue, and promoting regeneration of normal tissue structure.

Rehabilitation professionals treat a variety of inflammatory conditions resulting from trauma, surgical procedures, or problematic healing. The clinician called on to manage such injuries needs to understand the physiology of inflammation and healing and how it can be modified. The clinician can enhance healing by applying the appropriate physical agents, therapeutic exercises, or manual techniques. A successful rehabilitation program requires an understanding of biomechanics; the phases of tissue healing; and the effects of immobilization, therapeutic interventions, and nutritional status on the healing process.

Phases of Inflammation and Healing

This chapter provides readers with information on the processes involved in inflammation and tissue repair so that they can understand how physical agents may be used to modify these processes and improve patient outcomes. The process of inflammation and repair consists of three phases: inflammation, proliferation, and maturation. The **inflammation phase** prepares the wound for healing, the **proliferation phase** rebuilds damaged structures and strengthens the wound, and the **maturation phase** modifies scar tissue into its mature form (Fig. 3.1). The duration of each phase varies to some degree, and the phases generally overlap. Thus, the timetables for the various phases of healing provided in this chapter are only general guidelines, not precise definitions (Fig. 3.2).

> **◎ Clinical Pearl**
>
> The process of regeneration and repair after injury consists of three phases: inflammation, proliferation, and maturation.

INFLAMMATION PHASE (DAYS 1 TO 6)

Inflammation, from the Latin *inflamer,* meaning "to set on fire," begins when the normal physiology of tissue is altered by disease or trauma.[1] This immediate protective response attempts to destroy, dilute, or isolate the cells or agents that may be at fault. It is a normal and necessary prerequisite to healing. If no inflammation occurs, healing cannot take place. Inflammation can also be harmful, particularly when it is directed at the wrong tissue or is overly exuberant. For example, inappropriately directed inflammatory reactions that underlie autoimmune diseases such as rheumatoid arthritis can damage and destroy joints. Although the inflammatory process follows the same sequence of events regardless of the cause of injury, some causes result in exaggeration or prolongation of certain events.

Nearly 2000 years ago, Cornelius Celsus characterized the inflammatory phase by the four cardinal signs of calor, rubor, tumor, and dolor (Latin terms for "heat," "redness," "swelling," and "pain"). A fifth cardinal sign, functio laesa ("loss of function"), was added to this list by Virchow (Table 3.1).

> **◎ Clinical Pearl**
>
> Inflammation is characterized by heat, redness, swelling, pain, and loss of function.

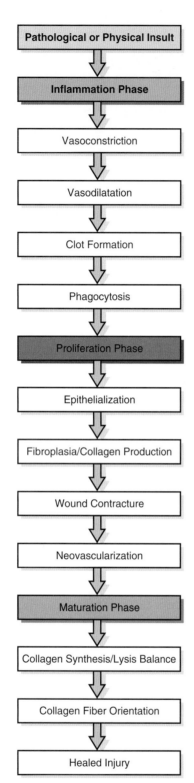

Pathological or Physical Insult

↓

Inflammation Phase

↓

Vasoconstriction

↓

Vasodilatation

↓

Clot Formation

↓

Phagocytosis

↓

Proliferation Phase

↓

Epithelialization

↓

Fibroplasia/Collagen Production

↓

Wound Contracture

↓

Neovascularization

↓

Maturation Phase

↓

Collagen Synthesis/Lysis Balance

↓

Collagen Fiber Orientation

↓

Healed Injury

FIGURE 3.1 Flow diagram of the normal phases of inflammation and repair.

An increase in blood in a given area, known as **hyperemia,** accounts primarily for the increased temperature and redness in the area of **acute inflammation.** The onset of hyperemia at the beginning of the inflammatory response is controlled by neurogenic and chemical mediators.[2] Local swelling results from increased permeability and vasodilation of local blood

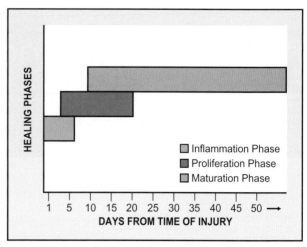

FIGURE 3.2 Timeline of the phases of inflammation and repair.

TABLE 3.1	Cardinal Signs of Inflammation	
Sign (English)	Sign (Latin)	Cause
Heat	Calor	Increased vascularity
Redness	Rubor	Increased vascularity
Swelling	Tumor	Blockage of lymphatic drainage
Pain	Dolor	Physical pressure or chemical irritation of pain-sensitive structures
Loss of function	Functio laesa	Pain and swelling

vessels and infiltration of fluid into interstitial spaces of the injured area. Pain results from the pressure of swelling and from irritation of pain-sensitive structures by chemicals released from damaged cells.[2] Both pain and swelling may result in loss of function.

There is some disagreement in the literature about the duration of the inflammation phase. Some investigators state that it is relatively short, lasting for fewer than 4 days[3,4]; others believe it may last for up to 6 days.[5,6] This discrepancy may be the result of individual and injury-specific variation, or it may reflect the overlapping nature of phases of inflammation and tissue healing.

The inflammatory phase involves a complex sequence of interactive and overlapping events, including vascular, cellular, hemostatic, and immune processes. **Humoral mediators** and **neural mediators** act to control the inflammatory phase. Evidence indicates that immediately after injury, **platelets** and **neutrophils** predominate and release a number of factors that amplify the platelet aggregation response, initiate a coagulation cascade, or act as chemo-attractants for cells involved in the inflammatory phase.[7] Neutrophil infiltration ceases after a few days, and neutrophils are replaced by **macrophages** starting 2 days after injury.[8] This shift in cell type at the site of injury correlates with a shift from the inflammation phase to the proliferation phase of healing.

Vascular Response

Alterations in the anatomy and function of the microvasculature, including capillaries, postcapillary venules, and lymphatic vessels, are among the earliest responses noted in the inflammatory phase.[9] Trauma such as a laceration, sprain, or contusion physically disrupts these structures and may produce bleeding, fluid loss, cell injury, and exposure of tissues to foreign material, including bacteria. Damaged vessels respond rapidly with transient constriction to minimize blood loss. This response, which is mediated by norepinephrine, generally lasts for 5 to 10 minutes but can be prolonged in small vessels by serotonin released from mast cells and platelets.

After the transient vasoconstriction of injured vessels, uninjured vessels near the injured area dilate. Capillary permeability is also increased by injury to the capillary walls and in response to chemicals released from injured tissues (Fig. 3.3). The vasodilation and increase in capillary permeability are initiated by histamine, Hageman factor, bradykinin, prostaglandins, and complement fractions. Vasodilation and increased capillary permeability last for up to 1 hour after tissue damage.

Histamine is released primarily by mast cells, as well as by platelets and basophils at the injury site.[10] Histamine causes vasodilation and increased vascular permeability in venules, which contribute to local **edema** (swelling). Histamine also attracts **leukocytes** (white blood cells) to the damaged tissue area.[11] The ability of a chemical to attract cells is known as **chemotaxis.** Histamine is one of the first inflammatory mediators released after tissue injury and is active for approximately 1 hour after injury (Fig. 3.4).[12]

Hageman factor (also known as *clotting factor XII*), an enzyme found in the blood, is activated by contact with negatively charged surfaces of the endothelial lining of vessels that are exposed when vessels are damaged. The role of Hageman factor is twofold. First, it activates the coagulation system to stop local bleeding. Second, it causes vasoconstriction and increased vascular permeability by activating other **plasma** proteins. It converts plasminogen to plasmin and prekallikrein to kallikrein, and it activates the alternative complement pathway (Fig. 3.5).[13]

Plasmin augments vascular permeability in both skin and lungs by inducing the breakdown of fibrin and by cleaving components of the **complement system.** Plasmin also activates Hageman factor, which initiates the cascade that generates bradykinin.

Plasma kallikrein attracts neutrophils and cleaves kininogen to generate several kinins, such as bradykinin. Kinins are biologically active peptides that are potent inflammatory substances derived from plasma. Kinins, particularly bradykinin, function similarly to histamine, causing a marked increase in permeability of the microcirculation. They are most prevalent

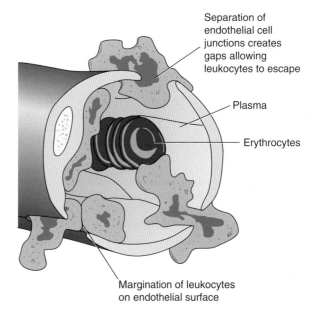

FIGURE 3.3 Vascular response to wound healing.

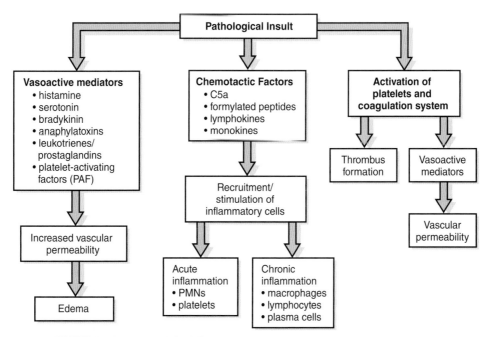

FIGURE 3.4 Mediators of the inflammatory response. *PMNs,* Polymorphonucleocytes.

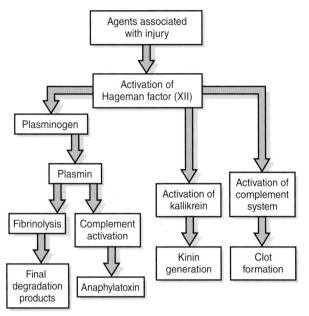

FIGURE 3.5 Hageman factor activation and inflammatory mediator production.

TABLE 3.2	Mediators of the Inflammatory Response
Response	**Mediators**
Vasodilation	Histamine
	Prostaglandins
	Serotonin
Increased vascular permeability	Bradykinin
	C3a, C5a
	PAF
	Histamine
	Serotonin
	Prostaglandins
Chemotaxis	Histamine
	C5a
	Monokines
	Kallikrein
	Lymphokines
Fever	Prostaglandins
Pain	Prostaglandins
	Hageman factor
	Bradykinin

PAF, Platelet-activating factor.

in the early phases of inflammation, after which they are rapidly destroyed by tissue proteases or kininases.[14]

Prostaglandins are produced by nearly all cells in the body and are released when the cell membrane is damaged. Two prostaglandins affect the inflammatory phase: prostaglandin E_1 (PGE_1) and PGE_2. PGE_1 increases vascular permeability by antagonizing vasoconstriction, and PGE_2 attracts leukocytes and synergizes the effects of other inflammatory mediators, such as bradykinin. Proinflammatory prostaglandins are also thought to be responsible for sensitizing pain receptors and **hyperalgesia.** In the early stages of the healing response, prostaglandins may regulate the repair process; they are also responsible for the later stages of inflammation.[15] Nonsteroidal antiinflammatory drugs (NSAIDs) specifically work by inhibiting prostaglandin synthesis, whereas **corticosteroids** inhibit inflammation through this and other mechanisms. Because prostaglandins are responsible for febrile states, these medications are also effective in reducing fever. More recent studies suggest that proinflammatory growth factors, including fibroblast growth factor and platelet-activating factor, also contribute to hyperalgesia.[16,17]

The anaphylatoxins C3a, C4a, and C5a are important products of the complement system. These complement fractions cause increased vascular permeability and induce mast cell and basophil degranulation, causing further release of histamine and further increasing vascular permeability.

Aside from chemically mediated vascular changes (Table 3.2), changes in physical attraction between blood vessel walls also alter blood flow. During the initial vasoconstriction, the opposing walls of the small vessels become approximated, causing the linings of blood vessels to stick together. Under normal physiological conditions, the cell membranes of inflammatory cells and the basement membranes have mutually repulsive negative charges; however, after injury, this repulsion decreases, and polarity may be reversed. This results in decreased repulsion between circulating inflammatory cells and vessel walls and contributes to the adherence of inflammatory cells to blood vessel linings.

As vasoconstriction of the postcapillary venules and increased permeability of the microvasculature cause blood flow to slow, an increase in cellular concentration occurs in the vessels, resulting in increased viscosity. Blood viscosity also increases as blood velocity slows because blood has shear-thinning properties.[18] In the normal physiological state, cellular components of blood within the microvasculature are confined to a central axial column, and the blood in contact with the vessel wall is relatively cell-free plasma.

Early in the inflammatory response, neutrophils, a type of leukocyte in the circulating blood, begin to migrate to the injured area. Within a few hours of injury, the bulk of neutrophils in the wound transmigrate across the capillary endothelial cell walls. The sequence of events in the journey of these cells from inside the blood vessel to the tissue outside the blood vessel is known as **extravasation.** Neutrophils break away from the central cellular column of blood and start to roll along the blood vessel lining (the endothelium) and adhere. They line the walls of the vessels in a process known as **margination.** Within 1 hour, the endothelial lining of the vessels can be completely covered with neutrophils. As these cells accumulate, they are laid down in layers in a process known as **pavementing.** Certain mediators control the adherence of leukocytes to the endothelium, enhancing or inhibiting this process. For example, fibronectin, a glycoprotein present in plasma and basement membranes, has an important role in the modulation of cellular adherence to vessel walls. After injury to the vessels, increased amounts of fibronectin are deposited at the injury site. Adherence of leukocytes to the endothelium or the vascular basement membrane is critical for their recruitment to the site of injury.

After margination, neutrophils begin to squeeze through the vessel walls in a process known as **diapedesis.** Endothelial

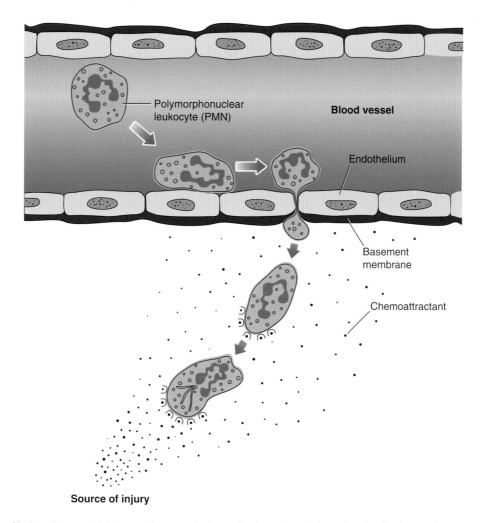

FIGURE 3.6 Illustration of leukocytic events in inflammation: margination, adhesion, diapedesis, and emigration in response to a chemoattractant emanating from the source of the injury.

P-selectin and E-selectin and intercellular adhesion mole-cule-1 (ICAM-1) and ICAM-2 are adhesion molecules crucial to diapedesis. These adhesion molecules interact with integrins on the surfaces of neutrophils as they insert their pseudopods into junctions between endothelial cells, crawl through widened junctions, and assume a position between the endothelium and the basement membrane. Then, attracted by chemotactic agents, they escape to reach the interstitium. This process of leukocyte migration from blood vessels into perivascular tissues is known as **emigration** (Fig. 3.6). Receptors on white blood cells and endothelial cells that allow rolling, margination, and diapedesis have been identified, and drugs that affect these functions have been developed. In the future, these drugs may play an important role in treating severe inappropriate inflammation.[19,20]

Edema is an accumulation of fluid within the extravascular space and interstitial tissues. Edema is the result of increased capillary hydrostatic pressure, increased interstitial osmotic pressure, increased venule permeability, and an overwhelmed lymphatic system that is unable to accommodate this substantial increase in fluid and plasma proteins. The clinical manifestation of edema is swelling. Edema formation and its control are discussed in detail in Chapter 19.

◯ Clinical Pearl

Edema is swelling caused by fluid accumulation outside the vessels.

Transudate, the fluid that first forms edema during inflammation, has very few cells and very little protein. This fluid is predominantly composed of dissolved electrolytes and water and has a specific gravity of less than 1.0. As the permeability of the vessels increases, more cells and lower-molecular-weight plasma proteins cross the vessel wall, making the extravascular fluid more viscous and cloudy. This cloudy fluid, known as **exudate,** has a specific gravity greater than 1.0. It is also characterized by a high content of lipids and cellular debris. Exudate is often observed early in the acute inflammatory process and forms in response to minor injuries such as blisters and sunburn.

Loss of protein-rich fluid from the plasma reduces osmotic pressure within the vessels and increases the osmotic pressure of interstitial fluids, which increases the outflow of fluid from the vessels, resulting in an accumulation of fluid in the interstitial tissue. When the exudate concentration of leukocytes increases, it is known as **pus** or suppurative exudate. Pus consists of neutrophils, liquefied digestion products of underlying tissue, fluid exudate, and often bacteria if an infection is present. When localized, suppurative exudate occurs within a solid tissue and results in an abscess, which is a localized collection of pus buried in a tissue, organ, or confined space. Pyogenic bacteria produce abscesses.

Four mechanisms are responsible for the increased vascular permeability seen in inflammation. The first mechanism is endothelial cell contraction, which leads to a widening of intercellular junctions or gaps. This mechanism affects venules while sparing capillaries and arterioles. It is controlled by chemical mediators and is relatively short-lived,

lasting for only 15 to 30 minutes.[21] The second mechanism is a result of direct endothelial injury and is an immediate, sustained response that potentially affects all levels of the microcirculation. This effect is often seen in severe burns or lytic bacterial infections and is associated with platelet adhesion and thrombosis or clot formation. The third mechanism is leukocyte-dependent endothelial injury. Leukocytes bind to the area of injury and release various chemicals and enzymes that damage the endothelium, thus increasing permeability. The fourth mechanism is leakage by regenerating capillaries that lack a differentiated endothelium and therefore do not have tight gaps. This may account for the edema characteristic of later-healing inflammation (Fig. 3.7).

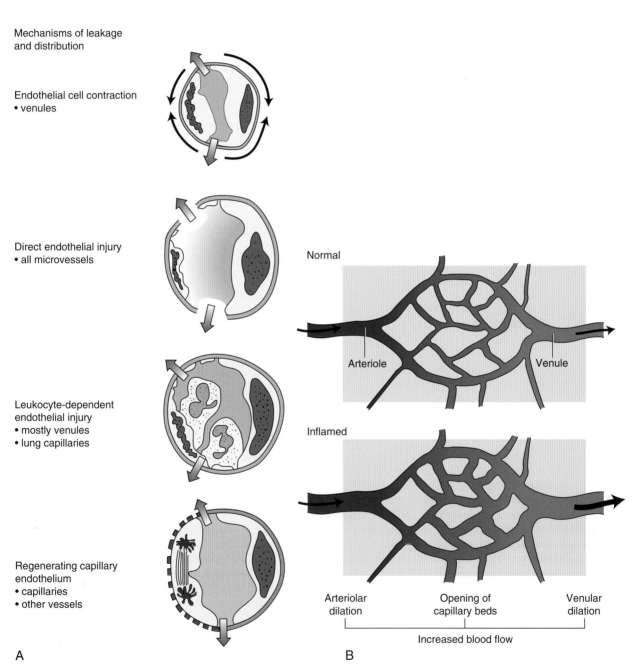

FIGURE 3.7 (A) Illustration of four mechanisms of increased vascular permeability in inflammation. (B) Vascular changes associated with acute inflammation.

Hemostatic Response

The hemostatic response to injury controls blood loss when vessels are damaged or ruptured. Immediately after injury, platelets enter the area and bind to the exposed subendothelial **collagen,** releasing fibrin to stimulate clotting. Platelets also release a regulatory protein known as **platelet-derived growth factor (PDGF),** which is chemotactic and mitogenic to **fibroblasts** and may also be chemotactic to macrophages, **monocytes,** and neutrophils.[22] Thus, platelets not only play a role in hemostasis, but they also contribute to the control of fibrin deposition, fibroblast proliferation, and angiogenesis.

When fibrin and fibronectin enter the injured area, they form cross-links with collagen to create a fibrin lattice. This tenuous structure provides a temporary plug in the blood and lymph vessels, limiting local bleeding and fluid drainage. The lattice seals off damaged vessels and confines the inflammatory reaction to the area immediately surrounding the injury. The damaged, plugged vessels do not reopen until later in the healing process. The fibrin lattice serves as the wound's only source of tensile strength during the inflammatory phase of healing.[23]

Cellular Response

Circulating blood is composed of specialized cells suspended in a fluid known as *plasma.* These cells include **erythrocytes** (red blood cells), leukocytes (white blood cells), and platelets. Erythrocytes play only a minor role in the inflammatory process, although they may migrate into tissue spaces if the inflammatory reaction is intense. Oxygen transport, the primary role of erythrocytes, is carried out within the confines of the vessels. An inflammatory exudate that contains blood usually indicates severe injury to the microvasculature. The accumulation of blood in a tissue or organ is referred to as a **hematoma;** bloody fluid in a joint is called a **hemarthrosis.** Hematomas in muscle can cause pain and can limit motion or function; they can also increase scar tissue formation. Hemoglobin-derived iron from phagocytosed red blood cells also contributes to tissue damage through increased generation of reactive oxygen species.[24]

A critical function of inflammation is to deliver leukocytes to the area of injury via the circulatory system. Leukocytes are classified according to their structure into **polymorphonucleocytes (PMNs)** and mononuclear cells (Fig. 3.8). PMNs have nuclei with several lobes and contain cytoplasmic granules. They are further categorized as neutrophils, basophils, and eosinophils by their preference for specific histological stains. Monocytes are larger than PMNs and have a single nucleus. In the inflammatory process, leukocytes have the important role of clearing the injured site of debris and microorganisms to set the stage for tissue repair.

Migration of leukocytes into the area of injury occurs within hours of the injury. Each leukocyte is specialized and has a specific purpose. Some leukocytes are more prominent in early inflammation, whereas others become more important during

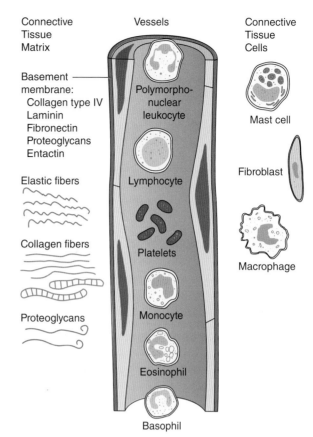

FIGURE 3.8 Connective tissue matrix, intravascular cells, and connective tissue cells involved in the inflammatory response.

later stages. Initially, the number of leukocytes at the injury site is proportionate to their concentration in the circulating blood.

Because neutrophils have the highest concentration in the blood, they predominate in the early phases of inflammation. Chemotactic agents released by other cells, such as mast cells and platelets, attract leukocytes at the time of injury. Neutrophils rid the injury site of bacteria and debris by **phagocytosis.** When lysed, lysosomes of the neutrophils release proteolytic enzymes (proteases) and collagenolytic enzymes **(collagenases),** which begin the debridement process. Neutrophils remain at the site of injury for only 24 hours, after which time they disintegrate. However, they help to perpetuate the inflammatory response by releasing chemotactic agents to attract other leukocytes into the area.

Basophils release histamine after injury and contribute to early increased vascular permeability. Eosinophils may be involved in phagocytosis to some degree, although they are classically involved in allergic inflammation or extra-gastrointestinal parasitic disease.[25]

For 24 to 48 hours after an acute injury, monocytes predominate. Monocytes make up 4% to 8% of the total white blood cell count. The predominance of these cells at this stage of inflammation is thought to result in part from their longer life span. Lymphocytes supply antibodies to mediate the body's immune response. They are prevalent in chronic inflammatory conditions.

Monocytes are converted into macrophages when they migrate from the capillaries into the tissue spaces. The macrophage is considered the most important cell in the

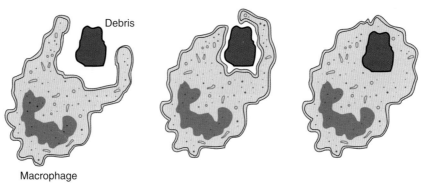

Debris

Macrophage

FIGURE 3.9 Diagrammatic representation of the process of phagocytosis.

Box 3.1 Macrophage Products

- Proteases
- Elastase
- Collagenase
- Plasminogen activator
- Chemotactic factors for other leukocytes
- Complement components of alternative and classical pathways
- Coagulation factors
- Growth-promoting factors for fibroblasts and blood vessels
- Cytokines
- Arachidonic acid metabolites

---

inflammatory phase and is essential for wound healing. Macrophages are important because they produce a wide range of chemicals (Box 3.1). They play a major role in phagocytosis by producing enzymes such as collagenase (Fig. 3.9). These enzymes facilitate the removal of necrotic tissue and bacteria. Macrophages also produce factors that are chemotactic for other leukocytes and growth factors that promote cell proliferation and the synthesis of extracellular matrix molecules by resident skin cells.[26]

Macrophages probably play a role in localizing the inflammatory process and attracting fibroblasts to the injured area by releasing chemotactic factors such as fibronectin. Macrophages activated by type 2 cytokines chemically influence the number of fibroblastic repair cells activated; therefore, in the absence of macrophages, fewer, less mature fibroblasts migrate to the injured site. More recent data suggest that a specific population of activated CD301b+ macrophages regulates a population of fibroblasts that proliferate at the wound site. High numbers of these CD301+ macrophages have been found in keloid scars—a pathological proliferation of scar tissue—which supports a profibrotic function of this macrophage and may be a possible future target for clinical intervention.[27]

In the later stages of **fibroplasia,** macrophages may enhance collagen deposition by causing fibroblasts to adhere to fibrin. Two distinct subsets of macrophages, M1 and M2, have been characterized.[28] Over the course from injury to repair, macrophages switch their phenotype from M1 to M2. In skeletal muscle and renal tissues, M1 macrophages promote inflammation, whereas M2 macrophages promote fibrosis. However, in the liver, M1 macrophages promote inflammation and fibrosis, whereas M2 macrophages promote resolution with matrix degradation and debris clearance, contributing to scar resolution. These functional differences in M1 and M2 macrophages in different tissues highlight the diversity of macrophages in different microenvironments.

As macrophages phagocytose organisms, they release a variety of substances, such as hydrogen peroxide, ascorbic acid, and lactic acid, that enhance the killing of microorganisms.[29] Hydrogen peroxide inhibits anaerobic microbial growth. The other two products signal the extent of damage in the area, and their concentration is interpreted by the body as a need for more macrophages in the area.[30] This interpretation causes increased production of these substances, which results in an increased macrophage population and a more intense and prolonged inflammatory response.

Macrophages are most effective when oxygen is present in injured tissues. However, they can tolerate low-oxygen conditions, as is apparent by their presence in chronic inflammatory states. Adequate oxygen tension in the injured area is also necessary to minimize the risk of infection. Tissue oxygen tension depends on the concentration of atmospheric oxygen available for breathing, the amount of oxygen absorbed by the respiratory and circulatory systems, the volume of blood available for transportation, and the state of the tissues. Local topical application of oxygen to an injured area does not influence tissue oxygen tension as much as the level of oxygen brought to the injured area by the circulating blood.[31–33]

Immune Response

The immune response is mediated by cellular and humoral factors. On a cellular level, macrophages present foreign antigens to T lymphocytes to activate them. Activated T lymphocytes elaborate a host of inflammatory mediators and activate B cells, causing them to evolve into plasma cells, which make antibodies that specifically bind foreign antigens. These antibodies can coat bacteria and viruses, inhibiting their function and opsonizing them so that they are more readily ingested and cleared from the system by phagocytic cells. Antibodies bound to antigens, bacteria, and viruses also activate the complement system, an important source of vasoactive mediators. The complement system is one of the most important plasma protein systems of inflammation because its components participate in virtually every inflammatory response.

The complement system is a series of enzymatic plasma proteins that is activated by two different pathways: classical and alternative.[34] Activation of the first component of either pathway of the cascade results in the sequential enzymatic activation of downstream components of the cascade (Fig. 3.10).

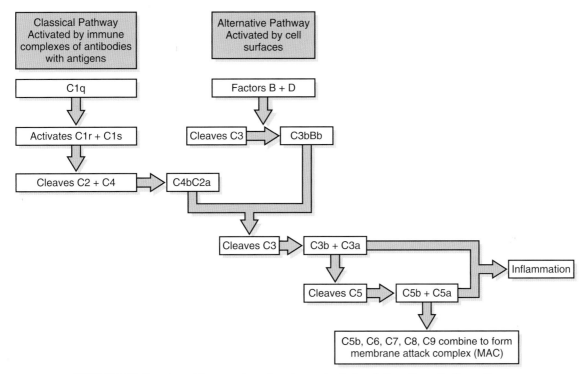

FIGURE 3.10 Overview of the complement system—classical and alternative activation pathways.

The classical pathway is activated by an antibody-antigen association, and the alternative pathway is activated by cellular or microbial substances. The end product of the cascade, by either pathway, is a complex of C5b, C6, C7, C8, and C9, which form the membrane attack complex (MAC). The MAC creates pores in plasma membranes, thereby allowing water and ions into the cell, leading to cell lysis and death.

The subcomponents generated earlier in the cascade also have important functions. Activation of components C1 to C5 produces subunits that enhance inflammation by making bacteria more susceptible to phagocytosis (known as **opsonization**), attracting leukocytes by chemotaxis, and acting as anaphylatoxins. Anaphylatoxins induce mast cell and basophil degranulation, causing the release of histamine, platelet-activating factor, and leukotrienes. These further promote increased vascular permeability.

In summary, the inflammatory phase has three major purposes. First, fibrin, fibronectin, and collagen cross-link to form a fibrin lattice that limits blood loss and provides the wound with some initial strength. Second, neutrophils followed by macrophages begin to remove damaged tissue. Third, endothelial cells and fibroblasts are recruited and stimulated to divide. This sets the stage for the proliferation phase of healing. Table 3.3 summarizes the events of the inflammatory phase of healing.

> **◎ Clinical Pearl**
>
> The inflammatory phase has three major purposes: (1) to form a fibrin lattice that limits blood loss and provides some initial strength to the wound, (2) to remove damaged tissue, (3) to recruit endothelial cells and fibroblasts.

PROLIFERATION PHASE (DAYS 3 TO 20)

The second phase of tissue healing is known as the *proliferation phase*. This phase generally lasts for up to 20 days and involves both **epithelial cells** and **connective tissues**.[23] Its purpose is to cover the wound and impart strength to the injury site.

> **◎ Clinical Pearl**
>
> During the proliferation phase, the wound is covered, and the injury site starts to regain some of its initial strength.

Epithelial cells form the covering of mucous and serous membranes and the epidermis of the skin. Connective tissue consists of fibroblasts, ground substance, and fibrous strands and provides the structure for other tissues. The structure, strength, and elasticity of connective tissue vary, depending on the type of tissue it comprises. Four processes occur simultaneously in the proliferation phase to achieve coalescence and closure of the injured area: **epithelialization,** collagen production, **wound contraction,** and **neovascularization.**

Epithelialization

Epithelialization, the reestablishment of the epidermis, is initiated early in proliferation when a wound is superficial, often within a few hours of injury.[35] When a wound is deep, epithelialization occurs later, after collagen production and neovascularization. Epithelialization provides a protective barrier to prevent fluid and electrolyte loss and to decrease the risk of infection. Healing of the wound surface by epithelialization alone does not provide adequate strength to

TABLE 3.3	Summary of Events of the Inflammatory Phase
Response	**Changes in the Injured Area**
Vascular	Vasodilation followed by vasoconstriction at the capillaries, postcapillary venules, and lymphatics
	Vasodilation mediated by chemical mediators—histamine, Hageman factor, bradykinin, prostaglandins, complement fractions
	Slowing of blood flow
	Margination, pavementing, and ultimately, emigration of leukocytes
	Accumulation of fluid in the interstitial tissues resulting in edema
Hemostatic	Retraction and sealing off of blood vessels
	Platelets form clots and assist in building of fibrin lattice, which serves as the source of tensile strength for the wound in the inflammatory phase
Cellular	Delivery of leukocytes to the area of injury to rid the area of bacteria and debris by phagocytosis
	Monocytes, the precursors of macrophages, are considered the most important cell in the inflammatory phase
	Macrophages produce a number of products essential to the healing process
Immune	Mediated by cellular and humoral factors
	Activation of the complement system via alternative and classical pathways, resulting in components that increase vascular permeability, stimulate phagocytosis, and act as chemotactic stimuli for leukocytes

meet the mechanical demands placed on most tissues. Such strength is provided by collagen produced during fibroplasia.

During epithelialization, uninjured epithelial cells from the margins of the injured area reproduce and migrate over the injured area, covering the surface of the wound and closing the defect. It is hypothesized that the stimulus for this activity is the loss of contact inhibition that occurs when epithelial cells are normally in contact with one another. Migrating epithelial cells stay connected to their parent cells, thereby pulling the intact epidermis over the wound edge. When epithelial cells from one edge meet migrating cells from the other edge, they stop moving because of contact inhibition (Fig. 3.11). Although clean, approximated wounds can be clinically resurfaced within 48 hours, larger open wounds take longer to resurface.[36] It then takes several weeks for this thin layer to become multilayered and to differentiate into the various strata of normal epidermis.

Collagen Production

Fibroblasts make collagen. Fibroblast growth, known as *fibroplasia,* takes place in connective tissue. Fibroblasts develop from undifferentiated mesenchymal cells located around blood vessels and in fat. They migrate to the injured area along fibrin strands, in response to chemotactic influences, and are present throughout the injured area.[37] For fibroplasia to occur, adequate supplies of oxygen; ascorbic acid; and other cofactors, such as zinc, iron, manganese, and copper,

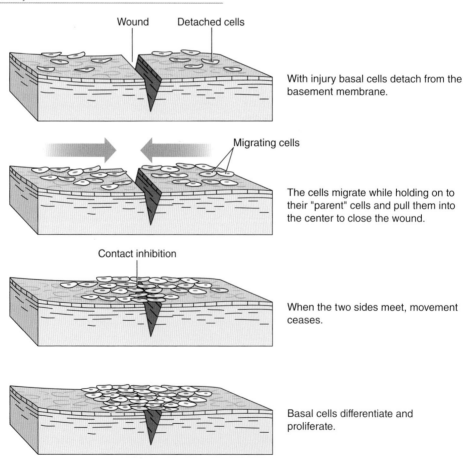

Wound   Detached cells

With injury basal cells detach from the basement membrane.

Migrating cells

The cells migrate while holding on to their "parent" cells and pull them into the center to close the wound.

Contact inhibition

When the two sides meet, movement ceases.

Basal cells differentiate and proliferate.

FIGURE 3.11 Schematic diagram of epithelialization.

are necessary.[38] As the number of fibroblasts increases, they begin to align themselves perpendicular to the capillaries.

Fibroblasts synthesize procollagen, which is composed of three polypeptide chains coiled and held together by weak electrostatic bonds into a triple helix. These chains undergo cleavage by collagenase to form tropocollagen. Multiple tropocollagen chains then coil together to form collagen microfibrils, which make up collagen fibrils and ultimately combine to form collagen fibers (Fig. 3.12). Cross-linking between collagen molecules provides further tensile strength to the injured area. Ascorbic acid (vitamin C) is an essential cofactor in collagen synthesis and resultant wound tissue quality.[39] Collagen serves a dual purpose in wound healing, providing increased strength and facilitating the movement of other cells, such as endothelial cells and macrophages, while they participate in wound healing.[40,41]

Tissue containing newly formed capillaries, fibroblasts, and **myofibroblasts** is referred to as **granulation tissue.** As the amount of granulation tissue increases, a concurrent reduction in the size of the fibrin clot allows for the formation of a more permanent support structure. These events are mediated by chemotactic factors that stimulate increased fibroblastic activity and by fibronectin that enhances the migration and adhesion of the fibroblasts. Fibroblasts initially produce a thin, weak-structured collagen with no consistent organization, known as **type III collagen.** This period is the most tenuous time during the healing process because of the limited tensile strength of the tissue. During the proliferation

phase, an injured area has the greatest amount of collagen, yet its tensile strength can be as low as 15% of the tensile strength of normal tissue.[42]

> ### ◎ Clinical Pearl
>
> During the proliferation phase, an injured area has the greatest amount of collagen, yet its tensile strength can be as low as 15% of the tensile strength of normal tissue.

Fibroblasts also produce hyaluronic acid, a glycosaminoglycan (GAG), which draws water into the area, increases the amount of intracellular matrix, and facilitates cellular migration. It is postulated that the composition of this substance is related to the number and location of the cross-bridges, thereby implying that the relationship between GAG and collagen dictates the scar architecture.[29,43]

The formation of cross-links allows the newly formed tissue to tolerate early, controlled movement without disruption. However, infection, edema, or excessive stress on the healing area may cause further inflammation and additional deposition of collagen. Excessive collagen deposition results in excessive scarring that may limit function.

By the seventh day after injury, a significant increase in the amount of collagen causes the tensile strength of the injured area to increase steadily. By day 12, the initial immature type III collagen starts to be replaced by **type I collagen,** a more mature and stronger form.[23,44,45] The ratio of type I to type III collagen increases steadily from this point forward. The production of collagen is maximal at day 21 of healing, but wound strength at this time is only approximately 20% of that of the normal dermis. By about 6 weeks after injury, when a wound is healing well, it has approximately 80% of its long-term strength.[46]

Wound Contraction

Wound contraction is the final mechanism for repairing an injured area. In contrast to epithelialization, which covers the wound surface, contraction pulls the edges of the injured site together, in effect shrinking the defect. Successful contraction results in a smaller area to be repaired by the formation of a scar. Contraction of the wound begins approximately 5 days after injury and peaks after about 2 weeks.[47] Myofibroblasts are the primary cells responsible for wound contraction. Myofibroblasts, identified by Gabbiani and associates in 1971,[48] are derived from the same mesenchymal cells as fibroblasts. Myofibroblasts are like fibroblasts except that they possess the contractile properties of smooth muscle. Myofibroblasts attach to the margins of intact skin and pull the entire epithelial layer inward. The rate of contraction is proportional to the number of myofibroblasts at and under the cell margins and is inversely proportional to the lattice collagen structure.

According to the "picture frame" theory, the wound margin beneath the epidermis is the location of myofibroblast action.[49] A ring of myofibroblasts moves inward from the wound margin. Although contractile forces are initially equal, the shape of the picture frame predicts the resultant speed of closure (Fig. 3.13). Linear wounds with one narrow dimension contract rapidly; square or rectangular wounds, with no edges close to each other, progress at a moderate pace; and circular wounds contract most slowly.[50]

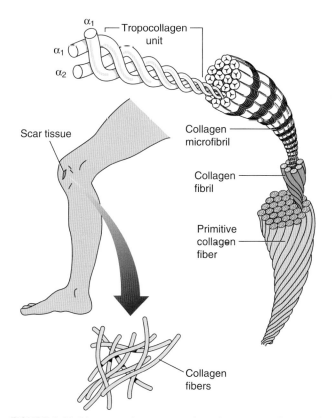

FIGURE 3.12 Diagrammatic representation of one tropocollagen unit joining with others to form collagen filaments and, ultimately, collagen fibers.

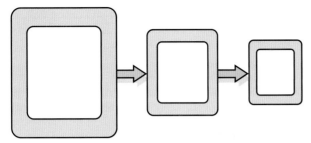

FIGURE 3.13 Illustration of the "picture frame" theory of wound contraction.

If wound contraction is uncontrolled, **contractures** can form. Contractures are conditions of fixed shortening of soft tissues that have high resistance to passive stretch.[51] Contractures may result from adhesions, muscle shortening, or tissue damage. Contractures are discussed further in Chapter 6.

When the initial injury causes minimal tissue loss and minimal bacterial contamination, the wound can be closed with sutures and thus can heal without wound contraction. This is known as **healing by primary intention** (also known as *primary union*) (Fig. 3.14). However, when the initial injury causes significant loss of tissue or bacterial contamination, the wound must first undergo the process of wound contraction to close the wound; this is known as **healing by secondary intention** (also known as *indirect union*) (see Fig. 3.14).[52] Later approximation of wound edges with sutures or the application of skin grafts can reduce wound contraction and is known as **healing by delayed primary intention.**[53,54] To minimize contraction, grafts must be applied early in the inflammatory phase, before the process of contraction begins.[55]

As scar tissue matures, it develops pressure-sensitive and tension-sensitive nerve endings to protect the immature vascular system, which is weak and can bleed easily with any insult. During the proliferation phase, the scar is red and swollen as a result of the increase in vascularity and fluid, the innervation of the healing site, and the relative immaturity of the tissue. The tissue can be damaged easily and is tender to tension or pressure.

Neovascularization

Neovascularization, the development of a new blood supply to the injured area, occurs as a result of **angiogenesis,** the growth of new blood vessels. Healing cannot occur without angiogenesis. These new vessels are needed to supply oxygen and nutrients to injured and healing tissue. It is thought that macrophages signal the initiation of neovascularization through the release of growth factors.[46] Angiogenesis can occur by one of three different mechanisms: (1) generation of a new vascular network, (2) anastomosis to preexisting vessels, or (3) coupling of vessels in the injured area.[56]

Vessels in the wound periphery develop small buds that grow into the wound area. These outgrowths eventually meet and join other arterial or venular buds to form a capillary loop. These vessels fill the injured area, giving it a pinkish to bright-red hue. As the wound heals, many of these capillary loops cease to function and retract, giving the mature scar a more whitish appearance than adjacent tissues. Initially, the walls of these capillaries are thin, making them prone to injury. Therefore, immobilization at this stage may help protect these vessels and permit further regrowth, whereas excessive early motion can cause microhemorrhaging and can increase the likelihood of infection.

MATURATION PHASE (DAY 9 FORWARD)

As the transition from the proliferation to the maturation stage of healing is made, changes in the size, form, and strength of the scar tissue occur. The maturation phase is the longest phase in the healing process. It can persist longer than a year after the initial injury. During this time, the numbers of fibroblasts, macrophages, myofibroblasts, and capillaries decrease, and the water content of the tissue declines. The scar becomes whiter in appearance as collagen matures and vascularity decreases. The goal of this phase is restoration of the prior function of injured tissue.

> **Clinical Pearl**
>
> The goal of the maturation phase is restoration of the prior function of injured tissue. This phase can last longer than a year after the initial injury.

Several factors determine the rate of maturation and the final physical characteristics of the scar, including fiber orientation and the balance of collagen synthesis and lysis. Throughout the maturation phase, synthesis and lysis of collagen occur in a balanced fashion. Hormonal stimulation that results from inflammation causes increased collagen destruction by the enzyme collagenase. Collagenase is derived from polymorphogranular leukocytes, the migrating epithelium, and the granulation bed. Collagenase can break the strong cross-linking bonds of the tropocollagen molecule, causing it to become soluble. It is then excreted as a waste by-product. Although collagenase is most active in the actual area of injury, its effects can be noticed to a greater extent in areas adjacent to the injury site. Thus, remodeling occurs through a process of collagen turnover.

Collagen, a glycoprotein, provides the extracellular framework for all multicellular organisms. Although more than 27 types of collagen have been identified, the following discussion is limited to types I, II, and III (Table 3.4).[57] All collagen molecules are made up of three separate polypeptide chains wrapped tightly together in a triple left-handed helix. Type I collagen is the primary collagen in bone, skin, and **tendon**

TABLE 3.4	Collagen Types
Type	**Distribution**
I	Most abundant form of collagen: skin, bone, tendons, most organs
II	Major cartilage collagen, vitreous humor
III	Abundant in blood vessels, uterus, skin
IV	All basement membranes
V	Minor component of most interstitial tissues
VI	Abundant in most interstitial tissues
VII	Dermal-epidermal junction
VIII	Endothelium
IX	Cartilage
X	Cartilage

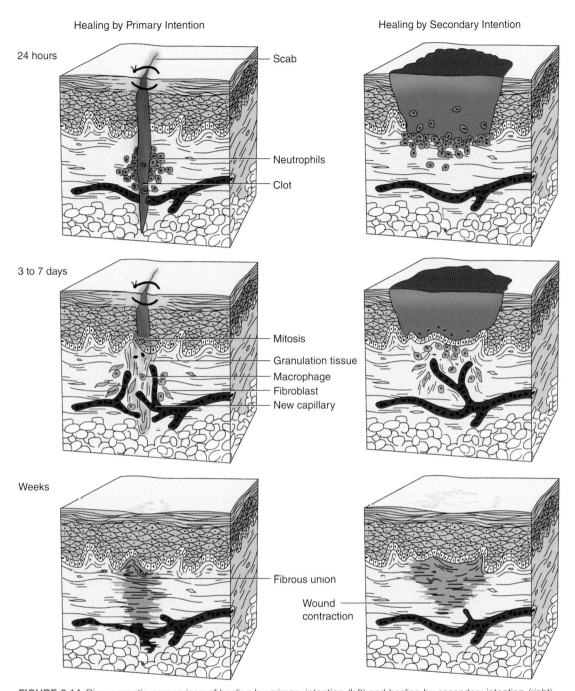

FIGURE 3.14 Diagrammatic comparison of healing by primary intention *(left)* and healing by secondary intention *(right)*.

and is the predominant collagen in mature scars. **Type II collagen** is the predominant collagen in **cartilage.** Type III collagen occurs in the gastrointestinal tract, uterus, and blood vessels of adults. It is also the first type of collagen to be deposited during the healing process.

During the maturation phase, the collagen synthesized and deposited is predominantly type I. Generally, the balance between synthesis and lysis slightly favors synthesis. Because type I collagen is stronger than the type III collagen deposited in the proliferation phase, tensile strength increases faster than mass. If the rate of collagen production is much greater than the rate of lysis, a keloid or hypertrophic scar can result. Keloids and hypertrophic scars are the result of excessive collagen

deposition caused by inhibition of lysis. It is believed that this inhibition of lysis is the result of a genetic defect. Keloids extend beyond the original boundaries of an injury and invade surrounding tissue, whereas hypertrophic scars, although raised, remain within the margins of the original wound. Treatment of keloids through surgery, medications, pressure, and irradiation has only limited success.[58–60]

Collagen synthesis is oxygen dependent, whereas collagen lysis is not.[61] Thus, when oxygen levels are low, the process of maturation is weighted toward lysis, resulting in a softer, less bulky scar. Hypertrophic scars can be managed clinically with prolonged pressure, which causes a decrease in oxygen, resulting in decreased overall collagen synthesis while maintaining the level of collagen lysis.[53] This is one of the bases for the use of pressure garments in the treatment of patients with burn injuries and for the use of elastomer in the management of scars in hand therapy. Eventually, balance is achieved when the scar bulk is flattened to approximate normal tissue.

Collagen synthesis and lysis may last for up to 12 to 24 months after an injury. The high rate of collagen turnover during this period can be viewed as both detrimental and beneficial. If scar tissue appears redder than surrounding tissue, remodeling is still occurring. Although a joint or tissue structure can lose mobility quickly during this stage, such a loss can be reversed through appropriate intervention.

The physical structure of collagen fibers is largely responsible for the final function of the injured area. Collagen in scar tissue is always less organized than collagen in surrounding tissue. Scars are inelastic because elastin, a normal skin component, is not present in scars,[46] so redundant folds are necessary to permit mobility of the structures to which they are attached. To understand this concept better, one may consider a spring, which, although made of an inelastic material, has a spiral form (like the redundant folds of a scar) that allows it to expand and contract. If short, dense adhesions are formed, these will restrict motion because they cannot elongate.

Two theories have been proposed to explain the orientation of collagen fibers in scar tissue: the induction theory and the tension theory. According to the induction theory, the scar attempts to mimic the characteristics of the tissue it is healing.[62] Thus, dense tissue induces a dense, highly cross-linked scar, whereas more pliable tissue results in a loose, less cross-linked scar. Dense tissue types have a preferential status when multiple tissue types are in proximity. Based on this theory, surgeons attempt to design repair fields that separate dense from soft tissues. If this is not possible, as in the case of repaired tendon that is left immobile over bone fractures, adhesions and poorly gliding tendons can result. In such cases, early controlled movement may be beneficial.

According to the tension theory, internal and external stresses placed on the injured area during the maturation phase determine the final tissue structure.[56] Muscle tension, joint movement, soft tissue loading and unloading, fascial gliding, temperature changes, and mobilization are forces that are thought to affect collagen structure. Thus, the length and mobility of the injured area may be modified by the application of stress during appropriate phases of healing. This theory has been supported by the work of Arem and Madden,[63] which has shown that the two most important variables responsible for successful remodeling are (1) the phases of the repair process in which mechanical forces were introduced and (2) the nature of the applied forces. For permanent changes to occur, scars need low-load, long-duration stretch during the appropriate phase.

Studies have shown that applying tension during healing increases tensile strength and that immobilization and stress deprivation reduce tensile strength and the organization of collagen structure. Recovery curves for tissue experimentally immobilized for 2 to 4 weeks reveal that these processes can take months to reverse and that reversal often is incomplete.

Physical loading of soft tissue produces an electrical current that can influence wound healing. This is known as the **piezoelectric** effect and can also be seen in bone. New bone can be formed when an electronegative force is applied and resorbed when an electropositive potential is applied.[64]

Each phase of the healing response is necessary and essential to the subsequent phase. In the optimal scenario, inflammation is a necessary aspect of the healing response and is the first step toward recovery, setting the stage for the other phases of healing. If repeated insult or injury occurs, however, a chronic inflammatory response can adversely affect the outcome of the healing process.

Acute inflammatory processes can have one of four outcomes. The first and most beneficial outcome is complete resolution and replacement of the injured tissue with like tissue. The second and most common outcome is healing by scar formation. The third outcome is the formation of an abscess. The fourth outcome is the possibility of progression to **chronic inflammation**.[12]

Chronic Inflammation

Chronic inflammation is the simultaneous progression of active inflammation, tissue destruction, and healing. Chronic inflammation can arise in one of two ways. The first follows acute inflammation and can be a result of the persistence of the injurious agent (e.g., cumulative trauma) or some other interference with the normal healing process. The second may be the result of an immune response to an altered host tissue or a foreign material (e.g., an implant or a suture), or it may be the result of an autoimmune disease (e.g., rheumatoid arthritis).

The normal acute inflammatory process lasts no longer than 2 weeks. If it continues for longer than 4 weeks, it is known as **subacute inflammation**.[3] Chronic inflammation is inflammation that lasts for months or years.

The primary cells present during chronic inflammation are mononuclear cells, including lymphocytes, macrophages, and monocytes (Fig. 3.15). Occasionally, eosinophils are also present.[13] Progression of the inflammatory response to a chronic state is a result of both immunological and nonimmunological factors. The macrophage is an important source of inflammatory and immunological mediators and is an important component in the regulation of their actions. The role of eosinophils is much less clear, although they are often present in chronic inflammatory conditions caused by an allergic reaction or a parasitic infection.[13]

Chronic inflammation results in increased fibroblast proliferation, which increases collagen production and ultimately increases scar tissue and adhesion formation. This may lead to loss of function as the delicate balance between the optimal tensile strength and mobility of involved tissues is lost.

Factors Affecting the Healing Process

Various local and systemic factors can influence or modify the processes of inflammation and repair (Box 3.2). Local factors such as the type, size, and location of the injury can affect wound healing, as can infection, blood supply, external physical forces, and movement.

> **◉ Clinical Pearl**
>
> Local factors that can affect wound healing include the type, size, and location of the injury; infection; blood supply; external physical forces; and movement. Systemic factors that can affect wound healing include age, disease, medications, and nutrition.

Leukocyte	Characteristics/Functions
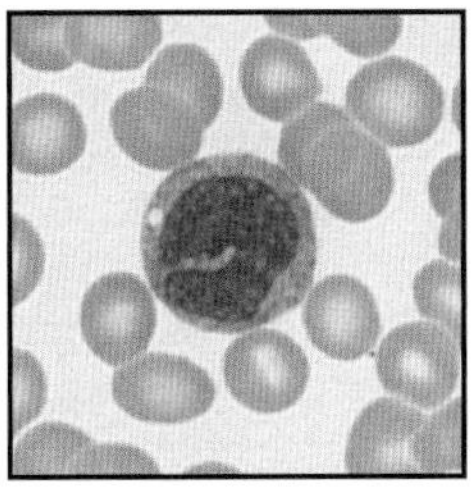 **A** Monocyte/Macrophage	Associated with • chronic inflammation • phagocytosis Regulates coagulation/fibrolytic pathways Regulates lymphocyte response Monocytes are converted to macrophages when they emigrate from capillaries into the tissue spaces.
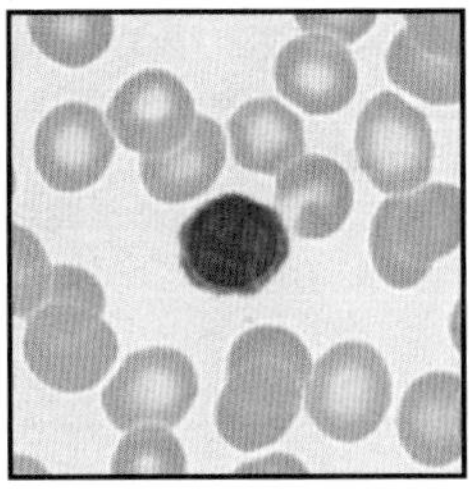 **B** Lymphocyte	Associated with • chronic inflammation Key cell in humoral and cell-mediated immune response
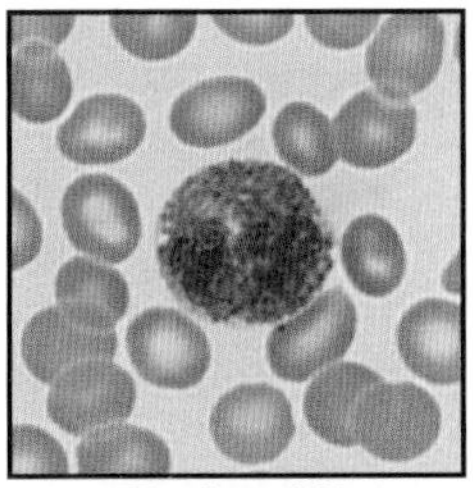 **C** Eosinophil	Associated with • allergic reactions • parasitic infections and associated inflammatory reactions Modulates mast cell-mediated reactions
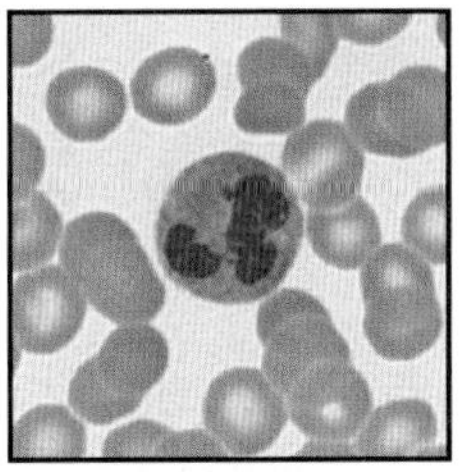 **D** Neutrophil	Associated with • acute inflammation • bacterial and foreign body phagocytosis
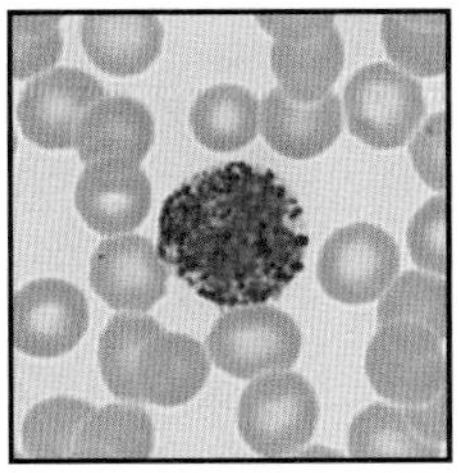 **E** Basophil	Associated with • allergic reactions Contains histamine, which causes increased vascular permeability Contains heparin, which slows blood clotting

Mononuclear cells (A, B)

Polymorphonuclear cells (C, D, E)

FIGURE 3.15 Cellular components of acute and chronic inflammation. (A) Monocyte/macrophage. (B) Lymphocyte. (C) Eosinophil. (D) Neutrophil. (E) Basophil. (Adapted from McPherson R, Pincus M: *Henry's clinical diagnosis and management by laboratory methods*, ed 21, Philadelphia, 2006, Saunders.)

Box 3.2	Factors Influencing Healing
LOCAL	**SYSTEMIC**
• Type, size, and location of injury	• Age
• Infection	• Infection or disease
• Vascular supply	• Metabolic status
• Movement/excessive pressure	• Nutrition
• Temperature deviation	• Hormones
• Topical medications	• Medication
• Electromagnetic energy	• Fever
• Retained foreign body	• Oxygen

LOCAL FACTORS

Type, Size, and Location of the Injury

Injuries located in well-vascularized tissue, such as the scalp, heal faster than injuries in poorly vascularized areas.[23] Injuries in areas of ischemia, such as injuries that may be caused by arterial obstruction or excessive pressure, heal more slowly.[23]

Smaller wounds heal faster than larger wounds, and surgical incisions heal faster than wounds caused by blunt trauma.[23] Soft tissue injuries over bones tend to adhere to the bony surfaces, preventing contraction and adequate opposition of the edges and delaying healing.[23]

Infection

Infection in an injured area is the most problematic local factor that can affect healing. Among the complications of wound healing, 50% are the result of local infection.[13] Infection can reduce collagen production and increase collagen lysis,[65] prevent or delay healing, and encourage excessive granulation tissue formation.[23]

Vascular Supply

The healing of injuries depends largely on the availability of a sufficient vascular supply. Nutrition, oxygen tension, and the inflammatory response all depend on the microcirculatory system to deliver their components.[66] Decreased oxygen tension resulting from a compromised blood supply can result in inhibition of fibroblast migration and collagen synthesis, leading to decreased tensile strength of the injured area and increased susceptibility to infection.[32]

External Forces

The application of physical agents, including thermal agents, electromagnetic energy, and mechanical forces, can influence inflammation and healing. Cryotherapy (cold therapy), thermotherapy (heat), therapeutic ultrasound, electromagnetic radiation, light, electrical currents, and mechanical pressure have all been used by rehabilitation professionals to modify the healing process. The impact of these physical agents on tissue healing is discussed in the chapters of Part II; each type of physical agent, its effects, and its clinical applications are described.

◎ Clinical Pearl

Physical agents used to modify the healing process include cryotherapy, thermotherapy, ultrasound, electromagnetic radiation, light, electrical currents, and compression.

Movement

Early movement of a newly injured area may delay healing. Therefore, immobilization may be used to aid early healing and repair. However, because immobility can result in adhesions and stiffness by altering collagen cross-linking and elasticity, continuous passive motion (CPM) with strictly controlled parameters is often used to remobilize and restore function safely.[67] CPM used in conjunction with short-term immobilization, compared with immobilization alone, has been shown to achieve a better functional outcome in some studies; however, other studies have found differences only in early range of motion (ROM).[68,69] It has been reported that patients using CPM during the inflammatory phase of soft tissue healing after anterior cruciate ligament reconstruction used significantly fewer pain-relieving narcotics than patients not using CPM.[70] Furthermore, CPM in conjunction with physical therapy after total knee arthroplasty resulted in improved knee ROM and decreased analgesic medication use.[71]

SYSTEMIC FACTORS

Systemic factors such as age, diseases, medications, and nutrition can also affect wound healing.

Age

Age should be considered because of variations in healing between pediatric, adult, and geriatric populations. Wound closure occurs more rapidly in pediatric patients than in adult patients because the physiological changes and cumulative sun exposure that occur with aging can reduce the healing rate.[72] In elderly adults, a decrease in the density and cross-linking of collagen reduces tensile strength, decreases numbers of mast cells and fibroblasts, and slows epithelialization.[72] The poor organization of cutaneous vessels in older patients also adversely affects wound healing.

Disease

A number of diseases can affect wound healing directly or indirectly. For example, poorly controlled diabetes mellitus impairs collagen synthesis, increases the risk of infection as a result of a dampened immune response, and decreases phagocytosis as a result of alterations in leukocyte function.[66,73] Peripheral vascular compromise is also prevalent in this population, leading to a decrease in local blood flow. Neuropathies, which are also common in patients with diabetes mellitus, can increase the potential for trauma and decrease the ability of soft tissue lesions to heal.

Patients who are immunocompromised, such as patients with acquired immunodeficiency syndrome (AIDS) or patients taking immunosuppressive drugs after organ transplantation, are prone to wound infection because they have an inadequate inflammatory response. AIDS also affects many other facets of the healing process through impairment of phagocytosis, fibroblast function, and collagen synthesis.[74]

Problems involving the circulatory system, including atherosclerosis, sickle cell disease, and hypertension, can have an adverse effect on wound healing because inflammation and healing depend on the cardiovascular system for the delivery of components to the local area of injury. Decreased oxygen tension caused by a reduced blood supply can inhibit fibroblast migration and decrease collagen synthesis, leading to decreased tensile strength and making the injured area susceptible to reinjury. Wounds with a decreased blood supply are also susceptible to infection.[32,75]

Medications

Patients with injuries or wounds often take medications with systemic effects that alter tissue healing. For example, antibiotics can prevent or fight off infection, which can help speed healing, but they may have toxic effects that inhibit healing. Corticosteroids, such as prednisone and dexamethasone, block the inflammatory cascade at a variety of levels, inhibiting many of the pathways involved in inflammation. It is thought that glucocorticoids act mainly by affecting gene transcription inside cells to inhibit the formation of inflammatory molecules, including cytokines, enzymes, receptors, and adhesion molecules.[76] They are thought to stimulate the production of antiinflammatory molecules. Corticosteroids decrease the margination, migration, and accumulation of monocytes at the site of inflammation.[77] They induce antiinflammatory actions by monocytes, such as phagocytosis of other inflammatory molecules, while repressing adhesion, apoptosis, and oxidative burst.[78] They severely inhibit wound contracture, decrease the rate of epithelialization, and decrease the tensile strength of closed, healed wounds.[79-81] Corticosteroids administered at the time of injury have a greater impact because decreasing the inflammatory response at this early stage delays subsequent phases of healing and increases the incidence of infection.

Compared with corticosteroids, NSAIDs, such as ibuprofen, are less likely to impair healing. They interrupt the production of prostaglandins from arachidonic acid but are not thought to adversely affect the function of fibroblasts or tissue macrophages.[82] NSAIDs can cause vasoconstriction and can suppress the inflammatory response[14]; some NSAIDs have been found to inhibit cell proliferation and migration during tendon healing.[83,84]

Nutrition

Nutrition can have a profound effect on healing tissues. Deficiency of a number of important amino acids, vitamins, minerals, or water, as well as insufficient caloric intake, can result in delayed or impaired healing. This occurs because physiological stress from the injury induces a hypermetabolic state. Thus, if insufficient "fuel" is available for the process of inflammation and repair, healing is slowed.

In most cases, healing abnormalities are associated with general protein-calorie malnutrition rather than with the depletion of a single nutrient.[85] Such is the case with patients with extensive burns who are in a prolonged hypermetabolic state. Protein deficiency can result in decreased fibroblastic proliferation, reduced proteoglycan and collagen synthesis, decreased angiogenesis, and disrupted collagen remodeling.[86] Protein deficiency can also adversely affect phagocytosis, which may lead to an increased risk of infection.[75]

Studies have shown that a deficiency of specific nutrients may also affect healing. Vitamin A deficiency can retard epithelialization, the rate of collagen synthesis, and cross-linking.[87] Thiamine (vitamin B_1) deficiency decreases collagen formation, and vitamin B_5 deficiency decreases the tensile strength of healed tissue and reduces the fibroblast number.[88,89]

Vitamin C deficiency impairs collagen synthesis by fibroblasts, increases the capillary rupture potential, and increases the susceptibility of wounds to infection.[90]

Many minerals also play an important role in healing. Insufficient zinc can decrease the rate of epithelialization, reduce collagen synthesis, and decrease tensile strength.[91,92] Magnesium deficiency may also cause decreased collagen synthesis, and copper insufficiency may alter cross-linking, leading to a reduction in tensile strength.[90]

ADJUNCTS TO PROMOTE WOUND HEALING

Negative-pressure wound therapy, as discussed in detail in Chapter 19 with hydrotherapy and other physical adjuncts to wound healing, promotes wound healing by decreasing seroma and hematoma formation and promoting the granulation process. Biological dressings containing silver reduce wound infection rates, allowing for a more normalized inflammatory response. Silicone-based wound dressings decrease hypertrophic scar formation by stimulating basic fibroblast growth factor.[93]

Immunonutrition, the use of specific nutrients to influence the immune system, can also improve wound healing. A few of the most common substances used for immunonutrition include l-arginine, glutamine, and omega-3 fatty acids. The impact of antioxidants such as selenium, zinc, vitamin C, vitamin E, and beta-carotene has also been studied and used to facilitate the healing of burn wounds and in the critical care setting. L-arginine, a nonessential amino acid under normal conditions, becomes an essential amino acid under stress. L-arginine can increase lymphocyte and monocyte proliferation through a nitric oxide mechanism.[94] Glutamine may be used as a fuel source in rapidly dividing cells under stress and when converted to glutathione, which is an antioxidant. Omega-3 fatty acids are major structural elements in cell membranes, and omega-3 fatty acid supplementation can reduce clotting and inflammation and increase cell surface activation.[95]

Healing of Specific Musculoskeletal Tissues

The primary determinants of the outcome of any injury are the type and extent of injury, the regenerative capacity of the tissues involved, the vascular supply of the injured site, and the extent of damage to the extracellular framework. The basic principles of inflammation and healing apply to all tissues; however, some tissue specificity applies to the healing response. For example, the liver can regenerate when more than half of it is removed, whereas even a thin fracture line in cartilage is unlikely to heal.

CARTILAGE

Cartilage has a limited ability to heal because it lacks lymphatics, blood vessels, and nerves.[96] However, cartilage reacts differently when injured alone than when injured in conjunction with the subchondral bone to which it is attached. Injuries confined to the cartilage do not form a clot or recruit neutrophils or macrophages, and cells adjacent to the injury show a limited capacity to induce healing. This limited response generally fails to heal the defect, and the lesions seldom resolve.[97]

With injuries that involve both articular cartilage and subchondral bone, vascularization of the subchondral bone allows for the formation of fibrin-fibronectin gel, giving access to the inflammatory cells and permitting the formation of granulation tissue. Differentiation of granulation tissue into chondrocytes can begin within 2 weeks. Normal-appearing cartilage can be seen within 2 months after the injury. However, this cartilage has a low proteoglycan content and therefore is predisposed to degeneration and erosive changes.[98] Recent research has explored the use of stem cells for cartilage repair.

TENDONS AND LIGAMENTS

Tendons and **ligaments** pass through similar stages of healing. Inflammation occurs in the first 72 hours, and collagen synthesis occurs within the first week. Fibroplasia occurs from intrinsic sources, such as adjacent cells, and from extrinsic sources, such as those brought in via the circulatory system.

The repair potential of tendon is controversial. Both intrinsic cells, such as epitendinous and endotendinous cells, and extrinsic peritendinous cells participate in tendon repair. The exact role of these cells and the final outcome depend on several factors, including the type of tendon, the extent of damage to the tendon sheath, the vascular supply, and the duration of immobilization. The first two stages of tendon healing, inflammation and proliferation, are similar to the healing phases of other tissues. The third phase, scar maturation, is unique to tendons in that this tissue can achieve a state of repair close to regeneration.

During the first 4 days after an injury, the inflammatory phase progresses with infiltration of both extrinsic and intrinsic cells. Many of these cells develop phagocytic capabilities, and others become fibroblastic. Collagen synthesis becomes evident by day 7 or day 8, with fibroblasts predominating at approximately day 14. Early in this stage, both cells and collagen are oriented perpendicularly to the long axis of the tendon.[99] This orientation changes at day 10, when new collagen fibers begin to align themselves parallel to the old longitudinal axis of the tendon stumps.[100] For the next 2 months, a gradual transition of alignment occurs, through remodeling and reorientation, parallel to the long axis. Ultimate maturation of the tissue depends on sufficient physiological loading.

If the synovial sheath is absent or uninjured, the relative contributions of intrinsic and extrinsic cells are balanced, and adhesions are minimal. If the synovial sheath is injured, the contributions of the extrinsic cells overwhelm the capacities of the intrinsic cells, and adhesions are common.

Factors affecting the repair of tendons are different from factors associated with the repair of ligaments.[101] Studies have shown that mobilization of tendons by controlled forces accelerates and enhances the strengthening of tendon repair, but mobilization by active contraction of the attached muscle less than 3 weeks after repair generally results in a poor outcome. The poor outcome may be a result of the fact that high tension can lead to ischemia and tendon rupture. Studies have found no significant difference in tendon strength when tendons are exposed to controlled low or high levels of passive force after repair.[102,103] It appears that mechanical stress is needed to promote the appropriate orientation of collagen fibrils and remodeling of collagen into its mature form and to optimize strength, but the amount of tension necessary to promote the optimal clinical response is not known.[104,105]

Many variables influence the healing of ligamentous tissue, the most important of which are the type of ligament, the size of the defect, and the amount of loading applied. For example, injuries to capsular and extracapsular ligaments generally stimulate an adequate repair response, whereas injuries to intracapsular ligaments often do not. Thus, in the knee, the medial collateral ligament often heals without surgical intervention, whereas the anterior cruciate ligament does not. These differences in healing may be a result of the synovial environment, limited neovascularization, or fibroblast migration from surrounding tissues. Treatments that stabilize the injury site and maintain the apposition of the torn ligament can help the ligament heal in its optimal length and can minimize scarring. Early, controlled loading of healing ligaments can also promote healing, although excessive loading may delay or disrupt the healing process.[106,107] Although mature ligamentous repair tissue is approximately 30% to 50% weaker than uninjured ligament,[108] this usually does not significantly impair joint function because the repaired tissue is usually larger than the original uninjured ligament.

SKELETAL MUSCLE

Muscles may be injured by blunt trauma causing a contusion, violent contraction, excessive stretch causing a strain, or muscle-wasting disease. Although skeletal muscle cells cannot proliferate, stem or reserve cells, known as *satellite cells*, can proliferate and differentiate in some circumstances to form new skeletal muscle cells after the death of adult muscle fibers.[98] It is believed that there are functional links between muscle regeneration and inflammation after muscle injury, and recent studies indicate that macrophages are essential to that interplay.[28] After a severe contusion, a calcified hematoma, known as *myositis ossificans*, may develop. Myositis ossificans is rare after surgery if hemostasis is controlled.

BONE

Bone is a specialized tissue that is able to heal itself with like tissue. Bone can heal by primary or secondary healing. Primary healing occurs with rigid internal fixation of the bone, whereas secondary healing occurs in the absence of such fixation. Bone goes through four histologically distinct stages in the healing process: (1) inflammation, (2) soft callus, (3) hard callus, and (4) bone remodeling. Some investigators also include the stages of **impaction** and **induction** before inflammation in this scheme.

Impaction is the dissipation of energy from an insult. The impact of an insult is proportional to the energy applied to the bone and is inversely proportional to the volume of the bone. Thus, a fracture is more likely to occur if the force is great or the bone is small. Energy dissipated by a bone is inversely proportional to its modulus of elasticity. Therefore, the bone of a person with osteoporosis, which has low elasticity, will fracture more easily. Young children have a more elastic bone structure that allows their bones to bend, accounting for the greenstick-type fractures seen in pediatric patients (Box 3.3).

Box 3.3   Stages of Fracture Healing

1. Impaction
2. Induction
3. Inflammation
4. Soft callus
5. Hard callus
6. Remodeling

Induction is the stage when cells that possess osteogenic capabilities are activated and is the least understood stage of bone healing. It is thought that cells may be activated by oxygen gradients, forces, bone morphogenetic proteins, or noncollagenous proteins. Although the timing of this process is not known exactly, it is thought to be initiated after the moment of impact. The duration of this stage is unknown, although the influence of induction forces seems to lessen with time. Therefore, optimizing early conditions for healing to minimize the potential for delayed union or nonunion is imperative.

Inflammation begins shortly after impact and lasts until some fibrous union occurs at the fracture site. At the time of fracture, the blood supply is disrupted, a fracture hematoma is formed, and oxygen tension and pH are decreased. This environment favors the growth of early fibrous or cartilaginous callus. This callus forms more easily than bone and helps stabilize the fracture site, decrease pain, and

lessen the likelihood of a fat embolism. It also rapidly and efficiently provides a scaffold for further circulation and for cartilage and endosteal bone production. The amount of movement at the fracture site influences the amount and quality of the callus. Small amounts of movement stimulate the formation of a callus, whereas excessive movement can disrupt the formation of a callus and can inhibit bony union.

The soft callus stage begins when pain and swelling subside and lasts until bony fragments are united by fibrous or cartilaginous tissue. This period is marked by a great increase in vascularity, growth of capillaries into the fracture callus, and increased cell proliferation. Tissue oxygen tension remains low, but pH returns to normal. The hematoma becomes organized with fibrous tissue cartilage and bone formation; however, no callus is visible radiographically. The callus is electronegative relative to the rest of the bone during this period. Osteoclasts remove the dead bone fragments.

The hard callus stage begins when a sticky, hard callus covers the ends of the fracture and ends when new bone unites with the fragments. This period corresponds to the period of clinical and radiological fracture healing. The duration of this period depends on the fracture location and the patient's age and can range from 3 weeks to 4 months.

The remodeling stage begins when the fracture is clinically and radiologically healed. It ends when the bone has returned to its normal state and the patency of the medullary canal is restored. Fibrous bone is converted to lamellar bone, and the medullary canal is revised. This process can take several months to several years to complete.[109]

CLINICAL CASE STUDIES

The following case studies summarize the concepts of inflammation and repair discussed in this chapter. Based on the scenario presented, an evaluation of clinical findings and goals of treatment is proposed.

CASE STUDY 3.1

Inflammation and Repair

Examination

History

JP is a 16-year-old high school student. She injured her right ankle 1 week ago playing soccer and was treated conservatively with crutches; rest, ice, compression, and elevation (RICE); and NSAIDs. She reports some improvement, although she is unable to play soccer because of continued right lateral ankle pain. Her x-ray showed no fracture, and her family physician diagnosed the injury as a grade II lateral ankle sprain. She comes to your clinic with an order to "evaluate and treat."

JP sustained this injury during a cutting motion while dribbling a soccer ball. She noted an audible pop, immediate pain

and swelling, and an inability to bear weight. She reports that her pain has decreased in intensity from 8/10 to 6/10, but the pain increases with weight bearing and with certain demonstrated movements.

Tests and Measures

The objective examination reveals moderate warmth of the skin of the anterolateral aspect of the right ankle. Moderate ecchymosis and swelling are also noted, with a girth measurement of 34 cm on the right ankle compared with 30 cm on the left. JP's ROM is restricted to 0 degrees dorsiflexion, 30 degrees plantar flexion, 10 degrees inversion, and 5 degrees eversion, with pain noted especially with plantar flexion and inversion. She exhibits a decreased stance phase on the right lower extremity. Pain and weakness occur on strength tests of the peroneals and gastrocnemius and soleus muscles. She also exhibits a marked decrease in proprioception, as evidenced by the single-leg balance test. Her anterior drawer test is positive, and her talar tilt is negative.

This patient is in what stage of healing? What kind of injury does she have? What physical agents could be useful for this patient?

Continued

CLINICAL CASE STUDIES—*cont'd*

Evaluation and Goals

ICF Level	Current Status	Goals
Body structure and function	Right ankle pain	Reduce inflammation to reduce pain and edema and increase ROM
	Loss of subtalar and talocrural motion	
	Increased girth	
	Decreased strength of evertors and plantar flexors	
	Decreased proprioception	
Activity	Difficulty ambulating	Increase ability to walk
Participation	Unable to play soccer	Return to playing soccer in next 2 to 3 months

ICF, International Classification of Functioning, Disability and Health; *ROM*, range of motion.

Prognosis

This patient has had a recent injury and is in the inflammatory phase of tissue healing, as evidenced by her signs of pain, edema, bruising, and warmth at the injured site. She is likely at the beginning of the proliferation phase of healing. Given her positive anterior drawer test, it is likely that the patient has injured her anterior talofibular ligament. The expected time of healing with a grade II ankle sprain and partial tear of the talofibular ligament is 2 to 3 months. At this stage of healing, the plan is to minimize the effects of inflammation and accelerate the healing process so that she can move on to the proliferation and maturation phases and regain normal function.

Intervention

Physical agents that may be used to help accelerate the acute inflammatory phase of healing include cryotherapy and compression. She should avoid applying heat. The patient should continue the RICE regimen accompanied by NSAIDs as needed for pain. Physical agents should be used as part of a rehabilitation program in which the patient slowly resumes passive motion followed by active motion and motion with weight bearing. Hydrotherapy may be used to facilitate non–weight-bearing movement.

CASE STUDY 3.2

Inflammation and Repair
Examination
History

HP is a 45-year-old man who sustained an on-the-job injury in which he had a severe abdominal wall strain while trying to stabilize a falling 200-lb metal object. He noted severe acute pain at his umbilicus. One week later, he noted a 3-cm defect and bulge that was painful. He could not reduce the bulge and sought medical attention. He underwent surgical repair of the abdominal wall defect and had what was thought to be a good repair. Six weeks later, the incision was well healed and the integrity of the repaired abdominal wall defect was good. He had increased his activity and was subsequently released to work, where he felt increasing discomfort and pain despite icing and ibuprofen, with no associated swelling at the repair site. There is no evidence of recurrent hernia with ultrasound. He is referred to your clinic for scar release, muscle strengthening, and mobility improvement.

Tests and Measures

There is a well-healed surgical scar with a palpable healing ridge under the scar but no areas of softness or infection. HP shows decreased ability to bend at the waist and pain with reaching overhead and squatting.

Evaluation and Goals

ICF Level	Current Status	Goals
Body structure and function	Anterior abdominal pain after umbilical hernia repair	Scar release, increased mobility, and rectus strengthening
Activity	Work activity including lifting, bending, and twisting	Improve ability to perform work activities
Participation	Cannot work at full duty	Return to full duty

ICF, International Classification for Functioning, Disability and Health.

Prognosis

This patient has an acute injury on top of an overuse injury. The wound is in the maturation phase of remodeling; therefore, techniques for improving function, muscle strengthening, and decreasing inflammation would be most effective.

Intervention

Suitable physical agents to release the patient's scar and improve functioning include heat and mechanical stress through stretching and ROM exercises. An exercise program to improve muscle strength and flexibility without reinjuring the area will help with his recovery and return to work. NSAIDs can be used to control muscular pain and swelling.

Chapter Review

1. The processes of inflammation and tissue repair involve a complex and dynamic series of events, the ultimate goal of which is restoration of normal function. In these events, the involved tissue progresses through three sequential but overlapping stages: (1) inflammation, (2) proliferation, and (3) maturation. This series of events follows a timely and predictable course.

2. The inflammation phase involves the interaction of hemostatic, vascular, cellular, and immune responses mediated by a number of neural and chemical factors. Characteristics of the inflammation phase include heat, redness, swelling, pain, and loss of function in the injured area.

3. The proliferation phase is characterized by epithelialization, fibroplasia, wound contraction, and neovascularization. During this phase, the wound appears red, and swelling decreases, but the wound is still weak and therefore is easily susceptible to damage from excessive pressure and tension.

4. The maturation phase involves balanced collagen synthesis and lysis to ultimately remodel the injured area. The optimal outcome of the maturation phase is new tissue that resembles the previously uninjured tissue. More frequently, scar tissue forms that is slightly weaker than the original tissue. Over time, the scar lightens in color.

5. If the normal healing process is disturbed, healing may be delayed, or chronic inflammation may result. Drugs such as corticosteroids, NSAIDs, and antibiotics are used to limit inflammation, but they can also hinder healing.

6. Physical agents may influence the progression of inflammation and tissue repair. Physical agents used at various stages of the healing process include thermotherapy, cryotherapy, electromagnetic radiation, light, electrical stimulation, ultrasound, and compression. The rehabilitation specialist must assess the stage of inflammation and repair to determine the appropriate agent to incorporate into the treatment plan for an optimal outcome.

7. The reader is referred to the Evolve website for additional resources and references.

Glossary

Acute inflammation: Inflammation that occurs immediately after tissue damage.

Angiogenesis: The growth of new blood vessels.

Cartilage: A fibrous connective tissue that lines the ends of the bones, forming the weight-bearing surface of joints, and the flexible parts of the nose and ears.

Chemotaxis: Movement of cells toward or away from chemicals.

Chronic inflammation: The simultaneous progression of active inflammation, tissue destruction, and healing. Chronic inflammation may last for months or years.

Collagen: The protein in the fibers of skin, tendon, bone, cartilage, and all other connective tissue. Collagen is made up of individual polypeptide molecules combined in triplets forming helical tropocollagen molecules that then associate to form collagen fibrils.

Collagenases: Enzymes that destroy collagen.

Complement system: A system of enzymatic plasma proteins activated by antigen-antibody complexes, bacteria, and foreign material that participates in the inflammatory response through cell lysis, opsonization, and the attraction of leukocytes by chemotaxis.

Connective tissues: Tissues consisting of fibroblasts, ground substance, and fibrous strands that provide the structure for other tissues.

Contractures: Conditions of fixed shortening of soft tissues that have high resistance to passive stretch, often producing deformity or distortion.

Corticosteroids: Drugs that decrease the inflammatory response through many mechanisms involving many cell types.

Diapedesis: The process by which leukocytes squeeze through intact blood vessel walls; a part of the process of extravasation.

Edema: Swelling that results from accumulation of fluid in the interstitial space.

Emigration: The process by which leukocytes migrate from blood vessels into perivascular tissues; a part of the process of extravasation.

Epithelial cells: Cells that form the epidermis of the skin and the covering of mucous and serous membranes.

Epithelialization: Healing by growth of epithelium over a denuded surface, thus reestablishing the epidermis.

Erythrocytes: Red blood cells.

Extravasation: The movement of leukocytes from inside a blood vessel to tissue outside the blood vessel.

Exudate: Wound fluid composed of serum with a high content of protein and white blood cells or solid materials from cells.

Fibroblasts: Cells in many tissues, particularly in wounds, that are the primary producers of collagen.

Fibroplasia: Fibroblast growth.

Granulation tissue: Tissue composed of new blood vessels, connective tissue, fibroblasts, and inflammatory cells that fills an open wound when it starts to heal; typically appears deep pink or red with an irregular, berry-like surface.

Healing by delayed primary intention: Healing in which wound contraction is reduced by delayed approximation of wound edges with sutures or application of skin grafts.

Healing by primary intention: Healing without wound contraction that occurs when wounds are rapidly closed with sutures with minimal loss of tissue and minimal bacterial contamination.

Healing by secondary intention: Healing with wound contraction that occurs when significant loss of tissue or bacterial contamination is present and wound edges are not approximated.

Hemarthrosis: Bloody fluid present in a joint.

Hematoma: The accumulation of blood in a tissue or organ.

Humoral mediators: Antibodies, hormones, cytokines, and a variety of other soluble proteins and chemicals that contribute to the inflammatory process.

Hyperalgesia: Increased sensitivity to painful stimuli.

Hyperemia: An excess of blood in a given area that causes redness and temperature increase in the area.

Impaction: Dissipation of energy resulting from an insult to bone.

Induction: The stage of bone healing when cells with osteogenic capabilities are activated.

Inflammation: The body's first response to tissue damage, characterized by heat, redness, swelling, pain, and often loss of function.

Inflammation phase: The first phase of healing after tissue damage.

Leukocytes: White blood cells.

Ligaments: Bands of fibrous tissue that connect bone to bone or cartilage to bone, supporting or strengthening a joint at the extremes of motion.

Macrophages: Phagocytic cells derived from monocytes and important for attracting other immune cells to a site of inflammation.

Margination: A part of the process of extravasation in which leukocytes line the walls of blood vessels.

Maturation phase: The final phase of tissue healing in which scar tissue is modified into its mature form.

Monocytes: Leukocytes that are larger than polymorphonucleocytes (PMNs), have a single nucleus, and become macrophages when in connective tissue and outside the bloodstream.

Myofibroblasts: Cells similar to fibroblasts that have the contractile properties of smooth muscles and are responsible for wound contraction.

Neovascularization: The development of a new blood supply to an injured area.

Neural mediators: Nerve-related contributions to the inflammatory process.

Neutrophils: White blood cells present early in inflammation that have the properties of chemotaxis and phagocytosis.

Opsonization: The coating of bacteria with protein that makes them more susceptible to phagocytosis.

Pavementing: A part of the process of extravasation in which leukocytes lie in layers inside the blood vessel.

Phagocytosis: Ingestion and digestion of bacteria and particles by a cell.

Piezoelectric: The property of being able to generate electricity in response to a mechanical force or being able to change shape in response to an electrical current.

Plasma: The acellular, fluid portion of blood.

Platelet-derived growth factor (PDGF): A protein produced by platelets that stimulates cell growth and division and is involved in normal wound healing.

Platelets: Small, anuclear cells in the blood that assist in clotting.

Polymorphonucleocytes (PMNs): Leukocytes whose nuclei have several lobes and contain cytoplasmic granules and that include neutrophils, basophils, and eosinophils.

Proliferation phase: The second phase of tissue healing, during which damaged structures are rebuilt and the wound is strengthened.

Pus: Opaque wound fluid that is thicker than exudate and contains white blood cells, tissue debris, and microorganisms; also called *suppurative exudate.*

Subacute inflammation: An inflammatory process that has continued for longer than 4 weeks.

Tendon: Fibrous band of tissue that connects muscle with bone.

Transudate: Thin, clear wound fluid composed primarily of serum.

Type I collagen: The most abundant form of collagen, found in skin, bone, tendons, and most organs.

Type II collagen: The predominant collagen in cartilage.

Type III collagen: A thin, weak-structured collagen with no consistent organization, initially produced by fibroblasts after tissue damage.

Wound contraction: The pulling together of the edges of an injured site to accelerate repair.

References

1. Stedman TL: *Stedman's medical dictionary*, ed 27, Philadelphia, 2000, Lippincott Williams & Wilkins.
2. Price SA, Wilson LM: *Pathophysiology: clinical concepts of disease processes*, ed 4, St Louis, 1992, Mosby Year Book.
3. Kellett J: Acute soft tissue injuries—a review of the literature. *Med Sci Sports Exerc* 18:489–500, 1986.
4. Garrett WE, Jr, Lohnes J: Cellular and matrix responses to mechanical injury at the myotendinous junction. In Leadbetter WB, Buckwalter JA, Gordon SL, editors: *Sports-induced inflammation*, Park Ridge, IL, 1990, American Academy of Orthopaedic Surgeons.
5. Andriacchi T, Sabiston P, DeHaven K, et al: Ligament: injury and repair. In Woo SL-Y, Buckwalter JA, editors: *Injury and repair of the musculoskeletal soft tissues*, Park Ridge, IL, 1988, American Academy of Orthopaedic Surgeons.
6. Garrett WE, Jr: Muscle strain injuries: clinical and basic aspects. *Med Sci Sports Exerc* 22:436–443, 1990.
7. Szpaderska A, Egozi E, Gamelli RL, et al: The effect of thrombocytopenia on dermal wound healing. *J Invest Dermatol* 120:1130–1137, 2003.
8. Eming SA, Krieg T, Davidson JM: Inflammation in wound repair: molecular and cellular mechanisms. *J Invest Dermatol* 127:514–525, 2007.
9. Fantone JC, Ward PA: Inflammation. In Rubin E, Farber JL, editors: *Pathology*, Philadelphia, 1988, JB Lippincott.
10. Wilkerson GB: Inflammation in connective tissue: etiology and management. *Athl Training* 20:298–301, 1985.
11. Christie AL: The tissue injury cycle and new advances toward its management in open wounds. *Athl Training* 26:274–277, 1991.
12. Kumar V, Abbas AK, Aster JC: *Robbins & Cotran pathologic basis of disease*, ed 9, Philadelphia, 2014, Saunders.
13. Fantone JC: Basic concepts in inflammation. In Leadbetter WB, Buckwalter JA, Gordon SL, editors: *Sports-induced inflammation*, Park Ridge, IL, 1990, American Academy of Orthopaedic Surgeons.
14. Peacock EE: *Wound repair*, ed 3, Philadelphia, 1984, WB Saunders.
15. Salter RB, Simmons DF, Malcolm BW, et al: The biological effects of continuous passive motion on the healing of full thickness defects in articular cartilage. *J Bone Joint Surg Am* 62:1232–1251, 1980.
16. Andres C, Hasenauer J, Ahn HS, et al: Wound-healing growth factor, basic FGF, induces Erk1/2-dependent mechanical hyperalgesia. *Pain* 154:2216–2226, 2013.
17. Morita K, Shiraishi S, Motoyama N, et al: Palliation of bone cancer pain by antagonists of platelet-activating factor receptors. *PLoS ONE* 9:e91746, 2014.
18. Yeom E, Kang YJ, Lee SJ: Changes in velocity profile according to blood viscosity in a microchannel. *Biomicrofluidics* 8:034110, 2014.
19. Egan BM, Chen G, Kelly CJ, et al: Taurine attenuates LPS-induced rolling and adhesion in rat microcirculation. *J Surg Res* 95:85–91, 2001.
20. Xia G, Martin AE, Besner GE: Heparin-binding EGF-like growth factor downregulates expression of adhesion molecules and infiltration of inflammatory cells after intestinal ischemia/reperfusion injury. *J Pediatr Surg* 38:434–439, 2003.
21. Majno G, Palade GE: Studies on inflammation. I. The effect of histamine and serotonin on vascular permeability: an electron microscopic study. *J Biophys Biochem Cytol* 11:571–605, 1961.
22. Pierce GF, Mustoe TA, Senia RM, et al: In vivo incisional wound healing augmented by PDGF and recombinant c-sis gene homodimeric proteins. *J Exp Med* 167:975–987, 1988.

23. Martinez-Hernandez A, Amenta PS: Basic concepts in wound healing. In Leadbetter WB, Buckwalter JA, Gordon SL, editors: *Sports-induced inflammation*, Park Ridge, IL, 1990, American Academy of Orthopaedic Surgeons.

24. Hooiveld MJ, Roosendaal G, van den Berg HM, et al: Haemoglobin-derived iron-dependent hydroxyl radical formation in blood-induced joint damage: an in vitro study. *Rheumatology (Oxford)* 42:784–790, 2003.

25. Bolognia J, Jorizzo JL, Schaffer JV, editors: *Dermatology*, Philadelphia, 2012, Elsevier Saunders.

26. DiPietro LA, Polverini PJ: Role of the macrophage in the positive and negative regulation of wound neovascularization. *Am J Pathol* 143:678–784, 1993.

27. Shook BA, Wasko RR, Rivera-Gonzalez GC, et al: Myofibroblast proliferation and heterogeneity are supported by macrophages during skin repair. *Science* 362(6417):eaar2971, 2018. https://doi.org/10.1126/science.aar2971.

28. Oishi Y, Manabe I: Macrophages in inflammation, repair and regeneration. *Int Immunol* 30(11):511–528, 2018. https://doi.org/10.1093/intimm/dxy054.

29. Hardy M: The biology of scar formation. *Phys Ther* 69:1014–1024, 1989.

30. Rutherford R, Ross R: Platelet factors stimulate fibroblasts and smooth muscle cells quiescent in plasma serum to proliferate. *J Cell Biol* 69:196–203, 1976.

31. Mathes S: Roundtable discussion: problem wounds. *Perspect Plast Surg* 2:89–120, 1988.

32. Whitney JD, Heiner S, Mygrant BI, et al: Tissue and wound healing effects of short duration postoperative oxygen therapy. *Biol Res Nurs* 2:206–215, 2001.

33. Tandara A, Mustoe T: Oxygen in wound healing—more than a nutrient. *World J Surg* 28:294–300, 2004.

34. Bellanti JA, editor: *Immunology*, ed 3, Philadelphia, 1985, WB Saunders.

35. Werb A, Gordon S: Elastase secretion by stimulated macrophages. *J Exp Med* 142:361–377, 1975.

36. Madden JW: Wound healing: biologic and clinical features. In Sabiston DC, editor: *Davis-Christopher textbook of surgery*, ed 11, Philadelphia, 1997, WB Saunders.

37. Clark RAF: Overview and general considerations of wound repair. In Clark RAF, Henson PM, editors: *The molecular and cellular biology of wound repair*, New York, 1988, Plenum Press.

38. Stotts NA, Wipke-Tevis D: Co-factors in impaired wound healing. *Ostomy Wound Manage* 42:44–56, 1996.

39. Kaplan B, Gönül B, Dinçer S, et al: Relationships between tensile strength, ascorbic acid, hydroxyproline, and zinc levels of rabbit full-thickness incision wound healing. *Surg Today* 34:747–751, 2004.

40. Monaco JL, Lawrence WT: Acute wound healing: an overview. *Clin Plast Surg* 30:1–12, 2003.

41. Lawrence WT: Physiology of the acute wound. *Clin Plast Surg* 25:321–340, 1998.

42. Levenson S: Practical applications of experimental studies in the care of primary closed wounds. *Am J Surg* 104:273–282, 1962.

43. Nemeth-Csoka M, Kovacsay A: The effect of glycosaminoglycans (GAG) on the intramolecular bindings of collagen. *Acta Biol Acad Sci Hung* 30:303–308, 1979.

44. Lachman SM: *Soft tissue injuries in sports*, St Louis, 1980, Mosby.

45. Hunt TK, Van Winkle W, Jr: Wound healing. In Heppenstall RB, editor: *Fracture treatment and healing*, Philadelphia, 1980, WB Saunders.

46. Baum CL, Arpey CJ: Normal cutaneous wound healing: clinical correlation with cellular and molecular events. *Dermatol Surg* 31:674–686, discussion 686, 2005.

47. Daly T: The repair phase of wound healing: re-epithelialization and contraction. In Kloth L, McCulloch J, Feeder J, editors: *Wound healing: alternatives in management*, Philadelphia, 1990, FA Davis.

48. Gabbiani G, Ryan G, Majeno G: Presence of modified fibroblasts in granulation tissue and their possible role in wound contraction. *Experientia* 27:549–550, 1971.

49. Watts GT, Grillo HC, Gross J: Studies in wound healing. II. The role of granulation tissue in contraction. *Ann Surg* 148:153–160, 1958.

50. McGrath MH, Simon RH: Wound geometry and the kinetics of the wound contraction. *Plast Reconstr Surg* 72:66–73, 1983.

51. Venes D, Taber CW: *Taber's cyclopedic medical dictionary*, ed 22, Philadelphia, 2013, FA Davis.

52. Billingham RE, Russell PS: Studies on wound healing, with special reference to the phenomena of contracture in experimental wounds in rabbit skin. *Ann Surg* 144:961–981, 1956.

53. Sawhney CP, Monga HL: Wound contracture in rabbits and the effectiveness of skin grafts in preventing it. *Br J Plast Surg* 23:318–321, 1970.

54. Stone PA, Madden JW: Biological factors affecting wound contraction. *Surg Forum* 26:547–548, 1975.

55. Rudolph R: Contraction and the control of contraction. *World J Surg* 4:279–287, 1980.

56. Alvarez OM: Wound healing. In Fitzpatrick T, editor: *Dermatology in general medicine*, ed 3, New York, 1986, McGraw-Hill.

57. Eyre DR: The collagens of musculoskeletal soft tissues. In Leadbetter WB, Buckwalter JA, Gordon SL, editors: *Sports-induced inflammation*, Park Ridge, IL, 1990, American Association of Orthopaedic Surgeons.

58. McPherson JM, Piez KA: Collagen in dermal wound repair. In Clark RAF, Henson PM, editors: *The molecular and cellular biology of wound repair*, New York, 1988, Plenum Press.

59. Kosaka M, Kamiishi H: New concept of balloon-compression wear for the treatment of keloids and hypertrophic scars. *Plast Reconstr Surg* 108:1454–1455, 2001.

60. Uppal RS, Khan U, Kakar S, et al: The effects of a single dose of 5-fluorouracil on keloid scars: a clinical trial of timed wound irrigation after extralesional excision. *Plast Reconstr Surg* 108:1218–1224, 2001.

61. Hunt TK, Van Winkle W: *Wound healing: normal repair—fundamentals of wound management in surgery*, South Plainfield, NJ, 1976, Chirurgecom, Inc.

62. Madden J: Wound healing: the biological basis of hand surgery. *Clin Plast Surg* 3:3–11, 1976.

63. Arem AJ, Madden JW: Effects of stress on healing wounds. I. Intermittent noncyclical tension. *J Surg Res* 20:93–102, 1976.

64. Kuzyk PRT, Schemitsch EH: The science of electrical stimulation therapy for fracture healing. *Indian J Orthop* 43:127–131, 2009.

65. Irvin T: Collagen metabolism in infected colonic anastomoses. *Surg Gynecol Obstet* 143:220–224, 1976.

66. Carrico T, Mehrhof A, Cohen I: Biology of wound healing. *Surg Clin North Am* 64:721–733, 1984.

67. Woo SL, Gelberman RM, Cobb NG, et al: The importance of controlled passive mobilization on flexor tendon healing: a biochemical study. *Acta Orthop Scand* 52:615–622, 1981.

68. Gelberman RH, Woo SL, Lothringer K, et al: Effects of early intermittent passive immobilization on healing canine flexor tendons. *J Hand Surg Am* 7:170–175, 1982.

69. Lau SK, Chiu KY: Use of continuous passive motion after total knee arthroplasty. *J Arthroplasty* 16:336–339, 2001.

70. McCarthy MR, Yates CK, Anderson MA, et al: The effects of immediate continuous passive motion on pain during the inflammatory phase of soft tissue healing following anterior cruciate ligament reconstruction. *J Orthop Sport Phys Ther* 17:96–101, 1993.

71. Brosseau L, Milne S, Wells G, et al: Efficacy of continuous passive motion following total knee arthroplasty: a meta-analysis. *J Rheumatol* 31:2251–2264, 2004.

72. Thomas DR: Age-related changes in wound healing. *Drugs Aging* 18:607–620, 2001.

73. Goodson W, Hunt T: Studies of wound healing in experimental diabetes mellitus. *J Surg Res* 22:221–227, 1997.

74. Peterson M, Barbul A, Breslin R, et al: Significance of T-lymphocytes in wound healing. *Surgery* 2:300–305, 1987.

75. Gogia PP: The biology of wound healing. *Ostomy Wound Manage* 38:12–22, 1992.

76. Adcock IM, Ito K, Barnes PJ: Glucocorticoids: effects on gene transcription. *Proc Am Thorac Soc* 1:247–254, 2004.

77. Behrens TW, Goodwin JS: Oral corticosteroids. In Leadbetter WB, Buckwalter JA, Gordon SL, editors: *Sports-induced inflammation*, Park Ridge, IL, 1990, American Academy of Orthopaedic Surgeons.

78. Ehrchen J, Steinmuller L, Barczyk K, et al: Glucocorticoids induce differentiation of a specifically activated, anti-inflammatory subtype of human monocytes. *Blood* 109:1265–1274, 2007.

79. Ehrlich H, Hunt T: The effect of cortisone and anabolic steroids on the tensile strength of healing wounds. *Ann Surg* 170:203–206, 1969.

80. Baker B, Whitaker W: Interference with wound healing by the local action of adrenocortical steroids. *Endocrinology* 46:544–551, 1950.

81. Stephens F, Dunphy J, Hunt T: The effect of delayed administration of corticosteroids on wound contracture. *Ann Surg* 173:214–218, 1971.

82. Abramson SB: Nonsteroidal anti-inflammatory drugs: mechanisms of action and therapeutic considerations. In Leadbetter WB, Buckwalter JA, Gordon SL, editors: *Sports-induced inflammation*, Park Ridge, IL, 1990, American Academy of Orthopaedic Surgeons.
83. Riley GP, Cox M, Harrall RL, et al: Inhibition of tendon cell proliferation and matrix glycosaminoglycan synthesis by non-steroidal anti-inflammatory drugs in vitro. *J Hand Surg Br* 26:224–228, 2001.
84. Tsai WC, Hsu CC, Chou SW: Effects of celecoxib on migration, proliferation and collagen expression of tendon cells. *Connect Tissue Res* 48:46–51, 2007.
85. Albina JE: Nutrition in wound healing. *JPEN J Parenter Enteral Nutr* 18:367–376, 1994.
86. Pollack S: Wound healing: a review. III. Nutritional factors affecting wound healing. *J Dermatol Surg Oncol* 5:615–619, 1979.
87. Freiman M, Seifter E, Connerton C: Vitamin A deficiency and surgical stress. *Surg Forum* 21:81–82, 1970.
88. Alverez OM, Gilbreath RL: Thiamine influence on collagen during granulation of skin wounds. *J Surg Res* 32:24–31, 1982.
89. Grenier JF, Aprahamian M, Genot C, et al: Pantothenic acid (vitamin B5) efficiency on wound healing. *Acta Vitaminol Enzymol* 4:81–85, 1982.
90. Pollack S: Systemic drugs and nutritional aspects of wound healing. *Clin Dermatol* 2:68–80, 1984.
91. Sandstead HH, Henriksen LK, Grefer JL, et al: Zinc nutriture in the elderly in relation to taste acuity, immune response, and wound healing. *Am J Clin Nutr* 36(Suppl 5):1046–1059, 1982.
92. Maitra AK, Dorani B: Role of zinc in post-injury wound healing. *Arch Emerg Med* 9:122–124, 1992.
93. van der Veer WM, Bloemen MC, Ulrich MM, et al: Potential cellular and molecular causes of hypertrophic scar formation. *Burns* 35:15–29, 2009.
94. Zhou M, Martindale RG: Arginine in the critical care setting. *J Nutr* 137(6 Suppl 2):1687S–1692S, 2007.
95. Codner P, Brasel K: Nutritional support. *Scientific American—Surgery* 2013.
96. Athanasiou KA, Shah AR, Hernandez RJ, et al: Basic science of articular cartilage repair. *Clin Sports Med* 20:223–247, 2001.
97. Gelberman R, Goldberg V, An K-N, et al: Tendon. In Woo SL-Y, Buckwalter JA, editors: *Injury and repair of musculoskeletal soft tissues*, Park Ridge, IL, 1988, American Academy of Orthopaedic Surgeons.
98. Caplan A, Carlson B, Faulkner J, et al: Skeletal muscle. In Woo SL-Y, Buckwalter JA, editors: *Injury and repair of musculoskeletal soft tissues*, Park Ridge, IL, 1988, American Academy of Orthopaedic Surgeons.
99. Strickland JW: Flexor tendon injuries. *Orthop Rev* 15:632–645. 701–721, 1986.
100. Lindsay WK: Cellular biology of flexor tendon healing. In Hunter JM, Schneider LH, Mackin EJ, editors: *Tendon surgery of the hand*, St Louis, 1987, Mosby.
101. Akeson WH, Frank CB, Amiel D, et al: Ligament biology and biomechanics. In Finnerman G, editor: *American Academy of Orthopaedic Surgeons symposium on sports medicine*, St Louis, 1985, Mosby.
102. Ketchum LD: Primary tendon healing: a review. *J Hand Surg Am* 2:428–435, 1977.
103. Goldfarb CA, Harwood F, Silva MJ, et al: The effect of variations in applied rehabilitation force on collagen concentration and maturation at the intrasynovial flexor tendon repair site. *J Hand Surg Am* 26:841–846, 2001.
104. Peacock EE, Jr: Biological principles in the healing of long tendons. *Surg Clin North Am* 45:461–476, 1965.
105. Potenza AD: Tendon healing within the flexor digital sheath in the dog. *J Bone Joint Surg Am* 44:49–64, 1962.
106. Long M, Frank C, Schachar N, et al: The effects of motion on normal and healing ligaments. *Trans Orthop Res Soc* 7:43, 1982.
107. Fronek J, Frank C, Amiel D, et al: The effects of intermittent passive motion (IPM) in the healing of medial collateral ligaments. *Trans Orthop Res Soc* 8:31, 1983.
108. Frank C, Woo SL-Y, Amiel D, et al: Medial collateral ligament healing: a multidisciplinary assessment in rabbits. *Am J Sports Med* 11:379–389, 1983.
109. McKibben B: The biology of fracture healing in long bones. *J Bone Joint Surg Br* 60:150–162, 1978.

Pain and Pain Management

William Rubine | Kimberly Jones

CHAPTER OBJECTIVES

After reading this chapter, the reader will be able to do the following:
* Define *pain*.
* Explain the types and mechanisms of pain.
* Measure pain.
* Describe the different ways to manage pain.

Pain is the most common reason people seek medical attention.[1] For patients, pain can be a distressing but dependable signal that something is wrong with their bodies. For rehabilitation providers, pain is often a reliable indicator of the condition of a patient's tissues and a motivation for patients to follow through with their treatment plans. However, there are also many patients for whom pain is a major barrier to rehabilitation; their pain can be severe, persistent, unpredictable, difficult to manage, and difficult to understand. When this occurs, patients and providers can both be confused and frightened. Providers don't know how to help. Patients don't do their exercises. Many people with severe or persistent pain end up disabled by decreased mobility, deconditioning, anxiety, depression, financial hardship, and in some cases, opioid use disorder.[2,3]

Disability from chronic pain is more common than most people realize. In the United States, chronic pain, loosely defined as pain that lasts longer than 3 to 6 months, is more prevalent and is more expensive to care for than diabetes, cardiovascular disease, and cancer combined.[4,5] Meanwhile, despite the publication of multiple guidelines for acute and chronic pain management,[6] a high percentage of patients, with a variable array of conditions and in a wide variety of settings, report inadequate pain management.[2] The need for a more informed understanding of pain and pain management, from a purely clinical perspective, is hard to overstate.[7] Recently, as discussed in Chapter 2, pain management has also become important from a public health perspective as health care providers of all specialties consider their responses to the opioid epidemic.[3,8]

One barrier to effective pain management is an incomplete understanding of the factors that influence how people experience pain—especially persistent pain. What causes people to experience pain for months or years after an injury that normally heals in weeks or months? What causes pain to spread or move around? Why does an activity such as a short walk not provoke pain one day but provoke a 3-day flare up on another?[9] This chapter provides an up-to-date explanation of the physiology of pain that should answer these questions and inform providers' clinical decision making as they use the physical agents described in the following chapters of this book.

Another current issue is that pain management and active therapy are sometimes seen as competing priorities in rehabilitation. Admonitions against "chasing pain" or using passive treatments appear in American Physical Therapy Association (APTA) guidelines, graduate programs, and postgraduate continuing professional education.[10] Passive use of physical agents can be considered to waste resources and provide minimal benefit to patients.[11] Active therapy can be considered to provide more benefit, and it demonstrates a higher level of skill on the part of the provider. However, pain management and active therapy, or functional restoration, can also be seen as complementary priorities. Treatment consisting of physical agents without functional restoration can be temporary and wasteful, but functional restoration without pain management can be impractical and unsustainable, particularly when the pain is severe, disabling, unpredictable, or persistent. The final part of this chapter provides a clinical reasoning framework for integrating pain management into active therapy in a way that empowers patients to understand their symptoms, minimize **flare-ups,** adhere to their treatment plan, take risks, and return to their normal life.

Terminology

The first step in understanding the neurophysiology of pain is to distinguish pain from **nociception.**

Nociception is defined as "the neural process of encoding **noxious stimuli.**"[12] A noxious stimulus can be anything mechanical, chemical, or thermal that is intense enough to potentially damage a body tissue. Nociception occurs when specialized nerve endings transduce noxious stimuli into series of action potentials, which are then propagated by sensory neurons to the central nervous system (CNS). Nociception is modulated by the nervous system at several sites such that some is facilitated, and some is inhibited. Most nociception never results in consciously perceived pain.

Pain is a conscious experience produced and perceived by the brain.[13] The exact characteristics of each specific pain experience are influenced by biological, psychological, and social factors. Whereas nociception is a simple physiological response to a noxious stimulus, pain is a complex conscious experience with sensory, emotional, and evaluative dimensions. The exact characteristics of a person's pain may or may not relate to the condition of their tissues. A person can even experience pain without any peripheral nociceptive input at all. However, whether or not the specific characteristics of a person's pain appear to match the condition of the tissues, pain should always be considered to be "real." In recognition of this, the International Association for the Study of Pain (IASP) defines pain as "an unpleasant sensory and emotional experience associated with, or resembling that associated with, actual or potential tissue damage."[12,14]

> ### ◎ Clinical Pearl
>
> Pain is not the same as nociception. Pain is an output of the brain triggered as part of the process of converting afferent action potentials into conscious awareness.

Two other important terms are **neuropathy** and **nociplasticity.**

Neuropathy is defined as "a disturbance of function or pathological change in a nerve."[12] The cause of neuropathy might be medical, as in diabetic neuropathy; mechanical, as in radiculopathy caused by a herniated lumbar disc; or idiopathic, without a known cause. Neuropathy will usually involve a lesion or disease that produces a neuroanatomically plausible distribution that is confirmed with imaging, nerve conduction tests, lab tests, or biopsy.[15] In cases where the cause of neuropathy can be resolved with treatment, the function of the affected nerves may return, but in many cases, neuropathic changes are permanent.

Nociplasticity is an aspect of bioplasticity. Nociplasticity describes the ability of the nervous and immune systems to undergo functional and structural changes that alter nociceptive processing.[16] Nociplastic changes are part of a normal and adaptive process initiated by noxious stimuli and typically resolve when the noxious stimuli resolve. But nociplastic changes can also persist with no, or only minimal, peripheral stimulus.[17] Neuropathy and nociplasticity both result in intense symptoms that can frighten patients and be challenging to manage. Unlike most neuropathies, however, nociplastic changes are perpetuated by repeated activity and reinforcement, rather than by a lesion or disease. Nociplastic changes are, theoretically[18] but not predictably, reversible with therapy.

The Nociceptive System
PHYSIOLOGY AND PATHOPHYSIOLOGY

The **nociceptive system** is made up of peripheral and central **afferent** neurons, as well as immune cells. The role of the nociceptive system is to detect noxious stimuli, transduce them into action potentials (known as *nociceptive input*), and modulate that input as it is transmitted to multiple areas in the brain, where it may or may not ultimately be perceived. The nociceptive system is often compared with an alarm system, like a car alarm. Unlike a car alarm, however, each element of the nociceptive system has the potential to undergo structural and functional changes that affect its sensitivity. Understanding the physiology of the nociceptive system and the adaptations it sometimes undergoes is key to effective pain management.

NOCICEPTORS AND PERIPHERAL SENSITIZATION

Nociceptors are **primary afferent neurons** that preferentially transmit noxious stimuli. They innervate mechano-, chemo-, and thermo-sensitive nerve endings present to a greater or lesser degree in all types of tissues. Each nociceptor has a cell body in a dorsal root or trigeminal ganglion, an axon that travels to the nerve endings in the neuron's target tissue, and proximal dendrites that synapse with the CNS.

Nociceptors also, generally, are sensitized following injury to their surrounding tissues[19] as part of the inflammatory and tissue healing process. This process, called **peripheral sensitization,** is driven by a wide variety of endogenous substances, including inflammatory mediators, neuropeptides, glutamate, and cytokines, that are produced in the tissues following an injury or surgical procedure. Peripheral sensitization usually increases sensitivity in the area of the tissue injury. For example, the pain that someone feels when they gently move or squeeze their thumb after hitting it with a hammer results from peripheral sensitization of nociceptors driven by the spread of inflammatory mediators and other endogenous substances in the soft tissues of the thumb. This localized sensitivity is called primary **hyperalgesia.**

Three types of primary afferent neurons are commonly discussed in relation to pain and nociception: **C fibers, A-delta fibers,** and **A-beta fibers.** C fibers and A-delta fibers are the most reactive to noxious stimuli and produce nociceptive input. A-beta fibers typically have a nonnociceptive sensory function, but these functions can be altered through nociplastic changes in the spinal cord.

Different peripheral nerve fibers have different functions. C fibers and A-delta fibers have nociceptive function. A-beta fibers transmit nonnociceptive input.

Peripheral Nerves

Peripheral nerves, such as a nerve root, cranial nerve, or the sciatic nerve, are made up of thousands of individual neurons separated from each other and from the rest of the body by three layers or sheaths of connective tissue. Each peripheral nerve has its own blood supply, and the connective tissue layers around the nerve are innervated by their own sensory nerves. Peripheral nerves channel action potentials, including nociception, into specific distributions called *neural zones.*

Dysfunction of peripheral nerve tissue may involve irritation of the connective tissue sheaths around the nerve, compromise of nerve conduction by disease or a lesion of the neurons (i.e., **peripheral neuropathy**), or a combination of the two. These conditions typically result in nerve trunk pain or dysesthetic pain. Nerve trunk pain is a deep, aching pain presumed to originate from irritation of the sheaths. Dysesthetic pain is a burning, tingling, lancinating, or electrical pain presumed to originate from damaged or regenerating neuronal fibers.[20] In either case, peripheral neuropathic pain will typically be distributed in a neural zone that corresponds to the affected nerves and may be accompanied by paresthesia, dysesthesia, or spasms. Neuropathic pain also commonly flares up hours or days after patients perform new or stressful activities.[21] If neuronal conduction is compromised to a great enough extent, then the patient may experience numbness or weakness in the relevant distribution as well. Research has found that many patients can reliably distinguish peripheral neuropathic pain from nociceptive pain by its electrical, burning, or lancinating quality.[21]

Initially, peripheral neuropathic pain may feel like a burning, tingling, shooting, or lancinating pain or like a deep ache approximating the course of the peripheral nerve. Over time, neuropathic pain may become nociplastic, altering the quality of pain descriptors.

The Dorsal Horn

Most primary afferent neurons, except the cranial nerves, project to the *substantia gelatinosa* of the dorsal horn of the spinal cord (Fig. 4.1), which is organized into distinct laminae that separate incoming signals according to nociceptive function. Laminae 1, 2, and 5 receive nociceptive input from C and A-delta fibers, whereas laminae 3 and 4 receive nonnociceptive input from A-beta fibers. This is one way the brain distinguishes between nociceptive and nonnociceptive inputs. Secondary afferent neurons, which receive the input from primary afferent neurons, are also differentiated according to nociceptive function: high-threshold neurons respond to noxious stimuli, low-threshold neurons respond

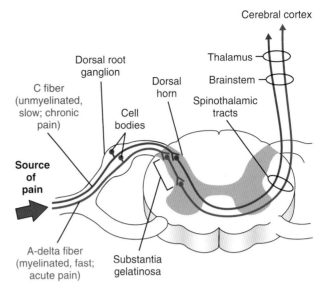

FIGURE 4.1 Ascending neural pathway of pain via A-delta and C fibers to the spinal cord and brain.

to nonnoxious stimuli, and wide-dynamic-range neurons respond to noxious and nonnoxious stimuli.[22]

The dorsal horn is the first site in the CNS where nociceptive signals are integrated with input from other primary afferents, local **interneurons** from different areas of the spinal cord, immune cells, and descending inhibition via the endogenous opioid system from the brain. This arrangement allows nociceptive input to be modulated by nonnociceptive sensory input, immune activity, and brain activity. This is where pain is "gated" (Fig. 4.2), as described in the **gate control theory of pain modulation**.[23] Many physical agents, as well as other interventions, are thought to control pain in part by supplying nonnociceptive input to the sensory nerves, inhibiting activation of nociceptive interneurons and "closing the gate" to nociceptive transmission at the spinal cord.[24]

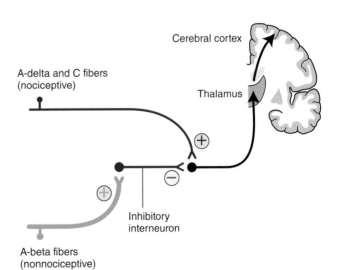

FIGURE 4.2 Simplified diagram of the gate control mechanism of pain modulation.

◎ **Clinical Pearl**

According to the classic gate control theory of pain modulation, nociceptive signals can be inhibited at the spinal cord by nonnociceptive input. Many physical agents are thought to control pain in part by supplying nonnociceptive input to the sensory nerves, "closing the gate" to the transmission of nociception at the spinal cord.

Nociplastic Changes in the Dorsal Horn. **Central sensitization** refers to nociplastic changes in the dorsal horn that facilitate nociceptive transmission. The main aspects of central sensitization include facilitation of synaptic transmission between primary and secondary afferents, inhibition of the endogenous opioid system, and facilitation of wide-dynamic-range neurons. Also, in some cases, C fibers die back from lamina 2 in the dorsal horn and are replaced by A-beta fibers, diverting nonnociceptive afferent input to the nociceptive ascending tracts.[17]

Like all nociceptive changes, central sensitization results in symptoms that no longer reliably reflect the state of the tissues. The pain can be widespread and inconsistent, not in any logical distribution. It can come and go for no apparent reason. It can flare up for days at a time. A sensitized nervous system can be compared with a malfunctioning car alarm that goes off unnecessarily throughout the day: the alarm (i.e., the pain) is real, but no one is really trying to steal the car.[25]

◎ **Clinical Pearl**

Central sensitization can cause pain that does not fit a typical anatomical or neurological distribution. Central sensitization is usually initiated by a nociceptive stimulus but can continue with no, or only minimal, ongoing peripheral stimulus. Pain associated with conditions driven may be widespread and constant, as with fibromyalgia, or may be regional and intermittent, as with irritable bowel syndrome.

The Brain

When nociceptive input reaches the brain, it is distributed throughout many sensory, motor, and emotional (or limbic) structures. There is no single "pain area" in the brain. Although there is variability among individuals, the areas of the brain most frequently involved in producing a pain experience include the primary and secondary somatosensory cortices, the motor and premotor cortices, the anterior cingulate cortex, the amygdala, the thalamus, and the prefrontal cortex.[9] When these areas act together to produce a pain experience, they are referred to as the **"pain matrix"** (Fig 4.3).[22,25]

Why are so many areas of the brain included in the pain neuromatrix? Because pain is more than a simple sensory perception of tissue health. According to the current theory, the **neuromatrix theory of pain,** the pain matrix unconsciously integrates nociceptive and nonnociceptive sensory input with biological, psychological, and social factors to determine the presence of threat and the need for protection.[13,16] When the presence of threat is detected and there is a need for protection,

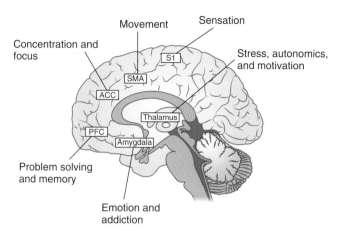

FIGURE 4.3 The pain matrix—a network of cells in the brain that, when activated, produce pain. *ACC,* Anterior cingulate cortex; *PFC,* prefrontal cortex; *S1,* primary somatosensory cortex; *SMA,* supplementary motor area.

a pain experience is produced as the conscious awareness of that process, intended to alert the person to danger and motivate them to protect the body tissues.

The neuromatrix theory of pain is just a theory, but it is supported by many observations of structural and functional changes in the brains of people with persistent pain. For example, chronic pain involves more activation of the prefrontal cortex than acute pain, implying a stronger influence of cognitive, emotional, and introspective influences.[26] Studies have also found specific patterns of global and focal atrophy in the gray matter of the brain of patients with chronic pain conditions that match their specific conditions.[9] Reduced specificity of neuronal activation in the sensory and motor homunculi, known as "smudging," has been found in patients with chronic pain[27] and has been found in one study to correlate with pain severity in patients with chronic low back pain.[28] A study in patients with chronic hip pain and osteoarthritis found that such morphological changes in the brain reversed when the pain resolved after total hip replacement.[29] When nociplastic changes such as these have occurred in a person's brain, the pain matrix becomes more sensitive to potential threats and less able to localize the stimuli. The person can experience unpredictable, inconsistent, widespread, and disproportionate levels of pain similar to that reported by patients with sensitization in the dorsal horn. The pain might be provoked by any kind of stimulus: visual, chemical, psychological, and so forth. The pain can even be provoked by stimuli without a direct effect on the tissues.

◎ **Clinical Pearl**

Nociplastic changes can cause pain that is out of proportion to the initiating stimulus and does not fit a typical anatomical or neurological distribution. The pain may be constant, as in fibromyalgia, or intermittent as in irritable bowel syndrome. All nociplastic changes are susceptible to flare-up for days. Nociplastic changes can also cause phantom sensations of swelling, stiffness, weakness, or pain. Nociplastic changes are usually initiated by a nociceptive stimulus but can continue with no ongoing peripheral stimulus or only a minimal stimulus.

Efferent Systems

When the pain matrix perceives a need for vigilance and protection, it doesn't just produce pain; it also triggers protective responses by the motor, autonomic, immune, and endocrine systems. These systems enable people to respond to the threat, whatever it is, and maintain homeostasis.[30] The motor system responds with voluntary and involuntary movements.[31] The **autonomic nervous system** adjusts the activity of the endocrine and immune systems, as well as of the smooth and cardiac muscles (Fig. 4.4), temperature, blood pressure, pH, and metabolite levels. One branch of the autonomic nervous system, called the **sympathetic nervous system,** prepares the body for "fight or flight" by increasing heart rate and blood pressure, constricting cutaneous blood vessels, and increasing sweating in the palms of the hands. Although stimulation of the sympathetic nervous system does not usually cause pain,[32] abnormal sympathetic activation can increase pain severity.[30] Nociceptors may also be directly stimulated by sympathetic **efferent** fibers or by **neurotransmitters** released by the sympathetic nerves. Inappropriate vasoconstriction, increased capillary permeability, or increased smooth muscle tone caused by sympathetic activity may also indirectly cause or exacerbate pain.[33] When the sympathetic nervous system is hyperactive, patients feel anxious and stressed.

The parasympathetic branch of the autonomic nervous system prepares the body to "rest and relax." Parasympathetic activity, primarily mediated by the vagus nerve, has been shown to reduce inflammation, sympathetic nervous system activation, oxidative stress, and the activity of the pain matrix and to enhance the analgesic effects of morphine.[34]

The endocrine system is made up of glands, including the hypothalamus, the pituitary, and the adrenals, which respond to threats by producing hormones. **Opiopeptins** are one such group of hormones. Opiopeptins inhibit nociception by binding to opioid receptors on many peripheral nerve endings and on neurons in several regions of the nervous system, including the periaqueductal gray matter (PAGM), the raphe nucleus of the brainstem, the superficial layers of the dorsal horn of the spinal cord (layers I and II), various areas of the limbic system, and the enteric nervous system.[35] Opiopeptins cause presynaptic inhibition by suppressing the inward flux of calcium ions and postsynaptic inhibition by promoting the outward flux of potassium ions. Opiopeptins also indirectly inhibit nociceptive transmission by inhibiting the release of gamma-aminobutyric acid (GABA) in the PAGM and the raphe nucleus.[36]

The release of opiopeptins is thought to play an important role in pain modulation during times of emotional stress. When stress is induced experimentally by the anticipation of

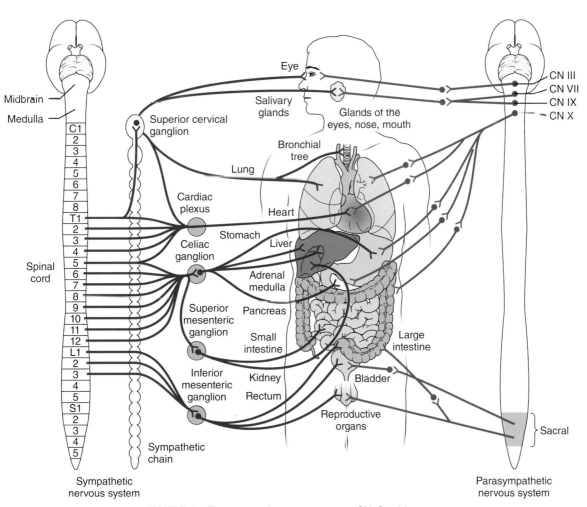

FIGURE 4.4 The autonomic nervous system. *CN,* Cranial nerve.

pain, opiopeptin levels in the brain and cerebrospinal fluid (CSF) become elevated, and pain thresholds are increased in both animals and humans.[37,38] Experimentally, animals have been shown to experience a diffuse **analgesia** when under stress. Humans demonstrate a naloxone-sensitive increase in the pain threshold and a parallel depression of the nociceptive flexion reflex when subjected to emotional stress.[38,39] These findings indicate that pain suppression in times of acute stress is most likely caused by increased opiopeptin levels at the spinal cord and higher CNS centers.

Opiopeptins provide a possible explanation for the paradoxical pain-relieving effects of painful stimulation such as high-intensity TENS, topical capsaicin, or acupuncture, all of which have been shown to produce analgesia, both where they are applied and in other areas.[39] Pain may be relieved by painful stimuli because the stimuli cause neurons in the PAGM of the midbrain and thalamus to produce and release opiopeptins.[40] Placebo analgesia is also thought to be mediated in part by opiopeptins. This claim is supported by observations that the opioid antagonist naloxone can reverse placebo analgesia and that placebos can also produce respiratory depression, a typical side effect of opioids.[41,42]

The hormones adrenaline, noradrenaline, and cortisol are also produced by the endocrine system. The endocrine system may be dysregulated in chronic pain. These hormones are generally produced in response to stress and have many beneficial effects in daily life, but persistently elevated levels, particularly of cortisol, can cause immunosuppression, osteoporosis, depression, altered sleep cycles, slow healing, and tissue degeneration. Although controversial, some authors have suggested that persistently elevated cortisol levels and immune system dysregulation may contribute to dysfunction and persistent inflammation in patients with chronic pain.[43]

Unlike the peripheral nervous system, which generally produces effects in specific neural zones, the immune system produces local, regional, and global effects. The role of local inflammation in acute pain is described in Chapter 3. The regional and global effects of the immune system include producing feelings of sickness and muscle aches and also contribute to the nociplastic changes described earlier in this chapter.[16] Histological studies have implicated immune activity in the development and maintenance of many chronic pain conditions, including the pain associated with rheumatoid arthritis, osteoarthritis, fibromyalgia, complex regional pain syndrome, multiple sclerosis, and diabetic neuropathy.[44]

All of the efferent stress response systems in the body are adapted to respond to temporary stresses but not to countering stressors that last for months or years. Under these conditions, the efferent systems can produce persistent stress, anxiety, and fatigue that contribute to chronic pain and disability but are often manageable to some extent by nonpharmacological techniques, including physical agents.[45]

Types of Pain

Pain is commonly categorized as **acute pain** or **chronic pain,** although the term *persistent pain* is also sometimes used in the place of *chronic pain*.[46] *Acute pain* usually refers to pain lasting less than 30 days. *Chronic pain* usually refers to pain that has outlasted the typical healing time of the involved tissues, often 3 to 6 months, depending on the tissues. Approximately 20% of the U.S. adult population has chronic pain, but not all

chronic pain is debilitating. Eight percent of U.S. adults have debilitating, high-impact chronic pain that frequently limits life or work activities. Understandably, those with high-impact chronic pain more often seek medical care.[47]

ACUTE PAIN

Acute pain is defined by the Department of Health and Human Services as "an expected physiologic experience to noxious stimuli that can become pathologic, is normally sudden in onset, time limited, and motivates behaviors to avoid actual or potential tissue injuries."[2] Acute pain generally occurs as a direct result of tissue injury caused by a wound, disease process, or invasive procedure and is associated with inflammation and tissue healing. In most cases, the pain and inflammation resolve as the tissues heal.

The first line of treatment for moderate or severe acute pain is usually pharmacological. An introduction to pharmacological approaches to pain management is provided later in this chapter. Nonpharmacological techniques can also help reduce acute pain and are recommended by the American College of Physicians, the IASP, and the American Pain Society.[48-50]

The priorities of nonpharmacological acute pain management are as follows: (1) to control inflammation, (2) to inhibit nociception, (3) to provide clear guidelines for activity (not too much, not too little) that encourage appropriate stress on the tissues, (4) to teach rest and relaxation, and (5) to repeatedly reassure the patient.[48,51] The most well-known nonpharmacological techniques for managing acute pain are summarized by *RICE:* rest, ice, compression, and elevation.[48] Rest allows damaged tissues to heal. Ice reduces pain by reducing inflammation and thereby reducing peripheral sensitization in the tissues. Compression and elevation reduce edema. Electrical stimulation also helps control acute pain, primarily by inhibiting nociception in the spinal cord in accordance with the gate control theory. Detailed reviews of the literature concerning physical agents for the control of acute pain, along with specific guidelines for applying these agents, are provided in later chapters of this book. The time spent applying physical agents also often provides an excellent opportunity to educate and reassure the patient, as well as to practice mindfulness-based techniques such as body scans or diaphragmatic breathing.

There are many published guidelines for patient education regarding pain in the acute setting, including the following examples:[6,51-53]

- Reinforce that pain is normal after an injury or surgery. Complete elimination of pain is usually not achievable in the short term, but this pain is not inherently dangerous and almost always resolves in time.[6,52]
- Review the numeric pain scale and how to communicate with all health care providers to follow a medication schedule and stay ahead of breakthrough pain.
- Detail the frequency and rationale for bed exercises, position changes, rest breaks, elevation, physical agents, and any other interventions.
- Set realistic expectations and build trust.

CHRONIC PAIN

Chronic pain has several definitions. One definition is based on time: pain present on at least half the days for longer than 6 months.[2,54] Another definition is based on tissue healing time: pain lasting longer than the expected healing time of the involved tissues.[9] Yet another definition is based on disability: pain leading to disability greater than would be expected by the injury.[12] Whatever the definition, chronic pain is more common than most people realize. One survey estimated that approximately 100 million U.S. adults have chronic pain.[54] Another found that spinal pain, probably the best-studied chronic pain condition, has a 19% annual prevalence in the United States and a 29% lifetime prevalence. Another study found that approximately 57% of all Americans reported recurrent or chronic pain in the previous year,[55,56] of whom 62% had been in pain for longer than 1 year, and 40% reported constant pain.

In conditions such as chronic low back pain and fibromyalgia, rehabilitation has only modest success.[57,58] One reason for this may be that these conditions represent a heterogeneous group of patients who cannot all be effectively treated in the same way. A patient with chronic neck pain resulting from the postural demands of their job cannot be managed in the same way as a patient with chronic neck pain, fibromyalgia, and kinesiophobia. Some chronic pain results from persistent nociception in the tissues, although psychosocial factors usually also play an important role. Most chronic conditions result from persistent neuropathy or nociplastic changes with psychosocial contributors. The wide variety of potential neuropathic and nociplastic issues is reflected by the wide variety of associated disorders, such as chronic spinal pain, fibromyalgia, neuropathy, **complex regional pain syndrome (CRPS),** phantom limb pain, poststroke pain, osteoarthritis and rheumatoid arthritis, headache, cancer pain, temporomandibular joint disorder, irritable bowel syndrome, and interstitial cystitis.[9,26,59] As confusing as this appears, from a pain management point of view, the signs and symptoms fall into patterns consistent with five pathophysiological pain

mechanisms: nociception, neuropathy, nociplasticity, movement systems, and psychosocial factors. All of these mechanisms are involved to some extent in acute pain, but they usually resolve. Chronic pain management begins with identifying and weighing the pathophysiological pain mechanisms that have not resolved.[60,61] In patients whose pain has lasted more than 3 months, nociplastic and psychosocial changes will almost always be present, but they may not be the only, or even the primary, perpetuators of the condition. A basic impression of which mechanisms dominate the symptoms in an individual patient can usually be inferred from a good subjective history and confirmed by a physical examination.[61] When the primary or dominant mechanism for a given patient has been determined, an effective pain management strategy is simpler to formulate.

The following sections provide brief descriptions of the typical symptoms associated with nociception, neuropathy, nociplasticity, and psychosocial issues and general suggestions for how to help manage pain resulting from these mechanisms. Evaluation of movement systems is outside the scope of this text.

Pain Mechanisms
PRIMARY CHRONIC NOCICEPTIVE PAIN
Nociceptive pain is defined by the IASP as "pain that arises from actual or threatened damage to non-neural tissue and is due to the activation of nociceptors."[12] A reliable stimulus-response relationship between movement or position and the patient's symptoms suggests that nociception is the primary mechanism. Also, nociceptive pain will usually be felt in an anatomically plausible distribution at or near the site of injury, although nociceptive pain may be referred (i.e., **referred pain**) to other areas of the body (Fig. 4.5).

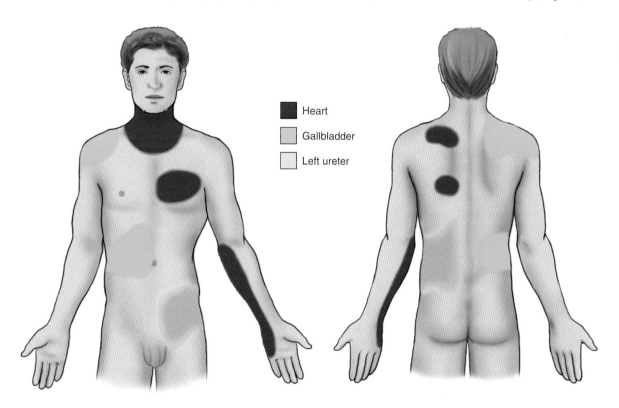

Heart
Gallbladder
Left ureter

FIGURE 4.5 Typical pain referral patterns.

When chronic nociceptive pain is perpetuated by ongoing inflammation, such as that caused by osteoarthritis or rheumatoid arthritis, pain may be reduced by antiinflammatory interventions such as rest, ice, and antiinflammatory medications.

When chronic nociceptive pain cannot be explained by an ongoing disease process, impairments of motor control, strength, or endurance should be suspected.[63] Treatment should then focus on strengthening and conditioning, mobilization of restrictions, and motor control. Pain or swelling can be used as a guide to when tissues are being irritated or fatigued, although some pain or soreness is not necessarily harmful and can usually be relieved with ice or rest. Even when nociceptive pain is the primary issue, patient education and reassurance are also important[64] because emotional and cognitive factors usually have a role. The clinician should avoid statements such as "you have the spine of an eighty-year-old" or "your knee is bone on bone" and focus on information that is factual but productive. Give advice that enables, not disables.

NEUROPATHIC PAIN

Neuropathic pain is defined as "pain arising as a direct consequence of a lesion or disease affecting the somatosensory system."[65] The range of painful neuropathic conditions is diverse, including peripheral neuropathies and diseases of the CNS such as stroke, spinal cord injury, Parkinson disease, or multiple sclerosis. This section details the signs and management strategies common to most painful neuropathies.

The clinical signs of neuropathic pain include **mechanosensitivity** of nerve tissues, sensory signs, and sympathetic signs. *Mechanosensitivty* means tenderness to palpation of the involved nerve or nerves or pain with active and passive movements that compress or stretch the nerves, such as Spurling's test or nerve tension tests.[66] Sensory signs include **allodynia,** paresthesia, or dysesthesia. Sympathetic signs include temperature changes, color changes, or trophic changes. If neuronal function is compromised, there may also be weakness or numbness. Validated screens for neuropathic pain have been developed, two of which are described later in this chapter in the section on measuring pain.

Managing neuropathic pain is more complex than managing nociceptive pain. Patients with neuropathy are often frightened or confused by the unusual, intense, and unpredictable nature of their symptoms and their sometimes-uncertain prognosis. Management should include extensive pain education that explains their specific symptoms. Many of these patients will be particularly likely to benefit from a multidisciplinary approach to pain management that includes psychological treatment such as cognitive-behavioral therapy.[67] Some will experience substantial relief with medications.[68]

In cases of peripheral neuropathic pain, physical agents that gate nociception, such as electrical stimulation, cold, or heat, are often effective.[69] Nerve trunk pain and paresthesia are sometimes reduced by gentle movements without undue tension on the nerve tissue, known as "flossing" or "sliders."[27,66] If there is a local mechanical dysfunction affecting the nerve, such as a herniated disc, then specific exercises or manual therapy can also be effective. In cases of central neuropathic pain, allodynia, hyperpathia, and dysesthesia can be managed with tactile desensitization, tactile discrimination training, or compression garments, as well as heat and TENS. Severe pain with movement, as seen in CRPS, can often be managed with graded motor imagery.

Patients with neuropathic pain have flare-ups. Therefore, pain management for patients with neuropathic pain should include a "flare-up plan."[70] Typical elements of a flare-up plan include the following:

- Active rest: The patient should plan 20- to 30-minute rests in a position of comfort three to four times per day. During these rests, they can apply ice, heat, or TENS for pain relief. Relaxation techniques, including diaphragmatic breathing and body scans, can also be helpful in these periods, as can distractions such as music, aroma therapy, or coloring books.
- Pacing: Between rests, they should continue their normal activities but not add new ones.
- Positivity: The patient should work hard to stay positive. Avoid negative thinking or verbiage. "Don't flare up, but don't freak out when you do."[16]

When neuropathic pain is accompanied by negative symptoms such as hypoesthesia or weakness, then nerve conduction may be compromised.[20] Cervical or lumbar traction may be indicated, depending on the location of the compromise. For example, one study[71] on the use of traction for cervical radicular pain found a greater than 79% likelihood of benefit from traction in patients with at least three of the following characteristics: peripheralization with C4 to C7 mobility testing, a positive shoulder abduction sign on the involved side, age older than 55 years, positive upper-limb neural tension testing, and relief with a manual distraction test.

NOCIPLASTIC PAIN

Nociplasticity is an important factor in a wide range of diagnoses, including fibromyalgia, osteoarthritis and rheumatoid arthritis, temporomandibular disorders, whiplash, low back pain, pelvic pain, and many other disorders.[9,17,59,72] These associated disorders are often called *functional somatic syndromes*. In addition to severe or widespread pain, nociplasticity is also associated with fatigue and sleep disturbance, impaired mental functioning, phantom (i.e., perceived but not physically apparent) swelling or stiffness, digestive dysfunction, sexual dysfunction, chemical sensitivity, and depression.[73] Like people with neuropathic pain, people with nociplastic pain are apt to experience flare-ups seemingly out of proportion to the activity that triggered them[16] or of longer duration.

Clinical signs of nociplastic pain include sensitivity to normally innocuous stimuli such as brushing or light touch (allodynia), pain from noxious stimuli that has an intensity or duration out of proportion to the stimulus (hyperalgesia), pain perceived in an area beyond the area typically affected by the stimulus (secondary hyperalgesia), unpleasant sensations besides pain (dysesthesia), and pain from repeated subthreshold stimuli (hyperpathia).[59] These patients' pain is also commonly, but not always, worsened by cold temperatures, loud noises, bright lights, and strong odors.[74,75] Patients with nociplastic pain will often have multiple positive neural tension tests on both sides or in both the upper and lower limbs. They may have mechanical impairments, but these often will not be severe enough to explain the associated symptoms. They might experience pain when watching people move or imagining movement or might have impaired tactile discrimination. Nijs and colleagues provide a detailed description of a recommended clinical examination to distinguish nociplastic from neuropathic and nociceptive pain.[73] The Central Sensitization Index[76] and the proposed 2010/2016 American College of Rheumatology (ACR) criteria for fibromyalgia[77] are also validated screens for identifying patients whose symptoms are dominated by nociplastic changes. These screens are described in more detail later in this chapter.

Once nociplastic changes are recognized as the dominant mechanism, the rehabilitation approach should be conceived of as desensitization to threat combined with graded exposure to feared or valued activities.[78,79] Patient education is important in the beginning. There are many published guidelines and resources for educating patients about nociplastic pain.[16,52,70,80] Points to be covered might include the following:
1. The problem is one of CNS sensitivity that developed as a result of neuroplasticity and can resolve in the same way, although it may take a long time.[18]
2. The nociceptive system is overly sensitive—"the car alarm is malfunctioning." A certain amount of pain is to be expected.
3. The pain that follows from walking or sitting is real pain, but it is not an indication of tissue damage or of irreversible lesions or disease of the CNS.

Nonpharmacological pain management should include physical agents that are comfortable and gate pain sensations, such as heat and TENS. Mindfulness-based stress, anxiety, and fatigue management are supported by the literature. Sensorimotor reeducation has some support. All of these should be integrated into a carefully designed and paced graded activity or graded exposure programs.[16,79,81,82] Suggestions for these are made in a later section of this chapter.

Because occasional flare-ups are likely, it helps to forewarn the patient and prepare a flare-up management plan that includes short-term treatment options. Specific suggestions for this are given in the earlier section on neuropathic pain.

PSYCHOSOCIAL FACTORS

Psychosocial factors such as catastrophizing, depression, kinesiophobia, fear avoidance, homelessness, food insecurity, and work- and family-related stresses can provoke pain, trigger flare-ups, or interfere with patients' ability to follow through with their treatment plan. Some of these factors will be present for most patients whose pain has lasted for more than a few months, although they may not predominate. Some patients with predominant psychosocial features will report symptoms similar to those of patients with nociplastic pain, such as spreading or inconsistent pain, pain without a clear anatomical correlate, pain that is significantly affected by mood or environment, or pain that flares up for days for no apparent reason, but they will not show sensory signs such as allodynia or hyperpathia. Also, patients with psychosocial pain are usually not as sensitive to cold as patients with central sensitization or peripheral neuropathic pain.[73]

To the extent that psychosocial factors contribute, rehabilitation providers should emphasize stress management as well as pain management and progressively return patients to their valued or feared activities through graded exposure.[83–85] Almost any physical agent could be helpful or unhelpful to these patients, depending on how it is used. Physical agents that help patients challenge their expectations and improve their function are helpful. Passive treatments that distract from that process may be wasteful at best and might be considered harmful if they perpetuate the patient's beliefs that their tissues are more inflamed or damaged than they really are.

Preventing Acute Pain From Becoming Chronic

It is unclear why some acute pain becomes chronic. One review found the incidence of persistent pain following common surgeries to be between 10% and 50%.[86] Another review identified pain intensity, pain duration, and the presence of severe depression as possible risk factors, although genetic predisposition was suspected to be more important.[9] A 2011 systematic review of studies evaluating psychosocial risk factors for chronic low back pain identified patients' judgments and beliefs regarding their acute low back pain as relatively powerful predictors for the development of chronic pain. Passive coping strategies and fear-avoidance behaviors in the first few months of a condition influenced disability but not pain.[87]

During the early phases of healing, physical agents or other nonpharmacological techniques that help reduce pain intensity, and any communication that reassures patients, may help prevent the development of chronic pain. Specific techniques such as RICE, TENS, tactile desensitization, breathing, relaxation, mirror therapy, or other modalities could all be appropriate depending on the patient and their situation. Care should be taken to minimize verbal and non-verbal messages that may exacerbate fear.[88] Clinicians should monitor their patients with acute pain for signs that peripheral sensitivity and nociplastic changes are not resolving as expected or that unhelpful psychological factors are developing. Examples of these would be aberrant movement patterns, secondary hyperalgesia, allodynia, hyperpathia, trophic changes, anxiety, depression, catastrophizing, kinesiophobia, and fear avoidance.[56,79] Clinicians should also watch for post-operative neuropathic pain because this is a leading cause of postoperative chronic pain.[48] If any of these develop, they should be communicated as early as possible to all members of the treatment team.

For example, a man fractures his tibia and fibula in a motorcycle accident. He requires surgery. In the days after surgery, he reports constant pain and all other cardinal signs of inflammation (calor, rubor, tumor, and functio laesa). He is reassured that his pain is normal; that he will be okay. But over the next few days, his leg pain starts to worsen. His ankle gets darker, and he develops allodynia. He limits movement of the ankle and avoids letting anything touch his lower leg. At this point, the therapist communicates their concerns to the whole team. The medical provider may do further examination or imaging to make sure nothing was missed. The therapist slows down the exercise progression but discourages the patient from stopping movement altogether and starts educating the patient about nociplasticity—for example: "Your nervous system is trying to protect you, but it is trying too hard"; "Sensitivity means that little things that should not hurt, do hurt, and things that should hurt a little, hurt a lot; but gentle motion and touch are not damaging your tissues"; and "Motion is lotion." The therapist teaches the patient tactile desensitization for the knee and perhaps does a trial of TENS. The patient may believe that as long as the leg is hurting like this, he should not move it or put any pressure on it at all. The therapist strongly encourages the patient that as long as he maintains any weight-bearing precautions set by the surgeon and the activity does not provoke a marked increase in swelling or a lasting pain (a flare-up), he should continue all his therapeutic exercise. He should do what he can, several times a day, on a non–pain-contingent basis. Also, he should follow a specific pain management plan, including rest and physical agents such as TENS and compression stockings.

Palliative Care

What is palliative care? Palliative care is focused on supporting quality of life for patients and their families through the prevention and relief of suffering by early identification and impeccable assessment and treatment of pain and other problems—physical, psychosocial, and spiritual. Patients receiving palliative care generally have a life-threatening illness such as cancer, heart disease, chronic lung disease, or AIDS, but they may also have other serious progressive disorders that affect quality of life, such as Alzheimer, multiple sclerosis, or amyotrophic lateral sclerosis (ALS). These patients' most common problems are pain, symptoms arising from skeletal metastases, weakness and deconditioning, neurological symptoms, pulmonary secretions, dyspnea, lymph-edema, and venous thrombosis. In palliative care, patients'

and care teams' priorities differ from those in typical rehabilitation. The emphases of palliative care are choice, symptom management (including pain management), and quality of life. Passive therapies, including physical agents, are not discouraged if they help meet these goals.

PAIN CAUSED BY MALIGNANCY

The treatment of pain caused by malignancy may differ from the treatment of pain from other causes because particular care must be taken to consider whether agents that could promote the growth or metastasis of malignant tissue should be avoided. Because the growth of some malignancies can be accelerated by increasing local circulation, agents such as ultrasound and diathermy, which are known to increase deep tissue temperature and circulation, generally should not be used in an area of malignancy.[89,90] However, in patients with end-stage malignancies, pain-relieving interventions that can improve the patient's quality of life but may adversely affect disease progression may be used with the patient's informed consent.

Measuring Pain

Pain measurement is one of the first steps in pain management. Comprehensive measurement of a person's pain experience allows for (1) improved communication between patients and providers, (2) targeted treatments, (3) goal setting, and (4) monitoring of treatment effectiveness.[91] A person's pain experience can be described as having three dimensions: sensory discriminative (what they feel and where they feel it), emotional affective (how they feel about it), and evaluative (what they think and expect). Each of these can be measured with an appropriate tool or scale. The techniques for pain measurement are the interview, the clinical exam, and written scales and questionnaires. This section focuses on useful scales and questionnaires for measuring pain. One caveat in measuring pain is that most people with chronic pain have multiple pain locations. When questioning patients about their chronic pain, be clear regarding whether you are asking about their "background" pain or a new pain area.

◎ Clinical Pearl

When evaluating pain, consider the location, intensity, and duration of the pain. Also consider how the pain affects the patient's function, activity, and participation.

VISUAL ANALOG AND NUMERICAL SCALES

With a visual analog scale (VAS), patients indicate their present level of pain on a horizontal or vertical line, on which one end represents no pain and the other end represents the most severe pain the patient can imagine (Fig. 4.6). With a numerical rating scale (NRS), patients note the severity of their pain on a scale from 0 to 10 or 0 to 100, with 0 representing no pain and 10 or 100, depending on the scale, representing the most severe pain the patient can imagine.[92]

VASs and NRSs are frequently used to assess the severity of a patient's clinical pain because they are quick and easy to

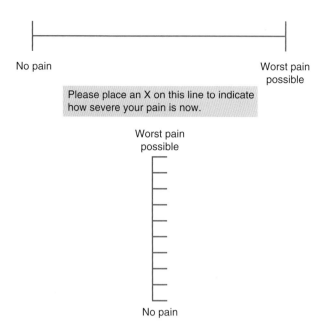

FIGURE 4.6 Visual analog scales for rating pain severity.

administer, are easily understood, and provide readily quantifiable data.[92] However, VASs and NRSs only reflect the intensity of pain in the sensory-discriminative dimension and do not provide information about the patient's thoughts and feelings about their pain or the effects of the pain on function and activity. The reliability of VASs and NRSs vary among patients and with the patient group examined, although the two types of scales have a high degree of agreement between them.[93] VASs and NRSs may also be used together to measure different dimensions of pain, for example, pain intensity, pain frequency, or level of distress.[94]

Alternative simple quantitative scales have been developed to use with patients who have difficulty using numerical scales or standard VASs. For example, young children who understand words or pictures but do not yet understand numerical representations of pain can use a scale with faces with expressions representing different experiences of pain (Fig. 4.7). This type of scale can also be used to assess pain in patients with limited comprehension due to language barriers or cognitive deficits. Pain scales based on the clinician's observation of a child's expression and behavior can also be used to rate pain in very young children and infants (Table 4.1).

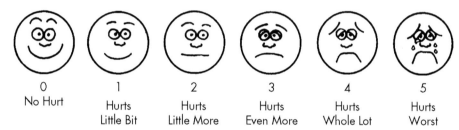

0	1	2	3	4	5
No Hurt	Hurts Little Bit	Hurts Little More	Hurts Even More	Hurts Whole Lot	Hurts Worst

FIGURE 4.7 Face scale for rating pain severity in children age 3 years and older and other patients with limited numerical communication ability. The patient uses this tool by pointing to each face and using the brief word instructions under it to describe pain intensity. (From Wong-Baker FACES Foundation: *Wong-Baker FACES® Pain Rating Scale*. 2020. Retrieved May 18, 2021, with permission from www.WongBakerFACES.org. Originally published in Whaley & Wong's *Nursing Care of Infants and Children*. © Elsevier Inc.)

TABLE 4.1	Neonatal Infant Pain Scale (NIPS) Operational Definitions	
	Score: Behavior	**Description**
Facial expression	0: Relaxed muscles	Restful face, neutral expression
	1: Grimace	Tight facial muscles, furrowed brow, chin, jaw (negative facial expression—nose, mouth, and brow)
Cry	0: No cry	Quiet, not crying
	1: Whimper	Mild moaning, intermittent
	2: Vigorous cry	Loud screams, rising, shrill, continuous (*Note:* Silent cry may be scored if baby is intubated, as evidenced by obvious mouth, facial movement.)
Breathing patterns	0: Relaxed	Usual pattern for this baby
	1: Change in breathing	Indrawing, irregular, faster than usual, gagging, breath-holding
Arms	0: Relaxed/restrained	No muscular rigidity, occasional random movements of arms
	1: Flexed/extended	Tense, straight arms; rigid or rapid extension, flexion
Legs	0: Relaxed/restrained	No muscular rigidity, occasional random leg movement
	1: Flexed/extended	Tense, straight legs; rigid or rapid extension, flexion
State of arousal	0: Sleeping/awake	Quiet, peaceful, sleeping, or alert and settled
	1: Fussy	Alert, restless, and thrashing

Score 0 = no pain likely; maximum score 7 = severe pain likely.
From Lawrence J, Alcock D, McGrath DP, et al: The development of a tool to assess neonatal pain. *Neonatal Network* 12:59–65, 1993.

The best timing to use a VAS or NRS depends on the specific situation. Patients with acute pain should be monitored multiple times throughout the day, especially if their pain is moderate or severe. Patients with chronic pain need not be questioned as often unless there is a reason to expect their pain to have changed. Too much focus on pain intensity in people with chronic pain can prove detrimental if this increases their overall focus on pain and their feeling of being at risk. Clinicians should balance the need for thorough pain measurement with the need to promote a message of safety and a focus on non–pain-contingent treatment.

> ### ⦿ Clinical Pearl
>
> - Visual analog and numerical pain scales are best used for quickly estimating pain severity.
> - Avoid repeatedly asking patients to rate their pain if there is no logical reason that it might have substantially changed.

SEMANTIC DIFFERENTIAL SCALES

Semantic differential scales consist of word lists and categories that represent sensory, emotional, or evaluative aspects of the pain experience. Patients are asked to select from these lists the words that best describe their pain. If you have ever asked a person to rate their pain on a scale of 0 to 10 and had them roll their eyes and say that "the numbers don't mean anything," then you have encountered the need for a semantic differentiation scale. These scales are designed to collect a broad range of qualitative information about the sensory, affective, and evaluative aspects of a patient's pain experience and to provide quantifiable data for intrasubject and intersubject comparisons. The long and short forms of the McGill Pain Questionnaire are commonly used for this type of pain assessment (Fig. 4.8).[95-97] They include descriptors across multiple categories, including temporal, spatial, pressure, and thermal, to describe sensory aspects of the pain; fear, anxiety, and tension to describe affective aspects of the pain; and cognitive experience of pain based on past experience and learned behaviors to describe evaluative aspects of the pain. The patient circles the one word in each of the applicable categories that best describes their present pain.[95,97]

Semantic differential scales have several advantages and disadvantages compared with other types of pain measures. They allow the scope, quality, and intensity of pain to be assessed and quantified. Counting the total number of words chosen provides a quick gauge of pain severity. A more sensitive assessment of pain severity can be obtained by adding the rank sums of all words chosen to produce a pain rating index (PRI). For greater specificity with regard to the most problematic area, an index for the three major categories of the questionnaire can also be calculated.[97] The primary disadvantages of these types of scales are that they are time consuming to administer, and they require the patient to have an intact cognitive state and a high level of literacy. Given these advantages and limitations, this type of scale is used most appropriately when detailed information about a patient's pain is needed, as in a chronic pain treatment program or in clinical research. For example, in patients with chronic wounds, the McGill Pain Questionnaire was more sensitive to the pain experience than a single rating of pain intensity and was positively correlated with wound stage, affective stress, and symptoms of depression.[98]

> ### ⦿ Clinical Pearl
>
> Semantic differential pain scales should be used for a detailed pain description.

The McGill Pain Questionnaire first demonstrated that pain quality descriptors could be useful in indicating probable pain mechanisms, but the specificity of the scale was insufficient[99] to fully elucidate pain mechanisms. The 12-item Neuropathic Pain Questionnaire[100] (NPQ); the Leeds Assessment of Neuropathic Symptoms and Signs (LANSS),[100] which includes a 7-item patient-completed questionnaire and a brief clinical assessment; and the Central Sensitization Inventory (CSI),[76] which includes a 25-item patient-completed questionnaire and assessment of whether the patient has been diagnosed with central sensitivity syndromes, are more recently developed screening tools specifically designed to identify patients with pain with predominantly neuropathic or nociplastic characteristics. These tools make it easier for clinicians to identify patients with neuropathic pain, but they do miss some cases. One study found that the NPQ failed to identify 10% to 20% of patients who were later found to have neuropathic pain.[101] The STarT Back Screening Tool is a 9-question patient questionnaire designed specifically to screen patients with low back pain for strong emotional-affective and evaluative features to stratify their risk, as for chronicity, as low, medium, or high. A different treatment plan is recommended for each risk group. In one randomized controlled trial, the use of the STarT Back screen by primary care physicians to guide treatment was associated with improved outcomes in the high-risk group and cost savings in the low-risk group without worsening of outcomes.[102]

OTHER MEASURES

In addition to screens, daily activity/pain logs indicating which activities ease or aggravate the pain; body diagrams on which the patient can indicate the location and nature of the pain (Fig. 4.9); and open-ended, structured interviews may also provide additional useful information.[103-105]

In selecting measures to assess pain, consider symptom duration, the patient's cognitive abilities, and the time needed to assess the patient's report of pain. For example, a simple VAS may be sufficient to track the progressive decrease in pain as a patient recovers from an acute injury. However, in more complex or prolonged cases, detailed measures such as semantic differential scales or combinations of several measures are more appropriate. For example, in patients with chronic pain, the numerical rating of pain severity often does not change, although function and mobility have improved.

What does your pain feel like?

Some of the words below describe your *present* pain. Indicate which words describe it best. Leave out any word group that is not suitable. Use only a single word in each appropriate group—the one that applies *best*.

1	2	3	4
1 Flickering	1 Jumping	1 Pricking	1 Sharp
2 Quivering	2 Flashing	2 Boring	2 Cutting
3 Pulsing	3 Shooting	3 Drilling	3 Lacerating
4 Throbbing		4 Stabbing	
5 Beating		5 Lancinating	
6 Pounding			

5	6	7	8
1 Pinching	1 Tugging	1 Hot	1 Tingling
2 Pressing	2 Pulling	2 Burning	2 Itchy
3 Gnawing	3 Wrenching	3 Scalding	3 Smarting
4 Cramping		4 Searing	4 Stinging
5 Crushing			

9	10	11	12
1 Dull	1 Tender	1 Tiring	1 Sickening
2 Sore	2 Taut	2 Exhausting	2 Suffocating
3 Hurting	3 Rasping		
4 Aching	4 Splitting		
5 Heavy			

13	14	15	16
1 Fearful	1 Punishing	1 Wretched	1 Annoying
2 Frightful	2 Grueling	2 Blinding	2 Troublesome
3 Terrifying	3 Cruel		3 Miserable
	4 Vicious		4 Intense
	5 Killing		5 Unbearable

17	18	19	20
1 Spreading	1 Tight	1 Cool	1 Nagging
2 Radiating	2 Numb	2 Cold	2 Nauseating
3 Penetrating	3 Drawing	3 Freezing	3 Agonizing
4 Piercing	4 Squeezing		4 Dreadful
	5 Tearing		5 Torturing

FIGURE 4.8 Semantic differential scale from the McGill Pain Questionnaire. (From Melzack R: The McGill Pain Questionnaire: major properties and scoring methods. *Pain* 1:277–299, 1975.)

Pain Management

In the previous four sections of this chapter, pain management techniques have been outlined for each of the pain mechanisms (except movement), but many patients one sees in rehabilitation, especially patients with chronic pain, will have multifactorial pain, and the relative priority of the different mechanisms will change over time. The suggestions made previously will have to be adapted, combined, and progressed. This section discusses considerations and priorities for pain management and for integrating physical agents into multimodal, active therapy programs.

First, good pain management is not passive. Patients have a lot of work to do. They learn about their condition so that they can "make sense of their pain."[82] They modify their behavior to protect weak or healing tissues, if necessary, and to minimize flare-ups. They apply physical agents to themselves, with supervision at first, then independently, to manage inflammation and modulate nociception.[22] They follow graded activity or graded exposure programs and flare-up plans. Also, because pain is just one part of a multisystem response, they adopt techniques to manage stress,[45] anxiety, and fatigue.[106] In therapy, these techniques should be emphasized, supervised, practiced, and reinforced just like any other therapeutic activities. To assess if a patient is independent with their pain management program, ask them to describe when and how they do it in detail. When a flare-up

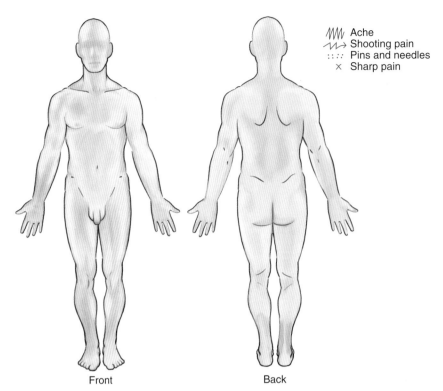

	Ache
	Shooting pain
	Pins and needles
×	Sharp pain

Front   Back

FIGURE 4.9 Body diagrams for marking the location and nature of pain. (From Cameron MH, Monroe LG: *Physical rehabilitation: evidence-based examination, evaluation, and intervention,* St Louis, 2007, Saunders.)

occurs in a patient with chronic pain, as they inevitably do, review the management plan with the patient and revise as necessary. Reinforce the pain education: "The pain flared up, but your body was okay." Flare-ups provide the best opportunities to adjust and reinforce pain management plans; don't let those opportunities go to waste.

Second, pain management should be multifactorial. Recall the pain matrix in Fig. 4.3, which shows that pain is processed by many different areas of the brain that serve a diverse set of functions, including emotion, learning, concentration, problem solving, and movement. Pain management and exercise in rehabilitation should target all the same areas. Ask patients about their thoughts, feelings, living situations, and goals, and include those considerations in their rehabilitation.

The following sections discuss indications and strategies for physical agents, pharmacological agents, and cognitive-behavioral strategies for pain management. Clinicians working in all types of settings should have a wide variety of pain management strategies, including physical agents, at their disposal, as well as expertise in their application.

PHYSICAL AGENTS

Physical agents can relieve pain directly by moderating the release of inflammatory mediators, modulating nociception at the spinal cord level, altering nerve conduction, or increasing opiopeptin levels. Physical agents may also indirectly reduce pain by decreasing the sensitivity of the muscle spindle system, thereby reducing muscle spasms, or by modifying vascular tone and the rate of blood flow, thereby reduc-

ing edema or ischemia.[107–109] Physical agents provide patients with an opportunity to stimulate their sensory and motor cortices by interacting with their injured body parts. Stimulating the brain in this way may help prevent the development or progression of chronic pain.[110] Physical agents also give patients an opportunity to practice independent pain management skills and develop self-efficacy, and sometimes provide a therapeutic window in which to perform exercises, including stretching or strengthening, which they would not otherwise be willing or able to tolerate.

Different physical agents control pain in different ways. For example, cryotherapy—the application of cold—controls acute pain in part by reducing the metabolic rate and thus reducing the production and release of inflammatory mediators such as histamine, bradykinin, substance P, and prostaglandins.[111] These inflammatory mediators cause pain directly by stimulating nociceptors and indirectly by altering the local microcirculation; they can damage tissue and impair tissue repair. Reducing the release of inflammatory mediators can thus directly relieve pain caused by acute inflammation and may indirectly limit pain by controlling edema and ischemia. These short-term benefits can optimize the rate of tissue healing and recovery.

Cryotherapy, thermotherapy, electrical stimulation, and traction, which provide thermal, mechanical, or other non-nociceptive sensory stimuli, are thought to alleviate pain in part by inhibiting pain transmission at the spinal cord. Physical agents that act by this mechanism can be used for the treatment of acute and chronic pain because they do not generally produce significant adverse effects or adverse interactions with medications, and they do not produce physical dependence with prolonged use. They are effective and appropriate for pain caused by conditions that cannot be directly modified, such as pain caused by surgery or a recent fracture, and for pain caused by peripheral nervous system pathology, such as peripheral neuropathy, but not necessarily phantom pain.[112,113] Electrical stimulation (ES) is thought to control pain in part by stimulating the release of opiopeptins at the spinal cord and at higher levels.[40] This is supported by studies showing that pain relief attained by certain types of ES is reversed by naloxone.[40]

Physical agents offer many advantages over other pain-modifying interventions. They are generally associated with fewer and less severe side effects than pharmacological agents. Adverse effects associated with physical agents are typically localized to the area of application and usually are avoided with care in applying treatment. When used appropriately, attending to all contraindications and dose recommendations, the risk of further injury from the use of physical agents is minimal. For example, an excessively warm hot pack may cause a burn in the area of application, but this risk can be minimized by carefully monitoring the temperature of the hot pack, by using adequate insulation between the hot pack and the patient, by not applying hot packs to individuals with impaired sensation or an impaired ability to report pain, and by checking with the patient for any sensation of excessive heat. Patients do not develop a dependence on physical agents, although they may wish to continue to use them even after they are no longer effective because they enjoy the sensation or attention associated with their application. For example, patients may wish to continue to be treated with ultrasound even though they have reached a stage of recovery where they would benefit more from active exercise. Physical agents do not generally cause a degree of sedation that would impair an individual's ability to work or drive safely.

Many physical agents can and should be used independently by patients to treat themselves. For example, a patient can learn to apply a pain-controlling agent, such as heat, cold, or TENS, when needed and so can become more independent of the health care practitioner and of pharmacological agents. Application of such physical agents at home can be an effective component of the treatment for acute and chronic pain.[114] This type of self-treatment can also help contain the costs of medical care.

Physical agents, used alone or in conjunction with other interventions, such as pharmacological agents, manual therapy, patient education, and exercise, can help remediate the underlying cause of pain while controlling the pain itself. For example, cryotherapy applied to an acute injury controls pain; however, this treatment also controls inflammation, limiting further tissue damage and pain. In this case, the use of nonsteroidal antiinflammatory drugs (NSAIDs) and rest, elevation, and compression in conjunction with cryotherapy could prove beneficial, although it may make assessment of the benefits of any one of these interventions more difficult. The selection of physical agents and their specific mechanisms of action and modes of application for controlling pain are discussed in the later parts of this book.

PHARMACOLOGICAL APPROACHES

Pharmacological analgesic agents control pain by modifying inflammatory mediators at the periphery, altering pain transmission from the periphery to the cortex, or altering the central perception of pain. The selection of a particular pharmacological analgesic agent depends on the cause of the pain, the length of time the individual is expected to need the agent, and the side effects of the agent. Pharmacological agents may be administered systemically by mouth, by injection, or transdermally or locally by injection into structures surrounding the spinal cord or into painful or inflamed areas. These different routes of administration allow the concentration of the drug at different sites of pain transmission to optimize the control of symptoms with varying distributions.

Systemic Analgesics

Administration of a systemic analgesic is often the primary method to manage pain. This type of treatment is easy to administer and inexpensive, and it can be an effective and appropriate pain-relieving intervention for many patients. A wide range of analgesic medications can be systemically administered orally or by other routes. These medications include NSAIDs (e.g., ibuprofen, naproxen), acetaminophen, opioids, anticonvulsants, and antidepressants.

Nonsteroidal Antiinflammatory Drugs

NSAIDs have both analgesic and antiinflammatory properties and therefore can relieve pain from both inflammatory and noninflammatory sources. They inhibit peripheral pain and inflammation by inhibiting the conversion of arachidonic acid to prostaglandins by cyclooxygenase; however, much lower doses and blood levels are required to reduce pain than to reduce inflammation.[115]

Clinical Pearl

Lower doses of NSAIDs are required to reduce pain than to reduce inflammation.

NSAIDs have been shown to reduce spontaneous and mechanically evoked activity in C and A-delta fibers in acute and chronic models of joint inflammation. Evidence suggests that NSAIDs exert central analgesic effects at the spinal cord and at the thalamus.[116-120]

Although NSAIDs have excellent short-term to medium-term applications in controlling moderately severe pain caused by musculoskeletal disorders, particularly when pain is associated with inflammation, side effects can limit their long-term use. The primary long-term complication of most NSAIDs is gastrointestinal irritation and bleeding.[121,122] NSAIDs decrease platelet aggregation and thus prolong bleeding time. They can cause kidney damage, edema, bone marrow suppression, rashes, and anorexia.[123,124] Combining multiple NSAIDs increases the risk of adverse effects.

Clinical Pearl

Gastrointestinal irritation and bleeding are the main long-term complications of NSAID use.

The first NSAID was aspirin. Many other NSAIDs, such as ibuprofen (Motrin, Advil), naproxen sodium (Naprosyn, Aleve), and piroxicam (Feldene), are now available both over the counter (OTC) and by prescription. The principal advantages of these newer NSAIDs over aspirin are that some have a longer duration of action, allowing less frequent dosing and better compliance, and some cause fewer gastrointestinal side effects. However, for most patients, aspirin effectively relieves pain at considerably less expense, although with a slightly greater risk of gastrointestinal bleeding, than the newer NSAIDs.

In the late 1990s, selective cyclooxygenase type 2 (COX-2) inhibitor NSAIDs, such as celecoxib (Celebrex, Celebra), rofecoxib (Vioxx), and valdecoxib (Bextra), were developed with the goal of producing fewer gastrointestinal side effects than older NSAIDs that inhibit both COX-1 and COX-2. However, because of an increased risk of heart attack and stroke associated with rofecoxib and valdecoxib use, both have been withdrawn from the U.S. market.[125–129] Celecoxib is still available but is required to have a black-box warning regarding its risks on the label.

NSAIDs are primarily administered orally, although ketorolac is available for administration by injection (Toradol)[130] and by nasal spray (Sprix). The mode of systemic administration does not alter the analgesic or adverse effects of these drugs. Diclofenac, another NSAID, is available topically as Flector patches or Voltaren gel. Topical administration is associated with less systemic absorption and therefore is expected to cause fewer systemic side effects, although the potential for skin reactions is associated with topical administration. Unfortunately, NSAIDs are largely ineffective in nociplastic pain states such as fibromyalgia, irritable bowel syndrome, and temporomandibular joint pain.[131]

> ### ◎ Clinical Pearl
> Gastrointestinal irritation and bleeding are the main long-term complications of NSAID use.

Acetaminophen

Acetaminophen (Tylenol) is an effective analgesic for mild to moderately severe pain; however, unlike NSAIDs, it has no clinically significant antiinflammatory activity.[132] Taken in the same dosage as aspirin, it provides analgesic and antipyretic effects comparable with those of aspirin.[132] Acetaminophen is administered primarily by the oral route, although administration by suppository or intravenous injection is effective for patients who are unable to take medications by mouth. Acetaminophen is useful for patients who cannot tolerate NSAIDs because of gastric irritation or when the prolonged bleeding time caused by NSAIDs would be a disadvantage. Prolonged use or large doses of acetaminophen can damage the liver; this risk is elevated in patients with chronic alcoholism. Skin rashes are an occasional side effect of this medication. When used in healthy adults for a short period, the suggested maximum daily dose is 4 g.[133]

Opioids

Opioids are drugs that contain opium, derivatives of opium, or any of several semisynthetic or synthetic drugs with opium-like activity. Morphine, hydromorphone, fentanyl, oxymorphone, codeine, hydrocodone, oxycodone, and methadone are examples of opioids used clinically. Tramadol is a commonly prescribed opioid-like medication. Although these drugs have slightly different mechanisms of action, all bind to opioid-specific receptors, and their effects are reversed by naloxone.[134] The various opioids differ primarily in their potency, duration of action, and restriction of use as a result of variations in pharmacodynamics and pharmacokinetics.

Opioids provide analgesia by mimicking the effects of endorphins and binding to opioid-specific receptors in the CNS.[135] They relieve pain by inhibiting the release of presynaptic neurotransmitters and inhibiting the activity of interneurons early in the nociceptive pathways to reduce or block C-fiber inputs into the dorsal horn.[136]

When given in sufficient doses, opioids often control severe acute pain with tolerable side effects. They may control pain that cannot be relieved by nonopioid analgesics. Side effects of opioids include nausea, vomiting, and sedation and the suppression of cough, gastrointestinal motility, and respiration. With long-term use, opioids are associated with physical dependence and depression. Respiratory suppression limits the dose that can be used even for short-term administration. People taking opioids can exhibit tolerance, dependence, or addiction. Tolerance may manifest as a need for increasing drug doses to maintain the same level of pain control or decreased pain control with the same dose. Physical dependence is a normal adaptation of the body to opioid use that causes withdrawal symptoms and a consequent rebound increase in pain when long-term use of the drug is decreased or discontinued. Addiction is the compulsive use of a drug despite physical harm; the presence of tolerance or dependence does not predict addiction.

Opioids generally are used to relieve postoperative pain or pain caused by malignancy. In recent years, opioid use has increased greatly, primarily as a result of more aggressive treatment of chronic pain.[137] Approximately 90% of patients with chronic pain receive opioids.[138] Long-term opioid use may result in tolerance, hormonal changes, and immunosuppression.[139]

Opioids can be administered by mouth, nose, or rectum; intravenously; transdermally; subcutaneously; epidurally; intrathecally; or by direct intraarticular injection. A popular and effective means of administration, particularly for hospitalized patients, is patient-controlled analgesia (PCA) (Fig. 4.10). With PCA, patients use a pump to self-administer

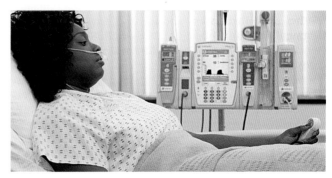

FIGURE 4.10 Patient-controlled analgesia. (Courtesy © Becton, Dickinson and Company.)

small, repeated intravenous opioid doses. The amount of medication delivered is limited by preestablished dosing intervals and maximum doses within a defined period. Pain control is more effective and adverse effects are less common with PCA than with more conventional provider-controlled opioid-administration methods.[140,141]

There is growing evidence that the long-term use of opioids for chronic pain is associated with multiple medical complications, including unintended overdose and death.[142] As a result, scientists from the United States and Canada authored guidelines urging that opioid use in people with chronic non-cancer pain be substantially reduced or discontinued.[143,144] Based on these guidelines, many clinicians have tapered opioid prescriptions in their patients with chronic pain.[145] As a result, physical therapists are providing care to patients who may be increasingly frightened, angry, and in need of better pain control.

Antidepressants

Some antidepressants, including tricyclics such as amitriptyline (Elavil), have been found to be effective adjunctive components of chronic pain treatment, with smaller doses than those typically used to treat depression being effective for this application.[146,147] Serotonin–norepinephrine reuptake inhibitors (SNRIs), including duloxetine (Cymbalta), milnacipran (Savella), and venlafaxine (Effexor), are antidepressants thought to decrease pain by mediating descending inhibitory pathways of the brainstem and spinal cord. Duloxetine and venlafaxine have been shown to reduce the pain associated with diabetic peripheral neuropathy, as well as other types of neuropathic pain.[148,149] Milnacipran and duloxetine are indicated for the treatment of chronic pain associated with fibromyalgia, and duloxetine is indicated for the treatment of chronic musculoskeletal pain. Studies have shown that patients with chronic pain who are depressed report much higher levels of pain and show more pain-related behaviors than patients who are not depressed.[150-152] In addition, antidepressants may exert an antinociceptive effect independent of the presence of depression.[153] It is still uncertain if the higher level of pain in depressed patients is a cause or a product of their depression; the use of antidepressants may prove beneficial in either situation.

Anticonvulsants

Anticonvulsants alter nerve conduction and are used primarily to treat neuropathic pain.[154] Gabapentin (Neurontin) and carbamazepine (Tegretol) are anticonvulsants that reduce chronic neuropathic pain,[155,156] and pregabalin (Lyrica), another anticonvulsant, was specifically developed for the treatment of neuropathic pain and has been shown to relieve pain associated with postherpetic neuralgia.[148,157] Pregabalin is also indicated to treat fibromyalgia.

Spinal Analgesia

Pain relief may be achieved by the administration of drugs such as opioids, local anesthetics, and corticosteroids into the epidural or subarachnoid space of the spinal cord.[158] This route of administration provides analgesia to areas innervated by segments of the cord receiving the drug and therefore is most effective when the pain has a spinal distribution, such as a dermatomal distribution in a single limb. The primary advantages of this route of administration are that the drug bypasses the blood-brain barrier and that high concentrations reach the spinal cord at sites of nociceptive transmission, thus increasing the analgesic effects while reducing adverse side effects.

Opioids administered spinally exert their effects by stimulating opioid receptors in the dorsal horn of the spinal cord.[159] When administered spinally, fat-soluble opioids have a rapid onset and a short duration of action, whereas water-soluble opioids have a slow onset and a more prolonged duration of action.[160] Local anesthetics delivered spinally have the unique ability to completely block nociceptive transmission; however, with increasing concentration, these drugs block sensory and then motor transmission, causing numbness and weakness.[161] High doses of these drugs can also cause hypotension. The side effects of local anesthetics limit their application to the short-term control of pain and to diagnostic testing. Catabolic corticosteroids, such as cortisone and dexamethasone, can be administered into the epidural or subarachnoid space to relieve pain caused by inflammation of spinal nerve roots or surrounding structures, although the safety of administering steroids intrathecally has yet to be determined.[157] These drugs inhibit the inflammatory response to tissue injury; however, because of side effects of repeated or prolonged use, including fat and muscle wasting, osteoporosis, and symptoms of Cushing syndrome, these drugs are not suitable for long-term application.

Local Injection

Local injection of corticosteroid, opioid, or local anesthetic can be particularly effective for relieving the pain associated with local inflammation. Such injections can be administered into joints, bursae, or trigger points or around tendons and can be used for therapeutic purposes, for pain relief, or for diagnostic purposes in identifying the structures causing pain.[162] Although this type of treatment can be very effective, repeated local injections of corticosteroids are not recommended because they can cause tissue breakdown and deterioration. Direct local injections of corticosteroids after acute trauma are not recommended because these drugs reduce the inflammatory response and thus may impair healing. Local injections of anesthetics generally provide only short-term pain relief and are used primarily during painful procedures or diagnostically.

Topical Analgesics

Capsaicin, a botanical compound found in chili peppers, can be applied topically to reduce pain by depleting substance P; it has been shown to be effective for diabetic neuropathy, osteoarthritis, and psoriasis.[163] Topical lidocaine has been used successfully in the treatment of postherpetic neuralgia.[157]

Multiple-Drug Therapies

Not surprisingly, no single drug class exerts adequate pain control for most patients with chronic pain. The overarching principle of medication use for chronic pain is to combine drugs from different classes to act on different mechanisms while producing minimal side effects. The average patient with chronic pain is taking four medications for pain.[164] Physical therapists may provide strategies for managing pain and promoting independence through exercise and physical agents rather than relying exclusively on medications.

COGNITIVE-BEHAVIORAL THERAPY

With the acceptance of the biopsychosocial model of pain, the practice of rehabilitation and pain management has come to include cognitive-behavioral interventions such as pacing, cognitive restructuring (including patient education), and graded exposure.[48,165,166] These treatments may alter pain directly by changing how pain is interpreted in the brain or indirectly by redirecting problematic behaviors that perpetuate painful conditions.[167,168] Most rehabilitation professionals are not trained to provide cognitive-behavioral therapy. However, they can use cognitive-behavioral principles to guide their treatments.

The primary objectives of applying a cognitive-behavioral approach to pain management are to help patients perceive their pain as manageable and to provide them with strategies and techniques for coping with pain and its consequent problems. Patients should learn to identify their dysfunctional automatic reactions to thoughts and to redirect their behavior. This increases patients' confidence as they see that they can successfully solve problems and maintain an active lifestyle. Some of the techniques used in the cognitive-behavioral approach to pain management are described in the following paragraphs.

Pacing

Poor pacing is a common problem. Patients do too much. Eventually they have a pain flare-up and react by becoming sedentary and remorseful. Then, when the pain begins to subside, they again engage in too much or too-vigorous physical activity. This leads them directly into another episode of pain and remorse, and the cycle continues. Good pacing skills include scheduling activities, consciously performing activities more slowly, taking breaks, and breaking tasks down into manageable parts.[73,169]

Cognitive Restructuring

Cognitive restructuring includes patient education and any other information that can alter maladaptive thoughts and emotions related to an individual's pain.[170] The most commonly heard phrase used in this regard is "hurt does not necessarily equal harm." The kind of education provided to patients may be important. Two studies have found that education about the physiology of pain and nociception (such as that provided in this chapter) was more effective at improving physical performance and decreasing pain catastrophizing compared with education about spinal anatomy and physiology.[166,171,172] Another randomized controlled trial found that pain neuroscience education combined with cognition-targeted exercise training was more effective than usual care for reducing pain and improving function and pain cognitions[173] in patients with chronic spinal pain.

Graded Exposure

Graded exposure involves a patient practicing (i.e., exposing themselves to) feared or valued activities that have become limited as a result of pain, fear, or deconditioning. Exposure should begin at a tolerable level called a **baseline** and follow a gradual, self-determined progression toward a predetermined goal.[81] The priorities are safety, non–pain contingency, and self-efficacy.

Returning to the example of the patient with ankle pain, assume that several months have passed. He now reports that he cannot walk for more than 5 minutes because of pain. His goal is to walk for 20 minutes. The referring provider and treating therapist have determined that the tibia and fibula are structurally sound. The pain is severe, but it is not distributed in a neural zone, and there is no reason in the patient's history to suspect neuropathy, so the primary mechanisms are hypothesized to be nociplasticity and psychosocial factors.

In the first step, pain neurophysiology is reviewed. The patient understands that his system is sensitized. Hurt does not equal harm. He and the therapist agree to start graded exposure. Although flare-ups are to be avoided, the plan is non–pain contingent. Some pain is to be expected. The patient's goal is to walk for 20 minutes. The next step is finding a starting point, or baseline. The patient is asked to "see what he *can* do" by taking three walks over the next several days and recording his time in minutes. He can stop whenever he chooses to. If he feels he did too much in one trial, he can do less in the next. If he feels he could have done more in one trial, he can do more in the next. At the next therapy session, the average of three trials is calculated, and that is his baseline.

Once the patient has self-determined a goal and a baseline, he should determine a date for his goal. In this example, his baseline is 5 minutes, and his goal is 20 minutes. How long does he want to spend working up to 20 minutes? Whatever time frame he chooses, the therapist and the patient use this to determine his progression. The patient follows the progression. If he feels better than usual, he should not do more. If he feels worse than usual, he should not do less.

Patients learning graded exposure can benefit from physical agents and other nonpharmacological pain management techniques before, during, or after they perform the activity. A physical agent is not passive if it helps a patient stick to their activity plan, even if they happen to sit or lie down when they apply it. Meanwhile, graded exposure conditions tissues and generates new memories of safety in the pain matrix. Studies of graded exposure programs show that they are associated with reduced pain catastrophizing and perceived harmfulness of activities,[84] decreased fear, improved function,[85] and reduced pain.[173]

CLINICAL CASE STUDIES

The following case studies summarize the concepts of pain discussed in this chapter. Based on the scenario presented, an evaluation of the clinical findings and goals of treatment is proposed. This is followed by a discussion of the factors to be considered in treatment selection.

CASE STUDY 4.1

Severe Acute Central Low Back Pain
Examination
History

MP is a 45-year-old woman who has been referred to physical therapy with a diagnosis of low back pain and a physician's order to evaluate and treat. MP complains of severe central low back pain that is aggravated by any movement, particularly forward bending. Her only current treatment is 600 mg of ibuprofen, which she is taking three times a day. She reports no previous diagnosis of back pain or other musculoskeletal conditions.

Systems Review

MP is accompanied to the clinic today by her husband. She is alert and attentive, and her overall affect is positive. MP reports no radiation of pain or other symptoms into her extremities. Pain disturbs her sleep, and she is unable to work at her usual secretarial job or perform her usual household tasks such as grocery shopping and cleaning. She reports that the pain started about 4 days ago, when she reached to pick up a suitcase, and has gradually decreased since its initial onset from a severity of 8, on a scale of 1 to 10, to a severity of 5 or 6. She complains of no weakness, numbness, or incoordination. Her score on the STarT Back Screening Tool is 2/9, indicating that she is in the low-risk group.

Tests and Measures

The objective examination is significant for restricted lumbar range of motion (ROM) in all planes. Forward bending is restricted to approximately 20% of normal, backward bending is restricted to approximately 50% of normal, and side bending is restricted to approximately 30% of normal in both directions. Palpable muscle guarding and tenderness in the lower lumbar area occur when the patient is standing or prone. All neurological testing, including straight leg raise and lower-extremity sensation, strength, and reflexes, is within normal limits.

Does this patient have acute or chronic pain? Is inflammation contributing to this patient's pain?

Evaluation and Goals

ICF Level	Current Status	Goals
Body structure and function	Low back pain	Decrease pain to zero in next week
	Limited lumbar ROM in all directions	Increase lumbar ROM to 100% of normal
	Muscle guarding and tenderness in lower lumbar area	Prevent recurrence of symptoms
Activity	Cannot sleep	Return to normal sleeping pattern
Participation	Unable to work, clean, or go grocery shopping	Return to secretarial job in 1 week
		Return to 100% of household activities in 2 weeks

ICF, International Classification for Functioning, Disability and Health model; *ROM,* range of motion.

Prognosis

This patient's back pain had an acute onset with a mechanism of injury traceable to her lifting her suitcase 4 days ago. Her pain, although at first severe, gradually improved. These observations indicate a good prognosis, as her pain is expected to continue to improve. Aside from treating her current pain, a successful long-term plan of care includes restoring the patient's previous level of function, improving her sleep, and educating her on good lifting mechanics and preventing future injury through exercises that increase the strength and flexibility of her back.

Intervention

The optimal intervention would address the acute symptom of pain and the underlying inflammation and, if possible, would help to resolve any underlying structural tissue damage or changes. Although a single treatment may not be able to address all these issues, treatments that address as many of these issues as possible and that do not adversely affect the patient's progress are recommended. As is explained in greater detail in Parts III through VI, a number of physical agents, including cryotherapy and ES, may be used to control this patient's pain and reduce the probable acute inflammation of lumbar structures; lumbar traction may also help to relieve her pain while modifying the underlying spinal dysfunction.

Continued

CASE STUDY 4.2

Chronic Low Back Pain

Examination

History

TJ is a 45-year-old woman who has been referred for therapy with a diagnosis of low back pain and an order to evaluate and treat, with a focus on developing a home program. Over the last several years, she has had multiple diagnostic tests that have not revealed any significant anatomical pathology, and she has received multiple treatments, including narcotic analgesics and physical therapy consisting primarily of hot packs, ultrasound, and massage, without significant benefit. Her only current treatment is 600 mg of ibuprofen, which she is taking three times a day.

Systems Review

TJ is unaccompanied in the clinic and seems burdened by her diagnosis. She complains of stiffness and general aching of her lower back that is aggravated by sitting for longer than 30 minutes. She reports occasional radiation of pain into her left lateral leg but no other symptoms in her extremities. The pain occasionally disturbs her sleep, and she is unable to work at her usual office job because of her limited sitting tolerance. She can perform most of her usual household tasks, such as grocery shopping and cleaning, although she frequently receives help from her family. She reports that the pain started about 4 years ago, when she reached to pick up a suitcase. Although the pain was initially severe—a level of 10 on a scale of 1 to 10—and subsided to some degree over the first few weeks, it has not changed significantly in the past 2 to 3 years and is now usually at a level of 9 or greater. Her StarT Back Screening Tool score is 8/9, indicating that she does not believe it is safe for her to be physically active, she worries a lot about her condition, and she feels that her pain is never going to improve and prevents her from enjoying herself. This score confirms that her treatment should include evaluation and treatment of psychosocial factors that probably contribute to her overall condition of chronic pain and disability.

Tests and Measures

The objective examination is significant for restricted lumbar ROM in all planes. Forward bending is restricted to approximately 40% of normal, backward bending is restricted to approximately 50% of normal, and side bending is restricted to approximately 50% of normal in both directions. Palpation reveals stiffness of the lumbar facet joints at L3 through L5 and tenderness in the lower lumbar area. All neurological testing, including lower-extremity sensation, strength, and reflexes, is within normal limits, although straight leg raising is limited to 40 degrees bilaterally by hamstring tightness, and prone knee bending is limited to 100 degrees bilaterally by quadriceps tightness. TJ is 5 feet 3 inches tall and reports her weight to be 180 lb. She reports that she has gained 50 lb since her initial back injury 4 years ago.

Does this patient have acute or chronic pain? What factors are contributing to the patient's pain?

Evaluation and Goals

ICF Level	Current Status	Goals
Body structure and function	Low back pain	Reduce pain to tolerable level
	Restricted lumbar ROM	Increase lumbar ROM
	Hamstring and quadriceps tightness	Normalize hamstring and quadriceps lengths
Activity	Impaired sleep	Improve to normal sleeping patterns in 1 month
	Cannot sit for >30 minutes	Improve sitting tolerance to 1 hour in 2 weeks
Participation	Unable to work	Return to at least 50% of work activities in 1 month
	Impaired ability to do cleaning and shopping	Return to 100% ability to clean and grocery shop
		Reduce dependence on medical personnel and medical treatment

ICF, International Classification for Functioning, Disability and Health model; *ROM,* range of motion.

Prognosis

Although further analysis may help identify the specific structures causing this patient's pain, the long duration of the pain is well beyond the normal time needed for a minor back injury to resolve. Lack of change in her pain over previous years and its lack of response to multiple treatments indicate that her pain may have a variety of contributory factors beyond local tissue damage, including deconditioning, psychological dysfunction, or social problems.

Intervention

The optimal intervention would ideally address the functional limitations caused by this patient's chronic pain and would provide her with independent means to manage her symptoms without adverse consequences. Thus, the focus of care should be on teaching TJ coping skills and improving her physical condition, including strength and flexibility. Physical agents probably would be restricted to independent use for pain management or as an adjunct to promote progression toward functional goals. As is explained in greater detail in Parts III through VI of this book, a number of physical agents, including cryotherapy, thermotherapy, and ES, may be used by patients independently to control pain, whereas thermotherapy may also be used to help increase the extensibility of soft tissues to allow more effective and rapid recovery of flexibility.

Chapter Review

1. Pain is the result of a complex interaction of mechanical and neurological processes, generally experienced when specialized receptors (nociceptors) at the periphery are stimulated by noxious thermal, chemical, or mechanical stimuli.

2. Nociceptive transmission may be modulated at the nerve ending, in the spinal cord, or in the brain. It can be facilitated or inhibited. It is possible for the brain to filter out nociceptive input and have no pain despite tissue damage or to produce a pain experience without any nociceptive input at all.

3. Because nociception is so modifiable at so many sites in the nervous system, and because pain can be experienced without nociception, pain cannot be considered a reliable indicator of the state of the tissues, particularly if it has persisted beyond the subacute phase.

4. Chronic pain is usually perpetuated by one or more of five mechanisms: nociception, peripheral sensitization, central sensitization, movement systems, and psychosocial factors. Each patient with chronic pain should be assessed for which mechanisms are primary or dominant. The treatment plan should then be tailored to those mechanisms.

5. The characteristics of a patient's pain can be assessed using a variety of measures, including visual analog and numerical scales, comparison with a predefined stimulus, or selection of words from a given list. These measures can help to direct care and indicate patient progress, especially early in the pain process.

6. Approaches that relieve or control pain include pharmacological agents, nonpharmacological agents (including physical agents), and patient education. Pharmacological agents may alter inflammation or peripheral nociceptor activation or may act centrally to alter pain transmission. Nonpharmacological agents can also modify nociceptor activation and may alter endogenous opioid levels. Patient education reduces stress and fear-avoidant behavior and helps patients follow through with rehabilitation.

7. A good understanding of the mechanisms underlying pain transmission and control, the tools available for measuring pain, and the various approaches available for treating pain is required to select and direct the use of physical agents appropriately within a comprehensive treatment program for a patient with pain.

8. In many people, pain diagnoses and characteristics evolve over time (e.g., acute pain becomes chronic; chronic pain becomes high-impact chronic pain; nociplastic pain may develop in persons initially diagnosed with neuropathic pain).

Glossary

A-beta fibers: Large, myelinated nerve fibers with receptors located in the skin, bones, and joints that transmit sensation related to vibration, stretching of skin, and mechanoreception. When working abnormally, these fibers can contribute to the sensation of pain.

Acute pain: "An expected physiologic experience to noxious stimuli that can become pathologic, is normally sudden in onset, time limited, and motivates behaviors to avoid actual or potential tissue injuries."[8]

A-delta fibers: Small, myelinated nerve fibers that transmit pain quickly to the central nervous system in response to high-intensity mechanical stimulation, heat, or cold. Pain transmitted by these fibers usually has a sharp quality.

Afferent: Conducting into the central nervous system.

Allodynia: Pain that occurs in response to stimuli that do not usually produce pain.

Analgesia: Reduced sensibility to pain.

Autonomic nervous system: The division of the nervous system that controls involuntary activities of smooth and cardiac muscles and glandular secretion. The autonomic nervous system is composed of the sympathetic and parasympathetic systems.

Baseline: A starting point for graded activity that a patient can perform with confidence without flaring up.

Central sensitization: A process of central nervous system (CNS) adaptation to nociceptive input that changes transmission from peripheral nerves to the CNS, increasing the magnitude and duration of the response to noxious stimuli (causing primary hyperalgesia) or repeated noxious stimuli (causing hyperpathia), enlarging the receptor fields of the nerves (causing secondary hyperalgesia), and reducing the pain threshold so that normally nonnoxious stimuli become painful (causing allodynia).

C fibers: Small, unmyelinated nerve fibers that transmit pain slowly to the central nervous system in response to noxious levels of mechanical, thermal, and chemical stimulation. Pain transmitted by these fibers is usually dull, long lasting, and aching.

Chronic pain: Pain that persists beyond the usual or expected length of time for tissue healing or pain present on at least half the days for longer than 6 months.[8]

Complex regional pain syndrome (CRPS): A chronic disease characterized by severe pain, usually in an arm or leg, associated with dysregulation of the sympathetic nervous system and central sensitization, usually following trauma (previously called *reflex sympathetic dystrophy*).

Efferent: Conducting away from the central nervous system.

Flare-up: Prolonged period of severe symptoms, seemingly out of proportion to the activity that triggered it,[173] that can last for several days.

Gate control theory of pain modulation: The theory that pain is modulated at the spinal cord level by inhibitory effects of innocuous afferent input.

Hyperalgesia: Increased sensitivity to noxious stimuli. Primary hyperalgesia: caused by changes in the tissues in the place where tenderness is perceived; secondary hyperalgesia: increased sensitivity in healthy tissues mediated by changes in the central nervous system.

Interneurons: A neuron that is neither purely sensory nor motor but that connects other neurons.

Mechanosensitivity: Responsiveness to mechanical stimuli.

Neuromatrix theory of pain: The theory that the pain matrix unconsciously integrates nociceptive and nonnociceptive sensory input with biological, psychological, and social factors to determine the presence of threat and need for protection.

Neuropathy: A disturbance of function or pathological change in a nerve.

Neurotransmitters: Substances released by presynaptic neurons that activate postsynaptic neurons.

Nociception: The neural process of encoding noxious stimuli.

Nociceptive system: The parts of the somatosensory nervous system responsible for transmitting and processing nociceptive impulses.

Nociceptors: High-threshold sensory receptors of the peripheral somatosensory nervous system that are capable of transducing and encoding noxious stimuli.

Nociplasticity: The ability of the nervous and immune systems to undergo functional and structural changes that amplify nociceptive processing[18] in the absence of a disease or lesion of the somatosensory system.

Noxious stimulus: A stimulus that is damaging or threatens damage to normal tissues.

Opiopeptins: Endogenous opioid-like peptides that reduce the perception of pain by binding to opioid receptors (previously called *endorphins*).

Pain: An unpleasant sensory and emotional experience associated with actual or potential tissue damage or described in terms of such damage.

Pain matrix: A variable group of cortical and subcortical regions in the brain involved in the processing of nociception and the perception of pain, usually including the anterior cingulate cortex, insular cortex, thalamus, and sensorimotor cortex.

Peripheral neuropathy: Dysfunction of peripheral nerve tissue that may involve irritation of the connective tissue sheaths or compromise of nerve conduction by a disease or lesion of the neurons.

Peripheral sensitization: Lowering of the nociceptor firing threshold in response to the release of various substances, including substance P, neurokinin A, and calcitonin gene–related peptide (CGRP), from nociceptive afferent fibers. Peripheral sensitization causes an increased magnitude of response to stimuli and an increase in the area from which stimuli can evoke action potentials.

Primary afferent neurons: Peripheral nerve cells responsible for transmitting sensory input.

Referred pain: Pain experienced in one area when the actual or threatened tissue damage has occurred in another area.

Sympathetic nervous system: The part of the autonomic nervous system involved in the "fight-or-flight" response of the body, causing increased heart rate, blood pressure, and sweating and dilation of the pupils.

References

1. Tompkins DA, Hobelmanna JG, Compton P: Providing chronic pain management in the "fifth vital sign" era: historical and treatment perspectives on a modern-day medical dilemma. *Drug Alcohol Depend* 173(Suppl 1):S11–S21, 2017. doi:10.1016/j.drugalcdep.2016.12.002.
2. Apfelbaum JL, Chen C, Mehta SS, et al: Postoperative pain experience: results from a national survey suggest postoperative pain continues to be undermanaged. *Anesth Analg* 97:534–540, 2003.
3. George SZ, Greenspan AI: Nonpharmacological management of pain: convergence in priorities fuels the drive for more evidence. *Phys Ther* 98(5):287–289, 2018. https://doi.org/10.1093/ptj/pzy034.
4. U.S. Institute of Medicine Committee on Advancing Pain Research, Care, and Education: *Relieving pain in America: a blueprint for transforming prevention, care, education, and research*, Washington, DC, 2011, National Academies Press.
5. Gaskin DJ, Richard P: The economic costs of pain in the United States. *J Pain* 13:715–724, 2012.
6. Wells N, Pasero C, McCaffery M: Improving the quality of care through pain assessment and management. In Hughes RG, editor: *Patient safety and quality: an evidence-based handbook for nurses*, Rockville, MD, 2004, Agency for Healthcare Research and Quality, 469–486.
7. Interagency Pain Research Coordinating Committee: *National pain strategy: a comprehensive population health-level strategy for pain*. https://iprcc.nih.gov/sites/default/files/HHSNational_Pain_Strategy_508C.pdf.
8. Kerr K, St. Marie B, Gordon DB, et al: An interprofessional consensus of core competencies for prelicensure education in pain management: curriculum application for physical therapy. *Phys Ther* 94(4):452–465, 2015. doi:10.3928/01484834-20150515-02.
9. Apkarian V, Baliki MN, Geha PY: Towards a theory of chronic pain. *Prog Neurobiol* 87:81–97, 2009.
10. American Physical Therapy Association: *Exclusive use or use of multiple biophysical agents HOD P06-18-17-27*. Last updated 30 August 2018. https://www.apta.org/uploadedFiles/APTAorg/About_Us/Policies/Practice/ExclusiveUse.pdf. (Accessed 17 August 2019).
11. Bemis-Dougherty A, Smith MH: "Five Things Physical Therapists and Patients Should Question" update. *Phys Ther* 96(1):121–122, 2016. doi:10.2522/ptj.2015.96.1.121.
12. International Association for the Study of Pain: *Classification of chronic pain, second edition (revised)*. https://www.iasp-pain.org/PublicationsNews/Content.aspx?ItemNumber=1673. (Accessed June 28, 2020).
13. Melzack R: Evolution of the neuromatrix theory of pain. The Prithvi Raj Lecture: presented at the Third World Congress of World Institute of Pain, Barcelona 2004. *Pain Pract* 5:85–94, 2005.
14. Raja SN, Carr DB, Cohen M, et al: The revised International Association for the Study of Pain definition of pain. *Pain* 161:1976–1982, 2020. doi:10.1097/j.pain.0000000000001939.
15. Finnerup NB, Haroutounian S, Kamerman P, et al: Neuropathic pain: an updated grading system for research and clinical practice. *Pain* 157(8):1599–1606, 2016.
16. Lorimer MG, Butler DS: *Explain pain supercharged*, Adelaide City West, 2017, NOI Group Publishers.
17. Woolf CJ: Central sensitization: implications for the diagnosis and treatment of pain. *Pain* 152(3 Suppl):1–31, 2011.
18. Kregel J, Coppieters I, Depauw R, et al: Does conservative treatment change the brain in patients with chronic musculoskeletal pain? A systematic review. *Pain Physician* 20:129–134, 2017. doi:10.36076/ppj.2017.154.
19. Gold MS: Peripheral pain mechanisms and nociceptor sensitization. In Fishman S, Ballantyne JC, editors: *Bonica's pain management*, ed 4, Philadelphia, 2010, Lippincott Williams & Wilkins, 25–34.
20. Nee RJ, Butler D: Management of peripheral neuropathic pain: integrating neurobiology, neurodynamics, and clinical evidence. *Phys Ther Sport* 7:36–49, 2006.
21. Smart KM, Blake C, Staines A, et al: Clinical indicators of "nociceptive," "peripheral neuropathic" and "central" mechanisms of musculoskeletal pain. A Delphi survey of expert clinicians. *Man Ther* 15:80–87, 2010.
22. Sluka KA: Central nociceptive pathways. In Sluka KA, editor: *Mechanisms and management of pain for the physical therapist*, ed 2, St Louis, 2016, Wolters Kluwer.
23. Melzack JD, Wall PD: Pain mechanisms: a new theory. *Science* 150:971–979, 1965.
24. Vance CG, Dailey DL, Rakel BA, et al: Using TENS for pain control: the state of the evidence. *Pain Manag* 4:197–209, 2014.
25. Moseley GL: Reconceptualising pain according to modern pain science. *Phys Ther Rev* 12:169–178, 2007.
26. Apkarian VA, Hashmi JA, Baliki MN: Pain and the brain: specificity and plasticity of the brain in clinical chronic pain. *Pain* 152:S49–S64, 2011.
27. Butler D: *The sensitive nervous system*, Adelaide, 2000, NOIgroup Publications.
28. Schabrun SM, Elgueta-Cancino EL, Hodges PW: Smudging of the motor cortex is related to the severity of low back pain. *Spine* 42(15):1172–1178, 2017. doi:10.1097/BRS.0000000000000938.
29. Gwilym SE, Filippini N, Douaud G, et al: Thalamic atrophy associated with painful osteoarthritis of the hip is reversible after arthroplasty: a longitudinal voxel-based morphometric study. *Arthritis Rheum* 62:2930–2940, 2010.
30. Chapman CR, Tuckett RP, Song CW: Pain and stress in a systems perspective: reciprocal neural, endocrine, and immune interactions. *J Pain* 9:122–145, 2008.

31. Hodges PW, Tucker K: Moving differently in pain: a new theory to explain the adaptation to pain. *Pain* 152(3 Suppl):S90–S98, 2011. doi:10.1016/j.pain.2010.10.020.

32. Janig W, McLachlan EM: The role of modification in noradrenergic peripheral pathways after nerve lesions in the generation of pain. In Fields HL, Liebeskind JC, editors: *Pharmacologic approaches to the treatment of chronic pain: new concepts and critical issues: progress in pain research and management*, 1, Seattle, WA, 1994, IASP Press.

33. Zimmerman M: Basic concepts of pain and pain therapy. *Drug Res* 34:1053–1059, 1984.

34. De Couck M, Nijs J, Gidron Y: You may need a nerve to treat pain the neurobiological rationale for vagal nerve activation in pain management. *Clin J Pain* 30(12):1099–1105, 2014. doi:10.1097/AJP.0000000000000071.

35. Willer JC: Endogenous, opioid, peptide-mediated analgesia. *Int Med* 9:100–111, 1988.

36. Hao JX, Xu XJ, Yu YX, et al: Baclofen reverses the hypersensitivity of dorsal horn wide dynamic range neurons to mechanical stimulation after transient spinal cord ischemia: implications for a tonic GABAergic inhibitory control of myelinated fiber input. *J Neurophysiol* 68:392–396, 1992.

37. Terman GW, Shavit Y, Lewis JW, et al: Intrinsic mechanisms of pain inhibition: activation by stress. *Science* 226:1270–1277, 1984.

38. Willer JC, Dehen H, Cambrier J: Stress-induced analgesia in humans: endogenous opioids and naloxone-reversible depression of pain reflexes. *Science* 212:689–691, 1981.

39. Willer JC, Roby A, Le Bars D: Psychophysical and electrophysiological approaches to the pain-relieving effects of heterotopic nociceptive stimuli. *Brain Res* 107:1095–1112, 1984.

40. Bassbaum AI, Fields HL: Endogenous pain control mechanisms: review and hypothesis. *Ann Neurol* 4:451–462, 1978.

41. Levine JD, Gordon NC, Fields HL: The mechanism of placebo analgesia. *Lancet* 2:654–657, 1978.

42. Bendetti F, Amanzio M, Baldi S, et al: Inducing placebo respiratory depressant responses in humans via opioid receptors. *Eur J Neurosci* 11:625–631, 1999.

43. Hannibal KE, Bishop MD: Chronic stress, cortisol dysfunction, and pain: a psychoneuroendocrine rationale for stress management in pain rehabilitation. *Phys Ther* Dec 94(12):1816–1825, 2014.

44. Totsch SK, Sorge RE: Immune system involvement in specific pain conditions. *Mol Pain*, 2017. doi:10.1177/1744806917724559.

45. Carson JW, Carson KM, Jones KD, et al: A pilot randomized controlled trial of the Yoga of Awareness program in the management of fibromyalgia. *Pain* 151(2):530–539, 2010. doi:10.1016/j.pain.2010.08.020.

46. Barker KL, Reid M, Minns Lowe CJ: Divided by a lack of common language? A qualitative study exploring the use of language by health professionals treating back pain. *BMC Musculoskelet Disord* 10:123, 2009.

47. Dahlhamer J, Lucas J, Zelaya C, et al: Prevalence of chronic pain and high-impact chronic pain among adults—United States, 2016. *MMWR Morb Mortal Wkly Rep* Sep 14 67(36):1001–1006, 2018. doi:10.15585/mmwr.mm6736a2.

48. Chou R, Gordon DB, de Leon-Casasola OA, et al: Management of postoperative pain: a clinical practice guideline from the American Pain Society, the American Society of Regional Anesthesia and Pain Medicine, and the American Society of Anesthesiologists' Committee on Regional Anesthesia, Executive Committee. *J Pain* 17(2):131–157, 2016.

49. Fishman SM, Young HM, Lucas Arwood E, et al: Core competencies for pain management: Results of an interprofessional consensus summit. *Pain Med (United States)* 14(7):971–981, 2013.

50. Fregoso G, Wang A, Tseng K, et al: Transition from acute to chronic pain: evaluating risk for chronic postsurgical pain. *Pain Physician* 22(5):479–488, 2019.

51. Schug SA, Palmer GM, Scott DA, et al: Acute pain management: Scientific evidence, fourth edition, 2015. *Med J Aust* 204(8):315–317, e1, 2016. doi:10.5694/mja16.00133.

52. Louw A, Puentedura E: *Therapeutic neuroscience education: teaching patients about pain, a guide for clinicians*, Minneapolis, MN, 2013, OPTP.

53. Katz J, Weinrib A, Fashler S, et al: The Toronto General Hospital Transitional Pain Service: development and implementation of a multidisciplinary program to prevent chronic postsurgical pain. *J Pain Res* 695, 2015. doi:10.2147/JPR.S91924.

54. Simon LS: Relieving pain in America: a blueprint for transforming prevention, care, education, and research. *J Pain Pall Care Pharmacother* 26(2):197–198, 2012. doi:10.3109/15360288.2012.678473.

55. Von Korf M, Crane P, Lane M, et al: Chronic spinal pain and physical-mental comorbidity in the United States: results from the national comorbidity survey replication. *Pain* 113:331–339, 2005.

56. Gatchel R, Okifuji A: Evidence-based scientific data documenting the treatment and cost-effectiveness of comprehensive pain programs for chronic nonmalignant pain. *J Pain* 7:779–793, 2006.

57. Scascighini L, Toma V, Dober-Spielmann S, et al: Multidisciplinary treatment for chronic pain: a systematic review of interventions and outcomes. *Rheumatol* 47(5):670–678, 2008. doi:10.1093/rheumatology/ken021.

58. Keller A, Hayden J, Bombardier C, et al: Effect sizes of non-surgical treatments of non-specific low-back pain. *Eur Spine J*, 2007. doi:10.1007/s00586-007-0379-x.

59. Latmoliere A, Woolf CJ: Central sensitization: a generator of pain hypersensitivity by central neural plasticity. *J Pain* 10:895–926, 2009.

60. Chimenti RL, Frey-law LA, Sluka KA: A mechanism-based approach to physical therapist management of pain. *Phys Ther* 98(5):302–314, 2018.

61. Nijs J, Apeldoorn A, Hallegraeff H, et al: Low back pain: guidelines for the clinical classification of predominant neuropathic, nociceptive, or central sensitization pain. *Pain Physician* 18(3):333–346, 2015.

62. Vardeh D, Mannion RJ, Woolf CJ: Towards a mechanism-based approach to pain diagnosis. *J Pain* 17(9, Suppl 2):T50–T69, 2016.

63. Comerford MJ, Mottram SL: Functional stability re-training: principles and strategies for managing mechanical dysfunction. *Man Ther* 6:3–14, 2001.

64. Louw A, Diener I, Butler DS, et al: The effect of neuroscience education on pain, disability, anxiety, and stress in chronic musculoskeletal pain. *Arch Phys Med Rehabil* 92:2041–2056, 2011.

65. Treede R-D, Jensen TS, Campbell JN, et al: Neuropathic pain: redefinition and a grading system for clinical and research purposes. *Neurology* 70(18):1630–1635, 2008. doi:10.1212/01.wnl.0000282763.29778.59.

66. Schmid A, Nee R, Coppieters M: Reappraising entrapment neuropathies–mechanisms, diagnosis and management. *Man Ther* 18:449–457, 2013.

67. Williams A, Eccleston C, Morley S: Psychological therapies for the management of chronic pain (excluding headache) in adults. *Cochrane Database Syst Rev* 11:CD007407, 2012.

68. Ohgi KA, Hunter T, Pillus L, et al: Pharmacotherapy for neuropathic pain in adults: systematic review, meta-analysis and updated NeuPSIG recommendations. *Lancet Neurol* 516:267–271, 2015.

69. DeSantana J, Walsh D, Vance C: Effectiveness of transcutaneous electrical nerve stimulation for treatment of hyperalgesia and pain. *Curr Rheumatol* 10(6):492–499, 2008.

70. O'Connor A, Kolski MC: *A world of hurt: a guide to classifying pain*, Webster Groves, MO, 2015, Thomas Land Publishers.

71. Raney NH, Petersen EJ, Smith TA, et al: Development of a clinical prediction rule to identify patients with neck pain likely to benefit from cervical traction and exercise. *Eur Spine J* 18:382–391, 2009.

72. Kindler LL, Bennett RM, Jones KD: Central sensitivity syndromes: mounting pathophysiologic evidence to link fibromyalgia with other common chronic pain disorders. *Pain Manag Nurs* 12(1):15–24, 2011. doi:10.1016/j.pmn.2009.10.003.

73. Nijs J, Torres-Cueco R, van Wilgen CP, et al: Applying modern pain neuroscience in clinical practice: criteria for the classification of central sensitization pain. *Pain Physician* 18:447–457, 2014.

74. Martenson ME, Halawa OI, Tonsfeldt KJ, et al: A possible neural mechanism for photosensitivity in chronic pain. *Pain* 157(4):868–878, 2016. doi:10.1097/j.pain.0000000000000450.

75. Bennett RM, Friend R, Jones KD: The Revised Fibromyalgia Impact Questionnaire (FIQR): validation and psychometric properties. *Arthritis Res Ther* 11:R120, 2009. doi:10.1186/ar2783.

76. Neblett R, Cohen H, Choi Y, et al: The Central Sensitization Inventory (CSI): establishing clinically-significant values for identifying central sensitivity syndromes in an outpatient chronic pain sample. *J Pain* March:1–8, 2013. doi:10.1016/j.jpain.2012.11.012.

77. Wolfe F, Clauw DJ, Fitzcharles M, et al: 2016 Revisions to the 2010/2011 fibromyalgia diagnostic criteria. *Semin Arthritis Rheum* 46(3):319–329, 2016. doi:10.1016/j.semarthrit.2016.08.012.

78. O'Sullivan PB, Caniero JP, O'Keeffe M, et al: Cognitive functional therapy: an integrated behavioral approach for the targeted management of disabling low back pain. *Phys Ther* 985(5):408–423, 2018.

79. Nijs J, Van Houdenhove B: From acute musculoskeletal pain to chronic widespread pain and fibromyalgia: application of pain neurophysiology in manual therapy practice. *Man Ther* 14:3–12, 2009.

80. Wijma AJ, van Wilgen CP, Meeus M, et al: Clinical biopsychosocial physiotherapy assessment of patients with chronic pain: the first step in pain neuroscience education. *Physiother Theory Pract* 32(5):368–384, 2016. doi:10.1080/09593985.2016.1194651.

81. Nijs J, Lluch Girbes E, Lundberg M, et al: Exercise therapy for chronic musculoskeletal pain: Innovation by altering pain memories. *Man Ther* 20(1):216–220, 2015. doi:10.1016/j.math.2014.07.004.

82. Gill JR, Brown CA: A structured review of the evidence for pacing as a chronic pain intervention. *Eur J Pain* 13:214–216, 2009.

83. George SZ, Wittmer VT, Fillingim RB, et al: Comparison of graded exercise and graded exposure clinical outcomes for patients with chronic low back pain. *J Orthop Sports Phys Ther* 40:694–704, 2010.

84. Leeuw M, Goossens ME, Van Breukelen GJ, et al: Exposure in vivo versus operant graded activity in chronic low back patients: results of a randomized controlled trial. *Pain* 138:192–207, 2008.

85. Linton SJ, Boersma K, Janson M, et al: A randomized controlled trial of exposure in vivo for patients with spinal pain reporting fear of work-related activities. *Eur J Pain* 12:722–730, 2008.

86. Kehlet H, Jensen TS, Woolf CJ: Persistent post surgical pain: risk factors and prevention. *Lancet* 367:1618–1625, 2006.

87. Ramond A, Bouton C, Richard I, et al: Psychosocial risk factors for chronic low back pain in primary care—a systematic review. *Fam Pract* 28:12–21, 2011.

88. Traeger AC, Moseley GL, Hübsche M: Pain education to prevent chronic LBP. *BMJ Open* 4:e005505, 2014.

89. Adams JE: Naloxone reversal of analgesia produced by brain stimulation in the human. *Pain* 2:161–166, 1976.

90. Akil H, Mayer DJ, Liebeskind JC: Antagonism of stimulation-produced analgesia by naloxone, a narcotic antagonist. *Science* 191:961–962, 1976.

91. Main CJ: Pain assessment in context: A state of the science review of the McGill pain questionnaire 40 years on. *Pain* 157(7):1387–1399, 2016. doi:10.1097/j.pain.0000000000000457.

92. Downie W, Leatham PA, Rhind VM, et al: Studies with pain rating scales. *Ann Rheum Dis* 37:378–388, 1978.

93. Grossman SA, Shudler VR, McQuire DB, et al: A comparison of the Hopkins Pain Rating Instrument with standard visual analogue and verbal description scales in patients with chronic pain. *J Pain Symptom Manage* 7:196–203, 1992.

94. Shillam CR, Dupree Jones K, Miller L: Fibromyalgia symptoms, physical function, and comorbidity in middle-aged and older adults. *Nurs Res* Sep-Oct; 60(5):309–317, 2011. doi:10.1097/NNR.0b013e31822bbdfa.

95. Melzack R: The McGill Pain Questionnaire: major properties and scoring methods. *Pain* 1:277–299, 1975.

96. Byrne M, Troy A, Bradley LA, et al: Cross-validation of the factor structure of the McGill Pain Questionnaire. *Pain* 13:193–201, 1982.

97. Prieto EJ, Hopson L, Bradley LA, et al: The language of low back pain: factor structure of the McGill Pain Questionnaire. *Pain* 8:11–19, 1980.

98. Roth RS, Lowery JC, Hamill JB: Assessing persistent pain and its relation to affective distress, depressive symptoms, and pain catastrophizing in patients with chronic wounds: a pilot study. *Am J Phys Med Rehabil* 83:827–834, 2004.

99. Cruccu G, Sommer C, Anand P, et al: EFNS guidelines on neuropathic pain assessment: revised 2009. *Eur J Neurol* 17(8):1010–1018, 2010. doi:10.1111/j.1468-1331.2010.02969.x.

100. Morgan KJ, Anghelescu DL: A review of adult and pediatric neuropathic pain assessment tools. *Clin J Pain* 33(9):844–852, 2017. doi:10.1097/AJP.0000000000000476.

101. Bennett MI, Attal N, Backonja MM, et al: Using screening tools to identify neuropathic pain. *Pain*, 2007. doi:10.1016/j.pain.2006.10.034.

102. Hill JC, Whitehurst DGT, Lewis M, et al: Comparison of stratified primary care management for low back pain with current best practice (STarT Back): A randomised controlled trial. *Lancet* 378(9802):1560–1571, 2011. doi:10.1016/S0140-6736(11)60937-9.

103. Ransford AO, Cairns D, Mooney V: The pain drawing as an aid to the psychological evaluation of patients with low-back pain. *Spine* 1:127–134, 1976.

104. Quinn L, Gordon J: *Functional outcomes documentation for rehabilitation*, St Louis, 2003, Saunders.

105. Fillingim RB, Loeser JD, Baron R, et al: Assessment of chronic pain: domains, methods, and mechanisms. *J Pain* 17(9 Suppl):T10–T20, 2016. doi:10.1016/j.jpain.2015.08.010.

106. Mairesse O, Neu D, Cagnie B, et al: Sleep disturbances in chronic pain: neurobiology, assessment, and treatment in physical therapist practice. *Phys Ther* 98(5):325–335, 2018.

107. Ernst E, Fialka V: Ice freezes pain? A review of the clinical effectiveness of analgesic cold therapy. *J Pain Symptom Manage* 9:56–59, 1994.

108. Crockford GW, Hellon RF, Parkhouse J: Thermal vasomotor response in human skin mediated by local mechanisms. *J Physiol* 161:10–15, 1962.

109. McMaster WC, Liddie S: Cryotherapy influence on posttraumatic limb edema. *Clin Orthop Relat Res* 150:283–287, 1980.

110. Allen RJ, Hulten JM: Effects of tactile desensitization on allodynia and somatosensation in a patient with quadrilateral complex regional pain syndrome. *Neurol Rep* 25:132–133, 2001.

111. Hocutt JE, Jaffe R, Rylander CR: Cryotherapy in ankle sprains. *Am J Sports Med* 10:316–319, 1982.

112. Winnem MF, Amundsen T: Treatment of phantom limb pain with transcutaneous electrical nerve stimulation. *Pain* 12:299–300, 1982.

113. Johnson MI, Mulvey MR, Bagnall AM: Transcutaneous electrical nerve stimulation (TENS) for phantom pain and stump pain following amputation in adults. *Cochrane Database Syst Rev* 8(8):CD007264, 2015. doi:10.1002/14651858.CD007264.pub3.

114. Bigos S, Bowyer O, Braen G, et al: *Acute low back problems in adults*, Clinical Practice Guideline No. 14, AHCPR Publication No. 95-0642, Rockville, MD, 1994, Agency for Health Care Policy and Research, Public Health Service, U.S. Department of Health and Human Services.

115. Tuman KJ, McCarthy RJ, March RJ, et al: Effects of epidural anesthesia and analgesia on coagulation and outcome after major vascular surgery. *Anesth Analg* 73:696–704, 1991.

116. Heppleman B, Pfeffer A, Stubble HG, et al: Effects of acetylsalicylic acid and indomethacin on single groups III and IV sensory units from acutely inflamed joints. *Pain* 26:337–351, 1986.

117. Grubb BD, Birrell J, McQueen DS, et al: The role of PGE2 in the sensitization of mechanoreceptors in normal and inflamed ankle joints of the rat. *Exp Brain Res* 84:383–392, 1991.

118. Malmberg AB, Yaksh TL: Hyperalgesia mediated by spinal glutamate or substance P receptor block by cyclo-oxygenase inhibition. *Science* 257:1276–1279, 1992.

119. Carlsson KH, Monzel W, Jurna I: Depression by morphine and the non-opioid analgesic agents, metamizol (dipyrone), lysine acetylsalicylate, and paracetamol, of activity in rat thalamus neurones evoked by electrical stimulation of nociceptive afferents. *Pain* 32:313–326, 1988.

120. Jurna I, Spohrer B, Bock R: Intrathecal injection of acetylsalicylic acid, salicylic acid and indomethacin depresses C-fibre-evoked activity in the rat thalamus and spinal cord. *Pain* 49:249–256, 1992.

121. Semble EL, Wu WC: Anti-inflammatory drugs and gastric mucosal damage. *Semin Arthritis Rheum* 16:271–286, 1987.

122. Griffin MR, Piper JM, Daugherty JR, et al: Nonsteroidal anti-inflammatory drug use and increased risk for peptic ulcer disease in elderly persons. *Ann Intern Med* 114:257–259, 1991.

123. Ali M, McDonald JWD: Reversible and irreversible inhibition of platelet cyclo-oxygenase and serotonin release by nonsteroidal anti-inflammatory drugs. *Thromb Res* 13:1057–1065, 1978.

124. Patronon C, Dunn MJ: The clinical significance of inhibition of renal prostaglandin synthesis. *Kidney Int* 31:1–12, 1987.

125. Juni P, Nartey L, Reichenbach S, et al: Risk of cardiovascular events and rofecoxib: cumulative meta-analysis. *Lancet* 364:2021–2029, 2004.

126. Bombardier C, Laine L, Reicin A, et al: Comparison of upper gastrointestinal toxicity of rofecoxib and naproxen in patients with rheumatoid arthritis. *N Engl J Med* 343:1520–1528, 2000.

127. Solomon SD, McMurray JV, Pfeffer MA, et al: Cardiovascular risk associated with celecoxib in a clinical trial for colorectal adenoma prevention. *N Engl J Med* 352:1071–1080, 2005.

128. Bresalier RS, Sandler RS, Quan H, et al: Cardiovascular events associated with rofecoxib in a colorectal adenoma chemoprevention trial. *N Engl J Med* 352:1092–1102, 2005.

129. Nussmeier NA, Whelton AA, Brown MT, et al: Complications of COX-2 inhibitors parecoxib and valdecoxib after cardiac surgery. *N Engl J Med* 352:1081–1091, 2005.

130. Toradol package insert, Nutley, NJ, 1995, Hoffmann-La Roche.
131. Phillips K, Clauw DJ: Central pain mechanisms in chronic pain states—maybe it is all in their head. *Best Pract Res Clin Rheumatol* 25(2):141–154, 2011.
132. Ameer B, Greenblatt DJ: Acetaminophen. *Ann Intern Med* 87:202–209, 1977.
133. McNeil: Regular Strength Tylenol Acetaminophen Tablets; Extra Strength Tylenol Acetaminophen Gelcaps, Geltabs, Caplets, Tablets; Extra Strength Tylenol Acetaminophen Adult Liquid Pain Reliever; Tylenol Acetaminophen Arthritis Pain Extended-Relief Caplets. In *Physicians' desk reference*, ed 56, Montvale, NJ, 2002, Medical Economics Company.
134. Hyleden JLK, Nahin RL, Traub RJ, et al: Effects of spinal kappa-aged receptor agonists on the responsiveness of nociceptive superficial dorsal horn neurons. *Pain* 44:187–193, 1991.
135. Hudson AH, Thomson IR, Cannon JE, et al: Pharmacokinetics of fentanyl in patients undergoing abdominal aortic surgery. *Anesthesiology* 64:334–338, 1986.
136. Mao J, Price DD, Mayer DJ: Mechanisms of hyperalgesia and morphine tolerance: a current view of their possible interactions: review article. *Pain* 62:259–274, 1995.
137. Trescot AM, Chopra P, Abdi S, et al: Opioid guidelines in the management of chronic non-cancer pain. *Pain Physician* 9:1–439, 2006.
138. Manchikanti L, Damron KS, McManus CD, et al: Patterns of illicit drug use and opioid abuse in patients with chronic pain at initial evaluation: a prospective, observational study. *Pain Physician* 7:431–437, 2004.
139. Anderson G, Sjøgren P, Hansen SH, et al: Pharmacological consequences of long-term morphine treatment in patients with cancer and chronic non-malignant pain. *Eur J Pain* 8:263–271, 2004.
140. Camp JF: Patient-controlled analgesia. *Am Fam Physician* 44:2145–2149, 1991.
141. Egbert AM, Parks LH, Short LM, et al: Randomized trial of postoperative patient-controlled analgesia vs. intramuscular narcotics in frail elderly men. *Arch Intern Med* 150:1897–1903, 1990.
142. Gomes T, Mamdani MM, Dhalla IA, et al: Opioid dose and drug-related mortality in patients with nonmalignant pain. *Arch Intern Med* 171:686–691, 2011.
143. Dowell D, Haegerich TM, Chou R: CDC guideline for prescribing opioids for chronic pain—United States, 2016. *MMWR Recomm Rep* 65(1):1–49, 2016.
144. Busse J, editor: *The 2017 Canadian guideline for opioids for chronic non-cancer pain*. 2010. http://nationalpaincentre.mcmaster.ca/opioid. (Accessed July 15, 2020).
145. Klimas J, Gorfinkel L, Fairbairn N, et al: strategies to identify patient risks of prescription opioid addiction when initiating opioids for pain: a systematic review. *JAMA Network Open* 2(5):e193365, 2019. doi:10.1001/jamanetworkopen.2019.3365.
146. Watson CP, Evans RJ, Rood K, et al: Amitriptyline versus placebo in postherpetic neuralgia. *Neurology* 32:671–673, 1983.
147. Von Korff M, Wagner EH, Dworkin SF, et al: Chronic pain and use of ambulatory health care. *Psychosom Med* 53:61–79, 1991.
148. Attal N, Nurmikko TJ, Johnson RW, et al: EFNS Task Force. EFNS guidelines on pharmacological treatment of neuropathic pain. *Eur J Neurol* 13:1153–1169, 2006.
149. Raskin J, Pritchett YL, Wang F, et al: A double-blind, randomized multicenter trial comparing duloxetine with placebo in the management of diabetic peripheral neuropathic pain. *Pain Med* 6:346–356, 2005.
150. Parmalee PA, Katz IB, Lawton MP: The relation of pain to depression among institutionalized aged. *J Gerontol* 46:15–21, 1991.
151. Keefe FJ, Wilkins RH, Cook WA, et al: Depression, pain, and pain behavior. *J Consult Clin Psychol* 54:665–669, 1986.
152. Kudoh A, Katagai H, Takazawa T: Increased postoperative pain scores in chronic depression patients who take antidepressants. *J Clin Anesth* 14:421–425, 2002.
153. Fishbain D: Evidence-based data on pain relief with antidepressants. *Ann Med* 32:305–316, 2000.
154. Wheeler AH, Stubbart J, Hicks B: *Pathophysiology of chronic back pain*. Last updated 13 April 2006. http://www.emedicine.com/neuro/topic516.htm. (Accessed 23 October 2006).
155. Wiffen PJ, McQuay HJ, Edwards JE, et al: Gabapentin for acute and chronic pain. *Cochrane Database Syst Rev* 2005(3):CD005452, 2005.
156. Wiffen PJ, McQuay HJ, Moore RA: Carbamazepine for acute and chronic pain. *Cochrane Database Syst Rev* 2005(3):CD005451, 2005.
157. Hempenstall K, Nurmikko TJ, Johnson RW, et al: Analgesic therapy in postherpetic neuralgia: a quantitative systematic review. *PLoS Med* 2:e164, 2005.
158. Coombs DW, Danielson DR, Pagneau MG, et al: Epidurally administered morphine for postceasarean analgesia. *Surg Gynecol Obstet* 154:385–388, 1982.
159. Yaksh TL, Noveihed R: The physiology and pharmacology of spinal opiates. *Ann Rev Pharmacol Toxicol* 25:443–462, 1975.
160. Sjostrum S, Hartvig P, Persson MP, et al: The pharmacokinetics of epidural morphine and meperidine in humans. *Anesthesiology* 67:877–888, 1987.
161. Gissen AJ, Covino BG, Gregus J: Differential sensitivity of fast and slow fibers in mammalian nerve. III. Effect of etidocaine and bupivacaine on fast/slow fibres. *Anesth Analg* 61:570–575, 1982.
162. McAfee JH, Smith DL: Olecranon and prepatellar bursitis: diagnosis and treatment. *West J Med* 149:607–612, 1988.
163. Zhang WY, Li Wan Po A: The effectiveness of topically applied capsaicin: a meta-analysis. *Eur J Clin Pharmacol* 46:517–522, 1994.
164. Giummarra MJ, Gibson SJ, Allen AR, et al: Polypharmacy and chronic pain: harm exposure is not all about the opioids. *Pain Med* 16(3):472–479, 2015. doi:10.1111/pme.12586. Epub 2014 Oct 3.
165. Eccleston C, Palermo TM, Williams AC, et al: Psychological therapies for the management of chronic and recurrent pain in children and adolescents. *Cochrane Database Syst Rev* 2009(2):CD003968, 2009.
166. Moseley GL: Evidence for a direct relationship between cognitive and physical change during an education intervention in people with chronic low back pain. *Eur J Pain* 8:39–45, 2004.
167. Moseley GL, Butler DS: Fifteen years of explaining pain: the past, present, and future. *J Pain* 16(9):807–813, 2015.
168. Butler AC, Chapman JE, Forman EM, Beck AT: The empirical status of cognitive-behavioral therapy: a review of meta-analyses. *Clin Psychol Rev* 26:17–31, 2006.
169. Butler DS, Moseley GL: *Explain pain*, Adelaide, 2003, NOIgroup Publications.
170. Turk DC, Gatchel RJ: *Psychological approaches to pain management: a practitioner's handbook*, ed 2, New York, 2003, The Guilford Press.
171. Moseley GL, Nicholas MK, Hodges PW: A randomized controlled trial of intense neurophysiology education in chronic low back pain. *Clin J Pain* 20:324–330, 2004.
172. Van Oosterwijck J, Meeus M, Paul L, et al: Pain physiology education improves health status and endogenous pain inhibition in fibromyalgia: a double-blind randomized controlled trial. *Clin J Pain* 29:873–882, 2013.
173. Malfliet A, Kregel J, Coppieters I, et al: Effect of pain neuroscience education combined with cognition-targeted motor control training on chronic spinal pain a randomized clinical trial. *JAMA Neurol* 75(7):808–817, 2018. doi:10.1001/jamaneurol.2018.0492.

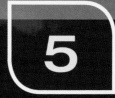

Managing Abnormal Muscle Tone

Diane D. Allen | Gail L. Widener | Dana F. Lindberg

CHAPTER OBJECTIVES

After reading this chapter, the reader will be able to do the following:
- Define *muscle tone* and terms used to differentiate types of abnormal muscle tone: flaccidity, spasticity, rigidity.
- Describe the biomechanical, neural, and pathological influences on muscle tone.
- Identify common impairments and adverse functional effects of abnormal muscle tone.
- Select the appropriate approach for measuring abnormal muscle tone.
- Evaluate and select physical agents that meet patient or caregiver goals when muscle tone is hypotonic, hypertonic, or fluctuating.

Muscle tone reflects the state of stiffness or slackness of a muscle as the muscle rests or prepares to move. Although voluntary muscle contraction is readily observed and measured as force or torque, muscle tone can be difficult to isolate from active contraction, making it less easily observed and measured. In addition, normal muscle tone can vary widely, from very slack to very stiff, as the body rests or prepares to move under various psychological, physical, and environmental conditions. However, pathological factors can make muscle tone less responsive to desired muscle relaxation or contraction, with too much stiffness, slackness, or involuntary fluctuations.

Neuromuscular and musculoskeletal disorders can result in muscle tone abnormalities and associated pain or dysfunction. Therefore, clinicians dealing with these disorders must learn effective ways to observe, assess, and manage abnormal muscle tone. The objective is to work with clients or patients to intervene where needed to improve movement and function. This chapter presents current definitions of *muscle tone* and its related concepts, ways of assessing muscle tone, biomechanical and neural factors that influence muscle tone, and some of the issues that arise when tone is abnormal. The examples, problems, and interventions discussed in this chapter focus on conditions that may be affected by physical agents.

What Is Muscle Tone?

Clinicians and researchers define *muscle tone* in various ways. In general, *tone* is the underlying tension in muscle that enables contraction. Common definitions of *muscle tone* include muscle tension or stiffness at rest,[1] readiness to move or hold a position, priming, tuning of the muscles,[2] or the degree of activation before movement. Muscle tone can also be described as passive or involuntary resistance in response to stretching a muscle. *Passive resistance* means that a person does not actively contract against the applied stretch, so the resistance noted can be attributed to underlying muscle tone rather than to voluntary muscle contraction. Muscle tone results from a combination of (1) involuntary resistance generated by neural input and (2) the length and tension of muscle and connective tissue at the joint position at which the muscle is tested.[3] Physical agents used by rehabilitation professionals may affect the neural or biomechanical components of muscle tone or both.

In thinking about muscle tone, consider the following scenario. A runner's quadriceps muscles have lower tone when the runner is relaxed, reclining with the feet propped up, than when the runner gets ready to meet an imminent challenge, positioned at the starting block of a race (Fig. 5.1). At the starting block, both biomechanical and neural components increase the runner's muscle tone. From the biomechanical standpoint, the muscles are stretched over flexed knees so that any slack is taken up in the muscles and soft tissue, and the contractile elements are positioned for the most efficient muscle shortening when the nerves signal the muscles to contract. From the neural standpoint, when the runner is poised to compete, neural activity increases in anticipation of beginning the race. The neural activation of the quadriceps is greater than when the runner was reclining and relaxed; neural activation presets the muscles for imminent contraction. The difference in muscle tone between the runner's relaxed and ready states can be

High tone in quadriceps muscle

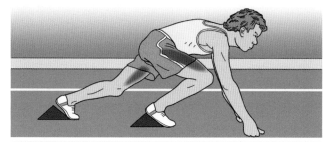

Low tone in quadriceps muscle

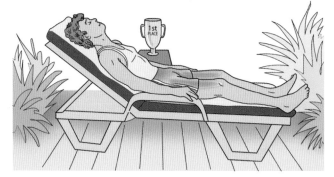

FIGURE 5.1 Normal variations in muscle tone.

palpated as a qualitative difference in resistance to a finger pressed into the quadriceps. In the relaxed state, a palpating finger will sink into the muscle slightly because the muscle provides little resistance to that deforming pressure. The deforming pressure places a small stretch on the muscle fibers. The finger will register relative softness at lower muscle tone compared with the hardness or resistance to stretch that is felt in the runner's ready state or during active contraction of the muscles when the race begins.

CHALLENGES WHEN DISCUSSING MUSCLE TONE

Some of the difficulties with describing and assessing muscle tone include (1) the similarities in a muscle's tone when actively contracting versus unconsciously preparing for activity and (2) the differences in a muscle's tone depending on the individual's situation or environment during observation or assessment. The difficulty separating muscle tone from muscle contraction becomes apparent when considering palpation of muscles in the previously described running scenario: finger pressure on the quadriceps muscles will meet resistance whether a runner contracts the muscles voluntarily or unconsciously prepares to contract them at the start of a race. A key to assessing muscle tone is that the individual must not actively contract the muscle while the muscle is tested. If an individual cannot avoid actively resisting a passive muscle stretch, the tonal quality assessed will be a combination of muscle tone and voluntary contraction.

◎ Clinical Pearl

To isolate muscle tone from voluntary contraction, assess when the muscle is at rest.

In addition, factors associated with the individual's situation or emotional state can affect muscle tone. The neural components of muscle tone can change not only with muscle contraction but also with posture (head and body position in relation to each other or to gravity), psychosocial factors, pain, and environmental conditions such as heat or cold. The biomechanical components can change with the muscle's length relative to its total excursion when tested and with the length of time a body part remains in a specific position. Is the individual under stress generally or maintaining contraction in other muscles to hold a position against gravity? Even people who have normal muscle control may have difficulty relaxing a target muscle in these situations. Has the individual been holding a relatively fixed position for an extended time just before testing? Many body tissues are thixotropic, meaning that substances stiffen in one position and become less stiff with movement.[1] Initial stiffness noted during passive stretching of muscles eases with repeated movements. If the runner in the previous scenario had stayed in the "ready" position—crouched at the starting block—for an extended time, any neural and biomechanical advantages of that position could have diminished. The runner's anticipation of the run may have wavered, and some stiffness in the soft tissues may have inhibited movement. Another key to assessing muscle tone, then, is to standardize the situation and positioning as much as possible, preferably with the individual relaxed and positioned for comfort and with the muscle moved through its full range at least once immediately before testing.

◎ Clinical Pearl

Match testing situations and conditions when repeating or comparing assessments of muscle tone.

Even with standardized testing, observing or scoring muscle tone at a single point in time may not adequately convey whether muscle tone is normal or abnormal. One reason is that normal tone is a spectrum rather than a precise point on a scale (Fig. 5.2). For example, the runner in the previously presented scenario had palpably different muscle tone in the relaxed and ready states (see Fig. 5.1); the difference is appropriate to each situation, and both palpable conditions reflect normal muscle tone. In other words, normal muscle tone includes a range of tension that allows an array

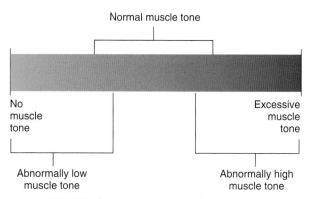

FIGURE 5.2 Normal muscle tone is a spectrum.

of postures, voluntary movement, and rest as the individual desires.

Another reason why single observations of muscle tone cannot be interpreted in isolation is that measures of abnormal muscle tone may overlap with normal muscle tone at either end of the tone spectrum. With abnormal tone, the individual has less ability to change tone as desired. Lower tone is not abnormal unless an individual cannot increase it sufficiently to prepare for movement or holding a position; higher tone is not abnormal unless an individual cannot alter it for function or it produces discomfort, as in muscle spasms or cramps. Thus, a particular amount of resistance to stretch could be normal or abnormal, with "normality" determined by any related impairments or dysfunction the individual encounters. Further, like normal muscle tone, abnormal tone can vary somewhat under normally occurring conditions; any changes to "abnormal" tone seemingly apparent after intervention, then, must be carefully distinguished from variations related to inadvertent differences in conditions during testing. Thus, although standardization of the testing position and environment is essential, understanding the impact of abnormal tone on the individual requires consideration of any functional deficits present, along with observations of tone. Functional deficits associated with abnormal muscle tone can include limitations of active movement during reaching, transfers, or gait; passive movement during handling of limbs or body parts for hygiene, dressing, or positioning; or elements of quality of life.[4]

Categories and Definitions of Abnormal Muscle Tone

HYPOTONICITY

Hypotonicity, or low muscle tone, means that the muscle has less resistance to stretch compared with normal muscles. Down syndrome and poliomyelitis are examples of conditions that can result in hypotonicity. The term **flaccidity** denotes extreme hypotonicity, with a total lack of tone or the absence of resistance to stretch within the middle range of the muscle's length. Flaccidity occurs with total muscle **paralysis,** the complete loss of voluntary muscle contraction. Paralysis is a movement disorder and not a tone disorder, although it will be associated with abnormalities of muscle tone.

HYPERTONICITY

Hypertonicity, or high tone, means that the muscle has more resistance to stretch compared with normal muscles. Rigidity and spasticity are two types of hypertonicity. **Rigidity** is an abnormal, hypertonic state in which involuntary muscle hyperactivity contributes to muscle stiffness, immovability, and resistance to stretch, regardless of the velocity of the stretch.[5] **Akinesia,** or the movement system diagnosis of "hypokinesia,"[6] is a lack, paucity, or arrest of ongoing voluntary movement sometimes coincident with, but distinct from, rigidity. Rigidity and akinesia are most frequently observed in disorders that affect the **basal ganglia,** such as Parkinson disease. **Spasticity** is another type of abnormal hypertonicity. Researchers and clinicians have sometimes used the term *spasticity* loosely to indicate various abnormal hypertonic muscle qualities; most, however, have agreed to

Box 5.1	Differentiating Spasticity From Other Entities
SPASTICITY IS	**SPASTICITY IS NOT**
A type of abnormal muscle tone	Paralysis
One type of hypertonicity	Abnormal posturing
Velocity-dependent resistance to passive muscle stretch	A particular diagnosis or neural pathology
	Hyperactive stretch reflex[a]
	Muscle spasm
	Voluntary movement restricted to movement in flexor or extensor synergy

[a]A component of spasticity but not an equivalent term.

Note: Spasticity, when present, does not always cause motor dysfunction.

define *spasticity* specifically as velocity-dependent involuntary resistance to stretch,[7,8] meaning that resistance is greater when the stretch occurs at higher velocities (Box 5.1). Spasticity may occur in any disorder that affects **upper motor neurons** at the supraspinal or spinal level, such as stroke, spinal cord injury (SCI), or cerebral palsy.[5] Spasticity itself does not necessarily inhibit function, although most people with spasticity also have some paralysis or **paresis** (indicating weakness rather than a complete loss of voluntary muscle contraction), as in *spastic paralysis* or *spastic hemiparesis.*[9,10] Because the specific effect of spasticity on patients' function varies, clinical assessment must include testing of both abnormal tone and the functional tasks that may show limitations.

Additional terms indicate particular muscle conditions that fit the category of hypertonicity. **Clonus** describes multiple rhythmic oscillations or beats of involuntary muscle contraction in response to a quick stretch, observed particularly with quick stretching of the ankle plantar flexors or wrist flexors. The **clasp-knife phenomenon** consists of initial resistance followed by a sudden release of resistance in response to the stretching of a hypertonic muscle, much like the resistance felt when closing a pocketknife.[7] A **muscle spasm** is an involuntary neurogenic shortening or holding of a muscle, typically in response to a noxious stimulus. For example, individuals with low back pain may have muscle spasms in the paraspinal musculature, creating hypertonicity that they cannot relax voluntarily. A **contracture** is a chronic shortening of muscle and other soft tissue resulting in loss of range of motion (ROM) at a particular joint; if the shortened tissue is within the muscle itself, as a result of a reduction in the number of sarcomeres[1] and/or shortening of connective tissue around the muscle, hypertonicity may result. **Dystonia** is involuntary sustained muscle hyperactivity occurring spontaneously and sometimes simultaneously in antagonistic muscle groups.[5] Dystonia usually results in abnormal postures or repetitive twisting movements.[11] Dystonia is seen in *spasmodic torticollis,* or wry neck, in which the individual's neck musculature is continuously contracted on one side and the individual involuntarily holds the head asymmetrically

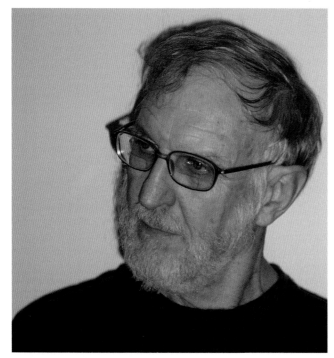

FIGURE 5.3 Spasmodic torticollis, with involuntary posturing of the neck because of dystonia.

(Fig. 5.3).[12] Dystonia can also occur sporadically, as in focal dystonia. For example, an individual has focal dystonia if the fingers cramp into abnormal postures whenever attempting a particular well-practiced task.[13]

Some muscle conditions require further clarification to avoid confusion with hypertonicity or its subcategories. Voluntary muscle contraction also results in resistance to stretch, but hypertonicity is only present if the resistance remains when the individual stops contracting voluntarily. Some movements and postures may suggest that hypertonia is present, but voluntary movement and habitual posture are distinct from muscle tone. The muscles must be tested to confirm the presence of resistance to passive stretch of varying velocities. For example, an individual with hemiparesis after a stroke may have "fractionated movement deficit," lacking isolated control over movement[6] such that raising the paretic arm depends on the use of a flexor **synergy** pattern, or the individual may hold the arm in a flexed posture, with the hand close to the abdomen, an adducted and internally rotated shoulder, a flexed elbow, and a flexed wrist and fingers. However, neither the synergy movement nor the flexed posture necessarily indicates spasticity in the elbow, wrist, and finger flexors. Because spasticity and synergy patterns of movement tend to appear at approximately the same time, clinicians may equate the two, but only testing of the muscle groups can confirm whether spasticity or hypertonicity is present (see Box 5.1). **Muscle stretch reflexes** may be hyperactive in muscles with abnormal tone,[9,14–16] but they do not distinguish spasticity from rigidity unless the muscles' resistance to passive stretch is observed at faster versus slower velocities. To reiterate the use of terms in this chapter, *hypertonicity* reflects abnormally heightened resistance to passive

muscle stretch, distinct from voluntary contraction, voluntary movement, posture, or muscle stretch reflex. The subcategory *spasticity* indicates that the resistance to stretch is greater when the stretch is faster[7]; *rigidity* indicates that the resistance to stretch is not velocity dependent.

FLUCTUATING ABNORMAL TONE

Muscle tone may fluctuate between hypotonic and hypertonic within the same muscles. Abnormally fluctuating muscle tone is most frequently observed in disorders such as Huntington disease that affect cortical areas that influence movement. Muscle tone is especially difficult to assess when it fluctuates widely, with involuntary movements that greatly restrict the individual's ability to relax individual muscles for a passive stretch. Thus, it is common to describe fluctuating tone qualitatively, based on visible involuntary movement rather than clinical tests of muscle tone. The term commonly used to describe any type of abnormal movement that is involuntary and has no purpose is **dyskinesia**. Specific types of dyskinesia include choreiform movement or **chorea** (dance-like, sharp, jerky movements), **ballismus** (ballistic or large throwing-type movements), **tremor** (low-amplitude, high-frequency oscillating movements), and **athetoid movement** (worm-like writhing motions).

Measuring Muscle Tone

Researchers and clinicians have used various quantitative and qualitative methods to assess muscle tone.[17–19] All assessment methods have limitations, so the interpretation of measurement findings requires caution. The methods described in this section for measuring muscle tone should be used with two caveats in mind: (1) the examiner should avoid generalizing the results of a single test, or even multiple tests, to all situations for the target muscle, and (2) the examiner should include measures of movement or function to obtain a more complete picture of the subject's ability to modify muscle tone appropriately to enhance or limit function.[20] For all assessment techniques, examiners must carefully observe and record the specific posture and state of the muscle group in question, whether shortened, elongated, voluntarily contracted, or relaxed. For example, ankle plantar-flexor hypertonicity assessed at rest in the supine position may or may not limit ankle dorsiflexion while walking; one way to improve the assessment would be to complete testing while the client is upright and moving the leg forward during the swing phase of gait.

> ◎ **Clinical Pearl**
>
> Assess movement and function along with muscle tone to get a more complete picture of the patient's ability to modify muscle tone appropriately.

QUANTITATIVE MEASURES

Most of the quantitative measures described for assessing muscle tone have been used in research rather than clinically. They are included here to provide options for clinicians wanting a more objective assessment of muscle tone.

The resistance to stretch provided by muscle tone can be quantified by tools similar to those used to quantify the force generated by a voluntarily contracting muscle. When measuring a voluntary contraction, the individual is asked to "push against the device with all your strength." When measuring muscle tone, the individual is asked to "relax and let me move you with this device." Most measures assess muscles that are reasonably accessible to the examiner and easy to isolate by the patient to contract or relax on command. Muscles at the knee, elbow, wrist, and ankle, for example, are easier to position and isolate than trunk muscles.

Dynamometer or Myometer

A handheld dynamometer or myometer may be used to assess muscle tone.[17] One example comes from a protocol for assessing tone in the plantar flexors: the patient is seated and positioned with the feet dangling and unsupported. The head of the dynamometer or myometer is placed at the metatarsal heads on the sole of the foot (Fig. 5.4). After determining that the ROM is relatively normal, the examiner passively dorsiflexes the ankle to a neutral position with pressure through the device several times at different velocities. The examiner controls the velocity by counting seconds, completing the movement in 3 seconds for a slow velocity and in less than half a second for a fast velocity. One study using this protocol reports high reproducibility for both the high-velocity and the low-velocity conditions (intraclass correlation coefficients, $r = 0.79$ and 0.90).[21] When testing tone, comparing high-velocity and low-velocity conditions enables the examiner to distinguish between spasticity and other forms of hypertonicity.

Myotonometer

An alternative handheld device for measuring muscle tone is the myotonometer. When held against the skin and perpendicular to a muscle, the myotonometer can apply a force of 0.25 to 2.0 kg and electronically record tissue displacement per unit force, as well as the amount of tissue resistance. A

study that quantified muscle tone in children with cerebral palsy and in a control group of healthy children showed the myotonometer to have good to excellent intrarater and interrater reliability when assessing tone of the rectus femoris muscle in relaxed and contracted states.[22] The study's authors recommended force levels between 0.75 and 1.50 kg as most reliable. Other force/torque measuring devices have also been used, including computer-controlled step motors and combinations of force transducers and electrogoniometers to record the resistance and joint angles when muscles are stretched.[17]

Isokinetic Testing Systems

Resistive torque can be measured by an isokinetic machine moving a body part at various speeds. The control of speed can be used to account for the biomechanical components of muscle tone and to determine the overall spasticity of muscles crossing the joint being moved. Quantitative tone in elbow flexors and extensors has been recorded for patients after stroke. The isokinetic machine was adapted to allow the forearm to move parallel to the ground (so that the effect of gravity was constant throughout the movement).[23] The reliability of this quantitative measure of biceps and triceps spasticity was 0.90 in six tests performed over 2 days.[19] Isokinetic testing has also been reported at the knee[24] and the ankle. In addition, this approach has been used to assess trunk rigidity in patients with Parkinson disease.[25]

Electromyography

Electromyography (EMG) is a diagnostic tool sometimes used to quantify muscle tone in research studies (Fig. 5.5). EMG can reflect and record the electrical activity of muscles using surface or fine wire/needle electrodes. During neurogenic muscle activation, the record will show deviations away from a straight isoelectric line (Fig. 5.6). The number and size of the deviations (peaks and valleys) represent the amount of muscle tissue electrically active during the voluntary contraction. When a relaxed muscle demonstrates

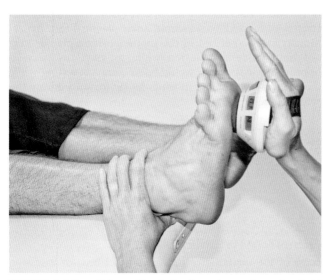

FIGURE 5.4 Quantifying ankle plantar flexor tone using a handheld dynamometer. (Image courtesy Hoggan Scientific, LLC, Salt Lake City, UT.)

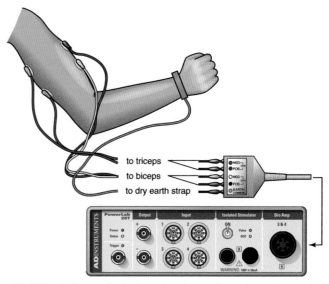

FIGURE 5.5 Components in performing surface electromyography (EMG). (Image courtesy AD Instruments, Sydney, Australia.)

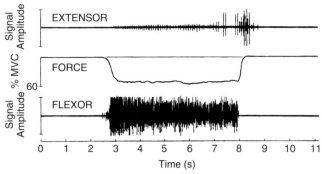

FIGURE 5.6 Example of an electromyographic (EMG) tracing from the extensor pollicis longus (upper tracing) and flexor pollicis (lower tracing) muscles during an isometric contraction of the flexor pollicis longus muscle. The middle tracing is the force output produced with a 60% maximum voluntary contraction (MVC). (From Basmajian JV, De Luca CJ: *Muscles alive: their functions revealed by electromyography,* ed 5, Baltimore, 1985, Williams & Wilkins.)

electrical activity when stretched, that activity is a measure of neurally derived muscle tone at that moment. Various protocols for assessing muscle tone using EMG have been suggested, including combinations of electrogoniometry to record the joint angle along with the EMG response to manual stretch at various fast speeds, providing sinusoidal muscle stretches at various speeds, and comparing the EMG amplitude with that obtained with a maximal voluntary contraction.[17]

Using EMG to evaluate muscle tone has several advantages. EMG is sensitive to low levels of muscle activity that may not be readily palpable by an examiner. In addition, the timing of muscle activation or relaxation can be detected by EMG and precisely matched to a command to contract or relax. Because of these features, EMG can also be used to provide **biofeedback** to a patient who is trying to learn how to initiate contraction or relaxation in a particular muscle group.[26] Further detailed information on surface EMG and EMG biofeedback is provided in Chapter 15. An additional advantage of EMG is that it can differentiate in some cases between neural and biomechanical components of muscle tone, which palpation alone cannot do. If a relaxed muscle shows no electrical activity via EMG when stretched but still provides resistance to passive stretch, its tone may be attributed to biomechanical rather than neural components of the muscle involved.

Disadvantages of EMG include its ability to monitor only a local area of muscle tissue directly adjacent to (within about 1 cm of) the electrode.[1] EMG requires specialized equipment and training beyond the resources of many clinical facilities. In addition, muscle tone and active muscle contraction cannot be distinguished from each other by looking at an EMG record. A label must indicate when the subject was told to contract and relax and when the muscle was stretched. Although EMG can record the amount of muscle activation, it measures force only indirectly via a complex relationship between activity and force output.[27] To compensate for some of the drawbacks of EMG testing, some authors recommend using both isokinetic and EMG testing to measure the effectiveness of therapeutic interventions addressing muscle tone.[24]

Pendulum Test

Some measures of muscle tone have been developed to test particular types of abnormalities, not merely muscle tone in general. The **pendulum test,** for example, is intended to test spasticity. This test consists of holding an individual's limb so that when it is dropped, gravity provides a quick stretch to the muscle in question.[1] Resistance to the quick stretch from spasticity will stop the limb from falling before it reaches the end of its range. The amount of spasticity, sometimes quantified via an electrogoniometer,[28] isokinetic dynamometer,[29] or magnetic sensing device,[30] is the difference between the angle at which the spastic muscle "catches" the movement and the angle that the limb would reach at the end of its normal range. Bohannon[29] reported high test–retest reliability of the pendulum test when the quadriceps muscle was tested in 30 consecutive participants with spasticity from a stroke or head injury. A limitation of the pendulum test is that some muscle groups cannot be tested by dropping a limb and watching it swing (e.g., the muscles of the trunk and neck).[6] A modification of the pendulum test is to have a limb drop into the clinician's hand after passively or actively lifting the limb against gravity. For example, with the individual in a supine position, the examiner or the individual could passively or actively flex the elbow to 90 degrees, then "drop" the forearm back to the starting position, comparing the speed of the drop with that of the opposite arm.

Near-Infrared Spectroscopy

Near-infrared spectroscopy (NIRS) uses optical sensors, muscle hemodynamics, and metabolism to examine muscle activity noninvasively. NIRS can measure tissue perfusion and oxygen consumption, which are related to muscle activation, for a given muscle by evaluating the ratio of oxygenated to deoxygenated hemoglobin in the blood.[31] Because muscle tone normally fluctuates depending on a range of biopsychosocial contextual factors, to determine if muscle tone is abnormal with NIRS, if there is concern for tone abnormalities, the affected limb should be compared with the contralateral normally functioning paretic limb. In a 2020 systematic review, McDougall and colleagues reported that NIRS can differentiate between spastic and nonspastic muscles and track changes in physiological function in response to interventions. The authors also concluded that NIRS may correlate with other established tone measures, including the Modified Ashworth Scale (see description in Qualitative Measures). Although promising, NIRS is a relatively novel approach to measuring muscle tone, and more high-quality research is needed to develop a valid, standardized approach to interpreting the data.[31]

Shear Wave Ultrasound Elastography

Shear wave ultrasound elastography (SWE) has been applied to measure muscle tone based on the theory that a muscle with abnormal tone responds differently to applied stress than a normally functioning muscle. For SWE, ultrasound is used to deliver a dynamic stress to the tissue. This stress deforms the tissue and produces shear waves perpendicular to the applied force. The device then quantifies tissue deformation to measure the viscoelastic properties of the muscle.[32] A 2020 literature review concluded that SWE results correlated with commonly used clinical measures of muscle tone;

however, the clinical utility of SWE is limited by high variability in its application and its inability to differentiate between biomechanical sources of resistance to stretch and neurological inputs that influence muscle viscoelasticity.[33]

QUALITATIVE MEASURES
Clinical Tone Scale

In the clinical setting, muscle tone is assessed qualitatively more often than quantitatively. The *clinical tone scale* is a common qualitative method for describing overall muscle tone. It is a 5-point ordinal scale, scored 0 to 4, that rates normal tone as 2 (Table 5.1). Absence of tone and hypotonicity are given scores of 0 and 1, respectively, and moderate hypertonicity and severe hypertonicity are given scores of 3 and 4, respectively.[34] The scores are given based on manual testing of muscles, with the individual positioned at rest and asked to relax. The clinician passively moves the body part smoothly throughout the muscle's available range before scoring to get a sense of the ROM. The clinician then moves the body part again to feel for resistance. The ratings on the clinical tone scale do not distinguish among types of hypertonicity; qualitative descriptors must be added to identify hypertonicity as spasticity or rigidity, for example. To differentiate among types of hypertonicity, the clinician may then position the target muscle in its midrange and move it at a faster and slower velocity to feel any difference in resistance to stretch. When muscle tone is normal, movement through the ROM feels light and easy. When muscle tone is hypotonic, passively moving through the muscle's range will still feel easy and unrestricted, but the body part typically feels heavy, as if it is dead weight, and the joint may be hypermobile. When tone is hypertonic for a particular muscle, the passive movement that stretches that muscle feels stiff or unyielding, or the muscle may catch, resisting the passive movement. When spasticity is identified, clinicians typically rate the muscle tone using a spasticity-specific scale like the Modified Ashworth Scale described later in the chapter. No specific scale has been rigorously tested for quantifying or describing other types of hyper- or hypotonicity[19]; clinicians commonly report findings with the clinical tone scale, adding qualitative descriptors as needed.

Muscle Stretch Reflex Test

Another commonly used qualitative method for assessing muscle response to stretch is to observe the response elicited by tapping on the muscle's tendon, activating the muscle stretch reflex. Sometimes confused with the clinical tone scale, in this 5-point scale, 2 (sometimes indicated in a chart as two plus signs, or ++) is also considered normal. Zero means no reflex activity is observed, 1+ means the reflex is diminished,

3+ means the reflex is brisker than average, and 4+ means very brisk or hyperactive reflex.[34] The muscle stretch reflex is not the same as muscle tone, although they are typically related.

Ashworth and Modified Ashworth Scales

The Ashworth Scale[35] and the Modified Ashworth Scale[36] are ordinal scales of *spasticity;* they are useful if the type of resistance to stretch is already known to be velocity dependent. The patient is usually positioned supine. For any specific muscle group to be tested, the clinician starts with the limb joint in a position to minimize the length of the target muscle group, then applies a stretch by moving the limb through the whole excursion of the muscle in 1 second (approximated by counting "one thousand one").[36] For example, to test the elbow flexors, the starting position would be maximal elbow flexion, and the stretch would move the joint into maximal elbow extension in 1 second. The starting position for the elbow extensors would be maximal elbow extension, and the stretch would move the joint into maximal elbow flexion. The resistance to stretch for any one muscle group is then qualitatively graded by assigning the appropriate number on the scale.

> ◎ **Clinical Pearl**
>
> The Modified Ashworth Scale is used to describe the level of spasticity, whereas the commonly used 5-point clinical tone scale describes low, normal, and high muscle tone.

The Ashworth Scale includes five grades from 0 (no increase in muscle tone) to 4 (rigidly held in flexion or extension). The intermediate grade of 1+ was added to the original Ashworth Scale to produce the Modified Ashworth Scale (Table 5.2), which is now used almost exclusively. The grade

TABLE 5.1	Commonly Used Clinical Tone Scale
Grade	**Description**
0	No tone
1	Hypotonicity
2	Normal tone
3	Moderate hypertonicity
4	Severe hypertonicity

TABLE 5.2	Modified Ashworth Scale[a] for Grading Spasticity
Grade	**Description**
0	No increase in muscle tone
1	Slight increase in muscle tone manifested by a catch and release or by minimal resistance at the end of the ROM when the affected part(s) is moved in flexion or extension
1+	Slight increase in muscle tone manifested by a catch, followed by minimal resistance throughout the remainder (less than half) of the ROM
2	More marked increase in muscle tone through most of the ROM, but affected part(s) easily moved
3	Considerable increase in muscle tone, passive movement difficult
4	Affected part(s) rigid in flexion or extension

ROM, Range of motion.

[a]Instructions: with the muscle at rest, move the joint so that the muscle is at its shortest length. Then, apply a stretch by moving the limb through the whole excursion of the muscle in 1 second (approximated by repeating "one thousand one") to the muscle's longest length. Grade the muscle's resistance to stretch using the numbers on the scale.

From Bohannon RW, Smith MB: Interrater reliability of a Modified Ashworth Scale of Muscle Spasticity. *Phys Ther* 67:207, 1987.

of 1+ is defined by a slight catch and continued minimal resistance through the range. Bohannon and Smith[36] reported 86.7% interrater agreement for the Modified Ashworth Scale when used to test 30 patients with spasticity of the elbow flexor muscles. Based on a systematic review and meta-analysis, Meseguer-Henarejos and colleagues determined the interrater reliability for the Modified Ashworth Scale to be between 56% and 78%, with an intraclass correlation coefficient (ICC) of 0.69, for the lower extremities and between 68% and 85%, with an ICC of 0.78, for the upper extremities.[37] The Modified Ashworth Scale had 0.50 sensitivity and 0.92 specificity for detecting muscle activity at the wrist as recorded by EMG in patients following stroke.[38] Recent literature supports that key variables, such as the speed of the applied resistance, should be standardized to optimize interrater reliability and the interpretation of test results for the Modified Ashworth Scale.[39]

Other Scales Used to Measure Tone

The Tardieu Scale[40] and multiple versions of a Modified Tardieu Scale[41,42] rate spasticity by having an examiner move the patient's body part at slow, moderate, and fast velocities, or sometimes using the slow and one of the faster velocities. A common scoring method in modified versions of the scale records the joint angle where there is any "catch" in resistance to movement before the muscle releases, designated R1, and then compares that angle with the angle where movement stops and the resistance does not release, designated R2. Calculating R2 – R1 is then defined as the dynamic component of spasticity. The original Tardieu Scale also grades the muscle's resistance to movement on a 0- to 5-point scale, noting, for instance, any clonus at the joint and whether clonus continues for more or less than 10 seconds. Some authors investigating hypertonicity after traumatic brain injury prefer a Modified Tardieu Scale over the Modified Ashworth Scale because it incorporates testing at different speeds rather than assuming that muscles' resistance to stretch will be velocity dependent.[43] A systematic review of the Tardieu Scale/Modified Tardieu Scale for the measurement of spasticity noted that evidence of reliability or validity for this scale is lacking and that the reliability for determining the angle of "catch" during passive movement,[42] R1, is particularly low.

The Ankle Plantar Flexors Tone Scale rates spasticity by the examiner moving the patient's ankle at fast velocities to determine midrange resistance and at slow velocities to determine end-range resistance through joint ROM.[44] The Tone Assessment Scale is a 12-item scale grouped into three sections recording resting posture, response to passive movement, and associated reactions.[17]

In both adults and children, the original or Modified Ashworth and Tardieu Scales are the most commonly used qualitative measures of spasticity across diagnoses.[17,18] For hypotonia, a systematic review of measures used in children revealed no common standardized instruments, with "clinical observation" as the most common tool among studies.[19]

Self-report questionnaires that ask about the patient's experience of tone, either generically or specific to a particular diagnosis, are also available. For example, the Multiple Sclerosis Spasticity Scale-88[45] (MSSS-88) provides respondents with 88 items spanning eight domains that they might perceive as affected by spasticity: muscle stiffness, pain or discomfort, muscle spasms, activities of daily living, walking, body movements, emotional health, and social functioning. The separate subscales can be used in isolation. The MSSS-88 has been translated into multiple languages and demonstrates good reliability and validity.[46] Some researchers compare self-report scales for usefulness in particular diagnostic groups: a review of self-report spasticity scales in SCI noted positive clinical features of the Patient-Reported Impact of Spasticity Measure (PRISM) and the Spinal Cord Injury-Spasticity Evaluation Tool (SCI-SET).[47] Other researchers focus on spasticity in a particular body region; for example, the self-report Leg Ability measure (LegA) has been shown to have good psychometric properties across its three domains of passive function, active function, and impact on quality of life.[4]

GENERAL CONSIDERATIONS WHEN MEASURING MUSCLE TONE

Choosing which measure, or measures, to use to assess muscle tone can be difficult. One systematic review of measures of spasticity in patients following stroke determined that none of the 15 standardized qualitative, EMG-related, or force-/torque-measuring protocols showed adequate reliability and validity evidence to be a gold standard.[17] Similarly, a systematic review of measures of spasticity in children and adolescents with cerebral palsy determined that none of the 17 standardized tools showed excellent psychometric properties across all factors assessed, with a particular lack in responsiveness (evidence of ability to change with intervention).[18] Thus, when measuring muscle tone, the examiner should consider and standardize the factors most likely to be influential.

The relative positions of the limb, body, neck, and head with respect to one another and to gravity can affect muscle tone. For example, asymmetrical and symmetrical tonic neck reflexes (ATNR and STNR, respectively) are known to influence the tone of flexors and extensors of the arms and legs, depending on the position of the head (Fig. 5.7), both in infants during early development and in patients with **central nervous system (CNS)** disorders.[48] Even in subjects with mature and intact nervous systems, subtle differences in muscle tone can be detected by palpation when the head position changes and initiates one of these reflexes. Likewise, the impact of gravity on a limb to stretch muscles or on the **vestibular system** to trigger responses to keep the head upright will change muscle tone according to the position of the head and the body. Therefore, the testing position must be reported for accurate interpretation and replication of any measurement of muscle tone.

Additional general guidelines for measuring muscle tone include standardization of touch and consideration of the muscle length at which a muscle or group of muscles is tested. The examiner must be aware that touching the patient's skin with a hand or with an instrument can influence muscle tone. For instance, a cold hand or stethoscope can change muscle tone, especially when the touch is unexpected. Temperature and placement of manual contacts and instruments must be consistent for accurate interpretation and replication. The length at which the tone of a specific muscle is tested must also be standardized. Because resistance to stretch differs with passive biomechanical differences at the extremes of range, and because ROM can be altered as a result of long-term

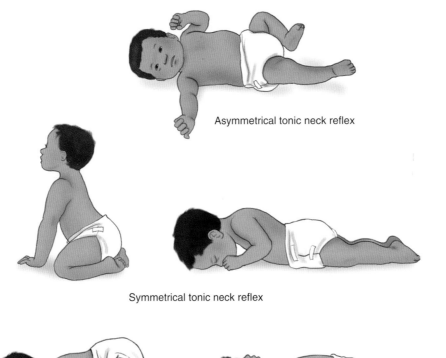

Asymmetrical tonic neck reflex

Symmetrical tonic neck reflex

Tonic labyrinthine reflex

FIGURE 5.7 Reflex responses to head or neck position.

changes in tone, the most consistent length to measure muscle tone is at the midrange of the available length of the muscle tested.

> ⊚ **Clinical Pearl**
>
> Muscle tone is measured most accurately at the midrange of the muscle's length.

Mechanisms Underlying Muscle Tone

Muscle tone originates from interactions between nervous system input and the biomechanical and biochemical properties of the muscle and its surrounding connective tissue. The practitioner must understand the underlying mechanisms that produce muscle tone to determine which physical agents to apply when tone is dysfunctional. The neural and biomechanical contributions to muscle tone are reviewed in this section.

BIOMECHANICAL CONTRIBUTIONS TO MUSCLE TONE

Muscle cells are also called *muscle fibers* or *fibrils*. Muscles have various components, including (1) contractile elements in the muscle fibers, (2) cellular elements providing structure, (3) connective tissue covering the fibers and the entire muscle, and (4) tendons attaching muscle to bone. When the contractile elements are activated, they slide past each other; their attachments to cellular elements shape the muscle as it shortens or lengthens, connective tissue coverings provide support and lubrication while the muscle changes length, and the tendons transfer forces to act on bones. All of these structures can also play a role in influencing muscle tone.

When neural input signals the muscle to contract or relax, the biochemical activity of the contractile elements changes force development in muscle fibers. The contractile elements of muscle fibers are called **myofilaments** and are housed within contractile units called **sarcomeres** (Fig. 5.8). With neural stimulation of the muscle fiber, storage sites in the muscle release calcium ions that allow **actin** and **myosin** protein molecules on different myofilaments to bind together. Binding of these specific protein molecules forms cross-bridges linking the myofilaments in a four-step cross-bridge cycle (Fig. 5.9). Step 1: Adenosine triphosphate (ATP) binds to myosin heads, causing detachment of the actin from the myosin molecules, undoing previous cross-bridges. Step 2: ATP hydrolyzes into adenosine diphosphate (ADP) and inorganic phosphate (Pi). Step 3: Myosin binds to the actin molecule, forming a *weakly bound state*. Step 4: In the presence of calcium ions, Pi is released from the myosin head, causing a *strong bond* between actin and myosin. Simultaneously, the cross-bridge swivels, moving the actin past the myosin mol-

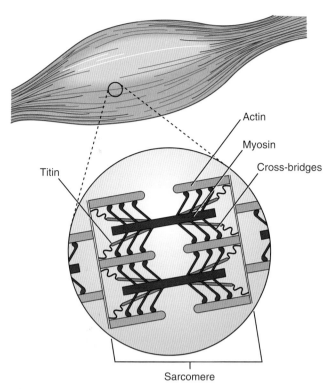

FIGURE 5.8 Sarcomere with contractile proteins (actin and myosin) and the structural protein titin.

ecule; this is the force-generating step. At this point, ADP is released from the myosin head, leaving the actin and myosin bound together. It is only when ATP binds to the myosin head (step 1) that myosin detaches from actin and the cycle starts again. As bonds are formed, broken, and formed again, the length of the sarcomere changes. The cycle of binding and releasing continues as long as calcium ions and ATP are present. Calcium ions are taken back into storage when activation of muscle ceases. Sources within the muscle supply an adequate amount of ATP for short-duration activities, but the muscle must depend on fuel delivered by the circulatory system for long-duration activities.

Actin and myosin myofilaments must overlap for cross-bridges to form (Fig. 5.10). When the muscle is elongated too far, cross-bridges cannot form because there is no overlap. When the muscle is in its most shortened position, actin and myosin run into the structural elements of the sarcomere, and no further cross-bridges can be formed. In the midrange of the muscle, actin and myosin can form the greatest number of cross-bridges. Therefore, muscles can generate the greatest amount of force at the midrange of their length. This length-tension relationship is one of the biomechanical properties of muscles.

Other biomechanical properties of muscles include friction and elasticity. Friction between sliding elements may increase with pressure on the tissues and viscosity of the fluids they contain. Elasticity of tissues may vary with different lengths of the muscle. When tissue becomes taut, as occurs when a muscle is fully lengthened, structural proteins that hold the sarcomeres in alignment contribute more to the overall resistance of the muscle to stretch. One specific structural protein is called **titin**; it has a springy component and

attaches to the center of the myosin molecule and the end of the sarcomere.[49,50] When muscles are elongated, titin is stretched and provides passive tension. In addition, at any given muscle length, titin and actin molecules interact and form weak attachments while the muscle is at rest[51]; the longer the rest, the more bonds are formed. These attachments provide an initial resistance to any movement away from the resting muscle length. This helps explain why leg muscles feel stiff when first standing up after a long car or plane ride. These forces have functional importance in helping maintain normal ankle stability during static standing. Thus, both the presence of weak actin-myosin bonds and titin attachments to actin molecules resist stretch of the muscle away from its resting position.

Both active contractile elements and passive properties of the muscle contribute to muscle tone. However, muscle tone can be generated from passive elements alone, especially near the end range of a muscle's length. High resistance to passive movement that increases near the end of the ROM in the elongated position typically indicates a biomechanical cause for the resistance, such as a shortened muscle or a tight joint capsule. Additional information about the soft tissue and joint contributions to motion restrictions can be found in Chapter 6.

Physical agents can change the muscular contributions to muscle tone. Heat increases the availability of ATP to myofilaments through improved circulation. Heat and cold can change the elasticity or friction of tissues, and physical agents such as electrical stimulation (ES) can activate muscle fibers directly, even without a neural connection to the muscle.

NEURAL CONTRIBUTIONS TO MUSCLE TONE

Neural inputs contributing to muscle tone come from the periphery, the spinal cord, and **supraspinal** brain centers (Fig. 5.11). Although multiple areas of the nervous system may participate, they all must work through **alpha motor neurons** to stimulate muscle fibers to contract (Fig. 5.12). This section provides a brief overview of the neural contributions to muscle tone. For a more complete description of the **peripheral nervous system (PNS)** and CNS and how they influence muscle tone, refer to a neurophysiology textbook.[52]

Alpha Motor Neurons

Muscle tone and activation depend on alpha motor neurons for neural stimulation. An alpha motor neuron, sometimes called a **lower motor neuron,** transmits signals from the CNS to muscles. The lower motor neuron cell body is in the ventral horn of the spinal cord (Fig. 5.13), and its axon exits the spinal cord and thus the CNS through the ventral nerve root. Each axon eventually reaches muscle, where it branches and innervates between 5 (in the eye muscles) and more than 1900 (in the gastrocnemius muscle) muscle fibers at motor end plates.[53] All of the muscle fibers innervated by a single axon with its branches constitute one **motor unit** (Fig. 5.14), which all get activated together whenever an action potential is transmitted down that axon. When sufficient motor units are recruited, the muscle visibly contracts. More forceful contraction of the muscle requires an increased number or rate of action potentials down the same axons or recruitment of additional motor units.

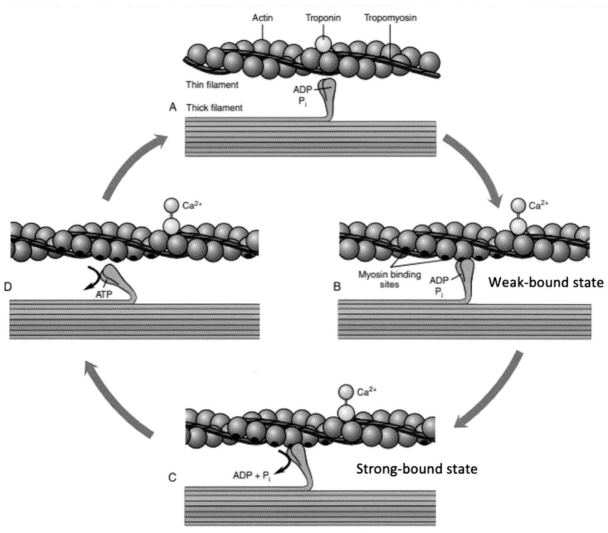

FIGURE 5.9 Steps in the cross-bridge cycle showing weak actin-myosin bonds (step 3) and strong actin-myosin bonds (step 4). (Modified from Banasick JL: Copstead LC: Pathophysiology, ed 6, St. Louis, 2018, Elsevier Inc.) *ADP*, Adenosine diphosphate; *ATP*, adenosine triphosphate; *Pi*, inorganic phosphate.

Activation of a particular motor unit depends on the sum of excitatory and inhibitory input to that alpha motor neuron (Fig. 5.15). Excitation or inhibition depends on sources and amounts of input from the thousands of neurons that synapse on that one particular alpha motor neuron. Understanding the sources of input to alpha motor neurons is essential for understanding the control of motor unit activation and thus alteration of muscle tone by physical agents or other means (Table 5.3).

Peripheral Sources of Input to Alpha Motor Neurons. The PNS includes all of the **neurons,** also called *nerve cells,* that project outside of the CNS, even if the cell bodies are located within the CNS. The PNS is composed of alpha motor neurons, gamma motor neurons, some autonomic nervous system effector neurons that carry information away from the CNS, and all the sensory neurons that carry information from the periphery to the CNS.

Peripheral inputs to motor neurons include signals from muscle, joint, and cutaneous receptors that provide the nervous system with critical information about the external and internal environment and body position. Incoming sensory signals travel in neurons that vary in size. The speed of information carried by neurons depends on both the size and the amount of myelin, a fatty coating on the outside of the axons of neurons. Larger neurons transmit faster than smaller neurons, and myelinated neurons transmit faster than unmyelinated neurons. Nerve conduction velocity is also affected by temperature, increasing with heat and decreasing with cooling.[54] When axons are cooled, as with the application of ice packs, nerve conduction velocity slows by approximately 2 m/second for every 1°C decrease in temperature.[55]

> **◎ Clinical Pearl**
>
> In general, cold slows nerve conduction velocity, and heat accelerates nerve conduction velocity.

Sensory input from peripheral receptors can have direct effects on alpha motor neurons. Direct effects of peripheral input may appear as relatively stereotyped motor responses called *spinal reflexes.* At their simplest, reflexes involve only

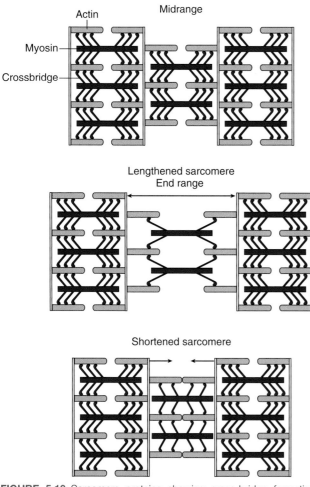

FIGURE 5.10 Sarcomere proteins showing cross-bridge formation between actin and myosin at different lengths.

one synapse between a sensory neuron and a motor neuron, as in the monosynaptic stretch reflex (also called *muscle stretch reflex;* see Fig. 5.13). However, most reflexes involve multiple **interneurons** in the spinal cord between sensory and motor neurons (Fig. 5.16). Because of the volume of input from multiple neurons and sources, the motor response to a specific sensory input can be modulated according to the context of the action.[56]

The normally functioning nervous system has multiple peripheral sources of input in order to protect the body, counter obstacles, or adapt to unexpected occurrences in the environment during volitional movement. Because of its direct connections in the spinal cord, peripheral input can assist function even before the brain has received or processed information about the success or failure of the movement. Peripheral input also influences muscle tone and is frequently the medium through which physical agents effect change.

Muscle Spindles

Inside the muscle, lying parallel to muscle fibers, are sensory organs called **muscle spindles** (Fig. 5.17). When a muscle is stretched, as it is when a tendon is tapped to stimulate a stretch reflex, the muscle spindles are also stretched. Receptors wrapped around the equatorial regions of the spindles

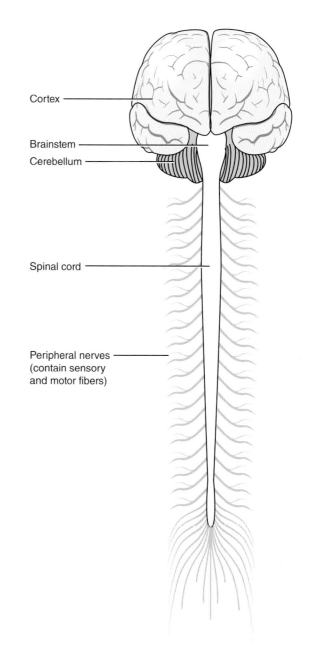

FIGURE 5.11 Schematic drawing of the nervous system, view from the front.

sense this lengthening, stimulating action potentials that carry the signal via **Ia sensory neurons** into the spinal cord. The signal goes both to the pool of alpha motor neurons for the muscle that was stretched (the agonist muscle) and to the cerebral cortex and other locations in the CNS to register the change in muscle length.[57] If excitatory input to the alpha motor neurons is sufficiently greater than inhibitory input from elsewhere, the alpha motor neurons will generate a signal to contract their associated muscle fibers via the muscle stretch reflex. Several traditional facilitation techniques for increasing muscle tone take advantage of the muscle stretch reflex, including quick stretch, tapping, resistance, high-frequency vibration, and positioning a limb so that gravity can provide stretch or resistance.

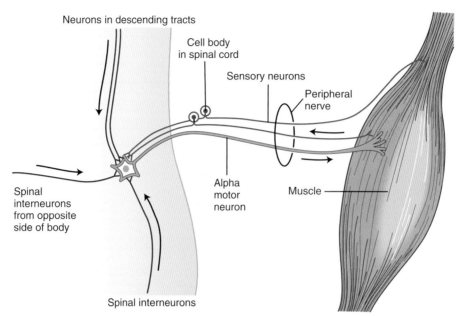

FIGURE 5.12 Alpha motor neuron: the final common pathway of neural signals to muscles.

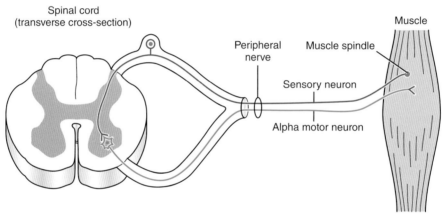

FIGURE 5.13 Monosynaptic muscle stretch reflex.

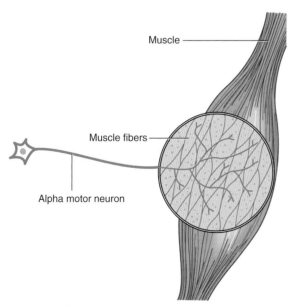

FIGURE 5.14 One motor unit: alpha motor neuron and muscle fibers innervated by it.

Another destination for signals transmitted by type Ia sensory neurons from the muscle spindle is the pool of alpha motor neurons for the antagonist muscle to inhibit activity on the opposite side of the joint. For example, signals from muscle spindles in the biceps *excite* alpha motor neurons of the biceps and *inhibit* those of the triceps (Fig. 5.18). This **reciprocal inhibition** helps prevent a muscle from working against its antagonist when activated.

Because muscles shorten as they contract and because muscle spindles register muscle stretch only if they are taut, spindles must be continually reset to eliminate sagging in the center portion of the spindles. **Gamma motor neurons** innervate muscle spindles at the end contractile regions and, when stimulated, cause the equatorial region of the spindle to tighten (see Fig. 5.17). Thus gamma motor neurons sensitize the spindles to changes in muscle length.[57] Gamma motor neurons are typically activated at the same time as alpha motor neurons during voluntary movement through a process called **alpha-gamma coactivation.**[58] Gamma motor neurons can also be activated independently of alpha motor

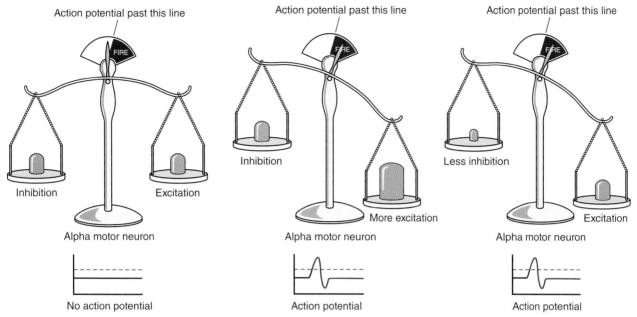

FIGURE 5.15 Balance of excitatory and inhibitory input to the alpha motor neuron at rest and when activated.

TABLE 5.3	Input to Alpha Motor Neurons (Simplified)	
Peripheral Receptors: *Pathways*; Function	Spinal Sources: *Pathways*; Function	Supraspinal Sources: *Descending Motor Tracts*; Function
Muscle spindles: *Ia sensory neurons*; sense change in muscle length and speed of change	Propriospinal interneurons: *tracts within and between spinal levels*; communicate between muscles in an extremity and between extremities	Sensorimotor cortex, cerebellum, basal ganglia: *corticospinal tracts*; volitional movement of trunk and extremities, distal extremities
Golgi tendon organs: *Ib sensory neurons*; sense muscle contraction and tension		Sensorimotor cortex, cerebellum, red nucleus: *rubrospinal tract*; volitional movement, automatic movements of upper extremities
Cutaneous receptors: *smaller sensory neurons*; sense proprioception, vibration, pain and temperature, touch		Vestibular system, cerebellum: *vestibulospinal tracts*; postural tone and alignment, align head and body with respect to gravity
Joint receptors: *smaller sensory neurons*, sense end range of joint position, pressure		Limbic system, autonomic nervous system, reticular formation: *Reticulospinal tracts*; postural and muscle tone, initiate locomotion, send input to trunk, both extremities

neurons via peripheral afferent nerves in the muscle, skin, and joints[59] and via descending tracts from the brainstem.[60] Mechanoreceptors and chemoreceptors in the homonymous muscles send excitatory input to gamma motor neurons during contraction,[59] ensuring that the muscle spindles retain high sensitivity to stretch as the muscle shortens. Functionally, one purpose of gamma motor neuron activation is to respond quickly to perturbations—that is, to prepare the muscle spindle to sense potential changes in length that might occur if perturbations interrupt a voluntary movement. For example, when someone walks across an icy sidewalk, knowing that a slip is probable, gamma motor neurons increase spindle sensitivity so that the spindles will detect the stretch and respond particularly quickly if one foot starts to slip on the ice.

Golgi Tendon Organs

Golgi tendon organs (GTOs) are sensory organs located at the musculotendinous junction (Fig. 5.19). GTOs are arranged in series with muscle fibers, and in contrast to muscle spindles, they detect muscle contraction or tension. Because of this organization, GTOs were thought to protect against muscle damage from overly strong contraction.[61] However, the current understanding is that GTOs respond throughout the total range of muscle contraction and provide continuous information about levels of muscle force to help maintain a steady level of muscle activation.[62]

GTOs transmit signals to the spinal cord via Ib sensory neurons. The signals reach both excitatory and inhibitory Ib spinal interneurons that relay signals to agonist and antagonist motor neuron pools. When the muscle contracts, GTO

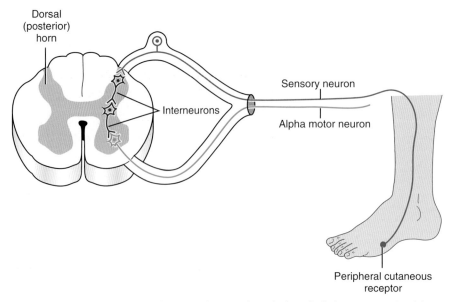

FIGURE 5.16 Sensorimotor reflex pathway, with sensory input to the spinal cord, via interneurons, to alpha motor neurons.

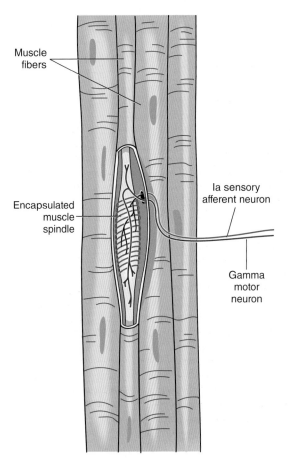

FIGURE 5.17 Muscle spindle within a muscle.

Both excitatory and inhibitory Ib spinal interneurons receive substantial input from other peripheral receptors (cutaneous, joint, muscle) and other spinal interneurons, and they receive descending input from supraspinal pathways. This additional input to the Ib interneurons provides flexibility to modulate movement when GTO receptors are activated. Ib interneurons can either inhibit or excite alpha motor neurons according to the task requirements.[63] For example, during the stance phase of gait, activation of GTO receptors in the hip and knee extensors results in facilitation of extensor muscles—a role opposite that expected from reflex activation as described previously.[64]

Forces elongating a muscle or tendon provide complementary input to an alpha motor neuron. Quick stretch stimulates the spindles to register a change in length, facilitating muscle contraction. Prolonged stretch initially may facilitate contraction but ultimately inhibits contraction, perhaps because GTOs register tension at the tendon and inhibit homonymous alpha motor neurons. Prolonged stretch is traditionally used to inhibit abnormally high tone in agonists and to facilitate antagonist muscle groups.[65] Inhibitory pressure on the tendon of a hypertonic muscle is thought to stimulate GTOs to inhibit abnormal muscle tone in the agonists while facilitating antagonists.[65] These techniques should be considered when positioning a patient for the application of physical agents or other interventions.

> ◎ **Clinical Pearl**
>
> Prolonged stretch and pressure on the tendon of a hypertonic muscle can inhibit high tone in agonist muscles and facilitate antagonist muscles.

input to homonymous muscles is inhibitory to signal the muscle fibers to relax (put the brakes on contraction). This reflex response is called **autogenic inhibition.** Input to alpha motor neurons of antagonist muscles is excitatory to signal the opposing muscles to contract.

Cutaneous Receptors

Stimulation of cutaneous sensory receptors occurs with every interaction of a person's skin with the external world. Temperature, texture, pressure, stretch, and potentially damaging stimuli are all transmitted through these receptors.

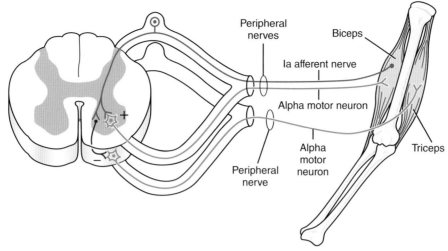

FIGURE 5.18 Reciprocal inhibition: muscle spindle input excites agonist muscles and inhibits antagonist muscles.

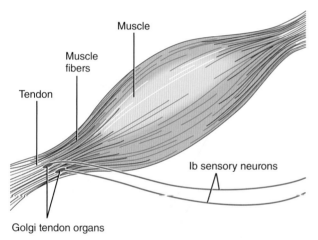

FIGURE 5.19 Golgi tendon organs (GTOs) within a muscle.

Cutaneous reflex responses tend to be more complex than muscle responses and involve multiple muscles. Potentially damaging stimuli that occur at the skin, such as stepping on a tack or touching a hot iron, ultimately facilitate withdrawal from the stimulus through activation of the appropriate alpha motor neurons and muscles. In a flexor withdrawal reflex, hip and knee flexors or elbow or wrist flexors are signaled to pull the foot or hand away from the potentially damaging stimulus. If the body is upright when a painful stimulus occurs at the foot, a crossed extension reflex occurs. Alpha motor neurons of the extensor muscles of the opposite hip and knee are facilitated so that when one foot is withdrawn from the painful stimulus, the other leg can support the individual's weight (Fig. 5.20).

Because muscles are linked to each other neurally via spinal interneurons for more efficient functioning, activation of an agonist frequently affects additional muscles. For example, when the biceps muscle is facilitated during a withdrawal reflex, the triceps muscle of the same arm is inhibited. Likewise, if a muscle is contracting strongly, many of its synergists will be facilitated to contract to help the function of the original muscle.

Intervention techniques that use cutaneous receptors to increase muscle tone include quick light touch, dynamic manual contacts, brushing, and quick icing. Techniques that use cutaneous receptors to decrease muscle tone include slow stroking, maintained manual contacts, neutral warmth, and prolonged icing. These facilitative and inhibitory techniques take advantage of motor responses to cutaneous stimulation as reported by researchers[66] and developed for clinical use by sensorimotor therapists.[67-69] The difference between facilitative and inhibitory techniques in clinical use usually lies in the speed and novelty of the stimulation. The nervous system stays alert when rapid changes are perceived, preparing the body to respond with movement, which necessitates increased muscle tone. Inhibitory techniques begin in a similar way as facilitative techniques, but the slow, repetitive, or maintained nature of the stimuli leads to adaptation by cutaneous receptors. The nervous system ignores what it already knows is there, and general relaxation is possible, with diminution of muscle tone.

Because cutaneous receptors can affect muscle tone, any physical agent that touches the skin can change tone, whether the touch is intentional or incidental. It is necessary to consider the location and type of cutaneous input provided whenever physical agents are used, particularly because the effect on muscle tone may counter the effect desired from the agent itself.

Clinical Pearl

Any physical agent that touches the skin can affect muscle tone.

Input From Spinal Sources

Circuits of neurons within the spinal cord also contribute to patterns of excitation and inhibition in alpha motor neurons. *Propriospinal* interneurons communicate intersegmentally via tracts within the spinal cord, between muscles within an extremity, and among different extremities. Propriospinal

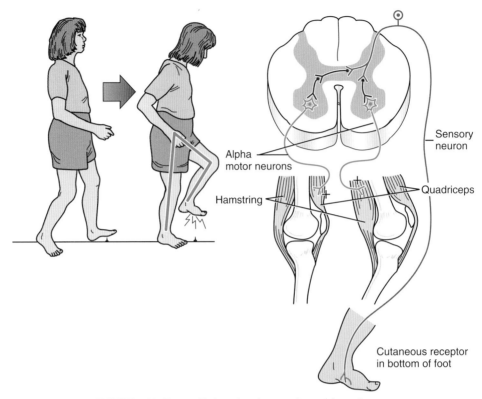

FIGURE 5.20 Flexor withdrawal and crossed extension reflexes.

interneurons receive input from peripheral afferents, as well as from many of the descending motor tracts discussed in the next section, and help produce synergies or particular patterns of muscle activation or movement.[65]

For example, when a person flexes their elbow forcefully against resistance, *propriospinal tracts* assist in communication between neurons at multiple spinal levels. The result is coordinated recruitment of synergistic muscles that add force to the movement. That same resisted arm movement facilitates flexor muscle activity in the opposite arm via propriospinal tracts that cross to the opposite side of the spinal cord.[70] Both of these pathways have been used in therapeutic exercises to increase tone and facilitate force output from muscles in patients with neurological dysfunction.[67,71]

Input From Supraspinal Sources

The term *supraspinal* refers to CNS areas that originate above the spinal cord in the upright human (see Fig. 5.11). Ultimately, these areas influence alpha motor neurons and spinal interneurons by sending signals down axons through a variety of descending motor tracts. Inputs to alpha motor neurons, either directly or indirectly, arising from the cerebrum or brainstem are referred to as *upper motor neurons.* Any voluntary, subconscious, or pathological change in the amount of input from descending motor pathways alters excitatory and inhibitory input to alpha and gamma motor neurons. Such changes alter muscle tone and activation, depending on the individual and the pathway or tract involved. Several of the major descending motor pathways and their influence on motor neurons are discussed in relation to the brain areas to which they are most closely related.

Sensorimotor Cortices. Volitional movement originates in response to a sensation, an idea, a memory, or an external stimulus to move, act, or respond. The decision to move is initiated in the cortex, with signals moving rapidly among neurons in various brain areas until they reach the motor cortex. Axons from neurons in the sensorimotor cortices form the corticospinal tracts (CSTs; from cortex to spinal cord) that run through the brain, most often crossing at the pyramids in the base of the brainstem and descending to synapse on appropriate interneurons and alpha motor neurons on the opposite side of the spinal cord (Fig. 5.21). Corticospinal input to interneurons and alpha motor neurons in the spinal cord is primarily responsible for voluntary contraction, particularly for fine motor functions of the distal parts of the upper extremities. As such, CST neurons tend to limit their activation to several muscles within an extremity.

Cerebellum. For every set of movement instructions that descends through the CST to signal posture or movement, a copy is routed to the **cerebellum** (see Fig. 5.21). Neurons in the cerebellum compare the intended movement with sensory input received from sensory afferents in the spinal cord about the actual movement. The cerebellum registers any discrepancies between the signal from the motor cortex and accumulated sensory input from the body via muscle spindles, GTOs, joints, and skin during movement. In addition, the cerebellum receives input from spinal pattern generators about ongoing rhythmical alternating movements. Cerebellar output helps correct for movement errors or unexpected obstacles to movement via the motor cortices and the red nuclei in the brainstem. The **red nucleus** sends

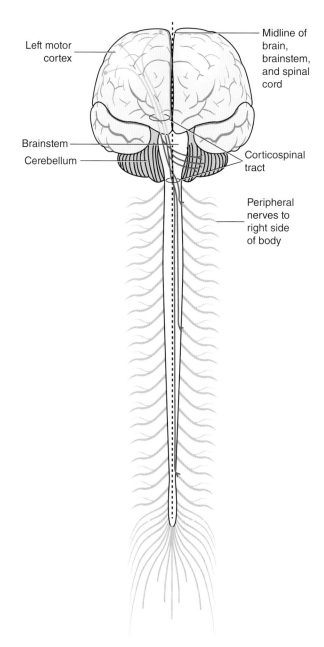

Left motor
cortex

Midline of
brain,
brainstem,
and spinal
cord

Brainstem
Cerebellum

Corticospinal
tract

Peripheral
nerves to
right side
of body

FIGURE 5.21 Corticospinal tract: schematic pathway from cortex to cerebellum and spinal cord.

signals to alpha motor neurons through the *rubrospinal tracts* (RuSTs) to the muscles of the neck and upper extremities to facilitate volitional movement. Ongoing correction is successful only during slower movement; if a movement is completed too quickly to be altered, information about success or failure of the movement can improve subsequent trials. Corticospinal and rubrospinal inputs to interneurons and alpha motor neurons function primarily to activate muscles voluntarily. Cerebellar influences on muscle tone and posture are mediated through connections with the *vestibulospinal tracts* (VSTs) and *reticulospinal tracts* (RSTs).[72,73] Damage to the cerebellum results in a loss of both alpha and gamma activation of motor neurons, typically with resultant hypotonia.

Vestibular System. The VSTs help regulate posture by transmitting signals from the vestibular system to interneurons that influence alpha motor neuron pools in the spinal cord. The vestibular system consists of receptors in the inner ear that receive ongoing information about the position of the head and the way it moves in space with respect to gravity, and vestibular nuclei in the brainstem that integrate information from the vestibular receptors with signals from joint, muscle, and skin receptors of the head and neck. Responses to the integrated information transmit through VSTs to facilitate extensor (antigravity) alpha motor neurons of the lower extremities and trunk to keep the body and head upright against gravity.

Reticular Formation. The RSTs transmit signals from the **reticular formation**—a group of nuclei located in the central region of the brainstem, the mesencephalon—to the spinal cord. These nuclei connect with the cerebral cortex, basal ganglia, and cerebellum.[73] In addition, the reticular formation receives input from all sensory systems, the autonomic nervous system (ANS), the hypothalamus, and the **limbic system,** reflecting the individual's emotions, motivation, and alertness. Differences in muscle tone mediated through these tracts may result in postural slumping in someone who is sad or lethargic or more erect posture in someone who is happy and energetic. The RSTs are also responsible for producing anticipatory postural responses that precede voluntary movement, for example, moving the body slightly posteriorly just before the arm is raised. This anticipatory postural response shifts the body mass to compensate for the forward movement of the body's center of mass when the arm is raised. The RSTs can also help modulate responses to reflexes according to the context of current movement. For example, while walking, someone may step on a sharp object with the right foot, noticing it only when the left foot is leaving the ground. Instead of allowing the expected flexor withdrawal reflex on the right (which would cause the person to fall), the RSTs help increase input to the motor neurons of extensor muscles on the right, momentarily permitting weight bearing on that sharp object until the left foot can be positioned to bear weight. Whereas the corticospinal tracts produce patterns of muscle activation in a single joint, the reticulospinal tracts produce bilateral patterns of muscle activation (synergies).[74]

Basal Ganglia. The basal ganglia modulate movement and tone. Similar to the cerebellum, the basal ganglia do not make direct connections to alpha motor neurons but work through connections to other descending pathways. Any volitional movement involves processing through connections in the basal ganglia (Fig. 5.22). Multiple chains of neurons looping through these nuclei, back and forth to the brainstem and motor cortical areas, influence the planning and postural adaptation of motor behavior.[73] In addition, the basal ganglia send signals to the RSTs that can influence underlying motor neuron activity. Dysfunction of any of the nuclei of the basal ganglia is associated with abnormal tone and disordered movement. For example, the rigidity, akinesia, and postural instability associated with Parkinson disease result primarily from basal ganglia pathology in one area, the substantia nigra pars compacta, whereas the excess muscle activation and tone

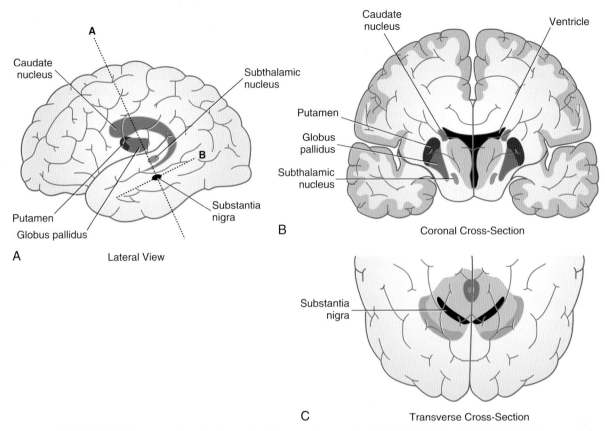

FIGURE 5.22 Basal ganglia within the brain: (A) lateral, (B) coronal, and (C) transverse cross-sectional views.

seen in conditions such as Huntington disease result from basal ganglia pathology in different areas, primarily the striatum.

Limbic System. The limbic system is composed of cortical areas and deep hemispheric nuclei involved in mediating emotions, memory, and motivation. These areas influence movement and muscle tone through connections with the hypothalamus and reticular formation in the brainstem. Circuits of neurons in the limbic system provide the ability to generate memories and attach meaning to them. Changes in muscle tone or activation can occur as a result of emotions recalled with particular memories of real or imagined events. For example, fear associated with a prior experience may heighten one's awareness when walking into a dark parking lot, activating the sympathetic nervous system (SNS) to plan the "fight-or-flight" response. The SNS activates the heart and lungs to work faster, dilates the pupils, and decreases the amount of blood pulsing through internal organs while diverting blood flow to the muscles. Muscle tone is increased to get ready for "fight or flight" in response to any potential danger in the parking lot. Muscle tone may further increase with a sudden unexpected noise but then may decrease again to an almost limp state when the noise is quickly identified as two good friends approaching from behind. Individuals may note similar changes in muscle tone with emotional responses to pain or fear of falling.

SUMMARY OF NORMAL MUSCLE TONE

Normal muscle tone depends on normal composition and functioning of muscles, the PNS, and the CNS. The motor units, with both alpha motor neurons and muscle fibers, must be functioning normally and be receiving normal input from all sources (see Table 5.3). Ultimately, the sum of all neural input and biomechanical factors determines the tone of a muscle. When pathology or injury affects muscles, alpha motor neurons, or any of the sources of input to alpha motor neurons, abnormal muscle tone may result.

Managing Abnormal Muscle Tone and Its Effects on Function

Various injuries or pathologies can result in abnormal muscle tone; some of these are considered in this section. Fig. 5.23 shows one example of pathology, nerve root compression, that can affect muscle tone and function. Abnormal muscle tone is considered an impairment of body function that may or may not lead to activity limitations and participation restrictions or effects on quality of life. Examination of muscle tone before and after an intervention can indicate if and how effectively the intervention modified muscle tone or its precipitating condition. Decisions about managing abnormal muscle tone depend on the role that abnormal muscle tone plays in limiting body function, activity, or participation and on the likelihood that the abnormality will cause problems, such as joint injury or muscle contracture, in the future.

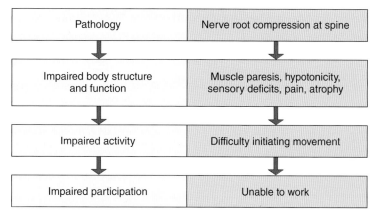

FIGURE 5.23 Example of the effect of pathology on body structure and function, activity, and participation.

Abnormal muscle tone, particularly hypertonia, can result from changes in neural activation of alpha motor neurons and changes in the muscle itself as it undergoes *myoplasticity*. When pathology affects output from descending pathways, the size of muscle fibers and level of myosin-actin bonding can change. Contractures with increased numbers of weak actin-myosin cross-bridges can occur, providing resistance to stretch of individual muscles. In addition, maladaptive neural connections, usually following CNS injury, can lead to tightness or co-contraction of agonist and antagonist muscles.[75]

In this section, some functional effects of muscle tone abnormalities are listed, and rehabilitation interventions are discussed (Table 5.4). The functional effects of abnormal tone depend on individual circumstances, which must be considered when muscle tone is examined. Circumstances can include additional impairments in body function and personal and environmental resources available to the patient. A young, active, or optimistic patient in a supportive environment tends to have less severe activity limitations than an older, sedentary, or depressed patient with the same degree of impairment in a less supportive environment. Just as the effects of abnormal tone depend on the individual's circumstances, so should rehabilitation depend on the individual's values and preferences, with goals set collaboratively.[76] Unfortunately, the patient's or caregiver's goals are not always highlighted in research on muscle tone rehabilitation. In the future, clinicians should examine not only the muscle tone itself but also the impact of tone abnormalities on the patient's function and caregivers' burden. Clinical suggestions for interventions to influence abnormal muscle tone should consider both immediate change that enhances subsequent muscle activation and any long-term impacts on function.

Any changes in muscle tone resulting from pathology or abnormal initial development will depend on the remaining muscle tissue and neurological input available to alpha motor neurons of that muscle. Remaining neural input may include partial or aberrant information from sources damaged by the pathology, normal information from undamaged sources, and altered input from undamaged sources in response to the pathology. When individuals have a movement problem, their nervous system will use whatever resources are readily available to solve it. For example, some patients may use their increased quadriceps tone to allow weight bearing on an otherwise weak leg. In such cases, eliminating the abnormal tone may diminish function rather than enhance it.

LOW MUSCLE TONE

Abnormally low muscle tone, or hypotonicity, generally results from loss or reduction of normal alpha motor neuron input to otherwise normal muscle fibers. Losses may result from damage to alpha motor neurons themselves or from motor endplate pathology that prohibits the muscle from responding to stimulation from alpha motor neurons. Loss of neural stimulation to the muscles may also result from conditions that increase inhibitory input or decrease excitatory input to alpha and gamma motor neurons (Fig. 5.24).

Clinical Pearl

Abnormally low muscle tone is usually a result of decreased neural excitation of otherwise normal muscles.

Hypotonicity makes the muscle less prepared for holding a position or performing a movement. Functional effects include (1) difficulty developing enough force to maintain posture or movement and (2) poor posture caused by frequent support of weight through tension on the ligaments, as in a hyperextended knee. Poor posture can result in cosmetically undesirable changes in appearance, such as a slumped spine or drooping facial muscles. Stretched ligaments can also compromise joint integrity, leading to pain (Box 5.2).

Alpha Motor Neuron Damage

If alpha motor neurons are no longer functioning, signals from the periphery, spinal cord, or supraspinal centers will not reach the muscle fibers and provide sufficient muscle tone to prepare for activation. Disease or injury of the alpha motor neurons that removes neuronal input to the muscle is called **denervation**. Denervation of a muscle or a group of muscles may be whole or partial. If all motor units of a muscle are affected, muscle tone is flaccid, and voluntary muscle activation is not possible: the muscle has **flaccid paralysis**. Examples of processes that may result in denervation include poliomyelitis, which affects the alpha motor neuron cell bodies; Guillain-Barré syndrome, which attacks

TABLE 5.4	Common Physical Agents for Managing Abnormal Muscle Tone	
Condition: Goal	Application Method; Example	Proposed Physiological Mechanism
Thermal Agents		
Hypertonicity: Reduce Tone	Moist hot pack (superficial heat); trapezius muscle spasm after whiplash injury	Increased elasticity of soft tissue, less energy required to deform/lengthen. Promotes relaxation, calming. Increased circulation provides more ATP to allow cross-bridge detachment.
	Ultrasound (deep heat); biceps brachii biomechanical stiffness after elbow immobilization	Increased temperature promotes blood flow, extensibility of tissue, and reduced viscosity of fluid elements in the tissue. May also increase tissue metabolism through cellular transport mechanisms.
	Prolonged cold via cold towel/ice bath; cold towel on plantar flexors for spasticity in MS	Decreased nerve conduction velocity (sensory and motor). Initial reduction in circulation limits available ATP for muscle contraction. May reduce inflammation and associated pain.
Hypotonicity: Increase Tone	Quick ice; paretic wrist extensors after stroke	Novel stimulus to cutaneous receptors, increases attention and consequent nervous system activity.
Hypertonicity/ Fluctuating Tone: Normalize Tone	Neutral warmth; swaddling or compression garments for tension, emotional lability	Promotes relaxation, calming. Decreases viscosity of fluids in tissues, increases extensibility of tissues.
Mechanical Agents		
Hypertonicity: Reduce Tone	Orthosis; serial splinting to stretch ankle plantarflexors	Prolonged tension on Golgi tendon organs inhibits hyperactive neural activation of agonist muscle.
	Mechanical traction; overactive muscles in painful lumbar spine	Prolonged tension on Golgi tendon organs. Repetitive traction may also promote relaxation and decrease guarding.
	Whole-body vibration; stand on vibrating platform preparing for gait training in CP	Modulation of synaptic transmission from Ia sensory neurons to motor neurons. May also increase perfusion to soft tissues and promote enhanced viscoelastic extensibility.
	Extracorporeal shock wave therapy (ESWT); to hypertonic quadriceps to assist positioning in sitting	Delivery of sonic waves may reduce motor neuron excitability through pressure on Golgi tendon organs. May increase nitric oxide delivery to surrounding tissues, enhance perfusion, and induce temporary dysfunction of neuromuscular junction.
	Continuous passive motion; flexing and extending knee in SCI to prepare for transfers	Movement in pain-free range may relax contractile tissue by breaking weak actin-myosin bonds and attachments between titin and actin. Decreases pain, reduces guarding.
Hypotonicity: Increase Tone	Focal vibration; to prepare paretic hip flexors post-stroke for swing phase of gait	High-frequency vibration activates the muscle stretch reflex, resulting in agonist muscle activation.
	Orthosis/splint; paretic wrist and finger extensors after stroke	Prevents overstretching of tissue while muscle lacks activation.
	Resistance; apply to agonist muscles with elastic bands, manual resistance, weights	Activates cross-bridge formation.
	Gravity; prop upright on extended arm to promote paretic triceps after stroke	Altering input to motor neurons through the vestibulospinal tract; also holding a position against the force of gravity.
Hypotonicity; Hypertonicity: Normalize Tone	Hydrotherapy; practice exercises in cool pool for person with MS and spasticity	Water temperature affects tissues/nerve conduction; buoyancy provides support; water resistance may stimulate muscle spindles and lead to additional motor neuron recruitment.
Electrical Agents		
Hypertonicity: Reduce Tone	Transcutaneous electrical stimulation (TENS); wrist/finger flexors to reduce spasticity, release grasp	Enhances presynaptic inhibition of the hyperactive stretch reflexes in spastic muscles and decreases co-contraction of the spastic antagonist muscles.
Hypotonicity: Increase Tone	Electrical stimulation: to paretic dorsiflexors for toe clearance in gait	Directly stimulates muscle to assist with isolated activation. May be applied during activity as functional electrical stimulation (FES).
Hypertonicity/ Hypotonicity: Normalize Tone	EMG biofeedback; auditory feedback signals hypertonic trapezius/improves control and scapulohumeral rhythm	Supraspinal inhibition or activation of descending motor pathways to facilitate desired motor neurons. May improve feedback during task practice.

ATP, Adenosine triphosphate; *CP*, cerebral palsy; *EMG*, electromyography; *MS*, multiple sclerosis; *SCI*, spinal cord injury.

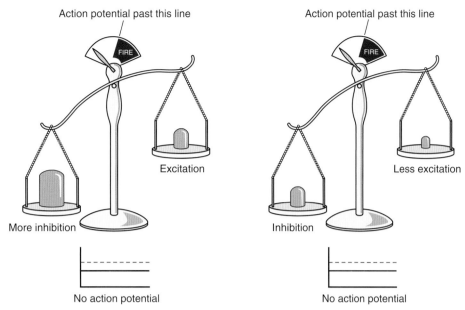

FIGURE 5.24 Inhibition of alpha motor neuron: inhibitory input exceeds excitatory input.

Box 5.2   Possible Consequences of Abnormally Low Muscle Tone

1. Difficulty developing adequate force output for normal posture and movement
   - Motor dysfunction
   - Secondary problems resulting from lack of movement (e.g., pressure sores, loss of cardiorespiratory endurance)
2. Poor posture
   - Reliance on ligaments to substitute for muscle holding eventual stretching of ligaments, compromised joint integrity, pain
   - Cosmetically undesirable changes in appearance (e.g., slumping of spine, drooping of facial muscles)
   - Pain

---

the Schwann cells so that the axons become demyelinated; crush or cutting types of trauma to the nerves; idiopathic damage to a nerve, as in Bell palsy that affects the facial nerve[77]; and nerve compression, similar to nerve root compression but affecting the more distal portion of the peripheral nerve.

When poliomyelitis eliminates functioning alpha motor neurons, recovery is limited by the number of intact motor neurons remaining. The remaining alpha motor neurons may increase the number of muscle fibers they innervate by increasing their number of terminal axonal branches. Intact neurons may thereby reinnervate muscle fibers that lost their innervation with destruction of associated alpha motor neurons (Fig. 5.25). This creates giant motor units in which many muscle fibers are innervated by a single alpha motor neuron.[78] Denervated muscle fibers that are not close enough to an intact alpha motor neuron for reinnervation die, causing loss of muscle bulk (atrophy). Passive and active-assisted ROM exercises may help maintain the length and viability of muscle fibers while potential reinnervation takes place.[78]

An injury that cuts or compresses the axons of alpha motor neurons can wholly or partially denervate a muscle. Recovery may occur if sufficient numbers of axons regrow from an intact cell body through any remaining myelin sheaths toward the muscle fibers.[78] Regrowth is slow, however, proceeding at a rate of 1 to 2 mm/day,[79] and may be less successful if the distance is long. Again, passive and active-assisted ROM exercises may help maintain the muscle fiber length or viability while regrowth takes place.[78] Recovery after Guillain-Barré syndrome and other conditions that damage myelination of peripheral nerves depends on remyelination of the axons, which can be fairly rapid, and on the slower process of regrowing any axons that were damaged during the demyelinated period.[80,81]

Rehabilitation After Alpha Motor Neuron Damage. Interventions used after alpha motor neuron damage typically focus on ROM exercise and therapeutic exercises to maintain muscle length and joint mobility and to strengthen the remaining musculature. For example, a systematic review of physical therapy after Bell palsy at acute and chronic stages reported low- and moderate-quality evidence that exercise is effective for improving facial disability.[77] Electrically stimulated muscle contractions may retard muscle atrophy, a consequence of alpha motor neuron damage, but the effect on axon regeneration is controversial.[78]

Rehabilitation after alpha motor neuron damage may also include functional training that teaches patients to compensate for movement losses after injury. Orthotic devices may be prescribed to support a limb for function while the muscle is flaccid or to protect the nerve, muscle, soft tissues, or joints from being overstretched. Such positioning devices may be required for several months if the nerve damage is severe and recovery of muscle tone is protracted.

Hydrotherapy and quick ice can help foster recovery after alpha motor neuron damage.[65,82] Hydrotherapy, in the form

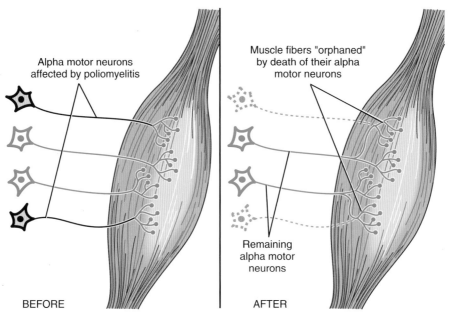

Alpha motor neurons
affected by poliomyelitis

Muscle fibers "orphaned"
by death of their alpha
motor neurons

Remaining
alpha motor
neurons

BEFORE

AFTER

FIGURE 5.25 Modification of remaining axons to innervate orphaned muscle fibers after polio eliminates some alpha motor neurons.

of aquatic therapy, may be used to support the body or limbs and to resist movement with ROM exercises in the water.[82] The combination of buoyancy and resistance can help strengthen remaining or returning musculature (see Chapter 19). Quick ice (see Chapter 8) or light touch on the skin over a particular muscle group adds excitatory input to any intact alpha motor neurons via cutaneous sensory neurons.[65] Clinicians must monitor the skin integrity of the affected region when applying physical agents because peripheral nerve damage can result in sensory loss, along with loss of intact alpha motor neurons.

Insufficient Excitation of Alpha Motor Neurons

Any condition that prohibits alpha motor neurons from receiving sufficient excitatory input to stimulate muscle fibers will result in decreased muscle tone and activation. Hypotonicity may occur whenever excitation through peripheral, spinal, or supraspinal sources is insufficient to result in alpha motor neuron firing.

> ### Clinical Pearl
>
> Clinicians must monitor skin integrity when applying physical agents because potential sensory loss along with motor deficits can reduce the patient's own response to imminent tissue damage.

Altered Peripheral Input: Immobilization. One condition that reduces peripheral sources of excitation to the alpha motor neuron is the application of a cast or brace to maintain immobility during fracture healing or recovery after ligament surgery. The immobilization device applies a fairly constant stimulus to cutaneous receptors but reduces reception of the various other inputs ordinarily encountered. Alpha

motor neurons are thus deprived of normal alterations in muscle spindle, GTO, cutaneous, or joint-receptor input. The immobilization device also inhibits movement at one or more joints, restricting the lengthening or shortening of local muscles. When the device is removed, there is usually measurable loss of muscle strength and bulk and reduced joint ROM. Muscle tone may also be affected, both by decreased activation of motor units and by increased biomechanical stiffness. These neural and biomechanical changes have opposing impacts on muscle tone, so the impact of this type of immobilization on passive stretch response can vary. On the other hand, if immobilization in a cast or splint places a hypertonic muscle in its lengthened position for several days at a time, it can apply a prolonged stretch. When used to stretch a muscle, the goal is to lower excessive muscle tone and increase passive ROM in a patient with severe hypertonicity.[73]

Altered Supraspinal Input: Stroke, Multiple Sclerosis, or Head Injury. Supraspinal input to the alpha motor neurons may be affected by a loss of blood supply (stroke) or direct injury to cortical or subcortical neurons (head injury) or through pathology that affects neurons or supporting cells (multiple sclerosis [MS]). Resultant muscle tone changes depend on the remaining proportions of excitatory and inhibitory input to alpha motor neurons.[83] For example, if all the descending motor tracts are destroyed, volitional movement may be absent in associated muscles. However, few, if any, pathologies affect all tracts equally; even traumatic SCIs commonly leave some proportion of intact connections. Most of the alpha motor neuron groups do not lose all descending input and must subsequently adapt to a new balance of excitatory and inhibitory input.[68]

Many supraspinal pathologies, such as stroke or SCI, may initially result in flaccidity, with no excitation of alpha motor neurons for hours to weeks. Immediately after an SCI, for example, the nervous system is typically in a state called *spinal shock*, in which the nerves shut down at and below the level of injury. This condition is marked by the flaccid tone of affected muscles and loss of spinal level reflex activity, such as the muscle stretch reflex. Positioning, with bolsters or splints, is typically used to prevent further injury while limbs are flaccid or hypotonic. However, as spinal shock wears off, the intact tract may begin to transmit excitatory or inhibitory input to the alpha motor neurons, resulting in a potential for voluntary and automatic movements. At this stage, rehabilitation generally focuses on muscle activation.

Rehabilitation to Increase Muscle Tone. Physical agents can increase muscle tone in patients with supraspinal lesions. For example, dynamic orthotics[84] and ES have moderate-level evidence of effectiveness for patients with a flaccid arm[14] or footdrop in patients with CNS injury.[85,86] Hydrotherapy and quick ice may help to increase muscle tone when used in conjunction with therapeutic exercise.[65]

> ◎ **Clinical Pearl**
>
> Physical agents used for hypotonicity caused by decreased input to the alpha motor neuron include ES, hydrotherapy, and quick ice.

The intent of any rehabilitation of patients with hypotonicity is to stimulate alpha motor neurons via remaining intact peripheral, spinal, and supraspinal sources of input. Many authors have described in detail the options available to the rehabilitation specialist for increasing muscle tone and motor output in patients who have had a stroke or a head injury.[10,65,67,87] For example, quick icing, tapping, and focal vibration[88] are facilitative techniques that can increase tone via cutaneous and muscle spindle receptors, respectively, and, when paired with voluntary movement, can increase functional motor output. ES might be combined with resistance of the muscle being stimulated or of synergistic muscles to increase tone and activation via interneurons of the spinal cord. Box 5.3 summarizes management options to increase low muscle tone and improve functional activation.

HIGH MUSCLE TONE

Many pathological conditions eventually result in abnormally high muscle tone. Hypertonicity may develop with any of the supraspinal lesions mentioned in the previous

---

Box 5.3   Interventions for Low Muscle Tone

- Hydrotherapy
- Quick ice
- Electrical stimulation (when muscle fibers are innervated)
- Biofeedback
- Light touch
- Tapping
- Resistive exercises
- Range-of-motion exercises
- Therapeutic exercises
- Functional training
- Orthotics
- Vibration therapy

---

section, as well as Parkinson disease. Hypertonicity occurs when an otherwise intact alpha motor neuron receives abnormally high excitatory input compared with inhibitory input (see Fig. 5.15). Changes in muscle can also lead to abnormally stiff muscle and connective tissue that contribute to hypertonicity.

Researchers and clinicians debate about the effects of hypertonicity, particularly spasticity, on function. Some have pointed out that spasticity of the antagonist does not necessarily interfere with voluntary movement of the agonist.[9,83] During walking, for example, it has been assumed that spasticity in the ankle plantar flexors prevents adequate dorsiflexion during the swing phase of gait, resulting in toe drag. However, EMG studies of patients with hypertonicity (both spasticity and rigidity) have shown essentially absent activity in the plantar flexors during swing, which is the same response seen in patients with normal gait.[16] Another study of upper-extremity function found deficits resulting from inadequate recruitment of agonists, not from increased activity in spastic antagonist muscles.[89] It appears that, rather than excessive antagonist activation impairing agonist function, voluntary movement is hindered by slowed and inadequate recruitment of the agonist and then delayed termination of agonist contraction. In other words, the timing and quantity of agonist muscle activation are directly altered.[9] In addition, biomechanical changes within the muscles can influence hypertonicity in patients with CNS lesions.[90]

On the other side of the argument, some researchers have shown that coactivation of spastic antagonists increases with faster movements, substantiating the claim that abnormal resistance to stretch inhibits voluntary motor control.[91] Additionally, a review of multiple drug studies revealed improved function in 60% to 70% of patients receiving intrathecally administered baclofen, a drug that reduces spasticity. The authors stated that "spasticity reduction can be associated with improved voluntary movement," although it is also possible that a decrease in tone will have no measurable effect or will even adversely affect function.[92]

Because of this controversy, it cannot be stated unequivocally that hypertonicity itself always impairs functional voluntary movement. However, other effects of hypertonicity must not be ignored. These include the potential for (1) muscle spasms that contribute to discomfort or pain; (2) contractures (shortened resting length) or other soft tissue changes caused by hypertonicity in a muscle group on one side of a joint; (3) abnormal postures that can lead to skin breakdown or pressure ulcers; (4) resistance to passive movement of a nonfunctioning limb that results in difficulties with assisted dressing, transfers, hygiene, and other activities; and (5) possibly a stereotyped movement pattern that could inhibit alternative movement solutions (Box 5.4). On the plus side, hypertonicity in the form of spasticity and muscle spasms may facilitate weight-bearing transfers and contribute to the maintenance of bone mineral density for people with SCI, although a review across studies showed equivocal results.[93]

Noxious Stimuli, Cold, and Stress

A noxious stimulus is an example of a peripheral source of input that can lead to hypertonicity. Cutaneous reception of imminently damaging stimuli and the consequent withdrawal and crossed-extension reflexes have already been discussed. Noxious stimuli to muscles or joints can result in increased tension in muscles around the area, although not necessarily in the muscle in which the stimulus originates, which may show no heightened EMG activity.[1] For example, in patients with back pain, the buildup of muscle tension may manifest as muscle spasms in the paraspinal musculature. Such spasms, called **guarding,** are thought to be a way to protect against further muscle damage. Guarding can have both supraspinal and peripheral origins due to the heavy involvement of the limbic system in the interpretation of and response to discomfort and pain.

The human body responds to cold via peripheral and supraspinal systems. When homeostasis is threatened, muscle tone increases, and the body may begin to shiver. Muscle tone also tends to increase with other threats, registered as stress. Hypertonicity may be palpable in various muscle groups, such as muscles in the shoulders and neck, when an individual registers more general discomfort or perceives a situation as threatening to the body or to self-esteem. The muscles prepare for "fight or flight" as the rest of the body engages in other SNS responses.

Managing Hypertonicity as a Result of Noxious Stimuli, Cold, or Stress.
Patients with hypertonicity resulting from noxious stimuli, cold, or stress can decrease muscle tone in several ways. The first and most effective solution is to remove the source of the hypertonicity; this can be done by eliminating biomechanical sources of imminent tissue damage, warming the body, and alleviating stress. When these solutions are not possible, applicable, or effective, management to decrease muscle tone resulting from noxious stimuli may include education on relaxation techniques, EMG biofeedback (see Chapter 15), and the use of neutral warmth or heat (see Part III), hydrotherapy (see Chapter 19), or cold.

Spinal Cord Injury

After a complete SCI, alpha motor neurons below the level of the lesion lack inhibitory and excitatory input from supraspinal sources. When spinal shock resolves, the alpha motor neurons will still receive input from sensory, propriospinal, and other interneurons below the level of the lesion. Further, the lack of inhibition from descending motor tracts allows alpha motor neurons below the level of injury to respond more readily to sensory inputs from the muscle spindle, GTO, joint, or cutaneous receptors. The hypertonicity is spasticity because quick stretch elicits greater resistance than does slow stretch.

Quick stretch may occur not only when the muscles are specifically tested for tone but also whenever the patient moves and gravity suddenly exerts a different pull on the muscles, depending on the mass of the limb. For example, patients who have a complete thoracic level injury may use their arms to manage leg and foot placement on the footrest of their wheelchair. When the leg is lifted, the foot hangs down with the ankle in a plantar-flexed position. When the leg is positioned on the footrest, weight lands on the ball of the foot, and the ankle moves passively into relative dorsiflexion. If foot placement is quick, the plantar flexors are quickly stretched, and sustained clonus may result until the feet are repositioned.

Frequently, hypertonicity is greater on one side of a joint than on the other because when people are upright, the force of gravity is unidirectional on the mass of a limb. Because a patient with a complete SCI has no active movement that can counter unidirectional forces, muscle shortening tends to occur in the muscles that are relatively more hypertonic. The biomechanical stiffness of hypertonic muscles increases, and contractures can develop. Such contractures can inhibit functions such as dressing, transfers, and positioning for pressure relief.

Managing Hypertonicity After Spinal Cord Injury.
A wide range of rehabilitation interventions may be helpful for managing spasticity after SCI. However, spasticity in patients with SCI may manifest as spasms triggered by noxious stimuli. Noxious stimuli can include restrictive clothing, a distended bladder, or some other internal irritation. The clinician should first look for and resolve noxious stimuli before trying other approaches to reduce spasticity.[94] When severe spasticity inhibits function and is without identifiable and removable causes, directed rehabilitation or pharmaceutical interventions should be tried.

Directed rehabilitation to reduce hypertonicity or resultant contractures in SCI typically includes selective ROM exercises,[94,95] positioning or orthotics to maintain functional muscle length, local or systemic medications,[96] and surgery.[94] Prolonged stretching has been associated with improved muscle tone and passive ROM in other populations, but the minimal research in SCI suggests that stretch may need to be an adjunct to other modalities or interventions to be effective in this population.[97] Heat can be used before stretching of hypertonic muscles to increase the effectiveness of stretching (see Part III), but this requires careful monitoring because patients with SCI generally have reduced or absent sensation below the level of the injury, so they will be less able to tell if applied heat gets too hot. Some clinicians use vibration to reduce hypertonicity, but currently, the evidence to support its efficacy in this population is rated low level.[98] Functional electrical stimulation (FES) has proved helpful: a recent systematic review reported that FES reduced spasticity in patients with SCI by 45% to 60% and also reduced EMG activity and increased ROM[99] (see Chapter 12). Transcranial magnetic stimulation is one of the more recently explored interventions; a recent meta-analysis supports its efficacy in reducing spasticity for patients with SCI.[100]

Cerebral Lesions

CNS lesions from stroke, cerebral palsy, tumors, CNS infections, MS, or head injury may change the balance of inputs to alpha motor neurons and result in hypertonicity (see Fig. 5.15).

The location and extent of the pathology determine the extent of muscle involvement and whether a muscle group loses all or only some of its supraspinal input.

Hypertonicity: Primary Impairment or Adaptive Response. The neurophysiological mechanism of hypertonicity is disputed. Various management approaches address hypertonicity based on assumptions about its significance. With one approach, developed by Bobath,[10] the nervous system is assumed to function as a hierarchy in which supraspinal centers control the spinal centers of movement, and "abnormal tonus" results from loss of inhibitory control from higher centers. The resultant therapeutic sequence involves normalizing the hypertonicity before, or along with, facilitating normal movement. Alternatively, the systems-based task-oriented approach considers that the primary goal of the nervous system in producing movement is to accomplish the desired task.[101] After a lesion develops, the nervous system uses its remaining resources to perform movement tasks. Hypertonicity, rather than being a primary result of the injury itself, may be the best adaptive response the nervous system can make, given the system's available resources after injury.

An example of task-oriented reasoning is as follows. Patients with paresis are sometimes able to use trunk and lower-extremity extensor hypertonicity to hold an upright posture. In this case, hypertonicity is an adaptive response to accomplish the task of maintaining an upright posture.[101,102] Eliminating the hypertonicity in such a case would decrease function, unless concurrent increases in controlled voluntary movement are elicited. Controlled movement, if it can be elicited, is always preferable to hypertonicity. Control implies the ability to change responses according to environmental and task demands, whereas the hypertonic extensor response is relatively stereotyped. The use of a stereotyped hypertonic response for function seems to block spontaneous development of more normal control.[10,103]

Evidence that hypertonicity may be an adaptive response includes the fact that it is not an immediate sequela of injury but instead develops over time and in only some individuals with a particular pathology.[104] After a cortical stroke, for example, recovery of muscle tone and voluntary movement follows a fairly predictable course.[68,105] At first, muscles may be flaccid on the side of the body opposite the lesion, without elicitable stretch reflexes. By day 3 after the stroke, about 25% of patients show signs of spasticity,[104] with increasing response of the muscles to quick stretch and the beginning of voluntary motor output that is limited to movement in flexor or extensor patterns, called *synergies*. Further recovery may include progression to full-blown spasticity, followed by a decrease in hypertonicity as controlled movement increases.[68] A particular patient's course of recovery may stall, skip, or plateau anywhere along this progression, but it does not regress. According to some studies, the prevalence of spasticity may increase to about 37% by 1 month after a stroke but decreases to 15% by about 6 months. Those who develop spasticity are more likely to have severe motor and sensory loss compared with those who have mild or moderate deficits.[104]

Managing Hypertonicity Due to Cerebral Lesions. Rehabilitation to address hypertonicity after a stroke resulting from upper motor neuron dysfunction depends on whether the hypertonicity inhibits function or care of the involved limb. The emphasis is on the return of independent function, whether that necessitates tone reduction and/or reeducation of controlled, voluntary movement patterns.

Various treatment options have been documented for addressing spasticity in patients who have had a stroke. Although not as well documented, many options may also apply to people who have had a traumatic brain injury. Choice of treatment will depend on patient preferences, comorbidities, and other contextual factors, such as resources available. When spasticity is severe, treatment often consists of a combination of pharmacological options, including botulinum toxin or baclofen,[106] along with nonpharmacological options, the emphasis of this section.[107]

Best-practice recommendations for addressing spasticity after a stroke include positioning in antispastic patterns, active ROM exercises,[108,109] stretching, electrical stimulation, and extracorporeal shock wave therapy[110-114] (ESWT), although some of these methods have low-level evidence to support their effectiveness.[14] The effectiveness of positioning and stretching may be enhanced with prolonged icing, inhibitory pressure, prolonged stretch, inhibitory casting, or continuous passive motion.[65,115-117] Active ROM exercises may help reeducate muscle control in isolated movements or along with functional task practice. Task practice along with biofeedback or EMG biofeedback[26] can improve passive ROM, addressing biomechanical components of hypertonicity. Reeducation of controlled voluntary movement patterns could include weight bearing to facilitate normal postural responses or training with directed practice of functional movement patterns. Reduction of hypertonicity may be a byproduct of improved motor control in the following example. If a patient feels insecure when standing upright, muscle tone will increase commensurate with the anxiety level. If balance and motor control are improved so that the patient feels more confident in the upright position, hypertonicity will be reduced. Positioning for comfort and for reduced anxiety is a critical component of any intervention intended to reduce muscle tone. Electrical stimulation as used in TENS has been shown in a number of systematic reviews to be effective at reducing spasticity on the Modified Ashworth Scale, either as a stand-alone intervention or combined with physiotherapy, although optimal parameters have yet to be determined.[118-121] Recent systematic reviews of ESWT, with between 140 and 385 participants, have documented significant improvements in spasticity of both upper- and lower-extremity musculature as measured by the Modified Ashworth Scale and include both an immediate and longer-term reduction in muscle tone[110-114]; one study reported decreased tone up to 12 weeks after application of shock waves.[114]

Management to reduce hypertonicity after stroke could also include[122-124] vibration training.[65] Studies on whole-body vibration and focal muscle vibration therapy to reduce spasticity in individuals after a stroke report positive outcomes. However, heterogeneity of the application of the vibratory stimulus and the methodological quality of studies are variable, and more research is required to determine its role in the treatment of spasticity.[122-124] Other novel interventions include transcranial magnetic stimulation,[125] electroacupuncture,[126] kinesiotaping,[127] and robot-assisted therapy.[128] In one study of robot-assisted therapy, participants received robot-applied or manually applied active-assisted to resistive ROM to the upper extremity for about 1 hour a day, 5 days a week, for 3 months, with improvements in Modified Ashworth Scale score and strength in both groups.[129] The frequency and duration guaranteed that the volume of movement was high, much higher than most patients get in standard rehabilitation, but improvement in muscle tone and strength may require that dose.

Individuals with increased muscle tone associated with MS or cerebral palsy may also benefit from a mixed treatment approach consisting of pharmacological[130] and nonpharmacological interventions.[131,132] Recent systematic reviews comprising 799 to 2720 subjects with MS have asserted that a treatment plan consisting of exercise therapy and TENS enhances the efficacy of pharmacological agents, including baclofen, botulinum toxin, or medical cannabinoids.[131,132] As in patients after a stroke, recent literature supports the use of robot-assisted gait training,[133] ESWT,[134] or a combination of FES with cycling[135] to reduce spasticity in patients with MS. Stretching and cold packs are also beneficial in temporarily reducing the spasticity of MS; hydrotherapy, particularly in cool water, allows ROM exercises with diminished influence of gravity, thus avoiding resistance-triggered spasms.[102] Cold has been applied in the form of garments, including jackets, head caps, or neck wraps with ice or other cooling elements. Evidence of change in hypertonicity with application of such cooling devices is equivocal: patients with MS reported reduced spasticity after a single use of a cooling garment, but the change in spasticity after cold application was not statistically significant.[136] Some therapeutic benefits are specific to the diagnosis; although the use of medical cannabinoids for reduction of hypertonicity is not yet well understood, available evidence so far reveals that it is most efficacious for those with MS-related spasticity.[137]

Knott and Voss[67] described a twofold approach to decreasing the tone of a hypertonic muscle group. Muscles can be approached directly, with verbal cues to relax or by applying cold towels to elicit muscle relaxation. Alternatively, muscles can be approached indirectly by stimulating the antagonists, which results in reciprocal inhibition of agonists and consequent lowering of agonist muscle tone. Antagonists can be stimulated with resisted exercise or ES (see Chapter 12).

> **◎ Clinical Pearl**
>
> EMG biofeedback of agonist muscle groups or electrical stimulation of antagonist muscle groups can be used to reduce muscle hypertonicity.

If a patient has severe hypertonicity or if many muscle groups are affected, techniques that influence the parasympathetic nervous system to decrease arousal or calm the individual generally might be used. Such techniques include soft lighting or music, slow rocking, neutral warmth, slow stroking, maintained touch, rotation of the trunk, and hydrotherapy (see Chapter 19), as long as the patient feels safely supported. For example, hydrotherapy in a cool water pool is advocated for patients with MS to reduce spasticity.[67] To address emotional states most effectively, therapies must be patient centered—for example, recent findings suggest that the effect of listening to music for tone reduction may largely depend on the musical preferences of the listener.[138]

Rigidity: A Consequence of Central Nervous System Pathology

Some cerebral lesions are associated with rigidity rather than spasticity. Head injuries, for example, may result in one of two specific patterns of rigidity, decorticate or decerebrate, either of which may be constant or intermittent. Both patterns include hypertonicity in the neck and back extensors; the hip extensors, adductors, and internal rotators; the knee extensors; and the ankle plantar flexors and invertors. The elbows are held rigidly at the sides, with wrists and fingers flexed in both patterns, but in decorticate rigidity, the elbows are flexed, and in decerebrate rigidity, they are extended (Fig. 5.26). The two types are thought to indicate the level of the lesion: above (decorticate) or below (decerebrate) the red nuclei in the brainstem. In most patients with head injury, however, the lesion is diffuse, and this designation is not helpful. Two positioning principles can diminish rigidity in either case and should be considered along with any other therapies: (1) reposition the patient in postures opposite to those listed, with emphasis on slight neck and trunk flexion and hip flexion past 90 degrees, and (2) avoid the supine position, which promotes extension in the trunk and limbs via the symmetrical tonic labyrinthine response (see Fig. 5.7).

Rigidity, similar to spasticity, can result in biomechanical muscle stiffness after sustained posturing in the shortened position. The longer the period of time without ROM exercises or positioning to elongate a muscle group, the greater the biomechanical changes that occur. Prevention is the best cure for biomechanical components of hypertonicity, but orthotics[117] or serial casting[115] can also help reduce muscle stiffness related to hypertonicity, and heat may be used to increase ROM temporarily before a cast or orthotic is applied.

Parkinson disease typically causes rigidity throughout the skeletal musculature rather than just of the extensors. In addition to pharmacological replacement of dopamine,[139] management can include temporary reduction of hypertonicity through heat,

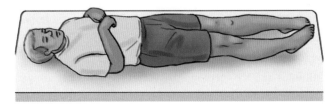

A

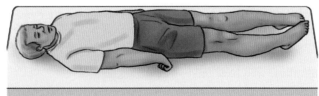

B

FIGURE 5.26 (A) Decorticate posture. (B) Decerebrate posture.

passive to active ROM, and rotational trunk movements, along with general inhibiting techniques to allow patients to accomplish particular functions. Box 5.5 summarizes management suggestions to decrease high muscle tone.

FLUCTUATING MUSCLE TONE

Commonly, pathology of the basal ganglia results in disorders of muscle tone and activation. Not only is voluntary motor output difficult to initiate, execute, and control, but also the variations in muscle tone seen in this population can be so extreme as to be visible with movement. The resting tremor of a patient with Parkinson disease is an example of a fluctuating tone that results in involuntary movement. A child with athetoid-type cerebral palsy, for whom movement is a series of involuntary writhings, also demonstrates fluctuating tone.

When an individual has fluctuating tone that moves the limbs through large ROMs, contractures usually are not a problem, but inadvertent self-inflicted injuries sometimes occur. As a hand or a foot flails around, it sometimes will run into a hard, immovable object. Patients and caregivers can be educated to alter the environment, padding necessary objects or removing unnecessary obstacles to avoid harm. If the fluctuating tone does not result in movement of large amplitude, positioning and ROM interventions should be considered. Neutral warmth has been advocated to reduce excessive movement resulting from muscle tone fluctuations in athetosis.[65]

Box 5.5 | Interventions for High Muscle Tone

Interventions for Pain, Cold, or Stress

Remove the source:
- Eliminate pain.
- Warm the patient.
- Alleviate stress.

Relaxation techniques
EMG biofeedback
Neutral warmth
Heat
Hydrotherapy
Cold towels or cooling garments
Stimulation of antagonists
- Resisted exercise
- Electrical stimulation

Interventions for Spinal Cord Injury

Selective ROM exercises
Prolonged stretch
Positioning
Orthotics
Medication
Surgery
Heat
Prolonged ice

Interventions for Cerebral Lesions

Prolonged ice
Inhibitory pressure

Prolonged stretch
Inhibitory casting
Continuous passive motion
Positioning
Reeducation of voluntary movement patterns
Stimulation of antagonists
- Resisted exercise
- Electrical stimulation

General relaxation techniques
- Soft lighting or music
- Slow rocking
- Neutral warmth
- Slow stroking
- Maintained touch
- Rotation of the trunk
- Hydrotherapy

Interventions for Rigidity

Positioning
ROM exercises
Orthotics
Serial casting after head injury
Heat
Medication
General relaxation techniques (as listed previously)

EMG, Electromyographic; *ROM*, range of motion.

CLINICAL CASE STUDIES

The following case studies summarize and apply the approaches to the management of muscle tone abnormalities discussed in this chapter and are not intended to be exhaustive. For each scenario presented, evaluation of clinical findings and goals of management are proposed. These are followed by a discussion of factors to be considered in intervention selection. Note that any technique used to alter tone abnormalities must be followed by voluntary activation of the musculature involved if the patient is to improve the ability to hold or move functionally. All plans of care should be developed in collaboration with the patient or client to ensure that issues of most value to the individual are prioritized.

CASE STUDY 5.1

Bell Palsy
Examination
History

GM is a 37-year-old businessman who states that the first signs of Bell palsy appeared 2 days ago after a long airplane flight during which he slept with his head resting against the window. GM states that the left side of his face feels as though it is being pulled downward; the muscles show a visible droop. He also currently notes some nasal congestion that inhibits

Continued

CLINICAL CASE STUDIES—*cont'd*

breathing through his nose. He is having trouble controlling saliva and eating properly because he cannot close his lips. He is concerned that this may not go away and that it may affect his ability to interact with people in his business.

Systems Review

GM is accompanied to this visit by his wife. His vital signs are normal. He denies any facial pain, visual loss, or dizziness. He reports feeling mildly to moderately sad, although he is eager to receive treatment. Symptoms of a presumed upper respiratory infection include enlarged nodes and nasal congestion but no fever. GM's wife has noted a lopsided smile since symptoms began.

Tests and Measures

On examination, muscles on the left side of GM's face do not respond voluntarily or automatically for facial expression, and the patient is unable to close his lips or his left eye tightly. The left corneal reflex is absent.

What is the muscle tone in the left facial muscles? What techniques would be appropriate for changing the muscle tone for this patient?

Evaluation and Goals

ICF Level	Current Status	Goals
Body structure and function	Left facial hypotonicity	Prevent overstretching or tightening of soft tissues
	Absent protective reflex for left eye	Protect left eye
	Facial muscle paralysis	Strengthen facial muscles as reinnervation occurs in 1 to 3 months
Activity	Inability to close lips and eat normally	Normalize function of lips, mouth
Participation	Difficulty conducting normal business transactions	Return to normal business activity

ICF, International Classification for Functioning, Disability and Health.

Prognosis

Bell palsy is paralysis of the facial muscles caused by dysfunction of the facial nerve (cranial nerve VII), usually on only one side, with varied causes. If the entire facial nerve on the left is affected, none of the muscle fibers on the left side of the face will be able to receive signals from any alpha motor neurons in this peripheral nerve, and the muscles will be flaccid. If the facial nerve is only partially affected, some muscles might be hypotonic. Spontaneous reinnervation of the muscle fibers is common after a facial palsy—usually within 1 to 3 months. Muscle tone can be expected to normalize as reinnervation

occurs if the muscle and the connective tissues have been maintained so that secondary biomechanical changes do not interfere.

Intervention

Gentle passive movement of the facial musculature may be indicated to counter soft tissue changes resulting from lack of active movement. Otherwise, GM may be left with a cosmetically unacceptable facial droop when the muscles are reinnervated. A patch or other form of protection over the left eye may be required to prevent eye injury while the motor component of the corneal reflex is paralyzed. As the muscle fibers are reinnervated, emphasis will be on performing exercises to elicit voluntary contraction rather than on improving muscle tone. Quick icing or light touch on the skin over a particular muscle that is beginning to be innervated may help GM isolate a muscle to move it voluntarily. Practice of facial movements while looking in a mirror may provide extra feedback for GM as he attempts to reestablish normal activation of the facial muscles. ES with biofeedback to focus voluntary activation on the appropriate muscles may be used to help GM resume function once muscles are reinnervated.

CASE STUDY 5.2

Intermittent Low Back Pain
Examination
History

SP is a 24-year-old woman who has had intermittent back pain over the past several months. The pain began when her lifestyle changed from that of an athlete training regularly to that of a student sitting for long periods. The pain in her lower back increased dramatically yesterday while she was bowling for the first time in 2 years. This pain is exacerbated by movement and long periods of sitting and alleviated somewhat by over-the-counter antiinflammatory medication and ice. SP complains of fatigue and unrelenting exhaustion that is not relieved by rest; pain wakes her up at night and makes it hard to go back to sleep. She reports low energy that has negatively affected her emotional well-being. Today, she rates her pain as 8/10. SP is distressed; she has been unable to study for her final examinations because of pain.

Systems Review

Her vital signs are normal.

Tests and Measures

SP has palpable muscle spasm in the paraspinal muscles at the lumbar level. Spinal ROM is limited in all directions because of pain. Transitional movements are slow and cautious, and posture is stiff during gait.

What is the underlying stimulus causing the muscle spasm? What intervention is appropriate to alleviate the spasm?

CLINICAL CASE STUDIES—*cont'd*

Evaluation and Goals

ICF Level	Current Status	Goals
Body structure and function	Low back pain	Diagnose source and identify movements and positions that do not increase pain
	Lumbar paraspinal muscle spasm	Alleviate muscle spasm by identifying and removing painful stimulus if present, limit guarding, increase circulation to help muscles relax
	Limited spinal ROM	Regain normal spinal ROM
Activity	Limited movement	Return to normal movement
	Inability to sit for prolonged periods	Regain ability to sit for at least 1 hour at a time
Participation	Inability to study for examinations	Return to studies

ICF, International Classification for Functioning, Disability and Health; *ROM*, range of motion.

Prognosis

Muscle spasms typically originate from painful stimuli, even if the stimuli are subtle. Possible stimuli in SP's case include injury to muscle fibers or other tissue while engaging in vigorous but unaccustomed activity, pain signals from a facet joint, and nerve root irritation. Consequent tension in surrounding muscles may hold or splint the injured area to avoid local movement that could irritate and exacerbate the pain. If persistent, the muscle spasm itself can contribute to the pain and discomfort by inhibiting local circulation and setting up its own painful feedback loop.

Intervention

Diagnosing the source of the painful stimulus is beyond the scope of this chapter, but many texts are devoted to the subject.[140-142] Once the stimulus is identified and removed, the muscle spasm may diminish by itself, or it may require separate intervention. Heat, ultrasound, or massage can increase local circulation (see Part III of this textbook). Prolonged icing, neutral warmth, or EMG biofeedback could be used to diminish hypertonicity directly, thus allowing restoration of more normal local circulation. Once the painful feedback loop of the muscle spasm is broken, patient education is necessary. Education should include instructions on how to strengthen local musculature and how to avoid postures and movements that aggravate the initial injury. Progression of activities must be guided by the patient's tolerance.

CASE STUDY 5.3

Recent Stroke
Examination
History

RB is a 74-year-old man who had a stroke 3 months ago. He initially had left hemiplegia, which has progressed from an initial flaccid paralysis to his current status that includes hemiparesis with hypertonicity in the biceps brachii and ankle plantar flexors. He has little control of movement on the left side of his body and requires assistance with movement in bed, transfers, and dressing. He is able to stand with assistance but has difficulty maintaining his balance and taking steps with a quad cane. He does not report any pain and exhibits no visible discomfort with passive ROM of the extremities.

Systems Review

RB presents a positive affect, and he reports being highly motivated to regain function and spend time with his several grandchildren. His vital signs are within normal limits. He denies any chest pain, shortness of breath, or dizziness.

Tests and Measures

During clinical observation, RB rests his left forearm in his lap while sitting with his back supported, but on standing, gravity quickly stretches his biceps once the weight of his forearm is unsupported and the left elbow responds by flexing to approximately 80 degrees. Full elbow extension is never observed during bed mobility, transfers, or standing. His left ankle shows plantar flexion with several beats of clonus when he first stands up, ending with weight mostly on the ball of his foot, unless the left foot is carefully positioned to bear most weight through the heel during static standing.

On examination, RB has a hyperactive stretch reflex in both the left biceps and the triceps, but muscle tone in the triceps is hypotonic, with a 1 on the clinical tone scale. The left biceps and plantar flexors tone show spasticity graded 1+ on the Modified Ashworth Scale, approximately equal to a 3 on the clinical tone scale. Spasticity is graded 1 on the Modified Ashworth Scale in the left quadriceps and 2 in the plantar flexors. During quick stretch of the left plantar flexors, clonus is apparent, lasting for three beats. When asked to lift his left arm, RB is unable to fractionate or isolate movements but can accomplish limited voluntary antigravity movement by elevating and retracting his scapula, abducting and externally rotating his shoulder, and flexing and supinating at the elbow—all consistent with a flexor synergy pattern of movement. When standing, he tends to position his left hip in internal rotation and slight adduction, along with a retracted pelvis and a hyperextended knee; this is consistent with the lower-extremity extensor synergy pattern of movement.

Continued

CLINICAL CASE STUDIES—cont'd

What measures of muscle tone are appropriate in evaluating RB? Which intervention is appropriate, given RB's hypertonicity?

Evaluation and Goals

ICF Level	Current Status	Goals
Body structure and function	Changes in muscle tone on the left side Muscle weakness in left upper and lower extremities Potential for loss of ROM in left extremities	Improve muscle tone and activation Maintain ROM of left upper and lower extremities
Activity	Abnormal voluntary movement of left upper extremity and left lower extremity Inability to stand and function without assistance	Regain ability to isolate muscle activation and move voluntarily Stand and move independently
Participation	Inability to play with grandchildren	Return to playing with grandchildren

ICF, International Classification for Functioning, Disability and Health; *ROM*, range of motion.

Prognosis

Goals are focused on improving RB's function and preventing secondary problems. Other possible tests for RB's muscle tone include the pendulum test for the biceps, a dynamometer or myometer test for the plantar flexors, and EMG studies to compare muscle activity on the two sides of RB's body. These quantitative measures would be especially useful for research that requires more precise measurement than the qualitative measures already performed.

Intervention

Appropriate interventions for RB may come from multiple sources and theoretical backgrounds. Only a few techniques that influence muscle tone are discussed here. Prolonged stretch of the biceps or the plantar flexors may be incorporated into functional activities such as standing with weight on the heels or weight-bearing on the hand in a position to recruit triceps as the agonist and inhibit biceps muscle tone as the antagonist. Prolonged icing (see Chapter 8) or prolonged stretch with an orthotic device may be added if soft tissue or muscle shortening is inhibiting full passive ROM at the shoulder, elbow, wrist, fingers, or ankle. Exercises may be used to facilitate activity of the antagonists to inhibit the biceps or the plantar flexors. ES of triceps and dorsiflexors would provide the dual benefit of inhibiting hypertonic musculature and strengthening muscles that are currently weak (see Chapter 12). EMG biofeedback might be used during a specific task to train RB in more appropriate activation patterns for the biceps or plantar flexors.

Increased hypertonicity as seen during standing could be alleviated by techniques to increase RB's alignment, balance, and confidence while standing. If he is better able to relax in this posture, his muscle tone will decrease as well. Discussion of specific therapeutic exercises to enhance RB's balance and function is beyond the scope of this chapter.

Chapter Review

1. Muscle tone is the passive resistance of a muscle to stretch. This resistance is affected by neural and biomechanical phenomena. Neural input involves subconscious or involuntary activation of motor units via alpha and gamma motor neurons. Biomechanical properties of muscle and myoplastic factors that affect muscle tone include contracture, weak myosin-actin bonds, titin-actin attachments, and abnormal muscle development.
2. Normal muscle tone and activation depend on normal functioning of the muscles, the PNS, and the CNS. The neural component of muscle tone is a result of input from peripheral, spinal, and supraspinal neurons. Summation of their excitatory and inhibitory signals determines whether an alpha motor neuron will send a signal to the muscle to contract or increase tone.
3. Neurally mediated tone abnormalities (hypotonicity, hypertonicity, and fluctuating tone) result from abnormal inhibitory or excitatory input to the alpha motor neuron. Abnormal input may occur as a result of pathologies that affect the alpha and gamma motor neurons or their input.
4. *Hypotonicity* refers to low muscle tone. For patients with hypotonicity, rehabilitation interventions are directed toward increasing tone to promote easier activation of muscles, improving posture, and restoring an acceptable cosmetic appearance. Physical agents that may be used to assist with this include hydrotherapy, quick ice, and ES.
5. *Hypertonicity* refers to high muscle tone. For patients with hypertonicity, rehabilitation interventions are often directed toward decreasing tone to decrease discomfort, increase ROM, allow normal positioning, and prevent contractures. Physical agents used to achieve these goals include heat, prolonged ice, cooling garments, hydrotherapy, biofeedback, and ES.
6. For patients with fluctuating muscle tone, rehabilitation interventions are directed toward normalizing tone to maximize function and prevent injury.

Glossary

Ia sensory neurons: Afferent nerves that carry stretch signals about muscle stretch from muscle spindles to the alpha motor neuron and provide excitatory stimuli for the stretched muscle to contract; these sensory signals are also sent to supraspinal centers.

Actin: A protein found in myofilaments of the sarcomere that participates in muscle contraction when it binds to the myosin protein.

Akinesia: Lack, paucity, or involuntary arrest of movement in general or intermittently occurring in continuous movements such as gait; may be noted in Parkinson disease.

Alpha-gamma coactivation: The activation of gamma motor neurons at the same time as alpha motor neurons during voluntary movement, which allows muscles to respond to perturbations during contraction. Alpha-gamma coactivation sensitizes the muscle spindle to changes in muscle length.

Alpha motor neuron: A neuron that stimulates muscle cells to contract. The cell body is in the central nervous system and the axon is located in the peripheral nervous system.

Athetoid movement: A type of dyskinesia that consists of worm-like writhing movements.

Autogenic inhibition: The mechanism by which type Ib sensory fibers from the Golgi tendon organs send simultaneous signals to inhibit agonist (homonymous) muscles while stimulating antagonist muscles to contract.

Ballismus: A type of dyskinesia that consists of large, throwing-type movements.

Basal ganglia: Groups of neurons (nuclei) located in the brain that modulate volitional movement, locomotion, postural tone, and cognition.

Biofeedback: The technique of making unconscious or involuntary body processes perceptible to the senses to facilitate manipulation of them by conscious mental control.

Central nervous system (CNS): The part of the nervous system consisting of the brain and the spinal cord.

Cerebellum: The part of the brain that coordinates movement by comparing intended movements with actual movements and correcting for movement errors or unexpected obstacles to movement.

Chorea: A type of dyskinesia that consists of dance-like, sharp, jerky movements.

Clasp-knife phenomenon: Initial resistance followed by sudden release of resistance in response to quick stretch of a hypertonic muscle.

Clonus: Multiple rhythmical oscillations or beats in the resistance of a muscle responding to quick stretch.

Contracture: Chronic shortening of muscle and soft tissue resulting in a loss of range of motion.

Denervation: Removal of neural input to an end organ.

Dyskinesia: Abnormal movement that is involuntary and without purpose.

Dystonia: A type of hypertonicity that consists of involuntary sustained muscle contraction, sometimes in antagonistic muscle groups.

Electromyography (EMG): Record of the electrical activity of muscles using surface or fine wire/needle electrodes.

Flaccidity: Lack of tone or absence of resistance to passive stretch within the middle range of the muscle's length.

Flaccid paralysis: A state characterized by loss of both muscle contraction (paralysis) and muscle tone (flaccidity).

Gamma motor neurons: Neurons that innervate muscle spindles at the polar end regions to cause the central region of the spindle to tighten, making muscle spindles more sensitive to muscle stretch.

Golgi tendon organs (GTOs): Sensory organs at the musculotendinous junction that detect muscle contraction or tension.

Guarding: A protective, involuntary increase in muscle tension in response to pain that manifests itself as muscle spasms.

Hypertonicity: High tone or increased resistance to stretch compared with normal muscles.

Hypotonicity: Low tone or decreased resistance to stretch compared with normal muscles.

Interneurons: Neurons that connect other neurons by transmitting signals between them.

Limbic system: A collection of neurons in the brain involved in generating emotions, memories, and motivation; can affect muscle tone through connections with the hypothalamus, reticular system, and basal ganglia.

Lower motor neuron: Another term for *alpha motor neuron.*

Motor unit: A single alpha motor neuron, or lower motor neuron, plus all the muscle fibers innervated by any of its branches.

Muscle spasm: Involuntary, neurogenic muscle shortening or holding, usually in response to a noxious stimulus.

Muscle spindles: Sensory organs that lie within muscle; they sense when muscle is stretched and send sensory signals via type Ia sensory neurons.

Muscle stretch reflex: Fast contractions of the muscle in response to stretch, mediated by the monosynaptic connection between the Ia sensory neurons and alpha motor neurons and usually tested by tapping on the tendon; also called the *deep tendon reflex.*

Muscle tone: The underlying tension in a muscle that serves as a background for contraction.

Myofilaments: Contractile and regulatory proteins of sarcomeres, including actin and myosin.

Myosin: One of the myofilaments in sarcomeres that have binding sites for adenosine triphosphate (ATP) and actin; when stimulated, these proteins bind with actin and help develop muscle force.

Neurons: Nerve cells, including the body (soma), nucleus, and all its projections (dendrites and axon)

Paralysis: Complete loss of voluntary muscle contraction.

Paresis: Incomplete paralysis; weakness because of partial loss of voluntary muscle contraction.

Pendulum test: A test for spasticity that uses gravity to provide a quick stretch for a particular muscle group; measured by observing the resistance to stretch in the swing of the limb after the stretch.

Peripheral nervous system (PNS): The part of the nervous system that lies outside the central nervous system (i.e., outside the brain and spinal cord).

Reciprocal inhibition: A mechanism by which agonist muscles are excited while antagonist muscles are simultaneously inhibited so that they do not work against each other; also called *reciprocal innervation.*

Red nucleus: Brainstem nucleus from which the rubrospinal tract arises.

Reticular formation: A group of neurons located in the central brainstem that receive sensory, autonomic, and hypothalamic input and influence muscle tone to reflect the individual's emotions, motivation, and alertness.

Rigidity: An abnormal, hypertonic state in which involuntary muscle hyperactivity contributes to muscle stiffness, immovability, and resistance to stretch, regardless of the velocity of the stretch.

Sarcomere: The contractile unit of muscle fibers, consisting of the contractile proteins actin and myosin, along with many structural proteins, including titin.

Spasticity: An abnormal, hypertonic muscle response in people with upper motor neuron dysfunction in which quicker passive muscle stretches elicit greater resistance than is elicited by slower stretches.

Supraspinal: Central nervous system areas that originate above the spinal cord in the upright human. Supraspinal neurons that synapse with either alpha motor neurons or spinal interneurons that connect to alpha motor neurons are called *upper motor neurons.*

Synergy: Pattern of muscle contraction in which several muscles work together to produce a movement. Abnormal synergies may occur when the individual lacks the motor control to contract the muscles in isolation.

Titin: Large intramuscular protein primarily responsible for the elastic quality of muscle.

Tremor: A type of dyskinesia that consists of low-amplitude, high-frequency oscillating movements.

Upper motor neuron: Supraspinal neurons that make connections either directly or indirectly through interneurons with lower motor neurons.

Vestibular system: The parts of the inner ear and brainstem that receive, integrate, and transmit information about the position of the head in relation to gravity and rotation of the head and contribute to maintenance of upright posture.

References

1. Simons DG, Mense S: Understanding and measurement of muscle tone as related to clinical muscle pain. *Pain* 75:1–17, 1998.
2. Davidoff RA: Skeletal muscle tone and the misunderstood stretch reflex. *Neurology* 42:951–963, 1992.
3. Gao F, Zhang L-Q: Altered contractile properties of the gastrocnemius muscle post stroke. *J Appl Physiol* 105:1802–1808, 2008.
4. Ashford SA, Siegert RJ, Williams H, et al: Psychometric evaluation of the leg activity measure (legA) for outcome measurement in people with brain injury and spasticity. *Disabil Rehabil* 43(7):976–987, 2021. doi:10.1080/09638288.2019.1643933.
5. Dressler D, Bhidayasiri R, Bohlega S, et al: Defining spasticity: a new approach considering current movement disorders terminology and botulinum toxin therapy. *J Neurol* 265:856–862, 2018.
6. Scheets PL, Sahrmann SA, Norton BJ: Use of movement system diagnoses in the management of patients with neuromuscular conditions: a multiple-patient case report. *Phys Ther* 87(Suppl. Appendices 1 and 2):654–669, 2007.
7. Sanger TD, Delgado MR, Gaebler-Spira D, et al: Classification and definition of disorders causing hypertonia in childhood. *Pediatrics* 111:89–97, 2003.
8. Malhotra S, Pandyan AD, Day CR, et al: Spasticity, an impairment that is poorly defined and poorly measured. *Clin Rehabil* 23:651–658, 2009.
9. Sahrmann SA, Norton BJ: The relationship of voluntary movement to spasticity in the upper motor neuron syndrome. *Ann Neurol* 2:460–465, 1977.
10. Bobath B: *Adult hemiplegia: evaluation and treatment*, ed 2, London, 1978, Heinemann.
11. Albanese A: The clinical expression of primary dystonia. *J Neurol* 250:1145–1151, 2003.
12. Claypool DW, Duane DD, Ilstrup DM, et al: Epidemiology and outcome of cervical dystonia (spasmodic torticollis) in Rochester, Minnesota. *Mov Disord* 10:608–614, 1995.
13. Peterson DA, Berque P, Jabusch H-C, et al: Rating scales for musician's dystonia: the state of the art. *Neurology* 81:589–598, 2013.
14. Hebert D, Lindsay MP, McIntyre A, et al: Canadian stroke best practice recommendations: stroke rehabilitation practice guidelines, update 2015. *Int J Stroke* 11:459–484, 2016.
15. Teasell R: Musculoskeletal complications of hemiplegia following stroke. *Semin Arthritis Rheum* 20:385–395, 1991.
16. Dietz V, Quintern J, Berger W: Electrophysiological studies of gait in spasticity and rigidity: evidence that altered mechanical properties of muscle contribute to hypertonicity. *Brain* 104:431–449, 1981.
17. Aloraini SM, Gaverth J, Yeung E, et al: Assessment of spasticity after stroke using clinical measures: a systematic review. *Disabil Rehabil* 37:2313–2323, 2015.
18. Flamand VH, Masse-Alarie H, Schneider C: Psychometric evidence of spasticity measurement tools in cerebral palsy children and adolescents: a systematic review. *J Rehabil Med* 45:14–23, 2013.
19. Naidoo P: Towards evidence-based practice—a systematic review of methods and tests used in the clinical assessment of hypotonia. *South African J Occup Ther* 43:2–8, 2013.
20. Giuliani C: Dorsal rhizotomy for children with cerebral palsy: support for concepts of motor control. *Phys Ther* 71:248–259, 1991.
21. Boiteau M, Malouin F, Richards CL: Use of a hand-held dynamometer and a Kin-ComR dynamometer for evaluating spastic hypertonicity in children: a reliability study. *Phys Ther* 75:796–802, 1995.
22. Lidstrom A, Ahlsten G, Hirchfeld H, et al: Intrarater and interrater reliability of myotonometer measurements of muscle tone in children. *J Child Neurol* 24:267–274, 2009.
23. Starsky AJ, Sangani SG, McGuire JR, et al: Reliability of biomechanical spasticity measurements at the elbow of people poststroke. *Arch Phys Med Rehabil* 86:1648–1654, 2005.
24. Grippo A, Carrai R, Hawamdeh Z, et al: Biomechanical and electromyographic assessment of spastic hypertonus in motor complete traumatic spinal cord-injured individuals. *Spinal Cord* 49:142–148, 2011.
25. Cano-de-la-Cuerda R, Vela-Desojo L, Mingolarra-Page JC, et al: Axial rigidity and quality of life in patients with Parkinson's disease: a preliminary study. *Qual Life Res* 20:817–823, 2011.
26. Oonagh MG, Persson UM, Caulfield B: Biofeedback in rehabilitation. *J Neuroeng Rehabil* 10, 2013. https://jneuroengrehab.biomedcentral.com/articles/10.1186/1743-0003-10-60.
27. Basmajian JV, De Luca CJ: *Muscles alive: their functions revealed by electromyography*, ed 5, Baltimore, 1985, Williams & Wilkins.
28. Jamshidi M, Smith AW: Clinical measurement of spasticity using the pendulum test: comparison of electrogoniometric and videotape analyses. *Arch Phys Med Rehabil* 77:1129–1132, 1996.
29. Bohannon RW: Variability and reliability of the pendulum test for spasticity using a Cybex II Isokinetic Dynamometer. *Phys Ther* 67:659–661, 1987.
30. Bohannon RW, Harrison S, Kinsella-Shaw J: Reliability and validity of pendulum test measures of spasticity obtained with the Polhemus tracking system from patients with chronic stroke. *J Neuroeng Rehabil* 6, 2009. https://doi.org/10.1186/1743-0003-6-30.
31. McDougall J, Chow E, Harris LR, et al: Near-infrared spectroscopy as a quantitative spasticity assessment tool: A systematic review. *J Neurol Sci* 412, 2020. doi:10.1016/j.jns.2020.116729.
32. Sigrist RMS, Liau J, Kaffas AE, et al: Ultrasound elastography: review of techniques and clinical applications. *Theranostics* 7(5):1303–1329, 2017.
33. Lehoux MC, Sobczak S, Cloutier F, et al: Shear wave elastography potential to characterize spastic muscles in stroke survivors: literature review. *Clin Biomech* 72:84–93, 2020.
34. O'Sullivan SB, Portney LG: Examination of motor function: motor control and motor learning. In O'Sullivan SB, Schmitz TJ, editors: *Physical rehabilitation,* ed 7, Philadelphia, 2019, FA Davis.
35. Ashworth B: Preliminary trial of carisoprodol in multiple sclerosis. *Practitioner* 192:540–542, 1964.
36. Bohannon RW, Smith MB: Interrater reliability of a modified Ashworth scale of muscle spasticity. *Phys Ther* 67:206–207, 1987.
37. Meseguer-Henarejos AB, Sanches-Meca J, Lopez-Pina JA, et al: Inter- and intra-rater reliability of the Modified Ashworth Scale: a systematic review and meta-analysis. *Eur J Phys Rehabil Med* 54:576–590, 2018.
38. Malhotra S, Cousins E, Ward A, et al: An investigation into the agreement between clinical, biomechanical and neurophysiological measures of spasticity. *Clin Rehabil* 22:1105–1115, 2008.
39. Banky M, Ryan HK, Clark R, et al: Do clinical tests of spasticity accurately reflect muscle function during walking: a systematic review. *Brain Inj* 31(4):440–455, 2017.
40. Tardieu G, Shentoub S, Delarue R: A la recherche d'une technique de mesure de la spasticité. *Rev Neurol* 91:143–144, 1954. In French.
41. Boyd R, Graham HK: Objective measurement of clinical findings in the use of botulinum toxin type A for the management of children with CP. *Eur J Neurol* 6(Suppl 4):S23–S35, 1999.
42. Haugh AB, Pandyan AD, Johnson GR: A systematic review of the Tardieu Scale for the measurement of spasticity. *Disabil Rehabil* 28:899–907, 2006.

43. Synnot A, Chau M, Pitt V, et al: Interventions for managing skeletal muscle spasticity following traumatic brain injury. *Cochrane Database Syst Rev* 2017:CD008929, 2017.

44. Takeuchi N, Kuwabara T, Usuda S: Development and evaluation of a new measure for muscle tone of ankle plantar flexors: the Ankle Plantar Flexors Tone Scale. *Arch Phys Med Rehabil* 90:2054–2061, 2009.

45. Hobart JC, Riazi A, Thompson J, et al: Getting the measure of spasticity in multiple sclerosis: the Multiple Sclerosis Spasticity Scale (MSSS88). *Brain* 129:224–234, 2006.

46. Rodic SZ, Knezevic TI, Kisic-Tepavcevic DB, et al: Validation of the Serbian version of Multiple Sclerosis Spasticity Scale 88 (MSSS-88). *PLoS ONE* 11:e0147042, 2016.

47. Ertzgaard P, Nene A, Kiekens C, et al: A review and evaluation of patient-reported outcome measures for spasticity in persons with spinal cord damage: Recommendations from the Ability Network – an international initiative. *J Spinal Cord Med* 43(6):813–823, 2019. doi:10.1080/10790268.2019.1575533.

48. Bohannon RW, Andrews AW: Influence of head-neck rotation on static elbow flexion force of paretic side in patients with hemiparesis. *Phys Ther* 69:135–137, 1989.

49. Linke WA: Titin elasticity in the context of the sarcomere: force and extensibility measurements on single myofibrils. *Adv Exp Med Biol* 481:179–206, 2000.

50. Granzier H, Labeit S: Structure-function relations of the giant elastic protein titin in striated and smooth muscle cells. *Muscle Nerve* 36:740–755, 2007.

51. Stubbs PW, Walsh LD, D'Souza A, et al: History-dependence of muscle slack length following contraction and stretch in the human vastus lateralis. *J Physiol* 596(11):2121–2129, 2018. doi:10.1113/JP275527.

52. Kandel ER, Schwartz JH, Jessell TM, et al: *Principles of neural science*, ed 5, New York, 2013, McGraw-Hill.

53. Enoka RM: *Neuromechanics of human movement*, ed 5, Champaign, IL, 2015, Human Kinetics.

54. Dhavalikar M, Gupta N: Effect of skin temperature on nerve conduction velocity and reliability of temperature correction formula in Indian females. *J Exerc Sci Phys* 5:24–29, 2009.

55. De Jesus P, Housmanowa-Petrusewicz I, Barchi R: The effect of cold on nerve conduction of human slow and fast nerve fibers. *Neurology* 23:1182–1189, 1973.

56. Nashner LM: Adapting reflexes controlling the human posture. *Exp Brain Res* 26:59–72, 1976.

57. Banks RW: The innervation of the muscle spindle: a personal history. *J Anat* 227:115–135, 2015.

58. Ellaway PH, Taylor A, Durbaba R: Muscle spindle and fusimotor activity in locomotion. *J Anat* 227:157–166, 2015.

59. Knutson GA: The role of the gamma-motor system in increasing muscle tone and muscle pain syndromes: a review of the Johansson/Sojka hypothesis. *J Manipulative Physiol Ther* 23:564–573, 2000.

60. Takakusaki K, Saitoh K, Harada H, et al: Role of basal ganglia-brainstem pathways in the control of motor behaviors. *Neurosci Res* 50:137–151, 2004.

61. Moore JC: The Golgi tendon organ: a review and update. *Am J Occup Ther* 38:227–236, 1984.

62. Chalmers G: Do Golgi tendon organs really inhibit muscle activity at high force levels to save muscles from injury, and adapt with strength training? *Sports Biomech* 1:239–249, 2002.

63. Pearson KG: Role of sensory feedback in the control of stance duration in walking cats. *Brain Res Rev* S7:222–227, 2008.

64. Rossignol S, Dubuc R, Gossard J-P: Dynamic sensorimotor interactions in locomotion. *Physiol Rev* 86:89–154, 2006.

65. O'Sullivan SB: Strategies to improve motor function. In O'Sullivan SB, Schmitz TJ, Fulk GD, editors: *Physical rehabilitation*, ed 7, Philadelphia, 2019, FA Davis.

66. Hagbarth KE: Spinal withdrawal reflexes in human lower limb. In Brunnstrom S, editor: *Movement therapy in hemiplegia: a neurophysiological approach*, Hagerstown, MD, 1970, Harper & Row.

67. Knott M, Voss DE: *Proprioceptive neuromuscular facilitation: patterns and techniques*, ed 2, New York, 1968, Harper & Row.

68. Brunnstrom S, editor: *Movement therapy in hemiplegia: a neurophysiological approach*, Hagerstown, MD, 1970, Harper & Row.

69. Sawner KA, LaVigne JM: *Brunnstrom's movement therapy in hemiplegia: a neurophysiological approach*, ed 2, Philadelphia, 1992, JB Lippincott.

70. Gracies JM, Meunier S, Pierrot-Deseilligny E, et al: Patterns of propriospinal-like excitation to different species of human upper limb motor neurons. *J Physiol* 434:151–167, 1990.

71. McDonald-Williams MF: Exercise and postpolio syndrome. *Neurol Rep* 20:37–44, 1996.

72. Shinodea Y, Sugiuchi Y, Izawa Y, et al: Long descending motor tract axons and their control of neck and axial muscles. *Prog Brain Res* 151:527–563, 2006.

73. Takakusaki K, Chiba R, Nozu T, et al: Brainstem control of locomotion and muscle tone with special reference to the role of the mesopontine tegmentum and medullary reticulospinal systems. *J Neural Transm (Vienna)* 123:695–729, 2015.

74. Davidson AG, Buford JA: Bilateral actions of the reticulospinal tract on arm and shoulder muscles in the monkey: stimulus triggered averaging. *Exp Brain Res* 173:25–39, 2006.

75. Lundy-Ekman L: Motor system: motor neurons and spinal motor function. In Neuroscience: fundamentals for rehabilitation, ed 5, St Louis, 2018, Elsevier.

76. Turner-Stokes L, Ashford S, Esquenazi A, et al: A comprehensive person-centered approach to adult spastic paresis: a consensus-based framework. *Eur J Phys Rehabil Med* 54:605–617, 2018.

77. Teixeira LJ, Valbuza JS, Prado GF: Physical therapy for Bell's palsy (idiopathic facial paralysis). *Cochrane Database Syst Rev* 2011(12):CD006283, 2011.

78. Recknor JB, Mallapragada SK: Nerve regeneration: tissue engineering strategies. In Bronzino JD, editor: *The biomedical engineering handbook: tissue engineering and artificial organs*, New York, 2006, Taylor & Francis.

79. Pfister BJ, Gordon T, Loverde JR, et al: Biomedical engineering strategies for peripheral nerve repair: surgical applications, state of the art, and future challenges. *Crit Rev Biomed Eng* 39:81–124, 2011.

80. Bassile CC: Guillain-Barré syndrome and exercise guidelines. *Neurol Rep* 20:31–36, 1996.

81. White CM, Pritchard J, Turner-Stokes L: Exercise for people with peripheral neuropathy. *Cochrane Database Syst Rev* 2010(1):43, 2010.

82. Morris DM: Aquatic neurorehabilitation. *Neurol Rep* 19:22–28, 1995.

83. Dietz V: Supraspinal pathways and the development of muscle-tone dysregulation. *Dev Med Child Neurol* 41:708–715, 1999.

84. Winstein, et al: Guidelines for adult stroke rehabilitation and recovery: a guideline for healthcare professionals from the American Heart Association/American Stroke Association. *Stroke* 47;e1–e72, 2016.

85. Dunning K, O'Dell MW, Kluding P, et al: Peroneal stimulation for foot drop after stroke: a systematic review. *Am J Phys Med Rehabil* 94:649–664, 2015.

86. Esnouf JE, Taylor PN, Mann GE, et al: Impact on activities of daily living using a functional electrical stimulation device to improve dropped foot in people with multiple sclerosis, measured by the Canadian Occupational Performance Measure. *Mult Scler* 16:1141–1147, 2010.

87. Lehmkuhl LD, Krawczyk L: Physical therapy management of the minimally-responsive patient following traumatic brain injury: coma stimulation. *Neurol Rep* 17:10–17, 1993.

88. Sitjà RM, Rigau CD, Fort Vanmeerhaeghe A, et al: Whole-body vibration training for patients with neurodegenerative disease. *Cochrane Database Sys Rev* 2012(2):CD009097, 2012.

89. Gowland C, deBruin H, Basmajian JV, et al: Agonist and antagonist activity during voluntary upper-limb movement in patients with stroke. *Phys Ther* 72:624–633, 1992.

90. Dietz V: Spastic movement disorder. *Spinal Cord* 38:389–393, 2000.

91. Knutsson E, Martensson A: Dynamic motor capacity in spastic paresis and its relation to prime mover dysfunction, spastic reflexes and antagonist co-activation. *Scand J Rehabil Med* 12:93–106, 1980.

92. Campbell SK, Almeida GL, Penn RD, et al: The effects of intrathecally administered baclofen on function in patients with spasticity. *Phys Ther* 75:352–362, 1995.

93. Biering-Sørensen F, Hansen B, Lee BSB: Non-pharmacological treatment and prevention of bone loss after spinal cord injury: a systematic review. *Spinal Cord* 47:508–518, 2009.

94. Fulk GD, Behrman AL, Schmitz TJ: Traumatic spinal cord injury. In O'Sullivan SB, Schmitz TJ, Fulk GD, editors: *Physical rehabilitation*, ed 7, Philadelphia, 2019, FA Davis.

95. Somers MF: *Spinal cord injury: functional rehabilitation*, Norwalk, CT, 1992, Appleton & Lange.

96. Wiener J, Hsieh J, McIntyre A, Teasell R: Effectiveness of 4-aminopyridine for the management of spasticity in spinal cord injury: a systematic review. *Top Spinal Cord Inj Rehabil* 24(4):353–362, 2018.

97. Bani-Ahmed A: The evidence for prolonged muscle stretching in ankle joint management in upper motor neuron lesions: considerations for rehabilitation—a systematic review. *Top Stroke Rehabil* 26(2):153–161, 2019.

98. Khan F, Amatya B, Bensmail D, et al: Non-pharmacological interventions for spasticity in adults: an overview of systematic reviews. *Ann Phys Rehabil Med* 62:265–273, 2019.

99. Bekhet AH, Bochkezanian V, Saab IM, et al: The effects of electrical stimulation parameters in managing spasticity after spinal cord injury: a systematic review. *Am J Phys Med Rehabil* 98(6):484–499, 2019.

100. Korzhoova J, Sinitsyn D, Chervyakov A, et al: Transcranial and spinal cord magnetic stimulation in treatment of spasticity: a literature review and meta analysis. *Eur J Phys Rehabil Med* 54(1):75–84, 2018.

101. Shumway-Cook A, Woollacott MH: *Motor control: translating research into clinical practice*, ed 5, Philadelphia, 2016, Wolters Kluwer.

102. Rosner LJ, Ross S: *Multiple sclerosis*, New York, 1987, Prentice Hall.

103. Bobath B: *Abnormal postural reflex activity caused by brain lesions*, ed 2, London, 1971, Heinemann.

104. Triccas LT, Kennedy N, Smith T, et al: Predictors of upper limb spasticity after stroke? A systematic review and meta-analysis. *Physiotherapy* 105:163–173, 2019.

105. Duncan PW, Badke MB: Therapeutic strategies for rehabilitation of motor deficits. In Duncan PW, Badke MB, editors: *Stroke rehabilitation: the recovery of motor control*, Chicago, 1987, Year Book Medical Publishers.

106. Buizer AI, Marens BH, van Ravenhorst CG, et al: Effect of continuous intrathecal baclofen therapy in children: a systematic review. *Dev Med Child Neurol* 61(2):128–135, 2019.

107. Intiso D, Santamato A, Di Rienzo F: Effect of electrical stimulation as an adjunct to botulinum toxin type A in the treatment of adult spasticity: a systematic review. *Disabil Rehabil* 39(21):2123–2133, 2017.

108. Salazar AP, Pinto C, Mossi JVR, et al: Effectiveness of static stretching positioning on post-stroke upper limb spasticity and mobility: systematic review with meta-analysis. *Ann Phys Rehabil Med* 62:274–282, 2019.

109. Veldema J, Jansen P: Ergometer training in stroke rehabilitation: systematic review and meta-analysis. *Arch Phys Med Rehabil* 101:674–689, 2020.

110. Dymarek R, Ptaszkowski K, Ptaszkowska L, et al: Shock waves as a treatment modality for spasticity reduction and recovery improvement in post-stroke adults—current evidence and qualitative systematic review. *Clin Interv Aging* 15:9–28, 2020.

111. Guo P, Gao F, Zhao T, et al: Positive effects of extracorporeal shock wave therapy on spasticity in poststroke patients: a meta-analysis. *J Stroke Cerebrovasc Dis* 26(11):2470–2476, 2017.

112. Jia G, Ma J, Wang S, et al: Long-term effects of extracorporeal shock wave therapy on poststroke patients: a meta-analysis of randomized controlled trials. *J Stroke Cerebrovasc Dis* 29(3), 2020. doi:10.1016/j.strokecerebrovasdis.2019.104591.

113. Xiang J, Wang W, Jiang W, et al: Effects of extracorporeal shock wave therapy on spasticity in post-stroke patients: a systematic review and meta-analysis of randomized controlled trials. *J Rehabil Med* 50:852–859, 2018.

114. Oh JH, Park HD, Han SH, et al: Duration of treatment effect of extracorporeal shock wave on spasticity and subgroup-analysis according to number of shocks and application site: a meta-analysis. *Ann Rehabil Med* 43(2):163–177, 2019.

115. Giorgetti MM: Serial and inhibitory casting: implications for acute care physical therapy management. *Neurol Rep* 17:18–21, 1993.

116. Lynch D, Ferraro M, Krol J, et al: Continuous passive motion improves shoulder joint integrity following stroke. *Clin Rehabil* 19:594–599, 2005.

117. McClure PW, Blackburn LG, Dusold C: The use of splints in the treatment of joint stiffness: biologic rationale and an algorithm for making clinical decisions. *Phys Ther* 74:1101–1107, 1994.

118. Mahmood A, Veluswamy SK, Hombali A, et al: Effect of transcutaneous electrical nerve stimulation on spasticity in adults with stroke: a systematic review and meta analysis. *Arch Phys Med Rehabil* 100:751–768, 2019.

119. Marcolino MAZ, Hauck M, Stein C, et al: Effects of transcutaneous electrical nerve stimulation alone or as additional therapy on chronic post-stroke spasticity: systematic review and meta-analysis of randomized controlled trials. *Disabil Rehabil* 42:623–635, 2020.

120. Kwong PWH, Ng GYF, Chung RCK, et al: Transcutaneous electrical nerve stimulation improves walking capacity and reduces spasticity in stroke survivors: a systematic review and meta-analysis. *Clin Rehabil* 32:1203–1219, 2018.

121. Lin S, Sun Q, Wang H, Xie G: Influence of transcutaneous electrical nerve stimulation on spasticity, balance, and walking speed in stroke patients: a systematic review and meta-analysis. *J Rehabil Med* 50:3–7, 2018.

122. Park YJ, Park SW, Lee HS: Comparison of the effectiveness of whole body vibration in stroke patients: a meta-analysis. *Biomed Res Int*, 2018. doi:10.1155/2018/5083634.

123. Huang M, Liao LR, Pang MYC: Effects of whole body vibration on muscle spasticity for people with central nervous system disorders: a systematic review. *Clin Rehabil* 31(1):23–33, 2017.

124. Alashram AR, Padua E, Romagnoli C, Annino G: Effectiveness of focal muscle vibration on hemiplegic upper extremity spasticity in individuals with stroke: a systematic review. *Neurorehabil* 45:471–481, 2019.

125. McIntyre A, Mirkowski M, Thompson A, et al: A systematic review and meta-analysis on the use of repetitive transcranial magnetic stimulation for spasticity poststroke. *PM&R* 10:293–302, 2018.

126. Cai Y, Zhang CS, Liu S, et al: Electroacupuncture for poststroke spasticity: a systematic review and meta-analysis. *Arch Phys Med Rehabil* 98:2578–2589, 2017.

127. Wang M, Pei ZW, Xiong BD, et al: Use of Kinesio taping in lower-extremity rehabilitation of post-stroke patients: a systematic review and meta-analysis. *Complement Ther Clin Pract* 35:22–32, 2019.

128. Veerbeek JM, Langbroek-Amersfoort AC, van Wegen EEH, et al: Effects of robot-assisted therapy for the upper limb after stroke: a systematic review and analysis. *Neurorehab Neural Rev* 3(2):107–121, 2017.

129. Serrezuela RR, Quezada MT, Zayas MH, et al: Robotic therapy for the hemiplegic shoulder pain: a pilot study. *J Neuroeng Rehabil* 17:54, 2020.

130. Yana M, Tutuola F, Westwater-Wood S, et al: The efficacy of botulinum toxin A lower limb injections in addition to physiotherapy approaches in children with cerebral palsy: a systematic review. *Neurorehabil* 44:175–189, 2019.

131. Etoom M, Khraiwesh Y, Lena F, et al: Effectiveness of physiotherapy interventions on spasticity in people with multiple sclerosis. *Am J Phys Med Rehabil* 97:793–807, 2018.

132. Fu X, Wang Y, Wang C, et al: A mixed treatment comparison on efficacy and safety of treatments for spasticity caused by multiple sclerosis: a systematic review and network meta-analysis. *Clin Rehabil* 32(6):713–721, 2018.

133. Yeh SW, Lin LF, Tam KW, et al: Efficacy of robot-assisted gait training in multiple sclerosis: a systematic review and meta-analysis. *Mult Scler Relat Dis* 41, 2020. doi:10.1016/j.msard.2020.102034.

134. Kim HJ, Park JW, Nam K: Effect of extracorporeal shockwave therapy on muscle spasticity in patients with cerebral palsy: systematic review and meta analysis. *Eur J Phys Rehabil Med* 55(6):761–771, 2019.

135. Scally JB, Baker JS, Rankin J, et al: Evaluating functional electrical stimulation (FES) cycling on cardiovascular, musculoskeletal and functional outcomes in adults with multiple sclerosis and mobility impairment: a systematic review. *Mult Scler Relat Disord* 37, 2020. doi:10.1016/j.msard.2019.101485.

136. Nilsagård Y, Denison E, Gunnarsson LG: Evaluation of a single session with cooling garment for persons with multiple sclerosis—a randomized trial. *Disabil Rehabil Assist Technol* 1:225–233, 2006.

137. Allan GM, Finley CR, Ton J, et al: Systematic review of systematic reviews for medical cannabinoids. *Can Fam Physician* 64:e78–e94, 2018.

138. Van Criekinge T, D'Aout K, O'Briend J, et al: Effect of music listening on hypertonia in neurologically impaired patients—a systematic review. *PeerJ* 7:e8228, 2019. doi:10.7717/peerj.8228.

139. Cutson TM, Laub KC, Schenkman M: Pharmacological and nonpharmacological interventions in the treatment of Parkinson's disease. *Phys Ther* 75:363–373, 1995.

140. Hengeveld K, Banks K, editors: *Maitland's vertebral manipulation: management of neuromusculoskeletal disorders*, vol 1, ed 8, London, 2013, Churchill Livingstone.

141. Grieve GP: *Common vertebral joint problems*, ed 2, Edinburgh, 1988, Churchill Livingstone.

142. Sahrmann S: *Diagnosis and treatment of movement impairment syndromes*, Philadelphia, 2002, Mosby.

Motion Restrictions

Linda G. Monroe

CHAPTER OBJECTIVES

After reading this chapter, the reader will be able to do the following:
- Define *range of motion* and the different types of motion.
- Describe the different types of motion restrictions and the pathologies that cause them.
- Select the appropriate treatment for each type of motion restriction.
- Safely and effectively apply treatment for motion restrictions.

This chapter discusses motion that occurs between body segments and factors that can restrict this motion. The amount of motion that occurs when one segment of the body moves in relation to an adjacent segment is known as **range of motion (ROM).** When a segment of the body moves through its available ROM, all tissues in that region, including bones, joint capsules, ligaments, tendons, intraarticular structures, muscles, nerves, fasciae, and skin, may be affected. If all these tissues function normally, full ROM can be achieved; however, dysfunction of any of these tissues may restrict available ROM. Many patients in rehabilitation seek medical treatment for motion restrictions. To restore motion most effectively, the therapist must understand the factors that influence normal motion and the factors that may contribute to motion restrictions. Accurately assessing motion restrictions and the tissues involved is necessary for the clinician to choose the best treatment modalities and parameters for optimal patient outcomes.

Motion restriction is an impairment that may directly or indirectly contribute to a patient's functional limitation and disability. For example, restricted shoulder ROM may impair an individual's ability to raise the arm above shoulder height and may prevent the individual from performing a job that involves overhead lifting. This impairment may contribute indirectly to further pathology by causing impingement of rotator cuff tendons, resulting in pain, weakness, and increased limitation in the ability to perform activities that require reaching.

In the absence of pathology, ROM is generally constrained by tissue length or the approximation (bringing together) of anatomical structures. The integrity and flexibility of the soft tissues surrounding a joint and the shapes and relationships of articular structures affect the amount of motion that can occur. When a joint is in the middle of its range, it can generally be moved by applying a small force because collagen fibers in the connective tissue surrounding the joint are in a relaxed state. The relaxed collagen fibers are loosely oriented in various directions and are only sparsely cross-linked with other fibers, allowing them to readily distend. As a joint approaches the end of its range, the collagen fibers begin to

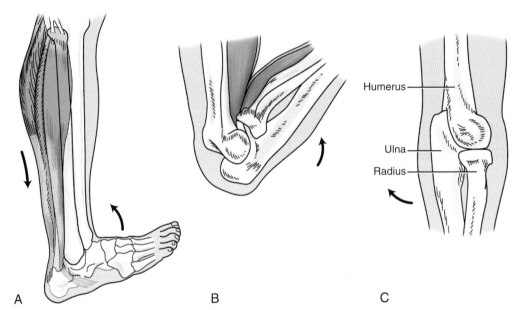

FIGURE 6.1 (A) Ankle dorsiflexion limited by soft tissue distention. (B) Elbow flexion limited by soft tissue approximation. (C) Elbow extension limited by bone approximation.

align in the direction of the stress and start to straighten. Motion ceases at the normal terminal range when fibers have achieved their maximum alignment or when soft or bony tissues approximate. For example, ankle dorsiflexion normally ends when fibers of the calf muscles have achieved maximum alignment and are fully lengthened (Fig. 6.1A), whereas elbow flexion normally ends when soft tissues of the anterior arm approximate with soft tissues of the anterior forearm (Fig. 6.1B), and elbow extension ends when the olecranon process of the ulna approximates with the olecranon fossa of the humerus (Fig. 6.1C).

Normal ROM for all human joints has been measured and documented.[1] However, these measures vary with the individual's sex, age, and health status.[2–4] ROM is generally greater in women than in men and decreases with age, although differences vary with different motions and joints and are not consistent for all individuals.[5–11] Because of this variability, normal ROM is determined by comparison with the motion of the contralateral limb, if available, rather than comparison with normative data. A motion is considered to be "restricted" when it is less than that of the same segment on the contralateral side of the same individual. When a normal contralateral side is not available—as occurs, for example, with the spine or when both shoulders are affected—motion is considered to be restricted when it is less than the normative data indicate for individuals of the same age and sex.

Types of Motion

The motion of body segments can be classified as active or passive.

ACTIVE MOTION

Active motion is the movement produced by contraction of the muscles crossing a joint. Examination of active ROM can provide information about an individual's functional abilities. Active motion may be restricted because of muscle weakness, abnormal muscle tone, pain, inability or unwillingness of the patient to follow directions, or restrictions in passive ROM.

PASSIVE MOTION

Passive motion is movement produced entirely by an external force without voluntary muscle contraction by the patient. The external force may be produced by gravity, a machine, another individual, or another part of the patient's own body. Passive motion may be restricted by soft tissue shortening, edema, **adhesion,** mechanical block, spinal disc herniation, or adverse neural tension.

Normal passive ROM is greater than normal active ROM when motion is limited by lengthening or approximation of soft tissue, but active and passive motion are equal when motion is limited by approximation of bone. For example, a few degrees of passive ankle dorsiflexion motion beyond the limits of active motion are possible because the limiting tissues are elastic and may be lengthened by an external force that is greater than that of active muscles when at terminal active ROM. A few degrees of additional passive elbow flexion beyond the limits of the active range are possible because limiting tissues are compressible by an external force greater than that of active muscles in that position and because approximating muscles may be less bulky when relaxed. This additional passive ROM may protect joint structures by absorbing external forces during activities performed at or close to the end of the active range.

PHYSIOLOGICAL AND ACCESSORY MOTION

Physiological motion is the motion of one segment of the body relative to another segment. For example, physiological knee extension is the straightening of the knee that occurs when the leg moves away from the thigh. **Accessory motion,** also called *joint play,* is the motion that occurs between joint surfaces during normal physiological motion.[12,13] For example,

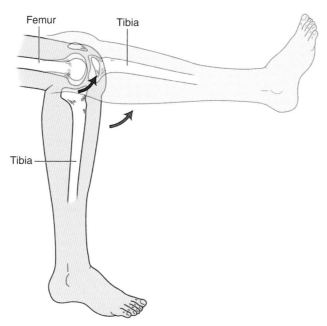

FIGURE 6.2 Accessory anterior gliding of the tibia on the femur *(red arrow)* during physiological knee extension *(blue arrow)*.

anterior gliding of the tibia on the femur is the accessory motion that occurs during physiological knee extension (Fig. 6.2). Accessory motions may be intraarticular, as in the prior example of anterior tibial gliding during knee extension, or extraarticular, as with upward rotation of the scapula during physiological shoulder flexion (Fig. 6.3). Although accessory motions cannot be performed actively in isolation from their associated physiological movement, they may be performed passively.

Normal accessory motion is required for normal active and passive joint motion to occur. The direction of normal accessory motion depends on the shape of the articular surfaces and the direction of physiological motion. Concave joint surfaces require accessory gliding to be available in the direction of the associated physiological motion of the segment, whereas convex joint surfaces require accessory gliding to be available in the opposite direction of the associated physiological motion of the segment.[12] For example, the tibial plateau, which has a concave surface at the knee, glides anteriorly during knee extension when the tibia is moving anteriorly, and the femoral condyles, which have convex surfaces at the knee, glide posteriorly during knee extension when the femur is moving anteriorly.

> ### ◎ Clinical Pearl
>
> With concave joint surfaces, accessory gliding occurs in the direction of the associated physiological joint motion. With convex joint surfaces, accessory gliding occurs in the direction opposite to the associated physiological joint motion.

Patterns of Motion Restriction

Restriction of motion at a joint can be classified as having a capsular or a noncapsular pattern.

CAPSULAR PATTERN OF MOTION RESTRICTION

A **capsular pattern of restriction** is the specific combination of motion loss that is caused by shortening of the joint capsule surrounding a joint. Each synovial joint has a unique capsular pattern of restriction.[14] Capsular patterns generally include restrictions of motion in multiple directions. For example, the capsular pattern for the glenohumeral joint involves restriction of external rotation, abduction, internal rotation, and flexion to progressively smaller degrees. Capsular patterns of restriction may be caused by the effusion, fibrosis, or inflammation commonly associated with degenerative joint disease, arthritis, immobilization, or acute trauma.[15]

NONCAPSULAR PATTERN OF MOTION RESTRICTION

A **noncapsular pattern of restriction** is motion loss that does not follow the capsular pattern. A noncapsular pattern of motion loss may be caused by a ligamentous adhesion, an internal derangement, or an extraarticular lesion.

Ligamentous adhesion will limit motion in directions that stretch the adhered ligament. For example, an adhesion of the talofibular ligament after an ankle sprain will restrict ankle inversion because this motion places the adhered ligament on stretch; however, this adhesion will not alter the motion of the ankle in other directions. Internal derangement, the displacement of loose fragments within a joint, will generally limit motion only in the direction that compresses the fragment. For example, a cartilage fragment in the knee generally will limit knee extension but will not limit knee flexion. Extraarticular lesions, such as muscle adhesions, hematomas, cysts, or inflamed bursae, may limit motion in the direction of stretch or compression, depending on the nature of the lesion. For example, adhesion of the quadriceps muscle to the shaft of the femur will limit stretching of the muscle, whereas a

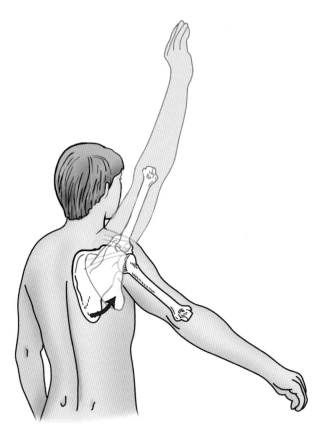

FIGURE 6.3 Extraarticular accessory motion (upward rotation of the scapula) accompanies shoulder flexion.

popliteal cyst will limit compression of the popliteal area. Both of these lesions will restrict motion in the noncapsular pattern of restricted knee flexion, with full, painless knee extension.

Tissues That Can Restrict Motion

Any of the musculoskeletal tissues in the area of a motion restriction may contribute to that restriction. These tissues are most readily classified as contractile or noncontractile (Box 6.1).

CONTRACTILE TISSUES

Contractile tissue is composed of the musculotendinous unit, which includes the muscle, the musculotendinous junction, the tendon, and the interface of the tendon with bone. Skeletal muscle is considered to be contractile because it can contract by forming cross-bridges of myosin proteins with actin proteins within its fibers. Tendons and their attachments to bone are considered contractile because contracting muscles apply tension directly to these structures. When a muscle contracts, it applies tension to its tendons, causing the bones to which it is attached and surrounding tissues to move through the available active ROM. When all components of the musculotendinous unit and the **noncontractile tissues** are functioning normally, available active ROM will be within normal limits. Injury or dysfunction of contractile tissue generally restricts active ROM in the direction of movement produced by contraction of the musculotendinous unit.

Box 6.1	Contractile and Noncontractile Sources of Motion Restriction	
CONTRACTILE TISSUE	**NONCONTRACTILE TISSUE**	
Muscle	Skin	
Musculotendinous junction	Ligament	
Tendon	Bursa	
Tendinous interface with bone	Capsule	
	Articular cartilage	
	Intervertebral disc	
	Peripheral nerve	
	Dura mater	

Dysfunction of contractile tissue may also result in pain or weakness on resisted testing of the musculotendinous unit. For example, a tear in the anterior tibialis muscle or tendon can restrict active dorsiflexion at the ankle and reduce the force generated by resisted testing of ankle dorsiflexion, but this lesion is not likely to alter passive plantar flexion or dorsiflexion ROM or active plantar flexion strength.

NONCONTRACTILE TISSUES

All tissues that are not components of the musculotendinous unit are considered noncontractile. Noncontractile tissues include skin, fascia, scar tissue, ligament, bursa, capsule,

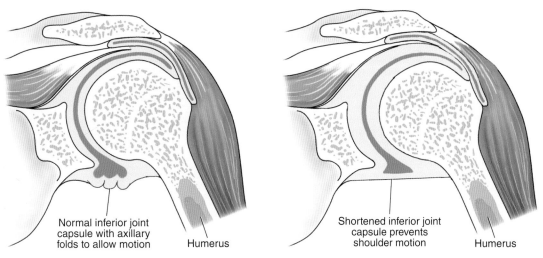

FIGURE 6.4 Joint capsule shortening and adhesion restricting shoulder range of motion.

articular cartilage, bone, intervertebral disc, nerve, and dura mater. When the noncontractile tissues in an area are functioning normally, passive ROM of the segments in that area will be within normal limits. Injury or dysfunction of noncontractile tissue can cause a restriction of passive ROM of joints in the area of the tissue in question and may contribute to restriction of active ROM. The direction, degree, and nature of the motion restriction depend on the type of noncontractile tissue involved, the type of tissue dysfunction, and the severity of involvement. For example, adhesive capsulitis of the shoulder, which involves shortening of the glenohumeral joint capsule and elimination of the inferior axillary fold, will restrict both passive and active shoulder ROM (Fig. 6.4).[16-22]

Pathologies That Can Cause Motion Restriction
CONTRACTURE
Motion may be restricted if any of the soft tissue structures in an area have become shortened. Such soft tissue shortening, known as a **contracture,** may occur in contractile or noncontractile tissues.[23,24] A contracture may be a consequence of external immobilization or lack of use. External immobilization usually is produced with a splint or a cast. Lack of use is usually the result of weakness, as may occur after poliomyelitis; poor motor control, as may occur after a stroke; or pain, as may occur after trauma. The pathophysiology of contracture is not well understood, despite the prevalence of contractures in patients who are immobilized for a prolonged period of time. This is due, in part, to the complex mix of tissues involved, the multiple circumstances that lead to immobilization, and the different changes that occur over time. It is believed that immobilization results in contracture because it allows anomalous cross-links to form between collagen fibers and because it causes fluid to be lost from fibrous connective tissue, including tendon, capsule, ligament, and fascia.[22,25-27] Anomalous cross-links can develop when tissues remain stationary because fibers remain in contact with each other for prolonged periods in the absence

of normal stress and motion and then start to adhere at their points of interception. These cross-links may prevent normal alignment of collagen fibers when motion is attempted. They increase the stress required to stretch the tissue, limit tissue extension, and result in contracture (Fig. 6.5). Fluid loss can also impair normal fiber gliding, causing collagen fibrils to have closer contact and limiting tissue extension.[28]

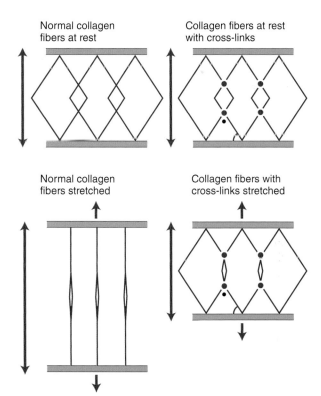

FIGURE 6.5 Normal collagen fibers and collagen fibers with cross-links. (Adapted from Woo SL, Matthews JV, Akeson WH, et al: Connective tissue response to immobility: correlative study of biomechanical measurements of normal and immobilized rabbit knees. *Arthritis Rheum* 18:262, 1975.)

The risk of contracture formation in response to immobilization is increased when the tissue has been injured because scar tissue, which is formed during the proliferation phase of healing, tends to have poor fiber alignment and a high degree of cross-linking between its fibers. Restriction of motion after an injury may be further aggravated if a concurrent problem, such as sepsis or ongoing trauma, amplifies the inflammatory response and causes excessive scarring.[24,26]

Permanent shortening of a muscle that produces deformity or distortion is termed a *muscle contracture*. A muscle contracture can be caused by prolonged muscle spasm, guarding, muscle imbalance, muscle disease, ischemic muscle necrosis, or immobilization. A muscle contracture may limit active and passive motion of joints that the muscle crosses and can cause deformity of joints normally controlled by the muscle.

When a joint is immobilized, structures that contribute to the limitation in ROM may change over time.[29] Trudel and Uhthoff[30] reported that restrictions in ROM during immobilization in an animal model were caused initially by changes in muscle, but articular structures from week 2 to week 32 contributed more to limitations in ROM.

EDEMA

Normally, a joint capsule contains fluid and is not fully distended when the joint is in midrange. This allows the capsule to fold or distend, altering its size and shape as needed for movement through full ROM. **Intraarticular edema** is excessive fluid formation inside a joint capsule. This type of edema distends the joint capsule and potentially restricts both passive and active joint motion in a capsular pattern. For example, intraarticular edema in the knee will limit knee flexion and extension, with flexion most affected.

Accumulation of fluid outside the joint, a condition known as **extraarticular edema,** may also restrict active and passive motion by causing soft tissue approximation to occur earlier in the range. Extraarticular edema generally restricts motion in a noncapsular pattern. For example, edema in the calf muscle may restrict knee flexion ROM but may have no effect on knee extension ROM.

> ### Clinical Pearl
>
> Intraarticular edema restricts motion in a capsular pattern. Extraarticular edema restricts motion in a noncapsular pattern.

ADHESION

Adhesion is the abnormal joining of parts to each other.[31] Adhesion may occur between different types of tissue and frequently causes restriction of motion. During the healing process, scar tissue can adhere to surrounding structures. Fibrofatty tissue may proliferate inside joints, and it may adhere between intraarticular structures as it matures into scar tissue.[32] Prolonged joint immobilization, even in the absence of local injury, can cause the synovial membrane surrounding the joint to adhere to the cartilage inside the joint. Adhesions can affect both the quality and the quantity of joint motion. For example, with adhesive capsulitis, adhesion of the joint capsule to the synovial membrane limits the quantity of motion. This adhesion also reduces, or even obliterates, the

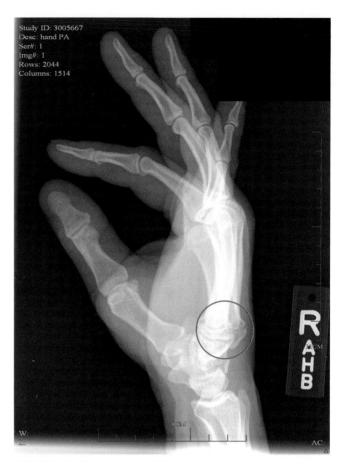

FIGURE 6.6 Osteophytes inhibiting carpal-metacarpal movement. (Courtesy J. Michael Pearson, MD, Oregon Health & Science University, Portland, OR.)

space between the cartilage and the synovial membrane, blocking normal synovial fluid nutrition and causing articular cartilage degeneration that can alter the quality of joint motion.[23,24,27]

MECHANICAL BLOCK

Motion can be mechanically blocked by bone or fragments of articular cartilage or by tears in intraarticular discs or menisci. Degenerative joint disease (and associated **osteophyte** formation) or malunion of bony segments after fracture healing frequently results in the formation of a bony block that restricts joint motion in one or more directions (Fig. 6.6). These pathologies cause extra bone to form in or around the joints. Loose bodies or fragments of articular cartilage, caused by avascular necrosis or trauma, can alter the mechanics of the joint, causing "locking" in various positions, pain, and other dysfunctions.[23,24,33] Tears in intraarticular fibrocartilaginous discs and menisci caused by high-force traumatic injury or by repetitive low-force strain generally block motion in one direction only.

SPINAL DISC HERNIATION

Spinal disc herniation may result in direct blockage of spinal motion if part of the disc material becomes trapped in a facet joint or if the disc compresses a spinal nerve root where it passes through the vertebral foramen. Spinal disc herniation is also often associated with other conditions that further limit spinal motion, including inflammation, hypertrophic changes, decreased disc height, or pain. Inflammation about the spinal facet joint or herniated segment can limit motion by narrowing the vertebral foramen and compressing the nerve root. Hypertrophic changes at the vertebral margins and facet joints, as well as decreased disc height, also narrow the vertebral foramen, making the nerve root more vulnerable to compression. Pain may limit motion by causing involuntary muscle spasms or by causing the individual to restrict movements voluntarily.

ADVERSE NEURAL TENSION

Under normal circumstances, the nervous system, including the spinal cord and the peripheral nerves, adapts to both mechanical and physiological stresses.[34] For example, during forward flexion of the trunk, the nervous system must adapt to the increased length of the spinal column without interruption of transmission.[35] Adverse neural tension, also described as *adverse mechanical tension of the nervous system*[36,37] or *nerve mechanosensitivity*,[38,39] is abnormal physiological and mechanical responses created by nervous system structures when their ROM and stretch capabilities are impaired.[40,41] Adverse neural tension may be caused by major or minor nerve injury or indirectly by extraneural adhesions that result in tethering of the nerve to surrounding structures. Nerve injury may be the result of trauma caused by friction, compression, or stretch. It may also be caused by disease, ischemia, inflammation, or a disruption in the axonal transport system. Ischemia can be caused by pressure exerted by extravascular fluid, blood, disc material, or soft tissues.

Adverse neural tension is most commonly caused by restricted nerve motion. Several structural features predispose nerve motion to restriction. Nerve motion is commonly restricted where nerves pass through tunnels, for example, where the median nerve passes through the carpal tunnel or where the spinal nerves pass through the intervertebral foramina. Peripheral nerve motion is likely to be restricted at points where the nerves branch, for example, where the ulnar nerve splits at the hook of the hamate or where the sciatic nerve splits into the peroneal and tibial nerves in the thigh. Places where the system is relatively fixed are also points of vulnerability, such as at the dura mater at L4 or where the common peroneal nerve passes the head of the fibula. The system is relatively fixed where nerves are close to unyielding interfaces, for instance, where the cords of the brachial plexus pass over the first rib or where the greater occipital nerve passes through the fascia in the posterior skull.[40]

WEAKNESS

When muscles are too weak to generate the force required to move a segment of the body through its normal ROM, active ROM will be restricted. Muscle weakness may result from changes in the contractile tissue, such as atrophy, injury, poor transmission to or along motor nerves, or poor synaptic transmission at the neuromuscular junction.

OTHER FACTORS

Motion restrictions may be caused by many other factors, including pain, psychological factors, and tone. Pain may restrict active or passive motion depending on whether contractile or noncontractile structures are the source of the pain. Psychological factors such as fear, poor motivation, or poor comprehension are most likely to cause restriction only of active ROM. Tone abnormalities, including spasticity, hypotonia, and flaccidity, may impair the control of muscle contractions, thus limiting active ROM.

Examination and Evaluation of Motion Restriction

Assessing motion requires examining the mobility of all structures in the area of restriction, including joints, muscles, intraarticular and extraarticular structures, and nerves. A thorough examination of all these structures is required to determine the pathophysiology underlying the motion restriction, to identify the tissues limiting motion, and to evaluate the severity and irritability of the dysfunction. A complete examination and evaluation can then direct treatment to the appropriate structures and will facilitate selecting the optimal intervention to meet the goals. Accurate assessments and reassessments of motion are essential for optimal use of physical agents to meet outcomes, and ongoing examination and evaluation of outcomes are required so that treatment is modified appropriately in response to changes in the dysfunction. Various tools and methods are available to quantitatively and qualitatively examine motion and motion restrictions.

QUANTITATIVE MEASURES

Goniometers, tape measures, and various types of inclinometers are commonly used in the clinical setting to quantitatively measure ROM (Fig. 6.7). These tools provide objective and moderately reliable measures of ROM and are practical and convenient for clinical use.[42–45] Radiographs, photographs, electrogoniometers, flexometers, and plumb lines may be used to enhance the accuracy and reliability of ROM measurement; these tools are often used for research purposes but are not available in most clinical settings. Different tools provide different information about available or demonstrated ROM. Most tools, including goniometers, inclinometers, and

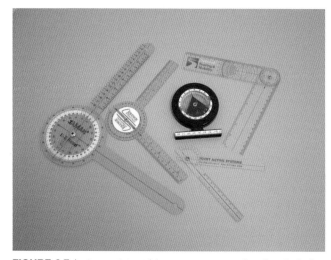

FIGURE 6.7 Instruments used to measure range of motion, including goniometers and an inclinometer.

electrogoniometers, measure the angle, or changes in angle, between body segments. Other tools, such as a tape measure, are used to measure girth or changes in the length of body segments.[46]

QUALITATIVE MEASURES

Qualitative assessment techniques, such as soft tissue palpation, accessory motion testing, and **end-feel,** provide valuable information about motion restrictions that can help guide treatment. Soft tissue palpation may be used to assess the mobility of skin or scar tissue, local tenderness, presence of muscle spasm, skin temperature, and quality of edema. Palpation is also used to identify bony landmarks before quantitative measurement of ROM.

TEST METHODS AND RATIONALE

Active, resisted, passive, and accessory motion and neural tension testing can be used to determine the tissues that restrict motion and to identify the nature of the pathologies contributing to motion restriction.

Active Range of Motion

Active ROM is tested by asking the patient to move the desired segment to its limit in a given direction. The patient is asked to report any symptoms or sensations, such as pain or tingling, experienced during this activity. The maximum motion is measured, and the quality or coordination of the motion and any associated symptoms are noted. Testing of active ROM yields information about the patient's ability and willingness to move functionally and is generally most useful for evaluating the integrity of contractile structures.

The following questions should be asked when active ROM is tested:
- Is the patient's ROM symmetrical, normal, restricted, or excessive?
- What is the quality of the available motion?
- Are any signs or symptoms associated with the motion?

Resisted Muscle Testing

Resisted muscle testing is performed by having the patient contract their muscle against a resistance strong enough to prevent movement.[47] Resisted muscle tests provide information about the ability of a muscle to produce force. This information may help the clinician determine whether contractile or noncontractile tissues are the source of a motion restriction because muscle weakness is commonly the cause of loss of active ROM.

Cyriax[14] identified four possible responses to resisted muscle testing and proposed interpretations for each of these responses (Table 6.1). When the force is strong and no pain is noted with testing, no pathology of contractile or nervous tissues is indicated. When the force is strong but pain is produced with testing, a minor structural lesion of the musculotendinous unit is usually indicated. When the force is weak and no pain is reported with testing, a complete rupture of the musculotendinous unit or a neurological deficit is indicated. When the force is weak but pain is produced with testing, a minor structural lesion of the musculotendinous unit with a concurrent neurological deficit or inhibition of contraction resulting from pain caused by pathology, such as inflammation, fracture, or neoplasm, is indicated.

TABLE 6.1	Cyriax's Interpretation of Resisted Muscle Tests
Finding	Interpretation
Strong and painless	No apparent pathology of contractile or nervous tissue
Strong and painful	Minor lesion of musculotendinous unit
Weak and painless	Complete rupture of musculotendinous unit
Weak and painful	Partial disruption of musculotendinous unit Inhibition by pain as a result of pathology such as inflammation, fracture, or neoplasm Concurrent neurological deficit

From Cyriax J: *Textbook of orthopedic medicine,* ed 8, London, 1982, Bailliere-Tindall.

Passive Range of Motion

Passive ROM is assessed when the tester moves the segment to its limit in a given direction. During passive ROM testing, the quantity of available motion is measured, and the quality of motion and symptoms associated with motion and the end-feel are noted. End-feel is the quality of resistance at the limit of passive motion as felt by the clinician. An end-feel may be physiological (normal) or pathological (abnormal). A physiological end-feel is present when passive ROM is full and the normal anatomy of the joint stops movement. Certain end-feels are normal for some joints but may be pathological at other joints or at abnormal points in the range. Other end-feels are pathological if felt at any point in the motion of any joint. Physiological and pathological end-feels for most joints are listed in Table 6.2.[12,48] Passive ROM is normally limited by stretching of soft tissues or by opposition of soft tissues or bone and may be restricted as a result of soft tissue contracture, mechanical block, or edema. The amount of passive motion available and the quality of the end-feel can assist the clinician in identifying the structures at fault and in understanding the nature of the pathologies contributing to motion restriction.

Combining the Findings of Active Range-of-Motion, Resisted Muscle Contraction, and Passive Range-of-Motion Testing

Combining the findings of active ROM, resisted muscle contraction, and passive ROM testing can help differentiate motion restrictions caused by contractile structures from restrictions caused by noncontractile structures. For example, the structures limiting motion are most likely to be contractile if active elbow flexion is restricted, if contraction of the elbow flexors is weak, and if the passive elbow flexion range is normal. In contrast, if both active and passive elbow flexion ROM are restricted but contraction of the elbow flexors is of normal strength, noncontractile tissues are probably involved. Other combinations of motion and contraction strength findings may indicate muscle substitution during active ROM testing, psychological factors limiting motion, use of poor testing technique, or pain that inhibits muscle contraction (Table 6.3). To definitely implicate a particular pathology or structure, the findings of these noninvasive tests may need to be correlated with the findings of other diagnostic procedures, such as radiographic imaging, diagnostic injection, or surgical exploration.

TABLE 6.2	Descriptions and Examples of Different Types of End-Feels		
Type	Description	Examples	Comments
Hard	Abrupt halt to movement when two hard surfaces meet	Physiological: elbow extension Pathological: result of malunion fracture or heterotopic ossification	May be physiological or pathological
Firm	Leathery, firm resistance when range is limited by joint capsule	Physiological: shoulder rotation Pathological: result of adhesive capsulitis	May be physiological or pathological
Soft	Gradual onset of resistance when soft tissue approximates or when range is limited by length of muscle	Approximation: knee flexion Muscle length: cervical side bending	May be physiological or pathological, depending on tissue bulk and muscle length
Empty	Movement is stopped by subject before tester feels resistance	Passive shoulder abduction is stopped by subject because of pain	Always pathological
Spasm	Movement stopped abruptly by reflex muscle contraction	Passive ankle dorsiflexion in subject with spasticity as a result of upper motor neuron lesion Active trunk flexion in subject with acute low back injury	Always pathological
Springy block	Rebound felt and seen at end of range	Caused by loose body or displaced meniscus	Always pathological
Boggy	Resistance by fluid	Knee joint effusion	Always pathological
Extended	No resistance felt within normal range expected for the particular joint	Joint instability or hypermobility	Always pathological

From Kaltenborn FM: *Mobilization of the extremity joints: examination and basic treatment techniques,* ed 3, Oslo, 1980, Olaf Norlis Bokhandel.

TABLE 6.3	Combining Findings of Active Range-of-Motion Assessment, Resisted Muscle Testing, and Passive Range-of-Motion Assessment		
Active ROM	Resisted Testing	Passive ROM	Probable Cause
Full	Strong	Full	No pathology restricting motion
Full	Strong	Restricted	Pathology beyond terminal active ROM Poor testing technique for passive ROM
Full	Weak	Restricted	Poor testing technique for passive ROM Strength at least 3/5 but less than 5/5
Full	Weak	Full	Strength at least 3/5 but less than 5/5
Restricted	Strong	Restricted	Noncontractile tissue restricting motion
Restricted	Weak	Full	Contractile tissue injury restricting motion
Restricted	Strong	Full	Poor testing techniques for active ROM or psychological factors limiting active ROM
Restricted	Weak	Restricted	Contractile and noncontractile tissues restricting motion

ROM, Range of motion.

Passive Accessory Motion

Passive accessory motion is tested using joint mobilization treatment techniques. The clinician can use these techniques to assess the motion of joint surfaces and the extensibility of major ligaments and portions of the joint capsule. During accessory motion testing, the clinician notes qualitatively whether the motion felt is greater than, less than, or similar to the normal accessory motion expected for that joint in that plane in that particular individual and whether pain is produced with testing.[13,49-51] Accessory motion testing may provide information about joint mechanics that is not available from other tests. For example, reduction of accessory gliding of the glenohumeral joint when passive shoulder flexion ROM is normal may indicate that glenohumeral joint motion is restricted and that motion of the scapulothoracic joint is excessive.

Muscle Length

Muscle length is tested by passively positioning muscle attachments as far apart as possible to elongate the muscle in the direction opposite to its action.[47] This technique will produce valid results only if the pathology of the noncontractile structures or muscle tone does not limit joint motion. When the length of muscles that cross only one joint is tested, passive ROM available at that joint will indicate their length. For example, the length of the soleus muscle can be assessed by measuring passive dorsiflexion ROM at the ankle. For testing the length of a muscle that crosses two or more joints, the muscle must first be elongated across one of the joints, and then that joint must be held in that position while the muscle is elongated as far as possible across the other joint it crosses.[47] Passive ROM available at the second joint will indicate the muscle's length. For example, the length of the gastrocnemius muscle can be tested by first elongating it across the knee while the knee is in full extension and then measuring the amount of passive dorsiflexion available at the ankle. Multijoint muscles must be fully extended across one joint before measurement is performed at the other joint to obtain a valid test of muscle length.

◎ Clinical Pearl

When measuring the length of a muscle that crosses two joints, first extend the muscle fully across one joint; then, while holding that joint in place, extend the muscle across the other joint.

Adverse Neural Tension

Adverse neural tension or nerve mechanosensitivity is usually tested by passive placement of neural structures in their position of maximum length. Evaluation is based on comparison with the contralateral side, comparison with norms, and assessment of symptoms produced in the position of maximum length.

Adverse neural tension or neurodynamic tests include passive straight leg raise (PSLR), prone knee bend, passive neck flexion, and upper-limb tension tests. PSLR, also known as *Lasègue sign,* is the most commonly used neural tension test and is intended to test for adverse neural tension in the sciatic nerve.

Because adverse neural tension tests may provoke symptoms in the presence of pathologies associated with muscles or joints, it is recommended that maneuvers that apply tension to the nervous system but do not additionally stress the muscles or joints be used to differentiate the sources of symptoms from this type of test. For example, the PSLR test can provoke symptoms in the presence of pathologies associated with the hamstring muscles or the sacroiliac, iliofemoral, or lumbar spinal facet joints. Therefore, at the onset of symptoms with this test, additional tension can be applied to the nervous system by passively dorsiflexing the ankle to increase tension on the sciatic nerve distally or by passively flexing the neck to tighten the dura proximally. If these maneuvers cause the patient's symptoms to worsen, adverse neural tension rather than joint or muscle pathology is probably the cause of the symptoms.[38,40,52]

Contraindications and Precautions to Range-of-Motion Techniques

ROM techniques are contraindicated when motion may disrupt the healing process. However, some controlled motion within the range, speed, and tolerance of the patient may be beneficial during the acute recovery stage or immediately after acute tears, fractures, and surgery. Limited, controlled motion is recommended to reduce the severity of adhesion and contracture and to reduce the decrease in circulation and loss of strength associated with complete immobilization.[53-56]

✶ CONTRAINDICATIONS

for the Use of Active and Passive ROM Techniques

Active and passive ROM examination techniques are contraindicated under the following circumstances:
- In the region of a dislocation or an unhealed fracture
- Immediately after surgical procedures to tendons, ligaments, muscles, joint capsules, or skin

✶ PRECAUTIONS

for the Use of Active and Passive ROM Techniques

Caution should be observed when motion of the part might aggravate the condition. This may occur in the following situations:
- When infection or an inflammatory process is present in or around the joint
- In patients taking analgesic medication that may cloud perception or communication of pain
- In the presence of osteoporosis or any condition that causes bone fragility
- With hypermobile joints or joints prone to subluxation
- In painful conditions where the techniques might reinforce the severity of symptoms
- In patients with hemophilia
- In the region of a hematoma
- If bony ankylosis is suspected
- Immediately after an injury in which disruption of soft tissue has occurred
- In the presence of myositis ossificans

In addition, neurodynamic testing should be performed with caution in the presence of inflammatory conditions; spinal cord symptoms; tumors; signs of nerve root compression; unrelenting night pain; neurological signs such as weakness, reflex changes, or loss of sensation; recent paresthesia or anesthesia; and reflex sympathetic dystrophy.[34,40] Detailed contraindications and precautions for each specific neurodynamic test are provided in other texts devoted to the assessment and treatment of adverse mechanical tension of the nervous system.[40]

Treatment Approaches for Motion Restrictions
STRETCHING

Currently, most noninvasive interventions for reestablishing soft tissue ROM involve stretching. Clinical and experimental evidence demonstrates that stretching can increase motion; however, results may be inconsistent, and recommended protocols vary.[57-62] When a stretch is applied to connective tissues within the elastic limit, these tissues may demonstrate **creep, stress relaxation,** and **plastic deformation** over time.[63,64] Creep is transient lengthening or deformation with the application of a fixed load. Stress relaxation is a decrease in the force required over time to hold a given

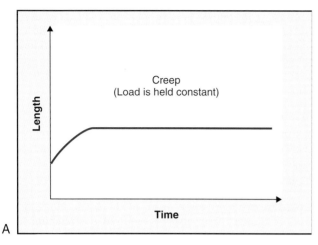

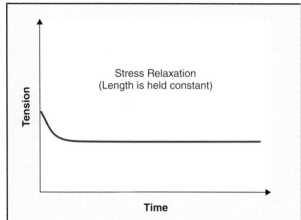

FIGURE 6.8 The relationships of time, tension, and length during (A) creep and (B) stress relaxation.

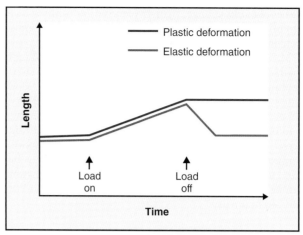

FIGURE 6.9 Plastic and elastic deformation.

length (Fig. 6.8). Creep and stress relaxation can occur in soft tissue in a short time and are thought to depend on viscous components of the tissue.[65] Plastic deformation is the elongation produced under loading that remains after the load is removed (Fig. 6.9). After plastic deformation, tissue will permanently increase its length. A controlled

stretch must be applied for a prolonged time—for at least 30 minutes a day in some conditions[66,67]—to cause plastic deformation. The length of time necessary to determine that no additional ROM gains are possible is unknown and probably varies with different pathologies[68] and tissues causing restriction, as well as with the duration of the restriction.[69] In addition to time, the force, direction, and speed of the stretch must be controlled to produce optimal lengthening of appropriate structures without damaging tissue or causing hypermobility.

Many stretching techniques may be used to increase soft tissue length. The most common are **passive stretching**, proprioceptive neuromuscular facilitation (PNF), and ballistic stretching (Table 6.4). When a passive stretch is performed, the limb is held in a position in which the patient feels a mild stretch. The force of gravity on the involved body part, the force of other limbs, or another individual can apply passive stretch. External devices such as progressive end-range splints, serial casts, or dynamic splints may be used to passively stretch tissue. Although optimal parameters for passively stretching normal and pathological tissues have not been established, it is generally recommended that low-load prolonged forces should be applied to minimize the risk of adverse effects.

TABLE 6.4	Types of Stretching		
Method	Description	Examples	Comments
Passive	Limb held passively in a position in which the subject feels a mild stretch	Manual progressive stretching Progressive end-range splinting Dynamic splinting	Pain perception is a factor Results in no motor learning Optimal parameters have not been established
PNF	Active muscle contraction followed by muscle relaxation in conjunction with passive stretch	Contract-relax Hold-relax Subject resists and aids	Requires assistance of an individual proficient in the technique May result in motor learning
Ballistic	Active, quick, short-amplitude movements at the end of subject's available ROM	Active stretching with "bounce" at end of range	Not generally used or recommended because this may increase tissue tightness by activating the stretch reflex in normal and spastic muscles

PNF, Proprioceptive neuromuscular facilitation; *ROM,* range of motion.

Studies of adults younger than 40 years old and without lower-extremity pathology found that passive hamstring muscle stretching performed for at least 30 seconds increased passive ROM. There was no consensus in the literature regarding the length of hold, interval of repetitions, frequency of stretch, or duration of stretch, but evidence suggests increased ROM with static stretching utilizing a longer duration,[70] increased repetitions,[71] fewer rest intervals,[72] or increased session frequency.[73,74] In adults older than 65 years, stretching protocols resulting in increased hamstring muscle ROM varied from 60 seconds to 20 minutes.[75-79] Passive stretching techniques have not been found to have long-term effects on contractures in individuals with neurological conditions[80-83] or with function in children with cerebral palsy.[84]

> ### ◎ Clinical Pearl
>
> To increase ROM in young adults, apply a low-load prolonged stretch for at least 30 to 60 seconds. To increase ROM in older adults, apply stretch for at least 60 seconds.

Manipulation of a joint while the patient is anesthetized involves high-force, passive stretching of the soft tissues to increase ROM. Manipulation under anesthesia can rapidly increase ROM because high forces that would otherwise be painful or cause muscles to spasm may be applied. These forces may cause greater increases in soft tissue length and may tear adhesions to increase motion; however, the risk of damaging structures or exacerbating inflammation may be greater with such techniques than with stretching while the patient is awake.

PNF techniques for muscle stretching inhibit contraction of the muscle being stretched and facilitate contraction of its opponent.[85,86] This is achieved by having the patient actively contract and then voluntarily relax the muscles to be stretched before the stretching force is applied. PNF techniques have the advantage over other stretching techniques of including a motor learning component from repeated active muscle contractions; however, their use is frequently limited by the requirement that a skilled individual must help the patient perform the technique.

Ballistic stretching is a technique in which the patient performs short, bouncing movements at the end of the available range. Although some people attempt to stretch in this manner, ballistic stretching is not generally used or recommended because it may increase tissue tightness by activating the stretch reflex.[87]

MOTION

The formation of contractures is a time-related process that may be inhibited by motion.[25] Motion can inhibit contracture formation by physically disrupting the adhesions between gross structures and/or by limiting intermolecular cross-linking. Active or passive motion stretches tissues, promotes their lubrication, and may alter their metabolic activity.[88] Because active ROM may be contraindicated during the early stages of healing, particularly after contractile tissue injury or surgery, gentle passive motion may be used to limit contracture formation at this stage.[89] For example, continuous passive motion (CPM) is used to prevent motion loss after joint trauma or surgery.[90] Research and clinical protocols for the use of CPM vary considerably, but adding CPM to physical therapy after total knee arthroplasty or rotator cuff repair has not been found to have clinically important effects.[55,91,92]

SURGERY

Noninvasive approaches of stretching and motion frequently resolve or prevent motion restrictions, but in some cases, surgery may be required to optimize motion. Surgery may be necessary if motion is restricted by a mechanical block, particularly if the block is bony. In such cases, the surgical procedure removes some or all of the tissue blocking the motion. Surgery may also be required if stretching techniques cannot lengthen a contracture adequately or if the functional length of a tendon is decreased because of hypertonicity. For example, Z-plasty procedures are frequently performed to lengthen the Achilles tendon in children with limited dorsiflexion caused by congenital plantar flexion contractures or by hypertonicity of the plantar flexor muscles. Z-plasty is generally performed when it can be expected to permit a more functional gait than is achieved with noninvasive techniques alone. Surgical procedures to increase ROM are also frequently performed in adults. For example, surgical release may be performed to restore motion limited by Dupuytren contracture, and tenotomy may be performed when tendon length limits motion. Surgery may also be performed to release adhesions and to lengthen scars that have formed after prolonged immobilization. For example, patients with extensive burns who have received limited medical intervention frequently develop contractures that cannot be stretched sufficiently to allow full function and therefore require surgical release. Surgery is more commonly performed to release adhesions that form after injury if scarring is exaggerated by prolonged inflammation or infection.

Role of Physical Agents in the Treatment of Motion Restrictions

Physical agents are most effectively used as adjuncts to treat motion restrictions. Combined with other interventions, they can enhance the functional recovery associated with regaining normal motion. Physical agents are used as components of the treatment of motion restrictions because they can increase soft tissue extensibility, control inflammation, control pain, and facilitate motion.

> ### ◎ Clinical Pearl
>
> Physical agents can help reduce motion restrictions by increasing soft tissue extensibility, controlling pain and inflammation, and facilitating motion.

INCREASE SOFT TISSUE EXTENSIBILITY

Physical agents that increase tissue temperature are used as components in the treatment of motion restriction because they can increase soft tissue extensibility, thereby decreasing the force required to increase tissue length and decreasing the risk of injury during the stretching procedure.[93] Applying physical agents to soft tissue before prolonged stretching can alter the viscoelasticity of the fibers, allowing greater plastic deformation to occur.[94,95] To achieve maximum benefit from physical agents that increase soft tissue extensibility, knowledge of the depth of the tissue and nature of the restriction to be treated is necessary. The appropriate thermal agents for heating superficial structures such as scar tissue or superficial tendons or deep structures such as the joint capsules of large joints or deep tendons are described in Part III.

CONTROL INFLAMMATION AND ADHESION FORMATION

Physical agents, particularly cryotherapy and certain types of electrical currents, are thought to control inflammation and its associated signs and symptoms after tissue injury.[96-98] Controlling inflammation may help prevent the development of motion restrictions by limiting edema during the acute inflammatory stage, thereby limiting the degree of immobilization. Controlling the severity and duration of inflammation also limits the duration and extent of the proliferative response and thus may limit adhesion as the tissue heals.

CONTROL PAIN DURING STRETCHING

Physical agents such as thermotherapy, cryotherapy, and electrical currents can help control pain.[99-101] Pain control may assist in the treatment of motion restrictions because if pain is decreased, tissues may be stretched for a longer period, and this may increase tissue length more effectively. If pain is controlled, motion may be initiated sooner after injury, limiting the loss of motion caused by immobilization.

FACILITATE MOTION

Some physical agents facilitate motion to assist in treating motion restrictions. Electrical stimulation of the motor nerves of innervated muscles or direct electrical stimulation of denervated muscle can make muscles contract. These muscle contractions may complement motion produced by normal physiological contractions or may substitute for such contractions if the patient does not or cannot move independently.[102-103] Immersion in water may also facilitate motion because it provides buoyancy, which assists with motion against gravity; this is particularly beneficial for treating patients who have active ROM restrictions caused by contractile tissue weakness.

CLINICAL CASE STUDIES

The following case studies summarize the concepts of motion restriction discussed in this chapter. Based on the scenario presented, an evaluation of the clinical findings and goals of treatment are proposed. These are followed by a discussion of the factors to be considered in treatment selection.

CASE STUDY 6.1

Low Back Pain With Radiculopathy
Examination
History

TR is a 45-year-old man who has been referred to physical therapy with a diagnosis of a right L5–S1 radiculopathy. The pain started about 6 weeks ago, the morning after TR spent a day stacking firewood, at which time he woke up with severe pain in his lower back and right lower extremity extending down to his lateral calf; he also had difficulty standing up straight. He has had similar problems in the past, but these have always resolved fully after a couple of days of bed rest and a few aspirin. TR first saw his doctor regarding his present problem 5 weeks ago. At that time, he was prescribed a nonsteroidal antiinflammatory drug (NSAID) and a muscle relaxant and was told to rest. His symptoms improved to their current level over the next 2 weeks but have not changed since. He has been unable to return to his job as a telephone installer since the onset of symptoms 6 weeks ago. A magnetic resonance imaging (MRI) scan last week showed a mild posterolateral disc bulge at L5–S1 on the right. The patient has not had previous physical therapy for his back problem.

Systems Review

TR reports constant mild to moderately severe (4/10 to 7/10) right low back pain that radiates to his right buttock and lateral

thigh after sitting for longer than 20 minutes that is relieved to some degree by walking or lying down. He reports no numbness, tingling, or weakness of the lower extremities. No signs of discomfort or weakness are visibly present.

Tests and Measures

The patient's weight is 91 kg (200 lb). The objective examination shows a significant (50%) restriction of lumbar ROM in forward bending and right side bending, both of which cause increased right, low back, and lower-extremity pain. Left side bending decreases his pain. Passive straight leg raising is 35 degrees on the right, limited by right-lower-extremity pain, and 60 degrees on the left, limited by hamstring tightness. Palpation reveals stiffness and tenderness to right unilateral posterior-anterior pressure at L5–S1 and no notable areas of hypermobility. All other tests, including lower-extremity sensation, strength, and reflexes, are within normal limits.
What is the likely cause of this patient's problem?
What symptoms point to this as the cause?

Evaluation and Goals

ICF Level	Current Status	Goals
Body function and structure	Right low back pain with radiation to right buttock and lateral thigh	Decrease pain to <3/10 in 1 week
	Restricted lumbar ROM	Eliminate pain completely in 3 weeks
	Restricted lumbar nerve root mobility on the right (limited right straight leg raise)	Return lumbar ROM and SLR to normal
	Bulging L5–S1 disc	

Continued

CLINICAL CASE STUDIES—cont'd

ICF Level	Current Status	Goals
Activity	Decreased sitting tolerance	Increase sitting tolerance to 1 hour in 1 week
	Unable to stand straight or lift	Stand straight in 1 week
		Lift 20 lb in 2 weeks
Participation	Unable to work	Return to limited work duties within 2 weeks
		Return to full work duties within 1 month

ICF, International Classification for Functioning, Disability and Health; *ROM,* range of motion; *SLR,* straight leg raise.

Prognosis

The distribution of TR's pain and its response to changes in loading indicate that his symptoms probably are related to the mild posterolateral disc bulge at L5–S1 on the right, as noted on his MRI scan.

Intervention

The optimal treatment for this patient would include interventions that could reduce disc protrusion and may also enhance relief of symptoms related to low back pain and sciatica. Therefore the preferred intervention to be considered at this time would be spinal traction. The type of traction and the parameters of treatment are discussed in Chapter 20, and this patient's case is further discussed in Case Study 20.3.

CASE STUDY 6.2

Adhesive Capsulitis
Examination
History

SJ is a 45-year-old female physical therapist. She has been diagnosed with adhesive capsulitis of the right shoulder and has been referred to physical therapy. SJ is right-hand dominant. She reports that her shoulder first began to hurt about 6 months ago with no apparent cause. Although the pain has almost completely resolved, her shoulder has gradually become stiffer, with a tight sensation at the end of the range. Although she is able to perform most of her work functions, she has difficulty reaching overhead, which interferes with placing objects on high shelves and with serving when playing tennis, and she has difficulty reaching behind her to fasten clothing.

Systems Review

SJ self-rates her right shoulder stiffness and pain today at 4/10. She notes fatigue in her left shoulder with compensation but no pain or stiffness. Her lower extremities are not affected.

Tests and Measures

The objective examination reveals restricted right shoulder active ROM (AROM) and passive ROM (PROM) and restricted passive glenohumeral joint inferior and posterior gliding. All other tests, including cervical and elbow ROM and upper-extremity strength and sensation, are within normal limits.

Active ROM	Right	Left
Flexion	120°	170°
Abduction	100°	170°
Hand behind back	Right 5 inches below left	

Passive ROM	Right	Left
Internal rotation	50°	80°
External rotation	10°	80°

ROM, Range of motion.

Glenohumeral passive inferior glide and posterior glide are both restricted on the right.

Is this patient's condition acute or chronic? Why is her shoulder movement restricted? What physical agents will best address this restriction?

Evaluation and Goals

ICF level	Current Status	Goals
Body structure and function	Capsular pattern of restricted right shoulder active and passive motion. Restricted right glenohumeral passive intraarticular gliding.	Restore normal active and passive ROM of right shoulder
Activity	Impaired reach overhead and behind back with right upper extremity	Improve ability to reach overhead and behind back for dressing and hair care without assist
Participation	Decreased tennis playing. Difficulty with reach overhead for housework and reach behind for dressing.	Return patient to prior level of playing tennis and performing housework without limitation from shoulder. Dressing with ease.

ICF, International Classification for Functioning, Disability and Health.

Prognosis

The goals of treatment at this time are to regain full AROM and PROM of the right shoulder and to return her to full sports participation and daily living activities. Loss of active and passive joint motion associated with adhesive capsulitis is thought to be a result of adhesion and loss of length of the anterior-inferior joint capsule. Effective treatment should attempt to increase the length of the joint capsule. Increasing tissue temperature before stretching will increase the extensibility of soft tissue, allowing the greatest increase in soft tissue length with the least force while minimizing the risk of tissue damage.

Intervention

Although there is disagreement concerning the optimal intervention for adhesive capsulitis, there are treatments that increase the extensibility and length of restricted soft tissues. Thermotherapy followed immediately by prolonged static stretching could be used to maximize ROM gain. Joint mobilization and strengthening later on may be necessary to regain full function of the shoulder. The types of thermotherapy and parameters for treatment are discussed in Part III. This patient's case is further discussed in Case Study 10.1.

CASE STUDY 6.3

Distal Radial Fracture With Weakness and Loss of Range of Motion
Examination
History

RS is a 62-year-old, right-handed housewife who fell and fractured her left distal radius 7 weeks ago. She underwent open reduction internal fixation (ORIF), and her cast was removed 1 week ago. While her cast was on, she was able to vacuum and cook simple meals, but she could not fold laundry, cook typical meals, shop independently for all groceries, perform her usual housecleaning activities, or play golf because she could not lift with her left hand. She has not yet returned to any of these activities. Her physician's prescription for therapy says "evaluate and treat." No limitations have been prescribed.

Systems Review

RS appears in clinic in no acute distress. She is attentive to questions and eager to begin treatment. Observation of the wrist reveals atrophy of the extensor and flexor muscles as a result of disuse because of cast immobilization. Pain severity is self-rated 0/10 at rest and 5/10 after 30 minutes of activity.

She reports no numbness or tingling in left or right upper extremities or weakness of the lower extremities.

Tests and Measures
Wrist ROM is as follows:

	Left		Right	
	AROM	**PROM**	**AROM**	**PROM**
Extension	30°	45°	70°	75°
Flexion	40°	60°	80°	85°
Ulnar deviation	10°	14°	30°	30°
Radial deviation	15°	15°	20°	20°
Pronation	15°	15°	85°	85°
Supination	8°	10°	80°	80°

AROM, Active range of motion; *PROM,* passive range of motion.

Strength is 3/5 in all directions within her pain-free range. RS has no history of heart disease, cancer, or any major medical problems.

What do you think is limiting wrist flexion and extension in this patient? What do you think is limiting pronation? How would your treatment plan to increase flexion ROM be different from your treatment plan to increase pronation? Why?

Evaluation and Goals

ICF Level	Current Status	Goals
Body structure and function	Left wrist pain and weakness and decreased ROM	Control pain Increase strength Increase ROM
Activity	Limited lifting capacity	Increase lifting capacity
Participation	Unable to cook, shop, clean, or play golf	Return to prior level of cooking, shopping, cleaning, and playing golf

ICF, International Classification for Functioning, Disability and Health; *ROM,* range of motion.

Prognosis
RS has reduced ROM and atrophy from her distal radius fracture and subsequent immobilization.

Intervention
The optimal treatment for this patient would include interventions that could help her regain strength and increase active ROM. The appropriate type of electrical stimulation and parameters of treatment to meet these goals are discussed in Chapter 12. This patient's case is further discussed in Case Study 12.2.

Chapter Review

1. There are multiple causes of motion restrictions. For a clinician to effectively use physical agents as an adjunct to treatment, the clinician must identify the cause or causes of restriction. Only after the tissue, area, depth, and stage of restriction have been assessed can the clinician choose an appropriate physical agent to enhance functional recovery.

Various physical agents are used as components in the treatment of motion restrictions to increase soft tissue extensibility, control inflammation, control pain, and facilitate motion.
2. The musculoskeletal and neural structures of the body are normally able to move. Active movement occurs when muscles contract, whereas passive movement occurs when

the body is acted on by an outside force. Physiological joint motion is the motion of one segment of the body relative to another, and accessory motion is the motion that occurs between joint surfaces during normal physiological motion.

3. Normal joint motion will vary with the joint, as well as with the patient's age, sex, and health status.

4. Motion may be restricted by a variety of pathologies, including contractures, edema, adhesions, mechanical blocks, spinal disc herniation, adverse neural tension, and weakness.

5. Various tests and measures may be used to determine the degree of motion restriction, the tissue involved, and the nature of the pathology contributing to motion restriction. Motion restrictions can be measured quantitatively using goniometers, tape measures, and inclinometers. Qualitative measures of motion restriction include manual tests of active, passive, resisted, and accessory motion and neurodynamic testing.

6. Motion restriction may be treated conservatively by stretching and movement, but sometimes invasive surgery is required for resolution. Physical agents may augment these interventions by increasing soft tissue extensibility before stretching, controlling inflammation and adhesion formation during tissue healing, controlling pain during stretching or motion, or facilitating motion.

Glossary

Accessory motion: The motion that occurs between joint surfaces during normal physiological motion; also called *joint play*.

Active motion: Movement produced by contraction of the muscles crossing a joint.

Adhesion: Binding together of normally separate anatomical structures by scar tissue.

Capsular pattern of restriction: A pattern of motion loss caused by shortening of the joint capsule.

Contractile tissue: Tissue that is able to shorten, such as muscle and tendon.

Contracture: Fixed shortening of soft tissue structures that restricts passive and active motion and can cause permanent deformity.

Creep: Transient lengthening or deformation of connective tissues with the application of a fixed load.

End-feel: The quality of resistance at the limit of passive motion as felt by the clinician.

Extraarticular edema: Excessive fluid outside of a joint.

Goniometers: Tools used to measure joint range of motion.

Intraarticular edema: Excessive fluid within a joint capsule.

Noncapsular pattern of restriction: A pattern of motion loss that does not follow the capsular pattern.

Noncontractile tissue: Tissue that cannot actively shorten, for example, skin, ligament, and cartilage.

Osteophyte: An abnormal bony outgrowth, as seen in arthritis.

Passive accessory motion: The motion between joint surfaces produced by an external force without voluntary muscle contraction.

Passive motion: Movement produced entirely by an external force without voluntary muscle contraction.

Passive stretching: A type of muscle stretching in which the limb is moved passively.

Physiological motion: The motion of one segment of the body relative to another segment.

Plastic deformation: The elongation of connective tissue produced under loading that remains after the load is removed.

Range of motion (ROM): The amount of motion that occurs when one segment of the body moves in relation to an adjacent segment.

Stress relaxation: A decrease in the amount of force required over time to maintain a certain length of connective tissue.

References

1. Greene WB, Heckman JD, editors: *Clinical measurement of joint motion*, Rosemont, IL, 1994, American Academy of Orthopedic Surgeons.
2. Kilgour GM, McNair PJ, Stott NS: Range of motion in children with spastic diplegia: GMFCS I-II compared to age and sex matched controls. *Phys Occup Ther Pediatr* 25:61–79, 2005.
3. Sauseng S, Kastenbauer T, Irsigler K: Limited joint mobility in selected hand and foot joints in patients with type 1 diabetes mellitus: a methodology comparison. *Diabetes Nutr Metab* 15:1–6, 2002.
4. Reichel LM, Hipp J, Fuentes A, et al: Quantitative analysis of cervical flexion-extension radiographs in rheumatoid arthritis patients. *J Spinal Disord Tech* 28(8):E478–E481, 2015. doi:10.1097/BSD.0b013e3182aa290f.
5. McKay MJ, Baldwin JN, Ferreira P, et al: Normative reference values for strength and flexibility of 1,000 children and adults. *Neurology* 88(1):36–43, 2017. doi:10.1212/WNL.0000000000003466.
6. Doriot N, Wang X: Effects of age and sex on maximum voluntary range of motion of the upper body joints. *Ergonomics* 49:269–281, 2006.
7. Soucie JM, Wang C, Forsyth A, et al: Range of motion measurements: reference values and a database for comparison studies. *Haemophilia* 17(3):500–507, 2011. doi:10.1111/j.1365-2516.2010.02399.x.
8. Intolo P, Milosavljevic S, Baxter DG, et al: The effect of age on lumbar range of motion: a systematic review. *Man Ther* 14:596–604, 2009.
9. Liu B, Wu B, Van Hoof T, et al: Are the standard parameters of cervical spine alignment and range of motion related to age, sex, and cervical disc degeneration? *J Neurosurg Spine* 23:274–279, 2015.
10. Einkauf DK, Gohdes ML, Jensen GM, et al: Changes in spinal mobility with increasing age in women. *Phys Ther* 67:370–375, 1987.
11. Pan F, Arshad R, Zander T, et al: The effect of age and sex on the cervical range of motion - a systematic review and meta-analysis. *J Biomech* 75:13–27, 2018. doi:10.1016/j.jbiomech.2018.04.047.
12. Kaltenborn F: *Manual mobilization of the joints, vol 1: the extremities*, ed 8, Minneapolis, 2014, Orthopedic Physical Therapy Products.
13. Hengeveld E, Banks K: *Maitland's vertebral manipulation*, vol 1, ed 8, London, 2014, Churchill Livingstone Elsevier.
14. Cyriax J: *Textbook of orthopaedic medicine*, ed 8, Baltimore, 1982, Williams & Wilkins.
15. Fritz JM, Delitto A, Erhard RE, et al: An examination of the selective tissue tension scheme, with evidence for the concept of a capsular pattern of the knee [published correction appears in *Phys Ther* 78(12):1339, 1998]. *Phys Ther* 78(10):1046–1061, 1998. doi:10.1093/ptj/78.10.1046.
16. Neviaser AS, Hannafin JA: Adhesive capsulitis: a review of current treatment. *Am J Sports Med* 38:2346–2356, 2010.
17. Ryan V, Brown H, Minns Lowe CJ, et al: The pathophysiology associated with primary (idiopathic) frozen shoulder: A systematic review. *BMC Musculoskelet Disord* 17(1):340, 2016. doi:10.1186/s12891-016-1190-9. .
18. Redler LH, Dennis ER: Treatment of adhesive capsulitis of the shoulder. *J Am Acad Orthop Surg* 27(12):e544–e554, 2019. doi:10.5435/JAAOS-D-17-00606.
19. Kelley MJ, Shaffer MA, Kuhn JE, et al: Shoulder pain and mobility deficits: adhesive capsulitis. *J Orthop Sports Phys Ther* 43(5):A1–A31, 2013. doi:10.2519/jospt.2013.0302.
20. Jain TK, Sharma NK: The effectiveness of physiotherapeutic interventions in treatment of frozen shoulder/adhesive capsulitis: a systematic review. *J Back Musculoskelet Rehabil* 27:247–273, 2014.

21. Rundquist PJ, Ludewig PM: Patterns of motion loss in subjects with idiopathic loss of shoulder range of motion. *Clin Biomech (Bristol, Avon)* 19:810–818, 2004.
22. Neviaser AS, Neviaser RJ: Adhesive capsulitis of the shoulder. *J Am Acad Orthop Surg* 19:536–542, 2011.
23. Born CT, Gil JA, Goodman AD: Joint contractures resulting from prolonged immobilization: etiology, prevention, and management. *J Am Acad Orthop Surg* 25(2):110–116, 2017. doi:10.5435/JAAOS-D-15-00697.
24. Evans PJ, Nandi S, Maschke S, et al: Prevention and treatment of elbow stiffness. *J Hand Surg Am* 34:769–778, 2009.
25. Woo SL, Matthews JV, Akeson WH, et al: Connective tissue response to immobility: correlative study of biomechanical and biochemical measurements of normal and immobilized rabbit knees. *Arthritis Rheum* 18:257–264, 1975.
26. Kwan PO: Tredget EE: Biological principles of scar and contracture. *Hand Clin* 33(2):227–264, 2017. doi:10.1016/j.hcl.2016.12.004.
27. Wong K, Trudel G, Laneuville O: Noninflammatory joint contractures arising from immobility: animal models to future treatments. *Biomed Res Int* 848290:2015, 2015.
28. Akeson WH, Amiel D, Woo SL-Y: Immobility effects on synovial joints, the pathomechanics of joint contracture. *Biorheology* 17:95–110, 1980.
29. Trudel G, Uhthoff HK, Goudreau L, et al: Quantitative analysis of the reversibility of knee flexion contractures with time: an experimental study using the rat model. *BMC Musculoskelet Disord* 15:338, 2014.
30. Trudel G, Uhthoff HK: Contractures secondary to immobility: is the restriction articular or muscular? An experimental longitudinal study in the rat knee. *Arch Phys Med Rehabil* 81:6–13, 2000.
31. *Dorland's illustrated medical dictionary*, ed 32, Philadelphia, 2012, Saunders.
32. Beck M: Groin pain after open FAI surgery: the role of intra-articular adhesions. *Clin Orthop Relat Res* 467:769–774, 2009.
33. Zhu F, Bao H, Yan P, et al: Do the disc degeneration and osteophyte contribute to the curve rigidity of degenerative scoliosis? *BMC Musculoskelet Disord* 18(1):128, 2017. doi:10.1186/s12891-017-1471-y.
34. Slater H, Butler DS: The dynamic central nervous system. In *Grieve's modern manual*, ed 2, New York, 1994, Churchill Livingstone.
35. Oliver J, Middleditch A: *Functional anatomy of the spine*, ed 2, London, 2005, Butterworth-Heinemann.
36. Butler DS: Adverse mechanical tension in the nervous system: a model for assessment and treatment. *Aust J Physiother* 35(4):227–238, 1989. doi:10.1016/S0004-9514(14)60511-0.
37. Shacklock M: Improving application of neurodynamic (neural tension) testing and treatments: a message to researchers and clinicians. *Man Ther* 10(3):175–179, 2005. doi:10.1016/j.math.2005.03.001.
38. Boyd BS, Wanek L, Gray AT, et al: Mechanosensitivity of the lower extremity nervous system during straight-leg raise neurodynamic testing in healthy individuals. *J Orthop Sports Phys Ther* 39:780–790, 2009.
39. Yılmaz S, Taş S, Tunca Yılmaz Ö: Comparison of median nerve mechanosensitivity and pressure pain threshold in patients with nonspecific neck pain and asymptomatic individuals. *J Manipulative Physiol Ther* 41(3):227–233, 2018. doi:10.1016/j.jmpt.2017.09.008.
40. Butler DS: *Mobilisation of the nervous system*, Edinburgh, 1991, Churchill Livingstone.
41. Rade M, Pesonen J, Könönen M, et al: Reduced spinal cord movement with the straight leg raise test in patients with lumbar intervertebral disc herniation. *Spine (Phila Pa 1976)* 42(15):1117–1124, 2017. doi:10.1097/BRS.0000000000002235.
42. Williams MA, McCarthy CJ, Chorti A, et al: A systematic review of reliability and validity studies of methods for measuring active and passive cervical range of motion. *J Manipulative Physiol Ther* 33:138–155, 2010.
43. Rondoni A, Rossettini G, Ristori D, et al: Intrarater and inter-rater reliability of active cervical range of motion in patients with nonspecific neck pain measured with technological and common use devices: a systematic review with meta-regression. *J Manipulative Physiol Ther* 40(8):597–608, 2017. doi:10.1016/j.jmpt.2017.07.002.
44. van Rijn SF, Zwerus EL, Koenraadt KL, et al: The reliability and validity of goniometric elbow measurements in adults: a systematic review of the literature. *Shoulder Elbow* 10(4):274–284, 2018. doi:10.1177/1758573218774326.
45. Kolber MJ, Hanney WJ: The reliability and concurrent validity of shoulder mobility measurements using a digital inclinometer and goniometer: a technical report. *Int J Sports Phys Ther* 7(3):306–313, 2012.
46. Norkin CC, White DJ: *Measurement of joint motion: a guide to goniometry*, ed 5, Philadelphia, 2016, FA Davis.
47. Kendall FP, McCreary EK, Provance PG: *Muscles: testing and function*, ed 5, Philadelphia, 2005, Lippincott Williams & Wilkins.
48. Magee DJ: *Orthopedic physical assessment*, ed 6, Philadelphia, 2013, Saunders.
49. Riddle DL: Measurement of accessory motion: critical issues and related concepts. *Phys Ther* 72:865–874, 1992.
50. Phillips DR, Twomey LT: A comparison of manual diagnosis with a diagnosis established by a uni-level lumbar spinal block procedure. *Man Ther* 1(2):82–87, 1996. doi:10.1054/math.1996.0254.
51. Hidalgo B, Hall T, Nielens H, et al: Intertester agreement and validity of identifying lumbar pain provocative movement patterns using active and passive accessory movement tests. *J Manipulative Physiol Ther* 37(2):105–115, 2014. doi:10.1016/j.jmpt.2013.09.006.
52. Bueno-Gracia E, Pérez-Bellmunt A, Estébanez-de-Miguel E, et al: Differential movement of the sciatic nerve and hamstrings during the straight leg raise with ankle dorsiflexion: implications for diagnosis of neural aspect to hamstring disorders. *Musculoskelet Sci Pract* 43:91–95, 2019. doi:10.1016/j.msksp.2019.07.011.
53. Hwang JH, Lee KM, Lee JY: Therapeutic effect of passive mobilization exercise on improvement of muscle regeneration and prevention of fibrosis after laceration injury of rat. *Arch Phys Med Rehabil* 87:20–26, 2006.
54. Järvinen TA, Järvinen TL, Kääriäinen M, et al: Muscle injuries: biology and treatment. *Am J Sports Med* 33(5):745–764, 2005. doi:10.1177/0363546505274714.
55. Harvey LA, Brosseau L, Herbert RD: Continuous passive motion following total knee arthroplasty in people with arthritis. *Cochrane Database Syst Rev* 2014(2):CD004260. doi:10.1002/14651858.CD004260.pub3.
56. Chang KV, Hung CY, Han DS, et al: Early versus delayed passive range of motion exercise for arthroscopic rotator cuff repair: a meta-analysis of randomized controlled trials. *Am J Sports Med* 43:1265–1273, 2015.
57. Glasgow C, Tooth LR, Fleming J: Mobilizing the stiff hand: combining theory and evidence to improve clinical outcomes. *J Hand Ther* 23:392–400, 2010. quiz 401.
58. Magnusson SP: Passive properties of human skeletal muscle during stretch maneuvers. A review. *Scand J Med Sci Sports* 8:65–77, 1998.
59. Sobolewski EJ, Ryan ED, Thompson BJ: Influence of maximum range of motion and stiffness on the viscoelastic stretch response. *Muscle Nerve* 48:571–577, 2013.
60. Freitas SR, Vaz JR, Bruno PM, et al: Stretching effects: high-intensity and moderate-duration vs. low-intensity and long-duration. *Int J Sports Med* 37:239–244, 2016.
61. Medeiros DM, Cini A, Sbruzzi G, et al: Influence of static stretching on hamstring flexibility in healthy young adults: systematic review and meta-analysis. *Physiother Theory Pract* 32(6):438–445, 2016. doi:10.1080/09593985.2016.1204401.
62. Freitas SR, Mendes B, Le Sant G, et al: Can chronic stretching change the muscle-tendon mechanical properties? A review. *Scand J Med Sci Sports* 28(3):794–806, 2018. doi:10.1111/sms.12957.
63. Taylor DC, Dalton JD, Seaber AV, et al: Viscoelastic properties of muscle-tendon units: the biomechanics of stretching. *Am J Sports Med* 18:300, 1990.
64. De Deyne PG: Application of passive stretch and its implications for muscle fibers. *Phys Ther* 81(2):819–827, 2001. doi:10.1093/ptj/81.2.819.
65. Ryan ED, Herda TJ, Costa PB, et al: Viscoelastic creep in the human skeletal muscle-tendon unit. *Eur J Appl Physiol* 108:207–211, 2010.
66. Harvey LA, Glinsky JA, Katalinic OM, et al: Contracture management for people with spinal cord injuries. *NeuroRehabilitation* 28:17–20, 2011.
67. Kim H, Cho S, Lee H: Effects of passive Bi-axial ankle stretching while walking on uneven terrains in older adults with chronic stroke. *J Biomech* 89:57–64, 2019. doi:10.1016/j.jbiomech.2019.04.014.
68. Farmer SE, James M: Contractures in orthopaedic and neurological conditions: a review of causes and treatment. *Disabil Rehabil* 23:549–558, 2001.
69. Wood KS, Daluiski A: Management of joint contractures in the spastic upper extremity. *Hand Clin* 34(4):517–528, 2018. doi:10.1016/j.hcl.2018.06.011.

70. Matsuo S, Suzuki S, Iwata M, et al: Acute effects of different stretching durations on passive torque, mobility, and isometric muscle force. *J Strength Cond Res* 27(12):3367–3376, 2013. doi:10.1519/JSC.0b013e318290c26f.

71. Boyce D, Brosky Jr JA: Determining the minimal number of cyclic passive stretch repetitions recommended for an acute increase in an indirect measure of hamstring length. *Physiother Theory Pract* 24(2):113–120, 2008. doi:10.1080/09593980701378298.

72. Freitas SR, Vaz JR, Bruno PM, et al: Are rest intervals between stretching repetitions effective to acutely increase range of motion? *Int J Sports Physiol Perform* 10(2):191–197, 2015. doi:10.1123/ijspp.2014-0192.

73. Marques AP, Vasconcelos AA, Cabral CM, et al: Effect of frequency of static stretching on flexibility, hamstring tightness and electromyographic activity. *Braz J Med Biol Res* 42(10):949–953, 2009. doi:10.1590/s0100-879 × 2009001000012.

74. Freitas SR, Mil-Homens P: Effect of 8-week high-intensity stretching training on biceps femoris architecture. *J Strength Cond Res* 29(6):1737–1740, 2015. doi:10.1519/JSC.0000000000000800.

75. Feland JB, Myrer JW, Schulthies SS: The effect of duration of stretching of the hamstring muscle group for increasing range of motion in people aged 65 years or older. *Phys Ther* 81:1110–1117, 2001.

76. Reid DA, McNair PJ: Effects of a six week lower limb stretching programme on range of motion, peak passive torque and stiffness in people with and without osteoarthritis of the knee. *N Z J Physiother* 39:5–12, 2011.

77. Davis DS, Ashby PE, McCale KL, et al: The effectiveness of 3 stretching techniques on hamstring flexibility using consistent stretching parameters. *J Strength Cond Res* 19:27–32, 2005.

78. Ryan ED, Herda TJ, Costa PB, et al: Acute effects of passive stretching of the plantarflexor muscles on neuromuscular function: the influence of age. *Age (Dordr)* 36(4):9672, 2014. doi:10.1007/s11357-014-9672-x.

79. Christiansen CL: The effects of hip and ankle stretching on gait function of older people. *Arch Phys Med Rehabil* 89(8):1421–1428, 2008. doi:10.1016/j.apmr.2007.12.043.

80. Katalinic OM, Harvey LA: Effectiveness of stretch for the treatment and prevention of contractures in people with neurological conditions: a systematic review. *Phys Ther* 91:11–24, 2011.

81. Moseley AM, Hassett LM: Serial casting versus positioning for the treatment of elbow contractures in adults with traumatic brain injury: a randomized controlled trial. *Clin Rehabil* 22:406–417, 2008.

82. Horsley SA, Herbert RD: Four weeks of daily stretch has little or no effect on wrist contracture after stroke: a randomized controlled trial. *Aust J Physiother* 53:239–245, 2007.

83. Rose KJ, Burns J: Interventions for increasing ankle range of motion in patients with neuromuscular disease. *Cochrane Database Syst Rev* 2010(2):CD006973, 2010.

84. Kalkman BM, Bar-On L, O'Brien TD, et al: Stretching interventions in children with cerebral palsy: why are they ineffective in improving muscle function and how can we better their outcome? *Front Physiol* 11:131, 2020. doi:10.3389/fphys.2020.00131.

85. Voss DE, Ionta MK, Myers BJ: *Proprioceptive neuromuscular facilitation*, ed 3, Philadelphia, 1985, Harper & Row.

86. Sharman MJ, Cresswell AG, Riek S: Proprioceptive neuromuscular facilitation stretching: mechanisms and clinical implications. *Sports Med* 36:929–939, 2006.

87. Lamontagne A, Maloun F, Richards CL: Viscoelastic behavior of plantar flexor muscle-tendon unit at rest. *J Orthop Sports Phys Ther* 26:244–252, 1997.

88. Frank C, Akeson WH, Woo SL-Y, et al: Physiology and therapeutic value of passive joint motion. *Clin Orthop Relat Res* 185:113–125, 1984.

89. Shen C, Tang ZH, Hu JZ, et al: Does immobilization after arthroscopic rotator cuff repair increase tendon healing? A systematic review and meta-analysis. *Arch Orthop Trauma Surg* 134:1279–1285, 2014.

90. Wright RW, Preston E, Fleming BC, et al: A systematic review of anterior cruciate ligament reconstruction rehabilitation. Part I: continuous passive motion, early weight bearing, postoperative bracing, and home-based rehabilitation. *J Knee Surg* 21:217–224, 2008.

91. Yi A, Villacis D, Yalamanchili R, et al: A comparison of rehabilitation methods after arthroscopic rotator cuff repair: a systematic review. *Sports Health* 7:326–334, 2015.

92. Yang X, Li GH, Wang HJ, et al: Continuous passive motion after total knee arthroplasty: a systematic review and meta-analysis of associated effects on clinical outcomes. *Arch Phys Med Rehabil* 100(9):1763–1778, 2019. doi:10.1016/j.apmr.2019.02.001.

93. Lentell G, Hetherington T, Eagan J, et al: The use of thermal agents to influence the effectiveness of low load prolonged stretch. *J Orthop Sports Phys Ther* 16:200–207, 1992.

94. Lehmann J, Masock A, Warren C, et al: Effect of therapeutic temperatures on tendon extensibility. *Arch Phys Med Rehabil* 51:481–487, 1970.

95. Draper DO, Castro JL, Feland B, et al: Shortwave diathermy and prolonged stretching increase hamstring flexibility more than prolonged stretching alone. *J Orthop Sports Phys Ther* 34(1):13–20, 2004. doi:10.2519/jospt.2004.34.1.13.

96. Hocutt JE, Jaffe R, Ryplander CR: Cryotherapy in ankle sprains. *Am J Sports Med* 10:316–319, 1982.

97. Dolan MG, Mychaskiw AM, Mendel FC: Cool-water immersion and high-voltage electrical stimulation curb edema formation in rats. *J Athl Train* 38:225–230, 2003.

98. Man IO W, Lepar GS, Morrissey MC, et al: Effect of neuromuscular electrical stimulation on foot/ankle volume during standing. *Med Sci Sports Exerc* 35(4):630–634, 2003. doi:10.1249/01.MSS.0000058432.29149.08.

99. Malanga GA, Yan N, Stark J: Mechanisms and efficacy of heat and cold therapies for musculoskeletal injury. *Postgrad Med* 127(1):57–65, 2015. doi:10.1080/00325481.2015.992719.

100. Algafly AA, George KP: The effect of cryotherapy on nerve conduction velocity, pain threshold and pain tolerance. *Br J Sports Med* 41(6):365–369, 2007. doi:10.1136/bjsm.2006.031237.

101. Zeng C, Li H, Yang T, et al: Electrical stimulation for pain relief in knee osteoarthritis: systematic review and network meta-analysis. *Osteoarthritis Cartilage* 23(2):189–202, 2015. doi:10.1016/j.joca.2014.11.014.

102. Yang JD, Liao CD, Huang SW, et al: Effectiveness of electrical stimulation therapy in improving arm function after stroke: a systematic review and a meta-analysis of randomised controlled trials. *Clin Rehabil* 33(8):1286–1297, 2019. doi:10.1177/0269215519839165.

103. Rosewilliam S, Malhotra S, Roffe C, et al: Can surface neuromuscular electrical stimulation of the wrist and hand combined with routine therapy facilitate recovery of arm function in patients with stroke? *Arch Phys Med Rehabil* 93(10):1715–21.e1, 2012. doi:10.1016/j.apmr.2012.05.017.

Introduction to Thermal Agents

7

CHAPTER OBJECTIVES

After reading this chapter, the reader will be able to do the following:
- Define *thermal agent*.
- Describe the different types of heat transfer: conduction, convection, conversion, radiation, and evaporation.
- Define *specific heat*.
- Describe the variables that affect heating by radiation, conversion, and convection.

This chapter reviews the basic physical principles and physiological effects of transferring heat to or from patients using superficial and deep thermal agents. Clinical applications of superficial cooling and superficial heating agents are discussed in Chapter 8. Clinical applications of deep-heating agents, ultrasound, and diathermy are discussed in Chapters 9 and 10. Superficial thermal agents are agents that primarily change the temperature of the skin and superficial subcutaneous tissues. In contrast, deep-heating agents increase the temperature of tissues to a depth of approximately 5 cm, heating large muscles and periarticular structures as well as skin and subcutaneous tissues.

The therapeutic application of thermal agents results in the transfer of heat to or from a patient's body as well as between tissues and fluids of the body. Heat transfer can occur by **conduction, convection, conversion, radiation,** or evaporation. Heating agents transfer heat to the body to increase temperature, whereas cooling agents transfer heat away from the body to decrease temperature. Thermoregulation by the body also uses the aforementioned processes to maintain core body temperature and to maintain equilibrium between internal metabolic heat production and heat loss or gain at the skin surface. The following section discusses the physical principles of heat transfer to, from, and within the body.

Specific Heat

Specific heat is the amount of energy required to raise the temperature of a unit mass of a material by 1°C. Materials with high specific heat require more energy to achieve the same temperature increase than materials with low specific heat. The specific heat of different materials and body tissues differs (Table 7.1). For example, skin has higher specific heat than fat or bone, and water has higher specific heat than air.

> ### ◎ Clinical Pearl
> Materials with high specific heat require more energy to heat up and hold more energy at a given temperature than materials with low specific heat.

In addition to requiring more energy to change their temperature, materials with high specific heat hold more energy than materials with low specific heat when both are at the same temperature. Therefore, to transfer the same amount of heat to a patient, thermal agents with high specific heat, such as those containing water (e.g., moist hot packs), are applied at lower temperatures than thermal agents with low specific heat, such as those containing air (e.g., **fluidized therapy**). The specific heat of a material is generally expressed in joules per gram per degree Celsius (J/g/°C).

Modes of Heat Transfer

Heat can be transferred to, from, or within the body by conduction, convection, conversion, radiation, or evaporation.

CONDUCTION

Heating by conduction is the result of energy exchange by direct collision between the molecules of two materials at different temperatures. Heating by conduction requires direct contact of the two materials. Heat is conducted from the material at the higher temperature to the material at the lower temperature as faster-moving molecules in the warmer material collide with molecules in the cooler material, causing them to accelerate. Heat transfer continues until the temperature and speed of molecular movement of both materials become equal. Heat may also transfer to or from a patient by conduction. If the physical agent used has a higher temperature than the patient's skin—for example, a hot pack or warm **paraffin**—heat will transfer from the agent to the patient, and the temperature of superficial tissues in contact with the heating agent will rise. If the physical agent used is colder than

TABLE 7.1	Specific Heat of Various Materials
Material	Specific Heat in J/g/°C
Water	4.19
Air	1.01
Average for human body	3.56
Skin	3.77
Muscle	3.75
Fat	2.30
Bone	1.59

TABLE 7.2	Thermal Conductivity of Various Materials
Material	Thermal Conductivity (cal/second)/ (cm^2 × °C/cm)
Silver	1.01
Aluminum	0.50
Ice	0.005
Water at 20°C	0.0014
Bone	0.0011
Muscle	0.0011
Fat	0.0005
Air at 0°C	0.000057

the patient's skin—for example, an ice pack—heat will transfer from the patient to the agent, and the temperature of the superficial tissues in contact with the cooling agent will fall.

Heat can also transfer from one area of the body to another by conduction. For example, when one area of the body is heated by an external thermal agent, the tissues adjacent to and in contact with that area will heat up by conduction.

◉ Clinical Pearl

Heat transfer by conduction occurs only between materials of different temperatures that are in direct contact with each other.

If air is present between a conductive thermal agent and the patient, the heat is conducted first from the thermal agent to the air and then from the air to the patient.

Rate of Heat Transfer by Conduction

The rate at which heat transfers by conduction between two materials depends on the temperature difference between the materials, their **thermal conductivity**, and their area of contact. The relationship among these variables is expressed by the following formula:

$$\text{Rate of heat transfer} = \frac{\begin{array}{c}\text{Area of contact} \times \\ \text{Thermal conductivity} \times \\ \text{Temperature difference}\end{array}}{\text{Tissue thickness}}$$

The thermal conductivity of a material describes the rate at which it transfers heat by conduction and is generally expressed in (cal/second)/(cm^2 × °C/cm) (Table 7.2). This is not the same as the specific heat of a material.

Several guidelines can be derived from the preceding formula.

Guidelines for Heat Transfer by Conduction

1. The greater the temperature difference between a heating or cooling agent and the body part it is applied to, the faster the rate of heat transfer. For example, the higher the temperature of a hot pack, the more rapidly the temperature of the area of the patient's skin in contact with the hot pack will increase. Generally, the temperatures of conductive physical agents are selected to achieve a fast but safe rate of temperature change. If a heating agent is only a few degrees warmer than the patient, heating will take too long; by contrast, if the temperature difference is large, heat transfer could be so rapid as to burn the patient.

2. Materials with high thermal conductivity transfer heat faster than materials with low thermal conductivity. Metals have high thermal conductivity, water has moderate thermal conductivity, and air has low thermal conductivity.

Heating and cooling agents are generally composed of materials with moderate thermal conductivity to provide a safe and effective rate of heat transfer. Materials with low thermal conductivity can be used as insulators to limit the rate of heat transfer. For example, some types of hot packs are kept hot by soaking in and absorbing water that is kept at approximately 70°C (175°F). The high temperature, high specific heat, and moderate thermal conductivity of the water allow efficient heat transfer; however, if the pack is applied directly to a patient's skin, the patient probably will soon feel uncomfortably hot and could burn. Therefore, towels or terry cloth hot-pack covers that trap air, which has low thermal conductivity, are placed between the pack and the patient to limit the rate of heat transfer. In general, six to eight layers of toweling are placed between a moist hot pack and a patient.

◉ Clinical Pearl

Place six to eight layers of toweling between a moist hot pack and the patient to limit the rate of heat transfer and avoid burns. Additional layers of toweling can be added to further decrease heat conduction.

If the patient becomes too hot, additional layers of toweling can be added to further limit the rate of heat conduction. Newer towels and covers are generally thicker and therefore act as more effective insulators than older ones. Because subcutaneous fat has low thermal conductivity, it also acts as an insulator, limiting the conduction of heat to or from the deeper tissues.

Because metal has high thermal conductivity, metal jewelry should be removed from any area that will be in contact with a conductive thermal agent. If metal jewelry is not removed, heat will transfer rapidly to and from the metal and may burn the skin in contact with it.

Ice causes more rapid cooling than water, even at the same temperature, partly because it has a higher thermal conductivity than water and partly because of the amount of energy it takes to convert ice to water. The thermal conductivities of different commercially available cold packs vary; some are higher than water or ice, and others are lower. Therefore, when changing the brand or type of cold pack used, one should not assume that the new pack can be applied in the same manner, for the same amount of time, or with the same number of layers of insulating material as the old pack.

3. The larger the area of contact between a thermal agent and the patient, the greater the total heat transfer. For example, when a hot pack is applied to the entire back, or when a patient is immersed up to the neck in a whirlpool, the total amount of heat transferred will be greater than if a hot pack is applied only to a small area overlying the calf.
4. The rate of temperature rise decreases in proportion to tissue thickness. When a thermal agent is in contact with a patient's skin, skin temperature increases the most, and deeper tissues are progressively less affected. The deeper the tissue, the less its temperature will change. Therefore, conductive thermal agents are well suited to heating or cooling superficial tissues but should not be used when the goal is to change the temperature of deeper tissues.

CONVECTION

Heat transfer by convection occurs as the result of direct contact between a circulating medium and another material of a different temperature. This contrasts with heating by conduction, in which contact between a stationary thermal agent and the patient is constant. During heating or cooling by convection, the thermal agent is in motion, so new parts of the agent at the initial treatment temperature keep coming into contact with the patient's body part. As a result, heat transfer by convection transfers more heat in the same period of time than heat transfer by conduction, when the same material at the same initial temperature is used. For example, immersion in a whirlpool will heat a patient's skin more rapidly than immersion in a bowl of water of the same temperature, and the faster the water moves, the more rapid the rate of heat transfer will be.

Blood circulating in the body also transfers heat by convection to reduce local changes in tissue temperature. For example, when a thermal agent is applied to an area of the body and produces a local change in tissue temperature, the circulation constantly moves the heated blood out of the area

and moves cooler blood into the area to return the local tissue temperature to a normal level. This local cooling by convection reduces the impact of superficial heating agents on the local tissue temperature. **Vasodilation** increases the rate of circulation, increasing the rate at which the tissue temperature returns to normal. Thus, the vasodilation that occurs in response to heat protects the tissues by reducing the risk of burning.

CONVERSION

Heat transfer by conversion involves the conversion of a nonthermal form of energy, such as mechanical, electrical, or chemical energy, into heat. For example, **ultrasound,** which is a mechanical form of energy, is converted into heat when applied at a sufficient intensity to a tissue that absorbs ultrasound waves. Ultrasound causes molecules in the tissue to vibrate; the friction between them generates heat, resulting in an increase in tissue temperature. When **diathermy,** an electromagnetic form of energy, is applied to the body, it causes rotation of polar molecules, which results in friction between the molecules and increases tissue temperature. Some types of cold packs cool by converting heat into chemical energy. Striking these chemical cold packs initiates a chemical reaction that extracts heat from the pack, causing it to become cold. Thermal energy is converted into chemical energy to drive this reaction.

In contrast to heating by conduction or convection, heating by conversion is not affected by the temperature of the thermal agent. When heat is transferred by conversion, the rate of heat transfer depends on the power of the energy source. The power of ultrasound and diathermy is usually measured in watts, which refers to the amount of energy in joules output per second. The amount of energy output by a chemical reaction depends on the reacting chemicals and is usually measured in joules. The rate at which tissue temperature increases depends on the volume and type of tissue being treated, the size of the applicator, and the efficiency of transmission from the applicator to the patient. Different types of tissues absorb different forms of energy to a variable extent and therefore heat differently.

Heat transfer by conversion does not require direct contact between the thermal agent and the body; however, it does require that any intervening material be a good transmitter of that type of energy. For example, transmission gel, lotion, or water must be used between an ultrasound transducer and the patient to transmit the ultrasound because air, which might otherwise come between the transducer and the patient, transmits ultrasound poorly.

Physical agents that heat by conversion may have other nonthermal physiological effects. For example, although the mechanical energy of ultrasound and the electrical energy of diathermy can produce heat by conversion, they are also thought to have direct mechanical or electrical effects on tissue. Full discussions of absorption and of the thermal and nonthermal effects of ultrasound and diathermy can be found in Chapters 9 and 10, respectively.

RADIATION

Heating by radiation involves the transfer of energy from a material with a higher temperature to one with a lower temperature without an intervening medium or contact. This contrasts with heat transfer by conversion, in which the medium and the patient may be at the same temperature, and with heat transfer by conduction or convection, which require the thermal agent to contact the tissue being heated. The rate of temperature increase caused by radiation depends on the intensity of the radiation, the relative sizes of the radiation source and the area being treated, the distance of the source from the treatment area, and the angle between the radiation and the tissue.

> ◎ **Clinical Pearl**
>
> Infrared lamps transfer heat by radiation.

EVAPORATION

A material must absorb energy to evaporate, that is, to change from a liquid to a gas (or vapor). This energy is absorbed in the form of heat derived from the material itself or an adjoining material, decreasing its temperature.

Evaporation of sweat acts to cool the body. The temperature of evaporation for sweat is a few degrees higher than the normal skin temperature; therefore, if the skin temperature increases as a result of exercise or an external source, and the humidity of the environment is low enough, the sweat produced in response to the increased temperature will evaporate, reducing the local body temperature. If the ambient humidity is high, evaporation will be impaired. Sweating is a homeostatic mechanism that serves to cool the body when it is overheated to help return body temperature toward the normal range.

A **vapocoolant spray** evaporates at an even lower temperature than water. When heated by the warm skin of the body, the spray very quickly changes from its liquid form to a vapor and cools the skin.

> ◎ **Clinical Pearl**
>
> Vapocoolant sprays transfer heat from the patient by evaporation.

Chapter Review

1. Thermal agents transfer heat to or from patients by conduction, convection, conversion, or radiation.
2. Materials with higher specific heat require more energy to heat up than materials with lower specific heat, and they hold more energy at a given temperature.
3. Materials with moderate thermal conductivity should be selected for an effective yet safe rate of heat transfer. The risk of injury is decreased by adding towels and removing jewelry.
4. Convection transfers more heat in the same period of time than is transferred by conduction. The rate of heat transfer by convection is related to the temperature and circulation speed of the medium.
5. Heating by conversion depends on the power of an energy source rather than its temperature and does not require direct contact between the thermal agent and the body but does require the intervening material to be a good transmitter of the energy.
6. Heating by radiation depends on the intensity, the relative sizes of the radiation source and the treated area, and the distance and angle of the applied radiation.

Glossary

Conduction: Heat transfer resulting from energy exchange by direct collision between molecules of two materials at different temperatures. Heat is transferred by conduction when the materials are in contact with each other.

Convection: Heat transfer through direct contact of a circulating medium with material of a different temperature.

Conversion: Heat transfer by conversion of a nonthermal form of energy, such as mechanical, electrical, or chemical energy, into heat.

Diathermy: The application of shortwave or microwave electromagnetic energy to produce heat within tissues, particularly deep tissues.

Fluidized therapy: A dry heating agent that transfers heat by convection. It consists of a cabinet containing finely ground particles of cellulose through which heated air is circulated.

Paraffin: A waxy substance that can be warmed and used to coat the extremities for thermotherapy.

Radiation: Transfer of energy from one material to another without the need for direct contact or an intervening medium.

Specific heat: The amount of energy required to raise the temperature of a given weight of a material by a given number of degrees, usually expressed in J/g/°C.

Thermal conductivity: The rate at which a material transfers heat by conduction, usually expressed in (cal/second)/(cm² × °C/cm).

Ultrasound: Sound with a frequency greater than 20,000 cycles per second that has thermal and nonthermal effects when applied to the body.

Vapocoolant spray: A liquid that evaporates quickly when sprayed on the skin, causing quick superficial cooling of the skin.

Vasodilation: An increase in blood vessel diameter. Heat generally causes vasodilation.

Superficial Cold and Heat

CHAPTER OBJECTIVES

After reading this chapter, the reader will be able to:

- Define *cryotherapy and thermotherapy.*
- Describe the physical effects of cryotherapy and thermotherapy.
- Explain the clinical indications for the use of cryotherapy and thermotherapy.
- Choose the best technique for treatment with cryotherapy or thermotherapy, and list the advantages and disadvantages of each.
- Select the appropriate equipment and optimal treatment parameters for treatment with cryotherapy and thermotherapy.
- Safely and effectively apply cryotherapy and thermotherapy.
- Accurately and completely document treatment with cryotherapy and thermotherapy.

Cryotherapy and thermotherapy are classified as deep or superficial based on the mode of application and depth of the resulting therapeutic temperature change. This chapter focuses on the application of superficial cooling and superficial heating agents. Physical agents that cool or heat by conduction, such as cold packs, hot packs, and **paraffin** wax; by convection, such as whirlpools and **Fluidotherapy**; or by radiation, such as infrared (IR) lamps, are all superficial heating or cooling agents. They exchange energy directly with the skin, and that temperature change penetrates a few millimeters deep by conduction from the skin to deeper tissues, gradually decreasing in effect because of absorption by the more superficial tissues. There are no deep-cooling agents used in rehabilitation. Deep-heating agents used in rehabilitation are ultrasound and diathermy, which both heat by conversion. Deep-heating agents are able to produce heat in deeper tissues, including muscle, because the energy that is converted into heat penetrates into the tissues and is then converted to heat as it is absorbed by the tissues. This chapter focuses on superficial heating agents. The deep-heating agents, ultrasound and diathermy, are covered in Chapters 9 and 10, respectively.

CRYOTHERAPY

Cryotherapy, the therapeutic use of cold, has clinical applications in rehabilitation and in other areas of medicine. This chapter discusses most uses of cryotherapy in rehabilitation. Outside of rehabilitation, cryotherapy is used primarily to destroy malignant and nonmalignant tissue growths. For these applications, very low-temperature cooling is generally applied directly to the tissue to be destroyed. In addition, whole-body therapeutic hypothermia is now commonly used after cardiac arrest and after severe stroke or neurological trauma. When used for these indications, the goal is generally to cool the body mildly to moderately to 32°C to 35°C (89.6 degrees Farenheit to 95 degrees Farenheit) in order to mitigate the severity of the destructive cascade following injury.[1] In rehabilitation, mild local cooling has traditionally been used to control inflammation, pain, and **edema;** to reduce **spasticity;** to control symptoms of multiple sclerosis; and to facilitate movement (Fig. 8.1). Although this type of cryotherapy is applied to the skin, it can produce clinically meaningful decreases in temperature deep beneath the area of application, including in intraarticular areas.[2–5] Recently, there has been growing interest in whole-body cryotherapy, using extremely cold air, for preventing and treating muscle soreness after exercise. This application is not covered in this book because it is not generally used in rehabilitation and because, to date, there is insufficient evidence to determine whether this intervention is effective, and if so, which specific protocols are likely to be effective.[6,7]

Effects of Cold
HEMODYNAMIC EFFECTS
Initial Decrease in Blood Flow

Cold applied to the skin causes an immediate reduction in skin temperature and **vasoconstriction** of the cutaneous vessels in the area of application. This vasoconstriction persists while the cooling is applied and may last for at least as long after cooling, even while the skin rewarms.[8,9] The vasoconstriction produced by cryotherapy results in an approximately 40% reduction in blood flow in the area where the cold is applied, where the tissue temperature decrease is greatest,

and is most effective when the placement is directly over an area of inflammation.[10]

> ◎ **Clinical Pearl**
>
> Cryotherapy causes vasoconstriction, which reduces local blood flow.

Cold causes cutaneous vasoconstriction by a combination of direct and indirect mechanisms (Fig. 8.2). Cooling activates cutaneous cold receptors, which directly stimulates the contraction of smooth muscles in blood vessel walls. Cooling also decreases the production and release of vasodilator mediators, such as histamine and prostaglandins, indirectly reducing vasodilation, and causes a reflex activation of sympathetic postsynaptic α-adrenergic neurons as well as activation of the rho-kinase pathway, resulting in cutaneous vasoconstriction in the area of application and, to a lesser extent, in areas distant from the area of application.[11–13] Cold is also thought to reduce circulation by increasing blood viscosity, thereby increasing resistance to blood flow.

It is thought that the body reduces blood flow in response to decreased tissue temperature to protect other areas from excessive cooling and to stabilize core body temperature.[14] The less blood that flows through an area being cooled, the smaller volume of blood that is cooled, and the less other areas in the circulatory system are affected. Reduced circulation results in a greater decrease in the temperature of the area where a cooling agent is applied because warmer blood is not being brought into the area to raise its temperature by convection. Correspondingly, a smaller decrease in temperature occurs in other areas of the body because little of the cold blood is circulated there.

Later Increase in Blood Flow

The immediate vasoconstriction response to cold is a consistent and well-documented phenomenon. When cold is applied for longer periods of time, or when the tissue temperature

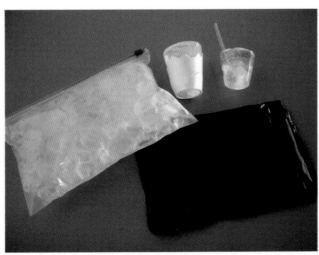

FIGURE 8.1 Cryotherapy agents.

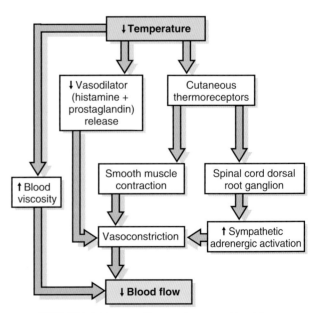

FIGURE 8.2 How cryotherapy decreases blood flow.

reaches less than 10°C (50°F), vasodilation may occur. This phenomenon is known as **cold-induced vasodilation (CIVD)** and was first reported by Lewis in 1930.[15] His findings were replicated in a number of later studies[16-18]; however, vasodilation is not a consistent response to prolonged cold application.[19,20] Lewis reported that when an individual's fingers were immersed in an ice bath, their temperature initially decreased, but after 15 minutes, their finger temperature cyclically increased and decreased (Fig. 8.3). Lewis correlated this temperature cycling with alternating vasoconstriction and vasodilation and called this the *hunting response*. Current literature generally refers to this phenomenon as *CIVD*. Various mechanisms have been proposed to underlie CIVD. CIVD may be mediated by an axon reflex in response to the pain of prolonged cold or very low temperatures. The contraction of smooth muscles of the blood vessel walls may be directly inhibited by extreme cold[21] or indirectly inhibited by sympathetic vasoconstrictor withdrawal.[22] Or sustained cold may decrease the release of neurotransmitters from the sympathetic nerves to the muscle walls of the arterio-venous anastomoses (AVAs).[23] AVAs are specific thermoregulatory organs present in the hands and feet that regulate blood flow in cold and heat.[24,25]

CIVD is most likely to occur in the distal extremities, such as the fingers or toes, and with applications of cold at temperatures below 1°C for longer than 15 minutes.[23] However, CIVD is almost absent during hypothermia, and people who are exposed to extreme cold frequently (e.g., fish filleters) develop an enhanced CIVD response that is thought to be protective. There are also ethnic differences in the CIVD response, with black people having the least CIVD response. Although the amount of vasodilation associated with CIVD is usually small, in clinical situations where vasodilation should be avoided, it is generally recommended that cold be applied for no more than 15 minutes to avoid CIVD, particularly when the distal extremities are treated. When vasodilation is the intended goal of the intervention, cryotherapy is not recommended because it does not consistently have this effect, and when it does, the effect is small.

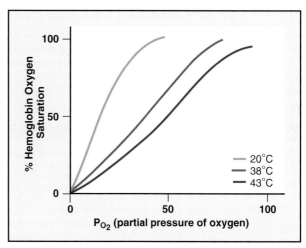

FIGURE 8.4 Effects of temperature on oxygen-hemoglobin dissociation curve. (Adapted from Barcroft J, King W: The effect of temperature on the dissociation curve of blood. *J Physiol* 39:374–384, 1909.)

Although the increase in skin redness seen with the application of cold may appear to be a sign of CIVD, this change is thought to be primarily the result of an increased concentration of oxyhemoglobin in the blood caused by a decrease in oxygen-hemoglobin dissociation that occurs at lower temperatures (Fig. 8.4). Because cooling decreases oxygen-hemoglobin dissociation, making less oxygen available to the tissues, CIVD is not an effective way to increase oxygen delivery to an area.

NEUROMUSCULAR EFFECTS

Cold has a variety of effects on neuromuscular function, including slowing nerve conduction velocity, elevating the pain threshold, altering muscle force generation, decreasing spasticity, and facilitating muscle contraction.

Decreased Nerve Conduction Velocity

When the temperature of a nerve is decreased, nerve conduction velocity decreases in proportion to the degree and duration of the temperature change.[26,27] Although decreased nerve conduction velocity can occur if a superficial cooling agent is applied to the skin for 5 minutes or longer,[28] this reduction fully reverses within 15 minutes in individuals with normal circulation. However, after 20 minutes of cooling, nerve conduction velocity may take 30 minutes or longer to recover because cooling for longer reduces the nerve's temperature more.[29]

Cold can decrease the conduction velocity of both sensory and motor nerves. Cold has the greatest effect on conduction by myelinated and small fibers and the least effect on conduction by unmyelinated and large fibers.[29] Therefore, A-delta fibers, which are small-diameter, myelinated, pain-transmitting fibers, undergo the greatest decrease in conduction velocity in response to cooling. Reversible nerve conduction block, which is when there is a failure of action potential propagation, can also occur when ice is applied superficially directly over major nerve branches, such as the peroneal nerve at the lateral aspect of the knee or the ulnar nerve at the elbow.[30]

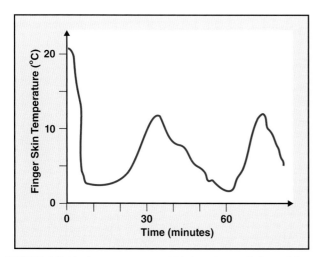

FIGURE 8.3 Hunting response, cold-induced vasodilation of finger immersed in ice water, measured by skin temperature change. (Adapted from Lewis T: Observations upon the reactions of the vessels of the human skin to cold. *Heart* 15:177–208, 1930.)

Reduced Pain and Increased Pain Threshold

Applying cryotherapy can increase the pain threshold and decrease the sensation of pain.[27,31-33] Proposed mechanisms for these effects include counterirritation via the gate control mechanism and reduction of muscle spasm, slowing of sensory nerve conduction velocity, or reduction of postinjury edema.[27,34]

> ### Clinical Pearl
>
> Cryotherapy can increase the pain threshold and decrease the sensation of pain.

Stimulation of cutaneous cold receptors by cold may provide sufficient sensory input to fully or partially block the transmission of painful stimuli to the brain cortex, increasing the pain threshold and decreasing pain sensation. Such gating of the pain sensation can reduce muscle spasm by interrupting the pain-spasm-pain cycle, as described in Chapter 4. Cryotherapy may reduce the pain associated with an acute injury by reducing the rate of blood flow in an area and by decreasing the rate of reactions related to acute inflammation, thus controlling postinjury edema formation. Reducing edema can also alleviate pain produced by compression of nerves or other pressure-sensitive structures.

Altered Muscle Strength

Depending on the duration of the intervention and the timing of measurement, cryotherapy may increase and decrease measures of muscle strength. Isometric muscle strength increases directly after applying ice massage for 5 minutes or less; however, the duration of this effect has not been documented.[35] Proposed mechanisms for this response to brief cooling include facilitation of motor nerve excitability and increased psychological motivation to perform. In contrast, after cooling for 15 minutes or longer, isometric muscle strength decreases immediately after cooling, adversely affecting speed, power, and agility-based running tasks and confounding measurement of progress.[36,37] This initial reduction in performance may reverse as quickly as 20 minutes later, when strength may be greater than precooling measures for the following 3 hours or longer (Fig. 8.5).[38-40] Proposed

mechanisms for reduced strength after prolonged cooling include reduced blood flow to the muscles, slowed motor nerve conduction, increased muscle viscosity, and increased joint or soft tissue stiffness.

It is important to be aware of these changes in muscle strength with cryotherapy because they can obscure accurate, objective assessment of muscle strength and of patient progress and may interfere with performance directly after cooling. Therefore, it is recommended that muscle strength be consistently measured before the application of cryotherapy, that precooling strength not be compared with postcooling strength, and that patients not return to activities with high-strength demands directly following local cryotherapy.[41] When immediate return to activity is desired after cryotherapy, the duration of cryotherapy should be short, or cryotherapy should be followed by progressive warm-up exercises.[40]

> ### Clinical Pearl
>
> Because muscle strength can be temporarily influenced by cryotherapy, strength testing should be performed before rather than after cryotherapy application.

Decreased Spasticity

When applied appropriately, cryotherapy is well known to temporarily decrease spasticity.[42,43] The amplitude of the Achilles tendon reflex and integrated electromyography (EMG) activity decrease within a few seconds of application of cold to the skin. This rapid response is most likely a reflex reaction to stimulation of cutaneous cold receptors reducing gamma motor neuron activity. This fast response must be related to the stimulation of cutaneous receptors because muscle temperature does not decrease after such a brief period of cooling.

After more prolonged cooling of 10 to 30 minutes, a temporary decrease in or elimination of spasticity and clonus, a depression of the Achilles tendon reflex, and a reduction in resistance to passive motion can also occur in patients with spasticity.[43-48] These changes are thought to be caused by decreased discharge from afferent spindles and Golgi tendon organs (GTOs) as a result of decreased muscle temperature.[49] These effects generally persist for 1 to 1.5 hours after cooling

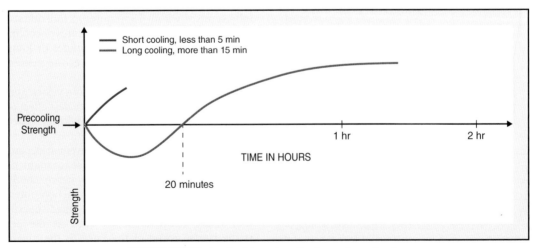

FIGURE 8.5 Effects of cold on strength of muscle contraction.

and therefore can be taken advantage of in treatment by applying cryotherapy to hypertonic areas for 10 to 30 minutes before employing other interventions to reduce spasticity during functional or therapeutic activities.

> ◎ **Clinical Pearl**
>
> Cryotherapy can temporarily reduce spasticity. Cooling for 10 to 30 minutes can reduce spasticity for the following 60 to 90 minutes, providing a window for other therapeutic or functional activities.

Facilitation of Muscle Contraction

Brief application of cryotherapy is thought to facilitate alpha motor neuron activity to contract a muscle that is flaccid because of prolonged upper motor neuron dysfunction.[43] This effect is observed in response to a few seconds of cooling and lasts for only a short time. With longer cooling for even a few minutes, a decrease in gamma motor neuron activity reduces the force of muscle contraction. This brief facilitation effect of cryotherapy is occasionally used clinically when attempting to stimulate the production of appropriate motor patterns in patients with upper motor neuron lesions.

METABOLIC EFFECTS
Decreased Metabolic Rate

Cold decreases the rate of all metabolic reactions, including reactions involved in inflammation and healing. Thus, cryotherapy can be used to control acute inflammation but is not recommended when healing is delayed because it may further impair recovery. The activity of cartilage-degrading enzymes such as collagenase, elastase, hyaluronidase, and protease, and the level of histamine, are reduced by decreases in joint temperature, with activity almost ceasing when joint temperatures reach 30°C (86°F) or lower.[50,51] Thus cryotherapy is recommended as an intervention to prevent or reduce inflammation and to prevent collagen destruction in inflammatory joint diseases such as osteoarthritis and rheumatoid arthritis.

> ◎ **Clinical Pearl**
>
> Cold decreases the local metabolic rate and therefore can reduce inflammatory activity.

Clinical Indications for Cryotherapy
INFLAMMATION CONTROL

Cryotherapy can be used to control acute inflammation, accelerating recovery from injury, trauma, or inflammatory joint disorders, without impeding tissue healing.[52] Cryotherapy reduces the heat, redness, edema, pain, and loss of function associated with the inflammatory phase of tissue healing. As noted previously, decreasing[33,53] the tissue temperature slows the rate of chemical reactions in the body. Cooling also reduces the release of inflammatory mediators during the acute inflammatory response. Cryotherapy directly reduces the heat associated with inflammation and decreases edema by decreasing the blood flow through vasoconstriction, increased blood viscosity, and decreased capillary permeability. It is thought that cryotherapy may also prevent microvascular damage in soft tissue injury by decreasing the activity of leukocytes, which damage vessel walls and increase capillary permeability,[54,55] and may decrease macrophage infiltration and the accumulation of inflammatory markers.[53] As described in greater detail in the following section, cryotherapy is thought to reduce pain by decreasing the activity of A-delta pain fibers and by gating at the spinal cord level. Controlling the edema and pain associated with inflammation limits the loss of function associated with this phase of tissue healing.

> ◎ **Clinical Pearl**
>
> Apply cryotherapy immediately after injury, during the acute inflammatory phase of healing, to help control bleeding, edema, and pain and accelerate recovery.

It is recommended that cryotherapy be applied immediately after an injury and throughout the acute inflammatory phase. Immediate application helps control injury-associated bleeding and edema; therefore, the sooner the intervention is applied, the greater and more immediate the potential benefits.[56] Local skin temperature can be used to estimate the stage of healing and to determine whether cryotherapy is indicated. If the local skin temperature of an area is elevated, the area is probably still inflamed, and cryotherapy is likely to be beneficial. Once the local skin temperature returns to normal, acute inflammation has probably resolved, and cryotherapy should be discontinued. Acute inflammation usually resolves within 48 to 72 hours following acute trauma but may be prolonged if the trauma is severe, the injuries are chronic, or the patient has an inflammatory disease such as rheumatoid arthritis. If the temperature of an area remains elevated for longer than expected, infection is possible, and the patient should be evaluated further. When acute inflammation has resolved, cryotherapy should be discontinued because continuing cryotherapy could impede recovery during the later proliferation and remodeling stages of healing by slowing chemical reactions or impairing circulation.

Cryotherapy is often recommended to treat acute inflammation caused by surgery or chronic inflammatory joint conditions such as osteoarthritis and rheumatoid arthritis. Applying cryotherapy for a number of days directly after surgery can reduce inflammation, edema, pain, and analgesic medication use after surgery and promote more rapid functional recovery (e.g., hip or knee replacement, shoulder surgery, abdominal surgery).[57–61] The lack of benefit, on average, found in trials of cryotherapy for patients with osteoarthritis is probably because the benefits associated with cryotherapy when applied during flares of inflammation are likely outweighed by the lack of benefit when applied between flares.[62,63]

Cryotherapy may reduce the severity of **delayed-onset muscle soreness (DOMS)**.[64] DOMS is thought to be caused by muscle inflammation and connective tissue damaged in response to exercise.[65,66] Two meta-analyses published in 2012, one that included 14 studies with a total of 239 subjects and another that included 17 studies with a total of 366 subjects, as well as a subsequent review in 2015 and later studies, have found that cryotherapy, particularly by immersion in cold water, is moderately effective in alleviating the symptoms of DOMS for up to 96 hours after exercise, particularly if the preceding exercise was high intensity and eccentric.[64,67–69] This effect is thought to be due to reductions in blood flow, inflammation, and metabolic enzymatic activity.

Although cryotherapy can reduce inflammation and its associated signs and symptoms, the cause of the inflammation may also need to be addressed directly to prevent recurrence. For example, if inflammation is caused by overuse of a tendon, the patient's use of that tendon must be limited to avoid recurrence of symptoms. However, if the inflammation is caused by surgery or acute trauma, the symptoms are not likely to recur.

When cryotherapy is applied to control inflammation, the treatment time is generally less than 15 minutes, particularly when treating the distal extremities, because longer applications may be associated with CIVD. The duration of cryotherapy in other areas is also generally limited to 20 minutes or less, and sessions should be at least 1 hour apart, to minimize the risk of cold-induced injuries as a result of excessive decreases in tissue temperature.

> ◎ **Clinical Pearl**
>
> When using cryotherapy to control inflammation, apply for no longer than 20 minutes, and keep applications at least 1 hour apart.

EDEMA CONTROL

Cryotherapy can be used to reduce edema, particularly edema associated with acute inflammation. During acute inflammation, edema is caused by increased intravascular fluid pressure and increased vascular permeability resulting in fluid extravasating into the interstitium. Cryotherapy reduces intravascular pressure by reducing blood flow into the area through vasoconstriction and increased blood viscosity. Cryotherapy also controls increases in capillary permeability by reducing the release of vasoactive substances such as histamine.

To most effectively minimize edema formation, cryotherapy should be applied as soon as possible after acute trauma, in conjunction with compression[70] and elevation of the affected area above the level of the heart (Fig. 8.6).[71] Compression and elevation reduce edema by pushing extravascular fluid out of the swollen area so that it can return to the venous and lymphatic drainage

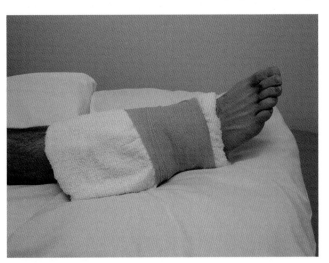

FIGURE 8.6 Cryotherapy with compression and elevation.

systems. The acronym **RICE** refers to the combined intervention of rest, ice, compression, and elevation.

> ◎ **Clinical Pearl**
>
> Cryotherapy, combined with rest, compression, and elevation, reduces postinjury edema.

Although cryotherapy can reduce edema associated with acute inflammation, it is not effective in controlling edema caused by immobility and poor circulation. In such cases, increased rather than decreased venous or lymphatic circulation is required to move fluid out of the affected area. This is best accomplished with compression, elevation, heat, exercise, and massage.[72] The mechanisms of action of this combination of treatments are discussed in detail in Chapter 20.

PAIN CONTROL

The decrease in tissue temperature produced by cryotherapy may directly or indirectly reduce the sensation of pain. Cryotherapy directly and rapidly modifies the sensation of pain by gating pain transmission through the activity of cutaneous thermal receptors. This immediate analgesic effect of cold is exploited when a **vapocoolant spray** or ice massage is used to cool the skin before stretching of the muscles below. The reduced sensation of pain allows the stretch to be more forceful and thus potentially more effective.

Applying cryotherapy for 10 to 15 minutes or longer can control pain for 1 hour or longer. This prolonged effect is thought to be the result of blocking conduction in deep, pain-transmitting A-delta fibers and gating of pain transmission by cutaneous thermal receptors.[29] The effect is thought to be prolonged because the temperature of the area remains lower than normal for 1 or 2 hours after the cooling modality is removed. Rewarming the area is slow because cold-induced vasoconstriction limits the flow of warm blood into the area, and subcutaneous fat insulates the deeper tissues from rewarming by conduction from ambient air.

Reducing pain through cryotherapy can also interrupt the pain-spasm-pain cycle by alleviating the muscle spasm even after the temperature of the treated area has returned to normal. Cryotherapy can also reduce pain indirectly by controlling its underlying cause, such as inflammation or edema.

MODIFICATION OF SPASTICITY

Cryotherapy can be used to temporarily reduce spasticity in patients with upper motor neuron dysfunction. Brief applications of cold lasting for approximately 5 minutes can almost immediately decrease deep tendon reflexes. Longer applications for 10 to 30 minutes decrease or eliminate clonus and may decrease the resistance of muscles to passive stretch. The decrease in spasticity produced by prolonged cooling generally lasts for an hour or longer after the intervention; this is sufficient to allow for a variety of therapeutic interventions, including active exercise, stretching, functional activities, or hygiene.

SYMPTOM MANAGEMENT IN MULTIPLE SCLEROSIS

Some patients with multiple sclerosis (MS) experience aggravation of their symptoms when they get hot, such as occurs in warm environments or with activity.[73] These patients can respond well to generalized cooling, showing improvements in both electrophysiological measures and clinical symptoms and function.[74] Cooling of the trunk with a vest, or cooling of the hand, can reduce a range of symptoms in people with MS, including fatigue, muscle weakness, visual dysfunction, tremor, and postural instability.[75-78]

> ### ◎ Clinical Pearl
>
> Many patients with multiple sclerosis are heat sensitive. Their symptoms worsen if they get warm, and these symptoms may be reduced by cooling.

FACILITATION

Rapid application of ice as a stimulus to elicit desired motor patterns, known as **quick icing,** is a technique developed by Rood. Although this technique may be used effectively in the rehabilitation of patients with flaccidity resulting from upper motor neuron dysfunction, it tends to have unreliable results and therefore is not commonly used.[79] The results of quick icing are unreliable because the initial phasic withdrawal pattern stimulated in the agonist muscles may lower the resting potential of the antagonists so that a second stimulus elicits activity in the antagonist muscles rather than in the agonists. This produces motion first in the desired direction, followed by a rebound movement in the opposite direction. Icing may also adversely affect motor control through dyssynchronization of the cortex as a result of increased sympathetic tone.

Contraindications and Precautions for Cryotherapy

Although cryotherapy is a relatively safe intervention, its use is contraindicated in some circumstances, and it should be applied with caution in others. Cryotherapy may be applied by a qualified clinician or by a properly instructed patient. Rehabilitation clinicians may use all forms of cryotherapy that are noninvasive and do not destroy tissue. Patients may use cold packs or ice packs, ice massage, or a **contrast bath** to treat themselves. If the patient's condition is worsening or does not improve after two or three treatments, the treatment approach should be reevaluated and changed, or the patient should be referred to a physician for further evaluation.

CONTRAINDICATIONS FOR THE USE OF CRYOTHERAPY

✳ CONTRAINDICATIONS

for the Use of Cryotherapy

- Cold hypersensitivity (cold-induced urticaria)
- Cold intolerance
- Cryoglobulinemia
- Paroxysmal cold hemoglobinuria
- Raynaud
- Over regenerating peripheral nerves
- Over an area with circulatory compromise or peripheral vascular disease

Cold Hypersensitivity (Cold-Induced Urticaria)

Some individuals have a familial or acquired hypersensitivity that causes them to develop a vascular skin reaction in response to cold exposure.[80] This reaction is marked by the transient appearance of smooth, slightly elevated patches, which are redder or paler than the surrounding skin and also often itch severely. This response is termed *cold hypersensitivity* or *cold-induced urticaria*. Symptoms may occur only in the area of cold exposure or all over the body.

Cold Intolerance

Cold intolerance in the form of severe pain, numbness, and color changes in response to cold can occur in patients with some types of rheumatic diseases or after severe accidental or surgical trauma to the digits.

Cryoglobulinemia

Cryoglobulinemia is an uncommon disorder characterized by the precipitation of serum proteins, cryoglobulins, in the circulation when below 37°C.[81] This disorder may be idiopathic but is more often associated with an underlying disorder, most often hepatitis C. Cryoglobulinemia can cause systemic vasculitis. Although the mainstay of treatment of cryoglobulinemia usually involves treatment of the underlying disorder and also often immunosuppression, cryotherapy should also be avoided in patients with cryoglobulinemia.

Paroxysmal Cold Hemoglobinuria

Paroxysmal cold hemoglobinuria is a rare autoimmune hemolytic anemia. In this disorder, an antibody against the P antigen on red cells attaches to the red cells at cold temperatures, causing red cell lysis when the blood recirculates to warmer parts of the body.[82] Cryotherapy should be avoided in patients with paroxysmal cold hemoglobinuria.

Raynaud

Raynaud, which is sometimes called a disease, syndrome, or phenomenon, is marked by brief episodes of vasospasm in the fingers and sometimes also the toes[83,84] and tips of the nose and ears. Raynaud may be classified as primary, when no underlying disease is found, or secondary, when there is an associated disease. Raynaud is characterized by sudden pallor and cyanosis of the skin of the digits, followed by redness, precipitated by cold or emotional upset, and relieved by warmth. Primary Raynaud is a common condition without severe sequelae. In contrast, secondary Raynaud can result in irreversible ischemia, causing digital necrosis, ulceration, and infection. Avoiding cold remains the most effective approach for managing any form of Raynaud. Therefore, cryotherapy should be avoided in patients with Raynaud.

> ### ▪ Ask the Patient
> - "Do you have any unusual responses to cold?" If the patient answers yes to this question, ask for further details, and include the following questions:
> - "Do you develop a rash when cold?" (a sign of cold hypersensitivity)
> - "Do you have severe pain, numbness, or color changes in your fingers when exposed to cold?" (signs of Raynaud)
> - "Do you see blood in your urine after being cold?" (a sign of paroxysmal cold hemoglobinuria)

If responses indicate that the patient may have cold hypersensitivity, cold intolerance, cryoglobulinemia, paroxysmal cold hemoglobinuria, or Raynaud, cryotherapy should not be applied.

Over Regenerating Peripheral Nerves

Cryotherapy should not be applied directly over a regenerating peripheral nerve because local vasoconstriction or altered nerve conduction may delay nerve regeneration.

> ### ▪Ask the Patient
> • "Do you have any nerve damage in this area?"
> • "Do you have any numbness or tingling in this limb? If so, where?"
>
> ### ▪Assess
> • Test sensation.

In the presence of sensory impairment or other signs of nerve dysfunction, cryotherapy should not be applied directly over an affected nerve.

Over an Area With Circulatory Compromise or Peripheral Vascular Disease

Cryotherapy should not be applied over an area with impaired circulation because cooling may aggravate the condition by causing vasoconstriction and increasing blood viscosity. Circulatory impairment may be the result of peripheral vascular disease, trauma to the vessels, or early healing and is often associated with edema resulting from inadequate venous return. When edema is present, it is important that its cause be determined—although edema resulting from inflammation can benefit from cryotherapy, edema resulting from impaired circulation may be exacerbated by cryotherapy. The causes of edema can be distinguished by observing the local skin color and temperature: edema caused by inflammation will make the skin warm and red, whereas edema caused by poor circulation will make the skin cool and pale.

> ### ◎ Clinical Pearl
> Avoid cooling when edema is caused by poor circulation (i.e., when the area is cool and pale).

> ### ▪Ask the Patient
> • "Do you have poor circulation in this limb?"
>
> ### ▪Assess
> • Skin temperature and color

If the patient has signs of impaired circulation, such as pallor and coolness of the skin in the area being considered for treatment, cryotherapy should not be applied.

PRECAUTIONS FOR THE USE OF CRYOTHERAPY

> ### ✱ PRECAUTIONS
> **for the Use of Cryotherapy**
> • Over the superficial main branch of a nerve
> • Over an open wound
> • Hypertension
> • Poor sensation or mentation
> • Very young and very old patients

Over the Superficial Main Branch of a Nerve

Applying cold directly over the superficial main branch of a nerve, such as the peroneal nerve at the lateral knee or the radial nerve at the posterolateral elbow, may cause a nerve conduction block.[26,30,85,86] Therefore, when applying cryotherapy to such an area, monitor signs of change in nerve conduction, such as distal numbness or tingling; if any of these occur, discontinue cryotherapy.

Over an Open Wound

It is generally recommended that cryotherapy not be applied directly over any deep, open wound because the reduced circulation and reduced metabolic rate may delay healing. Caution should be used if cryotherapy is applied to areas with superficial skin damage because if cutaneous thermal receptors are damaged, therapeutic vasoconstriction, pain control, and spasticity reduction may be diminished; in addition, the absence of skin reduces the insulating protection of subcutaneous layers and increases the risk of excessively cooling these tissues.

> ### ▪Assess
> • Inspect the skin closely for wounds, cuts, or abrasions.

Do not apply cryotherapy in the area of a deep wound. Use less intense cooling if cuts or abrasions are present.

Hypertension

Because cold can cause transient increases in systolic or diastolic blood pressure, patients with hypertension should be carefully monitored during the application of cryotherapy. Treatment should be discontinued if blood pressure increases beyond safe levels during treatment. Guidelines for safe blood pressures for individual patients should be obtained from the physician.

Poor Sensation or Mentation

If the patient cannot sense or report discomfort or other abnormal responses during cryotherapy, the clinician should use less intense cooling and monitor the patient carefully for any adverse effects.

Very Young and Very Old Patients

Caution should be used when applying cryotherapy to very young or very old patients because these individuals can have impaired thermal regulation and a limited ability to communicate.

Adverse Effects of Cryotherapy

Various adverse effects have been reported when cold is applied incorrectly or when contraindicated. The most severe adverse effect of cryotherapy is tissue death caused by prolonged vasoconstriction, ischemia, and thromboses in the smaller vessels. Tissue death may also result from freezing. Damage can occur when the tissue's temperature reaches 15°C (59°F); however, freezing (frostbite) does not occur until the skin temperature drops to between 4°C and 10°C (39°F and 50°F) or lower. Excessive exposure to cold may also cause temporary or permanent nerve damage, resulting in pain, numbness, tingling, hyperhidrosis, or abnormalities in nerve conduction.[87,88] To avoid damaging soft tissue or nerves, cold should be applied for no longer than 45 minutes, and the tissue temperature should be maintained above 15°C (59°F).

Application Techniques
GENERAL CRYOTHERAPY

Cryotherapy may be applied using a variety of materials, including cold or ice packs, ice cups, **controlled cold compression** units, vapocoolant sprays, frozen towels, ice water, or contrast baths.

Different materials cool the body at different rates and to different degrees and depths. For example, ice packs and packs containing a water/alcohol mixture cool the skin more, and more quickly, than gel packs or frozen peas at the same initial temperature.[89] Frozen peas applied for 20 minutes can reduce skin temperatures sufficiently to cause localized skin analgesia while reducing nerve conduction velocity and metabolic enzyme activity, but flexible frozen gel packs applied for the same duration do not cool to this level.[90] In general, applying frozen gel packs or ice packs for 20 minutes reduces the temperature of the skin and subcutaneous tissues up to 2 cm deep.[91] However, overlying adipose tissue and exercise performed while the ice is applied can lessen the cooling effect of this type of cryotherapy.[92,93] Submersion of the leg in a 10°C (50°F) whirlpool for 20 minutes prolongs tissue cooling more effectively than applying crushed ice directly to the calf muscle area for the same length of time.[94]

During the application of cryotherapy by any means, the patient will usually experience the following sequence of sensations: intense cold followed by burning, then aching, and finally analgesia and numbness. These sensations are thought to correspond to increasing stimulation of thermal receptors and pain receptors, followed by blocking of sensory nerve conduction as tissue temperature decreases.

APPLICATION TECHNIQUE 8.1 — GENERAL CRYOTHERAPY

Procedure

1. Evaluate the patient and set the goals of treatment.
2. Determine whether cryotherapy is the most appropriate intervention.
3. Determine that cryotherapy is not contraindicated for this patient or condition.

   Inspect the area to be treated for open wounds and rashes, and assess sensation. Check the patient's chart for any record of previous adverse responses to cold and for any diseases that would predispose the patient to an adverse response. Ask appropriate questions of the patient as described in preceding sections on contraindications and precautions.
4. Select the appropriate cooling agent according to the body part to be treated and the desired response.

   Select an agent that provides the desired intensity of cold, best fits the location and size of the area to be treated, is easily applied for the desired duration and in the desired position, is readily available, and is reasonably priced. An agent that conforms to the contours of the area being treated should be used to maintain good contact with the patient's skin. With agents that cool by conduction or convection, such as cold packs or a cold whirlpool, good contact must be maintained between the agent and the patient's body at all times to maximize the rate of cooling. For brief cooling, the best choice is an agent that is quick to apply and remove. Any of the cooling agents described in this text may be available for use in a clinical setting, and the patient can readily use ice packs, ice cups, and cold packs at

home. Ice packs and ice massage are the least expensive means of providing cryotherapy; controlled cold compression units are the most expensive.
5. Explain the procedure and the reason for applying cryotherapy, as well as the sensations the patient can expect to feel, as described previously.
6. Apply the appropriate cooling agent.

   Select from the following list (see applications for each cooling agent):
   - Cold packs or ice packs
   - Ice cups for ice massage
   - Controlled cold compression units
   - Vapocoolant sprays or brief icing
   - Frozen towels
   - Ice water immersion
   - Cold whirlpool
   - Contrast bath

   The next section of this chapter provides details on application techniques for different cooling agents and decisions to be made when a specific agent and application technique are selected.
7. Assess the outcome of the intervention.

   After completing cryotherapy with any of the preceding agents, reassess the patient, checking particularly for progress toward the set goals of treatment and for any adverse effects of the intervention. Remeasure quantifiable subjective conditions and objective limitations, and reassess function and activity.
8. Document the intervention.

COLD PACKS OR ICE PACKS

Cold packs are usually filled with a gel composed of silica or a mixture of saline and gelatin and are usually covered with vinyl (Fig. 8.7). The gel is formulated to be semisolid at between 0°C and 5°C (32°F and 41°F), so the pack conforms

to body contours when it is within this temperature range. The temperature of a cold pack is maintained by storing it in specialized cooling units (Fig. 8.8) or in a freezer at −5°C (23°F). Cold packs should be cooled for at least 30 minutes between uses and for 2 hours or longer before initial use.

Cool cold packs for at least 2 hours before initial use and for at least 30 minutes between uses.

Patients can use plastic bags of frozen vegetables at home as a substitute for cold packs, or they can make their own cold packs from plastic bags filled with a 4:1 ratio mixture of water and rubbing alcohol cooled in a home freezer. The addition of alcohol to the water decreases the freezing temperature of the mixture so that it is semisolid and flexible at −5°C (23°F).

Ice packs are made of crushed ice placed in a plastic bag. Ice packs provide more aggressive cooling than cold packs at the same temperature because ice has a higher specific heat than most gels and because ice absorbs a large amount of energy when it melts from a solid to a liquid. Cold packs and ice packs are applied in a similar manner; however, with an ice pack, more insulation should be used to protect the skin because an ice pack provides more aggressive cooling than a cold pack (Fig. 8.9).

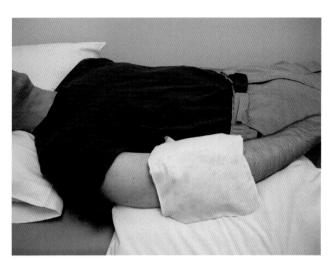

FIGURE 8.9 Application of a cold pack.

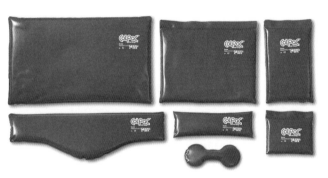

FIGURE 8.7 Cold packs. (Courtesy Chattanooga/DJO, Vista, CA.)

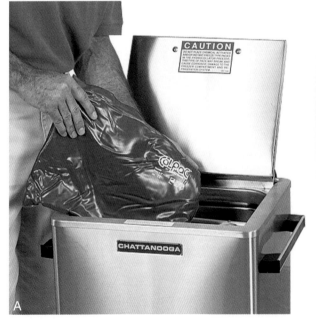

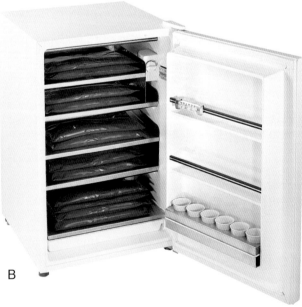

FIGURE 8.8 Cooling units for cold packs. (Courtesy Chattanooga/DJO, Vista, CA.)

APPLICATION TECHNIQUE 8.2   COLD PACKS OR ICE PACKS

Equipment Required

- Towels or pillow cases for hygiene and/or insulation
- For cold packs
  - Cold packs in a variety of sizes and shapes appropriate for different areas of the body
  - Freezer or specialized cooling unit
- For ice packs
  - Plastic bags
  - Ice chips
  - Ice chip machine or freezer

Procedure

1. Remove all jewelry and clothing from the area to be treated and inspect the area.
2. Wrap the cold pack or ice pack in a towel. Use a damp towel to cool more quickly. Dampen the towel with warm water so that the patient can gradually become accustomed to the cold sensation. Use a thin, dry towel to cool more slowly. A damp towel is generally appropriate for a cold pack, whereas a dry towel should be used for an ice pack because ice provides more intense cooling.
3. Position the patient comfortably, elevating the area to be treated if edema is present.
4. Place the wrapped pack on the area to be treated, and secure it well. Packs can be secured with elastic bandages or towels to ensure good contact with the patient's skin.
5. Leave the pack in place for 10 to 20 minutes to control pain, inflammation, or edema. Newer devices that allow more prolonged cooling are no more effective for reducing pain and analgesic medication use, or increasing range of motion (ROM), than cold or ice packs.[95] When cold is applied over bandages or a cast, increase the application time to allow the cold to penetrate through these insulating layers to the skin.[96] In this circumstance, the cold pack should be replaced with a newly frozen pack if the original pack melts during the course of the intervention.

If cryotherapy is being used to control spasticity, the pack should be left in place for up to 30 minutes. With these longer applications, check every 10 to 15 minutes for any signs of adverse effects.

1. Provide the patient with a bell or other means to call for assistance.
2. When the intervention is complete, remove the pack and inspect the treatment area for any signs of adverse effects, such as wheals or a rash. It is normal for the skin to be red or dark pink after icing.
3. Cold or ice pack application can be repeated every 1 to 2 hours to control pain and inflammation.

Advantages

- Easy to use
- Inexpensive materials and equipment
- Brief use of clinician's time
- Low level of skill required for application
- Can be applied by a patient at home
- Covers moderate to large areas
- Can be applied to an elevated limb

Disadvantages

- Pack must be removed from the treatment area to be visualized during treatment
- Patient may not tolerate the weight of the pack
- Pack may not be able to maintain good contact on small or contoured areas
- Long duration of treatment compared with massage with an ice cup

Ice Pack Versus Cold Pack

- Ice pack provides more intense cooling
- Ice pack is less expensive
- Cold pack is quicker to apply

ICE MASSAGE

Ice cups (Fig. 8.10) or frozen water ice pops (Fig. 8.11) can be used to apply ice massage. Frozen ice cups are made by freezing water in small paper or Styrofoam cups. To use these, the therapist holds on to the cup and gradually peels back one end to expose the surface of the ice, which is placed directly onto the patient's skin (Fig. 8.12). Ice pops are made by placing a stick or a tongue depressor into a paper cup of water before freezing. When frozen, the ice can be completely removed from the cup, and the stick can be used as a handle to apply the ice. Patients can easily make ice cups or ice pops for home use.

Ice massage may be applied for 5 to 10 minutes in the manner described in Application Technique 8.3 to control local pain, inflammation, or edema. Ice massage can also be used as a stimulus for facilitating the production of desired motor patterns in patients with impaired motor control. When applied for this purpose, the ice may be rubbed with pressure for 3 to 5 seconds or quickly stroked over the muscle bellies to be facilitated. This technique is termed *quick icing*.

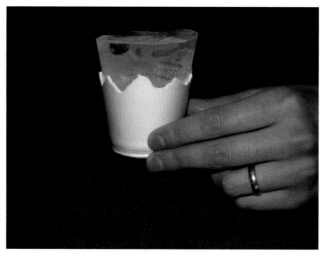

FIGURE 8.10 Ice cup.

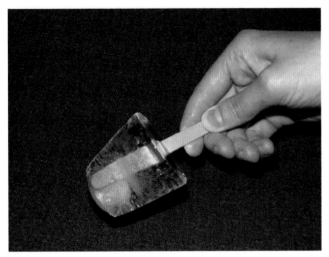

FIGURE 8.11 Ice pop.

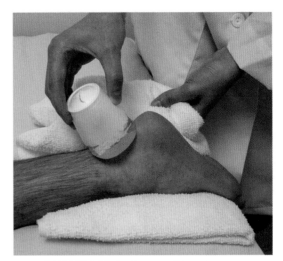

FIGURE 8.12 Application of ice massage.

APPLICATION TECHNIQUE 8.3   **ICE MASSAGE**

Equipment Required

- Small paper or Styrofoam cups
- Freezer
- Tongue depressors or Popsicle sticks (optional)
- Towels to absorb water

Procedure

1. Remove all jewelry and clothing from the area to be treated and inspect the area.
2. Place towels around the treatment area to absorb any dripping water and to wipe away water on the skin during treatment.
3. Prepare the ice cup or frozen ice pop by exposing the ice.
4. Rub ice over the treatment area using small, overlapping circles. Wipe away any water as it melts on the skin.
5. Continue ice massage application for 5 to 10 minutes, or until the patient experiences analgesia at the site of application.

6. When the intervention is complete, inspect the treatment area for any signs of adverse effects, such as wheals or a rash. It is normal for the skin to be red or dark pink after the application of ice massage.

Advantages

- Treatment area can be observed during application
- Technique can be used for small and irregular areas
- Short duration of treatment
- Inexpensive
- Can be applied by a patient at home
- Can be applied to an elevated limb

Disadvantages

- Too time-consuming for large areas
- Requires active participation by the clinician or the patient throughout application

---

CONTROLLED COLD COMPRESSION UNIT

Controlled cold compression units alternately pump cold water and air into a sleeve that is wrapped around a patient's limb (Fig. 8.13). The water's temperature should be between 10°C and 25°C (50°F and 77°F). Compression is applied by intermittently inflating the sleeve with air. Controlled cold compression units are most commonly used to control inflammation and edema directly after surgery and may also be used to control inflammation and related edema in other circumstances.[97]

When applied postoperatively, the sleeve is usually put on the patient's affected limb immediately after the surgery while the patient is in the recovery room, and the unit is sent home with the patient so that it can be used for a few days or weeks thereafter. Controlled cold compression is no more effective at cooling than a cold pack,[98] and conflicting study results make it unclear if applying cold together with compression after surgery in this manner is or is not more effective than ice or compression alone for reducing swelling, pain, or blood loss and in assisting the patient in regaining ROM and function.[99–102]

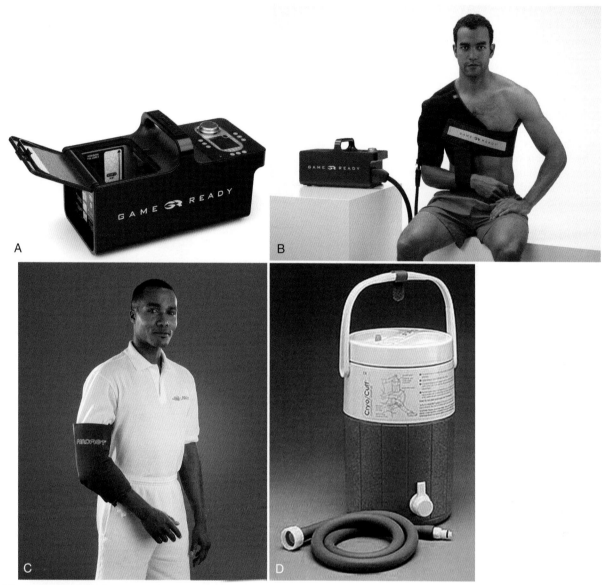

FIGURE 0.13 (A–D) Controlled cold compression units and their applications. (A–B, Courtesy Game Ready, Inc., Concord, CA. C–D, Courtesy Aircast, Vista, CA.)

APPLICATION TECHNIQUE 8.4 | CONTROLLED COLD COMPRESSION

Equipment Required

- Controlled cold compression unit
- Sleeves appropriate for areas to be treated
- Stockinette for hygiene

Procedure

1. Remove all jewelry and clothing from the area to be treated and inspect the area.
2. Cover the limb with a stockinette before applying the sleeve.
3. Wrap the sleeve around the area to be treated (see Fig. 8.13).
4. Elevate the area to be treated.
5. Set the temperature at 10°C to 15°C (50°F to 59°F).
6. Cooling can be applied continuously or intermittently. For intermittent treatment, apply cooling for 15 minutes every 2 hours.
7. Cycling intermittent compression may be applied at all times when the area is elevated.
8. When the intervention is completed, remove the sleeve and inspect the treatment area.

Advantages

- Allows simultaneous application of cold and compression
- Temperature and compression force are easily and accurately controlled
- Can be applied to large joints

Disadvantages

- Treatment site cannot be visualized during treatment
- Expensive
- Usable only for extremities
- Cannot be used for trunk or digits

VAPOCOOLANT SPRAYS AND BRIEF ICING

Various vapocoolant sprays, including ethyl chloride, Fluori-Methane, and a mixture of 1,1,1,3,3-pentafluoropropane and 1,1,1,2-tetrafluoroethane, can be used to achieve brief and rapid cutaneous cooling by evaporation before stretching. Although ethyl chloride is still available and used to temporarily control the pain associated with injections, starting intravenous (IV) lines, and venipuncture, as well as minor surgical procedures and minor sports injuries, its use is limited because it is volatile and flammable, can cause excessive decreases in skin temperature, and can have anesthetic effects when inhaled. Fluori-Methane is nonflammable and causes less reduction in temperature than ethyl chloride, but it is no longer commercially available because it is a volatile chlorofluorocarbon that can damage the ozone layer. The current commercially available, commonly used vapocoolant sprays, Spray and Stretch and Pain Ease (Gebauer Company, Cleveland, OH) (Fig. 8.14), are both made of a mixture of 1,1,1,3,3-pentafluoropropane and 1,1,1,2-tetrafluoroethane. Both of these products contain the same chemical components, but their delivery systems and U.S. Food and Drug Administration (FDA)–approved indications differ. Spray and Stretch has a fine-stream spray and is indicated for the treatment of myofascial pain syndromes, trigger points, restricted motion, and minor sports injuries. Pain Ease comes as a mist spray intended to control the pain associated with needles and minor surgical procedures and as a medium-stream spray intended for the treatment of musculoskeletal pain as part of the *spray and stretch* approach.

Rapid cutaneous cooling with a vapocoolant spray is generally used as a component of the approach known as *spray and stretch* to treat trigger points. This technique was developed by Janet Travell, who described it with the phrase, "Stretch is the action; spray is the distraction."[103] For this application, immediately before the muscles are stretched, the vapocoolant spray is applied in parallel strokes along the skin overlying the muscles with trigger points (Fig. 8.15).[104] Ice may also be stroked along the skin in the same area for this purpose (Fig. 8.16). This type of intervention is frequently applied directly after trigger-point injection. The rapid

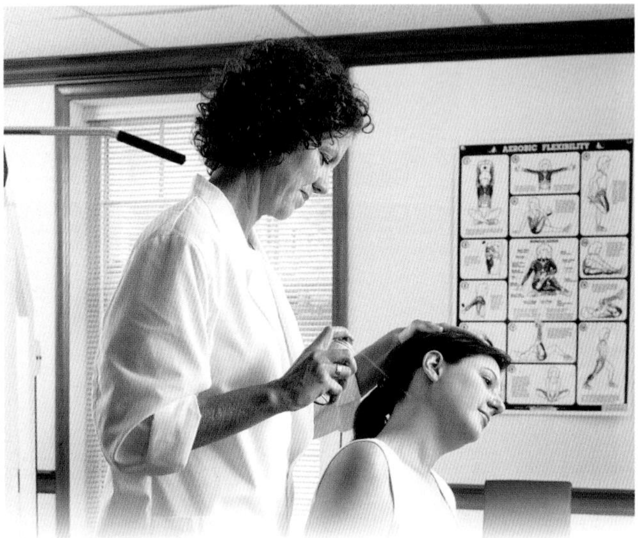

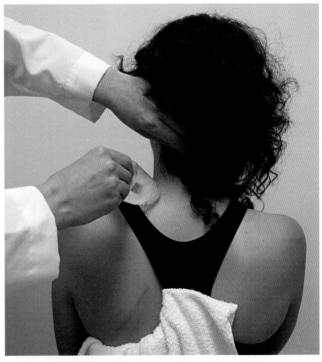

FIGURE 8.15 Application of vapocoolant spray. (Courtesy Gebauer Company, Cleveland, OH.)

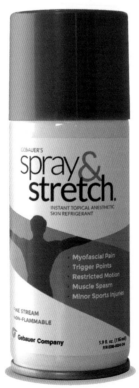

FIGURE 8.14 Vapocoolant spray. (Courtesy Gebauer Company, Cleveland, OH.)

FIGURE 8.16 Quick stroking with ice pop.

cooling provides a counterirritant stimulus to cutaneous thermal afferents overlying the muscles to cause a reflex reduction in motor neuron activity and thus a reduced resistance to stretch.[105] The "distraction" of rapid cutaneous cooling allows greater elongation of the muscle with passive stretching.

Clinical Pearl

Spray and stretch is used to treat trigger points by spraying a vapocoolant spray in parallel strokes along the skin overlying a muscle with trigger points and then immediately stretching the muscle.

APPLICATION TECHNIQUE 8.5 — VAPOCOOLANT SPRAYS AND BRIEF ICING[106,107]

Procedure

1. Identify trigger points and their related tight muscles.
2. Position the patient comfortably, with all limbs and the spine well supported and the area to be treated exposed and accessible.
3. Inspect the area to be treated.
4. Cover the patient's eyes, nose, and mouth if spraying near the face to minimize the patient's inhalation of the spray.
5. Apply two to five parallel sweeps of the spray or strokes of the ice 1.5 to 2 cm (0.5 to 1 inch) apart at a speed of approximately 10 cm (4 inches) per second along the direction of the muscle fibers. When using a spray, hold the can upright about 30 to 46 cm (12 to 18 inches) from the skin and angled so that the spray hits the skin at an angle of approximately 30 degrees. Continue until the entire muscle has been covered, including the muscle attachment and the trigger point.
6. During cooling, maintain gentle, smooth, steady tension on the muscle to take up any slack that may develop.
7. Immediately after cooling, have the patient take a deep breath and then perform a gentle passive stretch while exhaling. Contraction/relaxation techniques may be used to enhance the ROM increases obtained with this procedure.
8. Following this procedure, the skin should be rewarmed with moist heat, and the muscles should be moved through their full active ROM (AROM).

Advantages

- Brief duration of cooling
- Very localized area of application

Disadvantages

- Limited to use for brief, localized, superficial application of cold before stretching
- Requires skilled application

Documentation

The following should be documented:

- Area of the body treated
- Type of cooling agent used
- Treatment duration
- Patient positioning
- Response to the intervention

Documentation is typically written in the SOAP (subjective, objective, assessment, plan) note format. The following examples summarize only the modality component of the intervention and are not intended to represent a comprehensive plan of care.

EXAMPLES

When applying an ice pack (IP) to the patient's left knee to control postoperative swelling, document the following:

S: Pt reports postop L knee pain and swelling that increases with walking.

O: Pretreatment: Midpatellar girth 16½ inches. Gait "step to" when ascending stairs.

Intervention: IP L anterior knee for 15 min, L LE elevated.

Posttreatment: Midpatellar girth 15 inches. Gait "step through" when ascending stairs.

A: Decreased midpatellar girth, improved gait.

P: Instruct Pt in home program of IP to L anterior knee, 15 min, with L LE elevated, 3 × each day until next treatment session.

When applying ice massage (IM) to the area of the right lateral epicondyle to treat epicondylitis, document the following:

S: Pt reports pain in R lat elbow.

O: Pretreatment: 8/10 R lat elbow pain. R elbow unable to fully extend.

Intervention: IM R lat elbow for 5 min.

Posttreatment: Pain 6/10. Full elbow extension.

A: Pain decreased and elbow ROM improved.

P: Continue IM at end of treatment sessions until Pt has pain-free elbow function.

CLINICAL CASE STUDIES

The following case studies summarize the concepts of cryotherapy discussed in this chapter. Based on the scenarios presented, an evaluation of the clinical findings and goals of treatment are proposed. These are followed by a discussion of factors to be considered in the selection of cryotherapy as an indicated intervention and in selecting the ideal cryotherapy agent to promote progress toward the set goals.

CASE STUDY 8.1

Pain and Edema After Arthroscopic Knee Surgery

Examination

History

TF is a 20-year-old male accountant. He injured his right knee 4 months ago while playing football and was treated conservatively with nonsteroidal antiinflammatory drugs (NSAIDs) and physical therapy for 8 weeks. He experienced a moderate improvement in symptoms but was not able to return to sports because of continued medial knee pain. A magnetic resonance imaging (MRI) scan performed 3 weeks ago revealed a medial meniscus tear. TF underwent arthroscopic partial medial meniscectomy of his right knee 4 days ago. He has been referred to physical therapy with an order to evaluate and treat.

Systems Review

TF reports that the intensity of pain in his knee at rest has decreased from 9/10 directly after the surgery to 7/10 now, but his pain increases with weight bearing on the right lower extremity. He limits his ambulation to essential tasks and is using crutches. He also reports knee stiffness that is most noticeable when rising from his chair.

Tests and Measures

The objective examination reveals moderate warmth of the skin of TF's right knee, particularly at the anteromedial aspect, and his AROM is restricted to between –10 degrees of extension and 85 degrees of flexion. TF is ambulating with crutches, with a shorter stance phase on the right, and with his right knee held stiffly in approximately 30 degrees of flexion throughout the gait cycle. Knee girth at the midpatellar level is 17 inches on the right and 15.5 inches on the left.

What signs and symptoms in this patient can be addressed by cryotherapy? Which cryotherapy applications would be appropriate for this patient? Which would not be appropriate?

Evaluation and Goals

ICF Level	Current Status	Goals
Body structure and function	Right knee pain	Control pain
	Decreased right knee ROM	Increase right knee ROM to full
	Increased right knee girth	Control edema
	Warmth of the right knee consistent with inflammation	Accelerate resolution of the acute inflammation phase of healing
Activity	Limited ambulation	Have the patient tolerate ambulation up to ½ block in 2 weeks
Participation	Inability to play football	Return patient to playing noncontact sports in 1 month

ICF, International Classification for Functioning, Disability and Health; *ROM,* range of motion.

Key Studies or Reviews

1. Martimbianco AL, Gomes da Silva BN, de Carvalho AP, et al: Effectiveness and safety of cryotherapy after arthroscopic anterior cruciate ligament reconstruction. A systematic review of the literature. *Phys Ther Sport* 15(4):261–268, 2014.

   This systematic review evaluated the evidence from 10 trials in a total of 573 patients for the impact of cryotherapy primarily on pain edema and adverse events and secondarily on knee function, analgesic medication use, ROM, blood loss, hospital stay, quality of life, and patient satisfaction, following arthroscopic anterior cruciate ligament (ACL) reconstruction. There was only sufficient evidence to support that cryotherapy reduced pain more effectively than no cryotherapy.

2. Su EP, Perna M, Boettner F, et al: A prospective, multicenter, randomised trial to evaluate the efficacy of a cryopneumatic device on total knee arthroplasty recovery. *J Bone Joint Surg Br* 94(11 Suppl A):153–156, 2012.

   This study compared the effects of controlled cold compression to those of ice and static compression after total knee arthroplasty in a randomized controlled trial with 116 patients. The patients using the controlled cold compression device required significantly less pain medication in the first 2 weeks postoperatively, but there were no differences in ROM or knee girth between groups.

3. Schinsky MF, McCune C, Bonomi J: Multifaceted comparison of two cryotherapy devices used after total knee arthroplasty: cryotherapy device comparison. *Orthop Nurs* 35(5):309–316, 2016.

   This study compared the effects of controlled cold compression to those of an ice/gel wrap after total knee arthroplasty in a randomized controlled trial with 100 patients. The patients using the cryotherapy wrap reported significantly less pain at 6 weeks postoperatively, and hospital staff satisfaction was higher with the cryotherapy wrap. There were no significant differences between groups in swelling, ROM, blood loss, or adverse events.

Prognosis

Cryotherapy is an indicated intervention to control pain, edema, and inflammation and accelerate functional recovery after trauma or surgery. Cryotherapy alone can control the formation of edema, and this effect may be enhanced by the addition of compression and elevation. The presence of any contraindications to cryotherapy should be ruled out before cryotherapy is applied. Cryotherapy also should not be applied if infection is suspected. Because the peroneal nerve is superficial at the lateral knee, the patient should be monitored during the intervention for signs of nerve conduction block, such as tingling or numbness in the lateral leg. Although this patient has signs of inflammation, including heat, redness, pain, swelling, and loss of function, the fact that his signs and symptoms have decreased since the surgery was performed indicates that the course of recovery is appropriate and that there is probably no infection at the site. A progressive increase in the signs and symptoms of inflammation or complaints of fever and general malaise would suggest the presence of infection, requiring that a physician evaluate the patient before rehabilitation begins.

Intervention

To maximally cool the knee, cryotherapy should be applied to all skin surfaces surrounding the knee joint. A cold pack, an ice pack, or a controlled cold compression unit could adequately cover this area. Given that the evidence from key studies on this topic supports that cryotherapy can reduce pain after knee surgery and that an ice or cold pack together with compression is as effective as a controlled cold compression unit, at lesser expense and with greater satisfaction and less analgesic medication use, a cold or ice pack together with compression and elevation should be used. Ice massage would not be an appropriate intervention because it would take too long to apply to such a large area. Immersion in ice or cold water would not be appropriate either because this would require placing the swollen knee in a dependent position, potentially aggravating the edema and causing the additional discomfort of immersing the entire distal lower extremity in cold water. The cold or ice pack should be applied for approximately 15 to 20 minutes at a time to ensure adequate cooling of tissues and to minimize the possibility of excessive cooling or reactive vasodilation. This pack should be reapplied by the patient at home every 2 to 3 hours, when awake, while signs of inflammation are present (Fig. 8.17).

Documentation

S: *Pt reports R knee stiffness and pain that increases with weight bearing.*

O: Pretreatment: *R knee pain 7/10. Warm skin anteromedial R knee. R knee ROM −10 degrees extension and 85 degrees flexion. Gait: decreased stance phase on R LE and with R knee held at 30 degrees of flexion throughout gait cycle. R knee midpatellar girth 17 inches, L knee 15½ inches.*

Intervention: *IP R anterior knee × 15 min, R LE elevated.*

Posttreatment: *R knee pain 5/10. R midpatellar girth 16 inches. R knee ROM −10 degrees extension and 85 degrees flexion. Ambulates with knee moving through approximately 10 to 30 degrees of flexion.*

A: *Pt tolerated treatment well, with decreased pain and edema.*

P: *Pt to apply IP at home every 3 hours until edema and warmth of R knee resolve.*

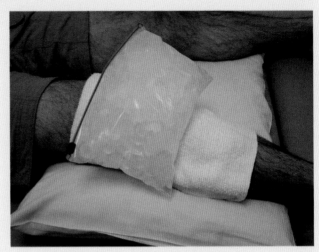

FIGURE 8.17 Application of ice pack to right knee.

CASE STUDY 8.2

Lateral Epicondylitis
Examination
History

SG is a 40-year-old female office worker. She has been referred to therapy with a diagnosis of lateral epicondylitis and an order to evaluate and treat. SG complains of constant moderate to severe pain (>5/10) at her right lateral elbow that prevents her from playing tennis. She has had similar symptoms previously after gardening or playing tennis, but these have always resolved within a couple of days, requiring no medical intervention. The pain started about 1 month ago on a morning after she spent a whole day pulling weeds and remained unchanged in severity and frequency until 3 days ago.

Systems Review

SG is a pleasant-appearing woman accompanied to the clinic by her husband. She is alert and cooperative with therapy testing and interventions. She reports a slight decrease in pain severity over the last 3 days, which she associates with starting to take an NSAID her physician prescribed. She reports no weakness or reduced ROM in the upper left or lower left or right extremities.

Tests and Measures

Objective examination reveals tenderness and mild swelling at the right lateral epicondyle and pain without weakness with resisted wrist extension. All other tests, including upper extremity sensation, ROM, and strength, are within normal limits.

What other interventions should be used with cryotherapy for this patient? What should you monitor for during cryotherapy application? How can this patient prevent a recurrence of her lateral epicondylitis?

Continued

CLINICAL CASE STUDIES—cont'd

Evaluation and Goals

ICF Level	Current Status	Goals
Body structure and function	Right elbow pain, tenderness, and swelling	Resolve inflammation Control pain Prevent recurrence
Activity	Difficulty using right arm when wrist extension is required	Able to extend right wrist against resistance without pain
Participation	Unable to play tennis	Return to playing tennis

ICF, International Classification for Functioning, Disability and Health.

◆ FIND THE EVIDENCE

PICO Terms	Natural Language Example	Sample PubMed Search
P (Population)	Patient with symptoms due to lateral epicondylitis	"Tennis Elbow" [MeSH] OR "lateral epicondylitis" [text word]
I (Intervention)	Cryotherapy	AND ("Cryotherapy" [MeSH] OR "cryotherapy" [title])
C (Comparison)	No cryotherapy	
O (Outcome)	Resolve inflammation; increase range of motion	

Key Studies

1. Manias P, Stasinopoulos D: A controlled clinical pilot trial to study the effectiveness of ice as a supplement to the exercise programme for the management of lateral elbow tendinopathy. *Br J Sports Med* 40:81–85, 2006.

    This small pilot study of 40 patients with lateral epicondylitis compared an exercise program five times per week for 4 weeks with ice against the same exercise program without ice. By the end of treatment, patients in both groups showed improvements in pain that were not significantly different. Although these conclusions would seem to argue against the use of ice for this patient, the study was likely underpowered to find an effect. Also, the benefits of ice are mostly realized early during recovery. Therefore, any differences in outcomes would occur far sooner than 4 weeks, and the continuing ice treatment throughout the full 4 weeks would probably provide no additional benefit. Further research is needed to assess the early effects of cryotherapy in the management of lateral epicondylitis.

Prognosis

Cryotherapy is an indicated intervention for the management of inflammation and pain and can be used prophylactically after exercise to prevent the onset of inflammation and soreness.

Advantages of cryotherapy over other interventions that can be effective for these indications, such as ultrasound, low-level laser therapy, shock-wave therapy, or electrical stimulation, are that it is quick, easy, and inexpensive to apply, and the patient can apply it at home. The presence of any contraindications to the application of cryotherapy should be ruled out before cryotherapy is applied. Cryotherapy alone is not likely to resolve the present symptoms and should be applied along with activity modification, manual therapy techniques, and exercises, as indicated, to achieve the goals of treatment. Because the radial nerve is superficial at the lateral elbow, the patient should be monitored during treatment for signs of nerve conduction block, such as tingling or numbness in her dorsal arm.

Intervention

Ice massage, an ice pack, or a cold pack can be used to apply cryotherapy to the area of the lateral epicondyle (Fig. 8.18). Because ice massage takes little time to apply to this small area and it allows signs and symptoms to be easily assessed throughout the intervention, this would be the most appropriate agent to use for this patient. Although an ice pack or a cold pack could also be used, these would be more appropriate if the symptomatic area were larger (e.g., if the area extended into the dorsal forearm). Cryotherapy should be applied until the treatment area is numb, which usually takes 5 to 10 minutes with ice massage or 15 to 20 minutes when an ice pack or a cold pack is used. Treatment should be discontinued sooner if numbness extends into the hand in the distribution of the radial nerve. Cryotherapy should be repeated until the signs and symptoms of inflammation have resolved but should be discontinued thereafter because vasoconstriction produced by the cryotherapy may retard the later stages of tissue healing. The patient should be instructed to apply cryotherapy prophylactically after activities that have previously resulted in elbow pain, such as tennis or gardening, to reduce the risk of recurrence of her present symptoms.

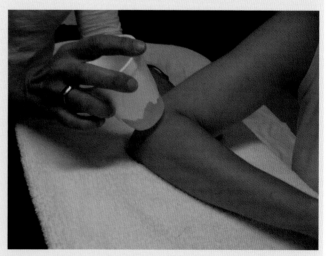

FIGURE 8.18 Application of ice massage to elbow.

CLINICAL CASE STUDIES—*cont'd*

Documentation

S: Pt reports R elbow pain, improved somewhat with NSAIDs.

O: Pretreatment: R lat epicondyle tenderness, mild edema, 8/10 pain with resisted wrist extension.

Intervention: IM to R lat epicondyle × 8 min.

Posttreatment: Decreased tenderness and edema. Pain 5/10 with resisted wrist extension.

A: Pt tolerated treatment well, with decreased pain and edema. Pt able to swing tennis racket without increasing pain above 5/10.

P: Pt to continue IM at home, as described, every 3 hours until edema and pain have resolved. Pt educated on prevention of future symptoms by applying IP or IM after gardening or tennis.

CASE STUDY 8.3

Delayed-Onset Muscle Soreness
Examination
History

FB is a 60-year-old male truck driver. He has been referred to physical therapy with a diagnosis of osteoarthritis of the left knee and an order to evaluate and treat. He reports that he has had arthritis in the left knee for the past 5 years and that he recently started performing exercises that have increased the strength, stability, and endurance of his legs but make his knee hurt and his thigh muscle sore the next day. His goals in therapy are to control this postexercise discomfort to allow him to continue his exercise program. He performed his exercises yesterday.

Systems Review

FB appears well and presents in the clinic without noticeable pain. He reports slight stiffness in his left knee, with no noticeable stiffness in his right knee. He reports 3/10 pain with resisted left knee extension, and he is eager to lessen pain to 0 or 1.

Tests and Measures

Palpation reveals a mild increase in the temperature of the left knee and tenderness of the anterior thigh. Knee girth and ROM are equal bilaterally.

In addition to using cryotherapy, how can this patient's postexercise pain be reduced? What should you monitor for during the application of cryotherapy in this patient?

Evaluation and Goals

ICF Level	Current Status	Goals
Body structure and function	Left knee and thigh pain after exercise	Control postexercise pain
Activity	Pain with resisted left knee extension	Pain-free resisted left knee extension
Participation	Decreased ability to do leg strengthening exercises	Return to full exercise program

ICF, International Classification for Functioning, Disability and Health.

◆ FIND THE EVIDENCE

PICO Terms	Natural Language Example	Sample PubMed Search
P (Population)	Patient with delayed-onset muscle soreness after exercise	("muscle soreness" [text word] AND "exercise" [text word])
I (Intervention)	Cryotherapy	AND ("Cryotherapy" [MeSH])
C (Comparison)	No cryotherapy	
O (Outcome)	Resolve postexercise pain	

Key Studies or Reviews

1. Bleakley C, McDonough S, Gardner E, et al: Cold-water immersion (cryotherapy) for preventing and treating muscle soreness after exercise. *Cochrane Database Syst Rev* (2):CD008262, 2012.

   This systematic review and meta-analysis evaluated the effect of immersion in cold water (<15°C) for minimizing DOMS after exercise. There were 17 small trials with 366 participants included, and pooled results showed statistically significant reduction of DOMS with this intervention at 24, 48, and 72 hours.

2. Hohenauer E, Taeymans J, Baevens JP, et al: The effect of post-exercise cryotherapy on recovery characteristics: A systematic review and meta-analysis. *Plos One* 10(9):e0139028, 2015.

   This systematic review and meta-analysis evaluated the effects of cooling compared with not cooling on recovery characteristics for up to 96 hours after exercise. Pooled data from 27 studies revealed that cooling, particularly immersion in cold water, significantly reduced DOMS 24, 48, and 96 hours after exercise.

Prognosis

Cryotherapy is an indicated treatment for DOMS and joint inflammation; however, the patient's exercise program should also be evaluated and possibly modified to reduce his discomfort after exercising. The presence of any contraindications should be ruled out before applying cryotherapy.

Intervention

As in Case Study 8.1, applying cryotherapy for 15 minutes with an ice pack or a cold pack would be appropriate to treat this patient. Given the findings of the recent systematic reviews, immersion in cold water should also be considered. The additional expense of controlled cold compression is not justified in this case because no edema is present, and therefore compression is not needed. The patient should apply the cryotherapy immediately after completing his exercise program. Because the peroneal nerve is superficial at the lateral knee, the patient should be monitored for signs of nerve conduction blockage, such as tingling or numbness in his lateral leg, during treatment.

Continued

Documentation

S: Pt reports knee and thigh pain lasting 1 day after performing leg strengthening exercises.

O: **Pretreatment:** L knee mild warmth. L anterior thigh tenderness. 3/10 pain with resisted L knee extension. Bilaterally equal knee girth and ROM.

Intervention: IP to L anterior thigh and knee × 15 min.

Posttreatment: Decreased L anterior thigh tenderness, 1/10 pain with L knee extension.

A: Pt tolerated treatment well, with decreased pain and tenderness.

P: Pt to apply IP immediately after completing exercise program. Exercise program should be reassessed and modified as needed to prevent pain.

THERMOTHERAPY

The therapeutic application of heat is called **thermotherapy.** Outside of the rehabilitation setting, thermotherapy is used primarily to destroy malignant tissue or to treat cold-related injuries. Within rehabilitation, thermotherapy is used primarily to control pain, increase soft tissue extensibility and circulation, and accelerate healing. Heat has these therapeutic effects because of its influence on hemodynamic, neuromuscular, and metabolic processes.

Effects of Heat

HEMODYNAMIC EFFECTS

Vasodilation

Therapeutic levels of heat cause vasodilation and thus increase blood flow.[108] When heat is applied to one area of the body, vasodilation occurs not only in the area of application, where the increase in tissue temperature is greatest, but also to a lesser degree in the more distal and deeper vessels that run through muscles, where temperature increases little if at all. Thermotherapy applied to the whole body can cause generalized vasodilation, increasing cardiac demand and potentially improving vascular endothelial function in the setting of cardiac risk factors and in chronic heart failure.[109-112]

> #### ◎ Clinical Pearl
>
> Heat causes vasodilation and thus increases blood flow.

Thermotherapy causes vasodilation by a variety of mechanisms, including rapid direct reflex activation of the smooth muscles of the blood vessels by cutaneous thermoreceptors and slower indirect activation of local spinal cord reflexes by cutaneous thermoreceptors and local release of chemical mediators of inflammation (Fig. 8.19).[113-115]

Superficial heating agents stimulate the activity of cutaneous thermoreceptors. Transmission from these cutaneous thermoreceptors, via their axons, directly to nearby cutaneous blood vessels causes the release of nitrous oxide, which then stimulates relaxation of the smooth muscles of the vessel walls, causing vasodilation in the area where the heat is applied.[114-117]

Cutaneous thermoreceptors also project via the dorsal root ganglion to synapse with sympathetic neurons in the

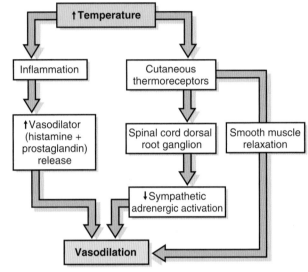

FIGURE 8.19 How heat causes vasodilation.

lateral gray horn of the thoracolumbar segments in the spinal cord, inhibiting their firing and thus decreasing sympathetic output.[118] This decrease in sympathetic activity reduces smooth muscle contraction, resulting in vasodilation at the site of heat application and in the cutaneous vessels of the distal extremities.[119] This distant vasodilatory effect of thermotherapy can be used to increase cutaneous blood flow to areas where it is difficult or unsafe to apply a heating agent directly.[120] For example, if a patient has an ulcer on the leg as a result of arterial insufficiency in the extremity, and the area is bandaged, does not tolerate pressure, or lacks sufficient circulation or sensation to safely tolerate the direct application of heat, thermotherapy could be applied to the low back to increase the circulation to the lower extremity to facilitate wound healing.

Because blood flow within skeletal muscles is influenced primarily by metabolic factors rather than by changes in sympathetic activity, and because superficial heating agents do not increase the temperature to the depth of most muscles, superficial thermotherapy produces much less pronounced increases in skeletal muscle blood flow than in cutaneous blood flow.[121,122] Therefore, exercise or deep-heating modalities such as ultrasound or diathermy, or a combination of these interventions, is recommended when the goal of treatment is increased skeletal muscle blood flow.

Superficial heating agents do not heat to the depth of most muscles. To heat deep muscles, use exercise or deep-heating modalities such as ultrasound or diathermy.

Cutaneous vasodilation and the increased blood flow that occurs in response to increased tissue temperature protect the body from excessive heating and tissue damage by convective cooling. When an area is heated with a thermal agent, it is simultaneously cooled by circulating blood, reducing the impact of the thermal agent on tissue temperature and thus the risk of burning.

NEUROMUSCULAR EFFECTS
Changes in Nerve Conduction Velocity and Firing Rate

Increased temperature increases nerve conduction velocity and decreases the conduction latency of sensory and motor nerves.[123-125] Nerve conduction velocity increases by approximately 2 m/second for every 1°C (1.8°F) increase in temperature. Although the clinical implications of these effects are not well understood, they may contribute to the reduced pain perception or improved circulation that occurs when tissue temperature increases. Although conduction velocity in normal nerves increases with heat, heating of demyelinated nerves can cause conduction block.[126-128] This occurs because heat shortens the duration of sodium channel opening at the nodes of Ranvier during neuronal depolarization, which can prevent the node from depolarizing.[129] Therefore, heat should be applied with caution to patients who have demyelinating conditions such as carpal tunnel syndrome or multiple sclerosis.

Changes in tissue temperature also affect the nerve firing rate (frequency). Elevating muscle temperature to 42°C (108°F) decreases the firing rate of type II muscle spindle efferents and gamma efferents and increases the firing rate of type Ib fibers from GTOs. The decreased gamma neuron activity decreases the stretch on the muscle spindles and thus reduces afferent firing from the spindles, which then decreases alpha motor neuron activity and may thus relax muscle spasms.[130]

Increased Pain Threshold

Several older and more recent studies demonstrate that local heat can increase the pain threshold and decrease pain.[131-135] Proposed mechanisms for these effects include a direct and immediate reduction of pain by increased activity of cutaneous thermoreceptors, which can have a gating effect on transmitting the pain sensation at the spinal cord level. This is followed by an indirect and more prolonged reduction of pain through decreased ischemia via increased blood flow and reduced spasm in the muscles that compress the blood vessels, as well as accelerated healing of damaged tissue.

Heat can increase the pain threshold and decrease the sensation of pain.

Changes in Muscle Strength

Muscle strength and endurance decrease during the initial 30 minutes after applying superficial or deep-heating agents.[136,137] This initial decrease in muscle strength is likely because heating of the motor nerves changes the firing rates of type II muscle spindle efferents, gamma efferents, and type Ib fibers from GTOs, which in turn decreases the firing rate of alpha motor neurons. Beyond 30 minutes and for the next 2 hours after the heat is applied, muscle strength gradually recovers to above pretreatment levels. There is also growing evidence for and interest in using heat before or during exercise to promote strength gains.[138,139] Delayed increases in strength are thought to be caused by an increase in the pain threshold and expression of heat shock proteins, upregulation of the expression of genes involved in muscle growth and differentiation, and attenuation of cellular damage and protein degradation during exercise.

It is important to be aware of how heat affects muscle strength when strength is being used to measure a patient's progress. Comparing preheating to postheating strength from the same or another session can be misleading. Therefore, muscle strength should always be measured before and not after a heating modality is applied. It is possible that applying heat during or before strengthening exercise will enhance the benefits of the exercise.

Measure muscle strength before applying heat, not after.

METABOLIC EFFECTS
Increased Metabolic Rate

Heat increases the rate of endothermic chemical reactions, including the rate of enzymatic biological reactions. Increased enzymatic activity has been observed in tissues at 39°C to 43°C (102°F to 109°F), with the reaction rate increasing by approximately 13% for every 1.0°C (1.8°F) increase in temperature and doubling for every 10°C (18°F) increase in temperature.[52] Enzymatic and metabolic activity rates continue to increase at tissue temperatures of up to 45°C (113°F). Beyond this, proteins begin to denature and enzyme activity rates decrease, ceasing completely at approximately 50°C (122°F).[140]

Any increase in the enzymatic activity rate will increase the rate of cellular biochemical reactions. Although this can increase oxygen uptake and accelerate healing, this can also increase the rate of destructive processes. For example, heat may accelerate the healing of a chronic wound, but heat can also increase the activity of collagenase and thus accelerate the destruction of articular cartilage in patients with rheumatoid arthritis.[50] This is one of the reasons thermotherapy should be avoided in areas of inflammation and should be used with caution in patients with inflammatory joint disorders.

Heat increases the local metabolic rate and therefore can exacerbate inflammation.

Increasing tissue temperature with thermotherapy also shifts the oxygen-hemoglobin dissociation curve to the right, making more oxygen available for tissue repair (see Fig. 8.4). Hemoglobin releases twice as much oxygen at 41°C (106°F) as it does at 36°C (97°F).[141] In conjunction with the increased rate of blood flow stimulated by increased temperature, and the increased enzymatic reaction rate, this increased oxygen availability may accelerate tissue healing.

ALTERED TISSUE EXTENSIBILITY
Increased Collagen Extensibility

Increasing the temperature of soft tissue increases its extensibility.[142-144] When soft tissue is heated before stretching, it achieves a greater increase in length when the stretching force is applied, less force is required to achieve the increased length, and the risk of tissue tearing is reduced. If heat is applied to collagenous soft tissue such as tendon, ligament, scar tissue, or joint capsule before prolonged stretching, plastic deformation can be achieved. With plastic deformation, gains in length produced by stretching are maintained after the stretching force stops. Plastic deformation is caused by changes in the organization and viscoelasticity of collagen fibers. In contrast, if collagenous tissue is stretched without prior heating, elastic deformation, in which the tissue lengthens while the force is applied but retracts when the force is removed, generally occurs.

For heat to increase the extensibility of soft tissue, the tissue temperature must be raised to the appropriate level. A maximum increase in residual length is achieved when the tissue is maintained at 40°C to 45°C (104°F to 113°F) for 5 to 10 minutes.[143,145,146] The superficial heating agents described subsequently can sufficiently heat superficial structures such as cutaneous scar tissue or superficial tendons. However, to adequately heat deeper structures, such as the joint capsules of large joints or deep tendons, deep-heating agents such as ultrasound or diathermy must be used.

Clinical Indications for Superficial Heat
PAIN CONTROL

Thermotherapy can be used clinically to control pain. This therapeutic effect may be mediated by gating of pain transmission through the activation of cutaneous thermoreceptors or may indirectly result from improved healing, decreased muscle spasm, or reduced ischemia. The indirect effects of thermotherapy on tissue healing and ischemia are primarily attributable to vasodilation and increased blood flow. Increasing skin temperature may also reduce the sensation of pain by altering nerve conduction or transmission. The experience of controlled heat being comfortable and relaxing may also influence the patient's perception of pain.

Continuous, low-level local heat (using a commercially available disposable pack inside a Velcro closure belt that heats up to 40°C [104°F] when exposed to air and maintains this heat for 8 hours), particularly when combined with exercise, has been shown to reduce pain and disability for patients with back pain, wrist pain, or DOMS.[147-149]

Although thermotherapy may reduce pain of any origin, thermotherapy is not recommended as an intervention for pain caused by acute inflammation because increasing tissue temperature may aggravate other signs and symptoms of inflammation, including heat, redness, and edema.[150]

INCREASED RANGE OF MOTION AND DECREASED JOINT STIFFNESS[151-153]

Thermotherapy can be used clinically when the goals are to increase joint ROM and decrease joint stiffness.[149,154-156] Both of these effects are thought to result from the increased soft tissue extensibility that occurs with increased soft tissue temperature. Increasing the soft tissue extensibility increases joint ROM because it enables greater increases in soft tissue length while reducing the likelihood of injury when a passive stretch is applied. A maximum increase in length with the lowest risk of injury is obtained if the tissue temperature is maintained at 40°C to 45°C (104°F to 113°F) for 5 to 10 minutes and a low-load, prolonged stretch is applied during the heating period and while the tissue is cooling (Fig. 8.20).[145,146] Therefore it is recommended that stretching be performed during and immediately after the application of thermotherapy because if the tissues are allowed to cool before being stretched, the effects of prior heating on tissue extensibility will be lost. In addition, because the effects of heat on tissue extensibility depend on increasing the temperature of the target tissues, it is important to consider whether the heating agent used will have a sufficient impact on the temperature of the target tissue. It is therefore unsurprising that application of a moist hot pack to the thigh until the muscle temperature at 1-inch depth increased by 0.4°C (32.72 degrees Farenheit) was not found to alter hamstring flexibility.[152]

Thermotherapy can decrease joint stiffness, which is a quality related to the amount of force and the time required to move a joint; as joint stiffness decreases, less force and time are required to produce joint motion. Proposed mechanisms for this effect include increased extensibility and viscoelasticity of periarticular structures, including the joint capsule and surrounding ligaments.

When a heating agent is used to increase soft tissue extensibility before stretching, an agent that can reach the shortened tissue must be used. Thus, superficial agents such as hot packs, paraffin, or infrared (IR) lamps are appropriate for use before stretching skin, superficial muscle, joints, or fascia,

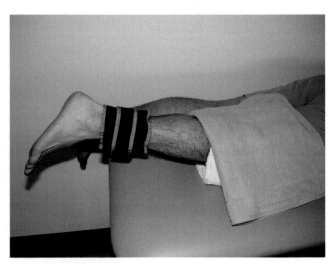

FIGURE 8.20 Low-load prolonged stretch with heat.

whereas deep-heating agents such as ultrasound or diathermy should be used before stretching deeper joint capsules, muscles, or tendons.

> ## ◎ Clinical Pearl
>
> To increase soft tissue extensibility before stretching, use an agent that will heat the size and depth of tissue that needs stretching.

ACCELERATED HEALING

Thermotherapy can accelerate tissue healing by increasing circulation, the enzymatic activity rate, and the availability of oxygen to the tissues. Increasing the rate of circulation accelerates the delivery of blood to the tissues, brings in oxygen and other nutrients, and removes waste products. Applying any physical agent that increases circulation can be beneficial during the proliferative or remodeling stage of healing or when chronic inflammation is present. However, because increasing circulation can also increase edema, thermotherapy should be applied with caution during the acute inflammation phase to avoid prolonging this phase and delaying healing.

By increasing the enzymatic activity rate, thermotherapy increases the rate of metabolic reactions, thus allowing the processes of inflammation and healing to proceed more rapidly. Increasing the temperature of the blood also increases the dissociation of oxygen from hemoglobin, making more oxygen available for the processes of tissue repair.

Because superficial heating agents increase the temperature of only the superficial few millimeters of tissue, they are best suited for accelerating the healing of shallow structures, such as skin, or of deeper tissue layers if they are exposed by skin ulceration. However, deeper effects may occur as the result of vasodilation in areas distant from or deep to the area of increased temperature.

INFRARED RADIATION FOR PSORIASIS

Although the ultraviolet (UV) frequency range of electromagnetic radiation is used most commonly to treat psoriasis (see Chapter 17), the IR range is occasionally used for this application.[157] IR radiation may reduce psoriatic plaques by increasing the temperature of the upper epidermis and the dermis in the region of plaques. Other applications of IR, particularly IR lasers, not related to heat are covered in Chapter 16.

Contraindications and Precautions for Thermotherapy

Although thermotherapy is a relatively safe intervention, its use is contraindicated in some circumstances, and it should be applied with caution in others. Thermotherapy may be applied by a qualified clinician or by a properly instructed patient. Clinicians may use all forms of thermotherapy, and patients may be shown how to use hot packs, paraffin, or IR lamps at home to treat themselves. When patients are taught to use these modalities at home, they should be instructed on how to use the modality, including the location at which it should be applied, the temperature to be used, safety precautions, and the duration and frequency of treatment. Patients must also be taught how to identify possible adverse effects and must be told to discontinue treatment should any of these occur. Even when thermotherapy is not contraindicated, as with all interventions, if the patient's condition worsens or does not improve after two or three treatments, the treatment approach should be reevaluated, or the patient should be reevaluated by a physician.

CONTRAINDICATIONS FOR THE USE OF THERMOTHERAPY

> ## ✳ CONTRAINDICATIONS
>
> ### for the Use of Thermotherapy
>
> * Recent or potential hemorrhage
> * Thrombosis
> * Impaired sensation
> * Impaired mentation
> * Malignant tumor
> * IR irradiation of the eyes[158]

Recent or Potential Hemorrhage

Heat causes vasodilation and increases the rate of blood flow. Because vasodilation may reopen a vascular lesion, increasing the rate of blood flow in an area of recent hemorrhage can restart or worsen the bleeding; in an area of potential hemorrhage, it can cause hemorrhage to start. Therefore, heat should not be applied to areas of recent or potential hemorrhage. Heat should also not be applied if the patient reports bruising or bleeding in the potential treatment area in the previous 48 to 72 hours or if recently formed red, purple, or blue ecchymosis is present.

> ### ▪ Ask the Patient
> * "When did this injury occur?"
> * "Did you have any bruising or bleeding?"
>
> ### ▪ Assess
> * Visually inspect for ecchymosis.

Thrombosis

The vasodilation and increased circulation caused by increased tissue temperature may cause a thrombus or a blood clot to become dislodged from the treatment and to move to the vessels of vital organs, resulting in morbidity or even death.

> ### ▪ Ask the Patient
> * "Do you have a blood clot in this area?"
>
> ### ▪ Assess
> * Check for calf swelling and tenderness (Homans sign) before applying heat to the leg.

Thermotherapy should not be applied if the patient says that there is a blood clot in the treatment area. Thermotherapy to the leg should not be applied if the calf is swollen or tender until the presence of a thrombus in the lower extremity has been ruled out.

Impaired Sensation or Impaired Mentation

A patient's sensation and a report of heat or pain are the primary indicators of the maximum safe temperature for thermotherapy; thus a patient who cannot feel or report the sensation of heat can easily be burned before the clinician realizes there is a problem. Therefore, heat should not be applied to areas where sensation is impaired or to patients who cannot readily let the therapist know when they are too hot.

> ◎ **Clinical Pearl**
>
> Use heat with caution in patients with diabetes because sensation is often impaired in their distal extremities.

▪ **Ask the Patient**
• "Do you have normal feeling in this area?"

▪ **Assess**
• Sensation in the area: A metal spoon placed under hot and then cold water can be used to test thermal sensation. If sensation is impaired solely in the treatment area, heat may be applied proximally to increase peripheral circulation via the spinal cord reflex, as described earlier. Note that sensation in the distal extremities is frequently impaired in patients with neuropathy caused by diabetes mellitus.
• Alertness and orientation: Thermotherapy should not be applied if the patient is unresponsive or confused.

Malignant Tissue

Thermotherapy may increase the growth rate or rate of metastasis of malignant tissue by increasing circulation to the area or by increasing the metabolic rate. Because a patient may not know if they have cancer or may be uncomfortable discussing this diagnosis directly, the therapist should both check the chart for a diagnosis of cancer and ask the patient the following questions.

▪ **Ask the Patient**
• "Are you under the care of a physician for any major medical problem? If so, what is the problem?"
• "Have you experienced any recent unexplained weight loss or gain?"
• "Do you have constant pain that does not change?" Note: If the patient has experienced recent unexplained changes in body weight or has constant pain that does not change, defer thermotherapy until a physician has performed a follow-up evaluation to rule out malignancy. If the patient is known to have cancer, ask the following question:
• "Do you know if you have a tumor in this area?" Note: Thermotherapy generally should not be applied in the area of a known or possible malignancy; however, for a terminally ill patient, with informed consent, such treatment may be given to relieve pain.

Infrared Irradiation of the Eyes

IR irradiation of the eyes should be avoided because such treatment may cause optical damage. To avoid irradiating the eyes, if applying IR, the patient should wear IR opaque goggles throughout treatment, and the therapist should also wear IR opaque goggles when near the lamp.

PRECAUTIONS FOR THE USE OF THERMOTHERAPY

> ✱ **PRECAUTIONS**
>
> **for the Use of Thermotherapy**
> • Acute injury or inflammation
> • Pregnancy
> • Impaired circulation
> • Poor thermal regulation
> • Edema
> • Cardiac insufficiency
> • Metal in the area
> • Over an open wound
> • Over areas where topical counterirritants have recently been applied
> • Demyelinated nerves

Acute Injury or Inflammation

Apply heat with caution to areas of an acute injury or acute inflammation because increasing tissue temperature can increase edema and bleeding as a result of vasodilation and increased blood flow. This may aggravate the injury, increase pain, and delay recovery.

▪ **Ask the Patient**
• "When did this injury occur?"

▪ **Assess**
• Skin temperature and color and local edema

Heat should not be applied within the first 48 to 72 hours after an injury. Elevated skin temperature, rubor, and local edema demonstrate the presence of acute inflammation and indicate that heat should not be applied to the area.

Pregnancy

A fetus may be damaged by maternal hyperthermia. Because this is unlikely to occur with superficial heating of the limbs, thermotherapy may be applied to such areas, but full-body heating, such as immersing most of the body in a whirlpool, should be avoided during pregnancy. Although maternal hyperthermia has not been demonstrated with the application of hot packs to the low back or abdomen, such application is also generally not recommended.

▪ **Ask the Patient**
• "Are you pregnant?"
• "Do you think you may be pregnant?"
• "Are you trying to get pregnant?"

If the patient is or may be pregnant, heat should not be applied to her abdomen or low back, and she should not be immersed in a warm or hot whirlpool.

Impaired Circulation or Poor Thermal Regulation

Areas with impaired circulation and patients having poor thermal regulation—particularly elderly and very young patients—may not vasodilate to a normal degree in response to increased tissue temperature, and therefore blood flow may not increase enough to protect the tissues from burning.

> ■ **Assess**
> • Check skin temperature and quality and nail quality, and look for tissue swelling or ulceration.

Lower-than-average skin temperature, thin skin, poor nails, swollen tissue, and skin ulcers are signs of impaired circulation. Mild, superficial heat or more insulation should be used in areas with poor circulation or in elderly or very young patients. Patients should be checked frequently for discomfort or signs of burning.

Edema

Applying thermotherapy to a dependent extremity can increase edema.[150] This effect is thought to result from the combination of the effects of gravity when the extremity is dependent and vasodilation, enhanced circulation, and increased inflammation caused by the increased metabolic rate that occurs with raised tissue temperature.

> ■ **Assess**
> • Measure the girth of the limb to be treated, and compare this with the contralateral side.
> • Palpate for pitting or brawny edema.
> • Check for other signs of inflammation, including heat, redness, and pain.

If edema is present in a limb, heat should not be applied to the limb in a dependent position.[159] Heat may be applied if the limb is elevated.

Cardiac Insufficiency

Heat causes both local and generalized vasodilation, which can increase cardiac demand. Because heat therapy may not be tolerated well by patients with cardiac insufficiency, these patients should be monitored closely, particularly if a large area is heated.

> ■ **Ask the Patient**
> • "Do you have any problems with your heart?"
>
> ■ **Assess**
> • In patients with heart problems, check heart rate and blood pressure before, during, and after intervention.

A slight decrease in blood pressure and an increase in heart rate are normal consensual responses to the application of heat. In patients with cardiac insufficiency, heat treatment should be discontinued if their heart rate falls or if they complain of feeling faint.

Metal in the Area

Metal has higher thermal conductivity and higher specific heat than body tissue and therefore may become very hot when conductive heating modalities are applied. For this reason, metal jewelry should be removed before applying superficial heating modalities, and caution should be taken if the superficial tissue in the treatment area contains metal, such as staples or bullet fragments.

> ■ **Ask the Patient**
> • "Do you have any metal inside of you in this area, such as staples or bullet fragments?"
> • "Can you remove your jewelry in the area to be heated?"

If metal is present that cannot be removed easily, apply heat with caution. Milder heat should be used at a lower temperature or intensity or with more insulation, and the area should be checked frequently during treatment for any signs of burning.

> ■ **Assess**
> • Inspect skin for scars that may cover metal.

Over an Open Wound

Paraffin should not be used over an open wound because it may contaminate the wound and is difficult to remove. All other forms of thermotherapy should be applied over open wounds with caution because the loss of epidermis reduces the insulation of subcutaneous tissues. If forms of thermotherapy other than paraffin are used in the area of an open wound, they should be applied at a lower temperature or intensity, or with more insulation, than would be used on areas with intact skin and checked frequently during treatment for signs of burning. When a heating agent is applied with the goal of increasing circulation and accelerating the healing of an open wound, hydrotherapy with clean, warm water may be applied directly to the wound. Other superficial heating agents may be applied close to but not directly over the wound to provide a therapeutic effect while reducing the risk of cross-contamination and burns.

Over Areas Where Topical Counterirritants Have Recently Been Applied

Topical counterirritants are ointments or creams that cause a sensation of heat when applied to the skin. These preparations generally contain substances, such as menthol, that simulate the sensation of heat by causing local superficial vasodilation and a mild inflammatory reaction in the skin. If a thermal agent is applied to an area where a topical counterirritant has been used, the blood vessels may not be able to vasodilate further to dissipate heat from the thermal agent, and a burn may result.

■ **Ask the Patient**
• "Have you applied any cream or ointment to this area today? If so, what type?"

If the patient has recently applied a topical counterirritant to an area, a superficial heating agent should not be applied. The patient should be instructed not to use this type of preparation before future treatment sessions and not to apply a superficial heating agent at home after using this type of preparation.

Demyelinated Nerves

Conditions associated with demyelination of peripheral nerves include carpal tunnel syndrome and ulnar nerve entrapment. Multiple sclerosis causes demyelination of central nerves. Apply heat with caution to areas with demyelinated nerves because heat can cause conduction block in both peripheral and central nerves.

■ **Ask the Patient**
• "Do you have carpal tunnel syndrome or ulnar nerve entrapment?"
• "Do you have multiple sclerosis?"

If the patient has a demyelinating condition, heat should be applied with caution to the affected areas.

Adverse Effects of Thermotherapy
BURNS

Excessive heating can cause **protein denaturation** and cell death. These effects may occur when heat is applied for too long, when the heating agent is too hot, or when heat is applied to a patient who does not have an adequate protective vasodilation response to increased tissue temperature. The effects of heat on cell viability are exploited in the medical treatment of malignancies, in which heat is applied with the goal of killing the malignant cells; however, during the application of heat in rehabilitation, cell death is to be avoided. Because protein begins to denature at 45°C (113°F) and cell death has been observed when cells were maintained at 43°C (109°F) for 60 minutes or at 46°C (115°F) for 7½ minutes, when applying heat in rehabilitation, the duration of application and tissue temperature should be kept below these levels.[160,161]

Overheating and tissue damage can be avoided by using superficial heating agents that cool during their application, by limiting the initial temperature of the agent, or by using insulation between the agent and the patient's skin (Box 8.1). For example, moist hot packs that are heated in hot water before being placed on the patient start to cool as soon as they are applied and therefore, if used with an appropriate number of layers of insulating towels, are unlikely to cause burns. In contrast, superficial heating agents attached to a power supply, such as plug-in electrical hot packs or IR lamps, are more likely to cause burns. The higher the temperature of a conductive superficial heating agent, the greater the rate of heat transfer to the patient and thus the greater the risk of burns; therefore, it is important not to overheat a conductive superficial heating agent and to always use adequate insulation.

Box 8.1   How to Avoid Tissue Damage When Using Thermal Agents
• Use superficial heating agents that get cooler during their application (e.g., hot pack, hot water bottle).
• Limit the initial temperature of the agent.
• Use enough insulation between the agent and the patient's skin.
• Provide a means for the patient to call you.

To avoid burns, heating agents should be applied in the manner recommended here. They should not be applied for longer periods or at higher temperatures, and the treatment time and temperature of the heating agent should be reduced if the patient has impaired circulation. Heating agents should not be applied where contraindicated, and all patients should be provided with a means of calling for assistance, such as a bell, if the clinician or another staff member is not in the immediate treatment area. During the intervention, the clinician should check to make sure that the patient has not fallen asleep. If the patient uses a superficial heating agent at home, they should use a timer that rings loudly at the end of the treatment time.

Clinical Pearl
To avoid burns, heating agents should not be applied for longer periods or at higher temperatures than recommended. The treatment time and temperature should be reduced if the patient has impaired circulation.

Superficial heating agents used at home should be the type that cools over time, such as a microwavable hot pack or a hot water bottle. If an electrical heating pad is used, it should have a switch that must be depressed at all times in order to stay on to ensure that the heating pad will turn off if the patient falls asleep.

It is recommended that the patient's skin be inspected for burns before initiating treatment because the patient may have been burned previously. The skin should also be inspected during and after thermotherapy. A recent superficial burn will appear red and may have blistering. As the burn heals, the skin will appear pale and scarred.

FAINTING

Occasionally, a patient may feel faint when heat is applied. Fainting, which is a sudden, transient loss of consciousness, is generally the result of inadequate cerebral blood flow and is most commonly caused by peripheral vasodilation and decreased blood pressure, generally associated with a decreased heart rate. Heating an area of the body generally causes vasodilation locally and, to a lesser extent, in areas distant from the site of application. This distant, or consensual, response can decrease cerebral blood flow sufficiently to cause a patient to faint. If a patient feels faint while heat is being applied, lower their head and raise their feet to bring more blood to the brain and help the patient recover. Heating as small an area as is clinically beneficial and removing excessive heavy clothing that insulates the whole body may help limit the consensual decrease in blood pressure associated with heating, reducing the probability of fainting.

Patients may also feel faint when getting up after thermotherapy. This feeling is caused by the additive hypotensive effects of postural (orthostatic) hypotension and the hypotensive effect of the heat, as described earlier. The patient's head should be kept elevated with a pillow during heat application to decrease post-treatment postural hypotension by reducing the extent of positional change at the completion of the intervention. It is also recommended that the patient remain in the position used during treatment for a few minutes after the thermal agent has been removed to allow blood pressure to normalize before rising.

BLEEDING

The vasodilation and increased blood flow caused by increasing tissue temperature may cause or aggravate bleeding in areas of acute trauma or in patients with hemophilia. Vasodilation may also cause reopening of any recent vascular lesion.

SKIN AND EYE DAMAGE FROM INFRARED RADIATION

IR radiation can produce adverse effects that are not produced by other superficial thermal agents. These include permanent damage to the eyes and permanent changes in skin pigmentation. Injury to the eyes, including corneal burning and retinal and lenticular damage, is the most likely and most severe hazard of IR radiation therapy.[158] Prolonged exposure to IR radiation may also cause epidermal hyperplasia.

Depending on the agent and the amount of insulation, warmth may not be felt for the first few minutes of treatment. The patient should not feel excessively hot and should not feel any sensation of increased pain or burning. If the patient reports any of these sensations, discontinue the treatment or reduce the intensity of the heat.

> **Clinical Pearl**
>
> The patient should feel a sensation of mild warmth when a heating agent is applied.

Application Techniques
GENERAL SUPERFICIAL THERMOTHERAPY

Superficial thermotherapy may be applied using a variety of materials, including hot packs, paraffin, Fluidotherapy, IR lamp, or contrast baths.

Different materials heat at different rates and to different degrees and depths. Moist hot packs heat the skin more, and more quickly, than paraffin or dry heating pads because water in the moist hot packs has higher specific heat and thermal conductivity. In addition, moist hot packs heat more effectively than a conductive thermal probe, both because the hot packs are moist and because they are much larger than the probe, allowing for more heat delivery by conduction.[162] When at the same temperature as a hot pack, Fluidotherapy heats more slowly than the hot pack because the air used by Fluidotherapy as its heating medium has a low thermal conductivity and specific heat. However, Fluidotherapy heats faster than stationary air at the same temperature because the moving air heats by convection, constantly replacing the cooled air adjacent to the patient's skin. Furthermore, the continual input of energy of Fluidotherapy maintains a constant air temperature, in contrast to moist hot packs, which cool over time. Although whirlpools have been used to provide superficial heating, particularly because they offer the advantages of heating by convection using a medium having high specific heat and thermal conductivity, they are rarely used today because they are difficult to keep clean and thus pose a risk of cross-contamination.

During the application of thermotherapy by any means, the patient will usually experience a sensation of gentle warmth. If at any time the patient feels burning or discomfort, discontinue use of the heating agent.

APPLICATION TECHNIQUE 8.6 — GENERAL SUPERFICIAL THERMOTHERAPY

Procedure

1. Evaluate the patient's problem and set the goals of treatment.
2. Determine whether thermotherapy is the most appropriate intervention.
3. Determine that thermotherapy is not contraindicated for this patient or this condition.

   Inspect the treatment area for open wounds and rashes, and assess sensation. Check the patient's chart for any record of previous adverse responses to heat or for any disease that may predispose the patient to an adverse response. Ask appropriate questions of the patient, as described in the preceding sections on contraindications and precautions.
4. Select the appropriate superficial heating agent according to the body part to be treated and the desired response.

   When applying superficial heat, select an agent that best fits the location and size of the area to be treated, is easily applied in the desired position, allows the desired amount of motion during application, is available, and is reasonably priced. Choose an agent that will conform to the area being treated so that it maintains good contact with the body. If edema is present, an agent that can be applied with the area elevated should be used. When applying thermotherapy with the goal of increasing ROM, it can be beneficial to allow active or passive motion while the treatment is being applied. Any of the heating agents described can be applied in the clinic; only hot packs and paraffin may be applied by patients at home.
5. Explain to the patient the procedure and the reason for applying thermotherapy, and describe the sensations that the patient can expect to feel.

   During the application of thermotherapy, the patient should feel a sensation of mild warmth.
6. Apply the appropriate superficial heating agent.

   Select from the following list (see applications for each superficial heating agent):

Continued

APPLICATION TECHNIQUE 8.6—cont'd

- Hot packs
- Paraffin
- Fluidotherapy
- IR lamp
- Contrast bath

7. Inspect the treated area and assess the outcome of treatment.

After completing thermotherapy with any of these agents, reevaluate the patient, checking particularly for progress toward the set goals of the intervention and for any adverse effects of the intervention. Remeasure quantifiable subjective complaints and objective impairments and disabilities.

8. Document the intervention.

HOT PACKS

Commercially available moist hot packs are usually made of bentonite, which is a type of clay, covered with canvas. Bentonite is used for this application because it can hold a large quantity of water for efficient delivery of heat and becomes pliable when hydrated. These types of hot packs are made in various sizes and shapes designed to fit different areas of the body (Fig. 8.21). They are stored in hot water kept at approximately 70°C to 75°C (158°F to 167°F) inside a purpose-designed, thermostatically controlled cabinet (Fig. 8.22) that stays on at all times. This type of hot pack takes 2 hours to heat initially and 30 minutes to reheat between uses.

◎ Clinical Pearl

Heat moist hot packs for at least 2 hours before initial use and for 30 minutes between uses.

Bentonite-filled moist hot packs are generally recommended for clinical use but are not suitable for home use because they need to be stored in hot water between applications. They cannot be reused if they dry out after they have become moist because they harden when dry and then will not rehydrate. A variety of other types of hot or warm packs are available for

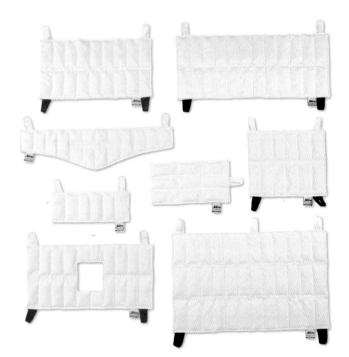

FIGURE 8.21 Hot packs of various shapes and sizes. (Courtesy Chattanooga/DJO, Vista, CA.)

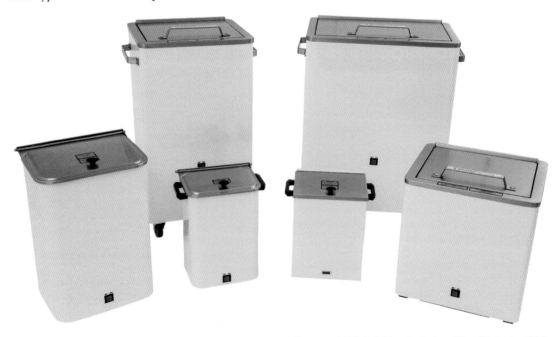

FIGURE 8.22 Thermostatically controlled hot pack containers. (Courtesy Whitehall Manufacturing, City of Industry, CA.)

home use, including chemical heating pads that are activated by mixing or contact of their contents with air; packs filled with rice or other dry materials that can be heated in a microwave; and electrical, plug-in heating pads. These heating pads generally provide dry rather than moist heat and therefore, because of the lower specific heat and thermal conductivity of air compared with water, produce milder and slower heating.[163]

Chemical heating pads are made from a variety of materials that warm up and maintain a therapeutic temperature range for 1 to 8 hours when exposed to air by opening the package, breaking an inner sealed bag, or mechanically agitating. Different chemicals are activated by different means, heat to slightly different temperatures, have different specific heats, and maintain their temperature for different lengths of time. Although none produces moist heat directly, most can be wrapped in a damp towel or cover to produce moist heat. Most chemical packs cannot be reused. Chemical packs come in a variety of shapes and sizes for application to different body areas; some are designed to be placed in a wrap, allowing

them to be worn during activity. The low-level, prolonged heating produced by wearing a heating pad during activity can reduce low back, neck, and wrist pain and the sensation of stiffness and can increase flexibility.[147–149,164,165]

Microwavable heating pads typically have a thick insulative cloth covering and are filled with grains that have a high specific heat. Caution should be applied when using this type of heating pad because microwaves heat unevenly.

Electrical, plug-in heating pads are not recommended for clinical use because they do not cool during application and therefore may burn the patient more easily. If patients wish to use an electrical heating pad at home, advise them to procure a pad that requires the switch to be held "on" the entire time for the pad to heat; to use only the medium or low setting; to limit application at the medium setting to 20 minutes; and to discontinue use if any sensation of pain, overheating, or burning occurs. Also, advise patients to inspect their skin for burns immediately after using the hot pack and for the following 24 hours.

APPLICATION TECHNIQUE 8.7   MOIST HOT PACKS

Equipment Required

- Hot packs in a variety of sizes and shapes appropriate for different areas of the body
- Specialized heating unit
- Towels
- Hot pack covers (optional)
- Timer
- Bell

Procedure

1. Remove clothing and jewelry from the area to be treated and inspect the area.
2. Wrap the hot pack in six to eight layers of dry towels. Hot pack covers, which come in various sizes to match the hot packs, can substitute for two to three layers of towels (Fig. 8.23). More layers should be used if the towels or hot pack covers are old and have become thin or if the patient complains of feeling too warm during treatment. The towels can be preheated to achieve

more uniform heating throughout the treatment period. More layers of towels should be used if the body part is on top of the hot pack than if the hot pack is placed over the body part. When the body part is on top of the pack, the towels are compressed, reducing insulation of the body, and the underlying table provides more insulation to the pack, causing it to cool more slowly.[166] If the patient complains of not feeling enough heat, fewer layers of towels may be used for the next treatment session; however, towels should not be removed during heating with hot packs because the increased skin temperature may decrease the patient's thermal sensitivity and ability to judge the tissue's heat tolerance accurately and safely.

3. Apply the wrapped hot pack to the treatment area and secure it well (Fig. 8.24).
4. Provide the patient with a bell or other means to call for assistance while the hot pack is on, and instruct the patient to call immediately if they experience any increase in discomfort. If the patient feels too hot, extra towels should be placed between the hot pack and the patient. If the patient does not feel hot

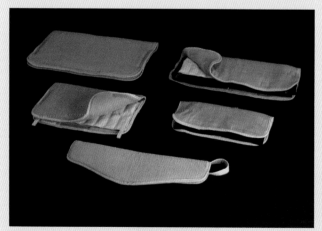

FIGURE 8.23 Hot pack covers. (Courtesy Whitehall Manufacturing, City of Industry, CA.)

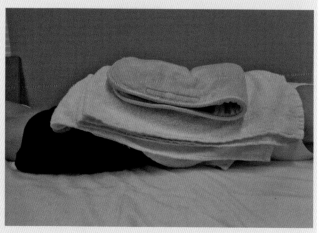

FIGURE 8.24 Application of a hot pack.

Continued

APPLICATION TECHNIQUE 8.7—*cont'd*

enough, fewer layers of towels should be used at the next treatment session.

5. After 5 minutes, check the patient's report and inspect the area being treated for excessive redness, blistering, or other signs of burning. Discontinue thermotherapy in the presence of signs of burning. If any signs of burning are noted, brief application of a cold pack or an ice pack is recommended to curtail the inflammatory response.

6. After 20 minutes, remove the hot pack and inspect the treatment area. It is normal for the area to appear slightly red and to feel warm to the touch.

Advantages

- Easy to use
- Inexpensive materials (packs and towels)

- Brief use of clinician's time
- Low level of skill needed for application
- Can be used to cover moderate to large areas
- Safe because packs start to cool on removal from the water cabinet
- Readily available for patient purchase and home use

Disadvantages

- Hot pack must be moved to allow observation of the treatment area during treatment
- Patient may not tolerate the weight of the hot pack
- Pack may not be able to maintain good contact with small or contoured areas
- Active motion is not practical during treatment
- Moderately expensive equipment (heated water cabinet) is needed

PARAFFIN

Warm, melted paraffin wax can be used for thermotherapy. To do this, paraffin wax is mixed with mineral oil in a 6:1 or 7:1 ratio of paraffin to oil to reduce its melting temperature from 54°C (129°F) to between 45°C and 50°C (113°F and 122°F). At this temperature, paraffin can be safely applied directly to the skin because its specific heat and thermal conductivity are low. To minimize heat loss, insulating mitts or layers of towel should be applied over the paraffin (Fig. 8.25). Paraffin is particularly good for heating the distal extremities because it can maintain good contact with these irregularly contoured areas. Paraffin may also be applied to more proximal areas such as the elbows and knees, or even the low back, by using the paint method described in Application Technique 8.8.

Paraffin is heated and stored in a thermostatically controlled container that maintains it at 52°C to 57°C (126°F to 134°F).[167] Such containers are available in large sizes for clinic use and smaller, portable sizes for home or clinic (Fig. 8.26). The manufacturers' safety and usage instructions for properly setting and adjusting these devices and for selecting appropriate paraffin wax products should be followed closely because some units are preset for specific products.

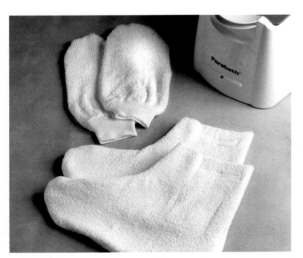

FIGURE 8.25 Mitts to wear over paraffin-coated hands or feet. (Courtesy The Hygenic Corporation, Akron, OH.)

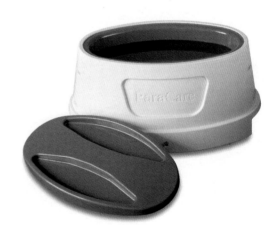

FIGURE 8.26 Thermostatically controlled paraffin bath. (Courtesy Medline Industries, Inc., Mundelein, IL.)

APPLICATION TECHNIQUE 8.8   PARAFFIN

Equipment Required

- Paraffin
- Mineral oil (or, more commonly, commercially available premixed paraffin with oil made specifically for this application)
- Thermostatically controlled container
- Plastic bags or paper
- Towels or mitts

Procedure

Paraffin may be applied by three different methods: dip wrap, dip immersion, and paint. The dip-wrap method is most commonly used. The dip-wrap and dip-immersion methods can only be used for treating the distal extremities. The paint method can be used for any area of the body. For all three methods, do the following:

1. Remove all jewelry from the area to be treated and inspect the area.
2. Thoroughly wash and dry the area to be treated to minimize contamination of the paraffin.

For the dip-wrap method (for the wrist and hand):

3. With fingers apart, dip the hand into the paraffin as far as possible and remove (Fig. 8.27). Advise the patient to avoid moving their fingers during the treatment because movement will crack the paraffin coating. Also, advise the patient to avoid touching the sides or the bottom of the tank because these areas may be hotter than the paraffin.
4. Wait briefly for the layer of paraffin to harden and become opaque.
5. Redip the hand, keeping the fingers apart. Repeat steps 3 through 5 six to ten times.
6. Wrap the patient's hand in a plastic bag, wax paper, or treatment-table paper and then in a towel or toweling mitt. The plastic bag or paper prevents the towel from sticking to the paraffin, and the toweling acts as insulation to slow the cooling of the paraffin. Caution the patient not to move their hand during dipping or the rest period because movement may crack the coating of paraffin. If this happens during dipping, hot paraffin may get trapped in the cracks, and if this happens during the rest period, air may penetrate, causing the paraffin to cool more rapidly.
7. Elevate the extremity.
8. Leave the paraffin in place for 10 to 15 minutes or until it cools.

9. When the intervention is complete, peel the paraffin off the hand and discard it (Fig. 8.28).

For the dip-immersion method:

3. With fingers apart, dip the hand into the paraffin and remove.
4. Wait 5 to 15 seconds for the layer of paraffin to harden and become opaque.
5. Redip the hand, keeping the fingers apart.
6. Allow the hand to remain in the paraffin for up to 20 minutes, and then remove it.

The temperature of the paraffin should be at the lower end of the recommended range for this method of application because the hand cools less during treatment than with the dip-wrap method. The heater should be turned off during treatment so that the sides and the bottom of the tank do not become too hot.

For the paint method:

3. Paint a layer of paraffin onto the treatment area with a brush.
4. Wait for the layer of paraffin to become opaque.
5. Paint on another layer of paraffin no larger than the first layer. Repeat steps 3 through 5 six to ten times.
6. Cover the area with plastic or paper and then with toweling. As with the dip-immersion method, the plastic or paper is used to prevent the towel from sticking to the paraffin, and the toweling acts as insulation to slow down the cooling of the paraffin. Caution the patient not to move during dipping or the rest period because movement may crack the coating of paraffin. If this happens during dipping, hot paraffin may get trapped in the cracks, and if this happens during the rest period, air may penetrate, causing the paraffin to cool more rapidly.
7. Leave the paraffin in place for 20 minutes or until it cools.
8. When the intervention is completed, peel off the paraffin and discard it.

For all methods:

When the intervention is complete, inspect the treatment area for any signs of adverse effects, and document the intervention.

In most clinics, the paraffin bath is left plugged in and on at all times. In this circumstance, it can be used by many patients, one after another, and its goal temperature can be maintained. If the unit is unplugged or turned off and the paraffin is allowed to cool, be sure that the paraffin has returned to between 52°C and 57°C (126°F and 134°F) before it is used again for treatment. Caution should be applied for the first 5 hours after turning a unit on because some units take up to 5 hours to heat the wax, and during this heating period, parts

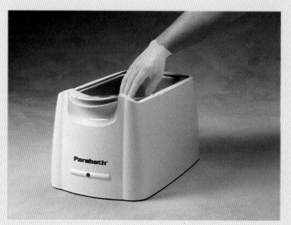
FIGURE 8.27 Application of paraffin by the dip-wrap method. (Courtesy The Hygenic Corporation, Akron, OH.)

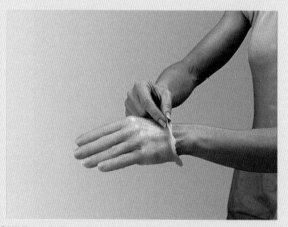
FIGURE 8.28 Removing paraffin from a patient's hand. (Courtesy HoMedics Inc., Commerce Township, MI.)

Continued

APPLICATION TECHNIQUE 8.8—cont'd

of the wax may be hotter than the recommended therapeutic temperature range. This could result in burning. Always follow the manufacturer's instructions to ensure safe use.

Advantages

- Maintains good contact with highly contoured areas
- Easy to use
- Inexpensive
- Body part can be elevated if dip-wrap method is used

- Oil lubricates and conditions the skin
- Can be used by the patient at home

Disadvantages

- Messy and time-consuming to apply
- Cannot be used over an open skin lesion because it may contaminate the lesion
- Risk of cross-contamination if the paraffin is reused
- Part in dependent position for dip-immersion method

FLUIDOTHERAPY

Fluidotherapy is a dry heating agent that transfers heat by convection.[168] It consists of a cabinet containing finely ground cellulose particles made from corn cobs (Fig. 8.29). Heated air is circulated through the particles, suspending and moving them so that they act like a liquid. The patient extends a body part into the cabinet, where it floats as if in water. Portals in the cabinet allow the therapist to access the patient's body part while it is being heated. Fluidotherapy units come in a variety of sizes suitable for treating different body parts. Both the temperature and the amount of particle agitation can be controlled by the clinician (Fig. 8.30).

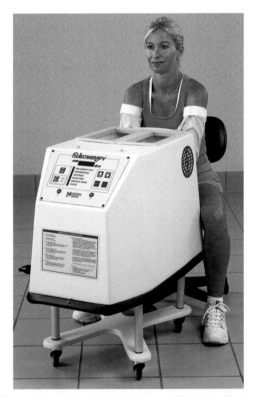

FIGURE 8.29 Application of Fluidotherapy. (Courtesy Chattanooga/DJO, Vista, CA.)

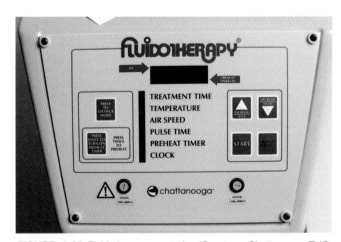

FIGURE 8.30 Fluidotherapy controls. (Courtesy Chattanooga/DJO, Vista, CA.)

APPLICATION TECHNIQUE 8.9   FLUIDOTHERAPY

Equipment Required

- Fluidotherapy unit of appropriate size and shape for areas to be treated

Procedure

1. Remove all jewelry and clothing from the area to be treated and inspect the area.
2. Cover any open wounds with a plastic barrier to prevent the cellulose particles from becoming lodged in the wound.
3. Extend the body part to be treated through the portal of the unit (see Fig. 8.29).
4. Secure the sleeve to prevent particles from escaping from the cabinet.
5. Set the temperature at 38°C to 48°C (100°F to 118°F).
6. Adjust the degree of agitation to achieve patient comfort.
7. The patient may move or exercise during the intervention.
8. Treat for 20 minutes.

Advantages

- Patient can move during the intervention to work on gaining AROM
- Minimal pressure applied to the area being treated
- Temperature well controlled and constant throughout intervention
- Easy to administer

Disadvantages

- Expensive equipment
- Limb must be in dependent position in some units, increasing the risk of edema formation
- The constant heat source may result in overheating
- If the corn cob particles spill onto a smooth floor, they will make the floor slippery

INFRARED LAMPS

IR lamps emit electromagnetic radiation within the frequency range that gives rise to heat when absorbed by matter (Fig. 8.31). IR radiation has a wavelength of 770 to 10^6 nm, lying between visible light and microwaves on the electromagnetic spectrum (see Fig. 16.6) and is emitted, along with visible light and UV radiation, by the sun. IR radiation is divided into three bands with differing wavelength ranges: IR-A, 770 to 1400 nm; IR-B, 1400 to 3000 nm; and IR-C, 3000 to 10^6 nm. IR lamps currently used in rehabilitation emit IR-A, generally with mixed wavelengths of approximately 780 to 1400 nm and peak intensity at approximately 1000 nm. Other sources of IR include sunlight, IR light-emitting diodes (LEDs), superluminous diodes (SLDs), and low-intensity lasers.

The increase in tissue temperature produced by IR radiation is proportional to the amount of radiation that penetrates the tissue, which is a function of the power and wavelength of the radiation, the distance between the radiation source and the tissue, the **angle of incidence** of the radiation, and the absorption coefficient of the tissue.

Most IR lamps deliver radiation with 50 to 1500 watts of power. Most IR radiation produced by today's lamps (780- to 1400-nm wavelength) is absorbed within the first few millimeters of human tissue, but at least 50% of IR radiation of 1200-nm wavelength penetrates beyond 0.8 mm and therefore is able to pass through the skin to interact with subcutaneous capillaries and cutaneous nerve endings.[169] Human skin allows maximum penetration of radiation with a wavelength of 1200 nm while being virtually opaque to IR radiation with a wavelength of 2000 nm or greater.[158]

The amount of energy reaching the patient from an IR radiation source is also related to the distance between the source and the tissue. As the distance of the source from the target increases, the intensity of radiation reaching the target decreases in proportion to the square of the distance. For example, if the source is moved from a position 5 cm from

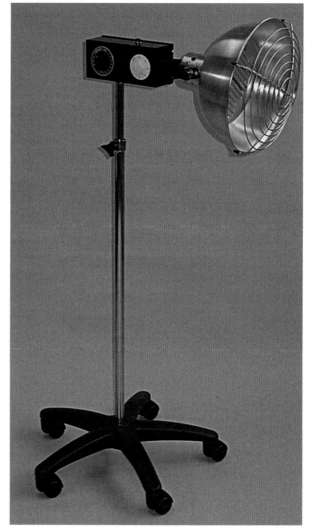

FIGURE 8.31 Infrared lamp. (Courtesy Brandt Industries, Bronx, NY.)

the target to 10 cm from the target—increasing by a factor of 2—the intensity of radiation reaching the target will fall to one-half or one-fourth of its prior level.

The amount of energy reaching the target is also related to the angle of incidence of the radiation; the angle of incidence is the angle between an incident ray and the normal to the surface. As the angle of incidence of the radiation changes, the intensity of the energy reaching the target decreases in proportion to the cosine of the angle of incidence. For example, if the angle of incidence changes from 0 degrees (i.e., perpendicular to the surface of the skin), with a cosine of 1, to 45 degrees, with a cosine of $\frac{1}{\sqrt{2}}$, the intensity of radiation will fall by a factor of $1 - 0.707 = 0.23$ or by about 23%. Thus, the intensity of radiation reaching the skin is greatest when the source is close to the patient's skin and the radiation beam is perpendicular to the skin surface.

IR radiation is absorbed the most by darker tissues having high IR absorption coefficients. With the same radiation and lamp positioning, dark skin will absorb more IR and therefore will increase in temperature more than light skin will.

A number of authors have provided formulae for calculating the exact amount of heat being delivered to a patient by IR radiation[170,171] or for measuring the increase in tissue temperature[172]; however, as with other thermal agents, in clinical practice, the patient's sensory report is the best gauge of skin temperature. The amount of heat transfer is adjusted by changing the power output of the lamp and/or the distance of the lamp from the patient so that the patient feels a comfortable level of warmth.

IR lamps for heating superficial tissues were popular during the 1940s and 1950s. Although IR produces expected effects of heat, including reducing pain in patients with chronic low back pain[173] and increasing joint flexibility and thus increasing ROM when combined with stretching,[155] the use of IR is not popular at this time. The decline in popularity appears to be the result of changes in practice style and concern about overheating patients if they are placed or move too close to the lamp, rather than excessive adverse effects or lack of therapeutic efficacy. Most current uses and literature regarding IR in therapy relate to low-intensity IR lasers with nonthermal effects, as discussed in detail in Chapter 16.

APPLICATION TECHNIQUE 8.10   INFRARED LAMPS

Equipment Required

- IR lamp
- IR opaque goggles
- Tape measure to measure distance of treatment area from IR source
- Towels

Procedure

1. Remove clothing and jewelry from the area to be treated and inspect the area. Drape the patient for modesty, leaving the area to be treated uncovered.
2. Put IR opaque goggles on the patient and the therapist if there is a possibility of IR irradiation of the eyes.
3. Allow the IR lamp to warm up for 5 to 10 minutes so it will reach a stable level of output.[166]
4. Position the patient with the surface of the area to be treated perpendicular to the IR beam and approximately 45 to 60 cm away from the source. Remember that the intensity of the IR radiation reaching the skin decreases, with an inverse square relationship, as the distance from the source increases and in proportion to the cosine of the angle of incidence of the beam. Adjust the distance from the source and wattage of the lamp output so that the patient feels a comfortable level of warmth. Measure and record the distance of the lamp from the target tissue.
5. Provide the patient with a means to call for assistance if discomfort occurs.
6. Instruct the patient to avoid moving closer to or farther from the lamp and to avoid touching the lamp because movement

toward or away from the lamp will alter the amount of energy reaching the patient.
7. Set the lamp to treat for 15 to 30 minutes. Generally, treatment times of about 15 minutes are used for subacute conditions, and treatment times of up to 30 minutes are used for chronic conditions. Most lamps have a timer that automatically shuts off the lamp when the treatment time has elapsed.
8. Monitor the patient's response during treatment. It may be necessary to move the lamp farther away if the patient becomes too warm. Be cautious in moving the lamp closer if the patient reports not feeling warm enough because the patient may have accommodated to the sensation and may not judge the heat level accurately once warm.
9. When the intervention is completed, turn off the lamp and dry any perspiration from the treated area.

Advantages

- Does not require contact of the medium with the patient, which reduces the risk of infection and the possible discomfort of the weight of a hot pack and avoids the problem of poor contact when highly contoured areas are treated
- The area being treated can be observed throughout the intervention

Disadvantages

- IR radiation is not easily localized to a specific treatment area
- It is difficult to ensure consistent heating in all treatment areas because the amount of heat transfer is affected by the distance of the skin from the radiation source and the angle of the beam with the skin, both of which vary with tissue contours and may be inconsistent between treatment sessions

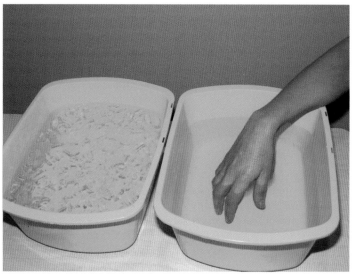

FIGURE 8.32 Contrast bath.

CONTRAST BATH

Contrast baths are applied by alternately immersing an area, generally a distal extremity, first in warm or hot water and then in cool or cold water (Fig. 8.32). Contrast baths have been shown to cause fluctuations in blood flow over a 20-minute treatment.[174] A 2009 systematic review of 28 studies from 1938 to 2009 found evidence that contrast baths may increase superficial blood flow and skin temperature, and a 2018 study found that contrast baths with a 4:1 heat:cold ratio increased circulation and oxygenation of the gastrocnemius muscle.[175,176] This form of thermotherapy is frequently used clinically when the treatment goal is to achieve the benefits of heat, including decreased pain and increased flexibility, while avoiding increased edema. The varying sensory stimulus is thought to promote pain relief and desensitization. Thus, treatment with a contrast bath may be considered when patients present with chronic edema; subacute trauma; inflammatory conditions such as sprains, strains, or tendinitis; or hyperalgesia or hypersensitivity caused by reflex sympathetic dystrophy or other conditions.

Clinical Pearl

Contrast baths are frequently used clinically when the treatment goal is to achieve the benefits of heat, including decreased pain and increased flexibility, while avoiding increased edema.

Contrast baths have been used to treat edema based on the rationale that the alternating vasodilation and vasoconstriction produced by alternating immersion in hot and cold water may help to train or condition the smooth muscles of the blood vessels. However, because no research data on the efficacy or mechanisms of this effect are available, it is recommended that clinicians carefully assess the effects of such treatment on the individual patient when considering using this treatment.

APPLICATION TECHNIQUE 8.11   CONTRAST BATH

Equipment Required

- Two water containers
- Thermometer
- Towels

Procedure

1. Fill two adjacent containers with water. The containers may be buckets or tubs. Fill one container with warm or hot water (38°C to 44°C [100°F to 111°F]) and the other with cold or cool water (10°C to 18°C [50°F to 64°F]). When contrast baths are used for the control of pain or edema, it is recommended that the temperature difference between the warm and cold water be large; when contrast baths are used for desensitization, it is recommended that the temperature difference between the two baths be small initially and then gradually increased as the patient's sensitivity decreases.

2. Immerse the area to be treated in warm water for 3 to 10 minutes; then immerse the area in cold water for 1 to 3 minutes.
3. Repeat this sequence five or six times to provide a total treatment time of 25 to 30 minutes.
4. When the treatment is completed, dry the area quickly and thoroughly.

Advantages

- May promote increased superficial blood flow
- Provides good contact with contoured distal extremities compared with other thermal agents
- May help to provide pain control without aggravating edema
- Allows movement in water for increased circulatory effects

Disadvantages

- Limb is in a dependent position, which may aggravate edema
- Some patients do not tolerate cold immersion

Documentation

The following should be documented:

- Area of the body treated
- Type of heating agent used
- Treatment parameters
  - Temperature or power of the agent
  - Number and type of insulation layers used
  - Distance of the agent from the patient
  - Patient's position or activity, if these can be varied with the agent used
  - Treatment duration
- Response to the intervention

Documentation is typically written in the SOAP note format. The following examples summarize only the modality component of intervention and are not intended to represent a comprehensive plan of care.

EXAMPLES

When applying a hot pack (HP) to low back pain (LBP), document the following:

S: Pt reports LBP that worsens with prolonged sitting when reading.
O: Pretreatment: LBP 7/10. Sitting tolerance 30 min when reading.
Intervention: HP low back, 20 min, Pt prone, six layers of towels.
Posttreatment: LBP 4/10 when reading.
A: Pain decreased from 7/10 to 4/10 when reading.
P: Continue use of HP as above before stretching and back exercises. Recheck sitting tolerance for reading at the beginning of next visit.

When applying paraffin to the right hand, document the following:

S: Pt reports R hand stiffness, especially with finger extension.
O: Pretreatment: Proximal interphalangeal (PIP) extension limited to −10 degrees. Unable to tie shoelaces without assistance.
Intervention: Paraffin R hand, 50°C (122°F), 10 min, dip wrap, seven dips.
Posttreatment: PIP extension 5 degrees after active and passive stretching. Able to tie shoelaces without assistance.
A: Decreased joint stiffness and improved ROM and function.
P: Continue use of paraffin as above to R hand before stretching and mobilization.

When applying Fluidotherapy to the left leg, ankle, and foot, document the following:

S: Pt reports L ankle stiffness.
O: Pretreatment: Ankle dorsiflexion 0 degrees.
Intervention: Fluidotherapy L LE, 42°C (108°F), 20 min. Ankle AROM during heating.
Posttreatment: Ankle dorsiflexion 5 degrees.
A: Ankle dorsiflexion increased from neutral to 5 degrees.
P: Discontinue Fluidotherapy. Progress to AROM and PROM and gait activities in weight-bearing position.

When applying IR radiation to the right forearm, document the following:

S: Pt reports R forearm pain with writing.
O: Pretreatment: Pain with motion associated with writing.
Intervention: IR R forearm, 1000 nm peak wavelength, 100 W at 50 cm for 20 min.
Posttreatment: Mild sensation of warmth at forearm; pain with writing decreased by 50%.
A: Tolerated well. Decreased pain with writing.
P: Continue IR as above 2 × per week before stretching.

CLINICAL CASE STUDIES

The following case studies summarize the concepts of superficial heat discussed in this chapter. Based on the scenarios presented, an evaluation of the clinical findings and the goals of the intervention are proposed. These are followed by a discussion of factors to be considered in the selection of superficial thermotherapy as the indicated treatment modality and in the selection of the ideal thermotherapy agent to promote progress toward set goals.

CASE STUDY 8.4

Osteoarthritis of the Hands
Examination
History

MP is a 75-year-old woman referred for therapy with a diagnosis of osteoarthritis of the hands and an order to evaluate and treat with a focus on developing a home program. MP complains of stiffness, aching, and pain in all her finger joints, making it difficult to grip cooking utensils, write, and perform

normal household tasks. She reports that these symptoms have gradually worsened over the past 10 years and have become much more severe in the past month since she stopped taking ibuprofen because of gastric side effects.

Systems Review

MP rates her hand joint pain and stiffness today at 5/10, equal bilaterally. Her lower extremities are not bothering her at this time.

Tests and Measures

Examination reveals stiffness and restricted flexion passive ROM (PROM) of the proximal interphalangeal (PIP) joints of fingers 2 to 5 to approximately 90 degrees and mild ulnar drift at the carpometacarpal (CMC) joints bilaterally. The joints are not warm or edematous, and sensation is intact in both hands. *Is this an acute or chronic condition? What must you consider before using heat in a patient with an inflammatory condition? What types of thermotherapy would be appropriate for this patient? Which type would not be appropriate?*

CLINICAL CASE STUDIES—*cont'd*

Evaluation and Goals

ICF Level	Current Status	Goals
Body structure and function	Restricted finger ROM	Increase finger ROM
	Pain, stiffness, and swelling of the finger joints	Decrease pain
	Abnormal ulnar drift of the CMC joints of the hands	Reduce joint stiffness
		Prevent further symptoms from developing
Activity	Gripping action difficult	Increase ability to grip
Participation	Difficulty with cooking, household tasks, writing	Optimize patient's ability to cook, do household tasks, and write

CMC, Carpometacarpal; *ICF,* International Classification for Functioning, Disability and Health; *ROM,* range of motion.

◆ FIND THE EVIDENCE

PICO Terms	Natural Language Example	Sample PubMed Search
P (Population)	Patients with pain and stiffness in the hands due to osteoarthritis	("Osteoarthritis/therapy" [MeSH] OR "osteoarthritis" [text word])
I (Intervention)	Thermotherapy	AND "thermotherapy" [text word] OR "thermal therapy" [text word] OR "hyperthermia, induced" [Mesh]
C (Comparison)	No thermotherapy	
O (Outcome)	Reduction of swelling; increased range of motion in hands; improved function	

Key Studies or Reviews

1. Valdes K, Marik T: A systematic review of conservative interventions for osteoarthritis of the hand. *J Hand Ther* 23:334–350, 2010.
   This systematic review that included 21 studies on hand therapy interventions for osteoarthritis of the hand dated between 1986 and 2009 concluded that "the literature supports the use of orthotics, hand exercises, application of heat, and joint protection education combined with provision of adaptive equipment to improve grip strength and function."
2. Kasapoglu Aksoy M, Altan L: Short-term efficacy of paraffin therapy and home-based exercise programs in the treatment of symptomatic hand osteoarthritis. *Turk J Phys Med Rehabil* 64(2):108–113, 2017.

This prospective, single-blind, randomized controlled study compared the effects of paraffin therapy and home-based exercise with home-based exercise alone on pain, quality of life, hand stiffness and function, and grip and pinch strength 2 and 6 weeks after the intervention. The paraffin therapy was delivered for five sessions/week for 2 weeks using the dip-wrap method. The exercises were handgrip strengthening, isometrics, and active resistive training to be performed for 15 minutes twice each day. Those who received paraffin therapy in addition to the exercises had significantly greater improvements in pain, quality of life, hand stiffness and function, and both grip and pinch strength at both 2 and 6 weeks compared with baseline.

Prognosis

Given the chronic, progressive nature of osteoarthritis, the intervention should focus on maintaining the patient's status, optimizing her function, and slowing the progression of her disabilities. Superficial heating agents can increase the extensibility of superficial soft tissue and therefore are indicated for the treatment of joint stiffness and restricted ROM. Superficial heating agents can also reduce joint-related pain. Although this patient has a diagnosis of osteoarthritis, which is an inflammatory disease, thermotherapy is not contraindicated at this time because her hands do not show signs of acute inflammation, such as increased temperature or edema of the finger joints. Her hands have intact sensation. Caution should be used, however, because at age 75 years, she may have impaired circulation or impaired thermal regulation. Therefore, the intensity of the thermal agent should be at the lower end of the range typically used.

Intervention

It is proposed that superficial heat be applied to the wrists, hands, and fingers of both hands. Paraffin, Fluidotherapy, and water are appropriate thermal agents; however, a hot pack is inappropriate because it would not provide good contact with these highly contoured areas. Fluidotherapy and water offer the advantage of allowing motion during their application; however, Fluidotherapy is generally too expensive and cumbersome for use at home or in many clinics, and water immersion may result in edema formation because the patient's hands must be in a dependent position while being heated. Warm water soaks, together with exercise, would be most appropriate if the patient does not develop edema with this intervention, and paraffin followed by exercise would be most appropriate if the patient develops edema with soaking in warm water. Paraffin is likely the preferred intervention. A recent study supports that paraffin improves pain, strength, stiffness, function, and quality of life in patients with hand osteoarthritis. The hands can also be elevated while paraffin is on, reducing the risk of edema formation. Paraffin is also inexpensive and safe enough to be used at home; however, it does not allow motion during application. Therefore, for optimal benefit, if paraffin is used to treat this patient, she

Continued

CLINICAL CASE STUDIES—cont'd

should perform AROM exercises immediately after removing the paraffin from her hands. If paraffin is used, it should be applied using the dip-wrap method rather than the dip-immersion method because the former allows elevation of the hand and is safer because it produces less intense and prolonged heating. Therefore, this method is least likely to cause edema formation and is safer for an older patient who may have impaired circulation or thermal regulation.

Documentation

S: Pt reports bilateral hand pain (7/10) and stiffness when cooking.

O: Pretreatment: PIP PROM approximately 90 degrees in fingers 2 to 5. Stiffness and pain with motion. Mild ulnar drift at bilateral CMC joints.

Intervention: Paraffin to bilateral hands, 50°C (108°F), 10 min, dip wrap, seven dips. ROM exercises after removing paraffin.

Posttreatment: PIP PROM 110 degrees in fingers 2 to 5. Pain (4/10) and decreased subjective stiffness. No visible edema. Pt prepared a pot of tea.

A: Increased ROM, decreased pain and stiffness without development of edema in response to paraffin. Pt able to fill and lift teapot without increasing pain level.

P: Continue paraffin application as above once daily at home before ROM exercises and meal preparation.

CASE STUDY 8.5

Low Back Pain
Examination

History

KB is a 45-year-old man with mild low back pain. Two months ago, he fell 10 feet from a ladder and sustained severe soft tissue bruising without any fractures. KB was referred for physical therapy 1 month ago with the diagnosis of a lumbar strain and with an order to optimize function to return to work. KB is currently participating in an active exercise program to improve his spinal flexibility and active stabilization, but he often feels stiff when starting to exercise. He has not returned to his job as a carpenter because of low back pain that is aggravated by forward bending and low back stiffness that is most intense during the first few hours of the day and that prevents him from lifting. He has also not yet returned to playing baseball with his children because he is scared that this will aggravate his back pain.

Systems Review

KB reports to the clinic with his wife, a registered nurse committed to her husband's rehabilitation. KB appears in good spirits and eager to begin a plan that will reduce his lower back pain. He reports that his pain is often worse at night when he lies still, making it difficult to fall asleep, and that it is alleviated to some degree by taking a hot shower. He had been making good progress, with increasing lumbar ROM, strength, and endurance, until the last 2 weeks, when his progress reached a plateau.

Tests and Measures

Palpation reveals spasms of the lumbar paravertebral muscles, and KB has 50% restriction of active forward bending ROM and 30% restriction of side bending bilaterally, with reports of a sensation of pulling in his low back at the end of the range and pain at a 7/10 level. Other objective measures including active backward bending, passive joint mobility, and lower extremity strength and sensation are within normal limits.

How may thermotherapy help this patient? What types of thermotherapy would be appropriate for this patient? Which type would not be appropriate? What types of activities should be combined with thermotherapy to help the patient achieve his goals?

Evaluation and Goals

ICF Level	Current Status	Goals
Body structure and function	Restricted trunk ROM in forward and side bending	Normalize lumbar forward and side bending ROM
	Low back pain	Control low back pain
	Paravertebral muscle spasms	Resolve paravertebral muscle spasms
Activity	Inability to bend forward to lift	Return lifting ability to prior baseline
	Difficulty falling asleep	Able to fall asleep within 15 minutes of going to bed
Participation	Inability to work as a carpenter or play baseball	Return to work Return to recreational sports

ICF, International Classification for Functioning, Disability and Health; *ROM,* range of motion.

◆ FIND THE EVIDENCE

PICO Terms	Natural Language Example	Sample PubMed Search
P (Population)	Patients with sustained lower back pain	("Low Back Pain" [MeSH] OR "low back pain" [text word])
I (Intervention)	Thermotherapy	AND ("hyperthermia, induced" [MeSH] OR "hyperthermia" [text word] OR "induced hyperthermia" [text word] OR "thermotherapy" [text word])
C (Comparison)	No thermotherapy	
O (Outcome)	Increased range of motion in lumbar; decreased pain; improved function	

Key Studies or Reviews

1. Qaseem A, Wilt TJ, McLean RM, et al: Noninvasive treatments for acute, subacute and chronic low back pain: A clinical practice guideline from the American College of Physicians. *Ann Intern Med* 166(7):514–530, 2017.

   This evidence-based clinical practice guideline is based on a systematic review of randomized controlled trials published through April 2015 on noninvasive treatments for low back pain. The guideline provides three recommendations. The first is that "most patients with acute or subacute low back pain will improve over time regardless of treatment and patients should select nonpharmacological treatment with superficial heat (moderate-quality evidence), massage, acupuncture, or spinal manipulation (low-quality evidence)." The other recommendations, which are for patients with chronic low back pain, are to first try nonpharmacological interventions, and if there is an inadequate response to these, to then consider nonopioid medications, and to only consider opioid medication in patients who have failed both of the aforementioned options and only if the benefits outweigh the risks.

2. French SD, Cameron M, Walker BF, et al: Superficial heat or cold for low back pain. *Cochrane Database Syst Rev* CD004750, 2006.

   This systematic review concludes that there is moderate evidence in a small number of trials that superficial heat provides a short-term reduction in pain and disability in patients with acute and subacute low back pain and that the addition of exercise further reduces pain and improves function.

Prognosis

Two months after his initial soft tissue back injury, KB now has subacute low back pain. Overall, his prognosis for recovery is good, with or without intervention. Current evidence-based guidelines support the use of nonpharmacological interventions, with moderate-quality evidence supporting benefits for superficial heat, with the addition of exercise further reducing pain and improving function. KB's rehabilitation program should likely focus on a program of stretching and strengthening exercises. Applying superficial heat before and between his exercises may improve performance and accelerate progress. Thermotherapy may reduce pain, stiffness, and soft tissue shortening. Furthermore, KB reports that a hot shower, which provides superficial heating, helps alleviate his symptoms. No contraindications to the use of thermotherapy for this patient are known.

Intervention

A deep-heating or superficial heating agent may provide appropriate thermotherapy for this patient. A deep-heating agent would have the advantage of increasing the temperature of both superficial tissues and the muscles of the low back; however, a superficial heating agent, likely with a hot pack, is recommended because the patient could readily use this independently at home at any time. In addition, there is more evidence that superficial heat is effective for reducing pain and improving function in patients with subacute low back pain.

A hot pack could be applied with the patient in a supine, prone, side lying, or sitting position. More insulating towels should be used if the patient is supine or sitting rather than prone or side lying because compression of the towels by the patient's body weight, and the insulating effect of the supporting surface, will slow the cooling of the pack. Treatment with a superficial heating agent generally would be applied for 20 to 30 minutes at a time, although longer use of a wearable heat wrap may also be effective. To optimize the benefit of increased soft tissue extensibility with heat, stretching should be performed immediately after the thermal agent is applied.

Documentation

S: Pt reports low back stiffness and pain with forward bending.

O: Pretreatment: LBP 4/10. Lumbar paravertebral muscle spasms. 30% restriction of active forward bending ROM. 30% restriction of bilateral side bending.

Intervention: HP low back, 20 min, Pt prone, six layers of towels.

Posttreatment: LBP 2/10, decreased paravertebral muscle spasms. 20% restriction of forward bending and minimal restriction of side bending.

A: Pt tolerated HP well, with decreased pain and increased ROM.

P: Continue use of HP as above twice daily before stretching and back exercises.

CASE STUDY 8.6

Foot Ulcer Caused by Arterial Insufficiency

Examination

History

BD is a 72-year-old woman with a 10-year history of non–insulin-dependent diabetes mellitus and a full-thickness ulcer on her lateral right ankle caused by arterial insufficiency. The ulcer has been present for 6 months and has been treated only with daily dressing changes. BD has poor arterial circulation in her distal lower extremities, but her physician has determined that she is not a candidate for lower extremity bypass surgery. She lives alone at home and is independent in all activities of daily living; however, her walking is limited to approximately 500 feet because of calf pain. Because of this, she has limited her participation in family activities such as taking her grandchildren to the park. BD has been referred to physical therapy for evaluation and treatment of her ulcer.

Systems Review

BD reports feeling saddened and discouraged by her health. She looks tired but reports willingness to begin therapeutic interventions to increase the distance that she can walk without pain.

Tests and Measures

The patient is alert and oriented. Sensation is impaired distal to the patient's knees and is intact proximal to the knees. A 2-cm-diameter, full-thickness ulcer is present on the right lateral ankle.

Continued

CLINICAL CASE STUDIES—cont'd

What concerns would you have about the use of thermo-therapy in this patient? On what part(s) of the body would you consider applying thermotherapy in this patient?

Evaluation and Goals

ICF Level	Current Status	Goals
Body structure and function	Loss of skin and underlying soft tissue on right lateral ankle	Decrease wound size
	Reduced sensation in bilateral distal lower extremities	Close wound
Activity	Walking is limited to 500 feet	Increase walking tolerance to 1 block
	Daily dressing changes	Decrease the need for dressing changes to one or two times per week and thus reduce risk of infection associated with open wounds
Participation	Decreased participation in family activities such as taking her grandchildren to the park	Patient able to take her grandchildren to the park. Participation in family activities not limited by calf pain

ICF, International Classification for Functioning, Disability and Health.

◆ FIND THE EVIDENCE

PICO Terms	Natural Language Example	Sample PubMed Search
P (Population)	Patient with calf pain due to ulcer	("ulcer" [MeSH] OR "ulcer" [text word])
I (Intervention)	Thermotherapy	AND ("hyperthermia, induced" [MeSH] OR "hyperthermia" [text word] OR "induced hyperthermia" [text word] OR "thermotherapy" [text word])
C (Comparison)	No thermotherapy	
O (Outcome)	Tissue healing; decreased size of ulcer; reduction in pain; increased function	

Key Studies

1. Tei C, Shinsato T, Kihara T, et al: Successful thermal therapy for end-stage peripheral artery disease. *J Cardiol* 47:163–164, 2006.

There are very few reports of successful nonsurgical treatment of arterial foot ulcers. This case report describes a patient with diabetes and a chronic nonhealing arterial foot ulcer 4.5 × 5.0 cm that healed completely with superficial heat therapy applied daily for 15 weeks.

2. Tei C, Shinsato T, Miyata M, et al: Waon therapy improves peripheral arterial disease. *J Am Coll Card* 50(22):2169–2171, 2007.

This article describes a case series of 20 patients with peripheral arterial disease (PAD), with a total of seven lower extremity ulcers, treated with 15 minutes of infrared at 60°C, 5 days/week for 10 weeks. All patients demonstrated improvements in their symptoms of PAD. Four of the ulcers healed completely, and the other three improved.

Prognosis

Thermotherapy may help achieve some of the proposed goals of treatment because it can improve circulation and thus facilitate tissue healing. Superficial heating agents can increase circulation both in the area to which the heat is applied and distally. Increasing tissue temperature can also increase oxygen-hemoglobin dissociation, increasing the availability of oxygen for tissue healing. Applying thermotherapy directly to the distal lower extremities of this patient would be contraindicated if she has impaired sensation in these areas. Application of thermotherapy proximal to the areas of sensory loss, possibly to her calf, thighs, or low back, may be a safe and effective way to promote wound healing without excessive risk.

Intervention

Thermotherapy using a deep or superficial heating agent would be appropriate for this patient. As with Case Study 8.5, deep heating would be ideal because it would affect both deep and superficial tissue temperatures; however, a superficial heating agent is more likely to be used because of its greater availability. A hot pack or an IR lamp could be used to heat this patient's low back or thighs and should be applied for about 20 minutes. If a hot pack is used, extra towels should be used because this patient's poor circulation puts her at increased risk for burns.

Documentation

S: Pt reports an ulcer on her R lateral ankle present for 6 months and calf pain limiting her walking to ~500 feet.

O: Pretreatment: Full-thickness ulcer right lateral ankle, 1 cm × 1 cm. Decreased sensation from ankle distally bilaterally.

Intervention: HP bilateral thighs, 20 min, Pt sitting, eight layers of towels.

Posttreatment: Skin in area of heat application intact without blistering or burns. Pt reports very mild warmth felt with this application.

A: Pt tolerated treatment without discomfort.

P: Continue application of HP to thighs, with six towels at next treatment, in conjunction with appropriate direct wound care.

CLINICAL CASE STUDIES—cont'd

CASE STUDY 8.7

Colles Fracture

Examination

History

FS is a 65-year-old woman who sustained a closed Colles fracture of her right arm 6 weeks ago. The fracture was initially treated with a closed reduction and cast fixation. This cast was removed 3 days ago, when radiographic reports indicated formation of callus and good alignment of the fracture site. FS has been referred to therapy with an order to evaluate and treat. She has not received any prior rehabilitation treatment for this injury.

Systems Review

FS reports severe pain, stiffness, and swelling of her right wrist and hand. She is wearing a wrist splint and is not using her right hand for any functional activities because she is afraid it may cause further damage. FS is retired and lives alone. She is unable to drive because of the dysfunction of her right hand and wrist.

Tests and Measures

The examination is significant for decreased active and passive ROM of the right wrist. Active wrist flexion is 30 degrees on the right and 80 degrees on the left. Wrist extension is 25 degrees on the right and 70 degrees on the left. Wrist ulnar deviation is 10 degrees on the right and 30 degrees on the left, and wrist radial deviation is 0 degrees on the right and 25 degrees on the left. Moderate nonpitting edema of the right hand is evident, and the skin of the right hand and wrist appears shiny. FS's functional grip on the right is limited by muscle weakness and restricted joint ROM. The patient is wearing a splint and is holding her hand across her abdomen. She reports severe pain when her hand is touched, even lightly. All other measures, including shoulder, elbow, and neck ROM; upper extremity sensation; and left upper extremity strength, are within normal limits for this patient's age and gender.

What type of hydrotherapy is best for this patient? What type of hydrotherapy would not be recommended?

Evaluation and Goals

ICF Level	Current Status	Goals
Body structure and function	Right hand and wrist: pain, weakness, hypersensitivity, restricted ROM, edema[a]	Control patient's pain, hypersensitivity, and fear
		Increase right wrist ROM by 20% to 50% in all planes in 2 to 4 weeks

ICF Level	Current Status	Goals
Activity	Avoiding all use of right hand and wrist	Short-term: Hold hand in normal position with normal swing during gait
		Long-term: Regain use of right hand for functional activities
Participation	Unable to drive	Return to driving

ICF, International Classification for Functioning, Disability and Health; *ROM,* range of motion.
[a]Although this patient's signs and symptoms are consistent with disuse after a fracture and immobilization, they are also consistent with acute complex regional pain syndrome (CRPS) type 1 (previously known as stage I reflex sympathetic dystrophy).

◆ FIND THE EVIDENCE

PICO Terms	Natural Language Example	Sample PubMed Search
P (Population)	Patients with complex regional pain syndrome due to Colles fracture	("reflex sympathetic dystrophy" [MeSH] OR "reflex sympathetic dystrophy" [text word])
I (Intervention)	Thermotherapy	AND ("hyperthermia, induced" [MeSH] OR "hyperthermia" [text word] OR "induced hyperthermia" [text word] OR "thermotherapy" [text word])
C (Comparison)	No thermotherapy	
O (Outcome)	Regain use of hand; increase strength	

1. Sezgin Ozcan D, Tatli HU, Polat CS, et al: The effectiveness of Fluidotherapy in poststroke complex regional pain syndrome: A randomized controlled study. *J Stroke Cerebrovasc Dis* 28(6):1578–1585, 2019.
   This randomized controlled trial compared conventional therapy 5 days/week without Fluidotherapy with conventional therapy with the addition of fifteen 20-minute sessions of Fluidotherapy at 40°C on edema, motor recovery, function, and pain in 30 patients with subacute CRPS type 1 of the upper extremity. After treatment, both groups showed improvements in almost all parameters, but improvements in edema volume and pain were significantly greater in those who also had Fluidotherapy.
2. Szerkes M, MacDermid JC, Birmingham T, et al: The effect of therapeutic whirlpool and hot packs on hand volume during rehabilitation after distal radius fracture: A blinded randomized controlled trial. *Hand* 12(3):265–271, 2017.

Continued

CLINICAL CASE STUDIES—cont'd

This randomized controlled trial compared the impact on hand volume of 15 minutes of therapeutic whirlpool at 40°C versus moist heat pack applied to the forearm, wrist, and hand for 3 consecutive visits in 60 patients with a recent distal radial fracture. The researchers found that patients receiving the whirlpool had a significantly greater volume increase after the treatment than those receiving the hot pack, but this difference was no longer significant 30 minutes later, after completing the therapy session, or 3 weeks later.

CRPS was an exclusion criterion for participation in this study, limiting generalizability to this patient case.

Prognosis

A contrast bath with warm and cool water of similar temperature, or Fluidotherapy with gentle agitation and warm temperature of 40°C, may reduce the hypersensitivity and hyperalgesia of this patient's hand while providing a suitable environment for active exercise to increase ROM and functional use of her hand. Hydrostatic pressure provided by water immersion and alternating vasoconstriction and vasodilation produced by a contrast bath may also help reduce edema in this extremity. A contrast bath is more likely to be used in most cases because the patient can also perform this treatment independently at home. A hot pack or warm or hot water whirlpool use are not recommended because the resulting increase in tissue temperature, particularly in conjunction with the dependent position of the extremity if a whirlpool is used, are likely to aggravate the edema already present in her hand. Although evaluation of this patient does not indicate any contraindication for the warm immersion, because higher temperatures may be used during later stages of treatment, her ability to sense temperature should be assessed before the use of a contrast bath or Fluidotherapy.

Intervention

A contrast bath is likely to be most effective for this patient because it may assist with desensitization and edema reduction while providing a comfortable environment for active exercise, and it can also be performed independently by the patient at home between therapy sessions. The temperature of the water in the two contrast baths should be similar initially, and as the patient progresses, the temperature difference may be gradually increased. The patient should also be encouraged to move her hand in the water.

Documentation

S: Pt reports R hand and wrist pain after a treated fracture.

O: Pretreatment: R wrist flexion 30 degrees, extension 25 degrees, ulnar deviation 10 degrees, radial deviation 0 degrees. L wrist flexion 80 degrees, extension 70 degrees, ulnar deviation 30 degrees, radial deviation 25 degrees. Restricted R grip. Nonpitting edema R hand.

Intervention: Contrast bath, 38°C (100°F) and 18°C (64°F). Warm × 4 min, then cold × 1 min. Sequence repeated 5 times.

Posttreatment: Decreased R hand edema, R wrist ROM improved with R wrist flexion 35 degrees, extension 30 degrees, ulnar deviation 20 degrees, radial deviation 5 degrees.

A: Pt tolerated contrast bath without pain or edema and gained increased ROM. Pt able to shift car from park to reverse and from reverse to park.

P: Continue contrast baths at home, gradually increasing the temperature difference. Pt given hand exercises to do at home.

Choosing Between Cryotherapy and Thermotherapy

Because some of the effects and clinical indications for the use of cryotherapy and thermotherapy are the same and others differ, there are some situations in which either may be used and others in which only one would be appropriate. Table 8.1 summarizes the effects of cryotherapy and thermotherapy to help the clinician choose between these options. Although both heat and cold can decrease pain and muscle spasm, they produce opposite effects on blood flow, edema formation, nerve conduction velocity, tissue metabolism, and collagen extensibility. Cryotherapy decreases these effects, and thermotherapy increases them.

Chapter Review

1. Cryotherapy is the transfer of heat from a patient with a cooling agent. Cryotherapy can decrease blood flow, decrease nerve conduction velocity, increase pain threshold, alter muscle strength, decrease the enzyme activity rate, temporarily decrease spasticity, and facilitate muscle contraction. These effects of cryotherapy are used clinically to control inflammation, pain, edema, and muscle spasm; to reduce spasticity temporarily; and to facilitate muscle contraction. Examples of physical agents used for cryotherapy include ice pack, cold pack, ice massage, and vapocoolant spray.

2. Thermotherapy is the transfer of heat to a patient with a heating agent. Thermotherapy can increase blood flow, increase nerve conduction velocity, increase pain threshold, alter muscle strength, and increase the enzyme activity rate. These effects of thermotherapy are used clinically to control pain, increase soft tissue extensibility, and accelerate healing. Examples of physical agents used for thermotherapy include hot pack, paraffin, Fluidotherapy, IR lamp, and contrast bath.

3. Thermal agents should not be applied when they may aggravate an existing pathology, such as a malignancy, or may cause damage, such as frostbite or burns.

TABLE 8.1	Effects of Cryotherapy and Thermotherapy	
Effect	**Cryotherapy**	**Thermotherapy**
Pain	Decrease	Decrease
Muscle spasm	Decrease	Decrease
Blood flow	Decrease	Increase
Edema formation	Decrease	Increase
Nerve conduction velocity	Decrease	Increase
Metabolic rate	Decrease	Increase
Collagen extensibility	Decrease	Increase
Joint stiffness	Increase	Decrease
Spasticity	Decrease	No effect

Glossary

Angle of incidence: The angle at which a beam (e.g., from an infrared lamp) contacts the skin.

Cold-induced vasodilation (CIVD): The dilation of blood vessels that occurs after cold is applied for a prolonged time or after tissue temperature reaches less than 10°C (50 degrees Farenheit). Also known as the *hunting response*.

Contrast bath: Alternating immersion in hot and cold water.

Controlled cold compression: Alternate pumping of cold water and air into a sleeve wrapped around a patient's limb; used most commonly to control pain and edema immediately after surgery.

Cryotherapy: The therapeutic use of cold.

Delayed-onset muscle soreness (DOMS): Soreness that often occurs 24 to 72 hours after eccentric exercise or unaccustomed training levels. DOMS probably is caused by inflammation as a result of tiny muscle tears.

Edema: Swelling resulting from accumulation of fluid in the interstitial space.

Fluidotherapy: A dry heating agent that transfers heat by convection. It consists of a cabinet containing finely ground particles of cellulose through which heated air is circulated.

Infrared (IR) lamp: A lamp that emits electromagnetic radiation in the IR range (wavelength approximately 750 to 1300 nm). IR radiation of sufficient intensity can cause an increase in superficial tissue temperature.

Paraffin: A waxy substance that can be warmed and used to coat the extremities for thermotherapy.

Protein denaturation: Breakdown of proteins that permanently alters their biological activity; it can be caused by excessive heat.

Quick icing: The rapid application of ice as a stimulus to elicit desired motor patterns in patients with reduced muscle tone or impaired muscle control.

RICE: An acronym for rest, ice, compression, and elevation. RICE is used to decrease edema formation and inflammation after an acute injury.

Spasticity: Muscle hypertonicity and increased deep tendon reflexes.

Thermotherapy: The therapeutic application of heat.

Vapocoolant spray: A liquid that evaporates quickly when sprayed on the skin, causing quick superficial cooling of the skin.

Vasoconstriction: A decrease in blood vessel diameter. Cold generally causes vasoconstriction.

References

1. Polderman KH: Mechanisms of action, physiological effects, and complications of hypothermia. *Crit Care Med* 37(7 Suppl):S186–S202, 2009. doi:10.1097/CCM.0b013e3181aa5241.
2. Martin SS, Spindler KP, Tarter JW, et al: Cryotherapy: an effective modality for decreasing intraarticular temperature after knee arthroscopy. *Am J Sports Med* 29:288–291, 2000.
3. Warren TA, McCarty EC, Richardson AL, et al: Intra-articular knee temperature changes: ice versus cryotherapy device. *Am J Sports Med* 32:441–445, 2004.
4. Glenn RE, Jr, Spindler KP, Warren TA, et al: Cryotherapy decreases intraarticular temperature after ACL reconstruction. *Clin Orthop Relat Res* 421:268–272, 2004.
5. Martin SS, Spindler KP, Tarter JW, et al: Does cryotherapy affect intraarticular temperature after knee arthroscopy? *Clin Orthop Relat Res* (400):184–189, 2002.
6. Costello JT, Baker PR, Minett GM, et al: Whole-body cryotherapy (extreme cold air exposure) for preventing and treating muscle soreness after exercise in adults. *Cochrane Database Syst Rev* (9), 2015:CD010789. doi:10.1002/14651858.CD010789.pub2.
7. Rose C, Edwards KM, Siegler J, et al: Whole-body cryotherapy as a recovery technique after exercise: a review of the literature. *Int J Sports Med* 38(14):1049–1060, 2017. doi:10.1055/s-0043-114861.
8. Khoshnevis S, Craik NK, Matthew Brothers R, et al: Cryotherapy-induced persistent vasoconstriction after cutaneous cooling: hysteresis between skin temperature and blood perfusion. *J Biomech Eng* 138(3), 2016:4032126. doi: 10.1115/1.4032126.
9. Khoshnevis S, Craik NK, Diller KR: Cold-induced vasoconstriction may persist long after cooling ends: an evaluation of multiple cryotherapy units. *Knee Surg Sports Traumatol Arthrosc* 23(9):2475–2483, 2015. doi: 10.1007/s00167.014-2911-y.
10. Foster D, Williams J, Forte AJ, et al: Application of ice for postoperative total knee incisions - does this make sense? A pilot evaluation of blood flow using fluorescence angiography. *Cureus* 11(7):e5126, 2019. doi:10.7759/cureus.5126.
11. Wolf SL: Contralateral upper extremity cooling from a specific cold stimulus. *Phys Ther* 51:158–165, 1971.
12. Christmas KM, Patik JC, Khoshnevis S, et al: Sustained cutaneous vasoconstriction during and following cryotherapy treatment: role of oxidative stress and Rho kinase. *Microvasc Res* 106:96–100, 2016. doi:10.1016/j.mvr.2016.04.005.
13. Christmas KM, Patik JC, Khoshnevis S, et al: Pronounced and sustained cutaneous vasoconstriction during and following cryotherapy treatment: role of neurotransmitters released from sympathetic nerves. *Microvasc Res* 115:52–57, 2018. doi:10.1016/j.mvr.2017.08.005 .
14. Palmieri RM, Garrison JC, Leonard JL, et al: Peripheral ankle cooling and core body temperature. *J Athl Train* 41:185–188, 2006.
15. Lewis T: Observations upon the reactions of the vessels of the human skin to cold. *Heart* 15:177–208, 1930.
16. Clark RS, Hellon RF, Lind AR: Vascular reactions of the human forearm to cold. *Clin Sci* 17:165–179, 1958.
17. Tyler CJ, Reeve T, Cheung SS: Cold-induced vasodilation during single digit immersion in 0°C and 8°C water in men and women. *PLoS One* 10(4):e0122592, 2015. doi:10.1371/journal.pone.0122592.
18. Keating WR: The effect of general chilling on the vasodilation response to cold. *J Physiol* 139:497–507, 1957.
19. Weston M, Taber C, Casagranda L, et al: Changes in local blood volume during cold gel pack application to traumatized ankles. *J Orthop Sports Phys Ther* 19:197–199, 1994.
20. Taber C, Countryman K, Fahrenbruch J, et al: Measurement of reactive vasodilation during cold gel pack application to nontraumatized ankles. *Phys Ther* 72:294–299, 1992.
21. Keating WR: *Survival in cold water*, Oxford, 1978, Blackwell.
22. Flouris AD, Cheung SS: Influence of thermal balance on cold-induced vasodilation. *J Appl Physiol* 106:1264–1271, 2009.
23. Daanen HAM: Finger cold-induced vasodilation: a review. *Eur J Appl Physiol* 89(5):411–426, 2003.
24. Heller HC, Grahn DA: Enhancing thermal exchange in humans and practical applications. *Disrupt Sci Technol* 1(1):11–20, 2012.
25. Diller KR: Heat transfer in health and healing. *J Heat Transfer* 137(10):11–12, 2015.
26. Lee JM, Warren MP, Mason SM: Effects of ice on nerve conduction velocity. *Physiotherapy* 64:2–6, 1978.
27. Algafly AA, George KP: The effect of cryotherapy on nerve conduction velocity, pain threshold and pain tolerance. *Br J Sports Med* 41:365–369, discussion 369, 2007.
28. Zankel HT: Effect of physical agents on motor conduction velocity of the ulnar nerve. *Arch Phys Med Rehabil* 47:787–792, 1966.
29. Douglas WW, Malcolm JL: The effect of localized cooling on cat nerves. *J Physiol* 130:53–54, 1955.
30. Bassett FH, Kirkpatrick JS, Engelhardt DL, et al: Cryotherapy induced nerve injury. *Am J Sports Med* 22:516–528, 1992.
31. Beaussier M, Sciard D, Sautet A: New modalities of pain treatment after outpatient orthopaedic surgery. *Orthop Traumatol Surg Res* 102(1 Suppl):S121–S124, 2016. doi:10.1016/j.otsr.2015.05.011.
32. Engelhard D, Hofer P, Annaheim S: Evaluation of the effect of cooling strategies on recovery after surgical intervention. *BMJ Open Sport Exerc Med* 5(1):e000527, 2019. doi:10.1136/bmjsem-2019-000527.
33. Hubbard TJ, Denegar CR: Does cryotherapy improve outcomes with soft tissue injury? *J Athl Train* 39(3):278–279, 2004.

34. Ernst E, Fialka V: Ice freezes pain? A review of the clinical effectiveness of analgesic cold therapy. *J Pain Symptom Manage* 9:56–59, 1994.

35. McGown HL: Effects of cold application on maximal isometric contraction. *Phys Ther* 47:185–192, 1967.

36. Bleakley CM, Costello JT, Glasgow PD: Should athletes return to sport after applying ice? A systematic review of the effect of local cooling on functional performance. *Sports Med* 42:69–87, 2012.

37. Torres R, Silva F, Pedrosa V, et al: The acute effect of cryotherapy on muscle strength and shoulder proprioception. *J Sport Rehabil* 26(6):497–506, 2017. doi:10.1123/jsr.2015-0215.

38. Oliver RA, Johnson DJ, Wheelhouse WW, et al: Isometric muscle contraction response during recovery from reduced intramuscular temperature. *Arch Phys Med Rehabil* 60:126–129, 1979.

39. Johnson J, Leider FE: Influence of cold bath on maximum handgrip strength. *Percept Mot Skills* 44:323–325, 1977.

40. Ruiz DH, Myrer JW, Durrant E, et al: Cryotherapy and sequential exercise bouts following cryotherapy on concentric and eccentric strength in the quadriceps. *J Athl Train* Winter 28(4):320–323, 1993.

41. Pritchard KA, Saliba SA: Should athletes return to activity after cryotherapy? *J Athl Train* 49:95–96, 2014.

42. Knuttsson E, Mattsson E: Effects of local cooling on monosynaptic reflexes in man. *Scand J Rehabil Med* 52:166–168, 1969.

43. Knuttsson E: Topical cryotherapy in spasticity. *Scand J Rehabil Med* 2:159–162, 1970.

44. Hartvikksen K: Ice therapy in spasticity. *Acta Neurol Scand* 38:79–83, 1962.

45. Miglietta O: Electromyographic characteristics of clonus and influence of cold. *Arch Phys Med Rehabil* 45:502–503, 1964.

46. Miglietta O: Action of cold on spasticity. *Am J Phys Med* 52:198–205, 1973.

47. Price R, Lehmann JF, Boswell-Bassette S, et al: Influence of cryotherapy on spasticity at the human ankle. *Arch Phys Med Rehabil* 74:300–304, 1993.

48. Harlaar J, Ten Kate JJ, Prevoœ AJH, et al: The effect of cooling on muscle co-ordination in spasticity: assessment with the repetitive movement test. *Disabil Rehabil* 23(11):453–461, 2001.

49. Wolf SL, Letbetter WD: Effect of skin cooling on spontaneous EMG activity in triceps surae of the decerebrate cat. *Brain Res* 91:151–155, 1975.

50. Harris ED, McCroskery PA: The influence of temperature and fibril stability on degradation of cartilage collagen by rheumatoid synovial collagenase. *N Engl J Med* 290:1–6, 1974.

51. Wojtecka-Lukasik E, Ksiezopolska-Orlowska K, Gaszewska E, et al: Cryotherapy decreases histamine levels in the blood of patients with rheumatoid arthritis. *Inflamm Res* 59(Suppl 2):S253–S255, 2010.

52. Hocutt JE, Jaffe R, Ryplander CR, et al: Cryotherapy in ankle sprains. *Am J Sports Med* 10:316–319, 1982.

53. Vieira Ramos G, Pinheiro CM, Peviani Messa S, et al: Cryotherapy reduces inflammatory response without altering muscle regeneration process and extracellular matrix remodeling of rat muscle. *Sci Rep* 6(1):18525, 2016.

54. Schaser KD, Stove JF, Melcher I, et al: Local cooling restores microcirculatory hemodynamics after closed soft-tissue trauma in rats. *J Trauma* 61:642–649, 2006.

55. Deal DN, Tipton J, Rosencrance E, et al: Ice reduces edema: a study of microvascular permeability in rats. *J Bone Joint Surg Am* 84:1573–1578, 2002.

56. Ohkoshi Y, Ohkoshi M, Nagasaki S: The effect of cryotherapy on intraarticular temperature and postoperative care after anterior cruciate ligament reconstruction. *Am J Sports Med* 27:357–362, 1999.

57. Ni SH, Jiang WT, Guo L, et al: Cryotherapy on postoperative rehabilitation of joint arthroplasty. *Knee Surg Sports Traumatol Arthrosc* 23:3354–3361, 2015.

58. Osbahr DC, Cawley PW, Speer KP: The effect of continuous cryotherapy on glenohumeral joint and subacromial space temperatures in the postoperative shoulder. *Arthroscopy* 18:748–754, 2002.

59. Saito N, Horiuchi H, Kobayashi S, et al: Continuous local cooling for pain relief following total hip arthroplasty. *J Arthroplasty* 19:334–337, 2004.

60. Singh H, Osbahr DC, Holovacs TF, et al: The efficacy of continuous cryotherapy on the postoperative shoulder: a prospective, randomized investigation. *J Shoulder Elbow Surg* 10:522–525, 2001.

61. Ravindhran B, Rajan S, Balachandran G, et al: Do ice packs reduce postoperative midline incision pain, NSAID or narcotic use? *World J Surg* 43(11):2651–2657, 2019. doi:10.1007/s00268-019-05129-1.

62. Dantas LO, Breda CC, da Silva Serrao PRM, et al: Short-term cryotherapy did not substantially reduce pain and had unclear effects on physical function and quality of life in people with knee osteoarthritis: a randomised trial. *J Physiother* 65(4):215–221, 2019.

63. Dantas LO, Moreira RFC, Norde FM, et al: The effects of cryotherapy on pain and function in individuals with knee osteoarthritis: a systematic review of randomized controlled trials. *Clin Rehabil* 33(8):1310–1319, 2019. doi:10.1177/0269215519840406.

64. Bleakley C, McDonough S, Gardner E, et al: Cold-water immersion (cryotherapy) for preventing and treating muscle soreness after exercise. *Cochrane Database Syst Rev* (2), 2012:CD008262. doi:10.1002/14651858.CD008262.pub2.

65. Lewis PB, Ruby D, Bush-Joseph CA: Muscle soreness and delayed-onset muscle soreness. *Clin Sports Med* 31:255–262, 2012.

66. Hyldahl RD, Hubal MJ: Lengthening our perspective: morphological, cellular, and molecular responses to eccentric exercise. *Muscle Nerve* 49:155–170, 2014.

67. Leeder J, Gissane C, van Someren K, et al: Cold water immersion and recovery from strenuous exercise: a meta-analysis. *Br J Sports Med* 46:233–240, 2012.

68. Hohenauer E, Taeymans J, Baeyens JP, et al: The effect of post-exercise cryotherapy on recovery characteristics: a systematic review and meta-analysis. *PLoS One* 10(9):e0139028, 2015. doi:10.1371/journal.pone.0139028.

69. Fonseca LB, Brito CJ, Silva RJ, et al: Use of cold-water immersion to reduce muscle damage and delayed-onset muscle soreness and preserve muscle power in jiu-jitsu athletes. *J Athl Train* 51(7):540–549, 2016. doi:10.4085/1062-6050-51.9.01.

70. Tomchuk D, Rubley MD, Holcomb WR, et al: The magnitude of tissue cooling during cryotherapy with varied types of compression. *J Athl Train* 45:230–237, 2010.

71. Wilkerson GB: Treatment of inversion ankle sprain through synchronous application of focal compression and cold. *Athl Train* 26:220–225, 1991.

72. Boris M, Wiedorf S, Lasinski B, et al: Lymphedema reduction by noninvasive complex lymphedema therapy. *Oncology* 8:95–106, 1994.

73. Marino FE: Heat reactions in multiple sclerosis: An overlooked paradigm in the study of comparative fatigue. *Int J Hyperthermia* 25(1):34–40, 2009.

74. Beenakker EA, Oparina TI, Hartgring A, et al: Cooling garment treatment in MS: clinical improvement and decrease in leukocyte NO production. *Neurology* 57:892–894, 2001.

75. Capello E, Gardella M, Leandri M, et al: Lowering body temperature with a cooling suit as symptomatic treatment for thermosensitive multiple sclerosis patients. *Ital J Neurol Sci* 16:533–539, 1995.

76. Schwid SR, NASA/MS Cooling Study Group: A randomized controlled study of the acute and chronic effects of cooling therapy for MS. *Neurology* 60:1955–1960, 2003.

77. Grahn DA, Murray JV, Heller HC: Cooling via one hand improved physical performance in heat-sensitive individuals with MS: A preliminary study. *BMC Neurology* 8(14), 2008.

78. Feys P, Helsen W, Liu X, et al: Effects of peripheral cooling on intention tremor in multiple sclerosis. *J Neurol Neurosurg Psychiatry* 76:373–379, 2005.

79. Umphred DA, Lazaro R: *Neurological rehabilitation*, ed 6, 2012, St Louis, Mosby.

80. Stepaniuk P, Vostretsova K, Kanani A: Review of cold-induced urticaria characteristics, diagnosis and management in a Western Canadian allergy practice. *Allergy Asthma Clin Immunol* 14:85, 2018. doi:10.1186/s13223-018-0310-5. PMID: 30574166.

81. Roccatello D, Saadoun D, Ramos-Casals M, et al: Cryoglobulinaemia. *Nat Rev Dis Primers* 4(1):11, 2018. doi:10.1038/s41572-018-0009-4.

82. Shanbhag S, Spivak J: Paroxysmal cold hemoglobinuria. *Hematol Oncol Clin North Am* 29(3):473–478, 2015. doi:10.1016/j.hoc.2015.01.004.

83. Wigley FM, Flavahan NA: Raynaud's phenomenon. *N Engl J Med* 375(6):556–565, 2016. doi:10.1056/NEJMra1507638.

84. Stringer T, Femia AN: Raynaud's phenomenon: current concepts. *Clin Dermatol* 36(4):498–507, 2018.

85. Parker JT, Small NC, Davis DG: Cold-induced nerve palsy. *Athl Train* 18:76–77, 1983.

86. Green GA, Zachazewski JE, Jordan SE: Peroneal nerve palsy induced by cryotherapy. *Phys Sportsmed* 17:63–70, 1989.

87. Covington DB, Bassett FH: When cryotherapy injures. *Phys Sportsmed* 21:78–93, 1993.

88. McGuire DA, Hendricks SD: Incidences of frostbite in arthroscopic knee surgery postoperative cryotherapy rehabilitation. *Arthroscopy* 22(10):1141, 2006.

89. Kanlayanaphotporn R, Janwantanakul P: Comparison of skin surface temperature during the application of various cryotherapy modalities. *Arch Phys Med Rehabil* 86:1411–1415, 2005.

90. Chesterton LS, Foster NE, Ross L: Skin temperature response to cryotherapy. *Arch Phys Med Rehabil* 83:543–549, 2002.

91. Enwemeka CS, Allen C, Avila P, et al: Soft tissue thermodynamics before, during, and after cold pack therapy. *Med Sci Sports Exerc* 34:45–50, 2002.

92. Myrer WJ, Myrer KA, Measom GJ, et al: Muscle temperature is affected by overlying adipose when cryotherapy is administered. *J Athl Train* 36:32–36, 2001.

93. Bender AL, Kramer EE, Brucker JB, et al: Local ice-bag application and triceps surae muscle temperature during treadmill walking. *J Athl Train* 40:271–275, 2005.

94. Myrer JW, Measom G, Fellingham GW: Temperature changes in the human leg during and after two methods of cryotherapy. *J Athl Train* 33:25–29, 1998.

95. Thienpont E: Does advanced cryotherapy reduce pain and narcotic consumption after knee arthroplasty? *Clin Orthop Relat Res* 472(11):3417–3423, 2014. doi:10.1007/s11999-014-3810-8.

96. Metzman L, Gamble JG, Rinsky LA: Effectiveness of ice packs in reducing skin temperature under casts. *Clin Orthop Relat Res* 330:217–221, 1996.

97. Mumith A, Pavlou P, Barrett M, et al: Enhancing postoperative rehabilitation following knee arthroplasty using a new cryotherapy product: a prospective study. *Geriatr Orthop Surg Rehabil* 6:316–321, 2015.

98. Ostrowski J, Purchio A, Beck M, et al: Effectiveness of salted ice bag versus cryocompression on decreasing intramuscular and skin temperature. *J Sport Rehabil* 28(2):120–125, 2019. doi:10.1123/jsr.2017-0173.

99. Schroder D, Passler HH: Combination of cold and compression after knee surgery: a prospective randomized study. *Knee Surg Sports Traumatol Arthrosc* 2:158–165, 1994.

100. Webb JM, Williams D, Ivory JP, et al: The use of cold compression dressings after total knee replacement: a randomized controlled trial. *Orthopedics* 21:59–61, 1998.

101. Alfuth M, Strietzel M, Vogler T, et al: Cold versus cold compression therapy after shoulder arthroscopy: a prospective randomized clinical trial. *Knee Surg Sports Traumatol Arthrosc* 24(7):2209–2215, 2016. doi:10.1007/s00167-015-3534-7.

102. Gatewood CT, Tran AA, Dragoo JL: The efficacy of post-operative devices following knee arthroscopic surgery: a systematic review. *Knee Surg Sports Traumatol Arthrosc* 25(2):501–516, 2017. doi:10.1007/s00167-016-4326-4.

103. Simons DG, Travell JG: Myofascial origins of low back pain. I. Principles of diagnosis and treatment. *Postgrad Med* 73:70–77, 1983.

104. Travell JG, Simons DG: *Myofascial pain and dysfunction: the trigger point manual*, Baltimore, 1983, Williams & Wilkins.

105. Travell JG: Myofascial trigger points: clinical view. In Bonica JJ, Albe-Fessard D, editors: *Advances in pain research and therapy*, New York, 1976, Raven Press.

106. Simons DG: Myofascial pain syndrome due to trigger points. *Int Rehabil Med Assoc Monogr* 1:1–3, 1987.

107. The Gebauer Company: Gebauer's spray and stretch indications and usage. http://www.gebauer.com/products/spray-and-stretch/gebauers-spray-and-stretch/. (Accessed 6 February 2007).

108. Horsman MR: Tissue physiology and the response to heat. *Int J Hyperthermia* 22(3):197–203, 2006.

109. Imamura M, Biro S, Kihara T, et al: Repeated thermal therapy improves impaired vascular endothelial function in patients with coronary risk factors. *J Am Coll Cardiol* 38:1083–1088, 2001.

110. Cider A, Svealv BG, Tang MS, et al: Immersion in warm water induces improvement in cardiac function in patients with chronic heart failure. *Eur J Heart Fail* 8:308–313, 2006.

111. Kihara T, Biro S, Imamura M, et al: Repeated sauna treatment improves vascular endothelial and cardiac function in patients with chronic heart failure. *J Am Coll Cardiol* 39:754–759, 2002.

112. Brunt VE, Howard MJ, Francisco MA, et al: Passive heat therapy improves endothelial function, arterial stiffness and blood pressure in sedentary humans. *J Physiol* 594(18):5329–5342, 2016. doi:10.1113/JP272453.

113. Crockford GW, Hellon RF, Parkhouse J: Thermal vasomotor response in human skin mediated by local mechanisms. *J Physiol* 161:10–15, 1962.

114. Kellogg DL, Jr, Liu Y, Kosiba IF, et al: Role of nitric oxide in the vascular effects of local warming of the skin in humans. *J Appl Physiol* 86:1185–1190, 1999.

115. Minson CT, Berry LT, Joyner MJ: Nitric oxide and neurally mediated regulation of skin blood flow during local heating. *J Appl Physiol* 91:1619–1626, 2001.

116. Fox HH, Hilton SM: Bradykinin formation in human skin as a factor in heat vasodilation. *J Physiol* 142:219, 1958.

117. Kellogg DL, Jr, Liu Y, McAllister K, et al: Bradykinin does not mediate cutaneous active vasodilation during heat stress in humans. *J Appl Physiol* 93:1215–1221, 2002.

118. Guyton AC: *Textbook of medical physiology*, ed 8, Philadelphia, 1991, WB Saunders.

119. Abramson DI: Indirect vasodilation in thermotherapy. *Arch Phys Med Rehabil* 46:412–415, 1965.

120. Wessman MS, Kottke FJ: The effect of indirect heating on peripheral blood flow, pulse rate, blood pressure and temperature. *Arch Phys Med Rehabil* 48:567–576, 1967.

121. Wyper DJ, McNiven DR: Effects of some physiotherapeutic agents on skeletal muscle blood flow. *Physiotherapy* 62:83–85, 1976.

122. Crockford GW, Hellon RF: Vascular responses in human skin to infra-red radiation. *J Physiol* 149:424–426, 1959.

123. Currier DP, Kramer JF: Sensory nerve conduction: heating effects of ultrasound and infrared radiation. *Physiother Can* 34:241–246, 1982.

124. Kelly R, Beehn C, Hansford A, et al: Effect of fluidotherapy on superficial radial nerve conduction and skin temperature. *J Orthop Sports Phys Ther* 35:16–23, 2005.

125. Franssen H, Wieneke GH: Nerve conduction and temperature: necessary warming time. *Muscle Nerve* 17(3):336–344, 1994.

126. Tilki HE, Stalberg E, Coskun M, et al: Effect of heating on nerve conduction in carpal tunnel syndrome. *J Clin Neurophysiol* 21:451–456, 2004.

127. Rutkove SB, Geffroy MA, Lichtenstein SH: Heat-sensitive conduction block in ulnar neuropathy at the elbow. *Clin Neurophysiol* 112:280–285, 2001.

128. Davis SL, Jay O, Wilson TE: Thermoregulatory dysfunction in multiple sclerosis. *Handb Clin Neurol* 157:701–714, 2018. doi:10.1016/B978-0-444-64074-1.00042-2.

129. Rasminsky M: The effect of temperature on conduction in demyelinated single nerve fibers. *Arch Neurol* 28:287–292, 1973.

130. Fischer M, Schafer SS: Temperature effects on the discharge frequency of primary and secondary endings of isolated cat muscle spindles recorded under a ramp-and-hold stretch. *Brain Res* 840:1–15, 1999.

131. Lehmann JF, Brunner GD, Stow RW: Pain threshold measurements after therapeutic application of ultrasound, microwaves and infrared. *Arch Phys Med Rehabil* 39:560–565, 1958.

132. Benson TB, Copp EP: The effects of therapeutic forms of heat and ice on the pain threshold of the normal shoulder. *Rheumatol Rehabil* 13:100–104, 1974.

133. Malanga GA, Yan N, Stark J: Mechanisms and efficacy of heat and cold therapies for musculoskeletal injury. *Postgrad Med* 127(1):57–65, 2015.

134. Petrofsky J, Laymon M, Loo H: Local heating of trigger points reduces neck and plantar fascia pain. *J Back Musculoskelet Rehabil*, 2019 Sep 20 [Epub ahead of print]. doi:10.3233/BMR-181222.

135. Petrofsky JS, Laymon MS, Alshammari FS, et al: Use of low level of continuous heat as an adjunct to physical therapy improves knee pain recovery and the compliance for home exercise in patients with chronic knee pain: a randomized controlled trial. *J Strength Cond Res* 30(11):3107–3115, 2016.

136. Chastain PB: The effect of deep heat on isometric strength. *Phys Ther* 58:543–546, 1978.

137. Edwards R, Harris R, Hultman E, et al: Energy metabolism during isometric exercise at different temperatures of m. quadriceps femoris in man. *Acta Physiol Scand* 80:17–18, 1970.

138. Freiwald J, Hoppe MW, Beermann W, et al: Effects of supplemental heat therapy in multimodal treated chronic low back pain patients on strength and flexibility. *Clin Biomech (Bristol, Avon)* 57:107–113, 2018. doi:10.1016/j.clinbiomech.2018.06.008.

139. McGorm H, Roberts LA, Coombes JS, et al: Turning up the heat: an evaluation of the evidence for heating to promote exercise recovery, muscle rehabilitation and adaptation. *Sports Med* 48(6):1311–1328, 2018. doi:10.1007/s40279-018-0876-6.

140. Miller MW, Ziskin MC: Biological consequences of hyperthermia. *Ultrasound Med Biol* 15:707–722, 1989.

141. Barcroft J, King W: The effect of temperature on the dissociation curve of blood. *J Physiol* 39:374–384, 1909.

142. Lentell G, Hetherington T, Eagan J, et al: The use of thermal agents to influence the effectiveness of low-load prolonged stretch. *J Orthop Sports Phys Ther* 16:200–207, 1992.

143. Draper DO, Castro JL, Feland B, et al: Shortwave diathermy and prolonged stretching increase hamstring flexibility more than prolonged stretching alone. *J Orthop Sports Phys Ther* 34(1):13–20, 2004. Jan.

144. Held M, Tweer S, Medved F, et al: Changes in the biomechanical properties of human skin in hyperthermic and hypothermic ranges. *Wounds* 30(9):257–262, 2018.

145. Lehmann JF, DeLateur BJ: Therapeutic heat. In Lehmann JF, editor: *Therapeutic heat and cold*, ed 4, Baltimore, 1990, Williams & Wilkins.

146. Lehmann J, Masock A, Warren C, et al: Effect of therapeutic temperatures on tendon extensibility. *Arch Phys Med Rehabil* 51:481–487, 1970.

147. French SD, Cameron M, Walker BF, et al: Superficial heat or cold for low back pain. *Cochrane Database Syst Rev* (1), 2006:CD004750.

148. Mayer JM, Mooney V, Matheson LN, et al: Continuous low-level heat wrap therapy for the prevention and early phase treatment of delayed-onset muscle soreness of the low back: a randomized controlled trial. *Arch Phys Med Rehabil* 87:1310–1357, 2006.

149. Michlovitz S, Hun L, Erasala GN, et al: Continuous low-level heat wrap therapy is effective for treating wrist pain. *Arch Phys Med Rehabil* 85:1409–1416, 2004.

150. Magness J, Garrett T, Erickson D: Swelling of the upper extremity during whirlpool baths. *Arch Phys Med Rehabil* 51:297–299, 1970.

151. Petrofsky JS, Laymon M, Lee H: Effect of heat and cold on tendon flexibility and force to flex the human knee. *Med Sci Monit* 19:661–667, 2013.

152. Sawyer PC, Uhl TL, Mattacola CG, et al: Effects of moist heat on hamstring flexibility and muscle temperature. *J Strength Cond Res* 17(2):285–290, 2003.

153. Funk D, Swank AM, Adams KJ, et al: Efficacy of moist heat pack application over static stretching on hamstring flexibility. *J Strength Cond Res* 15(1):123–126, 2001.

154. Knight CA, Rutledge CR, Cox ME, et al: Effect of superficial heat, deep heat, and active exercise warm-up on the extensibility of the plantar flexors. *Phys Ther* 81:1206–1214, 2001.

155. Usuba M, Miyanaga Y, Miyakawa S, et al: Effect of heat in increasing the range of knee motion after the development of a joint contracture: an experiment with an animal model. *Arch Phys Med Rehabil* 87:247–253, 2006.

156. Robertson VJ, Ward AR, Jung P: The effect of heat on tissue extensibility: a comparison of deep and superficial heating. *Arch Phys Med Rehabil* 86:819–825, 2005.

157. Zhang P, Wu MX: A clinical review of phototherapy for psoriasis. *Lasers Med Sci* 33(1):173–180, 2018. doi:10.1007/s10103-017-2360-1.

158. Moss C, Ellis R, Murray W, et al: *Infrared radiation, non-ionizing radiation protection*, ed 2, Geneva, 1989, World Health Organization.

159. Szekeres M, MacDermid JC, Birmingham T, et al: The effect of therapeutic whirlpool and hot packs on hand volume during rehabilitation after distal radius fracture: a blinded randomized controlled trial. *Hand (NY)* 12(3):265–271, 2017. doi:10.1177/1558944716661992.

160. Sapareto SA, Dewey WC: Thermal dose determination in cancer therapy. *Int J Radiat Oncol Biol Phys* 10:787–800, 1984.

161. Hornback NB: *Hyperthermia and cancer*, Boca Raton, FL, 1984, CRC Press.

162. Ostrowski J, Herb CC, Scifers J, et al: Comparison of muscle temperature increases produced by moist hot pack and thermostim probe. *J Sport Rehabil* 28(5):459–463, 2019. doi:10.1123/jsr.2017-0294.

163. Petrofsky J, Berk L, Bains G, et al: Moist heat or dry heat for delayed onset muscle soreness. *J Clin Med Res* 5(6):416–425, 2013. doi:10.4021/jocmr1521w.

164. Nadler SF, Steiner DJ, Erasala GN: Continuous low-level heat wrap therapy provides more efficacy than ibuprofen and acetaminophen for acute low back pain. *Spine* 27:1012–1017, 2002.

165. Petrofsky JS, Laymon M, Alshammari F, et al: Use of low level of continuous heat and Ibuprofen as an adjunct to physical therapy improves pain relief, range of motion and the compliance for home exercise in patients with nonspecific neck pain: a randomized controlled trial. *J Back Musculoskelet Rehabil* 30(4):889–896, 2017. doi:10.3233/BMR-160577.

166. Enwemeka CS, Booth CK, Fisher SL, et al: Decay time of temperature of hot packs in two application positions. *Phys Ther* 76:S96, 1996.

167. *Parabath paraffin heat therapy owner's guide*, Akron, OH, 2004, The Hygenic Corporation.

168. Borrell RM, Henley ES, Purvis H, et al: Fluidotherapy: evaluation of a new heat modality. *Arch Phys Med Rehabil* 58:69–71, 1977.

169. Hardy JD: Spectral transmittance and reflectance of excised human skin. *J Appl Physiol* 9:257–264, 1956.

170. Orenberg EK, Noodleman FR, Koperski JA, et al: Comparison of heat delivery systems for hyperthermia treatment of psoriasis. *Int J Hyperthermia* 2:231–241, 1986.

171. Selkins KM, Emery AF: Thermal science for physical medicine. In Lehmann JF, editor: *Therapeutic heat and cold*, ed 3, Baltimore, 1982, Williams & Wilkins.

172. Westerhof W, Siddiqui AH, Cormane RH, et al: Infra-red hyperthermia and psoriasis. *Arch Dermatol Res* 279:209–210, 1987.

173. Gale GD, Rothbart PJ, Li Y: Infrared therapy for chronic low back pain: a randomized, controlled trial. *Pain Res Manag* 11:193–196, 2006.

174. Fiscus KA, Kaminski TW, Powers ME: Changes in lower-leg blood flow during warm-, cold-, and contrast-water therapy. *Arch Phys Med Rehabil* 86:1404–1410, 2005.

175. Breger Stanton DE, Lazaro R, Macdermid JC: A systematic review of the effectiveness of contrast baths. *J Hand Ther* 22:57–69, 2009. quiz 70.

176. Shadgan B, Pakravan AH, Hoens A, et al: Contrast baths, intramuscular hemodynamics, and oxygenation as monitored by near-infrared spectroscopy. *J Athl Train* 53(8):782–787, 2018. doi:10.4085/1062-6050-127-17.

Ultrasound

CHAPTER OBJECTIVES

After reading this chapter, the reader will be able to do the following:
- Define *ultrasound*.
- Describe the physical effects of ultrasound.
- Explain the clinical indications for the use of ultrasound.
- Choose the best technique for treatment with ultrasound, and list the advantages and disadvantages of each.
- Select the appropriate equipment and optimal treatment parameters for treatment with ultrasound.
- Safely and effectively apply ultrasound.
- Accurately and completely document treatment with ultrasound.

Methods to generate and detect **ultrasound** first became available in the United States in the 19th century. The first large-scale application of ultrasound was for sound navigation and ranging (SONAR) in submarines during World War II. SONAR uses short pulses of ultrasound sent through water. When the ultrasound pulse reaches an object, it is reflected, and an ultrasound detector can pick up this returned echo. Because the time for the ultrasound wave to reach a reflecting surface and then echo back to the detector is proportional to the distance between the detector and the reflecting surface, this time can be used to calculate the distance to objects, such as other submarines, rocks, or the sea floor. This pulse-echo technology is still used today for underwater navigation and has been adapted for medical imaging applications for "viewing" a fetus or other soft tissue structures. Real-time ultrasound, which also uses this pulse-echo approach, can be used to assess deep muscle activity during exercise.[1,2] Early SONAR devices used high-intensity ultrasound for ease of detection, but the use of these devices was limited because they also heated and thereby injured sea life. Although this limited the utility of high-intensity ultrasound for SONAR, it led to the development of clinical ultrasound devices specifically intended for heating biological tissue. Ultrasound has a number of advantages over other heating agents. Ultrasound can penetrate more deeply than superficial heating agents. Ultrasound also heats tissue with high collagen content, such as tendons, ligaments, or fascia. Ultrasound has been widely used clinically for heating tissues for over 70 years.

> ### ◎ Clinical Pearl
> Ultrasound most effectively heats deep tissue with high collagen content, such as tendons, ligaments, joint capsules, and fascia.

Subsequently, ultrasound was found to also have nonthermal effects, and the clinical use of ultrasound in rehabilitation for these nonthermal effects now surpasses the use of ultrasound for its thermal effects. The most recent development in the therapeutic application of ultrasound is shock wave therapy. Shock waves are pulsed high-amplitude, short-duration sound waves. Shock wave therapy is discussed in detail in Chapter 18.

Ultrasound continues to be one of the most frequently used physical agents in rehabilitation practice today. A study of ultrasound use among orthopedic clinical specialist physical therapists in the United States published in 2007 reported up to 84% of respondents using this modality for specific conditions,[3] and a similar study of orthopedic and sports specialist physical therapists in Brazil reported that 98% of respondents believed ultrasound is an important tool in their practice and use ultrasound to treat 25% to over 90% of their patients.[4] Similarly, a survey of Australian physical therapists published in 2009 reported over 70% having access to ultrasound devices and 60% using ultrasound daily or monthly.[5] More recent studies have yielded similar results, with two surveys of Canadian physical therapists, both published in 2013, reporting that over 80% of Canadian physical therapists use ultrasound in their practice,[6,7] many of them daily.

Physical Properties of Ultrasound
ULTRASOUND DEFINITION
Ultrasound is a type of sound and, like all forms of sound, consists of waves that transmit energy by alternately compressing and rarefying material (Fig. 9.1). Ultrasound is sound with a **frequency** above 20,000 cycles per second (hertz [Hz]), exceeding the limits of normal human hearing. Humans can hear sound with a frequency of 16 to 20,000 Hz. Generally, therapeutic ultrasound has a frequency of 0.7 to 3.3 megahertz (MHz) (700,000 to 3,300,000 cycles/second) to maximize energy **absorption** at a depth of 2 to 5 cm of soft tissue.

Audible sound and ultrasound have many similar properties. For example, as ultrasound enters the body, it gradually decreases in intensity as a result of **attenuation,** in the same way that the sound we hear gradually becomes quieter farther from its source (Fig. 9.2). Ultrasound attenuation is tissue and frequency specific, increasing with the collagen content of tissues and with the frequency of the ultrasound (Table 9.1). Another way to quantify ultrasound attenuation is with the **half-depth.** The half-depth is the depth of tissue at which the ultrasound intensity is half the applied intensity. This depth is greatest when ultrasound attenuation is low, as it is for water or ultrasound gel, and is lowest when ultrasound attenuation is high, as for bone (Table 9.2).

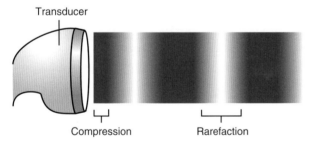

FIGURE 9.1 Ultrasound compression-rarefaction wave.

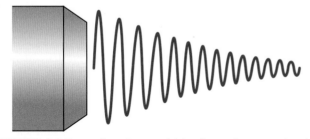

FIGURE 9.2 Decreasing ultrasound intensity as the wave travels through tissue.

TABLE 9.1	Attenuation of 1-MHz Ultrasound	
Tissue	Attenuation Coefficient, dB/cm	%/cm
Blood	0.1	3
Fat	0.61	13
Nerve	0.88	0
Muscle	0.7–1.4 (higher along the fibers than across the fibers)	24
Blood vessels	1.7	32
Skin	2.7	39
Tendon	4.9	59
Cartilage	5.0	68
Bone	13.9	96

TABLE 9.2	Ultrasound Half-Depths in Millimeters at 1 and 3 MHz	
Tissue	1 MHz	3 MHz
Water, ultrasound gel	11,500	3,833
Fat	50	16.5
Muscle (parallel)	24.6	8
Muscle (perpendicular)	9	3
Skin	11.1	4
Tendon	6.2	2
Cartilage	6	2
Bone	2.1	0
Air	2.5	0

Ultrasound waves cause a slight circular motion of the material they pass through, but they do not carry the material along with the wave. Similarly, when someone speaks, the audible sound waves of the voice reach across the room, but the air in front of the speaker's mouth is agitated only slightly and is not moved across the room.

This chapter describes the physical properties of ultrasound and its effects on the body to derive guidelines for the optimal clinical application of therapeutic ultrasound.

ULTRASOUND GENERATION
Ultrasound is generated by applying a high-frequency, alternating electrical current to the crystal in the **transducer** (also known as the *applicator* or *sound head*) of an ultrasound unit (Fig. 9.3). The crystal is made of a material with **piezoelectric** properties, causing it to expand and contract at the same frequency that the current changes polarity. When the crystal expands, it compresses the material in front of it, and when it contracts, it rarefies the material in front of it (Fig. 9.4). This alternating **compression** and **rarefaction** is the ultrasound wave.

The property of piezoelectricity—the ability to generate electricity in response to a mechanical force or to change shape in response to an electrical current—was first discovered by Paul-Jacques and Pierre Curie in the 1880s. A variety of materials are piezoelectric, including bone, natural quartz, synthetic plumbum zirconium titanate (PZT), and barium titanate. Ultrasound transducers are usually made of PZT

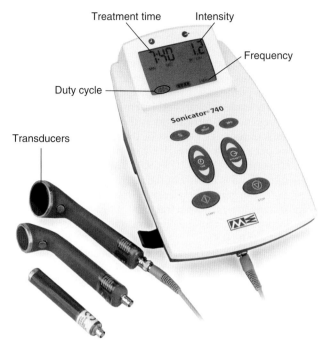

FIGURE 9.3 Ultrasound unit and transducers. (Courtesy Mettler Electronics, Anaheim, CA.)

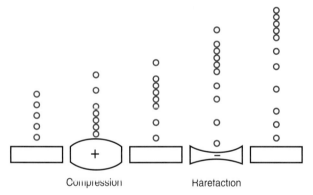

FIGURE 9.4 Ultrasound compression rarefaction wave production by piezoelectric crystal.

because this is presently the least costly and most efficient piezoelectric material.

To obtain a pure, single frequency of ultrasound, a single frequency of alternating current is applied to a piezoelectric crystal whose thickness resonates at this frequency. Resonance occurs when the ultrasound frequency and the crystal thickness conform to the following formula:

$$f = \frac{c}{2t}$$

where f is frequency, c is the speed of sound in the material, and t is the thickness of the crystal. Thus, thinner crystals are used to generate higher frequencies of ultrasound. All ultrasound crystals, particularly those that are used for higher-frequency ultrasound, are fragile and should be handled with care.

Multifrequency transducers used to be made with a single uniform crystal whose thickness was optimized for one of the frequencies but that could vibrate at other frequencies by applying those frequencies of alternating electrical currents; however, this may result in decreased efficiency, variability in output frequency, reduced **effective radiating area (ERA)**, and increased beam nonuniformity.[8] Therefore multifrequency transducers now use composite materials that can deliver multiple frequencies of ultrasound more accurately and efficiently.[9]

ULTRASOUND BEAM

The ultrasound beam delivered from an ultrasound transducer does not diverge like light from a flashlight but, rather, initially converges and then diverges (Fig. 9.5). The **near field,** also known as the *Fresnel zone,* is the convergent region, and the **far field,** also known as the *Fraunhofer zone,* is the divergent region. In the near field, interference of the ultrasound beam causes variations in ultrasound intensity. In the far field, there is little interference, resulting in a more uniform distribution of ultrasound intensity. The length of the near field (Table 9.3) depends on the ultrasound frequency and the ERA according to the following formula:

$$\frac{\text{Radius of transducer}^2}{\text{Wavelength of ultrasound}}$$

In most human tissue, most of the ultrasound intensity is attenuated within the first 2 to 5 cm of tissue depth, which lies within the near field for transducers of most frequencies and areas.

Ultrasound Parameters

Ultrasound is delivered to the body by the machine's transducer. Each transducer has an ERA. The ERA is the area of the transducer from which at least 5% of the peak ultrasound intensity radiates (Fig. 9.6).[10] This is essentially the size of the area of tissue to which ultrasound is delivered and is generally slightly smaller than the outside area of the treatment head. The U.S. Food and Drug Administration (FDA) requires that the ERA be marked directly on the sound head or on its cable or on the machine itself if the sound head is not detachable.[11]

Ultrasound transducers do not output the same intensity of ultrasound over their entire ERA. The ultrasound beam is never uniform, and it is usually the most intense near the middle of the ERA. This nonuniformity is described in terms of the **beam nonuniformity ratio (BNR).** The BNR is the

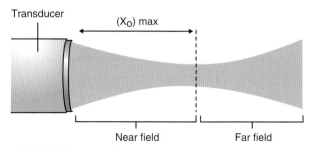

FIGURE 9.5 Longitudinal cross section of an ultrasound beam.

Ultrasound Frequency, MHz	ERA, cm²	Length of Near Field, cm
1	5	11
3	5	33
1	1	2.1
3	1	6.3

TABLE 9.3 Length of the Near Field for Different Frequencies of Ultrasound and Different Areas (ERAs) of Ultrasound Transducers

ERA, Effective radiating area.

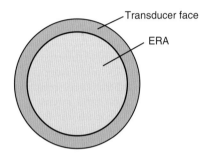

FIGURE 9.6 Effective radiating area (ERA).

ratio of the peak intensity within the ERA to the average intensity within the ERA (Fig. 9.7). For most units, this is usually around 5:1, although it can be as low as 2:1. The higher the BNR, the less uniform the beam and the higher the peak intensity within the ERA. For example, with a transducer with a BNR of 5:1, when the intensity is set at 2 W/cm², the peak intensity within the ERA could be as high as 10 W/cm². With a transducer with a BNR of 2:1, when the intensity is set at 1.5 W/cm², the peak intensity within the ERA could be as high as 3 W/cm². In the United States, the FDA requires that the maximum BNR be specified on the transducer,[11] and most units have a BNR below 5:1 or 6:1. Because the ultrasound beam is always nonuniform, even

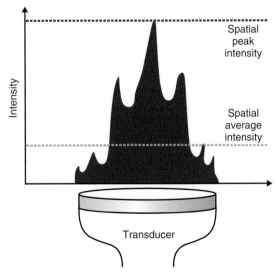

FIGURE 9.7 Beam nonuniformity.

with a fairly low BNR, clinicians are advised to always move the transducer during treatment to even out the intensity in the treatment area.

After selecting a transducer with given ERA and BNR, the clinician can also select certain features of the ultrasound known as its *parameters*. These include the ultrasound frequency, **duty cycle, power,** and **intensity.**[11]

The frequency of ultrasound is the number of compression-rarefaction cycles per unit of time, generally expressed in cycles per second (hertz [Hz]) or millions of cycles per second (megahertz [MHz]) (Fig. 9.8). The frequency of therapeutic ultrasound is usually in the range of 1 to 3.3 MHz, and the provider can generally select one of two frequency options for most transducers. Lower-frequency ultrasound penetrates more deeply. Higher-frequency ultrasound is absorbed more superficially (Fig. 9.9).

Ultrasound may be delivered continuously or in a pulsed mode. **Pulsed ultrasound** is produced when the high-frequency alternating electrical current is delivered to the transducer for only a limited proportion of the treatment time, as determined by the selected duty cycle. The duty cycle is the proportion of the total treatment time that ultrasound is being delivered. This can be expressed as a percentage or a ratio. **Continuous ultrasound** is being delivered throughout the treatment time and thus has a 100% duty cycle (Fig. 9.10). Pulsed ultrasound may have any duty cycle below 100%. For example, when ultrasound is delivered for 20% of the time and is not delivered for 80% of the time, this is described as a 20%, or 1:5, duty cycle. Although the length of the pulses to produce a given pulsed duty cycle can vary, in general, therapeutic ultrasound machines deliver pulsed ultrasound by dividing a 10-ms segment into the on and off time. Thus, 20% pulsed ultrasound is on for 2 ms, followed by being off for 8 ms, whereas 10% pulsed ultrasound is on for 1 ms, followed by being off for 9 ms (Fig. 9.11).

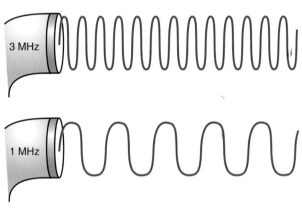

FIGURE 9.8 Ultrasound frequencies: 1 and 3 MHz.

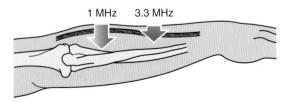

FIGURE 9.9 Frequency controls the depth of penetration of ultrasound; 1-MHz ultrasound penetrates approximately 3 times as far as 3.3-MHz ultrasound. (Courtesy Mettler Electronics, Anaheim, CA.)

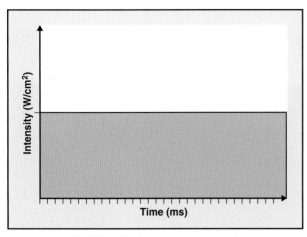

FIGURE 9.10 Continuous ultrasound.

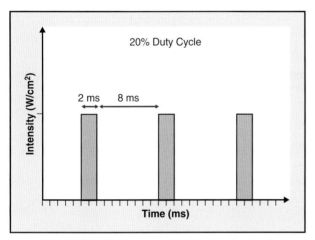

FIGURE 9.11 Twenty percent duty cycle ultrasound.

Ultrasound power is the amount of acoustic energy per unit time, expressed in watts (W). Ultrasound intensity is the power averaged over the ERA, expressed in watts per centimeter squared (W/cm^2). The World Health Organization limits the intensity output by therapeutic ultrasound units to 3 W/cm^2.[12] The intensity of pulsed ultrasound may be expressed in one of two ways, the **spatial average temporal peak (SATP) intensity** or the **spatial average temporal average (SATA) intensity** (Fig. 9.12). The SATP intensity is the intensity averaged over the ERA during the on time of the pulse. The SATA intensity is the intensity averaged over the ERA *and* averaged over the entire on and off time. For example, 20% pulsed ultrasound that is composed of 2-ms pulses at 1 W/cm^2 with 8 ms off between these pulses has an SATP intensity of 1 W/cm^2 and a SATA intensity of 0.2 W/cm^2 (1 W/cm^2 × 20%).

SATA is equal to SATP for continuous ultrasound. The therapeutic ultrasound units used in rehabilitation read out the SATP intensity of pulsed ultrasound. However, the intensity of ultrasound in units marketed for bone healing is described in terms of SATA. In this chapter, the intensity of pulsed ultrasound is always the SATP intensity, followed by the duty cycle, unless specifically stated otherwise. In general, therapeutic ultrasound devices deliver ultrasound with a frequency of 1 to 3.3 MHz, at 0% to 100% duty cycle, 0- to

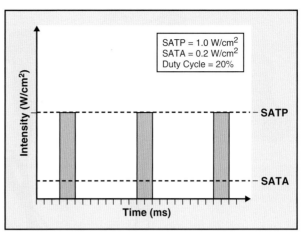

FIGURE 9.12 Spatial average temporal peak (SATP) and spatial average temporal average (SATA) intensity.

3-W/cm^2 intensity. This ultrasound is applied to the patient for around 5 to 15 minutes by a clinician in the clinic. There are also fixed very low-intensity ultrasound devices available that are intended for home use by the patient. One type of these, known as *low-intensity pulsed ultrasound* (LIPUS), is specifically intended for bone healing (Fig. 9.13). LIPUS devices generally deliver ultrasound at 1.5-MHz frequency, 20% duty cycle, at 0.15-W/cm^2 SATA intensity and are generally applied for 20 minutes daily. The other type of these, known as *low-intensity therapeutic ultrasound* (LITUS), intended for long-duration tissue heating, delivers ultrasound at 3-MHz frequency, continuous 100% duty cycle, at 0.132-W/cm^2 intensity, and is applied for up to 4 hours at a time (Fig. 9.14).[13-15]

Effects of Ultrasound

Ultrasound has a variety of biophysical effects. These can be classified as thermal or nonthermal effects. Increasing tissue temperature is the thermal effect of ultrasound. The effects of ultrasound that do not depend on an increase in tissue temperature are the nonthermal effects. Traditionally, the thermal and nonthermal effects of ultrasound are considered separately, although to some degree, both occur with all

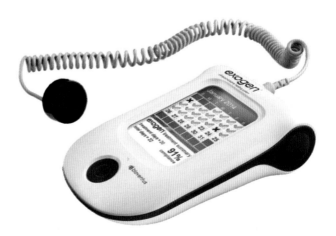

FIGURE 9.13 Low-intensity pulsed ultrasound (LIPUS) device intended for home use for fracture healing. (Courtesy Bioventus LLC, EXOGEN.)

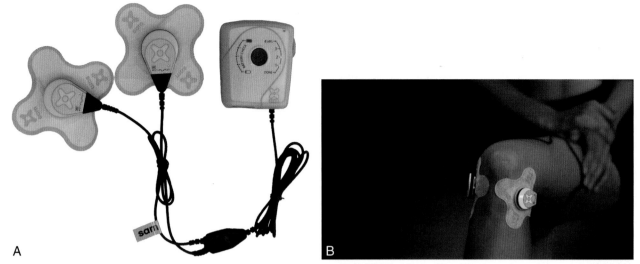

FIGURE 9.14 Low-intensity therapeutic ultrasound (LITUS) device intended for long-duration home use. (A) Device. (B) LITUS transducers in place. (Courtesy ZetrOZ Systems LLC.)

applications of ultrasound. Continuous ultrasound has the greatest effect on tissue temperature; however, nonthermal effects can also occur with continuous ultrasound. Additionally, although pulsed ultrasound is typically applied clinically, with a duty cycle of 20% and a low SATA intensity, and produces minimal sustained changes in tissue temperature, ultrasound with these parameters can cause brief localized heating during the on time of a pulse.[16,17] Both thermal and nonthermal effects of ultrasound can be used to accelerate the achievement of treatment goals when ultrasound is applied to the appropriate pathological condition with the appropriate parameters at the appropriate time.

THERMAL EFFECTS

The thermal effects of ultrasound are produced when ultrasound is absorbed by the tissues. **Absorption** is the conversion of the mechanical energy of ultrasound into heat. The amount of heat produced depends on the amount of energy delivered and the absorption coefficient. The amount of energy delivered depends on the ultrasound intensity and duty cycle, and the absorption coefficient depends on the ultrasound frequency and the tissue type (Table 9.4). As with attenuation coefficients, ultrasound absorption coefficients increase with the collagen content of tissues and with the frequency of the ultrasound. Ultrasound absorption coefficients are determined by measuring the rate of temperature rise in a homogeneous tissue model exposed to an ultrasound field of known intensity.

Ultrasound absorption accounts for about one-half of attenuation. The remainder of attenuation is due to **reflection** and **refraction.** Reflection and refraction also affect the distribution of the thermal effects of ultrasound.

Ultrasound reflection is the redirection of an incident ultrasound beam away from a surface at an angle equal and opposite to the angle of incidence (Fig. 9.15). Ultrasound is reflected at tissue interfaces, with most reflection occurring where there is the greatest difference between the acoustic impedance of adjacent tissues. Acoustic impedance is the resistance to the propagation of ultrasound waves. Air has

TABLE 9.4	Ultrasound Absorption Coefficients in Decibels/Centimeter for 1- and 3-MHz Ultrasound	
Tissue	1 MHz	3 MHz
Blood	0.025	0.084
Fat	0.14	0.42
Nerve	0.2	0.6
Muscle (parallel)	0.28	0.84
Muscle (perpendicular)	0.76	2.28
Blood vessels	0.4	1.2
Skin	0.62	1.86
Tendon	1.12	3.36
Cartilage	1.16	3.48
Bone	3.22	Too low to measure

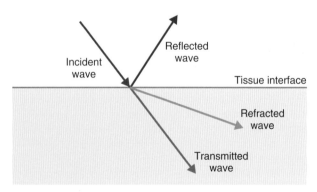

FIGURE 9.15 Ultrasound reflection and refraction.

high acoustic impedance, and skin has low acoustic impedance. Ultrasound reflection results in greater heating adjacent to the reflective surface. There is 100% reflection of ultrasound at the air-skin interface. This causes the ultrasound transducer to heat up substantially if there is air between the transducer and the patient's skin. A transmission medium, usually gel or water, with similar impedance to skin and soft tissue is therefore applied between the sound head and the skin to eliminate the air between the sound head and the body and thus avoid an air-skin interface with high reflection. There is no reflection at the transmission medium–sound head interface and only 0.1% reflection at the transmission medium–skin interface. In the body, most reflection—approximately 35%—occurs at soft tissue–bone interfaces. This results in more heat accumulation around bones.

Ultrasound refraction is the bending or redirection of waves when they pass from one tissue to another (see Fig. 9.12). When refraction occurs, the ultrasound wave enters the tissue at one angle and continues through the tissue at a different angle. Because the body is made up of various types of tissue, applied therapeutic ultrasound that is initially directed in one direction also spreads in the area as a result of refraction.

Tissues Affected

The earliest studies demonstrating that ultrasound can increase tissue temperature were published by Harvey in 1930.[18] The thermal effects of ultrasound, including acceleration of metabolic rate, reduction or control of pain and muscle spasm, alteration of nerve conduction velocity, increased circulation,[19] and increased soft tissue extensibility, are the same as effects obtained with other heating modalities, as described in Part III, except that the tissues heated are different.[20,21] Ultrasound generally reaches more deeply than superficial heating agents, such as hot packs and paraffin, and heats smaller areas than the other deep-heating agent, diathermy (see Chapter 10).[22]

> ◎ **Clinical Pearl**
>
> Ultrasound generally heats deeper areas than superficial heating agents and smaller areas than diathermy.

Ultrasound heats tissues with a high ultrasound **absorption coefficient** more than tissues with low absorption coefficients. As discussed previously, tissues with high absorption coefficients generally have higher collagen content, and tissues with low absorption coefficients generally have lower collagen content but higher water content. Thus, ultrasound is particularly well suited to heating tendons, ligaments, joint capsules, and fasciae while not overheating the overlying fat. Ultrasound can also be very effective for heating small areas of scar tissue in muscles because scar tissue has more collagen than uninjured muscle. Ultrasound generally is not the ideal physical agent for heating normal muscle tissue because muscle has a relatively low absorption coefficient, and most muscles are much larger than available ultrasound transducers.

Factors Affecting the Amount of Temperature Increase

The increase in tissue temperature produced by the absorption of ultrasound depends on the type, depth, and area of tissue to which the ultrasound is applied, as well as the frequency, average intensity, and duration of the ultrasound. The speed at which the ultrasound transducer is

moved, within the range of 2 to 8 cm/second, has been shown not to affect the increase in tissue temperature produced.[23]

> ◎ **Clinical Pearl**
>
> To avoid hotspots or uneven treatment when applying ultrasound, always keep the ultrasound sound head moving. Within the range of 2 and 8 cm/second, it does not matter how fast or slowly you move the sound head.

The rate of tissue heating by ultrasound is proportional to the ultrasound intensity and the absorption coefficient of the tissue at the applied ultrasound frequency.[24] Tissue heating is faster if the ultrasound intensity is higher and if the absorption coefficient is higher. Absorption coefficients increase with increased collagen content of the tissue and in proportion to the ultrasound frequency. Thus faster heating occurs with higher-intensity and higher-frequency ultrasound and in tissues with high collagen content. However, when the absorption coefficient is high, the temperature increase occurs only in a smaller volume of more superficial tissue than when the absorption coefficient is low. Changing the absorption coefficient alters the heat distribution but does not change the total amount of energy delivered (Fig. 9.16). Using higher-frequency ultrasound, 3 MHz rather than 1 MHz, and treating tissues with higher collagen content, reduces the depth of ultrasound penetration but produces a higher maximum tissue temperature. Ultrasound with 1-MHz frequency is considered best for heating tissues up to 5 cm deep, and ultrasound with 3-MHz frequency is considered best for heating tissues up to about 2 cm deep.[25,26]

Although theoretical models predict that 3-MHz ultrasound will increase tissue temperature 3 times faster than 1-MHz ultrasound, in vivo human research suggests that 3-MHz ultrasound produces an almost fourfold faster rate of temperature increase than 1-MHz ultrasound applied at 0.5 to 2.0 W/cm². Therefore clinically, an intensity that is 3 to 4 times lower may be needed to achieve a similar temperature

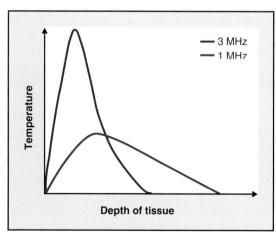

FIGURE 9.16 Temperature distribution for 1- and 3-MHz ultrasound at the same intensity.

increase using 3-MHz ultrasound as opposed to 1-MHz ultrasound.[27]

To increase the total amount of energy being delivered to the tissue, the duration of ultrasound applied or the average ultrasound intensity must be increased.[28] With all other ultrasound parameters and tissue characteristics kept the same, higher-intensity ultrasound produces greater temperature increases.[16,27,29] In addition, with all other ultrasound parameters and tissue characteristics kept the same, longer treatment times will also produce greater temperature increases. The LITUS device, which has a very low fixed intensity of 0.132 W/cm², takes advantage of this by applying low-intensity continuous ultrasound for a number of hours. This device has been shown to increase intramuscular temperature at 1.5-cm depth by up to 4°C within 80 to 90 minutes and up to 4.4°C within 2 to 3 hours. At 3-cm depth, it has been shown to reach maximal steady-state temperature increases of around 3°C.[30] During clinical ultrasound application, the resulting increase in tissue temperature is also affected by circulation and the presence of bone in the treatment area. As the ultrasound produces local heat, blood circulating through the tissues from other areas will moderate the increase in tissue temperature. In addition, reflection of ultrasound at soft tissue–bone interfaces will result in additional heating of the soft tissues directly around bones.[31]

On average, when ultrasound is delivered at 1-W/cm² intensity at 1-MHz frequency in vivo in healthy humans, soft tissue temperature increases by approximately 0.2°C per minute.[27,32] However, nonuniform intensity of ultrasound output, the variety of tissue types with different absorption coefficients in a clinical treatment area, and reflection at tissue boundaries can cause nonuniform temperature increases within the ultrasound field. The highest temperature is generally produced at soft tissue–bone interfaces, where reflection is greatest. Moving the sound head throughout the application helps equalize the heat distribution and minimize excessively hot or cold areas.

The number of unknown variables, including the thickness of each tissue layer, the amount of circulation, the distance to reflecting soft tissue–bone interfaces, and variability among machines,[33-35] makes it difficult to accurately predict the temperature increase that will be produced clinically when ultrasound is applied to a patient. Therefore, the initial treatment parameters are set according to theoretical and research predictions; however, when using ultrasound to heat tissues, the patient's report of warmth is used to determine the final ultrasound intensity.

> ◎ **Clinical Pearl**
>
> When applying ultrasound to heat tissues, the initial treatment parameters are set according to theoretical and research predictions, but because the patient's report of warmth is used to determine the final ultrasound intensity, the patient must be able to feel heat and be able to communicate effectively and reliably.

If the ultrasound intensity is too high, the patient will most likely complain of a deep ache from overheating of the periosteum. If this occurs, the ultrasound intensity must be reduced to avoid burning the tissue. If the ultrasound intensity

is too low, the patient will not feel any increase in temperature. More specific guidelines for the selection of optimal ultrasound treatment parameters for tissue heating are given later in the section "Application Technique." Because the patient's report is used to determine the maximum safe ultrasound intensity, thermal-level ultrasound should not be applied to patients who cannot feel or report discomfort caused by overheating.

Applying Other Physical Agents in Conjunction With Thermal-Level Ultrasound

Various physical agents can be applied together with, before, or after the application of ultrasound. Applying a hot pack before ultrasound increases the temperature of the superficial 1 to 2 mm of skin and subcutaneous tissue while not affecting the temperature of deeper tissue layers.[36] Applying ultrasound with cold water as the transmission medium cools the superficial skin by conduction and convection, thereby reducing the increase in superficial tissue temperature produced by ultrasound. Applying ice before ultrasound is applied also reduces the temperature increase produced by ultrasound in the deeper tissues.[37] Heating (39°C [102°F]) or cooling (18°C [64°F]) ultrasound conduction gel decreases the rate of heating with ultrasound, with the fastest rate of heating occurring with slightly warm (25°C [77°F]) conduction gel.[38] In addition, ice, or any other thermal agent, should be applied with caution before the application of ultrasound because the loss of sensation that these agents may cause can reduce the accuracy of patient feedback regarding deep tissue temperature.

Although some clinicians apply ultrasound in conjunction with electrical stimulation to combine the benefits of both modalities, there is little published research that evaluates the efficacy of this combination of interventions, and one study found that adding ultrasound to electrical stimulation, exercise, and superficial heat provided no additional benefit in the management of soft tissue disorders of the shoulder.[39] In general, one should analyze the effects of each physical agent independently when considering applying a combination of agents concurrently or in sequence.

NONTHERMAL EFFECTS

Ultrasound has a variety of effects on biological processes that are thought to be unrelated to any increase in tissue temperature. When ultrasound is delivered in a pulsed mode, with a 20% or lower duty cycle, heat generated during the on time of the cycle is dispersed during the off time, minimizing the net increase in temperature. Thus, pulsed ultrasound with a 20% duty cycle is generally used to apply and study the nonthermal effects of ultrasound, although some studies have used low intensities of continuous ultrasound to study these effects.

> ◎ **Clinical Pearl**
>
> Pulsed ultrasound, with a duty cycle of 20%, is most commonly used to produce the nonthermal benefits of ultrasound.

These nonthermal effects of ultrasound are the result of the mechanical events produced by ultrasound, including cavitation, microstreaming, and acoustic streaming. Cavitation is the formation, growth, and pulsation of gas-filled bubbles caused by ultrasound. During the compression phase of an ultrasound wave, bubbles in the tissue are made smaller, and during the rarefaction phase, they expand. Cavitation may be stable (also known as *inertial*) or unstable (also known as *transient*). With stable cavitation, the bubbles oscillate in size repeatedly but do not burst. With unstable cavitation, the bubbles grow over a number of cycles and then suddenly implode (Fig. 9.17). This implosion produces large, brief, local pressure and temperature increases and causes free radical formation. Stable cavitation has been proposed as a mechanism for the nonthermal therapeutic effects of ultrasound, whereas unstable cavitation is thought not to occur at the intensities of ultrasound used therapeutically.[40] Microstreaming is microscale eddying that occurs near any small, vibrating object. Microstreaming occurs around the gas bubbles set into oscillation by stable cavitation.[41] Acoustic streaming is the steady, circular flow of cellular fluids induced by ultrasound. This flow is larger in scale than the flow caused by microstreaming and is thought to alter cellular activity by transporting material from one part of the ultrasound field to another.[41]

Acoustic streaming, microstreaming, and cavitation are thought to produce biological effects by increasing cell membrane permeability. Cavitation can alter the cell membrane itself, and acoustic streaming and microstreaming can alter the movement of substances that cross the cell membrane. Low-intensity ultrasound increases intracellular calcium levels,[42] increases skin and cell membrane permeability,[43] and promotes the function of various types of cells. Ultrasound increases mast cell degranulation and the release of chemotactic factor and histamine,[44] promotes macrophage responsiveness,[45] increases the rate of protein synthesis by fibroblasts[46] and tenocytes,[47] and increases the rate of proteoglycan synthesis by chondrocytes.[48-51] Low-intensity ultrasound can also increase nitric oxide synthesis in endothelial cells[52,53] and increases blood flow.[54,55]

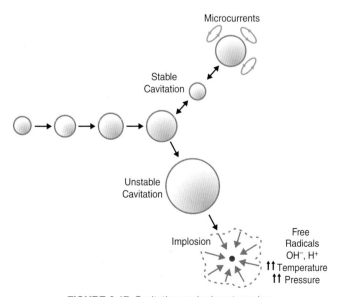

FIGURE 9.17 Cavitation and microstreaming.

Because the cellular and vascular processes caused by low-intensity ultrasound are essential components of tissue healing, they are thought to explain the enhanced recovery found to occur in patients with a variety of pathological conditions. For example, increasing intracellular calcium can alter the enzymatic activity of cells and can stimulate the synthesis and secretion of proteins, including proteoglycans.[56] Vasodilation from increased nitric oxide and the resulting increased blood flow may further enhance healing by promoting the delivery of essential nutrients to the area.

The fact that ultrasound can affect macrophage responsiveness partly explains why ultrasound is particularly effective during the inflammatory phase of repair, when the macrophage is the dominant cell type.

Clinical Indications for Ultrasound

The thermal and nonthermal effects of ultrasound can be used as components of the treatment of a wide variety of conditions. The thermal effects are used primarily before stretching of shortened soft tissue and to reduce pain. The nonthermal effects are used primarily to accelerate tissue healing, modify inflammation, and facilitate transdermal drug penetration (**phonophoresis**).

> **Clinical Pearl**
>
> The thermal effects of ultrasound are used primarily before stretching of shortened soft tissue and to reduce pain. The nonthermal effects of ultrasound are used primarily to accelerate tissue healing, modify inflammation, and facilitate transdermal drug penetration.

SOFT TISSUE SHORTENING

As discussed in detail in Chapter 6, soft tissue shortening can be caused by immobilization, inactivity, or scarring and can restrict joint range of motion (ROM), cause pain, and limit function. Shortening of the joint capsule, surrounding tendons, or ligaments is frequently responsible for these adverse consequences, and stretching of these tissues can help the tissues regain their normal length and promote functional patient recovery. Increasing the temperature of soft tissue temporarily increases its extensibility, which increases the length gained for the same force of stretch while reducing the risk of tissue damage.[17,57-59] The increased length of soft tissue is achieved more effectively if the stretching force is applied while the tissue temperature is elevated. This increased ease of stretching is thought to be due to altered viscoelasticity of collagen and of the collagen matrix.

Because ultrasound can penetrate to the depth of most joint capsules, tendons, and ligaments and because these tissues have high ultrasound absorption coefficients, ultrasound can be an effective physical agent for heating these tissues before stretching. For example, an early study found that when applied in conjunction with exercise, the deep heating produced by 1-MHz continuous ultrasound at 1.0 to 2.5 W/cm² was more effective in increasing hip joint ROM than the superficial heating produced by infrared (IR) radiation.[60] More recent studies support that continuous ultrasound at 1.5 W/cm² applied for 10 minutes before stretching results in greater increases in ROM static stretching alone or

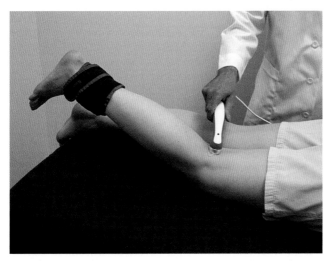

FIGURE 9.18 Ultrasound being applied to the posterior knee in conjunction with an extension stretching force.

stretching with placebo ultrasound.[17,57,61] Studies that have not found an increase in tissue extensibility have generally used too low of an ultrasound dose, because either the ultrasound intensity or the ultrasound treatment time was too low to effectively heat the tissues.[62] Overall, research supports that continuous ultrasound of intensity and duration sufficient to increase tissue temperature by 3°C to 8°C can increase soft tissue extensibility, thereby reducing soft tissue shortening and increasing joint ROM when applied in conjunction with stretching. The treatment parameters most likely to be effective for this application are 1- or 3-MHz frequency, depending on the tissue depth, at 0.5- to 1.0-W/cm^2 intensity when 3-MHz frequency is used and at 1.5- to 2.5-W/cm^2 intensity when 1-MHz frequency is used, applied for 5 to 10 minutes. For optimal effect, it is recommended that stretching be applied during heating by ultrasound and be maintained for 5 to 10 minutes after ultrasound is removed while the tissue is cooling (Fig. 9.18).

> ### ◎ Clinical Pearl
>
> For optimal effect, it is recommended that stretching be applied during heating by ultrasound and be maintained for 5 to 10 minutes after ultrasound is removed while the tissue is cooling.

PAIN CONTROL

Ultrasound may control pain by altering pain transmission or perception or by modifying the underlying condition causing pain. These effects may be the result of stimulation of cutaneous thermal receptors, increased soft tissue extensibility, or changes in nerve conduction, all of which may be caused by increased tissue temperature. The nonthermal effects of ultrasound may also reduce pain by modulating inflammation or neuronal pain signaling.[63,64]

Ultrasound can be more effective in controlling pain than placebo or treatment with other thermal agents, and the addition of ultrasound to an exercise program can augment pain relief.[65–68] These benefits have been found in randomized controlled trials in patients with acute (within 48 hours) soft tissue injuries,[65] recent onset of pain caused by prolapsed spinal discs and nerve root compression,[66] shoulder pain,[67,69] and both osteoarthritis[15] and rheumatoid arthritis.[68]

In general, the studies cited here support that continuous ultrasound may help reduce pain when applied at 1- or 3-MHz frequency, depending on the tissue depth, and 0.5- to 3.0-W/cm^2 intensity, continuous duty cycle, for 3 to 10 minutes, with some research supporting that much-lower-intensity continuous ultrasound applied for 4 hours daily may also be effective.[15]

SOFT TISSUE HEALING AND INFLAMMATION

The addition of ultrasound, particularly low-intensity ultrasound, to conservative care may accelerate soft tissue healing, including the healing of chronic wounds and the healing of acute muscle, ligament, and tendon injuries.[70–74] Early studies found that adding ultrasound (pulsed 20% duty cycle, 0.8- to 1.0-W/cm^2 intensity, 3-MHz frequency for 5 to 10 minutes), applied around the border of the wound, to conventional wound care for venous or pressure ulcers resulted in significantly greater reduction in wound area than adding sham ultrasound.[75,76] Not all studies have found such benefits, and overall, the size and quality of the current trials are insufficient to draw firm conclusions in many areas.[72,77–81] Differences in outcomes may be due to differences in the specific interventions, including the ultrasound parameters and the other treatments used. Most of the studies demonstrating benefit using standard rehabilitation ultrasound devices appear to have used 3-MHz ultrasound, at least 0.8-W/cm^2 intensity, pulsed at 20% duty cycle, applied for 5 to 10 minutes, and did not report using cytotoxic agents to clean the wounds. However, ultrasound parameters were not reported for all published studies.

Traditionally, megahertz-frequency, 0.5- to 1.0-W/cm^2 intensity, pulsed ultrasound has been used to promote wound healing, with the device contacting the wound or periwound area. Lower-frequency ultrasound, below 100 kHz, at less than 0.1-W/cm^2 intensity, applied using a saline mist as the ultrasound transmission medium, has gained some popularity for wound healing.[72,82–88] For this application, the applicator is held 5 to 15 mm from the wound and perpendicular to the wound, and multiple vertical and horizontal passes are made over the wound during the treatment. The treatment duration depends on the area of the wound. A wound smaller than 10 cm^2 is treated for 3 minutes; a wound 10 to 19 cm^2 is treated for 4 minutes; for each additional 10 cm^2, the time is increased by 1 minute.[84] Long-duration megahertz-frequency LITUS has also shown some promise for promoting soft tissue healing, although the focus of current studies has been on musculoskeletal injuries rather than chronic wounds.[73]

High-frequency and low-frequency ultrasound may also promote healing of surgical skin incisions[89,90] and can relieve pain from scars even when applied months or years after surgery. Fieldhouse[91] reported successful treatment of painful, thickened episiotomy scars with ultrasound at 0.5 to 0.8 W/cm^2 for 5 minutes three times a week for 6 to 16 weeks at 15 months to 4 years after the procedure. Earlier intervention was recommended for earlier relief of symptoms.

Overall, published studies support that ultrasound may facilitate wound healing. The treatment parameters that have generally been found to be effective for this application are pulsed 20% duty cycle, 0.5- to 1.0-W/cm² intensity, 3-MHz frequency for 3 to 10 minutes. Additional well-controlled studies with this range of ultrasound dosing are needed to ascertain the effectiveness of this intervention and to evaluate if other treatment parameters, such as lower frequency or longer application at a lower intensity, are more or less effective. Ultrasound can be applied to wounds or incisions by applying transmission gel to the intact skin around the wound perimeter and treating only over this area (Fig. 9.19), or the wound can be treated directly by covering it with an ultrasound coupling sheet or by placing it and the ultrasound transducer in water (Fig. 9.20).[73,92–94]

Studies in animals on the effect of ultrasound on tendon healing after surgical incision and repair have also demonstrated benefits, with almost all studies showing improved tendon healing after surgical incision despite the use of a wide range of ultrasound parameters, including different intensi-

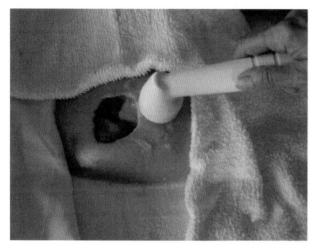

FIGURE 9.19 Ultrasound treatment of a wound: periwound application technique. (From McCulloch JM, Kloth LC. *Wound healing: evidence-based management,* ed 4, Philadelphia, 2010, FA Davis.)

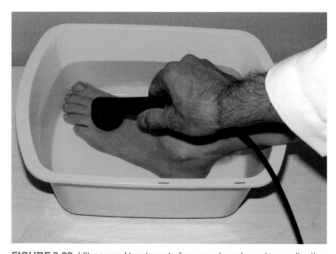

FIGURE 9.20 Ultrasound treatment of a wound: underwater application technique.

ties (0.5 to 2.5 W/cm²), modes (pulsed or continuous), and treatment durations (3 to 10 minutes). These studies have found that ultrasound promotes the formation of stronger tendons when applied starting as soon as 1 day postoperatively and has the greatest benefit when applied in the first 2 weeks.[92–99] Although most studies have found ultrasound to improve tendon healing, one early study published in 1982 suggested that ultrasound may impair healing. In this study, strength and healing appeared to be reduced in surgically repaired flexor profundus tendons in seven rabbits after treatment with pulsed ultrasound at 0.8 W/cm², 1 MHz for 5 minutes daily for 6 weeks compared with placebo-treated controls.[100] However, the authors of this study questioned the meaning of their findings because the strength of the tendons in both treated and untreated groups was more than 10 times lower than that reported in other studies for normal flexor tendon healing in rabbits. Immobilization was attempted throughout the postinjury period, but technical difficulties in maintaining cast fixation and thus apposition of the tendon ends may have resulted in gap formation and poor strength in all subjects. The small sample size and poor reporting of data also call into question the validity of this study. Furthermore, adverse effects of ultrasound on tendon healing have not been reported in other research. This study has been used by some to support recommendations to avoid using ultrasound for the first 6 weeks after tendon repair, but a recent study in humans supports that low-dose ultrasound applied starting 5 to 7 days after surgery, while maintaining immobilization for the first 3 weeks, promotes healing after flexor tendon (superficialis or profundus) repair in the hand.[101] Similarly, a recent study in rabbits that underwent patellar tendon harvest found that providing ultrasound as soon as 1 day after the lesion for the following 2 weeks improved the mechanical strength of the healing tendons when starting 2 or 4 weeks after the lesion was not effective.[99]

Overall, animal research supports the early use of ultrasound to promote tendon healing after rupture or lesion with surgical repair, and clinical trials in humans support this. The ultrasound doses found to be effective for this application are 0.5- to 2.5-W/cm² intensity, pulsed or continuous, 1- or 3-MHz frequency for 3 to 5 minutes. Although high-intensity ultrasound has been found to promote tendon healing, the lower end of the range is recommended to minimize the risk of adverse effects from heating acutely inflamed tissue postoperatively.

In addition to facilitating recovery from tissue injury, ultrasound has also been reported to reduce tendon inflammation (tendinitis/tendinosis).[73,93,102,103] A systematic review of physical therapy interventions for lateral epicondylitis found that the only intervention with sufficient evidence supporting its efficacy was ultrasound.[104] The most recent systematic review of the evidence for the effectiveness of electrophysical modalities for the treatment of medial and lateral epicondylitis was also supportive of the effectiveness of ultrasound compared with placebo.[105] This review also reported moderate evidence for ultrasound and friction massage being more effective than laser therapy. Specifically, Binder et al.[106] found significantly enhanced recovery in patients with lateral epicondylitis treated with ultrasound compared with patients treated with sham ultrasound. Pulsed ultrasound was applied with a 20% duty cycle, 1.0- to 2.0-W/cm² intensity, 1-MHz frequency for 5 to 10 minutes for 12 treatments over a 4- to 6-week period. Lundeberg et al.[107,108] reported significantly less pain in patients with lateral epicondylitis at 13 weeks and significantly greater global improvement at 5 and 13 weeks with ultrasound compared with rest, but there were no significant differences in outcomes between ultrasound-treated and sham ultrasound–treated groups.[107,108] A more recent randomized placebo-controlled trial of 30 people with lateral epicondylitis found that very low-intensity pulsed ultrasound (1.5 MHz, 0.15 W/cm^2 for 20 minutes daily, LIPUS) was associated with a nonsignificant trend in favor of ultrasound.[102] In addition, in 1999 Ebenbichler et al.[109] reported greater resolution of calcium deposits, less pain, and greater improvement in quality of life at 9 months in patients with calcific tendinitis of the shoulder treated with ultrasound compared with patients with the same disorder treated with sham ultrasound. For this study, ultrasound was applied for 24 15-minute sessions with a frequency of 0.89 MHz and an intensity of 2.5 W/cm^2 pulsed mode 1:4. In 2018, the same team published a 10-year long-term follow-up of the patients in this trial and found that those in the treatment group and the placebo group had similar long-term radiological and functional outcomes, supporting that ultrasound may accelerate recovery but not affect long-term outcome.

Some studies have not found ultrasound to help reduce symptoms associated with tendinitis, but variations in outcomes may be due to the use of different treatment parameters and the application of ultrasound at different stages of healing. Applying ultrasound with parameters that would increase tissue temperature may aggravate acute inflammation, and conversely, because pulsed ultrasound may be ineffective in the chronic, late stage of recovery if the tissue requires heating to promote stretching or increased circulation, applying ultrasound with the same parameters to all patients may obscure any treatment effect.

It is recommended that ultrasound be applied in a pulsed mode at low intensity (0.5 to 1.0 W/cm^2) during the acute phase of tendon inflammation to minimize the risk of aggravating the condition and accelerate recovery. It is also recommended that continuous ultrasound at high enough intensity to increase tissue temperature be applied in combination with stretching to assist in resolving chronic tendinitis if the problem is accompanied by soft tissue shortening as a result of scarring.

◎ Clinical Pearl

Apply ultrasound in a pulsed mode at low intensity to accelerate recovery from acute tendinitis. Consider applying continuous mode ultrasound at higher intensity along with stretching for chronic tendinitis if soft tissue shortening is contributing to the problem.

Some animal studies show that ruptured ligaments may also benefit from low-intensity ultrasound. Sparrow et al.[110] found that ultrasound applied to transected medial collateral ligaments of rabbits every other day for 6 weeks increased the proportion of type I collagen and improved biomechanics (ability to resist greater loads and absorb more energy) compared with ligaments treated with sham ultrasound. In this study,

researchers used continuous ultrasound with an intensity of 0.3 W/cm^2 at a frequency of 1 MHz for 10 minutes. Warden et al.[111] examined the effects of ultrasound (1-MHz frequency, 0.5-W/cm^2 intensity, pulsed at 20% duty cycle, for 20 minutes 5 days a week) and a nonsteroidal antiinflammatory drug (NSAID) on ligament healing at 2, 4, and 12 weeks and found that low-intensity, pulsed ultrasound alone accelerated ligament healing, whereas the NSAID alone delayed ligament healing. When used together, the effect of the NSAID canceled the positive effect of the ultrasound. Another study found that pulsed ultrasound within the first few days of ligament injury in rats increased the number of inflammatory mediators, amplifying inflammation in the early stages of healing but possibly accelerating the overall course of inflammatory and healing processes.[112]

Based on the few available studies specifically related to ligament healing and findings related to the healing of other soft tissues, it is recommended that low-dose (0.5 to 1.0 W/cm^2) pulsed ultrasound be considered for this application.

JOINT INFLAMMATION

A number of studies have examined the impact of ultrasound on joint inflammation. A 2010 Cochrane collaboration systematic review concluded that ultrasound may reduce pain and improve function and quality of life in patients with knee osteoarthritis (OA),[113] and more recent systematic reviews have come to similar conclusions.[114,115] These benefits have been found with both pulsed and continuous ultrasound, although pulsed ultrasound was found to be associated with both pain relief and functional improvements, whereas continuous ultrasound was only consistently associated with pain relief. Interestingly, LITUS (3-MHz frequency, continuous, for up to 4 hours each day), which applies very low-intensity (0.132 W/cm^2) continuous ultrasound for up to 4 hours each day, has also been found to be associated with reduced pain and improved function in patients with knee OA.[15]

BONE FRACTURES

Early texts recommended that ultrasound not be applied over unhealed fractures, likely because applying high-dose, continuous ultrasound over an unhealed fracture causes pain.[116–117] However, numerous studies over the past 25 years or more have not found LIPUS to adversely affect fracture healing in animals or humans, and some studies support that LIPUS may aid fracture healing. A device specifically designed to apply LIPUS to promote fracture healing was cleared by the FDA in 1994 for home use, and in 2000, the FDA expanded its clearance of this device to include the treatment of nonunion fractures.

The original LIPUS device for fracture healing has fixed preset treatment parameters of 1.5-MHz frequency, 0.15-W/cm^2 SATP intensity, and 20% duty cycle (i.e., 30-mW/cm^2 SATA) and a treatment duration of 20 minutes. Although most of the parameters available on the LIPUS devices can be replicated by standard clinical ultrasound units, with the original LIPUS device, the pulses are delivered differently than those provided by standard clinical ultrasound units. Standard clinical ultrasound units deliver 20% pulsed ultrasound with 2 ms on pulses separated by 8 ms of off time (i.e., 100-Hz pulse frequency), whereas the original LIPUS device delivers 20% pulsed ultrasound with 200 μs on pulses separated by 800 μs of off time (i.e., 1000-Hz pulse frequency). Although the impact of these differences in pulse lengths and frequency is not known, some research suggests that differences in ultrasound pulse lengths can affect the intensity of stable cavitation.[118] A LIPUS device produced in Japan and marketed outside the United States for bone healing (Osteotron IV, Ito Co. Ltd., Japan), but that is not available in the United States, allows more selection of parameters. It offers the original 1.5-MHz frequency, 0.15-W/cm^2 SATP intensity, and 20% duty cycle but also the option of 0.75-MHz frequency, 0.225- and 0.3-W/cm^2 SATP intensity, and treatment times of 20 or 30 minutes, and the pulses can be either 2-μs on pulses separated by 8 ms of off time or 200-μs on pulses separated by 800 μs of off time.

The popularity of LIPUS has varied over time. A study published in 2004 found that at that time, although most orthopedic surgeons believed that ultrasound can promote fracture healing in some cases, most were not using this modality, primarily because of a lack of evidence or a lack of availability.[119] However, in 2006, sales from LIPUS amounted to about $250 million in the United States alone,[120] and by 2008, 21% of trauma surgeons in Canada prescribed LIPUS for tibial fractures.[121] Additionally, in 2020, surgeons around the world reported using LIPUS for the treatment of nonunion fractures[122,123] and in fresh fractures in patients with compromised healing potential. Multiple studies and systematic reviews on the efficacy of LIPUS have reached conflicting conclusions, leading to changes in recommendations and national policies over time. As noted previously, in 1994, the FDA cleared a LIPUS device for use for fracture healing, and in 2000, the FDA expanded the clearance to nonunion fractures. Similarly, in 2010 the United Kingdom National Institute for Health and Care Excellence (NICE) supported the use of LIPUS to reduce fracture healing time and to provide clinical benefit, particularly for delayed or nonunion fractures.[124,125] A systematic review of 24 trials published as recently as 2016 supported this policy, concluding that "LIPUS treatment effectively reduces time to radiographic fracture union, but this does not directly result in a beneficial effect of accelerated functional recovery or the prevention of delayed union or nonunion."[120] However, a systematic review of 26 randomized controlled trials published in 2017 in the *British Medical Journal* concluded that "based on moderate to high quality evidence from studies in patients with fresh fracture, LIPUS does not improve outcomes important to patients and probably has no effect on radiographic bone healing."[126,127] The clinical practice guideline published concurrently by the authors of this review also recommended against the use of LIPUS, given the cost, current evidence, and the fact that further research was unlikely to alter the evidence. In 2018 NICE updated its LIPUS recommendations. NICE continued to find no safety concerns, but based on the efficacy-related evidence, NICE recommends *against* the use of LIPUS for promoting fresh fracture healing at low risk of nonhealing, noting that LIPUS should only be used in the context of research for promoting healing of fresh fractures at high risk of nonhealing and that LIPUS should only be used clinically to promote healing of delayed-union and nonunion fractures by specialists and with special oversight or in research.[128–130]

The reason for the mixed results of studies on LIPUS for fracture healing, and thus the optimal clinical recommendations, remain unclear.[131] Although the evidence supporting the safety of LIPUS for fracture healing is strong, the overall evidence for efficacy is mixed. It is possible that the increases in bone formation in response to LIPUS that are readily observed in animal models also occur in humans but do not translate into functional recovery or full healing consistently enough, particularly in mixed populations of patients, to reach statistical significance. It is currently this author's opinion, based on the current research, that LIPUS should not be used to treat fresh fractures without risk factors for delayed or nonunion. However, LIPUS should be considered, along with other treatment options such as electrical bone growth stimulation, for the treatment of delayed or nonunion fractures or fractures at high risk of delayed or nonunion.

If used for fracture healing, ultrasound should be applied at 0.15-W/cm^2 intensity and 20% duty cycle for 15 to 20 minutes daily.

CARPAL TUNNEL SYNDROME

There is controversy regarding the use of ultrasound for the treatment of carpal tunnel syndrome, likely because continuous ultrasound may adversely affect nerve conduction because of overheating.[132,133] However, systematic reviews published in 2010 and 2017 of various nonsurgical treatments for carpal tunnel syndrome concluded that there was strong evidence that ultrasound provides benefits in the short term and moderate evidence that ultrasound provides benefits in the midterm; however, there were no studies investigating long-term effects.[134,135] Overall, ultrasound was found to be more effective than placebo, corticosteroid injection, or other nonsurgical interventions, being associated with significantly reduced subjective complaints and improved hand grip and finger pinch strength, electromyographic variables (motor distal latency and sensory nerve conduction velocity),[136] function, and pain.[137,138] Proposed mechanisms for the potential benefit of ultrasound for patients with carpal tunnel syndrome include the antiinflammatory and tissue-stimulating effects of this intervention.[139] In general, ultrasound was applied either pulsed at 20% duty cycle, 1.0 W/cm^2 or continuous at 0.5 W/cm^2 in patients with carpal tunnel syndrome, but some evidence suggests that lower intensities, below 0.2 W/cm^2, may be even more effective.[139]

PHONOPHORESIS

Phonophoresis (also known as *sonophoresis*) is the application of ultrasound in conjunction with a topical drug preparation as the ultrasound transmission medium in order to enhance the delivery of the drug through the skin to produce local or systemic drug effects. Transcutaneous drug delivery has a number of advantages over oral drug administration.[140] Transcutaneous (also known as *transdermal*) drug delivery provides a higher initial drug concentration at the delivery site; avoids gastric irritation and first-pass metabolism by the liver; and avoids the pain, trauma, and infection risk associated with injection. Transcutaneous delivery also allows delivery to a larger area than is readily achieved by injection.

The first report on the use of ultrasound to enhance drug delivery across the skin was published in 1954 when ultrasound was applied with hydrocortisone cream as the transmission medium to treat arthritis in the fingers.[141] This was followed in the 1960s by a series of studies by Griffin et al.[142-145] performed to evaluate the location and depth of hydrocortisone delivery and the effects of varying ultrasound parameters on hydrocortisone phonophoresis. The authors of these initial studies proposed that ultrasound enhanced the delivery of the drug by exerting pressure that drove the drug through the skin. This is unlikely. Ultrasound exerts only a few grams of force, which would not be sufficient for this outcome. We now know that ultrasound can reversibly increase the permeability of the drug-diffusion barrier posed by the skin, primarily the stratum corneum layer of the skin.[140,146] The stratum corneum is the superficial cornified layer of the skin that acts as a protective barrier, preventing foreign materials from entering the body through the skin (Fig. 9.21).[147] Notably, ultrasound can enhance drug penetration if the ultrasound and drug are applied together or when ultrasound is applied before the drug is put on the skin. Furthermore, when ultrasound and the drug are applied at the same time, drug penetration continues to be enhanced for some time after the ultrasound application is complete.[148,149]

The exact mechanism underlying the effect of ultrasound on the skin is not understood.[140] Ultrasound may change the permeability of the stratum corneum through thermal and/or nonthermal mechanisms. Heat could increase drug diffusion and skin permeability, although in general, phonophoresis is performed with LIPUS, which does not cause any appreciable temperature changes.[150] The nonthermal effects of cavitation and microstreaming may produce channels in the lipid bilayer of the stratum corneum, and cavitation may physically disrupt this layer.

When the permeability of the stratum corneum is increased, a drug will diffuse across it because of the difference in concentration on either side of the skin. A drug is initially more concentrated at the delivery site, but once it diffuses across the stratum corneum, it is then distributed around the body via the vascular circulation. Therefore, therapists should be aware that although drugs delivered by phonophoresis initially have a higher concentration at the application site, they then become systemic, and therefore the contraindications for systemic delivery of these drugs also apply to this mode of delivery.

> **◉ Clinical Pearl**
>
> Although drugs delivered by phonophoresis are initially more concentrated at the delivery site, they are quickly distributed around the body by the vascular system.

Rehabilitation practitioners primarily use phonophoresis with a gel-based transmission medium to deliver the corticosteroid antiinflammatory medication dexamethasone through the skin for the treatment of pain and dysfunction associated with inflammatory conditions such as osteoarthritis, tendinitis, tenosynovitis, and carpal tunnel syndrome.[151,152] This intervention is usually limited to 6 treatments because 6 phonophoresis treatments with dexamethasone have been shown not to cause an increase in urinary free cortisol, which is a measure of adrenal suppression,[153] but the use of up to 10 treatments has been reported in the literature.[151] Some recent research also supports the use of phonophoresis with NSAID gel for inflammatory conditions,[154,155] and although this may not be as effective as phonophoresis with a corticosteroid,[156] phonophoresis with NSAIDs has gained popularity among some clinicians. Whatever the medication, for phonophoresis to potentially be effective, the medication must be dissolved in a gel-based rather than cream-based transmission medium because ultrasound is transmitted well by gels but poorly by creams.[157,158]

Current research supports using ultrasound to facilitate transdermal penetration of some medications. When using phonophoresis to treat inflammation, 20% pulsed ultrasound, to avoid heating of the inflammatory condition and to optimize the mechanical effects of the ultrasound,[159] at 0.5- to 1.0-W/cm^2 intensity for 5 to 10 minutes, is most likely to be effective. Ultrasound with a 3-MHz frequency is recommended to focus the ultrasound superficially and thus have the greatest impact at the level of the skin. The drug preparation used should also effectively transmit ultrasound. The LITUS described earlier has also been shown in in-vitro studies to be effective for phonophoresis. LITUS has been shown to increase the delivery of the antiinflammatory diclofenac by almost fourfold in a human skin model.[160]

In recent years, a wealth of research has explored the use of phonophoresis to deliver drugs other than antiinflammatory medications. Much of this research has focused on insulin, vaccines, and other drugs that can be given only by injection or infusion.[161-165] Although animal studies have been promising, this approach to drug delivery is hampered by difficulties with precise dose control.[166] Ultrasound is also being explored as a method for monitoring blood glucose levels.[167]

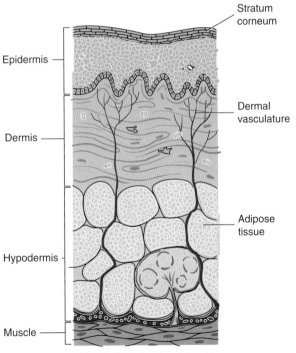

FIGURE 9.21 Layers of the skin.

Stratum corneum

Epidermis

Dermal vasculature

Dermis

Adipose tissue

Hypodermis

Muscle

Contraindications and Precautions for Ultrasound

Although ultrasound is a relatively safe intervention, it must be applied with care to avoid harming the patient.[168,169] Ultrasound with the range of parameters available on clinical devices may not be used by patients to treat themselves. These clinical therapeutic ultrasounds must be used by, or under the supervision of, a licensed practitioner. LIPUS and continuous LITUS ultrasound devices are available for use by patients to treat themselves at home, but these devices may also only be used at the recommendation of a licensed practitioner.

There is general agreement in the literature regarding recommended contraindications and precautions for the clinical application of therapeutic ultrasound, although all sources do vary to some degree.[170] Even when ultrasound is not contraindicated, if the patient's condition is worsening or is not improving within two or three treatments, reevaluate the treatment approach, and consider changing the intervention or referring the patient to a physician for reevaluation.

CONTRAINDICATIONS FOR ULTRASOUND

✱ CONTRAINDICATIONS

for Ultrasound

- Malignant tumor
- Pregnancy
- Central nervous system (CNS) tissue
- Joint cement
- Plastic components
- Pacemaker or implantable cardiac rhythm device
- Thrombophlebitis
- Eyes
- Reproductive organs

Malignant Tumor

Although no research data are available on the effects of applying therapeutic ultrasound to malignant tumors in humans, the application of continuous ultrasound at 1.0 W/cm^2, 1 MHz for 5 minutes for 10 treatments over a period of 2 weeks to mice with malignant subcutaneous tumors has been shown to be associated with significantly larger and heavier tumors, and more lymph node metastases, compared with untreated controls.[171] Because this study supports that therapeutic ultrasound may increase the rate of tumor growth or metastasis, it is recommended that therapeutic ultrasound not be applied to malignant tumors in humans. Caution should also be used when treating a patient with a history of a malignant tumor or tumors because it can be difficult to ascertain whether any malignant cells remain. It is recommended that the therapist consult with the referring physician before applying ultrasound to a patient with a history of malignancy within the past 5 years.

Ultrasound is sometimes used as a component of the treatment of certain types of malignant tumors; however, the devices used for this application are designed to produce a specific temperature range in the tumor, to either induce sensitization to chemotherapy and radiotherapy or to destroy tumor cells directly.[172] This can help destroy malignant tumors while not damaging healthy tissue. Because the therapeutic ultrasound devices generally available to physical therapists do not allow such precise determination and control of tissue temperature or localization, and because primary treatment of malignancy is outside the scope of practice of rehabilitation professionals, therapeutic ultrasound devices intended for rehabilitation applications should not be used for the treatment of malignancy.

▪ Ask the Patient
- "Have you ever had cancer? Do you have cancer now?"
- "Do you have fevers, chills, sweats, or night pain?"
- "Do you have pain at rest?"
- "Have you had recent unexplained weight loss?"

If the patient presently has cancer, ultrasound should not be used. If the patient has a history of cancer or signs of cancer, such as fevers, chills, sweats, night pain, pain at rest, or recent unexplained weight loss, the therapist should consult with the referring physician to rule out the presence of malignancy before applying ultrasound.

Pregnancy

Maternal hyperthermia has been associated with fetal abnormalities, including growth retardation, microphthalmia, exencephaly, microcephaly, neural tube defects, and myelodysplasia.[173,174] A published report also documents a case of sacral agenesis, microcephaly, and developmental delay in a child whose mother was treated 18 times with pulsed ultrasound for a left psoas bursitis between days 6 and 29 of gestation.[175] High-frequency (6.7-MHz), low-intensity (1.95-mW/cm^2) ultrasound applied for 30 minutes or longer to the abdomen of pregnant mice during late pregnancy (third trimester) has also been found to impair neuronal migration in the brain.[176] Therefore it is recommended that therapeutic ultrasound not be applied at any level in areas where it may reach a developing fetus. This includes the abdomen, low back, and pelvis.

In contrast to therapeutic ultrasound, diagnostic ultrasound frequently used during pregnancy to assess the position and development of the fetus and placenta, which has a much lower average intensity than therapeutic ultrasound, has been shown to be safe and without adverse consequences for the fetus and the mother.[177,178]

▪ Ask the Patient
- "Are you pregnant, might you be pregnant, or are you trying to become pregnant?"

The patient may not know if she is pregnant, particularly in the first few days or weeks after conception; however, because damage may occur at any time during fetal development, ultrasound should not be applied in any area where the beam may reach the fetus of a patient who is or might be pregnant.

Central Nervous System Tissue

Concern has arisen that ultrasound may damage CNS tissue. However, because CNS tissue is usually covered by bone both in the spinal cord and in the brain, this is rarely a problem. However, the spinal cord may be exposed if the patient has had a laminectomy above the L2 level; in such cases, ultrasound should not be applied over or near the area of the laminectomy.

Methyl Methacrylate Cement or Plastic

Methyl methacrylate cement and plastic are materials used for fixation or as components of prosthetic joints. Although very little ultrasound is able to reach to the depth of most prosthetic joints, some of these materials are rapidly heated by ultrasound,[179] so ultrasound should not be applied over areas where plastic components are used. Ultrasound may be used over areas with metal implants such as screws, plates, or all-metal joint replacements because metal is not rapidly heated by ultrasound, and ultrasound has been shown not to loosen screws or plates.[180]

> ■ **Ask the Patient**
> • "Do you have a joint replacement in this area?"
> • "Was cement used to hold it in place?"
> • "Does it have plastic components?"

If the patient has a joint replacement, ultrasound should not be applied in the area of the prosthesis until the therapist has determined that neither cement nor plastic was used.

Pacemaker or Implantable Cardiac Rhythm Device

Ultrasound can potentially affect a pacemaker or implantable cardioverter-defibrillator (ICD). In pacemakers, ultrasound can potentially cause single-beat inhibition of the pacing and components of a pacemaker, or the ICD can be damaged if ultrasound is aimed directly at the device. Therefore, pacemaker and ICD device manufacturers recommend that ultrasound should not be focused within 6 inches of the implanted device. Ultrasound may be applied to other areas in patients with pacemakers or ICDs. Should a patient with a pacemaker or ICD feel dizzy, lightheaded, or short of breath during an ultrasound treatment, the therapy should be discontinued immediately.

> ■ **Ask the Patient**
> • "Do you have a pacemaker?"

Thrombophlebitis

Because ultrasound may dislodge or cause partial disintegration of a thrombus, which could result in obstruction of the circulation to vital organs, ultrasound should not be applied over or near an area where a thrombus is or may be present.

> ■ **Ask the Patient**
> • "Do you have a blood clot in this area?"

Eyes

It is recommended that ultrasound not be applied over the eyes because cavitation in the ocular fluid may damage the eyes.

Reproductive Organs

Because ultrasound at the levels used for rehabilitation may affect gamete development, it should not be applied in the areas of the male or female reproductive organs.

PRECAUTIONS FOR ULTRASOUND

> ✱ **PRECAUTIONS**
>
> **for Ultrasound**
> • Acute inflammation
> • Epiphyseal plates
> • Fractures
> • Breast implants

Acute Inflammation

Because heat can exacerbate acute inflammation, causing increased bleeding, pain, and swelling; impaired healing; and delayed functional recovery, ultrasound at sufficient intensity to produce heat should be applied with caution in areas of acute inflammation.

Epiphyseal Plates

The literature regarding the application of ultrasound over epiphyseal plates supports that low-dose ultrasound appears to be safe but that high-dose ultrasound is not. Both an early study (1953)[181] and a more recent study (2003)[182] found that high-dose ultrasound, at greater than 3.0 W/cm^2 in the earlier study and at 2.2 W/cm^2 in the later study, can profoundly damage epiphyseal plates. However, a number of studies have found that low-dose ultrasound at up to 0.5 W/cm^2 does not damage the growth plates in skeletally immature rats[183,184] or rabbits,[182,185] and the LIPUS device specifically designed for use in fracture healing has proven effective in children.[186] Therefore, high-dose ultrasound (i.e., with intensity >0.5 W/cm^2) should not be applied over growing epiphyseal plates. Because the age of epiphyseal closure varies, radiographic evaluation rather than age should be used to determine whether epiphyseal closure is complete.

Fractures

Although low-dose ultrasound can accelerate fracture healing, the application of high-intensity ultrasound over a fracture generally causes pain and may impair fracture healing. Therefore, only low-dose ultrasound, as described in the section on fracture healing, and not high-dose ultrasound, should be applied over a fracture.

Breast Implants

Because heat may increase the pressure inside a breast implant and cause it to rupture, high-dose ultrasound should not be applied over breast implants.

Adverse Effects of Ultrasound

Ultrasound rarely causes adverse effects.[187] However, various adverse effects can occur if ultrasound is applied incorrectly or when contraindicated. The most common adverse effect of ultrasound is a burn. Burns can occur when high-intensity, continuous ultrasound is applied, particularly if a stationary application technique is used. The risk of burns is further increased in areas with impaired circulation or sensation and with superficial bone. To minimize the risk of burning a patient, always move the ultrasound head, and do not apply thermal-level ultrasound to areas with impaired circulation or sensation. Reduce the ultrasound intensity in areas with superficial bone or if the patient complains of any increase in discomfort with the application of ultrasound. Because ultrasound devices made by different manufacturers set with the same parameters may produce different temperature increases,[35] patient report must always be used to help gauge the degree of heating and safety.

Standing waves, with intensity maxima and minima at fixed positions one-half wavelength apart, can occur when the ultrasound transducer and a reflecting surface are exact multiples of wavelengths apart, allowing the reflected wave to superimpose on the incident wave entering the tissue. Ultrasound standing waves can cause blood cell stasis because of collections of gas bubbles and plasma at antinodes and collections of cells at nodes (Fig. 9.22).[188,189] This is accompanied by damage to the endothelial lining of the blood vessels. These effects have been demonstrated with ultrasound of 1- to 5-MHz frequency with intensity of 0.5 W/cm² for 0.1 second. Although the stasis is reversed when ultrasound application stops, endothelial damage remains. Standing waves can be avoided by moving the sound head throughout the treatment. Therefore, to prevent the adverse effects of standing waves, it is recommended that the ultrasound transducer be moved throughout treatment application.

Another concern is the possibility of cross-contamination and infection of patients. Studies have found that 27% to 35.5% of ultrasound transducer heads, 14.5% to 28% of ultrasound transmission gels, and 52.7% of gel bottle tips taken from various physical therapy practices were contaminated

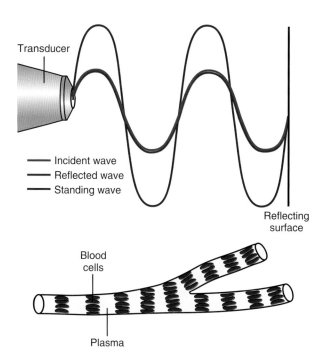

FIGURE 9.22 Ultrasound standing waves. (A) Formation of standing waves. (B) Banding of blood cells and plasma due to standing waves.

with bacteria.[190,191] Contamination of the transducer heads was generally with bacteria normally found on the skin, but some gels and gel bottle heads were contaminated with *Staphylococcus aureus,* including methicillin-resistant *S. aureus* (MRSA). Swabbing transducers and gel bottle heads with disinfectant significantly reduced the levels of contamination.

> ### Clinical Pearl
> Ultrasound transducers and gel bottle heads can harbor bacteria. Swab them with disinfectant to reduce the level of contamination.

Application Technique

This section provides guidelines for the sequence of procedures required for the safe and effective application of therapeutic ultrasound.

APPLICATION TECHNIQUE 9.1   ULTRASOUND

Equipment Required

- Ultrasound unit
- Gel, water, or other transmission medium
- Antimicrobial agent
- Towel

Procedure

1. Evaluate the patient's clinical findings and set the goals of treatment.
2. Determine whether ultrasound is the most appropriate intervention.
3. Confirm that ultrasound is not contraindicated for the patient or the condition. Check with the patient and check the patient's chart for contraindications or precautions regarding the application of ultrasound.
4. Remove all clothing and jewelry from the treatment area.
5. Apply an ultrasound transmission medium to the area to be treated. Before treatment of any area with a risk of cross-infection, swab the tip of the bottle or container of transmission medium with 0.5% alcoholic chlorhexidine, or use the antimicrobial approved for this use in the facility.[191,192] Apply enough medium to eliminate any air between the sound head

Continued

APPLICATION TECHNIQUE 9.1—*cont'd*

and the treatment area. Select a medium that transmits ultrasound well, does not stain, is not allergenic, is not rapidly absorbed by the skin, and is inexpensive. Gels or lotions meeting these criteria have been specifically formulated for use with ultrasound. If using ultrasound for phonophoresis, the medicated ultrasound transmission medium still needs to transmit ultrasound well. Topical agents in a gel form generally transmit ultrasound well, whereas topical agents in a cream-based medium generally do not transmit ultrasound well and should therefore be avoided for phonophoresis.[157,158] For the application of ultrasound underwater, place the area to be treated in a container of water (see Fig. 9.20).

6. Select a sound head with an ERA approximately half the size of the treatment area.

7. Select the optimal treatment parameters, including ultrasound frequency, intensity, duty cycle, and duration; the appropriate size of the treatment area; and the appropriate number and frequency of treatments. Parameters are generally determined by whether the intended effect is thermal or nonthermal. See

the next section for a general discussion of parameters. Detailed information on parameters for specific conditions is included in the previous section.

8. Before treatment of any area with a risk of cross-infection, swab the sound head with 0.5% alcoholic chlorhexidine, or use the antimicrobial approved for this use in the facility.[191,192]

9. Place the sound head on the treatment area.

10. Turn on the ultrasound machine.

11. Move the sound head within the treatment area. The sound head is moved to optimize the uniformity of ultrasound intensity delivered to the tissues and to minimize the risk of standing wave formation.[188,189] See "Moving the Sound Head" later in this chapter for a detailed description of how to move the sound head.

12. When the intervention is completed, remove the conduction medium from the sound head and the patient, swab the sound head and bottle tip with approved antimicrobial, and reassess the patient for any changes in status.

13. Document the intervention.

ULTRASOUND TREATMENT PARAMETERS

Specific recommendations for different clinical applications are given in the previous sections concerning specific clinical conditions. General guidelines for treatment parameters follow.

Frequency

The frequency is selected according to the depth of tissue to be treated. For tissue up to 5 cm deep, 1 MHz is used; for tissue 1 to 2 cm deep, 3 MHz is used. The depth of penetration is lower in tissues with high collagen content and in areas of increased reflection.

Duty Cycle

The duty cycle is selected according to the treatment goal. When the goal is to increase tissue temperature, a 100% (continuous) duty cycle should be used.[41] When ultrasound is applied where only the nonthermal effects without tissue heating are desired, pulsed ultrasound with a 20% or lower duty cycle should be used.[32] Many ultrasound machines allow the selection of other pulsed duty cycles, but almost all the research using therapeutic pulsed ultrasound has used a 20% duty cycle. Although the nonthermal effects of ultrasound are produced by continuous ultrasound, it is thought that they are not optimized with application at this level.

Intensity

Intensity is selected according to the treatment goal. When the goal is to increase tissue temperature, the patient should feel some warmth within 2 to 3 minutes of initiating ultrasound application and should not feel increased discomfort at any time during the treatment. When 1-MHz frequency ultrasound is used, an intensity of 1.5 to 2.0 W/cm^2 generally produces this effect. When 3-MHz frequency is used, an intensity of approximately 0.5 W/cm^2 is generally sufficient.

A lower intensity is effective at the higher frequency because energy is absorbed in a smaller, more superficial volume of tissue, resulting in a greater temperature increase with the same ultrasound intensity. Intensity is adjusted up or down from these levels according to the patient's report. The intensity is increased if no sensation of warmth is noted within 2 to 3 minutes and is decreased immediately if any discomfort is reported. If superficial bone is present in the treatment area, a slightly lower intensity will be sufficient to produce comfortable heating because the ultrasound reflected by the bone will cause a greater increase in temperature.

When ultrasound was applied for nonthermal effects, successful treatment outcomes have been documented for most applications using an intensity of 0.5- to 1.0-W/cm^2 SATP (0.1- to 0.2-W/cm^2 SATA), with 0.15-W/cm^2 SATP (0.03-W/cm^2 SATA) sufficient for the facilitation of bone healing.

Duration

Treatment duration is selected according to the treatment goal, the size of the area to be treated, and the ERA of the sound head. For most thermal or nonthermal applications, ultrasound should be applied for 5 to 10 minutes for each treatment area that is twice the ERA of the transducer. For example, when an area measuring 20 cm^2 is treated with a sound head that has an ERA of 10 cm^2, the treatment duration should be 5 to 10 minutes. When an area of 40 cm^2 is treated with the same 10 cm^2, the treatment duration should be extended to 10 to 20 minutes.

When the treatment goal is to increase tissue temperature, the treatment duration should be adjusted according to the frequency and intensity of the ultrasound. For example, if the goal is to increase tissue temperature from 37°C (98°F) to the minimal therapeutic level of 40°C (104°F) and if 1-MHz ultrasound at an intensity of 1.5 W/cm^2 is applied to an area twice the ERA of the transducer, the treatment duration must be at least 9 minutes, whereas if the intensity is increased to 2 W/cm², the treatment duration need be only 8 minutes.[21] If 3-MHz ultrasound is used at an intensity of 0.5 W/cm², the treatment duration must be at least 10 minutes to achieve the same temperature level. The LITUS device, which delivers 3-MHz continuous ultrasound at the very low intensity of 0.132 W/cm², increases tissue temperature by applying this low-intensity ultrasound for up to 4 hours.

In general, treatment duration should be increased when lower intensities or lower frequencies of ultrasound are used, when areas slightly larger than twice the ERA of the transducer are treated, or when higher tissue temperatures are desired. Treatment duration should be decreased when higher intensities or frequencies of ultrasound are used, when areas smaller than twice the ERA of the transducer are treated, or when lower tissue temperatures are desired.

Area to Be Treated

The size of the area that can be treated with ultrasound depends on the ERA of the transducer and the duration of treatment. As explained in the previous discussion of duration of treatment, a treatment area equal to twice the ERA of the sound head can be treated in 5 to 10 minutes. Smaller areas can be treated in proportionately shorter times; however, it is impractical to treat areas measuring less than 1½ times the ERA of the sound head and still keep the sound head moving within the area. Larger areas can be treated in proportionately longer times; however, ultrasound should not be used to treat areas larger than 4 times the ERA of the transducer, such as the whole low back, because this requires excessively long treatment durations and, when heating is desired, will not produce consistent heating (Figs. 9.23 and 9.24).

Number and Frequency of Treatments

The recommended number of treatments depends on the goals of treatment and the patient's response. If the patient is making progress at an appropriate rate toward established goals for this intervention, treatment should be continued. If the patient is not progressing appropriately, the intervention should be modified by changing the ultrasound parameters or

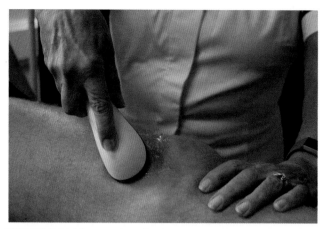

FIGURE 9.24 Ultrasound application to the medial knee for treatment of medial collateral ligament sprain. (Courtesy EMS Physio, Wantage, UK.)

by selecting a different intervention. In most cases, an effect should be detectable within one to three treatments. For problems in which progress is commonly slow, such as chronic wounds, or in which progress is hard to detect, such as fractures, treatment may need to be continued for a longer period. The frequency of treatments depends on the level of ultrasound being used and the stage of healing. Thermal-level ultrasound is usually applied only during the subacute or chronic phase of healing, when treatment three times a week is recommended; ultrasound at nonthermal levels may be applied at earlier stages, when treatment may be daily. These frequencies of treatment are based on current clinical standards of practice because no published studies at this time have compared the efficacy of different treatment frequencies.

Sequence of Treatment

In most cases, ultrasound may be applied before or after other interventions; however, when ultrasound is used to heat tissue, it should not be applied after any intervention that may impair sensation, such as ice. Also, when thermal-level ultrasound is used to increase collagen extensibility to maximize the increase in length produced by stretching, the ultrasound must be applied *directly* before and, if possible, during application of the stretching force. The clinician should not wait or apply another intervention between applying the ultrasound and stretching because the tissue starts to cool as soon as the ultrasound application ends.

Moving the Sound Head

Most authors recommend that the sound head be moved at approximately 4 cm/second—quickly enough to maintain motion and slowly enough to maintain contact with the skin—although studies have not found any difference in heating effects when the sound head is moved at 2, 4, 6, or 8 cm/second.[23,193] If the sound head is kept stationary or is moved too slowly, the area of tissue under the center of the transducer where the intensity is greatest will receive much more ultrasound than the areas under the edges of the transducer. This will be more pronounced with a higher-BNR transducer. With continuous ultrasound, this can result in

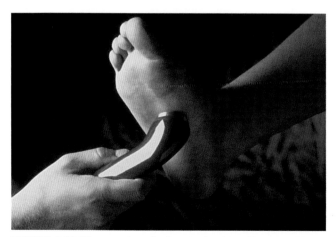

FIGURE 9.23 Ultrasound application to the foot. (Courtesy Mettler Electronics, Anaheim, CA.)

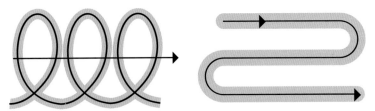

FIGURE 9.25 Stroking technique for ultrasound application.

overheating and burning of the tissues at the center of the field; with pulsed ultrasound, this can reduce the efficacy of the intervention. A stationary sound head should not be used when continuous or pulsed ultrasound is applied. If the sound head is moved too quickly, the therapist may not be able to maintain good contact of the sound head with the skin, and thus the ultrasound will not be able to enter the tissue, and the therapist may tend to inappropriately increase the overall size of the treatment area.

The sound head should be moved in a manner that causes the center of the head to change position so that all parts of the treatment area receive similar exposure. Strokes overlapping by half the ERA of the sound head are recommended (Fig. 9.25). The clinician should keep within the predetermined treatment area of generally 1½ to 2 times the ERA.

The surface of the sound head should be kept in constant parallel contact with the skin to ensure that ultrasound is transmitted to the tissues. Poor contact will impede the transmission of ultrasound because much of it will be absorbed by intervening air or will be reflected at the air–tissue interface. To promote more effective intervention, some clinical ultrasound units are equipped with a transmission sensor that gives a signal when contact is poor.

Documentation

The following should be documented:
- Area of the body treated
- Ultrasound frequency
- Ultrasound intensity
- Ultrasound duty cycle
- Treatment duration
- Whether the ultrasound was delivered underwater
- Patient's response to the intervention

Documentation is typically written in the SOAP note (Subjective, Objective, Assessment, Plan) format. The following examples summarize the modality component only of the intervention and are not intended to represent a comprehensive plan of care.

EXAMPLES

When applying ultrasound (US) to the left lateral knee over the lateral collateral ligament (LCL) to facilitate tissue healing, document the following:

S: *Pt reports L lateral knee pain with turning during activities has decreased from frequent 8/10 to occasional 5/10 since last week after therapy treatment.*

O: Intervention: *US L lateral knee, LCL, 0.5 W/cm², pulsed 20%, 3 MHz, 5 min.*

A: *Pt tolerated treatment well, with decreased knee pain since US initiated.*

P: *Reassess pain level next treatment; if pain resolved, discontinue US.*

When applying ultrasound to the R inferior anterior shoulder capsule, document the following:

S: *Pt notes slowly improving R shoulder ROM and now is able to use R UE when combing her hair since last treatment.*

O: Pretreatment: *R shoulder active abduction ROM 120 degrees, passive abduction ROM 135 degrees.*

Intervention: *US R inferior anterior shoulder, 2.0 W/cm², continuous, 1 MHz, 5 min, followed by joint mobility inferior glide grade IV.*

Posttreatment: *R shoulder passive abduction 150 degrees.*

A: *Improved shoulder PROM with thermal US and joint mobilization.*

P: *Continue US as above followed by mobilization and ROM to R shoulder to allow for upper body grooming and dressing.*

Ultrasound Machine Care and Calibration

Therapeutic ultrasound machines require appropriate care to function well and deliver ultrasound with the intended parameters. The accuracy of the ultrasound parameters varies among machines and manufacturers even when the machine is new.[194] Care should be used when transporting or moving the machine, particularly the transducer, because moving the machine and jostling or bumping it, as can happen when transporting from room to room or in and out of elevators, can worsen its calibration. Dropping the transducer can break the piezoelectric crystal inside it. If this happens, the crystal will no longer produce ultrasound and must be replaced. Ultrasound machines should also be tested at least annually for safe operation and calibration of output parameters. Some authors recommend monthly or even more frequently.[195] Ultrasound machine calibration can usually be performed either by the biomedical engineering department of the hospital or by the company that sold the machine. Unfortunately, in many settings, ultrasound machines are rarely calibrated, and the performance and accuracy of the devices in clinical use, including the ERA, BNR, timer, and intensity, are poor.[196,197]

CLINICAL CASE STUDIES

The following case studies summarize the concepts of applying therapeutic ultrasound as discussed in this chapter. Based on the scenarios presented, an evaluation of the clinical findings and goals of treatment are proposed. These are followed by a discussion of factors to be considered in the selection of ultrasound as the indicated intervention modality and in the selection of the ideal treatment parameters to promote progress toward the set goals (Fig. 9.26).

CASE STUDY 9.1

Soft Tissue Shortening
Examination
History

LR is a 22-year-old, right-handed man who injured his right hand 5 weeks ago. He struck his hand against a glass window and, on pulling his hand back, deeply lacerated the volar forearm approximately 1 inch proximal to the wrist crease. The median nerve was lacerated, as well as the flexor pollicis longus, flexor carpi radialis, flexor digitorum profundus to the index finger, and flexor digitorum superficialis to the middle and index fingers. He underwent surgical nerve and tendon repair and postoperatively was placed in a dorsal blocking splint. On discharge, he was incarcerated for 4 weeks. He has since been released and has returned for hand therapy services, having not been seen for therapy since his inpatient stay. LR has been

completing all unilateral self-care activities of daily living with his nondominant left hand and either seeks help for or avoids noncritical bimanual tasks. Although he has not returned to work, LR reports that his inability to perform most tasks with his dominant right hand will prevent him from returning to work.

Systems Review

LR is a young, well-appearing man. He is alert and cooperative with therapy testing and interventions. He reports that he continually wore the splint that was fabricated for him until 4 days ago. Before his injury, he worked intermittently in janitorial services, in lawn and yard maintenance, and as a delivery driver. He is eager to return to manual labor work. He has no atrophy and no self-reported weakness, ROM restrictions, or sensory changes in the left upper extremity or either lower extremity.

Tests and Measures

Active range of motion (AROM) in the right wrist is 0/80 degrees flexion and 0/20 degrees extension. Passive wrist extension is 0/28 degrees. LR can actively flex all digits, indicating that all tendons are intact, but the skin along the volar forearm pulls when he tries to flex the digits, and he cannot isolate digital flexion for the middle and index fingers. Specifically, digital ROM is as follows, with digital extension measured with the wrist in slight flexion. With the wrist in neutral, LR cannot fully extend the IP joints.

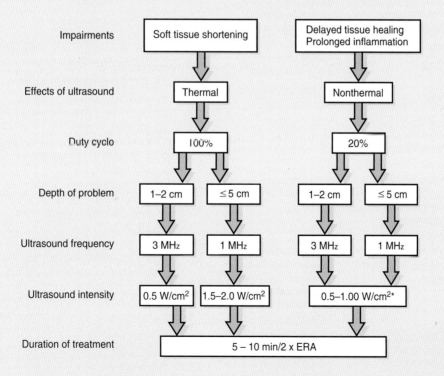

*0.2 W/cm² for fracture healing

FIGURE 9.26 Decision-making chart for ultrasound treatment parameters. *ERA*, Effective radiating area.

Continued

CLINICAL CASE STUDIES—cont'd

Joint		Thumb	Index	Middle	Ring	Small
MCP extension/flexion	AROM	0/50°	0/65°	0/50°	0/90°	0/90°
	PROM	0/50°	0/75°	0/75°	0/80°	0/85°
PIP extension/flexion	AROM	0/55°	0/35°	0/40°	0/80°	0/80°
	PROM	0/80°	0/90°	0/95°	0/90°	0/90°
DIP extension/flexion	AROM		0/25°	0/50°	0/75°	0/70°
	PROM		0/60°	0/70°	0/80°	0/75°

AROM, Active range of motion; *DIP,* distal interphalangeal; *MCP,* metacarpophalangeal; *PIP,* proximal interphalangeal; *PROM,* passive range of motion.

What does pulling of the skin along the volar forearm when this patient attempts to flex his fingers indicate? How may ultrasound help this patient? What studies should be performed before ultrasound is used on this patient?

Pain severity is 0/10 at rest and with activity. Tinel sign is noted at the level of the median nerve injury. Sensory testing with Semmes-Weinstein monofilaments revealed diminished protective sensation of the volar thumb, index finger, middle finger, and radial half of the ring finger but intact sensation more proximally along the forearm. Strength testing was deferred; however, he is likely weak owing to prolonged immobilization and low median nerve injury.

Evaluation and Goals

ICF Level	Current Status	Goals
Body structure and function	Decreased sensation, ROM, and likely strength	Mobilize nerve to avoid or reduce adhesion of nerve to scar
	Decreased ROM	Mobilize tendons to ensure tendon gliding for improved ROM
		Elongate soft tissue to increase ROM
	Decreased strength due to prolonged immobilization and low median nerve injury	Increase strength
Activity	Limited ability to simultaneously extend wrist and digits in preparation for grasping	Improve reach in preparation for grasp
Participation	No participation in bimanual ADLs and IADLs	Resume completion of unilateral tasks with dominant right hand, and participate fully in bimanual ADL and IADL tasks
	Not seeking employment owing to self-perceived inability to participate in bimanual work tasks	Return to employment and use of both hands in bimanual tasks

ADLs, Activities of daily living; *IADLs,* instrumental activities of daily living; *ICF,* International Classification for Functioning, Disability and Health; *ROM,* range of motion.

◆ FIND THE EVIDENCE

PICO Terms	Natural Language Example	Sample PubMed Search
P (Population)	Patients with symptoms due to soft tissue shortening	("Contracture*" [MeSH] OR "Contracture" [text word] OR "Therapy, Soft Tissue" [MeSH] OR "Tissue Shortening" [text word])
I (Intervention)	Ultrasound therapy	AND "Ultrasonic Therapy*" [MeSH] AND English [lang] AND "humans" [MeSH terms]
C (Comparison)	No ultrasound therapy	
O (Outcome)	Increased range of motion	

Key Studies or Reviews

1. Nakano J, Yamabayashi C, Scott A, et al: The effect of heat applied with stretch to increase range of motion: a systematic review. *Phys Ther Sport* 13:180–188, 2012.
   This systematic review of 12 studies concluded that stretching with heat, including heating with ultrasound, results in greater increases in ROM than stretching alone in healthy people.

2. Morishita K, Karasuno H, Yokoi Y, et al: Effects of therapeutic ultrasound on range of motion and stretch pain. *J Phys Ther Sci* 26:711–715, 2014.
   This study found that 3-MHz continuous ultrasound applied for 10 minutes to the upper trapezius in humans increased skin surface temperature and cervical lateral bending ROM more than placebo ultrasound or rest.

3. Usuba M, Miyanaga Y, Miyakawa S, et al: Effect of heat in increasing the range of knee motion after the development of a joint contracture: an experiment with an animal model. *Arch Phys Med Rehabil* 87:247–253, 2006.
   This study found that stretching with ultrasound was more effective than stretching without ultrasound for increasing ROM in an animal knee joint contracture model. Ultrasound treatment included 8 minutes of 1-MHz continuous ultrasound at 1 W/cm².

CLINICAL CASE STUDIES—cont'd

4. Bleakley C, Costello JT: Do thermal agents affect range of movement and mechanical properties in soft tissues? A systematic review. *Arch Phys Med Rehabil* 94:149–163, 2013.

   This systematic review of 36 studies found that heat increases ROM, and a combination of heat and stretching is more effective than heating alone.

Prognosis

LR has reduced ROM, likely because of tendon adhesions and soft tissue shortening. Additionally, he likely has reduced hand strength because of prolonged immobilization and low median nerve injury. Thermotherapy over the volar wrist, particularly combined with stretching, may help elongate the tendons and scar tissue. Continuous ultrasound would likely be more effective than other thermotherapy options because ultrasound penetrates deeply and can reach the flexor digitorum profundus. Ultrasound is also absorbed more by tissues with more collagen, such as scar tissue. Given the level of injury, that he is in his fifth postoperative week, that all tendons appear to be intact, and that abundant scar and adhesions are evident, he likely can withstand more active tensile loads along the flexor tendons without great risk of tendon rupture.

Intervention

Continuous ultrasound (i.e., 100% duty cycle), 3 MHz frequency, and intensity of 0.8 W/cm^2 for 10 minutes, is recommended. Ultrasound may initially be applied with the wrist in slight extension and the fingers in relaxed flexion, followed by gentle muscle and tendon stretch and tendon gliding exercises. Eventually, because composite wrist and digital extension is deemed safe, ultrasound can be applied with the flexor tendons on stretch to gain the maximum effect of heat application on mobility and ROM.

Documentation

S: Pt stated, "I can't straighten my wrist and fingers at the same time."

O: Pt was seen for activities to improve hand function, specifically, tissue elongation to promote maximal composite extension in preparation for grasp and tendon excursion to reduce effects of tendon adhesions, thus promoting full digital closure during grasp. US was applied to volar wrist with wrist in extension and digits in relaxed flexion as follows: 100% duty cycle, 3 MHz, 0.8 W/cm^2 for 10 min. This was followed by gentle tendon (FPL, FDS, FDP, FCR, and PL) stretching and tendon gliding exercises. At the end of treatment:
1. Digital extension was full at all joints simultaneously with wrist in 5° of extension.
2. IP flexion for thumb IP joint was 0/65°.
3. PIP flexion of index and middle fingers was 50° and 45°, respectively.

A: Previously, Pt could not maintain simultaneous extension of digits with wrist in neutral. He can now do so and more with additional 5° of extension. PIP flexion improved in index finger more than in middle finger. Pt appears to benefit from application of thermotherapy with US.

P: Continue treatment twice weekly using US and stretching for tissue elongation to maximize functional use of dominant hand in activities. Consider electrical stimulation to facilitate tendon excursion through scar. Because Pt has been essentially immobilized for longer than 4 weeks, dorsal blocking splint will be discontinued. Volar-based wrist and digital extension splint will be fabricated to elongate flexor tendons and volar wrist capsule.

CASE STUDY 9.2

Tendon Healing

Examination

History

BJ is an 18-year-old female college student. She sustained a complete rupture of her left Achilles tendon 2 weeks ago while playing basketball, and the tendon was surgically repaired 3 days ago. She has been referred for physical therapy to attain a pain-free return to sports as quickly as possible. She reports mild discomfort at the surgical incision site that increases with walking. Her leg is in a walking boot for immobilization.

Systems Review

BJ is a well-appearing young woman walking readily with a heeled "boot." She is alert, cooperative, and eager to engage in therapy and return to full activity. She has no atrophy or self-reported weakness, ROM restrictions, or sensory changes in either upper extremity or the right lower extremity.

Tests and Measures

The patient has restricted passive dorsiflexion ROM of −15 degrees on the left compared with +10 degrees on the right. Mild swelling, tenderness, and redness are noted in the area of the surgical repair, along with atrophy of the calf muscles on the left. All other measures are within normal limits.

What do tenderness, swelling, and erythema indicate? Would ultrasound help this patient? What studies should be performed before ultrasound is used on this patient?

Evaluation and Goals

ICF Level	Current Status	Goals
Body structure and function	Restricted left ankle dorsiflexion PROM	Resolve inflammation and limit scar tissue formation
	Tenderness, swelling, and erythema at site of surgical repair	Maximize tendon strength in shortest time possible
	Atrophy of left calf muscles	In the longer term, normalize left ankle ROM, normalize left calf size and strength

Continued

CLINICAL CASE STUDIES—cont'd

ICF Level	Current Status	Goals
Activity	Limited ambulation	Return to normal ambulation
Participation	Unable to participate in sports	Return to sports in 2 months

ICF, International Classification for Functioning, Disability and Health; *PROM,* passive range of motion; *ROM,* range of motion.

◆ FIND THE EVIDENCE

PICO Terms	Natural Language Example	Sample PubMed Search
P (Population)	Patients with tendon and ligament injuries	("Tendon Injuries" [MeSH]) OR "Ligaments/injuries" [MeSH] OR "Tendinopathy" [MeSH])
I (Intervention)	Ultrasound therapy	AND "Ultrasonic Therapy*" [MeSH]
C (Comparison)	No ultrasound therapy	
O (Outcome)	Tendon and ligament healing	AND English[lang] AND "humans" [MeSH terms]

Key Studies or Reviews

1. Tsai WC, Tang ST, Liang FC: Effect of therapeutic ultrasound on tendons. *Am J Phys Med Rehabil* 90:1068–1073, 2011.
   This review concludes that there is "strong supporting evidence from animal studies about the positive effects of ultrasound on tendon healing. In vitro studies also demonstrate that ultrasound can stimulate cell migration, proliferation, and collagen synthesis of tendon cells that may benefit tendon healing. These positive effects of therapeutic ultrasound on tendon healing revealed by in vivo and in vitro studies help explain the physiologic responses to this physical modality and could serve as the foundation for clinical practice."
2. Fu SC, Shum WT, Hung LK, et al: Low-intensity pulsed ultrasound on tendon healing: a study of the effect of treatment duration and treatment initiation. *Am J Sports Med* 36:1742–1749, 2008.
   This randomized controlled trial compared the effects of LIPUS (1 MHz, 20% duty cycle, 0.15 W/cm^2 for 20 minutes daily) at different time points and for different amounts of time after surgical patellar tendon donor site harvest in 60 rats. The authors found that ultrasound improved the ultimate strength of the tendons and collagen alignment when it was applied for 2 weeks starting the day after surgery but was not effective if applied later or for longer.
3. Geetha K, Hariharan NC, Mohan J: Early ultrasound therapy for rehabilitation after zone II flexor tendon repair. *Indian J Plast Surg* 47:85–91, 2014.

This observational study compared outcomes in 100 patients with 139 digits with zone II flexor tendon repairs. In total, 99 digits in 72 of these patients were treated with pulsed ultrasound, starting 3 to 7 days after surgery, with the dorsal splint in place. The remainder were only immobilized. Excellent to good results were achieved in 72% to 77% of those treated with ultrasound and in only 25% of those treated with immobilization.

Prognosis

Therapeutic ultrasound may be used at this time to promote tendon repair and the development of greater strength in the repaired tendon by nonthermal mechanisms. Therapeutic ultrasound may also promote completion of the inflammation stage of tissue healing and progression to the proliferation and remodeling stages. As the signs of inflammation resolve, thermal-level ultrasound may be used to increase the temperature of the tendon to facilitate stretching and recovery of normal ankle ROM.

Because ultrasound should be used with caution over unclosed epiphyseal plates and because this patient is at an age when epiphyseal closure may or may not be complete, radiographic studies of skeletal maturity should be performed before ultrasound is applied. If studies indicate that the epiphyseal plates are closed, ultrasound may be applied in the usual manner. If studies indicate that the epiphyseal plates are not closed, thermal-level ultrasound should not be used; however, most authors agree that low-level pulsed ultrasound may be used.

Intervention

Ultrasound will be applied over the area of the tendon repair. A frequency of 3 MHz is selected to maximize absorption in the Achilles tendon, which is a superficial structure. For the initial treatment, a 20% pulsed duty cycle is used to avoid increasing the tissue temperature, thereby potentially aggravating the inflammatory reaction, and an intensity of 0.5 W/cm^2 is selected, consistent with studies demonstrating improved tendon repair with this intensity of ultrasound. Because the treatment area probably will be in the range of 5 cm^2, a small sound head with an ERA of 2 to 3 cm^2 should be used. Given this relationship of the sound head ERA to the treatment area, ultrasound should be applied for 5 to 10 minutes. Treatment would generally be applied three to five times per week, depending on the availability of resources and the importance of a rapid functional recovery. In studies demonstrating enhanced tendon healing with the application of therapeutic ultrasound, ultrasound was applied daily; however, treatment three times per week is more consistent with present practice patterns. Because of contouring of this area and its accessibility, treatment may be applied underwater.

When signs of inflammation resolve and it is expected that tendon strength is sufficient to tolerate stretching, ultrasound may be used to increase dorsiflexion ROM. At that time the duty cycle should be increased to 100%, and the intensity may be increased to between 0.5 and 0.75 W/cm^2 to heat the tendon before stretching.

CLINICAL CASE STUDIES—cont'd

Documentation

S: Pt reports L ankle swelling, tenderness, and decreased ROM 3 days after Achilles tendon repair.

O: Pretreatment: Mild swelling, tenderness, erythema over surgical repair site. L calf muscle atrophy (midcalf girth 37 cm L, 42 cm R).

Intervention: US applied to left Achilles tendon underwater × 5 min. Sound head ERA 2 cm². Frequency 3 MHz, 20% pulsed duty cycle, intensity 0.5 W/cm².

Posttreatment: Decreased tenderness over surgical site.

A: Pt tolerated treatment well.

P: Continue treatment as above 5 × weekly for 2 weeks. Initiate stretching with continuous US when cleared by MD.

CASE STUDY 9.3

Wound Healing
Examination
History

JG is an 80-year-old woman with a 10-cm² stage IV infected pressure ulcer over her left greater trochanter. She is bedridden, minimally responsive, and completely dependent on others for feeding and bed mobility as a result of having had three strokes over the past 5 years. She developed the present ulcer 6 months ago after experiencing a loss of appetite because of an upper respiratory infection. JG is turned every 2 hours, avoiding left side lying; has been placed on systemic antibiotics; and is receiving conventional wound care. However, her wound has not improved in the last month. She has been referred to physical therapy with the hope that the addition of other interventions may promote tissue healing.

Systems Review

JG is accompanied to the clinic by her caregiver. The patient is not responsive to questions but appears to be visibly aching from pain in the lower left extremity. Avoidance of contact near the wound has resulted in severely weakened upper left extremity. The function of her upper and lower right extremities, impaired since her last stroke, has not been restored.

Tests and Measures

A stage IV pressure ulcer measuring 3 × 3.5 cm with purulent drainage is seen over her left greater trochanter.

Is this an acute or chronic wound? Is ultrasound a good choice for intervention? Does this patient have any contraindications for the use of ultrasound?

Evaluation and Goals

ICF Level	Current Status	Goals
Body structure and function	Soft tissue ulceration and infection	Resolution of wound infection
	Delayed tissue healing	Decreased wound size
		Wound closure
		Prevention of reulceration

ICF Level	Current Status	Goals
Activity	Decreased strength	Increased strength and mobility
	Limited mobility	
Participation	Dependent on others for moving and eating	Decreased dependence on others for ADLs

ADLs, Activities of daily living; *ICF,* International Classification for Functioning, Disability and Health.

◆ FIND THE EVIDENCE

PICO Terms	Natural Language Example	Sample PubMed Search
P (Population)	Patients with pressure ulcers	("Pressure ulcer*" [MeSH])
I (Intervention)	Ultrasound therapy	AND "Ultrasonic Therapy*" [MeSH] AND English [lang] AND "humans" [MeSH terms]
C (Comparison)	No ultrasound therapy	
O (Outcome)	Reduced size or closure of ulcer	

Key Studies or Reviews

1. Maeshige N, Fujiwara H, Honda H, et al: Evaluation of the combined use of ultrasound irradiation and wound dressing on pressure ulcers. *J Wound Care* 19:63–68, 2010.
   This study in five patients with seven pressure ulcers suggests that ultrasound used alongside conventional wound care may promote healing of pressure ulcers.
2. Baba-Akbari Sari A, Flemming K, Cullum NA, et al: Therapeutic ultrasound for pressure ulcers. Therapeutic ultrasound for pressure ulcers. *Cochrane Database Syst Rev* (3):CD001275, 2006.
   This systematic review found no evidence of benefit of ultrasound in the treatment of pressure ulcers from well-controlled randomized controlled trials but could not rule out a benefit because there were so few trials, some with methodological limitations and small numbers of participants.

Prognosis

Therapeutic ultrasound has been shown in some studies to facilitate the healing of chronic wounds, including pressure ulcers and infected wounds. Because conventional modes of treatment have failed to promote any improvement in wound status over the past month, it is appropriate to consider the addition of adjunctive treatments such as ultrasound or other physical agents to the treatment regimen at this time. The use of ultrasound is not contraindicated in this patient, although thermal-level ultrasound should not be used because the

Continued

patient is minimally responsive and therefore would not be able to report excessive heating by ultrasound.

Intervention

In most studies demonstrating improved healing with the application of ultrasound to chronic wounds, ultrasound was applied to the periwound area alone; therefore, it is recommended that treatment of this patient should focus on the area of intact periwound skin using a gel conduction medium. A frequency of 3 MHz is selected in accordance with research findings regarding the use of ultrasound for wound healing and to maximize absorption in the superficial tissues surrounding the wound. A 20% pulsed duty cycle is used to produce the nonthermal effects of ultrasound while avoiding increased tissue temperature. An intensity of 0.5 to 1.0 W/cm^2 is selected, consistent with studies demonstrating improved wound healing with ultrasound. Because the treatment area is in the range of 10 cm^2, a medium-sized sound head with an ERA of approximately 5 cm^2 should be used. Given this relationship of the sound head ERA to the treatment area, ultrasound should be applied for 5 to 10 minutes, and treatment should

be provided three to five times per week, depending on the availability of resources. Treatment with ultrasound should be continued until the wound closes or progress plateaus. One can expect an approximate 30% reduction in wound size per month. It is important that standard wound care procedures be continued when ultrasound is added to the treatment regimen for a chronic wound.

Documentation

S: Minimally responsive Pt with nonhealing (6 months) pressure ulcer.

O: Pretreatment: 3 × 3.5 cm stage IV ulcer with purulent drainage over L greater trochanter.

Intervention: US to periwound area with gel transmission medium × 5 min. Sound head ERA 5 cm^2. Frequency 3 MHz, 20% pulsed duty cycle, intensity 0.5 W/cm^2.

Posttreatment: Same as before treatment.

A: Pt appeared to be comfortable during US application.

P: Apply US as above 5 × weekly until wound closes or stops healing. Monitor wound size. Continue standard wound care. Coordinate pressure relief with nursing.

Chapter Review

1. Ultrasound is sound with a frequency higher than that audible by the human ear. Ultrasound is a mechanical compression-rarefaction wave that travels through tissue, producing thermal and nonthermal effects.
2. Ultrasound can increase the temperature of deep tissue, particularly tissue with high collagen content; can increase the extensibility of this tissue; and can reduce pain.
3. Ultrasound can increase the permeability of cell membranes by nonthermal mechanisms and thereby facilitate tissue healing and transdermal drug penetration.
4. To achieve intended treatment outcomes, the appropriate ultrasound frequency, intensity, duty cycle, and treatment duration must be selected and applied.
5. Ultrasound should not be applied when it may aggravate an existing pathological condition, such as a malignancy, or when it may burn or otherwise damage tissue.
6. When evaluating an ultrasound device for clinical application, one should consider the appropriateness of the available frequencies, pulsed duty cycles, sizes of sound heads, and BNRs for the types of problems expected to be treated with the device.

Glossary

Absorption: Conversion of the mechanical energy of ultrasound into heat.

Absorption coefficient: The degree to which a material absorbs ultrasound, generally expressed in decibels/cm. Absorption coefficients are tissue and frequency specific and are highest for tissues with the highest collagen content and with higher ultrasound frequencies (see Table 9.4).

Acoustic streaming: The steady, circular flow of cellular fluids induced by ultrasound.

Attenuation: The decrease in ultrasound intensity as ultrasound travels through tissue (see Table 9.1).

Beam nonuniformity ratio (BNR): The ratio of the **spatial peak intensity** to the **spatial average intensity.**

Cavitation: The formation, growth, and pulsation of gas-filled bubbles caused by ultrasound.

Compression: Increase in density of a material as ultrasound waves pass through it.

Continuous ultrasound: Continuous delivery of ultrasound throughout the treatment period.

Duty cycle: The proportion of the total treatment time that the ultrasound is on.

Effective radiating area (ERA): The area of the transducer from which at least 5% of the peak ultrasound intensity radiates.

Frequency: The number of compression-rarefaction cycles per unit of time, expressed in cycles per second, or hertz (Hz).

Half-depth: The depth of tissue at which the ultrasound intensity is half its initial intensity (see Table 9.2).

Intensity: The power per unit area of the sound head, expressed in watts per centimeter squared (W/cm^2).

Microstreaming: Microscale eddying that occurs near any small, vibrating object.

Near field/far field: The near field (the Fresnel zone) is the region closest to the ultrasound transducer where the beam converges and varies in intensity. The far field (the Fraunhofer zone) is the region further from the ultrasound transducer where the beam diverges and is more uniform. Therapeutic ultrasound is generally attenuated within the near field during applications in humans (see Table 9.3).

Phonophoresis: The application of ultrasound with a topical drug to facilitate transdermal drug delivery. Also known as *sonophoresis*.

Piezoelectric: The property of being able to generate electricity in response to a mechanical force or being able to change shape in response to an electrical current (as in an ultrasound transducer).

Power: The amount of acoustic energy per unit time, expressed in watts (W).

Pulsed ultrasound: Intermittent delivery of ultrasound during the treatment period.

Rarefaction: Decrease in density of a material as ultrasound waves pass through it.

Reflection: The redirection of an incident beam away from a surface at an angle equal and opposite to the angle of incidence.

Refraction: The bending or redirection of waves when they pass from one tissue to another.

Spatial average intensity: The average intensity of the ultrasound output over the area of the transducer.

Spatial average temporal average (SATA) intensity: The spatial average intensity of the ultrasound averaged over the on time and the off time of the pulse.

Spatial average temporal peak (SATP) intensity: The spatial average intensity of the ultrasound during the on time of the pulse.

Spatial peak intensity: The peak intensity of the ultrasound output over the area of the transducer.

Standing waves: Intensity maxima and minima at fixed positions one-half wavelength apart that occur when the ultrasound transducer and a reflecting surface are exact multiples of wavelengths apart.

Transducer: A crystal that converts electrical energy into sound; also called **sound head**. This term is also used to describe the part of an ultrasound unit that contains the crystal.

Ultrasound: Sound with a frequency greater than 20,000 cycles per second that, when applied to the body, has thermal and nonthermal effects.

References

1. Jedrzejczak A, Chipchase LS: The availability and usage frequency of real time ultrasound by physiotherapists in South Australia: an observational study. *Physiother Res Int* 13:231–240, 2008.
2. Gluppe SB, Engh ME, Bo K: Immediate effect of abdominal and pelvic floor muscle exercises on interrecti distance in women with diastasis recti abdominis who were parous. [published online ahead of print, 2020 Apr 17]. *Phys Ther*, 2020 pzaa070. doi:10.1093/ptj/pzaa070.
3. Wong RA, Schumann B, Townsend R: A survey of therapeutic ultrasound use by physical therapists who are orthopaedic certified specialists. *Phys Ther* 87:986–994, 2007.
4. de Brito Vieira WH, Aguiar KA, da Silva KM, et al: Overview of ultrasound usage trends in orthopedic and sports physiotherapy. *Crit Ultrasound J* 4(1):11, 2012. doi:10.1186/2036-7902-4-11.
5. Chipchase LS, Williams MT, Robertson VJ: A national study of the availability and use of electrophysical agents by Australian physiotherapists. *Physiother Theory Pract* 25:279–296, 2009.
6. Armijo-Olivo S, Fuentes J, Muir I, et al: Usage patterns and beliefs about therapeutic ultrasound by Canadian physical therapists: an exploratory population-based cross-sectional survey. *Physiother Can* 65(3):289–299, 2013. doi:10.3138/ptc.2012-30BC.
7. MacIntyre NJ, Busse JW, Bhandari M: Physical therapists in primary care are interested in high quality evidence regarding efficacy of therapeutic ultrasound for knee osteoarthritis: a provincial survey. *Scientific World J* 2013, 2013:348014. doi:10.1155/2013/348014.
8. Pye SD, Milford C: The performance of ultrasound physiotherapy machines in Lothian Region, Scotland, 1992. *Ultrasound Med Biol* 20:347–359, 1994.
9. Chapelon JY, Cathignol D, Cain C, et al: New piezoelectric transducers for therapeutic ultrasound. *Ultrasound Med Biol* 26:153–159, 2000.
10. Žauhar G, Radojčić ĐS, Dobravac D, et al: Quantitative testing of physiotherapy ultrasound beam patterns within a clinical environment using a thermochromic tile. *Ultrasonics* 58:6–10, 2015.
11. U.S. Food and Drug Administration: Summary of the ultrasonic therapy performance standard requirements. https://www.fda.gov/media/75884/download. (Accessed July 12, 2020).
12. Hill CR, Ter Haar G: *Ultrasound and non-ionizing radiation protection*, Copenhagen, 1981, World Health Organization.
13. U.S. Food and Drug Administration: 510(k) premarket notification. https://www.accessdata.fda.gov/scripts/cdrh/cfdocs/cfpmn/pmn.cfm?ID=K130978. (Accessed August 15, 2020).
14. U.S. Food and Drug Administration: 510(k) premarket notification. https://www.accessdata.fda.gov/scripts/cdrh/cfdocs/cfpmn/pmn.cfm?ID=K191568. (Accessed August 15, 2020).
15. Draper DO, Klyve D, Ortiz R, et al: Effect of low-intensity long-duration ultrasound on the symptomatic relief of knee osteoarthritis: a randomized, placebo-controlled double-blind study. *J Orthop Surg Res* 13(1):257, 2018.
16. Atkins TJ, Duck FA: Heating caused by selected pulsed Doppler and physiotherapy ultrasound beams measured using thermal test objects. *Eur J Ultrasound* 16:243–252, 2003.
17. Acevedo B, Millis DL, Levine D, et al: Effect of therapeutic ultrasound on calcaneal tendon heating and extensibility in dogs. *Front Vet Sci* 6:185, 2019.
18. Harvey EN: Biological aspects of ultrasonic waves: a general survey. *Biol Bull* 59:306–325, 1930.
19. Morishita K, Karasuno H, Yokoi Y, et al: Effects of therapeutic ultrasound on intramuscular blood circulation and oxygen dynamics. *J Jpn Phys Ther Assoc* 17:1–7, 2014.
20. Lehmann JF, DeLateur BJ, Stonebridge JB, et al: Therapeutic temperature distribution produced by ultrasound as modified by dosage and volume of tissue exposed. *Arch Phys Med Rehabil* 48:662–666, 1967.
21. Lehmann JF, DeLateur BJ, Warren G, et al: Bone and soft tissue heating produced by ultrasound. *Arch Phys Med Rehabil* 48:397–401, 1967.
22. Smith K, Draper DO, Schulthies SS, et al: The effect of silicate gel hot packs on human muscle temperature. *J Athl Train* 30:S33, 1995.
23. Weaver SL, Demchak TJ, Stone MB, et al: Effect of transducer velocity on intramuscular temperature during a 1-MHz ultrasound treatment. *J Orthop Sports Phys Ther* 36:320–325, 2006.
24. Nyborg WN, Ziskin MC: Biological effects of ultrasound. *Clin Diagn Ultrasound* 16:24, 1985.
25. Hayes BT, Merrick MA, Sandrey MA, et al: Three-MHz ultrasound heats deeper into the tissues than originally theorized. *J Athl Train* 39:230–234, 2004.
26. Ohwatashi A, Ikeda S, Harada K, et al: Temperature changes caused by the difference in the distance between the ultrasound transducer and bone during 1 MHz and 3 MHz continuous ultrasound: a phantom study. *J Phys Ther Sci* 27:205–208, 2015.
27. Draper DO, Castel JC, Castel D: Rate of temperature increase in human muscle during 1 MHz and 3 MHz continuous ultrasound. *J Orthop Sports Phys Ther* 22:142–150, 1995.
28. Gallo JA, Draper DO, Brody LT, Fellingham GW: A comparison of human muscle temperature increases during 3-MHz continuous and pulsed ultrasound with equivalent temporal average intensities. *J Orthop Sports Phys Ther* 34(7):395–401, 2004. doi:10.2519/jospt.2004.34.7.395.
29. Levine D, Mills DL, Mynatt T: Effects of 3.3-MHz ultrasound on caudal thigh muscle temperature in dogs. *Vet Surg* 30:170–174, 2001.
30. Rigby JH, Taggart RM, Stratton KL, et al: Intramuscular heating characteristics of multihour low-intensity therapeutic ultrasound. *J Athl Train* 50(11):1158–1164, 2015.
31. Darlas Y, Solasson A, Clouard R, et al: Ultrasonothérapie: calcul de la thermogenèse. *Ann Readapt Med Phys* 32:181–192, 1989.
32. TerHaar G: Basic physics of therapeutic ultrasound. *Physiotherapy* 64:100–103, 1978.

33. Merrick MA, Bernard KD, Devor ST, et al: Identical 3-MHz ultrasound treatments with different devices produce different intramuscular temperatures. *J Orthop Sports Phys Ther* 33:379–385, 2003.

34. Johns LD, Demchak TJ, Straub SJ, et al: The role of quantitative Schlieren assessment of physiotherapy ultrasound fields in describing variations between tissue heating rates of different transducers. *Ultrasound Med Biol* 33:1911–1917, 2007.

35. Holcomb WR, Joyce CJ: A comparison of temperature increases produced by 2 commonly used ultrasound units. *J Athl Train* 38:24–27, 2003.

36. Lehmann JF, Stonebridge JB, DeLateur BJ, et al: Temperatures in human thighs after hot pack treatment followed by ultrasound. *Arch Phys Med Rehabil* 59:472–475, 1978.

37. Draper DO, Schulties S, Sorvisto P, et al: Temperature changes in deep muscle of humans during ice and ultrasound therapies: an in vivo study. *J Orthop Sports Phys Ther* 21:153–157, 1995.

38. Oshikoya CA, Shultz SJ, Mistry D, et al: Effect of coupling medium temperature on rate of intramuscular temperature rise using continuous ultrasound. *J Athl Train* 35:417–421, 2000.

39. Kurtais Gursel Y, Ulus Y, Bilgic A, et al: Adding ultrasound in the management of soft tissue disorders of the shoulder: a randomized placebo-controlled trial. *Phys Ther* 84:336–343, 2004.

40. Goodman CE, Al-Karmi AM, Joyce JM, et al: The biological effects of therapeutic ultrasound: frequency dependence. *Proceedings of the 14th annual meeting of the society for physical regulation in biology and medicine*, Washington, DC, 1994, Society for Physical Regulation in Biology and Medicine.

41. Kramer JF: Ultrasound: evaluation of its mechanical and thermal effects. *Arch Phys Med Rehabil* 65:223–227, 1984.

42. Mortimer AJ, Dyson M: The effect of therapeutic ultrasound on calcium uptake in fibroblasts. *Ultrasound Med Biol* 14:499–506, 1988.

43. Peruzzi G, Sinibaldi G, Silvani G, et al: Perspectives on cavitation enhanced endothelial layer permeability. *Colloids Surf B Biointerfaces* 168:83–93, 2018. doi:10.1016/j.colsurfb.2018.02.027.

44. Fyfe MC, Chahl LA: Mast cell degranulation: a possible mechanism of action of therapeutic ultrasound. *Ultrasound Med Biol* 8(Suppl 1):62, 1982.

45. Young SR, Dyson M: Macrophage responsiveness to therapeutic ultrasound. *Ultrasound Med Biol* 16:809–816, 1990.

46. Harvey W, Dyson M, Pond JB, et al: The stimulation of protein synthesis in human fibroblasts by therapeutic ultrasound. *Rheumatol Rehabil* 14:237, 1975.

47. Tsai WC, Pang JH, Hsu CC, et al: Ultrasound stimulation of types I and III collagen expression of tendon cell and upregulation of transforming growth factor beta. *J Orthop Res* 24:1310–1316, 2006.

48. Kopakkala-Tani M, Karjalainen HM, Karjalainen T, et al: Ultrasound stimulates proteoglycan synthesis in bovine primary chondrocytes. *Biorheology* 43:271–282, 2006.

49. Miyamoto K, An HS, Sah RL, et al: Exposure to pulsed low intensity ultrasound stimulates extracellular matrix metabolism of bovine intervertebral disc cells cultured in alginate beads. *Spine* 30:2398–2405, 2005.

50. Choi BH, Woo JI, Min BH, et al: Low-intensity ultrasound stimulates the viability and matrix gene expression of human articular chondrocytes in alginate bead culture. *J Biomed Mater Res A* 79:858–864, 2006.

51. Min BH, Woo JI, Cho HS: Effects of low-intensity ultrasound (LIUS) stimulation on human cartilage explants. *Scand J Rheumatol* 35:305–311, 2006.

52. Altland OD, Dalecki D, Suchkova VN, et al: Low-intensity ultrasound increases endothelial cell nitric oxide synthase activity and nitric oxide synthesis. *J Thromb Haemost* 2:637–643, 2004.

53. Hsu SH, Huang TB: Bioeffect of ultrasound on endothelial cells in vitro. *Biomol Eng* 21:99–104, 2004.

54. Rawool NM, Goldberg BB, Forsberg F, et al: Power Doppler assessment of vascular changes during fracture treatment with low-intensity ultrasound. *J Ultrasound Med* 22:145–153, 2003.

55. Barzelai S, Sharabani-Yosef O, Holbova R, et al: Low-intensity ultrasound induces angiogenesis in rat hind-limb ischemia. *Ultrasound Med Biol* 32:139–145, 2006.

56. Parvizi J, Parpura V, Greenleaf JF, et al: Calcium signaling is required for ultrasound-stimulated aggrecan synthesis by rat chondrocytes. *J Orthop Res* 20:51–57, 2002.

57. Morishita K, Karasuno H, Yokoi Y, et al: Effects of therapeutic ultrasound on range of motion and stretch pain. *J Phys Ther Sci* 26:711–715, 2014.

58. Nakano J, Yamabayashi C, Scott A, et al: The effect of heat applied with stretch to increase range of motion: a systematic review. *Phys Ther Sport* 13:180–188, 2012.

59. Petrofsky JS, Laymon M, Lee H: Effect of heat and cold on tendon flexibility and force to flex the human knee. *Med Sci Monit* 19:661–667, 2013.

60. Lehmann JF: Clinical evaluation of a new approach in the treatment of contracture associated with hip fracture after internal fixation. *Arch Phys Med Rehabil* 42:95–100, 1961.

61. Wessling KC, DeVane DA, Hylton CR: Effects of static stretch versus static stretch and ultrasound combined on triceps surae muscle extensibility in healthy women. *Phys Ther* 67:674–679, 1987.

62. Reed BV, Ashikaga T, Fleming BC, et al: Effects of ultrasound and stretch on knee ligament extensibility. *J Orthop Sports Phys Ther* 30:341–347, 2000.

63. Hsieh YL: Reduction in induced pain by ultrasound may be caused by altered expression of spinal neuronal nitric oxide synthase-producing neurons. *Arch Phys Med Rehabil* 86:1311–1317, 2005.

64. Hsieh YL: Effects of ultrasound and diclofenac phonophoresis on inflammatory pain relief: suppression of inducible nitric oxide synthase in arthritic rats. *Phys Ther* 86:39–49, 2006.

65. Middlemast S, Chatterjee DS: Comparison of ultrasound and thermotherapy for soft tissue injuries. *Physiotherapy* 64:331–332, 1978.

66. Nwuge VCB: Ultrasound in treatment of back pain resulting from prolapsed disc. *Arch Phys Med Rehabil* 64:88–89, 1983.

67. Munting E: Ultrasonic therapy for painful shoulders. *Physiotherapy* 64:180–181, 1978.

68. Robinson V, Brosseau L, Casimiro L, et al: Thermotherapy for treating rheumatoid arthritis. *Cochrane Database Syst Rev* 2012(2):CD002826, 2002.

69. Petterson S, Plancher K, Klyve D, et al: Low-intensity continuous ultrasound for the symptomatic treatment of upper shoulder and neck pain: a randomized, double-blind placebo-controlled clinical trial [published correction appears in *J Pain Res* Jul 27;13:1899–1900, 2020]. *J Pain Res* 13:1277–1287, 2020.

70. Flemming K, Cullum H: Therapeutic ultrasound for pressure sores. *Cochrane Database Syst Rev* 2000(4):CD001275, 2000.

71. Taradaj J, Franek A, Brzezinska-Wcislo L, et al: The use of therapeutic ultrasound in venous leg ulcers: a randomized, controlled clinical trial. *Phlebology* 23:178–183, 2008.

72. Cullum N, Liu Z: Therapeutic ultrasound for venous leg ulcers. *Cochrane Database Syst Rev* 2017(5):CD001180, 2017. doi:10.1002/14651858.CD001180.pub4.

73. Best TM, Wilk KE, Moorman CT, et al: Low intensity ultrasound for promoting soft tissue healing: a systematic review of the literature and medical technology. *Intern Med Rev (Wash DC)* 2(11):271, 2016.

74. Daniels S, Santiago G, Cuchna J, et al: The effects of low-intensity therapeutic ultrasound on measurable outcomes: a critically appraised topic. *J Sport Rehabil* 27(4):390–395, 2018.

75. Dyson M, Suckling J: Stimulation of tissue repair by ultrasound: survey of the mechanisms involved. *Physiotherapy* 63:105–108, 1978.

76. McDiarmid T, Burns PN, Lewith GT, et al: Ultrasound and the treatment of pressure sores. *Physiotherapy* 71:66–70, 1985.

77. Lundeberg T, Nordstrom F, Brodda-Jansen G, et al: Pulsed ultrasound does not improve healing of venous ulcers. *Scand J Rehabil Med* 22:195–197, 1990.

78. Eriksson SV, Lundeberg T, Malm M: A placebo-controlled trial of ultrasound therapy in chronic leg ulceration. *Scand J Rehabil Med* 23:211–213, 1991.

79. TerRiet G, Kessels AGH, Knipschild P: A randomized clinical trial of ultrasound in the treatment of pressure ulcers. *Phys Ther* 76:1301–1312, 1996.

80. Markert CD, Merrick MA, Kirby TE, et al: Nonthermal ultrasound and exercise in skeletal muscle regeneration. *Arch Phys Med Rehabil* 86:1304–1310, 2005.

81. Watson JM, Kang'ombe AR, Soares MO, et al: Use of weekly, low dose, high frequency ultrasound for hard to heal venous leg ulcers: the VenUS III randomised controlled trial. *BMJ* 342:d1092, 2011.

82. Samuels JA, Weingarten MS, Margolis DJ, et al: Low-frequency (<100 kHz), low-intensity (<100 mW/cm^2) ultrasound to treat venous ulcers: a human study and in vitro experiments. *J Acoust Soc Am* 134:1541–1547, 2013.

83. Beheshti A, Shafigh Y, Parsa H, et al: Comparison of high-frequency and MIST ultrasound therapy for the healing of venous leg ulcers. *Adv Clin Exp Med* 23:969–975, 2014.
84. Ennis WJ, Valdes W, Gainer M, et al: Evaluation of clinical effectiveness of MIST ultrasound therapy for the healing of chronic wounds. *Adv Skin Wound Care* 19:437–446, 2006.
85. Ennis WJ, Foreman P, Mozen N, et al: Ultrasound therapy for recalcitrant diabetic foot ulcers: results of a randomized, double-blind, controlled, multicenter study. *Ostomy Wound Manage* 51:24–39, 2005.
86. Kavros SJ, Miller JL, Hanna SW: Treatment of ischemic wounds with noncontact, low-frequency ultrasound: the Mayo Clinic experience, 2004–2006. *Adv Skin Wound Care* 20:221–226, 2007.
87. Maher SF, Halverson J, Misiewicz R, et al: Low-frequency ultrasound for patients with lower leg ulcers due to chronic venous insufficiency: a report of two cases. *Ostomy Wound Manage* 60:52–61, 2014.
88. Honaker JS, Forston MR, Davis EA, et al: Effects of non-contact low-frequency ultrasound on healing of suspected deep tissue injury: a retrospective analysis. *Int Wound J* 10:65–72, 2013.
89. Young SR, Dyson M: The effect of therapeutic ultrasound on angiogenesis. *Ultrasound Med Biol* 16:261–269, 1990.
90. Jeffers AM, Maxson PM, Thompson SL, et al: Combined negative pressure wound therapy and ultrasonic MIST therapy for open surgical wounds: a case series. *J Wound Ostomy Continence Nurs* 41:181–186, 2014.
91. Fieldhouse C: Ultrasound for relief of painful episiotomy scars. *Physiotherapy* 65:217, 1979.
92. Enwemeka CS: The effects of therapeutic ultrasound on tendon healing. *Am J Phys Med Rehabil* 6:283–287, 1989.
93. Enwemeka CS, Rodriguez O, Mendosa S: The biomechanical effects of low intensity ultrasound on healing tendons. *Ultrasound Med Biol* 16:801–807, 1990.
94. Frieder SJ, Weisberg B, Fleming B, et al: A pilot study: the therapeutic effect of ultrasound following partial rupture of Achilles tendons in male rats. *J Orthop Sports Phys Ther* 10:39–46, 1988.
95. Jackson BA, Schwane JA, Starcher BC: Effect of ultrasound therapy on the repair of Achilles tendon injuries in rats. *Med Sci Sports Exerc* 23:171–176, 1991.
96. Ng GY, Ng CO, See EK: Comparison of therapeutic ultrasound and exercises for augmenting tendon healing in rats. *Ultrasound Med Biol* 30:1539–1543, 2004.
97. Yeung CK, Guo X, Ng YF: Pulsed ultrasound treatment accelerates the repair of Achilles tendon rupture in rats. *J Orthop Res* 24:193–201, 2006.
98. da Cunha A, Parizotto NA, Vidal Bde C: The effect of therapeutic ultrasound on repair of the Achilles tendon (tendo calcaneus) of the rat. *Ultrasound Med Biol* 27:1691–1696, 2001.
99. Fu SC, Shum WT, Hung LK, et al: Low-intensity pulsed ultrasound on tendon healing: a study of the effect of treatment duration and treatment initiation. *Am J Sports Med* 36(9):1742–1749, 2008.
100. Roberts M, Rutherford JH, Harris D: The effect of ultrasound on flexor tendon repairs in rabbits. *Hand* 14:17–20, 1982.
101. Geetha K, Hariharan NC, Mohan J: Early ultrasound therapy for rehabilitation after zone II flexor tendon repair. *Indian J Plast Surg* 47(1):85–91, 2014.
102. Dvaz AP, Ostor AJK, Speed CA, et al: Pulsed low-intensity ultrasound therapy for chronic lateral epicondylitis: a randomized controlled trial. *Rheumatology* 45:566–670, 2006.
103. Warden SJ, Metcalf BR, Kiss ZS, et al: Low-intensity pulsed ultrasound for chronic patellar tendinopathy: a randomized, double blind, placebo-controlled trial. *Rheumatol Int* 47:467–471, 2008.
104. Smidt N, Assendelft WJ, Arola H, et al: Effectiveness of physiotherapy for lateral epicondylitis: a systematic review. *Ann Med* 35(1):51–62, 2003.
105. Dingemanse R, Randsdorp M, Koes BW, et al: Evidence for the effectiveness of electrophysical modalities for treatment of medial and lateral epicondylitis: a systematic review. *Br J Sports Med* 48:957–965, 2014.
106. Binder A, Hodge G, Greenwood AM, et al: Is therapeutic ultrasound effective in treating soft tissue lesions? *Br Med J* 290:512–514, 1985.
107. Lundeberg T, Abrahamsson P, Haker E: A comparative study of continuous ultrasound, placebo ultrasound and rest in epicondylalgia. *Scand J Rehabil Med* 20:99–101, 1988.
108. Haker E, Lundeberg T: Pulsed ultrasound treatment in lateral epicondylitis. *Scand J Rehabil Med* 23:115–118, 1991.
109. Ebenbichler GR, Erdogmus CB, Resch KL, et al: Ultrasound therapy for calcific tendinitis of the shoulder. *N Engl J Med* 340:1533–1538, 1999.
110. Sparrow KJ, Finucane SD, Owen JR, et al: The effects of low-intensity ultrasound on medial collateral ligament healing in the rabbit model. *Am J Sports Med* 33:1048–1056, 2005.
111. Warden SJ, Avin GA, Beck EM, et al: Low-intensity pulsed ultrasound accelerates and a nonsteroidal anti-inflammatory drug delays knee ligament healing. *Am J Sports Med* 34:1094–1102, 2006.
112. Leung MC, Ng GY, Yip KK: Effect of ultrasound on acute inflammation of transected medial collateral ligaments. *Arch Phys Med Rehabil* 85:963–966, 2004.
113. Rutjes AW, Nuesch F, Sterchi R, Juni P: Therapeutic ultrasound for osteoarthritis of the knee or hip. *Cochrane Database Syst Rev* 2010(1):CD003132, 2010.
114. Zeng C, Li H, Yang T, et al: Effectiveness of continuous and pulsed ultrasound for the management of knee osteoarthritis: a systematic review and network meta-analysis. *Osteoarthr Cartil* 22(8):1090–1099, 2014.
115. Zhang C, Xie Y, Luo X, et al: Effects of therapeutic ultrasound on pain, physical functions and safety outcomes in patients with knee osteoarthritis: a systematic review and meta-analysis. *Clin Rehabil* 30(10):960–971, 2016.
116. Griffin J, Karselis T: *Physical agents for physical therapists*, Springfield, IL, 1982, Charles C Thomas.
117. Hecox B, Mehreteab TA, Weisberg J: *Physical agents: a comprehensive text for physical therapists*, East Norwalk, CT, 1994, Appleton & Lange.
118. Cheng M, Li F, Han T, et al: Effects of ultrasound pulse parameters on cavitation properties of flowing microbubbles under physiologically relevant conditions. *Ultrason Sonochem* 52:512–521, 2019. doi:10.1016/j.ultsonch.2018.12.031.
119. Busse JW, Bhandari M: Therapeutic ultrasound and fracture healing: a survey of beliefs and practices. *Arch Phys Med Rehabil* 85:1653–1656, 2004.
120. Rutten S, van den Bekerom MP, Sierevelt IN, et al: Enhancement of bone-healing by low-intensity pulsed ultrasound: a systematic review. *JBJS Rev* 4(3):01874474-201603000-00006, 2016.
121. Busse JW, Morton E, Lacchetti C, et al: Current management of tibial shaft fractures: a survey of 450 Canadian orthopedic trauma surgeons. *Acta Orthop* 79:689–694, 2008.
122. Bawale R, Segmeister M, Sinha S, et al: Experience of an isolated use of low-intensity pulsed ultrasound therapy on fracture healing in established non-unions: a prospective case series [published online ahead of print, 2020 Apr 30]. *J Ultrasound*, 2020. doi:10.1007/s40477-020-00464-9.
123. Gopalan A, Panneerselvam E, Doss GT, et al: Evaluation of efficacy of low intensity pulsed ultrasound in facilitating mandibular fracture healing—a blinded randomized controlled clinical trial. *J Oral Maxillofac Surg* 78(6):997. e1–997.e7, 2020. doi:10.1016/j.joms.2020.01.036.
124. National Institute for Health and Care Excellence: Low-intensity pulsed ultrasound to promote fracture healing (Interventional Procedure Guidance 374). 2010. http://www.nice.org.uk/guidance/ipg374. (Accessed August 16, 2020).
125. Higgins A, Glover M, Yang Y, et al: EXOGEN ultrasound bone healing system for long bone fractures with non-union or delayed healing: a NICE medical technology guidance. *Appl Health Econ Health Policy* 12(5):477–484, 2014. doi:10.1007/s40258-014-0117-6.
126. Schandelmaier S, Kaushal A, Lytvyn L, et al: Low intensity pulsed ultrasound for bone healing: systematic review of randomized controlled trials. *BMJ* 356:j656, 2017. doi:10.1136/bmj.j656.
127. Poolman RW, Agoritsas T, Siemieniuk RA, et al: Low intensity pulsed ultrasound (LIPUS) for bone healing: a clinical practice guideline. *BMJ* 356:j576, 2017. doi:10.1136/bmj.j576.
128. National Institute for Health and Care Excellence: Low-intensity pulsed ultrasound to promote healing of fresh fractures at low risk of non-healing (Interventional Procedures Guidance IPG621). https://www.nice.org.uk/guidance/ipg621/chapter/1-Recommendations. (Accessed August 16, 2020).
129. National Institute for Health and Care Excellence: Low-intensity pulsed ultrasound to promote healing of fresh fractures at high risk of non-healing (Interventional Procedures Guidance IPG622). https://www.nice.org.uk/guidance/ipg622/chapter/1-Recommendations. (Accessed August 16, 2020).

130. National Institute for Health and Care Excellence: Low-intensity pulsed ultrasound to promote healing of delayed-union and non-union fractures (Interventional Procedures Guidance IPG623). https://www.nice.org.uk/guidance/ipg623/chapter/1-Recommendations. (Accessed August 16, 2020).

131. Nicholson JA, Tsang STJ, MacGillivray TJ, et al: What is the role of ultrasound in fracture management? Diagnosis and therapeutic potential for fractures, delayed unions, and fracture-related infection. *Bone Joint Res* 8(7):304–312, 2019. doi:10.1302/2046-3758.87.BJR-2018-0215.R2.

132. Herrick JF: Temperatures produced in tissues by ultrasound: experimental study using various technics. *J Acoust Soc Am* 25:12–16, 1953.

133. Oztas O, Turan B, Bora I, et al: Ultrasound therapy effect in carpal tunnel syndrome. *Arch Phys Med Rehabil* 79:1540–1544, 1988.

134. Huisstede BM, Hoogvliet P, Randsdorp MS, et al: Carpal tunnel syndrome. Part I: effectiveness of nonsurgical treatments—a systematic review. *Arch Phys Med Rehabil* 91:981–1004, 2010.

135. Huisstede BM, Hoogvliet P, Franke TP, et al: Carpal tunnel syndrome: effectiveness of physical therapy and electrophysical modalities. an updated systematic review of randomized controlled trials. *Arch Phys Med Rehabil* 99(8):1623–1634, 2018. doi:10.1016/j.apmr.2017.08.482. e23.

136. Ebenbichler GR, Resch KL, Nicolakis P, et al: Ultrasound treatment for treating the carpal tunnel syndrome: randomised "sham" controlled trial. *BMJ* 316:731–735, 1998.

137. Chang YW, Hsieh SF, Horng YS, et al: Comparative effectiveness of ultrasound and paraffin therapy in patients with carpal tunnel syndrome: a randomized trial. *BMC Musculoskelet Disord* 15:399, 2014.

138. Piravej K, Boonhong J: Effect of ultrasound thermotherapy in mild to moderate carpal tunnel syndrome. *J Med Assoc Thai* 87(Suppl 2):S100–S106, 2004.

139. Ito A, Wang T, Nakahara R, et al: Ultrasound therapy with optimal intensity facilitates peripheral nerve regeneration in rats through suppression of pro-inflammatory and nerve growth inhibitor gene expression. *PLoS One* 15(6):e0234691, 2020.

140. Seah BC, Teo BM: Recent advances in ultrasound-based transdermal drug delivery. *Int J Nanomedicine* 13:7749–7763, 2018. doi:10.2147/IJN.S174759.

141. Fellinger K, Schmid J: *Klinik und therapie des chronischen gelenkrheumatismus,* Vienna, 1954, Maudrich.

142. Griffin JE, Touchstone JC: Ultrasonic movement of cortisol into pig tissues. I: movement into skeletal muscle. *Am J Phys Med* 42:77–85, 1963.

143. Griffin JE, Touchstone JC, Liu ACY: Ultrasonic movement of cortisol into pig tissues. II: movement into paravertebral nerve. *Am J Phys Med* 44:20–25, 1965.

144. Griffin JE, Touchstone JC: Low intensity phonophoresis of cortisol in swine. *Phys Ther* 48:1336–1344, 1968.

145. Griffin JE, Touchstone JC: Effects of ultrasonic frequency on phonophoresis of cortisol into swine tissues. *Am J Phys Med* 51:62–78, 1972.

146. Oberli MA, Schoellhammer CM, Langer R, et al: Ultrasound-enhanced transdermal delivery: recent advances and future challenges. *Ther Deliv* 5(7):843–857, 2014. doi:10.4155/tde.14.32.

147. Wong TW: Electrical, magnetic, photomechanical and cavitational waves to overcome skin barrier for transdermal drug delivery. *J Control Release* 193:257–269, 2014.

148. Bommannan D, Okuyama H, Stauffer P, et al: Sonophoresis. I: the use of high frequency ultrasound to enhance transdermal drug delivery. *Pharm Res* 9:559–564, 1992.

149. Rosim GC, Barbieri CH, Lanças FM, et al: Diclofenac phonophoresis in human volunteers. *Ultrasound Med Biol* 31:337–343, 2005.

150. Ita K: Recent progress in transdermal sonophoresis. *Pharm Dev Technol* 22(4):458–466, 2017.

151. Bakhtiary AH, Fatemi E, Emami M, et al: Phonophoresis of dexamethasone sodium phosphate may manage pain and symptoms of patients with carpal tunnel syndrome. *Clin J Pain* 29:348–353, 2013.

152. Said Ahmed MA, Saweeres ESB, Abdelkader NA, et al: Improved pain and function in knee osteoarthritis with dexamethasone phonophoresis: a randomized controlled trial. *Indian J Orthop* 53(6):700–707, 2019. doi:10.4103/ortho.IJOrtho_639_18.

153. Franklin ME, Smith ST, Chenier TC, et al: Effect of phonophoresis with dexamethasone on adrenal function. *J Orthop Sports Phys Ther* 22:103–107, 1995.

154. Luksurapan W, Boonhong J: Effects of phonophoresis of piroxicam and ultrasound on symptomatic knee osteoarthritis. *Arch Phys Med Rehabil* 94:250–255, 2013.

155. Yildiz N, Atalay NS, Gungen GO, et al: Comparison of ultrasound and ketoprofen phonophoresis in the treatment of carpal tunnel syndrome. *J Back Musculoskelet Rehabil* 24:39–47, 2011.

156. Soyupek F, Yesildag A, Kutluhan S, et al: Determining the effectiveness of various treatment modalities in carpal tunnel syndrome by ultrasonography and comparing ultrasonographic findings with other outcomes. *Rheumatol Int* 32:3229–3234, 2012.

157. Cameron MH, Monroe LG: Relative transmission of ultrasound by media customarily used for phonophoresis. *Phys Ther* 72(2):142–148, 1992.

158. Cage SA, Rupp KA, Castel JC, et al: Relative acoustic transmission of topical preparations used with therapeutic ultrasound. *Arch Phys Med Rehabil* 94(11):2126–2130, 2013.

159. Ebrahimi S, Abbasnia K, Motealleh A, et al: Effect of lidocaine phonophoresis on sensory blockade: pulsed or continuous mode of therapeutic ultrasound? *Physiotherapy* 98:57–63, 2012.

160. Masterson J, Kluge B, Burdette A, Lewis G, Sr: Sustained acoustic medicine; sonophoresis for nonsteroidal anti-inflammatory drug delivery in arthritis. *Ther Deliv* 11(6):363–372, 2020. doi:10.4155/tde-2020-0009.

161. Andrade PC, Flores GP, Uscello Jde F, et al: Use of iontophoresis or phonophoresis for delivering onabotulinumtoxin A in the treatment of palmar hyperhidrosis: a report on four cases. *An Bras Dermatol* 86:1243–1246, 2011.

162. Feiszthuber H, Bhatnagar S, Gyöngy M, et al: Cavitation-enhanced delivery of insulin in agar and porcine models of human skin. *Phys Med Biol* 60(6):2421–2434, 2015.

163. Jabbari N, Asghari MH, Ahmadian H, et al: Developing a commercial air ultrasonic ceramic transducer to transdermal insulin delivery. *J Med Signals Sens* 5(2):117–122, 2015.

164. Yu ZW, Liang Y, Liang WQ: Low-frequency sonophoresis enhances rivastigmine permeation in vitro and in vivo. *Pharmazie* 70(6):379–380, 2015.

165. Pereira TA, Ramos DN, Lopez RF: Hydrogel increases localized transport regions and skin permeability during low frequency ultrasound treatment. *Sci Rep* 7:44236, 2017.

166. Smith NB, Lee S, Malone E, et al: Ultrasound-mediated transdermal transport of insulin in vitro through human skin using novel transducer designs. *Ultrasound Med Biol* 29:311–317, 2003.

167. Chuang H, Taylor E, Davison TW: Clinical evaluation of a continuous minimally invasive glucose flux sensor placed over ultrasonically permeated skin. *Diabetes Technol Ther* 6:21–30, 2004.

168. Miller DL, Smith NB, Bailey MR, et al: Overview of therapeutic ultrasound applications and safety considerations. *J Ultrasound Med* 31:623–634, 2012.

169. Electrophysical agents—contraindications and precautions: an evidence-based approach to clinical decision making in physical therapy. *Physiother Can* 62(5):1–80, 2010.

170. Batavia M: Contraindications for superficial heat and therapeutic ultrasound: do sources agree? *Arch Phys Med Rehabil* 85:1006–1012, 2004.

171. Sicard-Rosenbaum L, Lord D, Danoff JV, et al: Effects of continuous therapeutic ultrasound on growth and metastasis of subcutaneous murine tumors. *Phys Ther* 75:3–11, 1995.

172. Kok HP, Cressman ENK, Ceelen W, et al: Heating technology for malignant tumors: a review. *Int J Hyperthermia* 37(1):711–741, 2020.

173. Shista K: Neural tube defects and maternal hyperthermia in early pregnancy: epidemiology in a human embryo population. *Am J Med Genet* 12:281–288, 1982.

174. Kalter H, Warkany J: Congenital malformations: etiological factors and their role in prevention. *N Engl J Med* 308:424–431, 1983.

175. McLeod DR, Fowlow SB: Multiple malformations and exposure to therapeutic ultrasound during organogenesis. *Am J Med Genet* 34:317–319, 1989.

176. Ang ES, Jr Gluncic V, Duque A, et al: Prenatal exposure to ultrasound waves impacts neuronal migration in mice. *Proc Natl Acad Sci USA* 103:12903–12910, 2006.

177. Carstensen EL, Gates AH: The effects of pulsed ultrasound on the fetus. *J Ultrasound Med* 3:145–147, 1984.

178. National Council of Radiation Protection and Measurements: *Biological effects of ultrasound: mechanisms and clinical implications*, Bethesda, MD, 1983, The Council. NCRP Report No. 74.

179. Normand H, Darlas Y, Solassol A, et al: Etude expérimentale de l'effet thermique des ultrasons sur le matériel prothétique. *Ann Readapt Med Phys* 32:193–201, 1989.
180. Skoubo-Kristensen E, Sommer J: Ultrasound influence on internal fixation with rigid plate in dogs. *Arch Phys Med Rehabil* 63:371–373, 1982.
181. Deforest RE, Herrick JF, Janes JM: Effects of ultrasound on growing bone: an experimental study. *Arch Phys Med Rehabil* 34:21, 1953.
182. Lyon R, Liu XC, Meier J: The effects of therapeutic vs. high-intensity ultrasound on the rabbit growth plate. *J Orthop Res* 21:865–871, 2003.
183. Spadaro JA, Skarulis T, Albanese SA: Effect of pulsed ultrasound on bone growth in rats. *Trans Meet Soc Phys Reg Biol Med* 14:10, 1994.
184. Spadaro JA, Albanese SA: Application of low-intensity ultrasound to growing bone in rats. *Ultrasound Med Biol* 24:567–573, 1998.
185. Ogurtan Z, Celik I, Izci C, et al: Effect of experimental therapeutic ultrasound on the distal antebrachial growth plates in one-month-old rabbits. *Vet J* 164:280–287, 2002.
186. Ota T, Itoh S, Yamashita K: The efficacy and safety of combination therapy of low-intensity pulsed ultrasound stimulation in the treatment of unstable both radius and ulna fractures in children. *Biomed Mater Eng* 28(5):545–553, 2017. doi:10.3233/BME-171697.
187. Nyborg WL: Biological effects of ultrasound: development of safety guidelines. II: general review. *Ultrasound Med Biol* 27:301–333, 2001.
188. Dyson M, Pond JB, Woodward B, et al: The production of blood cell stasis and endothelial damage in blood vessels of chick embryos treated with ultrasound in a stationary wave field. *Ultrasound Med Biol* 63:133–138, 1974.
189. TerHaar GR, Dyson M, Smith SP: Ultrastructural changes in the mouse uterus brought about by ultrasonic irradiation at therapeutic intensities in standing wave fields. *Ultrasound Med Biol* 5:167–179, 1979.
190. Schabrun S, Chipchase L, Rickard H: Are therapeutic ultrasound units a potential vector for nosocomial infection? *Physiother Res Int* 11:61–71, 2006.
191. Spratt HG, Jr, Levine D, Tillman L: Physical therapy clinic therapeutic ultrasound equipment as a source for bacterial contamination. *Physiother Theory Pract* 30:507–511, 2014.
192. Ferguson HN: Ultrasound in the treatment of surgical wounds. *Physiotherapy* 67:43, 1981.
193. Liceralde P: *The effects of ultrasound transducer velocity on intramuscular tissue temperature across a treatment site*, Las Vegas, 2009, University of Nevada. Master's thesis.
194. Johns LD, Straub SJ, Howard SM: Variability in effective radiating area and output power of new ultrasound transducers at 3 MHz. *J Athl Train* 42(1):22–28, 2007.
195. Rivest M, Quirion-de Girardi C, Seaborne D, et al: Evaluation of therapeutic ultrasound devices: performance stability over 44 weeks of clinical use. *Physiother Can* 39(2):77–86, 1987.
196. Ferrari CB, Andrade MA, Adamowski JC, et al: Evaluation of therapeutic ultrasound equipment performance. *Ultrasonics* 50(7):704–709, 2010.
197. Shaw A, Hodnett M: Calibration and measurement issues for therapeutic ultrasound. *Ultrasonics* 48(4):234–252, 2008.

Diathermy

CHAPTER OBJECTIVES

After reading this chapter, the reader will be able to do the following:
- Define diathermy.
- Describe effects of diathermy.
- Compare and contrast thermal and nonthermal diathermy.
- Safely and effectively apply thermal and nonthermal diathermy.
- Choose the best technique for treatment with thermal and nonthermal diathermy, and list the advantages and disadvantages of each.
- Select the appropriate equipment and parameters for treatment with thermal and nonthermal diathermy.
- Accurately and completely document treatment with thermal and nonthermal diathermy.

Diathermy, from the Greek meaning "through heating," is the application of shortwave (approximately 1.8- to 30-MHz frequency and 3- to 200-m wavelength) or microwave (300-MHz to 300-GHz frequency and 1-mm to 1-m wavelength)

electromagnetic energy to produce heat and other physiological changes in tissues. An overview of the physics of electromagnetic radiation is provided in Chapter 16 of this book, along with information about therapeutic uses of lasers and light that utilize energy in the visible or near-visible frequency ranges of the electromagnetic spectrum. This chapter focuses on the thermal and nonthermal effects of electromagnetic radiation in the shortwave and microwave range.

Shortwave radiation is a band of electromagnetic radiation within the radiofrequency range (3 kHz to 300 MHz and 1-m to 100-km wavelength). Radiofrequency radiation lies between extremely **low-frequency electromagnetic radiation** and **microwave radiation** (Fig. 10.1). Microwave radiation has a shorter wavelength and higher frequency than shortwave radiation, lying between radiofrequency and infrared (IR) radiation on the electromagnetic spectrum. Both shortwave radiation and microwave radiation are nonionizing, being of longer wavelength and lower frequency than ultraviolet. This means they do not have enough energy to remove electrons from atoms and molecules but can heat substances.[1] At the present time, shortwave diathermy (SWD) devices are manufactured and available in the United States, whereas microwave diathermy (MWD) devices are not manufactured in the United States but can be obtained from abroad.

The use of diathermy dates back to 1892 when d'Arsonval used radiofrequency electromagnetic fields with 10-kHz frequency to produce a sensation of warmth without the muscular contractions that occur at lower frequencies. The clinical use of SWD became popular much later, in the early 20th century. SWD was popular in the United States during the 1930s for treating infections. However, by the 1950s, with the advent of antibiotics and with growing concerns about potential hazards to the patient and the operator if SWD equipment was applied inappropriately, the use of diathermy declined. Diathermy also lost popularity because, by its nature, the electromagnetic field cannot be readily contained to eliminate interference with other electronic equipment and because most diathermy devices were large, expensive, and cumbersome to use.

The radiation used for diathermy falls within the radiofrequency range and therefore can interfere with radiofrequency signals used for communications. To avoid this, the U.S. Federal Communications Commission (FCC) has assigned certain frequencies of shortwave and microwave radiation solely for medical applications. SWD devices have been allocated the three frequency bands centered on 13.56, 27.12, and 40.68 MHz, with ranges of ±6.78, 160, and 20 kHz, respectively.[2]

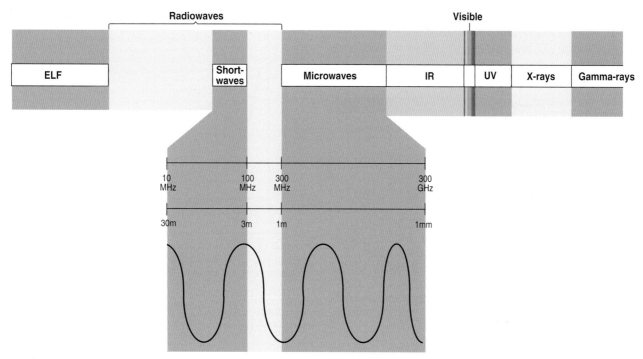

FIGURE 10.1 Shortwaves and microwaves in the electromagnetic spectrum. *ELF,* Extremely low frequency; *IR,* infrared; *UV,* ultraviolet.

The U.S. Food and Drug Administration (FDA) recognizes the 13.56- and 27.12-MHz bands as being used for SWD. The 27.12-MHz band is most commonly used for SWD devices because it has the widest bandwidth and therefore is the easiest and least expensive to generate. MWD devices for medical application have been allocated the frequency of 2450 MHz.

In recent years there has been renewed interest in diathermy because smaller, better-shielded devices have been developed and because there is now more evidence clarifying and supporting the benefits of this intervention.[3] Diathermy of sufficient power can produce heat in large areas,[4-7] and there is a growing body of evidence that low-average-power, pulsed diathermy has nonthermal effects that can help control pain and edema and promote wound and tissue healing.

Both SWD and MWD can be delivered in a continuous **(continuous shortwave diathermy)** or pulsed mode and, when delivered at a sufficient average intensity, can generate heat in the body.[8-10] When delivered in a pulsed mode at low average intensities, heat is dissipated before it can accumulate; however, pulsed low-intensity electromagnetic energy in the shortwave or microwave frequency range may produce physiological effects through nonthermal mechanisms. When applied at nonthermal levels, pulsed SWD is referred to by many terms, including *pulsed shortwave diathermy (PSWD), pulsed electromagnetic field (PEMF), pulsed radiofrequency (PRF),* and *pulsed electromagnetic energy (PEME).* In October 2015, the FDA issued an order to rename shortwave diathermy not used for heating as **nonthermal shortwave therapy (SWT)** with the specific indication of being "intended for adjunctive use in the palliative treatment of postoperative pain and edema of soft tissue."[11] Therefore, although much of the literature on this intervention uses the previously listed terms, in this edition of this text, SWD not used for heating is referred to as *SWT.*

Physical Properties of Diathermy

The most obvious effect of diathermy is that it can increase tissue temperature. The amount of temperature increase depends on the amount of energy absorbed by the tissue, which is determined by the average intensity of the electromagnetic field output by the device, the distance of the applicator from the tissue, and the type of tissue to which the field is applied.

> **◉ Clinical Pearl**
>
> When applying diathermy, the increase in tissue temperature is determined in large part by the intensity of the electromagnetic field, the distance of the applicator from the tissue, and the type of tissue.

A diathermy signal may be delivered either continuously or pulsed. Either can heat tissue if the signal's average intensity reaching the tissues is sufficiently high. In general, if the average power of the signal is greater than 38 W, tissue temperature will increase.[17] In clinical practice, the impact of diathermy on tissue temperature is also influenced by the type of tissue, the circulation within it, and the distance between the tissue and the applicator. Most currently available diathermy devices do not clearly indicate their output power; they deliver pulsed diathermy with a high fixed peak power, and the average power is adjusted by changing the pulse frequency and/or duration and to produce different "levels" (e.g., 1, 2, 3, and 4 or low, medium, and high). Therefore, clinicians must use a combination of the device's specific instructions and the patient's report to ascertain whether a particular diathermy application increases tissue temperature.

When applied at sufficient power to increase tissue temperature, diathermy has a number of advantages over other thermal agents. It can heat tissues more deeply than superficial thermal agents such as hot packs, and it can heat larger areas than ultrasound.

> ◎ **Clinical Pearl**
>
> Diathermy can heat more deeply than hot packs and heats larger areas than ultrasound.

SWD is not reflected by bones and therefore does not concentrate at the periosteum or pose a risk of periosteal burning, as does ultrasound; however, MWD is reflected at tissue interfaces, including interfaces between air and skin, skin and subcutaneous fat, and soft tissue and superficial bones, and therefore produces more heat close to these interfaces. Reflected microwaves can also form standing waves, resulting in hotspots in other areas. Both SWD and MWD treatments generally need little time to apply and do not require that the clinician be in direct contact with the patient throughout the treatment period.

Types of Diathermy Applicators

Three different types of diathermy applicators are available: inductive coils, capacitive plates, and a **magnetron**.[12] Inductive coils and capacitive plates can be used to apply SWD. A magnetron is used to apply MWD. SWT devices use an **inductive coil applicator** in the form of a drum or capacitive plate.

INDUCTIVE COIL

An inductive diathermy applicator consists of a coil through which an alternating electrical current flows. The current produces a magnetic field perpendicular to the coil, which induces electrical eddy currents in the tissues (Fig. 10.2). The eddy currents cause charged particles in the tissue to oscillate, causing friction that heats the tissue.

Heating with an inductive coil diathermy applicator is known as *heating by the magnetic field method* because the electrical current that heats the tissues is induced by a magnetic field. The amount of heat generated in an area of tissue is affected by the strength of the magnetic field reaching the tissue and by the strength and density of the induced eddy

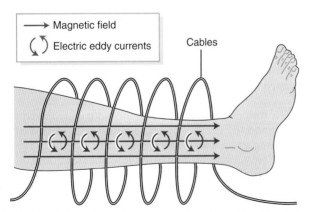

FIGURE 10.2 Generation of magnetic fields and induction of electrical fields by an inductive coil.

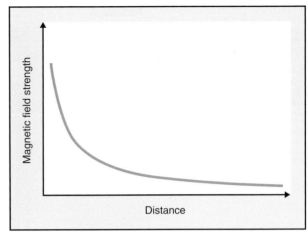

FIGURE 10.3 Typical behavior of magnetic field strength delivered by a shortwave diathermy device as the distance from the applicator increases. Note that this is an inverse square relationship.

currents. The strength of the magnetic field decreases in proportion to the square of the distance between the tissue and the applicator (inverse square law), but it does not vary with tissue type (Fig. 10.3). The strength of the induced eddy currents is determined by the strength of the incoming magnetic field and by the electrical conductivity of the tissue in the area, which is governed mainly by the type of tissue and the frequency of the applied signal. Metals and tissues having high water and electrolyte content, such as muscle or synovial fluid, have high electrical conductivity, whereas tissues with low water content, such as fat, bone, and collagen, have low electrical conductivity (Tables 10.1 and 10.2). Thus, inductive coils can heat both deep and superficial tissues, but they produce the most heat in tissues with the highest electrical conductivity.

> ◎ **Clinical Pearl**
>
> An inductive coil diathermy applicator produces the most heat in tissues with high electrical conductivity.

Inductive coil applicators used to be made with cables containing bundles of plastic-coated wires that were wrapped around the patient's limb (Fig. 10.4). An alternating electrical current flowing through the wires induced eddy currents inside the limb. Because these cables are so difficult to apply, cable diathermy applicators are no longer available. Modern

TABLE 10.1	Conductivity of Muscle at Different Frequencies
Frequency (MHz)	**Conductivity (siemens/meter)**
13.56	0.62
27.12	0.60
40.68	0.68
200	1.00
2450	2.17

From Durney CH, Massoudi H, Iskander MF: *Radiofrequency radiation dosimetry handbook, USAFSAM-TR-85-73,* Salt Lake City, 1985, University of Utah Electrical Engineering Department.

TABLE 10.2	Conductivity of Different Tissues at 25 MHz
Tissue	**Conductivity (siemens/meter)**
Muscle	0.7–0.9
Kidney	0.83
Liver	0.48–0.54
Brain	0.46
Fat	0.04–0.06
Bone	0.01

From Durney CH, Massoudi H, Iskander MF: *Radiofrequency radiation dosimetry handbook, USAFSAM-TR-85-73,* Salt Lake City, 1985, University of Utah Electrical Engineering Department.

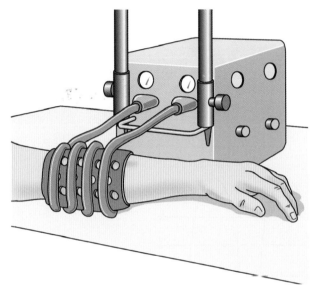

FIGURE 10.4 An inductive coil shortwave diathermy applicator setup with cables around the patient's limb. This type of applicator produces a uniform, incident electromagnetic field that induces an electrical field and current within the target tissue.

inductive coil diathermy applicators consist of a spiral coil wrapped flat inside a drum or a flat, conformable plate within plastic housing (Fig. 10.5A–B). The drum or plate is placed directly over the area being treated, or the garment is placed around the area being treated. Alternating electrical current flows in the coil, producing a magnetic field, which induces eddy currents within the tissues directly in front of a drum or plates (Fig. 10.5C).

CAPACITIVE PLATES
Capacitive plate diathermy applicators are made of metal encased in plastic housing or transmissive carbon rubber electrodes placed between felt pads. A high-frequency alternating electrical current flows from one plate or electrode to the other through the patient, producing an electrical field and a flow of current in the body tissue between them (Fig. 10.6A). Thus, the patient becomes part of the electrical circuit connecting the two plates or electrodes. As current flows through the tissue, it causes oscillation of charged particles, which heats the tissue (Fig. 10.6B).

Heating tissue using capacitive plate diathermy applicators is known as *heating by the electrical field method* because the electrical current that generates the heat is produced directly by an electrical field. The amount of heat generated in an area of tissue depends on the strength and density of the electrical current, with most heating occurring in tissues having the highest conductivity. Because an electrical current will always take the path of least resistance, when a capacitive plate applicator is used, the current will generally concentrate in the more conductive superficial tissues and will not effectively penetrate to deeper tissues if they are less conductive, such as fat or collagen. Thus, capacitive plates generally produce more heat in skin and less in deeper structures, in contrast to inductive applicators, which heat the deeper structures more effectively because the incident magnetic field can achieve greater penetration to induce the electrical field and current within the targeted tissue (Fig. 10.7).[13,14]

> ◎ **Clinical Pearl**
>
> Capacitive plate diathermy applicators produce more heat in the skin and superficial tissues, whereas inductive applicators produce more heat in deeper structures.

MAGNETRON (CONDENSER)
A magnetron delivers MWD using an antenna to produce a high-frequency alternating current. The current induces an electromagnetic field that is directed toward the tissue by a curved, reflecting director that surrounds the antenna. The short wavelength of the microwave and the presence of the director allow this type of diathermy to be focused and applied to small, defined areas. Therefore, these devices are particularly useful during rehabilitation when only small areas of tissue are involved.[15] MWD is also frequently used to medically treat malignant tumors by hyperthermia.[16] Magnetrons used clinically are similar to the magnetrons used in microwave ovens to cook food.

Microwaves produced by a magnetron penetrate to different depths and heat different tissue locations, depending on the microwave frequency and the tissue's composition.[9,17–20] They generate the most heat in tissues that have high electrical conductivity; however, because of its high frequency and short wavelength, MWD penetrates less deeply than SWD. Microwaves can reflect at tissue interfaces, forming standing waves that cause uneven heating within the field.

Effects of Diathermy
THERMAL EFFECTS
If applied at sufficient average intensity for sufficient time, SWD and MWD increase tissue temperature, leading to a sensation of heat in the patient and a range of physiological effects.[5–7,15,21,22] The physiological effects of increased tissue temperature include vasodilation, increased nerve conduction velocity, elevated pain threshold and reduced pain, altered muscle strength, accelerated enzymatic activity, and increased soft tissue extensibility. These are described in detail in Chapter 8. All of these have been observed in response to the application of diathermy.[23–28]

Diathermy is generally selected when the goal is to heat large, deep areas of soft tissue because it is the only physical

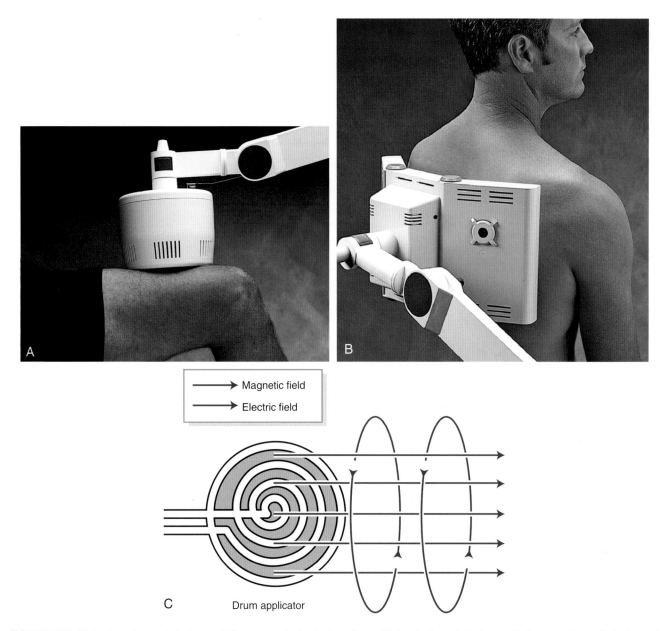

FIGURE 10.5 (A) An inductive coil shortwave diathermy applicator in drum form. (B) Application of shortwave diathermy using an inductive coil applicator that can conform to the body. (C) Magnetic field generated by an inductive drum shortwave diathermy applicator and the resultant induced electrical field. (A and B, Courtesy Mettler Electronics Corporation, Anaheim, CA.)

agent that will do this. Note that diathermy heats superficial tissues when it is heating underlying deep tissues. For example, diathermy increases circulation in the skin, subcutaneous tissues, and muscles[23,27,29,30] and increases deep tissue extensibility.[31,32] This is in contrast to superficial heating agents, as described in Chapter 8, which increase the temperature of only the superficial outer few millimeters of tissue. This is also in contrast to ultrasound,[22] discussed in Chapter 9, which heats small, deep areas of tissue.

NONTHERMAL EFFECTS

When diathermy is applied in a pulsed mode with a low average intensity, no maintained increase in tissue temperature is produced because any transient heating of tissues that may occur during a brief pulse is dissipated by blood perfusing the area

during the off time between pulses. This is similar to the lack of a maintained temperature increase produced with pulsed ultrasound. As discussed earlier in this chapter, the nonthermal application of shortwave electromagnetic radiation has been given many names (e.g., *PEMF, PEME*), but the current FDA recommended term is *nonthermal shortwave therapy (SWT)*.[11]

Although the mechanism by which SWT achieves physiological effects is uncertain, these effects are most likely produced by altering cell ion binding to cell membranes, thus changing membrane function and cellular activity.[33,34] This can then trigger a cascade of biological processes, including growth factor activation in fibroblasts, chondrocytes, and nerve cells; macrophage activation; changes in myosin phosphorylation; and increases in microvascular perfusion.[33,35–42] Increasing microvascular perfusion and thus local circulation

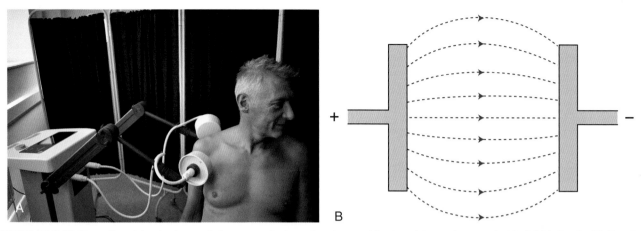

FIGURE 10.6 (A) Capacitive plate shortwave diathermy applicators placed around the target to produce an electrical field directly. (B) Electrical field distribution between capacitive shortwave diathermy plates. (A, Courtesy EMS Physio, Wantage, UK.)

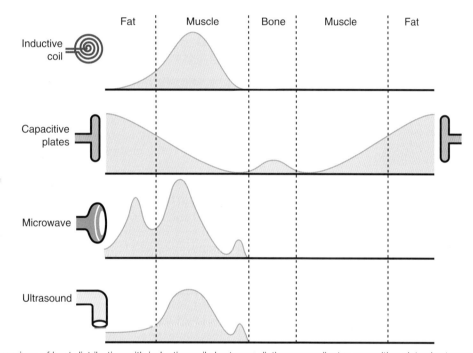

FIGURE 10.7 Comparison of heat distribution with inductive coil shortwave diathermy applicator, capacitive plate shortwave diathermy applicator, microwave diathermy, and ultrasound.

may increase local tissue oxygenation, nutrient availability, and phagocytosis, all of which contribute to accelerated tissue healing. SWT modulates pain, edema, and inflammation and improves tissue healing, likely at least in part by modifying the dynamics of nitric oxide via calcium-calmodulin–dependent constitutive nitric oxide synthase in the target tissue. The effects of SWT are probably somewhat specific to certain treatment parameters, including the frequency, pulse frequency, and power of the applied radiation.

Clinical Indications for Diathermy
THERMAL-LEVEL DIATHERMY

Thermal-level diathermy is indicated when achieving the goals of therapy can be facilitated by heating large, deep structures such as the knee joint, hip joint, or diffuse areas

of the spine. The clinical benefits of applying continuous or pulsed diathermy at intensities sufficient to increase tissue temperature are the same as the benefits of applying other thermal agents (see Chapter 8), except that diathermy uniquely affects large, deep areas. Benefits may include pain control, accelerated tissue healing, decreased joint stiffness, and if applied in conjunction with stretching, increased range of motion (ROM). Five studies, all performed by the same research group and all using pulsed SWD with an average output of 48 W, found that this intervention in conjunction with stretching resulted in greater increases in muscle length and ROM than did stretching alone.[43–46] Follow-up studies by other investigators also support that continuous thermal-level diathermy reduces pain and increases ROM in patients with chronic knee osteoarthritis.[28,47,48] Systematic reviews and meta-analyses also support that thermal-level diathermy significantly reduces pain and improves muscle performance in patients with knee osteoarthritis.[26,49]

NONTHERMAL SHORTWAVE THERAPY

The first documented clinical application in the United States of diathermy at a nonthermal level was reported in the 1930s, when Ginsberg used a pulsed form of SWD to fight infection without producing a significant temperature rise in tissue.[50] He reported successfully treating a variety of acute and chronic infections with this type of electromagnetic radiation and stated that this was the most effective treatment he had ever used. However, this was before antibiotics were commonly available. In 1965, Milinowski patented a device designed to deliver electrotherapy without generating heat. He stated that this device produced good clinical results in a range of conditions while eliminating the factors of patient heat tolerance and contraindications when treating with heat.[51] Numerous nonthermal SWT devices are now available for clinical and home use, primarily to control pain and promote tissue healing. Some novel ways to apply SWT have been developed. For example, an SWT device placed in a soft cervical collar has been designed for home use by patients with neck pain,[52,53] and a device that places the coil in a bandage is in development for the promotion of wound healing.[54] In addition, because the electromagnetic radiation of SWT can penetrate through a cast, this approach was evaluated in patients put in casts after Colles fracture and was found to help control edema during wrist immobilization.[55]

Pain Control

Numerous studies support that SWT improves or accelerates resolution of pain after soft tissue injury or surgery, including acute ankle sprains,[56,57] chronic low back pain,[58–61] recent foot surgery,[62] cesarean section,[63] lateral epicondylitis,[64] and other conditions.[65–70] A 2012 meta-analysis that included 25 controlled clinical trials with 1332 patients found strong statistical evidence that SWT performed in patients with postoperative and nonpostoperative pain and edema was associated with improvements in pain, reduction in edema, and improvements in wound healing outcomes,[71] and several more recent, although small, randomized controlled clinical trials continue to support these conclusions.[60,61,63]

Soft Tissue Healing

Some studies support that SWT increases the healing rate of soft tissue in incisional wounds,[72] chronic wounds,[73–75] burn-related injuries,[76] and tendon injuries[77,78] in animal and human subjects.[72–74,76,79] However, the small number and size of the studies, as well as limitations in study design, limit the ability to draw definitive conclusions about the efficacy of SWT for promoting soft tissue healing.[80–82] Mechanisms thought to underlie potential improvements in tissue healing with SWT include increased circulation, improved tissue oxygenation, and increased fibroblast and chondrocyte proliferation as a result of impacts on cell or cell membrane function.[77]

Nerve Healing

A 2019 systematic review that included 11 studies, 7 in animals and 4 in humans, of SWT for promoting nerve regeneration after peripheral nerve injuries concluded that this intervention can improve the electrophysiological parameters, myelinated fiber number, and axon diameter of the injured nerve.[83] The studies in humans were all related to carpal tunnel syndrome. A few animal studies have also found that SWT may have beneficial effects on motor function recovery and lesion volume size after acute spinal cord injury, potentially by modulating inflammation, oxidative stress, and heat shock protein 70.[84–86]

Bone Healing

Animal and human studies have shown accelerated bone healing with the application of electromagnetic fields, including SWT.[87–90] A 2014 systematic review and meta-analysis of randomized controlled trials found that the application of electromagnetic fields can accelerate the healing of acute fractures, but there was insufficient evidence that it reduced the incidence of nonunion acute fractures.[91] A more recent study also supports that early addition of pulsed electromagnetic field treatment during cast immobilization of distal radius fractures has beneficial effects on the pain, sensation, ROM, and daily functioning of patients.[92]

> ◎ **Clinical Pearl**
>
> Nonthermal SWT (i.e., nonthermal pulsed diathermy) does not increase tissue temperature but can accelerate edema resolution, reduce pain after injury, and accelerate soft tissue healing.

Osteoarthritis Symptoms

Several studies have evaluated the effectiveness of SWT for improving symptoms of osteoarthritis. These studies have examined the effects of this intervention on inflammation, ROM, pain, stiffness, functional ability, mobility, and synovial thickness. A 2013 systematic review of randomized controlled trials of electromagnetic fields for treating osteoarthritis that included nine studies with a total of 636 participants concluded that electromagnetic field treatment may provide moderate pain relief for patients with osteoarthritis.[93] Systematic reviews and meta-analyses examining the effects of electromagnetic fields on knee osteoarthritis published in 2012, 2013, and 2017 also all concluded that this intervention helps control pain associated with knee osteoarthritis, but more high-quality trials are still needed.[49,94,95] As with other indications, some studies suggest that the impact of this intervention may differ with different SWT frequencies.[96]

Contraindications and Precautions for Diathermy

Although diathermy is a safe treatment modality when applied appropriately, to avoid adverse effects, it should not be used when contraindicated, and appropriate precautions should be taken when necessary. When any form of diathermy is used at an intensity that may increase tissue temperature, all contraindications and precautions that apply to the use of thermotherapy apply (see Chapter 8). In addition, other contraindications and precautions apply uniquely to this type of physical agent, and some unique reasons have been put forth for these restrictions. These are described in detail in the boxes that follow.

CONTRAINDICATIONS FOR ALL FORMS OF DIATHERMY

> ✳ **CONTRAINDICATIONS**
>
> **for Diathermy**
>
> - Implanted or transcutaneous neural stimulators, including cardiac pacemakers
> - Pregnancy

Implanted or Transcutaneous Neural Stimulators, Including Cardiac Pacemakers

Diathermy of any sort should *never* be used in patients with implanted or transcutaneous stimulators, such as deep brain stimulators and cardiac pacemakers, because the electromagnetic energy of the diathermy may interfere with the functioning of the device and cause burns by heating its components. Two cases of severe brain injury have been reported when diathermy was applied to patients with implanted deep brain stimulators, essentially causing burns deep inside the brain.[97,98] In patients with pacemakers, the risk of adverse effects is greatest when the thorax is being treated. Although some authors state that the extremities may be treated in patients with pacemakers, we recommend that diathermy not be used in any area in a patient who has a pacemaker.[99]

> ◎ **Clinical Pearl**
>
> Diathermy of any sort, including SWT, should *never* be used in patients with implanted or transcutaneous stimulators, such as deep brain stimulators and cardiac pacemakers, because the electromagnetic energy of the diathermy may interfere with the functioning of the device and cause burns by heating its components.

Pregnancy

Application of diathermy during pregnancy is contraindicated because of concerns regarding the effects of deep heat and electromagnetic fields on fetal development. Maternal hyperthermia has been shown to increase the risk of abnormal fetal development, and SWD has been linked to increased rates of spontaneous abortion and abnormal fetal development in animals.[100–103] Diathermy, particularly of the lower abdominal and pelvic regions, should be avoided during pregnancy, and because the distribution of an electromagnetic field is not predictably constrained in the body, exposing any other part of the body to diathermy should also be avoided. A discussion of the risks and precautions for pregnant therapists applying diathermy to patients follows the section on precautions for applying diathermy to patients.

CONTRAINDICATIONS FOR THERMAL-LEVEL DIATHERMY

> ✳ **CONTRAINDICATIONS**
>
> **for Thermal-Level Diathermy**
>
> - Metal implants
> - Malignancy
> - Eyes
> - Testes
> - Growing epiphyses

Metal Implants

Metal is highly electrically conductive and can become very hot with the application of thermal-level diathermy, potentially leading to damaging heating of adjacent tissues. Because this applies to metal both inside and outside the patient, diathermy should not be applied to patients who have metal in them, such as from implants, screws, or shrapnel, and all jewelry should be removed before diathermy is applied. Care should be taken that no metal is present in furniture or other objects touching or close to the patient being treated.

The risk of extreme temperature increases is greatest when metal is present within the superficial tissues, as can occur with shrapnel fragments. Although it is generally recommended that diathermy be avoided in any areas close to or containing metal, the use of carefully controlled doses of pulsed thermal-level diathermy to facilitate gains in ROM after injury or surgery with implanted metal has been reported without adverse effects.[44,104]

Malignancy

The use of diathermy in an area of malignancy is contraindicated, unless treatment is being provided for the tumor itself. Diathermy is occasionally used by physicians, often in combination with other interventions, to treat malignant tumors by hyperthermia.[105] Doing so requires fine temperature control because cancer cells may die within certain narrow temperature ranges but proliferate at temperatures close to these ranges. Such treatment is outside the realm of the rehabilitation professional.

Over the Eyes

The eyes should not be treated with diathermy because heating the intraocular fluid may damage the internal structures of the eyes.

Over the Testes

It is recommended that diathermy not be applied over the testes because increasing local tissue temperature may adversely affect fertility.

Over Growing Epiphyses

Although the effects of diathermy on growing epiphyses are unknown, it should be avoided in these areas because diathermy may alter the rate of epiphyseal closure.

CONTRAINDICATIONS FOR NONTHERMAL SHORTWAVE THERAPY

✴ CONTRAINDICATIONS

for Nonthermal Shortwave Therapy

- Deep tissues such as internal organs
- Substitute for conventional therapy for edema and pain
- Pacemakers, electronic devices, or metal implants (warning)

Deep Tissues Such as Internal Organs

Although contraindicated for the treatment of internal organs, SWT can be used to treat soft tissue overlying an organ.

> ■ **Assess**
> - Check the patient's chart for any record of organ disease.
> - Check with the patient's physician before applying SWT in an area with organ disease present.

Substitute for Conventional Therapy for Edema and Pain

SWT should not replace conventional therapy for edema and pain, but it may be used as an adjunctive modality in conjunction with conventional methods, including compression, immobilization, and medications.

Implanted Pacemakers, Electronic Devices, or Metal Implants

The electromagnetic radiation of SWT may interfere with the functioning of cardiac pacemakers and other electromedical devices. Therefore, SWT should never be used over or near electronic medical devices, including pacemakers, and should be used with caution with and around patients with other external or implanted medical electronic devices.

SWT devices can be used to treat soft tissue adjacent to most metal implants without significantly heating the metal. However, if implanted metal forms closed loops, such as with the wires used to fasten rods and plates in surgically repaired fractures, current can flow in the wire loops, causing local heating. Therefore, if a patient has a metal implant, the clinician should determine its type and location before applying SWT.

> ■ **Ask the Patient**
> - "Do you have a pacemaker or any other metal in your body?"
>
> ■ **Assess**
> - Check the patient's chart for any information regarding a pacemaker or other metal implants.

If the patient has a pacemaker or is using other medical electronic devices, SWT should not be used except in extreme circumstances, such as when trying to save a limb from amputation. In such circumstances, when the use of SWT is being considered, the patient's physician should be consulted, and the clinician should try to shield all electronic medical devices from the electromagnetic field. If the patient has metal implants, an x-ray should be requested. If the metal implants are nonlooping, treatment with SWT may be applied with caution, but if the metal forms loops, SWT should be avoided.

PRECAUTIONS FOR ALL FORMS OF DIATHERMY

✴ PRECAUTIONS

for All Forms of Diathermy

- Near electronic or magnetic equipment
- Obesity
- Copper-bearing intrauterine contraceptive devices

Near Electronic or Magnetic Equipment

A number of studies and reports have demonstrated the presence of unwanted electrical and magnetic radiation around diathermy applicators.[106-111] Because the treatment field may interfere with electronic or magnetic equipment such as computers or computer-controlled medical devices, it is recommended that the leads and applicators of diathermy devices be at least 3 m and preferably 5 m from other electrical equipment. Precise guidelines are not available because interference depends on the power, wavelength, and exact arrangement and shielding of the diathermy device and the other equipment being used. In general, it is therefore recommended that diathermy devices not be used in proximity to computers or computer-controlled devices.

Obesity

Diathermy should be used with caution in obese patients because it may heat fat excessively. Capacitive plate applicators, which generally result in greater increases in the temperature of fat than other types of applicators, should be avoided with obese patients.[12]

Copper-Bearing Intrauterine Contraceptive Devices

Although copper-bearing intrauterine contraceptive devices do contain a small amount of metal, calculations and in vivo measurements have shown that these devices and the surrounding tissue increase in temperature only slightly when exposed to therapeutic levels of diathermy.[112,113] Therefore, diathermy may be used by therapists and by patients with such devices.

PRECAUTIONS FOR NONTHERMAL SHORTWAVE THERAPY

✱ PRECAUTIONS

for Nonthermal Shortwave Therapy

- Pregnancy
- Skeletal immaturity

The use of thermal-level diathermy is contraindicated during pregnancy. In addition, because the effects of electromagnetic energy on fetal or child development are unknown, SWT should be used with caution during pregnancy and in skeletally immature patients.

PRECAUTIONS FOR THERAPISTS APPLYING DIATHERMY

Concern has focused on potential hazards to therapists applying diathermy because of the high strength of electromagnetic fields close to the device and their repeated exposure from treating multiple patients, potentially multiple times each day. Diathermy devices produce diffuse radiation that can irradiate the therapist if they are standing too close to the machine. Therefore it is recommended that therapists stay at least 2 m (6 feet) away from all continuous diathermy applicators, at least 1.5 m (4.5 feet) away from all SWT applicators, and out of the direct beam of any MWD device during patient treatment.[114]

Some reports have noted above-average rates of spontaneous abortion and abnormal fetal development in therapists after the use of SWD equipment; however, other studies have failed to demonstrate a statistically significant correlation between SWD exposure and congenital malformation or spontaneous abortion.[115,116] One comparison of therapists exposed to SWD and MWD found that only MWD increased their risk of miscarriage.[117] However, a subsequent study found that shortwaves can have potentially harmful effects on pregnancy outcome, specifically low birth weight. This effect increased with dosage.[118] Although current research findings are inconsistent, given possible associated risks, it is recommended that pregnant therapists avoid exposure to SWD and MWD.[111,119,120]

Possible Effects of Electromagnetic Fields on Malignancy

Substantial controversy exists regarding the effects of electromagnetic fields on malignancy. The literature on this topic is primarily concerned with risks associated with living near and working with power lines because these also induce electromagnetic fields around them. Although some reports suggest that the electromagnetic fields generated from power lines may be linked to cancers and leukemia, others have failed to show such an association.[121-123] In 1995, the Council of the American Physical Society (APS) reviewed the literature on this topic and concluded that "the scientific literature and the reports of reviews by other panels show no consistent, significant link between cancer and power line fields. ... No plausible biophysical mechanisms for the systematic initiation or promotion of cancer by these power line fields have been identified." Their most recent review of the subsequent literature again supported this opinion, stating, "Since that time, there have been several large in vivo studies of animal populations subjected for their life span to high magnetic fields and epidemiological studies, done with larger populations and with direct, rather than surrogate, measurements of the magnetic field exposure. These studies have produced no results that change the earlier assessment by APS. In addition, no biophysical mechanisms for the initiation or promotion of cancer by electric or magnetic fields from power lines have been identified."[124]

The electromagnetic fields associated with power lines are of much lower frequency (50 to 60 Hz) than fields used in pulsed or continuous SWD devices (27.12 MHz); thus the application of data from the studies on power lines to the effects of SWD is unclear. At this time, no recommendations have been put forth against using nonthermal levels of SWT in the area of a malignancy, and there are no indications to suggest that SWT is carcinogenic.

Adverse Effects of Diathermy
BURNS

Diathermy can cause soft tissue burns when used at normal or excessive doses, and because the distribution of this type of energy varies significantly with the type of tissue, it can burn some layers of tissue while sparing others.[125,126] Fat layers are at greatest risk of burning when capacitive plate applicators are used because fat is heated more by this type of device and because fat is less well vascularized than muscle or skin and therefore is not cooled as effectively by vasodilation. All forms of diathermy also preferentially heat water. Therefore, during diathermy treatment, the patient's skin should be kept dry by wrapping with towels.

◎ Clinical Pearl

To avoid burns during diathermy treatments, keep the patient's skin dry by wrapping with towels.

Application Technique

Thermal-level diathermy is the most effective way to heat large areas of deep tissue. SWT can reduce pain and may accelerate tissue healing. Although SWT can be used at acute, subacute, and chronic stages of an injury, the literature and anecdotal reports suggest that better results are achieved when acute conditions are treated.

APPLICATION TECHNIQUE 10.1   DIATHERMY

Procedure

1. Evaluate the patient's problem and determine the goals of treatment.
2. Confirm that diathermy is the most appropriate intervention.

   Because diathermy induces an electrical current in the tissues without touching the patient's body, the use of this physical agent may be particularly appropriate when direct contact with the patient is not possible or desirable, for example, if infection may be present, if the patient cannot tolerate direct contact with the skin, or if the area is in a cast. Determine that diathermy is not contraindicated.
3. Select the most appropriate diathermy device.

   Choose either a thermal or a nonthermal application according to the desired effects of the treatment and contraindications. Choose the appropriate applicator (inductive coil, capacitive plate, or magnetron) according to the desired depth of penetration and the type of tissue to be treated.
4. Explain the procedure to the patient, the reason for applying diathermy, and the sensations the patient may feel.

   During the application of thermal-level diathermy, the patient should feel a comfortable sensation of mild warmth and no increase in pain or discomfort.

   The application of SWT is not generally associated with any change in the patient's sensation, although some patients report feeling slight tingling or mild warmth that may be due to increased local circulation in response to the treatment.
5. Remove all metal jewelry and clothing having metal fastenings or components, such as buttons, zippers, or clips, from the area to be treated.

   Nonmetal clothing, bandages, or casts do not need to be removed before treatment with diathermy because they do not alter the magnetic fields. However, when thermal-level diathermy is used, clothing should be removed from the area so that towels can be applied to absorb local perspiration.
6. Clean and dry the skin, and inspect it if necessary.
7. Position the patient comfortably on a chair or plinth with no metal components. Position the patient so that the area to be treated is readily accessible.
8. If applying thermal-level diathermy, wrap the area to be treated with toweling to absorb local perspiration. If applying SWT, it is not necessary to place towels between the applicator and the body, but a disposable cloth or plastic cover can be placed over the applicator if there is risk of cross-contamination or infection.
9. Position the device and applicator for effective and safe treatment. See later section for more information on positioning.
10. Tune the device.

    SWD devices require tuning the applicator to each particular load. Tuning adjusts the precise frequency of the device within the accepted range and optimizes coupling between the device and the load. Most modern diathermy devices tune automatically. To tune a device that requires manual tuning, first turn it on and allow it to warm up according to the manufacturer's directions, then turn up the intensity to a low level; adjust the tuning dial until a maximal reading on the power/intensity indicator is obtained.
11. Select the appropriate treatment parameters.

    When thermal-level diathermy is applied, the intensity should be adjusted to produce a sensation of mild warmth in the patient. The gauge of heating used in clinical practice is the patient's reported sensation because temperature increases are not consistently related to the amount of energy delivered. The patterns of energy and heat distribution by both SWD and MWD are difficult to predict because they are influenced by many factors, including the amount of reflection; the electrical properties of different types of tissue in the field; the size and composition of the tissue; the field frequency; and the applicator's type, size, geometry, distance, and orientation. This issue is further complicated by evidence that the thermal sensation threshold may be affected by the field frequency.[126] Thermal-level diathermy is generally applied for approximately 20 minutes.

    When applying SWT, most clinicians select the intensity, pulse frequency, and total treatment time based on the manufacturer's recommendations and on their individual experience because clinical research using these devices does not clearly indicate which parameters are most effective. Most manufacturers recommend using the maximum strength and frequency available on the device for all conditions, and many devices do not allow the parameters to be adjusted. If the patient reports any discomfort, it is recommended that the energy output be reduced until the discomfort resolves. This can be done by reducing the pulse rate, pulse duration, peak intensity, or numeric setting depending on the controls available on the specific device. Most SWT treatments are administered for 30 to 60 minutes once or twice a day, five to seven times a week.
12. Provide the patient with a bell or other means to call for assistance during treatment and a means to turn off the diathermy device. Instruct the patient to turn off the device and call immediately if they experience excessive heating or an increase in pain or discomfort.
13. After 5 minutes, check that the patient is not too hot or is not experiencing any increase in symptoms.
14. When the treatment is complete, turn off the device, remove the applicator and towels, and inspect the treatment area. It is normal for the area to appear slightly red; it may also feel warm to the touch.
15. Assess the outcome of the intervention.

    Reassess the patient, checking particularly for any signs of burning and for progress toward the goals of treatment. Remeasure quantifiable subjective complaints and objective impairments and disabilities.
16. Document the treatment.

POSITIONING
Inductive Applicator

Modern inductive diathermy applicators are available in a drum, conforming plate, or garment form (see Fig. 10.5). The drum or plate should be placed directly over and close to the skin or tissues to be treated, with a slight air gap to allow heat to dissipate. Avoid contact with the skin if infection may be present. Place the center of the applicator over the area facing and as parallel as possible to the tissues being treated. The garment is put on to surround the limb.

Advise the patient to remain still during treatment to maintain a constant distance between the applicator and the treatment area. If the distance between the surface of the applicator and the tissues being treated increases, the strength of the magnetic field will decrease in proportion to the square of that distance (see Fig. 10.3). For example, if the distance doubles, the field strength will decrease by a factor of four. Maintaining a consistent distance between the applicator and the treatment area is important to ensure consistent treatment.

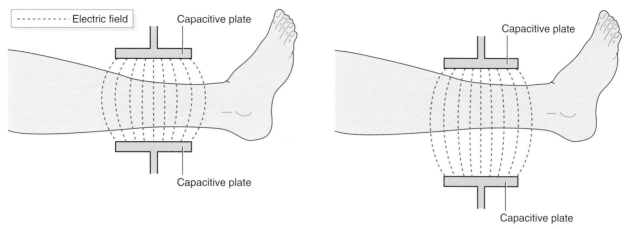

FIGURE 10.8 Electrical field distribution in tissue with evenly and unevenly placed capacitive shortwave diathermy plates.

Capacitive Applicator

A capacitive applicator has two plates that are placed approximately 2 to 10 cm (1 to 3 inches) from the skin surface at an equal distance on either side of the treatment area. By placing the plates close to the body, the maximum field strength in the treatment area is achieved because the field is most concentrated near the plates, and placing the plates at an even distance evens the field's distribution. Unequal placement will result in uneven heating, with the areas closest to the plate becoming hotter than areas farther from the plate (Fig. 10.8).

Magnetron Microwave Applicator

The magnetron microwave applicator should be placed a few inches from the area to be treated and directed toward the area, with the beam perpendicular to the patient's skin.

Documentation

The following should be documented:
- Area of the body treated
- Frequency range
- Average power or power setting
- Pulse rate
- Time of irradiation
- Type of applicator
- Treatment duration
- Patient positioning
- Distance of the applicator from the patient
- Patient's response to the treatment

Documentation is typically written in the SOAP (Subjective, Objective, Assessment, Plan) note format. The following examples summarize only the modality component of treatment and are not intended to represent a comprehensive plan of care.

EXAMPLES

When applying SWD to the low back, document the following:

S: Pt reports low back pain at level 7/10.
O: **Pretreatment:** Limited lumbar ROM in all planes, limited by pain.
Intervention: 27.12 MHz continuous SWD, power level 3, to low back, drum applicator 3 inches from Pt, Pt prone, 20 min.
Posttreatment: Report of mild warmth, pain decreased to 4/10.
A: Pt tolerated SWD well, with decreased low back pain.
P: Continue SWD as above before ther ex program.

When applying MWD to the posterior left knee, document the following:

S: Pt reports stiffness and pain with L knee extension.
O: **Pretreatment:** L knee extension ROM –40 degrees.
Intervention: 2450 MHz continuous MWD to posterior knee, 3 inches from skin surface, power level 4, 15 min. Pt prone with 3-lb cuff weight at ankle.
Posttreatment: Extension ROM increased to –30 degrees.
A: Pt tolerated MWD well, with increased ROM.
P: Continue MWD as above, followed by active ROM exercises into extension.

When applying pulsed SWD to an ulcer on the lateral aspect of the right distal leg, document the following:

S: Pt reports he is scheduled to have cardiac pacemaker implanted in 2 weeks.
O: **Pretreatment:** R distal LE lateral ulcer 9 × 5 cm.
Intervention: SWT intensity 6, pulse rate 600 pps, to R distal leg in area of venous insufficiency ulcer, applicator 3 inches from lateral leg, 45 min.
Posttreatment: Ulcer dimensions decreased to 7 × 4 cm over past week.
A: Pt tolerated SWT well, with decreased ulcer size.
P: Continue SWT as above 1 × per day. Discontinue SWT component of care after pacemaker is implanted.

CLINICAL CASE STUDIES

The following case studies summarize the concepts of diathermy discussed in this chapter. Based on the scenario presented, an evaluation of the clinical findings and goals of treatment are proposed. These are followed by a discussion of the factors to be considered in the selection of diathermy as the indicated intervention, the ideal diathermy device, and the parameters to promote progress toward the goals.

CASE STUDY 10.1

Adhesive Capsulitis

Examination

History

SJ is a 45-year-old female physical therapist. She has been diagnosed with adhesive capsulitis of the right shoulder and has been referred to physical therapy. She reports shoulder stiffness, with a tight sensation at the end of range. Although she is able to perform most of her work functions, she has difficulty reaching overhead, which interferes with placing objects on high shelves and serving when playing tennis; she also has difficulty reaching behind her to fasten clothing.

Systems Review

SJ self-rates her right shoulder stiffness and pain today at 4/10. Because she compensates with her left arm, she notes that her left shoulder has become fatigued but is not painful or stiff. Her lower extremities are not affected.

Tests and Measures

The objective examination reveals restricted right shoulder active ROM (AROM) and passive ROM (PROM) and restricted passive glenohumeral joint inferior and posterior gliding. All other tests, including cervical and elbow ROM and upper extremity strength and sensation, are within normal limits.

Shoulder ROM	Right	Left
Active ROM		
Flexion	120°	170°
Abduction	100°	170°
Hand behind back	Right 5 inches below left	
Passive ROM		
Internal rotation	50°	80°
External rotation	10°	80°

ROM, Range of motion.

Glenohumeral passive inferior and posterior glides are both restricted on the right.

What are some reasonable goals of treatment for this patient? What type of diathermy would be most appropriate? How would you position the patient during treatment? What should be done in addition to diathermy?

Evaluation and Goals

ICF Level	Current Status	Goals
Body structure and function	Restricted right shoulder ROM	Restore normal right shoulder passive and active ROM
	Restricted right glenohumeral passive intraarticular gliding	
Activity	Impaired reach overhead and lifting over her head and behind her back with right upper extremity	Improve ability to reach overhead and behind back and get dressed without assistance
Participation	Decreased tennis playing Difficulty dressing	Return patient to playing tennis and dressing with ease

ICF, International Classification for Functioning, Disability and Health; *ROM*, range of motion.

◆ FIND THE EVIDENCE

PICO Terms	Natural Language Example	Sample PubMed Search
P (Population)	Patients with pain and stiffness in the shoulder due to adhesive capsulitis	("Adhesive capsulitis" [text word] OR "frozen shoulder" [text word])
I (Intervention)	Diathermy	AND ("diathermy" [text word] OR "diathermy" [MeSH] OR "shortwave therapy" [text word] OR "short-wave therapy" [MeSH] OR "Pulsed Radiofrequency Treatment" [MeSH])
C (Comparison)	No diathermy	
O (Outcome)	Increased range of motion in shoulder; improved function	

Key Studies or Reviews

No studies clearly support or refute the effectiveness of diathermy to treat patients with reduced ROM and reduced function due to adhesive capsulitis. However, diathermy is recommended before stretching in patients with reduced ROM and reduced function due to adhesive capsulitis because diathermy uniquely heats large, deep areas[7] and because heating soft tissues increases their extensibility.[31]

Prognosis

The goals of treatment at this time are to regain full AROM and PROM of the right shoulder and to return her to full sports participation and daily living activities. Loss of active and passive joint motion associated with adhesive capsulitis is thought to be a result of adhesion and loss of length of the anterior-inferior joint capsule. Effective treatment should attempt to increase the length of the joint capsule. Increasing tissue temperature before stretching will increase the extensibility of soft tissue, allowing the greatest increase in soft tissue length with the least force while minimizing the risk of tissue damage. Diathermy is the optimal modality for heating the shoulder capsule because this thermal agent can reach large areas of deep tissue. A superficial heating agent, such as a hot pack, would be less effective because it would not increase the temperature of tissue at the depth of the joint capsule, and ultrasound would not generally be as effective because its ability to heat is limited by the effective radiating area of its sound head.

Intervention

A continuous diathermy device must be used to increase tissue temperature. An SWD device with an inductive coil applicator in a drum form is recommended because it provides deep, even heat distribution and is easy to apply. The device should be applied to the right shoulder, ideally with the shoulder positioned at end-of-range flexion and abduction to apply a gentle stretch to the anterior-inferior capsule. The diathermy should be applied for approximately 20 minutes, set to produce a sensation of mild, comfortable warmth. Diathermy should be followed immediately by a low-load, prolonged stretch to maximize ROM gains.

Documentation

S: Pt reports R shoulder stiffness and diagnosis of adhesive capsulitis causing difficulty donning and clasping bra.

O: **Pretreatment**; R shoulder decreased AROM and PROM compared with L shoulder for flexion, abduction, internal rotation, external rotation (see above for measurements).

Intervention: 27.12 MHz continuous SWD, power level 3, to R shoulder, drum applicator 3 inches from Pt, Pt sitting with R shoulder at end-of-range flexion and abduction x 20 min, followed by 10 min low-load prolonged stretch.

Posttreatment: R shoulder flexion PROM increased from 120 to 140 degrees, abduction increased from 100 to 120 degrees.

A: Pt tolerated SWD well, noting sensation of warmth, increased PROM after treatment.

P: Continue SWD three times weekly as above until patient regains full PROM and ability to don and clasp bra and returns to prior level of function.

CASE STUDY 10.2

Acute Ankle Inversion Sprain
Examination

History

MB is a 24-year-old female recreational soccer player who sustained a grade II left ankle inversion sprain approximately 48 hours ago. She has been applying ice and a compression bandage to the ankle, resting and elevating the ankle as much

as possible, and using a cane to reduce weight bearing when walking. Following examination and x-rays, her physician referred her to physical therapy to attain a pain-free return to sports as rapidly as possible.

Systems Review

MB's mother accompanied her to clinic. MB reports moderate pain at the lateral ankle that is aggravated by weight bearing and ankle swelling made worse when her ankle is in a dependent position.

Tests and Measures

Objective examination reveals a mild increase in superficial skin temperature at the left lateral ankle and edema of the left ankle, with a girth of 25.5 cm (10 inches) on the left compared with 21.5 cm (8.5 inches) on the right. Left ankle ROM is restricted in all planes, with 0 degrees dorsiflexion on the left and 10 degrees on the right; 20 degrees plantar flexion on the left and 45 degrees on the right; 10 degrees inversion on the left, with pain at the lateral ankle at the end of range, and 30 degrees on the right; and 20 degrees eversion on the left with 30 degrees on the right. Isometric testing of muscle strength against manual resistance at midrange revealed no abnormalities.

What are the goals of treatment at this time? What type of diathermy is appropriate? What type of diathermy is contraindicated for this patient? How would you position this patient during treatment? What else should this patient do?

Evaluation and Goals

ICF Level	Current Status	Goals
Body structure and function	Left ankle pain, swelling, increased temperature, decreased ROM	Decrease symptoms and regain normal ROM
Activity	Decreased weight-bearing tolerance, limited ambulation	Return to normal ambulation and weight bearing
Participation	Unable to play soccer	Return to playing soccer in 4 weeks

ICF, International Classification for Functioning, Disability and Health; *ROM*, range of motion.

◆ FIND THE EVIDENCE

PICO Terms	Natural Language Example	Sample PubMed Search
P (Population)	Patients with ankle swelling and pain	"ankle" [text word] AND ("edema" [text word] OR "Edema" [MeSH] OR "swelling" [text word])
I (Intervention)	Diathermy	AND ("diathermy" [text word] OR "shortwave therapy" [text word] OR "short-wave therapy" [MeSH] OR "Magnetic Field Therapy" [MeSH])

Continued

CLINICAL CASE STUDIES—cont'd

PICO Terms	Natural Language Example	Sample PubMed Search
C (Comparison)	No diathermy	
O (Outcome)	Reduction of ankle pain and swelling	

Key Studies or Reviews

1. Pasila M, Visuri T, Sundholm A: Pulsating shortwave diathermy: value in treatment of recent ankle and foot sprains. *Arch Phys Med Rehabil* 59:383–386, 1978.

This study found that two different SWT devices were each associated with improved walking ability and reduction of swelling compared with placebo in patients with recent ankle and foot sprains.

Prognosis

The goals of treatment at this time are to control pain, resolve edema, and restore normal ROM so that the patient can fully participate in sports. The diagnosis of a grade II ankle sprain indicates that there has been some damage to the ankle ligaments; therefore the goals of treatment should also include healing these soft tissues.

Nonthermal SWT is an indicated adjunctive treatment for pain and edema and has been shown to accelerate soft tissue healing. Because this patient is already applying rest, ice, compression, and elevation (RICE) to her ankle at home and desires a rapid return to full sports participation, the addition of SWT may help maximize her rate of recovery. Thermal-level diathermy should not be applied to this patient because the use of all thermal agents is contraindicated in the presence of acute injury or inflammation.

Intervention

It is proposed that nonthermal SWT be started immediately after the evaluation to reduce pain and swelling. The patient's limb should be placed in a comfortable elevated position to help reduce swelling. The SWT applicator should be positioned over the lateral aspect of the ankle as close to the skin as possible, with its center over the area of the ankle with the most marked swelling and as parallel as possible to the damaged tissues.

Daily application of SWT for 30 minutes, with power and pulse rate set at 6, is generally used to treat this type of acute injury. If the patient reports any increase in discomfort, the pulse rate should be decreased until the discomfort resolves. SWT can be followed by applying ice, after which the ankle should be wrapped in a compression bandage. The patient should continue with RICE and be instructed in appropriate ambulation, weight bearing, and ROM exercises. She may also need to wear a splint if the ankle is unstable.

Documentation

S: Pt sustained grade II L ankle inversion sprain 48 hours ago, has been applying RICE, and reports L ankle pain, swelling, and decreased weight-bearing tolerance.

O: **Pretreatment:** L ankle girth 25.5 cm, R ankle girth 21.5 cm. L ankle ROM restricted in all planes, with 0 degrees dorsiflexion, 20 degrees plantar flexion, 10 degrees inversion with pain at the lateral ankle at the end of range, and 20 degrees eversion.

Intervention: SWT to L lateral ankle, 3 inches from skin, power and pulse settings of 6, for 30 min. Ice and compression applied after SWT.

Posttreatment: Mildly improved L ankle ROM, ankle circumference unchanged.

A: Pt experienced no discomfort with treatment.

P: Continue daily SWT and RICE protocol at all other times. Pt will be instructed in ambulation, weight bearing, and ROM exercises.

CASE STUDY 10.3

Sacral Pressure Ulcer
Examination
History

FG is an 85-year-old man with a stage IV sacral pressure ulcer. He is bedridden, minimally responsive, and dependent for all bed mobility and feeding activities. He is able to swallow but eats poorly. Treatment until this time has consisted of sharp debridement and hydrocolloid dressings. Although this treatment has reduced the yellow slough, the wound has changed little over the past month.

Systems Review

FG is accompanied to the clinic by his full-time caregiver. His caregiver reports that FG reported earlier in the week that his pain was at a 9/10, and FG acknowledged in the clinic that this rating remains accurate.

Tests and Measures

The pressure ulcer is 15 × 8 cm and 3 cm deep in the deepest area. There is no tunneling or undermining. Approximately 70% of the wound bed is red and granulating, and 30% is covered with yellow slough.

What are reasonable goals of treatment for this patient? What type of diathermy should be used, and why? How often should diathermy be applied? What other aspects of wound care are important for this patient?

Evaluation and Goals

ICF Level	Current Status	Goals
Body structure and function	Sacral ulcer (impaired tissue integrity), reduced strength	Achieve a completely red wound base (short term), decrease ulcer size (long term), wound closure (long term)
Activity	Bedridden, poor appetite, at risk for infection	Prevent infection

CLINICAL CASE STUDIES—cont'd

ICF Level	Current Status	Goals
Participation	Dependent for bed mobility and eating	Decrease patient's medical care requirements

ICF, International Classification for Functioning, Disability and Health.

◆ FIND THE EVIDENCE

PICO Terms	Natural Language Example	Sample PubMed Search
P (Population)	Patients with sacral pressure ulcer and related pain	("pressure ulcer" [text word] OR "pressure ulcer" [MeSH])
I (Intervention)	Diathermy	AND ("diathermy" [text word] OR "diathermy" [MeSH] OR "shortwave therapy" [text word] OR "short-wave therapy" [MeSH] OR "Pulsed Radiofrequency Treatment" [MeSH] OR "Magnetic Field Therapy" [MeSH])
C (Comparison)	No diathermy	
O (Outcome)	Reduction of ulcer pain; healing of wound	

Key Studies or Reviews

1. Conner-Kerr T, Isenberg RA: Retrospective analysis of pulsed radiofrequency energy therapy use in the treatment of chronic pressure ulcers. *Adv Skin Wound Care* 25:253–260, 2012.

   This retrospective analysis of data from 89 patients found a median 51% reduction in wound surface area after 4 weeks of SWT, with 51% of wounds achieving at least 50% reduction in wound surface area, suggesting that SWT is a "beneficial adjuvant treatment option for healing chronic pressure ulcers."

2. Aziz Z, Bell-Syer SEM: Electromagnetic therapy for treating pressure ulcers, *Cochrane Database Syst Rev* 2015(9): CD002930, 2015.

   The authors of this systematic review of randomized controlled trials concluded that there is no strong evidence that electromagnetic therapy promotes complete healing of pressure ulcers, but these conclusions were limited because the review included only two individual trials with a total of 60 participants. This demonstrates the ongoing need for high-quality randomized controlled clinical trials in this important area.

Prognosis

Nonthermal SWT has been shown to accelerate the healing of chronic open wounds, including pressure ulcers. One advantage of this treatment modality over other adjunctive treatments is that it can be applied without removing the dressing, limiting the mechanical and temperature disturbance to the wound and reducing the time required to set up treatment. Also, because nonthermal SWT produces little sensation, it can be applied even if the patient is insensate or cognitively incapable of giving sensory feedback about the treatment. Limiting the mechanical disruption of the wound is particularly important in this case because 70% of the wound bed is covered with red granulation tissue that is fragile but does have the potential to heal.

Intervention

A comprehensive wound care program that addresses pressure relief, dressings, the patient's nutritional status, and debridement when necessary is required to optimize the healing of this patient's wound. Nonthermal SWT may be used as an adjunct to these interventions to facilitate healing and closure of the wound. The applicator's treatment surface should be positioned as close to and as parallel to the tissues to be treated as possible, with the center of the applicator over the deepest part of the wound. The wound dressing may be left in place. If tunneling is present, the center of the applicator should be positioned over the deepest part of the tunnel to promote its closure before the more superficial wound site closes. The applicator's head can be covered with a plastic bag or surgical covering if infection may be an issue. It is recommended that the wound be treated twice a day for 30 minutes or once a day for 45 to 60 minutes. If the patient feels discomfort, the pulse rate should be lowered. The pulse rate setting should also be reduced if the wound's surface appears to be closing before its depth has filled completely.

Documentation

S: Bedridden, poorly responsive Pt with stage IV sacral pressure ulcer.

O: **Pretreatment:** Sacral ulcer 15 × 8 cm and 3 cm deep in deepest area. No tunneling or undermining. 70% of wound bed is red and granulating, and 30% is covered with yellow slough.

Intervention: SWT twice daily for 30 min to sacral ulcer, power 6 and pulse rate 600 pps, Pt prone, applicator covered with sheath and 3 inches from wound.

Posttreatment: Wound appears unchanged after 2 treatments.

A: SWT applied with no noticeable adverse effects.

P: Continue SWT twice daily for 1 more week. Continue if wound improves, discontinue if no benefit appreciated.

Chapter Review

1. Diathermy is the application of shortwave or microwave electromagnetic energy to a person's body.
2. The effects of diathermy may be thermal or nonthermal. Continuous diathermy produces thermal effects and is used for heating large areas of deep tissue. Nonthermal diathermy is known as *SWT*. SWT may lessen pain; reduce edema; decrease symptoms of osteoarthritis; and accelerate wound, nerve, and bone healing.
3. Contraindications for the use of diathermy depend on whether the application is thermal or nonthermal. Both thermal and nonthermal diathermy are contraindicated if a patient has implanted or transcutaneous neural stimulators (including cardiac pacemakers and deep brain stimulators) or is pregnant. Contraindications for thermal diathermy include metal implants; malignancy; and application over the eyes, testes, and growing epiphyses. Also, thermal diathermy should not be applied to deep tissue such as organs or used as a substitute for conventional therapy for edema and pain.
4. Precautions for all forms of diathermy include electronic or magnetic equipment in the vicinity, patient obesity, and copper-bearing intrauterine contraceptive devices. Precautions for the use of SWT include pregnancy and skeletal immaturity.
5. The reader is referred to the Evolve website for additional resources and references.

Glossary

Continuous shortwave diathermy: The clinical application of continuous shortwave electromagnetic radiation to increase tissue temperature.

Diathermy: The application of shortwave or microwave electromagnetic energy to increase tissue temperature, particularly in deep tissues.

Inductive coil applicator: A coil through which an alternating electrical current flows, producing a magnetic field perpendicular to the coil and inducing electrical eddy currents in the tissue within or in front of the coil. This type of applicator can be used to apply shortwave diathermy.

Low-frequency electromagnetic radiation: Electromagnetic radiation that is nonionizing and that cannot break molecular bonds or produce ions. This includes extremely low-frequency waves, shortwaves, microwaves, infrared, visible light, and ultraviolet.

Magnetron: An applicator that produces a high-frequency alternating current in an antenna. This type of applicator is used to apply microwave diathermy.

Microwave radiation: Nonionizing electromagnetic radiation with a frequency range of 300 MHz to 300 GHz, which lies between the ranges of radiofrequency and infrared radiation.

Nonthermal shortwave therapy (SWT): The clinical application of pulsed shortwave electromagnetic radiation in which heating is not the therapeutic mechanism of action.

Shortwave radiation: Nonionizing electromagnetic radiation with a frequency range of approximately 3 to 30 MHz. Shortwave is a band within the radiofrequency range. The radiofrequency range lies between extremely low-frequency radiation and microwave radiation.

References

1. Centers for Disease Control and Prevention: The electromagnetic spectrum: non-ionizing radiation. https://www.cdc.gov/nceh/radiation/nonionizing_radiation.html. (Accessed February 29, 2020).
2. Hitchcock RT, Patterson RM: *Radio-frequency and ELF electromagnetic energies: a handbook for health professionals*, New York, 1995.
3. Silberstein N: Diathermy: comeback, or new technology? An electrically induced therapy modality enjoys a resurgence. *Rehab Manag* 21(30):32–33, 2008.
4. Mattsson MO, Simkó M: Emerging medical applications based on non-ionizing electromagnetic fields from 0 Hz to 10 THz. *Med Devices (Auckl)* 12:347–368, 2019. doi:10.2147/MDER.S214152.
5. Rhode AC, Lavelle LM, Berry DC: Efficacy of rebound diathermy as a thermal heating agent: a critically appraised topic. *J Sport Rehabil* 28(6):656–659, 2019. doi:10.1123/jsr.2018-0034.
6. Hawkes AR, Draper DO, Johnson AW, et al: Heating capacity of rebound shortwave diathermy and moist hot packs at superficial depths. *J Athl Train* 48(4):471–476, 2013. doi:10.4085/1062-6050-48.3.04.
7. Draper DO, Hawkes AR, Johnson AW, et al: Muscle heating with Megapulse II shortwave diathermy and ReBound diathermy. *J Athl Train* 48(4):477–482, 2013. doi:10.4085/1062-6050-48.3.01.
8. Silverman DR, Pendleton LA: A comparison of the effects of continuous and pulsed shortwave diathermy on peripheral circulation. *Arch Phys Med Rehabil* 49:429–436, 1968.
9. Conradi E, Pages IH: Effects of continuous and pulsed microwave irradiation on distribution of heat in the gluteal region of minipigs. *Scand J Rehabil Med* 21:59–62, 1989.
10. Draper DO, Knight K, Fujiwara T, et al: Temperature change in human muscle during and after pulsed short-wave diathermy. *J Orthop Sports Phys Ther* 29:13–18, 1999, discussion 19–22.
11. U.S. Food and Drug Administration and U.S: Department of Health and Human Services: Physical medicine devices; reclassification of shortwave diathermy for all other uses, henceforth to be known as nonthermal shortwave therapy. Final order; technical correction. *Fed Regist* 80:61298–61302, 2015.
12. Kloth LC, Zisken MC: Diathermy and pulsed radio frequency radiation. In Michlovitz SL, editor: *Thermal agents in rehabilitation*, Philadelphia, 1996, FA Davis.
13. Verrier M, Falconer K, Crawford SJ: A comparison of tissue temperature following two shortwave diathermy techniques. *Physiother Can* 29:21–25, 1977.
14. Leitgeb N, Omerspahic A, Niedermayr F: Exposure of non-target tissues in medical diathermy. *Bioelectromagnetics* 31:12–19, 2010.
15. Giombini A, Giovannini V, Di Cesare A, et al: Hyperthermia induced by microwave diathermy in the management of muscle and tendon injuries. *Br Med Bull* 83:379–396, 2007.
16. Cihoric N, Tsikkinis A, Van Rhoon G, et al: Hyperthermia-related clinical trials on cancer treatment within the ClinicalTrials.gov registry. *Int J Hyperther* 31(6):609–614, 2015.
17. McMeeken JM, Bell C: Effects of selective blood and tissue heating on blood flow in the dog hind limb. *Exp Physiol* 75:359–366, 1990.
18. Fadilah R, Pinkas J, Weinberger A, et al: Heating rabbit joint by microwave applicator. *Arch Phys Med Rehabil* 68:710–712, 1987.
19. Scott RS, Chou CK, McCumber M, et al: Complications resulting from spurious fields produced by a microwave applicator used for hyperthermia. *Int J Radiat Oncol Biol Phys* 12:1883–1886, 1986.
20. Goats GC: Microwave diathermy. *Br J Sports Med* 24(4):212–218, 1990.
21. Murray CC, Kitchen S: Effect of pulse repetition rate on the perception of thermal sensation with pulsed shortwave diathermy. *Physiother Res Int* 5:73–84, 2000.
22. Garrett CL, Draper DO, Knight KL: Heat distribution in the lower leg from pulsed short-wave diathermy and ultrasound treatments. *J Athl Train* 35:50–55, 2000.
23. McNiven DR, Wyper DJ: Microwave therapy and muscle blood flow in man. *J Microw Power* 11:168–170, 1976.
24. McMeeken JM, Bell C: Microwave irradiation of the human forearm and hand. *Physiother Theory Pract* 75:359–366, 1990.

25. Wyper DJ, McNiven DR: Effects of some physiotherapeutic agents on skeletal muscle blood flow. *Physiotherapy* 60:309–310, 1976.

26. Laufer Y, Dar G: Effectiveness of thermal and athermal short-wave diathermy for the management of knee osteoarthritis: a systematic review and meta-analysis. *Osteoarthritis Cartilage* 20:957–966, 2012.

27. Mitchell SM, Trowbridge CA, Fincher AL, et al: Effect of diathermy on muscle temperature, electromyography, and mechanomyography. *Muscle Nerve* 38:992–1004, 2008.

28. Teslim OA, Adebowale AC, Ojoawo AO, et al: Comparative effects of pulsed and continuous short wave diathermy on pain and selected physiological parameters among subjects with chronic knee osteoarthritis. *Technol Health Care* 21:433–440, 2013.

29. Chastain PB: The effect of deep heat on isometric strength. *Phys Ther* 58:543–546, 1978.

30. McMeeken JM, Bell C: Effects of microwave irradiation on blood flow in the dog hind limb. *Exp Physiol* 75:367–374, 1990.

31. Robertson VJ, Ward AR, Jung P: The effect of heat on tissue extensibility: a comparison of deep and superficial heating. *Arch Phys Med Rehabil* 86:819–825, 2005.

32. Oosterveld FG, Rasker JJ: Effects of local heat and cold treatment on surface and articular temperature of arthritic knees. *Arthritis Rheum* 37:1578–1582, 1994.

33. Pilla AA: Nonthermal electromagnetic fields: from first messenger to therapeutic applications. *Electromagn Biol Med* 32:123–136, 2013.

34. Pilla AA: Electromagnetic fields instantaneously modulate nitric oxide signaling in challenged biological systems. *Biochem Biophys Res Commun* 426:330–333, 2012.

35. Rozengurt E, Mendoza S: Monovalent ion fluxes and the control of cell proliferation in cultured fibroblasts. *Ann N Y Acad Sci* 339:175–190, 1980.

36. Boonstra J, Skaper SD, Varons SJ: Regulation of Na+, K+ pump activity by nerve growth factor in chick embryo dorsal root ganglia cells. *J Cell Physiol* 113:452–455, 1982.

37. Gemsa D, Seitz M, Kramer W, et al: Ionophore A23187 raises cyclic AMP levels in macrophages by stimulation of prostaglandin E formation. *Exp Cell Res* 118:55–62, 1979.

38. Hill J, Lewis M, Mills P, et al: Pulsed short-wave diathermy effects on human fibroblast proliferation. *Arch Phys Med Rehabil* 83:832–836, 2002.

39. Pasek J, Pasek T, Sieroń-Stołtny K, et al: Electromagnetic fields in medicine—the state of art. *Electromagn Biol Med* 35:170–175, 2016.

40. Markov MS: *Electromagnetic fields in biology and medicine*, Boca Raton, FL, 2015, CRC Press.

41. Mayrovitz HN, Larsen PB: A preliminary study to evaluate the effect of pulsed radio frequency field treatment on lower extremity peri-ulcer skin microcirculation of diabetic patients. *Wounds* 7:90–93, 1995.

42. Mayrovitz HN, Larsen PB: Effects of pulsed electromagnetic fields on skin microvascular blood perfusion. *Wounds* 4:197–202, 1992.

43. Draper DO, Castro JL, Feland B, et al: Shortwave diathermy and prolonged stretching increase hamstring flexibility more than prolonged stretching alone. *J Orthop Sports Phys Ther* 34:13–20, 2004.

44. Sieger C, Draper DO: Use of pulsed shortwave diathermy and joint mobilization to increase ankle range of motion in the presence of surgical implanted metal: a case series. *J Orthop Sports Phys Ther* 36:669–677, 2006.

45. Peres SE, Draper DO, Knight KL, et al: Pulsed shortwave diathermy and prolonged long-duration stretching increase dorsiflexion range of motion more than identical stretching without diathermy. *J Athl Train* 37:43–50, 2002.

46. Brucker JB, Knight KL, Rubley MD, et al: An 18-day stretching regimen, with or without pulsed, shortwave diathermy, and ankle dorsiflexion after 3 weeks. *J Athl Train* 40:276–280, 2005.

47. Ozen S, Doganci EB, Ozyuvali A, et al: Effectiveness of continuous versus pulsed short-wave diathermy in the management of knee osteoarthritis: a randomized pilot study. *Caspian J Intern Med Fall* 10(4):431–438, 2019. doi:10.22088/cjim.10.4.431.

48. Rabini A, Piazzini DB, Tancredi G, et al: Deep heating therapy via microwave diathermy relieves pain and improves physical function in patients with knee osteoarthritis: a double-blind randomized clinical trial. *Eur J Phys Rehabil Med* 48(4):549–559, 2012.

49. Wang H, Zhang C, Gao C, et al: Effects of short-wave therapy in patients with knee osteoarthritis: a systematic review and meta-analysis. *Clin Rehabil* 31(5):660–671, 2017.

50. Ginsberg AJ: Ultrasound radiowaves as a therapeutic agent. *Med Rec* 19:1–8, 1934.

51. Milinowski AS: Athermapeutic device, United States Patent No. 3181. 35, 1965.

52. Foley-Nolan D, Barry C, Coughlan RJ, et al: Pulsed high frequency (27 MHz) electromagnetic therapy for persistent neck pain: a double blind placebo-controlled study of 20 patients. *Orthopedics* 13:445–451, 1990.

53. Foley-Nolan D, Moore K, Codd M, et al: Low energy, high frequency, pulsed electromagnetic therapy for acute whiplash injuries. *Scand J Rehabil Med* 24:51–59, 1992.

54. Long Y, Wei H, Li J, et al: ACS effective wound healing enabled by discrete alternative electric fields from wearable nanogenerators. *Nano* 12(12):12533–12540, 2018. doi:10.1021/acsnano.8b07038.

55. Lazović M, Kocić M, Dimitrijević L, et al: Pulsed electromagnetic field during cast immobilization in postmenopausal women with Colles' fracture. *Srp Arh Celok Lek* 140:619–624, 2012.

56. Pilla AA, Martin DE, Schuett AM, et al: Effect of PRF therapy on edema from grades I and II ankle sprains: a placebo controlled randomized, multi-site, double-blind clinical study. *J Athl Train* 31:S53, 1996.

57. Pennington GM, Danley DL, Sumko MH: Pulsed, non-thermal, high frequency electromagnetic field (Diapulse) in the treatment of grade I and grade II ankle sprains. *Mil Med* 153:101–104, 1993.

58. Wagstaff P, Wagstaff S, Downey M: A pilot study to compare the efficacy of continuous and pulsed magnetic energy (shortwave diathermy) on the relief of low back pain. *Physiotherapy* 72:563–566, 1986.

59. Lee PB, Kim YC, Lim YJ, et al: Efficacy of pulsed electromagnetic therapy for chronic lower back pain: a randomized, double-blind, placebo-controlled study. *J Int Med Res* 34:160–167, 2006.

60. Sorrell RG, Muhlenfeld J, Moffett J, et al: Evaluation of pulsed electromagnetic field therapy for the treatment of chronic postoperative pain following lumbar surgery: a pilot, double-blind, randomized, sham-controlled clinical trial. *J Pain Res* 11:1209–1222, 2018. doi:10.2147/JPR.S164303.

61. Elshiwi AM, Hamada HA, Mosaad D, et al: Effect of pulsed electromagnetic field on nonspecific low back pain patients: a randomized controlled trial. *Braz J Phys Ther* 23(3):244–249, 2019. doi:10.1016/j.bjpt.2018.08.004.

62. Kaplan EG, Weinstock RE: Clinical evaluation of Diapulse as adjunctive therapy following foot surgery. *J Am Podiatry Assoc* 58:218–221, 1968.

63. Khooshideh M, Latifi Rostami SS, Sheikh M, et al: Pulsed electromagnetic fields for postsurgical pain management in women undergoing cesarean section: a randomized, double-blind, placebo-controlled trial. *Clin J Pain* 33(2):142–147, 2017. doi:10.1097/AJP.0000000000000376.

64. Babaei-Ghazani A, Shahrami B, Fallah E, et al: Continuous shortwave diathermy with exercise reduces pain and improves function in lateral epicondylitis more than sham diathermy: a randomized controlled trial. *J Bodyw Mov Ther* 24(1):69–76, 2020. doi:10.1016/j.jbmt.2019.05.025.

65. Barker AT, Barlow PS, Porter J, et al: A double blind clinical trial of low power pulsed shortwave therapy in the treatment of soft tissue injury. *Physiotherapy* 71:500–504, 1985.

66. McGill SN: The effects of pulsed shortwave therapy on lateral ankle sprains. *N Z J Physiother* 51:21–24, 1988.

67. Dziedzic K, Hill J, Lewis M, et al: Effectiveness of manual therapy or pulsed shortwave diathermy in addition to advice and exercise for neck disorders: a pragmatic randomized controlled trial in physical therapy clinics. *Arthritis Rheum* 53:214–222, 2005.

68. Osti L, Buono AD, Maffulli N: Pulsed electromagnetic fields after rotator cuff repair: a randomized, controlled study. *Orthopedics* 38:e223–e228, 2015.

69. Strauch B, Herman C, Dabb R, et al: Evidence-based use of pulsed electromagnetic field therapy in clinical plastic surgery. *Aesthet Surg J* 29:135–143, 2009.

70. Rawe IM, Lowenstein A, Barcelo CR, et al: Control of postoperative pain with a wearable continuously operating pulsed radiofrequency energy device: a preliminary study. *Aesth Plast Surg* 36:458–463, 2012.

71. Guo L, Kubat NJ, Nelson TR, et al: Meta-analysis of clinical efficacy of pulsed radio frequency energy treatment. *Ann Surg* 255:457–467, 2012.

72. Cameron BM: Experimental acceleration of wound healing. *Am J Orthop* 3:336–343, 1961.

73. Itoh M, Montemayor JS, Matsumoto E, et al: Accelerated wound healing of pressure ulcers by pulsed high peak power electromagnetic energy (Diapulse). *Decubitus* 2:24–28, 1991.

74. Salzberg CA, Cooper-Vastola SA, Perez FJ, et al: The effect of non-thermal pulsed electromagnetic energy (Diapulse) on wound healing of pressure ulcers in spinal cord injured patients: a randomized, double-blind study. *Wounds* 7:11–16, 1995.

75. Conner-Kerr T, Isenberg RA: Retrospective analysis of pulsed radiofrequency energy therapy use in the treatment of chronic pressure ulcers. *Adv Skin Wound Care* 25(6):253–260, 2012. doi:10.1097/01.ASW.0000415342.37554.

76. Ionescu A, Ionescu D, Milinescu S, et al: Study of efficiency of Diapulse therapy on the dynamics of enzymes in burned wound. *Proc Int Congr Burns* 6:25–26, 1982.

77. Strauch B, Patel MK, Rosen DJ, et al: Pulsed magnetic field therapy increases tensile strength in a rat Achilles tendon repair model. *J Hand Surg Am* 31:1131–1135, 2006.

78. Szlosek PA, Taggart J, Cavallario JM, et al: Effectiveness of diathermy in comparison with ultrasound or corticosteroids in patients with tendinopathy: a critically appraised topic. *J Sport Rehabil* 23:370–375, 2014.

79. Strauch B, Patel MK, Navarro JA, et al: Pulsed magnetic fields accelerate cutaneous wound healing in rats. *Plast Reconstr Surg* 120(2):425–430, 2007.

80. Aziz Z, Bell-Syer SEM: Electromagnetic therapy for treating pressure ulcers. *Cochrane Database Syst Rev* 2015(9):1–25, 2015. doi:10.1002/14651858.CD002930.pub6.

81. Aziz Z, Cullum N: Electromagnetic therapy for treating venous leg ulcers. *Cochrane Database Syst Rev* 2015(7):1–31, 2015. doi:10.1002/14651858.CD002933.pub6.

82. Game FL, Apelqvist J, Attinger C, et al: Effectiveness of interventions to enhance healing of chronic ulcers of the foot in diabetes: a systematic review. *Diabetes Metab Res Rev* 32(Suppl 1):154–168, 2016. doi:10.1002/dmrr.2707.

83. Fu T, Lineaweaver WC, Zhang F, et al: Role of shortwave and microwave diathermy in peripheral neuropathy. *J Int Med Res* 47(8):3569–3579, 2019. doi:10.1177/0300060519854905.

84. Wilson DH, Jagadeesh P: Experimental regeneration in peripheral nerves and the spinal cord in laboratory animals exposed to a pulsed electromagnetic field. *Paraplegia* 14:12–20, 1976.

85. Crowe MJ, Sun ZP, Battocletti JH, et al: Exposure to pulsed magnetic fields enhances motor recovery in cats after spinal cord injury. *Spine* 28:2660–2666, 2003.

86. Wang C, Liu Y, Wang Y, et al: Lowfrequency pulsed electromagnetic field promotes functional recovery, reduces inflammation and oxidative stress, and enhances HSP70 expression following spinal cord injury. *Molecular Med Rep* 19(3):1687–1693, 2019.

87. Cook HH, Narendan NS, Montgomery JC: The effects of pulsed, high-frequency waves on the rate of osteogenesis in the healing of extraction wounds in dogs. *Oral Surg Oral Med Oral Pathol* 32:1008–1016, 1971.

88. Pilla AA: 27.12 MHz pulsed radiofrequency electromagnetic fields accelerate bone repair in a rabbit fibula osteotomy model. *Presented at the Bioelectromagnetics Society Meeting*, Boston, MA, 1995.

89. Cook JJ, Summers NJ, Cook EA: Healing in the new millennium: bone stimulators: an overview of where we've been and where we may be heading. *Clin Podiatr Med Surg* 32:45–59, 2015.

90. Martinez-Rondanelli A, Martinez JP, Moncada ME, et al: Electromagnetic stimulation as coadjuvant in the healing of diaphyseal femoral fractures: a randomized controlled trial. *Colomb Med* 45:67–71, 2014.

91. Hannemann PF, Mommers EH, Schots JP, et al: The effects of low-intensity pulsed ultrasound and pulsed electromagnetic fields bone growth stimulation in acute fractures: a systematic review and meta-analysis of randomized controlled trials. *Arch Orthop Trauma Surg* 134:1093–1106, 2014.

92. Krzyżańska L, Straburzyńska-Lupa A, Rąglewska P, et al: Beneficial effects of pulsed electromagnetic field during cast immobilization in patients with distal radius fracture. *Biomed Res Int* 2020:6849352, 2020. doi:10.1155/2020/6849352.

93. Li S, Yu B, Zhou D, et al: Electromagnetic fields for treatment of osteoarthritis. *Cochrane Database Syst Rev* 2013(12):CD003523, 2013.

94. Ryang We S, Koog YH, Jeong KI, et al: Effects of pulsed electromagnetic field on knee osteoarthritis: a systematic review. *Rheumatology* 52:815–824, 2013.

95. Marks R: Pulsed electromagnetic fields and osteoarthritis: a case where the science and its application do not always concur. *EC Orthopaedics* 6(6):216–229, 2017.

96. Veronesi F, Torricelli P, Giavaresi G, et al: In vivo effect of two different pulsed electromagnetic field frequencies on osteoarthritis. *J Orthop Res* 32(5):677–685, 2014. doi:10.1002/jor.22584.

97. Ruggera PS, Witters DM, von Maltzahn G, et al: In vitro assessment of tissue heating near metallic medical implants by exposure to pulsed radio frequency diathermy. *Phys Med Biol* 48:2919–2928, 2003.

98. Nutt JG, Anderson VC, Peacock JH, et al: DBS and diathermy interaction induces severe CNS damage. *Neurology* 56:1384–1386, 2001.

99. Health Notice (Hazard) 80(10). *Implantable cardiac pacemakers: interference generated by diathermy equipment*, 1980.

100. McMurray RG, Katz VL: Thermoregulation in pregnancy: implications for exercise. *Sports Med* 10:146–158, 1990.

101. Edwards MJ: Congenital defects in guinea pigs following induced hyperthermia during gestation. *Arch Pathol Lab Med* 84:42–48, 1967.

102. Edwards MJ: Congenital defects due to hyperthermia. *Adv Vet Sci Comp Med* 22:29–52, 1978.

103. Brown-Woodman PD, Hadley JA, Waterhouse J, et al: Teratogenic effects of exposure to radiofrequency radiation (27.12 MHz) from a short wave diathermy unit. *Ind Health* 26:1–10, 1988.

104. Draper DO: Pulsed shortwave diathermy and joint mobilizations for achieving normal elbow range of motion after injury or surgery with implanted metal: a case series. *J Athl Train* 49:851–855, 2014.

105. Aiba H, Yamada S, Mizutani J, et al: Clinical outcomes of radio-hyperthermo-chemotherapy for soft tissue sarcoma compared to a soft tissue sarcoma registry in Japan: a retrospective matched-pair cohort study. *Cancer Med* 7(4):1560–1571, 2018. doi:10.1002/cam4.1366.

106. Tofani S, Agnesod G: The assessment of unwanted radiation around diathermy RF capacitive applicators. *Health Phys* 47:235–241, 1984.

107. Lau RW, Dunscombe PB: Some observations on stray magnetic fields and power outputs from shortwave diathermy equipment. *Health Phys* 46:939–943, 1984.

108. Lerman Y, Caner A, Jacubovich R, et al: Electromagnetic fields from shortwave diathermy equipment in physiotherapy departments. *Physiotherapy* 82:456–458, 1996.

109. Martin JC, McCallum HM, Strelley S, et al: Electromagnetic fields from therapeutic diathermy equipment: a review of hazards and precautions. *Physiotherapy* 77:3–7, 1991.

110. Gryz K, Karpowicz J: Environmental impact of the use of radiofrequency electromagnetic fields in physiotherapeutic treatment. *Rocz Panstw Zakl Hig* 65(1):55–61, 2014.

111. Shah SG, Farrow A: Systematic literature review of adverse reproductive outcomes associated with physiotherapists' occupational exposures to non-ionising radiation. *J Occup Health* 56(5):323–331, 2014.

112. Nielson NC, Hansen R, Larsen T: Heat induction in copper-bearing IUDs during short-wave diathermy. *Acta Obstet Gynecol Scand* 58:495, 1979.

113. Heick A, Espesen T, Pedersen HL, et al: Is diathermy safe in women with copper-bearing IUDs? *Acta Obstet Gynecol Scand* 70:153–155, 1991.

114. Shah SG, Farrow A: Assessment of physiotherapists' occupational exposure to radiofrequency electromagnetic fields from shortwave and microwave diathermy devices: a literature review. *J Occup Environ Hyg* 10(6):312–327, 2013. doi:10.1080/15459624.2013.782203.

115. Kallen B, Malmquist G, Moritz U: Delivery outcome among physiotherapists in Sweden: is non-ionizing radiation a fetal hazard? *Arch Environ Health* 37:81–84, 1982. Reprinted in Physiotherapy 78:15–18, 1992.

116. Larsen A, Olsen J, Svane O: Gender-specific reproductive outcome and exposure to high frequency electromagnetic radiation among physiotherapists. *Scand J Work Environ Health* 17:318–323, 1991.

117. Ouellet-Hellstrom R, Stewart WF: Miscarriages among female physical therapists who report using radio and microwave frequency electromagnetic radiation. *Am J Epidemiol* 10:775–785, 1993.

118. Lerman Y, Jacubovich R, Green MS: Pregnancy outcome following exposure to shortwaves among female physiotherapists in Israel. *Am J Ind Med* 39:499–504, 2001.

119. Takininen H, Kyyronene P, Hemminki K: The effects of ultrasound, shortwaves and physical exertion on pregnancy outcomes in physiotherapists. *J Epidemiol Community Health* 44:196–201, 1990.

120. Li DK, Chen H, Ferber JR, et al: Exposure to magnetic field non-ionizing radiation and the risk of miscarriage: a prospective cohort study. *Sci Rep* 7(1):17541, 2017. doi:10.1038/s41598-017-16623-8.

121. Werheimer N, Leeper E: Electrical wiring configurations and childhood cancer. *Am J Epidemiol* 109:273–284, 1979.

122. Milham Jr S: Mortality from leukemia in workers exposed to electrical and magnetic fields (letter). *N Engl J Med* 307:249, 1982.

123. Johansen C: Electromagnetic fields and health effects—epidemiologic studies of cancer, diseases of the central nervous system and arrhythmia-related heart disease. *Scand J Work Environ Health* 30(Suppl 1):1–30, 2004.

124. American Physical Society: National Policy Statement 05.3 electric and magnetic fields and public health, adopted April 15, 2005. http://www.aps.org/policy/statements/05_3.cfm. (Accessed April 12, 2020).

125. Surrell JA, Alexander RC, Cohle SD: Effects of microwave radiation on living tissues. *J Trauma* 27:935–939, 1987.

126. Ozen S, Helhel S, Bilgin S: Temperature and burn injury prediction of human skin exposed to microwaves: a model analysis. *Radiat Environ Biophys* 50(3):483–489, 2011. doi:10.1007/s00411-011-0364-y.

Introduction to Electrotherapy

11

Michelle H. Cameron | Michelle Ocelnik

CHAPTER OBJECTIVES

After reading this chapter, the reader will be able to do the following:
- Define *electrical current* and identify the different types.
- Describe the effects of electrotherapy.
- Compare and contrast the different techniques for electrotherapy.
- Safely and effectively apply electrotherapy.
- Choose the best technique for treatment with electrotherapy, and list the advantages and disadvantages of each.
- Select the appropriate equipment and parameters for treatment with electrotherapy.
- Accurately and completely document treatment with electrotherapy.

This chapter introduces the use of electrical currents in rehabilitation and discusses the history of electrical stimulation, the devices used, and the features of therapeutic electrical currents, including their waveforms and other parameters. This is followed by an overview of the clinical effects of electrical currents, contraindications and precautions for the application of electrical currents, and a summary of application techniques and documentation for electrical stimulation treatment. Specific clinical applications of electrical currents are discussed in greater detail in Chapters 12 through 15.

An **electrical current** is a flow of charged particles. The charged particles may be electrons or ions (charged molecules). Electrical currents have been applied to biological systems to change physiological processes since at least 2000 years ago, when it was recorded that the Romans used electrical discharge from torpedo fish to alleviate pain.[1,2]

There was a revival of interest in medical applications of electrical currents in the late 18th and early 19th centuries. In 1791, Galvani first recorded producing muscle contractions by touching metal to a frog's muscle. He called this effect "animal electricity." A few years later, after Volta constructed the first true battery in 1800, Galvani used the current put out by this device to produce muscle contractions. He named this continuous flow of current in one direction "Galvanic current." In an attempt to understand how electrical currents cause muscle contractions, Duchenne mapped out the locations on the skin where electrical stimulation most effectively caused specific muscles to contract. He called these locations "**motor points**."[3] During the 1830s, Faraday discovered that bidirectional electrical currents could be induced by a moving magnet. He called this current "Faradic current." Faradic current can also be used to produce muscle contractions. In 1905, Lapicque developed the "law of excitation," relating the intensity and duration of a stimulus to whether it would produce a muscle contraction. Lapicque introduced the concept of the strength-duration curve, which is described later in this chapter and continues to be the basis for most of the therapeutic uses of electrical currents today.

Electrical stimulation has a wide range of clinical applications in rehabilitation, including producing muscle contractions for strengthening and improving endurance and motor control, controlling pain, controlling spasticity, promoting tissue healing, enhancing transdermal drug delivery, and providing electromyographic biofeedback. These applications are explained in detail in Chapters 12 through 15.

Many professionals, including physical therapists, occupational therapists, athletic trainers, physicians, and chiropractors, find electrical stimulation to be a valuable and effective component of their therapeutic armamentarium. In an ongoing effort to provide evidence-based treatment, researchers have evaluated the efficacy and effectiveness of electrical stimulation for common clinical applications. The proliferation of more sophisticated machines has also increased interest in the use of electrical stimulation as a rehabilitation intervention. These machines have multiple waveforms, allow a wide variety of parameter selections, may include computer-generated images of body parts and electrode placement for specific diagnoses, and may be integrated into bracing devices to facilitate functional use. The availability of small, patient-friendly units that can be used at home has also enhanced the

225

effectiveness of electrical stimulation by allowing ongoing treatment between clinic visits.

Electrical stimulation can be applied to the body in a variety of ways. The electricity may be delivered by a stimulator implanted inside the body, such as with cardiac pacemakers and spinal cord stimulators, or by an external stimulator that delivers current to implanted or external surface transcutaneous electrodes. Alternatively, electrical stimulation can be applied percutaneously with acupuncture needles to acupuncture points. This application is termed *electroacupuncture* and is briefly discussed in Chapter 13. This book focuses on the application of electrical stimulation by external stimulators that deliver current transcutaneously via surface electrodes applied to the skin.

Electrical Current Devices, Waveforms, and Parameters

The external stimulation devices used to deliver current transcutaneously consist of a power source and controls to adjust features of the output current (Fig. 11.1). These devices can be small, portable electrical stimulators, about the size of a small camera or deck of cards, that are battery powered, or larger clinical stimulators, about the size of a toaster oven, which usually need to be plugged into the wall outlet. However, some smaller portable devices and larger clinical units are now available with rechargeable batteries. The stimulator delivers current to the patient via electrodes placed on the skin. In general, the stimulator is connected to the electrodes by lead wires. Recently, some devices come with wireless electrodes that do not use lead wires to connect them to the stimulator. With wireless electrodes, the signal generators either attach directly to pre-gelled electrodes and are controlled via an app or other wireless programmer, or the signal generators communicate with the electrodes using Bluetooth technology. However the electrodes connect with the signal generator, electrical current flows between the electrodes through the patient's skin and underlying tissues to produce a physiological and therapeutic effect.

The features of the electrical current that can be adjusted by the controls on the device are usually called *parameters.* The terminology used to describe these parameters can be confusing, in part because various synonymous terms are used to describe the same feature. For example, *rate* and *frequency* are used interchangeably to describe the number of pulses of electrical current that occur in a second, and *pulse width* and *pulse duration* are used interchangeably to describe how long a single pulse lasts. In an attempt to standardize the terminology used and promote more consistent use of terms describing therapeutic electrical currents, the Clinical Electrophysiology Section of the American Physical Therapy Association (APTA) published a guide to electrotherapeutic terminology that included recommended standard terminology and definitions. However, the guide has not been widely adopted and has not been reissued or revised since 2000.[4] In this text, we use the terminology and definitions most widely used clinically and by device manufacturers and provide commonly used alternatives, within the text in parentheses following the preferred term as well as in the glossary definitions. Following are descriptions and explanations of commonly available electrical current parameters used for clinical electrical stimulation. These parameters may be adjustable or preset, depending on the specific unit.

WAVEFORMS

An electrical current is a flow of charged particles. The shape of the current waveform is a graphic representation of the current flow over time. Waveforms can be of almost any shape, including square, rectangular, triangular, sinusoidal, or irregularly shaped, based on the velocity of current flow. The vertical axis represents the direction of current flow (positive or negative), and the horizontal axis represents time. The following section describes the waveforms commonly available on electrical stimulation devices used both in the United States and around the world. Various other waveforms in use outside the United States, such as exponential, diadynamic, and Trabert, are not described in this text.

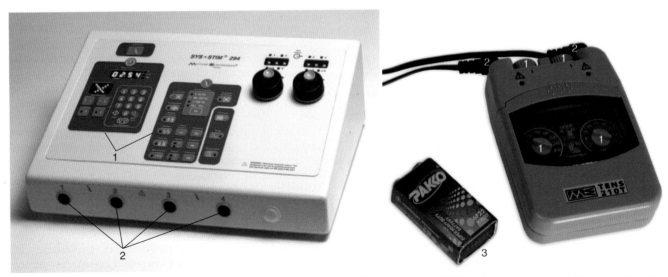

FIGURE 11.1 Electrical stimulation device with parts labeled. *(1)* Controls to adjust parameters. *(2)* Sockets for electrodes. *(3)* Power supply. Note that for clinical units, the power is supplied from the wall via a cord, usually inserted in the back. For portable units, the power is usually supplied by a 9V battery. (Courtesy Mettler Electronics, Anaheim, CA.)

Direct Current, Alternating Current, and Pulsed Current

Waveforms can be divided into three types: **direct current (DC)**, **alternating current (AC)**, and **pulsed current (PC)**. DC is a continuous stream of charged particles flowing in one direction (Fig. 11.2). DC is the type of current that comes out of a battery and was the earliest type of current ever used clinically, but DC is not the type of current that comes out of most battery-driven electrical stimulation devices, and DC is not commonly used for electrotherapy at this time because it is generally uncomfortable. DC is used for **iontophoresis** (the transcutaneous delivery of medications facilitated by an electrical current) and for stimulating contractions in denervated muscle because other types of currents are generally not effective for these applications.

AC is a continuous, sinusoidal, bidirectional flow of charged particles where the current is always flowing back and forth (Fig. 11.3). AC is the type of current that comes out of a wall socket, although it is not necessarily the type of current that comes out of an electrical stimulation device plugged into the wall. AC can be used for pain control and to produce muscle contractions.

PC is an interrupted flow of charged particles where the current flows in a series of pulses separated by periods where no current flows. PC may be produced by a battery-powered or wall current–powered device. PC is often used for pain control, for tissue healing, or to produce muscle contractions. PC may flow in only one direction during a pulse, which is known as **monophasic pulsed current** (Fig. 11.4A), or it may flow back and forth during a pulse, which is known as **biphasic pulsed current** (see Fig. 11.4B).

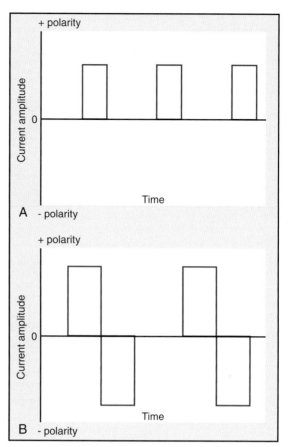

FIGURE 11.4 (A) Monophasic and (B) biphasic pulsed currents.

Monophasic pulsed currents may be used for any clinical application of electrical stimulation but are most commonly used to promote tissue healing and manage acute edema. The most commonly encountered monophasic pulsed current is high-volt pulsed current (HVPC), also known as *pulsed galvanic current*. This waveform is made up of pulses, each composed of a pair of short, exponentially decaying waves that travel in the same direction (Fig. 11.5).

Clinical Pearl

Biphasic pulsed currents are the most commonly used waveform in electrotherapy. This type of current can be used to produce muscle contractions or to control pain.

Biphasic pulsed currents are the most commonly used waveform in electrotherapy and are mainly used to control pain or to produce muscle contractions. A biphasic pulsed current is made up of two phases. During each pulse, the current flows in one direction during the first phase and in the opposite direction in the second phase. The waveform is called *biphasic symmetrical* when the speed and total amount of current flow are the same during the two phases. The waveform is called *biphasic asymmetrical* when the speed of current flow is different for each phase. A biphasic asymmetrical waveform is balanced if the total amount of current flow for the two phases is the same and is unbalanced if the total amount of current flow for the two phases

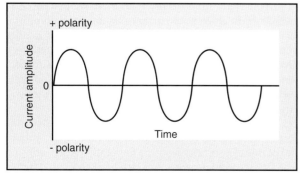

FIGURE 11.2 Direct current (DC).

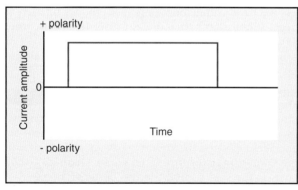

FIGURE 11.3 Alternating current (AC).

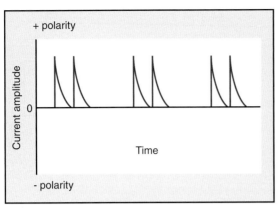

FIGURE 11.5 High-voltage pulsed current.

is different (Fig. 11.6). In general, the biphasic PC waveforms produced by electrotherapy devices are symmetrical (which are always balanced) or asymmetrical balanced. There is usually little, if any, clinical difference between the effects of symmetrical and asymmetrical balanced PC waveforms. However, when applied to small muscles such as in the face or hands or to children, an asymmetrical balanced PC waveform may be more comfortable than a symmetrical PC waveform of the same duration because the duration of the high-amplitude phase is shorter in the asymmetrical

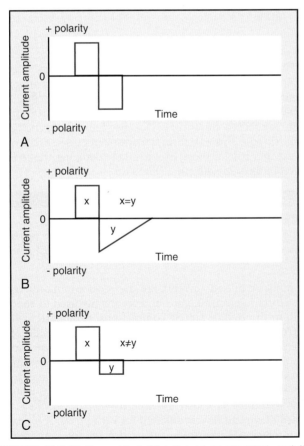

FIGURE 11.6 (A) Symmetrical, (B) balanced asymmetrical, and (C) unbalanced asymmetrical biphasic pulsed currents.

waveform. This is supported by a study in which subjects reported that asymmetrical biphasic waveforms were more comfortable when used to produce contractions of smaller muscle groups, such as the wrist flexors or extensors, and symmetrical biphasic waveforms were more comfortable when used to produce contractions of larger muscle groups, such as the quadriceps.[5]

Interferential Current, Premodulated Current, and Russian Protocol

Interferential current, premodulated current, and Russian protocol are all variations of AC waveforms, all with a frequency (number of waves per second) of between 1000 and 10,000 Hz. This frequency range is known as **medium-frequency AC.**

Interferential current is produced by the interference of two medium-frequency ACs where the frequencies are slightly different from each other. The lower of these frequencies is termed the *carrier frequency*. These two ACs are delivered through two pairs of electrodes, from the same stimulator but through separate channels, with the electrodes configured on the skin so that the two ACs intersect (Fig. 11.7A). Where they intersect, the currents interfere, producing higher amplitude when both currents are in the same phase (i.e., moving in the same direction) and lower amplitude when the two currents are in opposite phases (i.e., moving in opposite directions). This produces envelopes of pulses, known as *beats*, within the tissues where the ACs intersect. The frequency of the beats is equal to the difference between the carrier frequency and the other original AC. For example, when an AC with a carrier frequency of 5000 Hz interferes with an AC with a frequency of 5100 Hz, this will produce beats with a frequency of 100 Hz in the tissue (see Fig. 11.7B). Most electrical stimulation units that produce interferential current stimulation have a preset carrier frequency (usually 2500, 4000, or 5000 Hz) and allow the clinician to set only the beat frequency. Some units also allow the clinician to select the carrier frequency.

◎ Clinical Pearl

Interferential current is produced by the interference of two medium-frequency ACs with slightly different frequencies delivered through two pairs of electrodes from the same stimulator through separate channels configured on the skin so that the two currents intersect.

Interferential current is thought to be more comfortable and to penetrate more deeply than biphasic pulsed current waveforms.[6] Interferential current may be more comfortable because it allows a low-amplitude current to be delivered through the skin, where most discomfort is produced, while delivering a higher current amplitude to deeper tissues. Interferential current also delivers more total current than pulsed waveforms and may stimulate a larger area than other waveforms. However, although a 2010 systematic review and meta-analysis that included 22 studies supported that adding interferential current to standard interventions enhances relief of muscle, soft tissue, or postoperative pain,[7] only a few of the studies in that review or since have compared biphasic pulsed currents (as typically used for transcutaneous electrical

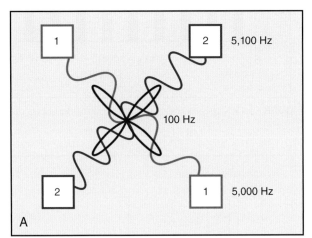
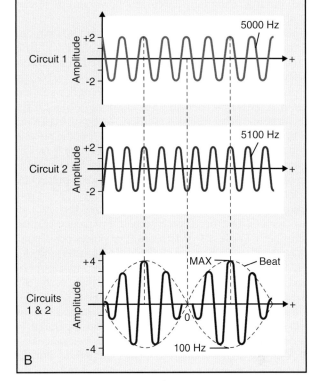

FIGURE 11.7 (A) Intersecting medium-frequency alternating currents producing an interferential current between two crossed pairs of electrodes. (B) An alternating current with a frequency of 5000 Hz interfering with an alternating current with a frequency of 5100 Hz to produce an interferential current with a beat frequency of 100 Hz. (Modified from May H-U, Hansjürgens A: *Nemectrodyn Model 7 manual of Nemectron GmbH,* Karlsruhe, Germany, 1984, Nemectron GmbH.)

nerve stimulation [TENS]) with interferential current,[8–12] and only one of these found interferential current to be more effective than biphasic currents for pain control.[11]

Premodulated current is an AC current in the medium-frequency range with sequentially increasing and decreasing current amplitude (Fig. 11.8). Premodulated current is produced with a single circuit and two electrodes but has the same waveform as the current that results from the two circuits used to produce interferential current, as just described. Although premodulated current is easier to set up than interferential current, because it only requires two electrodes rather than four, it does not have most of the theoretical advantages of interferential current, including delivery of lower-current amplitude to the skin and a larger area of stimulation.

Russian protocol uses a medium-frequency AC with a carrier frequency of 2500 Hz delivered in 10-ms-long **bursts** with 50 bursts per second, with a 10-ms interval between bursts (Fig. 11.9). This specific Russian protocol was developed by Yakov Kots for strengthening the quadriceps muscles in Russian Olympic athletes.[13] Today, the term *Russian stimulation* is applied to an AC delivered in bursts, where the carrier frequency of the AC is anywhere between 1000 and 10,000 Hz, known as *medium frequency,* and the burst frequency is generally in between 1 and 100 bursts per second.

PARAMETERS

For DC, the current flows continuously at the same speed throughout the stimulation time, so the only parameters are the current amplitude, also known as *strength* or *intensity,* and the total treatment time. However, for AC and PC, the current flow varies over time. These variations are described

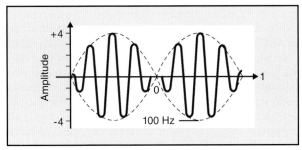

FIGURE 11.8 Premodulated current.

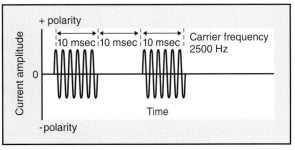

FIGURE 11.9 Russian protocol.

by their duration (how long the current flows) and frequency (how often the current flows).

A **phase** is the period when electrical current flows in one direction (Fig. 11.10). The **phase duration** (phase width) is how long a phase lasts and is usually measured in microseconds (10^{-6} seconds).

A **pulse** is the period when electrical current flows in any direction. A pulse may be made up of one or more phases. The **pulse duration** (pulse width) is how long each pulse lasts and is the time from the beginning of the first phase of the pulse to the end of the last phase of the pulse. Pulse duration is usually measured in microseconds (10^{-6} seconds) (see Fig. 11.10). The **interpulse interval** is the amount of time between pulses (see Fig. 11.10).

Frequency (rate) is the number of cycles (for AC) or pulses (for PC) that occur each second. Frequency is measured in hertz (1 Hz = 1 cycle/second) or pulses per second (pps), and although hertz should ideally be used only for cycles, as occurs with AC, and pulses per second should be applied only for pulses, as occurs with PC, these terms are often used interchangeably in practice (Fig. 11.11).

Amplitude (strength, intensity) is the magnitude of the current flow (Fig. 11.12). Amplitude can be measured in amps or volts and is most often just denoted by a range of 1 to 10, where a higher number is higher amplitude, but the actual number of amps or volts is not shown, similar to the way a volume control on an audio device increases the volume but does not show the decibels. Specific amplitude units are not shown on most electrotherapy devices because the

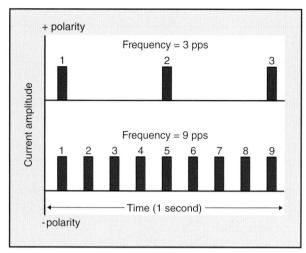

FIGURE 11.11 Monophasic pulsed currents with frequencies of 3 and 9 pps.

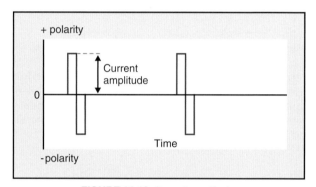

FIGURE 11.12 Current amplitude.

absolute amplitude on a battery-powered unit may vary as the battery wears down and because the amplitude of any clinical electrical stimulation should be adjusted according to the patient's response, not an absolute number.

Clinical Pearl

Pulse duration is how long a pulse lasts. Frequency is the number of pulses/second. Amplitude is the magnitude of the current flow.

In addition to the parameters already described, devices intended to stimulate muscle contractions with electrical currents allow the current to be programmed to turn on for a specified number of seconds during the treatment and then turn off for a specified number of seconds during the treatment. This is usually done to simulate the voluntary contract and relax phases of physiological exercise and to reduce muscle fatigue.

The seconds when the current is on are known as the **on time** (hold time), and the seconds when the current is off are known as the **off time** (relax time). The on time produces the muscle contraction, and the off time allows the muscle to relax. The relationship between on time and off time is often expressed as a ratio. For example, if the on time is 10 seconds and the off time is 50 seconds, this may be written as a 10:50 second on:off time or as a 1:5 on:off ratio (Fig. 11.13).

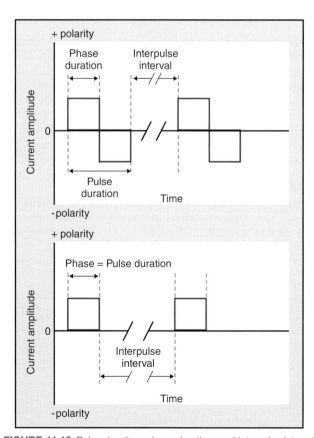

FIGURE 11.10 Pulse duration, phase duration, and interpulse interval for biphasic pulsed currents.

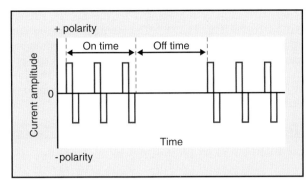

FIGURE 11.13 On:off times for a biphasic current.

To minimize the uncomfortable sensation that can occur when an electrical current suddenly comes on at the beginning of the on time and then suddenly turns off at the end of the on time, most devices with on:off times have the current ramp up slowly at the beginning of the on time and ramp down slowly at the end of the on time. The **ramp-up time** is the number of seconds it takes for the current amplitude to increase from zero during the off time to its maximum amplitude during the on time. The **ramp-down time** is the number of seconds it takes for the current amplitude to decrease from its maximum amplitude during the on time to zero during the off time (Fig. 11.14).

Additional electrical current parameters specific to certain clinical applications are discussed and included in the glossaries of Chapters 12 through 15.

Effects of Electrical Currents
STIMULATION OF ACTION POTENTIALS IN NERVES

For most clinical applications, electrical currents exert their physiological effects by depolarizing nerve membranes, thereby producing an **action potential (AP)**, the message unit of the nervous system. To stimulate an AP, an electrical current must have sufficient amplitude and duration. Once an AP is stimulated in a nerve, that AP will propagate from the location of stimulation all the way along the nerve's axon until it reaches its terminus. The terminus of a motor nerve is a muscle. The terminus of a sensory nerve is the spinal cord. The body will respond to an AP reaching its terminus in the same way as it responds to APs initiated by physiological stimuli, producing muscle contractions when a motor nerve is stimulated and a tingling sensation when a sensory nerve is stimulated.

⊙ Clinical Pearl

Electrical currents most often produce clinical results because they stimulate action potentials in sensory and/or motor nerves.

An AP is the basic unit of nerve communication. When a nerve is at rest, without physiological or electrical stimulation, the inside is more negatively charged than the outside by 60 to 90 mV. This charge difference at rest is known as the **resting membrane potential** (Fig. 11.15). The resting membrane potential is maintained by having more sodium ions outside the nerve and fewer potassium ions inside the nerve, making the inside negative relative to the outside. When a sufficient stimulus is applied, sodium channels in the nerve cell membrane open rapidly, whereas potassium channels open slowly. Because of the high extracellular concentration of sodium, sodium ions rush into the nerve through the open

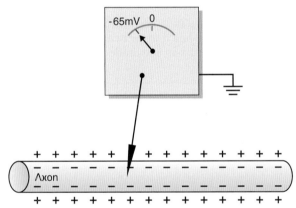

FIGURE 11.15 Resting membrane potential.

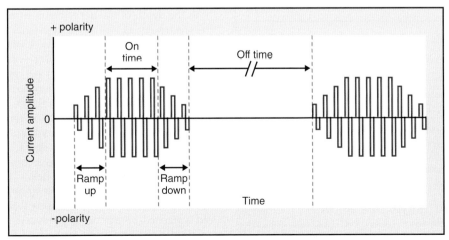

FIGURE 11.14 Ramp-up and ramp-down times.

sodium channels. This makes the inside of the nerve more positively charged, reversing the membrane potential. When the membrane potential reaches +30 mV, the permeability to sodium decreases, and potassium channels rapidly open, increasing the permeability to potassium. Because the intracellular concentration of potassium ions is high, potassium ions then flow out of the nerve, returning the membrane polarization to its resting state of −60 to −90 mV. This sequential **depolarization** and repolarization of the nerve cell membrane caused by the changing flow of ions across the cell membrane is the AP (Fig. 11.16).

A nerve AP generally lasts approximately 1 to 5 ms (1/1000th to 5/1000th of a second), and while an AP is occurring, no additional APs can occur in the same segment of the nerve. During this time, the nerve cannot be further excited, no matter how strong a stimulus is applied. This period is known as the **absolute refractory period.** Because additional APs cannot occur during the absolute refractory period, there is a limit to how many APs can occur in a second. In general, a maximum of 200 to 1000 APs can occur in a second. Directly after depolarization, before the nerve returns to its resting potential, there is a brief period of membrane hyperpolarization. During this period, a greater stimulus than usual is required to produce another AP. This period of hyperpolarization is known as the **relative refractory period.**

Strength-Duration Curve

The amplitude and duration of electrical current required to produce an AP depend on the type of nerve being stimulated. The combination of current amplitude and duration required

for depolarization is represented by the nerve's strength-duration curve (Fig. 11.17).[14] The strength-duration curve for a nerve is a graphic representation of the minimum combination of electrical current amplitude (strength) and pulse duration needed to produce an AP in that nerve. This interplay of amplitude and pulse duration forms the basis for the specificity of the effect of electrical stimulation.

> **◎ Clinical Pearl**
>
> The interplay of amplitude and pulse duration is the basis for the specificity of the effect of electrical stimulation. Selecting different values of these two parameters determines which nerves will be activated.

In general, lower-current amplitudes and shorter pulse durations can stimulate APs in sensory nerves, whereas higher-current amplitudes or longer pulses are needed to stimulate APs in motor nerves. Even higher-current amplitudes and longer pulses are needed to stimulate APs in pain-transmitting C fibers. Therefore, short pulses, with pulse durations of 50 to 100 μs (50 to 100×10^{-6} seconds), are usually used to produce sensory stimulation only, whereas longer pulses, with pulse durations of 150 to 350 μs, are usually used to produce muscle contractions. When stimulating very small muscles, such as muscles of the face or hand, pulse durations of 100 to 125 μs may be sufficient to produce a contraction and may be more comfortable. Pulse durations are usually kept well below 1 ms (10^{-3} seconds, 1000 μs) to avoid stimulating C fibers and thereby avoid causing pain with the stimulation. However, pulses of much longer duration—longer than 10 ms—are required to produce contractions of denervated muscle where the stimulus directly produces APs in muscles when there is no motor nerve. This type of stimulation is uncomfortable if pain-transmitting A-delta and C nerves are present.

The range of current strength and pulse duration predicted by the strength-duration curve to produce a response in a particular type of nerve is based on averages. Specific values may differ between individuals and for the same individual in different areas of the body or at different times or under different circumstances.[15] Furthermore, when the electrical current is applied through the skin using transcutaneous electrodes, the required current amplitude will be affected by both the depth of the nerve being stimulated and the size of the electrodes, as well as the resistance of the skin.[16] Higher-amplitude current will be needed when using larger electrodes, when stimulating an area with substantial adipose tissue[17,18] or to stimulate deeper nerves effectively. However, the order in which nerves are depolarized is the same for all individuals, in accordance with the strength-duration curve, with sensory nerves responding to shorter pulses than motor nerves and motor nerves responding to shorter pulses than pain-transmitting A-delta or C fibers.

When an applied current has a combination of amplitude and pulse duration that falls below the strength-duration curve for a particular nerve type, stimulation is considered to be subthreshold, and no response will occur. Once the threshold is reached, an AP will be produced. Increasing the current amplitude or pulse duration beyond that which is sufficient to stimulate an AP does not change the AP in any way. It does

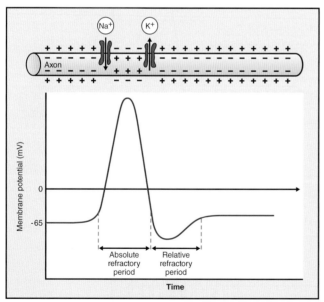

FIGURE 11.16 An action potential is the basic unit of nerve communication and is achieved by rapid sequential nerve depolarization and repolarization in response to stimulation. Nerve depolarization starts when the Na+ (sodium) gate opens and Na+ flows into the cell, causing a rapid change from the normal negative resting membrane potential to a positively charged state. Repolarization follows as permeability to sodium decreases, causing the K+ (potassium) channels to open and K+ to flow out of the cell, initially hyperpolarizing the nerve and then returning the nerve membrane to its resting potential.

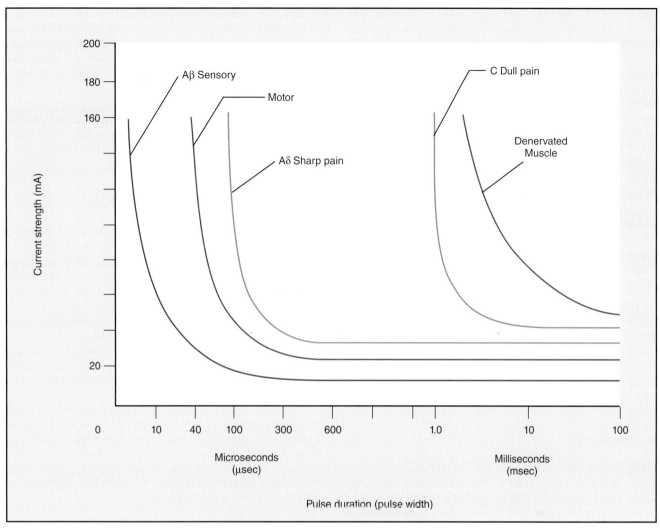

FIGURE 11.17 Strength-duration curve.

not make the AP larger or longer. APs in nerves are all the same. They occur in response to an adequate stimulus at or above the threshold. The same AP occurs with any stimulus above the threshold, and no AP occurs with any stimulus below the threshold level. There is no grading of APs, with weaker or stronger responses. Thus an AP is considered an all-or-none response.

> **Clinical Pearl**
>
> An AP occurs in a nerve when its threshold is reached. Further increasing the current amplitude or pulse duration does not make the AP larger or longer.

In addition to sufficient current amplitude and pulse duration, the current amplitude must rise quickly for an AP to be triggered. If the current rises too slowly, the nerve will accommodate the stimulus. **Accommodation** is the process by which a nerve gradually becomes less responsive to stimulation; a stimulus of sufficient amplitude and duration that *usually* produces a response no longer does so. Accommodation occurs with a slow rate of current rise because the pro-

longed subthreshold stimulation allows sufficient potassium ions to leak out of the nerve to prevent depolarization.

The electrical stimuli used for therapeutic electrical stimulation are similar to the electrical stimuli used for diagnostic nerve conduction studies. For these types of studies, an electrical pulse of 50 to 1000 μs in duration is applied to a sensory or motor peripheral nerve at one point along the nerve. The current amplitude is increased until a maximal signal is detected at another place along the nerve to evaluate the conduction speed and maximum current amplitude that can be transmitted along that segment of nerve. This type of test is often uncomfortable because a maximal stimulus is required to evaluate the health and integrity of the nerve.

Action Potential Propagation Along Nerves

Once an AP is generated, it triggers an AP in the adjacent area of the nerve membrane. This process is called **propagation** or *conduction* of the AP along the neuron. In general, with physiological stimulation, AP propagation occurs in only one direction. This normal physiological direction of propagation is known as *orthodromic.* With electrically stimulated APs, propagation occurs in both directions from the site of stimulation. Propagation in the opposite of normal direction is known as *antidromic propagation.*

The speed at which an AP travels depends on the diameter of the nerve along which it travels and whether the nerve is myelinated or not. **Myelin** is a fatty sheath that wraps around certain axons. The greater the diameter of the nerve, the faster the AP will travel. For example, large-diameter myelinated A-alpha motor nerves conduct at between 60 and 120 m/second, whereas smaller-diameter myelinated A-gamma and A-delta nerves conduct at only 12 to 30 m/second. APs also travel faster in myelinated nerves than in unmyelinated nerves.

> **◎ Clinical Pearl**
>
> Action potentials travel faster in large-diameter myelinated nerves than in small-diameter or unmyelinated nerves.

The nerve's myelin sheath has small gaps in it called **nodes of Ranvier.** APs propagate along myelinated nerve fibers by jumping from one node to the next node—a process called **saltatory conduction** (Fig. 11.18). Saltatory conduction accelerates the conduction of APs along a nerve. For example, unmyelinated C fibers that transmit slow pain and temperature sensations conduct at only 0.5 to 2 m/second, which is much slower than the 12- to 30-m/second conduction speed of similar-diameter myelinated A-delta nerves.[19]

DIRECT STIMULATION OF MUSCLE

Innervated muscles contract in response to electrical stimulation when a stimulated AP in the motor nerves reaches the muscle that nerve innervates. This is known as **neuromuscular electrical stimulation (NMES).** Denervated muscles, where the motor nerve is absent or has been injured or severed, require stimulation of much longer duration and do not contract in response to the pulses of electricity that readily produce APs in motor nerves. Electrical stimulation can produce contractions in denervated muscles when the electrical current produces APs directly in the muscle cells. This requires pulses of electricity lasting at least 10 ms, and generally substantially longer, and is known as **electrical muscle stimulation (EMS)** or *stimulation of denervated muscle.*[20,21] NMES and EMS are discussed in greater detail in Chapter 12.

> **◎ Clinical Pearl**
>
> Pulses lasting longer than 10 ms are needed to produce contractions in denervated muscle.

IONIC EFFECTS OF ELECTRICAL CURRENTS

Most electrical currents used clinically have balanced biphasic waveforms. Balanced biphasic waveforms leave no **charge** in the tissue and thus have no ionic effects. Electrical charge is the quantity of unbalanced electricity in a body. In contrast to balanced biphasic waveforms, DC, pulsed monophasic currents, and unbalanced biphasic waveforms, which are used occasionally for electrical stimulation, do leave a net charge in the tissue. This charge can produce ionic effects. The negative electrode (**cathode**) attracts positively charged ions and repels negatively charged ions, while the positive electrode (**anode**) attracts negatively charged ions and repels positively charged ions (Fig. 11.19).

The ionic effects of electrical currents can be exploited therapeutically. For example, for iontophoresis, DC is used to repel ionized drug molecules and thus increase transdermal drug penetration. The ionic effects of electricity are also exploited for the treatment of inflammation, to facilitate tissue healing, and to reduce the formation of edema, as described in detail in Chapter 14.

Contraindications and Precautions for Electrical Currents

The use and application of electrical currents are not without risks. Widely accepted contraindications and precautions have been established to ensure the best clinical practice and

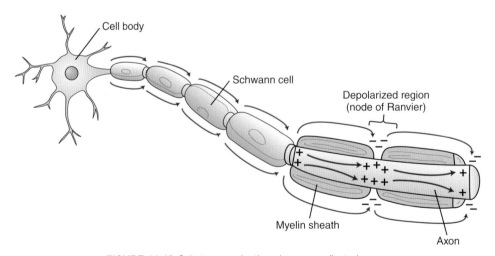

FIGURE 11.18 Saltatory conduction along a myelinated nerve.

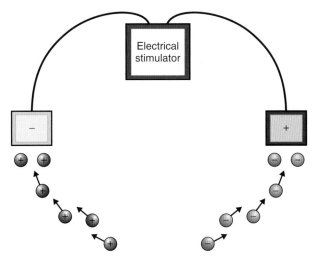

FIGURE 11.19 Ionic effects of electrical stimulation.

application of these tools. These contraindications and precautions are presented in the next section and apply to all uses of electrical stimulation.

CONTRAINDICATIONS FOR ELECTRICAL CURRENTS

★ CONTRAINDICATIONS

for Electrical Currents

- Demand cardiac pacemaker, implantable defibrillator, or unstable arrhythmia
- Placement of electrodes over carotid sinus
- Areas where venous or arterial thrombosis or thrombophlebitis is present
- Pregnancy—over or around the abdomen or low back (electrical stimulation may be used for pain control during labor and delivery, as discussed in Chapter 13)

Demand Pacemaker, Implantable Cardiac Defibrillator, or Unstable Arrhythmias

Electrical stimulation should be avoided in the thoracic, cervical, shoulder, upper lumbar, and chest areas in patients with demand cardiac pacemakers or implantable cardiac defibrillators. Electrical stimulation is not recommended in patients who are dependent on pacemakers because electrical stimulation may interfere with the functioning of these devices, potentially interfering with the heart rate monitoring and causing a change in the paced heart rate with a pacemaker[22] or[23] causing a defibrillator not to shock when it should or to shock when it should not.[24] Burst mode is most likely to cause these types of problems. Electrical stimulation on the limbs in patients with pacemakers or defibrillators is less likely to be unsafe but is not recommended at this time, given the limited data in this area.[25] Electrical stimulation may also aggravate an unstable arrhythmia that is not treated with a pacemaker.

▪ Ask the Patient
- "Do you have a cardiac pacemaker or an implanted cardiac defibrillator?"
- "Do you have a history of heart problems, or have you been treated for heart problems?"
- "What type of heart problems do you have?"
- "How recently has your doctor checked your heart?"

▪ Assess
- Check patient visually for surgical scar and feel for placement of a device under the skin.

Some patients may forget or not realize they have a pacemaker or an implanted cardiac defibrillator. These devices are usually implanted under the left clavicle but may be as lateral as the axilla (Fig. 11.20).

If the patient has a pacemaker or an implanted cardiac defibrillator, electrical stimulation should not be applied. If the patient is unsure of his or her cardiac status or has recently had episodes of cardiac arrhythmia or pain, the therapist should consult with the referring physician to rule out the possibility of cardiac compromise before using electrical stimulation as a treatment modality.

Over the Carotid Sinus

Care should be taken to avoid placing electrodes on the anterior or lateral neck in the areas over the carotid sinuses because stimulation to these areas may induce a rapid fall in blood pressure and heart rate that may cause the patient to faint.

Venous or Arterial Thrombosis or Thrombophlebitis

Stimulation should not be placed over areas of known venous or arterial thrombosis or thrombophlebitis because stimulation may increase circulation, increasing the risk of releasing emboli.

▪ Ask the Patient
- "Do you have a blood clot in this area?" (Be sure you have checked the chart or asked the nurse in charge.)

▪ Assess
- Check area for increased swelling, redness, and increased tenderness. If any of these are present, do not apply electrical stimulation until the possibility of a thrombus has been ruled out.

Pelvis, Abdomen, Trunk, and Low Back Area During Pregnancy

The effects of electrical stimulation on the developing human fetus and on the human pregnant uterus have not been determined.[26] Therefore it is recommended that stimulation electrodes not be placed in any way that the current may reach the fetus. Electrodes should not be applied to the low back, abdomen, or hips, where the path of the current might cross the uterus.

Occasionally, electrical stimulation is used to control back pain during labor and delivery as an alternative to general anesthesia or a spinal block. Although the evidence for the effectiveness of this intervention is mixed, no studies reported

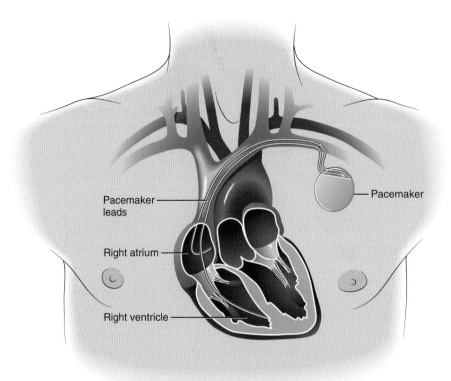

FIGURE 11.20 Location of pacemaker implanted under the left clavicle.

adverse effects of this intervention. A 2011 systematic review and meta-analysis that included nine studies involving a total of 1076 pregnant women concluded that there was no statistically significant effect of TENS on pain relief or the need for pharmacological analgesia during labor,[27] but a subsequent 2012 review noted that the inconsistent effectiveness of TENS during labor may be because of inconsistent and suboptimal application.[28] This is supported by a study published in 2018 in 63 women, which found that TENS with a frequency of 80 to 100 Hz and a long pulse duration (350 μs) significantly reduced pain during labor by an average of 2.9/10 points, and this was found to be more effective than either placebo TENS or TENS with 100-Hz frequency and 100-μs pulse duration.[29] More studies are needed to clarify the optimal parameters for the efficacy of this intervention. If applying TENS for control of low back pain during labor, electrodes can be placed on the low back or in the anterior lower abdominal region, depending on where the pain is felt. The patient increases the current amplitude during a contraction and turns the amplitude down or off between contractions.

■ **Ask the Patient**
• "Are you pregnant?"
• "Could you be pregnant?"
• "Are you trying to get pregnant?"

The patient may not know whether she is pregnant, particularly in the first few days or weeks after conception. Because damage may occur early during development, electrical stimulation should not be applied in any area where the current may reach the fetus of a patient who is or might be pregnant.

PRECAUTIONS FOR ELECTRICAL CURRENTS

★ **PRECAUTIONS**

for Electrical Currents

• Cardiac disease
• Impaired mentation
• Impaired sensation
• Malignant tumors
• Areas of skin irritation or open wounds

Cardiac Disease

Cardiac disease includes previous myocardial infarction or other specifically known congenital or acquired cardiac abnormalities.

■ **Ask the Patient**
• "Do you have a known history of cardiac disease?"
• "Have you had a previous myocardial infarction?"
• "Have you ever had rheumatic fever as a child or an adult?"
• "Are you aware of having any cardiac problems at this time?"

■ **Assess**
• Check for surgical incisions in thoracic area, both anteriorly and posteriorly.
• Check patient's resting pulse and respiratory rate before initiating treatment, and check for changes in these values during and after applying electrical stimulation.

Impaired Mentation or Impaired Sensation

The patient's sensation and reporting of pain are usually used to guide the selection of the current intensity and to keep the intensity within safe limits. If the patient cannot report or feel pain, electrical stimulation must be applied with caution, and close attention must be paid to any possible adverse effects. For example, caution should be used when applying electrical stimulation to the legs of patients with diabetic neuropathy. In addition, patients with impaired mentation may be agitated and may try to pull off the electrodes, resulting in unsafe increases in current density.

> ■ **Assess**
> • Sensation in the area
> • Patient orientation and level of alertness
> • Patient agitation

Electrical stimulation may be used to treat chronic open wounds in areas with decreased sensation by determining the appropriate current amplitude in an area with intact sensation.

Malignant Tumors

Although no research has explored the effects of applying electrical stimulation to malignant tumors in humans because electrical currents can enhance tissue growth, in most cases it is recommended that electrical stimulation not be applied to patients with known or suspected malignant tumors. Electrical stimulation should not be applied to any area of the body of a patient with a malignancy because malignant tumors can metastasize to areas beyond where they are first found or known to be. Occasionally, electrical stimulation is used to control pain in patients with known malignancy,[30] but this is done only when the improvement in quality of life afforded by this intervention is considered to be greater than the possible risks associated with the treatment.[31]

> ■ **Ask the Patient**
> • "Have you ever had cancer? Do you have cancer now?"
> • "Do you have fever, sweats, chills, or night pain?"
> • "Do you have pain at rest?"
> • "Have you had recent unexplained weight loss?"

Skin Irritation or Open Wounds

Electrodes should not be placed over abraded skin or known open wounds unless electrical stimulation is being used to treat the wound. Open or damaged skin should be avoided because it has lower **impedance** (resistance to AC) and less sensation than intact skin, and this may result in the delivery of too much current to the area. The skin should not be shaved immediately before stimulation because this can cause skin cuts or abrasions.

> ■ **Assess**
> • Inspect patient's skin carefully for cuts, scratches, or abrasions before placing electrodes.
> • Check for increased redness, swelling, warmth, rashes, or broken and abraded areas.

Adverse Effects of Electrical Currents

Very few potential adverse effects result from the clinical application of electrical currents. Careful evaluation of the patient and review of the patient's pertinent medical history and current medical status will minimize the likelihood of any adverse effects. In addition, patients should be monitored directly throughout the initial treatment with electrical stimulation and monitored by report for subsequent treatments for any adverse effects of the stimulation. If a patient is provided with an electrical stimulation unit for home use, the patient should be clearly instructed in its use and in the early identification of potential adverse effects.

Electrical currents can cause burns. This effect is seen most commonly when a DC or AC (including interferential current)[32] is being applied. With DC and AC, the current is always flowing, resulting in high total charge delivery; in contrast, with PC, current only flows during the pulses and does not flow during the long interpulse intervals. In addition, the chemical effects produced under DC electrodes can be caustic. If there is not enough conduction medium on an electrode, as can occur with repeated use of self-adhesive electrodes or poorly applied nonadhesive electrodes, the risk of burns also increases because of the increased **current density** in the areas where conduction is adequate. The risk of burns can be minimized by using at least 2- by 2-inch electrodes, and preferably 2- by 4-inch electrodes, for interferential currents and by using only electrodes that have been well taken care of and are not old and dry and therefore adhere well to the skin.

Skin irritation or inflammation may occur in the area where electrical stimulation electrodes are applied because the patient is allergic to the contact surface of the electrode, such as the adhesive, gel, or foam rubber. If this occurs, a different type of electrode should be tried.

Some patients find electrical stimulation to be painful. In such patients, using a shorter pulse duration and increasing the current amplitude slowly over a longer period of time, or using larger electrodes, may be better tolerated. In patients who find all forms of electrical stimulation painful, other treatment approaches should be used.

Application Technique

This section provides guidelines on the sequence of procedures required for safe and effective application of therapeutic electrical stimulation.

APPLICATION TECHNIQUE 11.1   ELECTRICAL STIMULATION

Procedure

1. Assess the patient and set treatment goals.
2. Determine whether electrical stimulation is the most appropriate intervention.
3. Confirm that electrical stimulation is not contraindicated for this patient or for the specific diagnosis you are treating. Check with the patient and review the patient's chart for contraindications or precautions regarding the application of electrical stimulation.
4. Select an electrical stimulation unit with the necessary waveform and adjustable parameters for the intervention (e.g., muscle contraction, pain modulation, tissue healing).
5. Explain the procedure to the patient, including an explanation of what the patient might expect to experience and any instructions or directions regarding patient participation with the electrical stimulation.
6. Position the patient appropriately and comfortably for the intervention.
7. Inspect the skin where the stimulation is to be applied for any signs of abrasion or skin irritation. Clean the skin with soap and water, and clip hair if necessary for good adhesion of the electrode to the skin and thus good current flow. Soap and water should be used for cleaning because this does not dry the skin and will remove any dirt, body oils, or topical applications remaining from surgery, such as iodine-based cleaners. Alcohol should not be used to clean the skin before electrical stimulation because this dries the skin excessively, reducing electrical conduction, and alcohol that remains on the skin can accelerate breakdown of the gel on electrodes.
8. Check electrodes and lead wires for continuity or signs of excessive wear, and replace any of those found faulty or of concern.
9. Apply the electrodes to the area being treated. Use conductive gel if electrodes are not pre-gelled. Use the appropriate size and number of electrodes to address the problem. For specific information on electrode selection and placement, see the sections on these topics.
10. Attach the lead wires to the electrodes and to the stimulation unit.
11. Set optimal parameters for treatment, including waveform, polarity, frequency, on:off time, ramp up and ramp down, and length of treatment time, as indicated for the goals of the intervention. For specific information on parameter selection for different treatment effects, refer to the sections on parameter selection within the clinical application discussions in Chapters 12 through 14.
12. Slowly advance the amplitude until the patient is just able to notice a sensation under the electrodes. If a muscle contraction is needed to achieve the treatment objectives, continue to increase the amplitude until the indicated strength of contraction is produced or to patient tolerance, whichever is reached first.
13. Observe the patient's reaction to stimulation over the first few minutes of the treatment. If the treatment includes muscle contraction, observe the amplitude, direction, and quality of the contraction. The parameters may need to be adjusted or the electrodes may need to be moved slightly if the expected outcome is not achieved.
14. When the treatment is complete, remove the electrodes and inspect the patient's skin for any signs of adverse reaction to the treatment.
15. Document the treatment, including all treatment parameters and the patient's response to the treatment.

PATIENT POSITIONING

Patient positioning is dictated by the area to be treated, the goal of treatment, and the device used. Attention to patient comfort and modesty is important. Upper extremity setups require short sleeves or a halter top for women, and some men may not be comfortable with their shirts off. When treating the neck, upper and lower back, or hips, the clinician should ask patients if they feel sufficiently covered by their clothing or the additional sheets or towels the clinician has placed. If in doubt, additional covering may add to a patient's comfort. For lower extremity setups, shorts are generally adequate and allow the patient to perform voluntary exercise with the stimulation in place.

ELECTRODE TYPE

Many different types of electrodes are available for use with electrical stimulation devices. The electrodes serve as the interface between the patient and the stimulator. Electrodes are connected to the machine by coated lead wires. Surgically implantable electrodes are also available, but because these are not placed by therapists, they are not discussed further in this book. A number of factors should be considered when selecting electrodes for electrical stimulation, including electrode material, size, and shape; the need for conductive gel; and the tissues to be treated.

The electrodes most commonly used today are disposable and flexible and have a self-adhesive gel coating that serves as the conduction medium (Fig. 11.21). The gel decreases the electrical **resistance** between the electrode and the skin. Self-adhesive electrodes may be designed for single use or for multiple uses over a period of 1 month or longer. Although many electrodes on the market may appear to be made of similar material and conductive gel, conductivity, impedance, and comfort may differ between and within types.[33,34] How many times an electrode can be used depends on the type and thickness of the gel coating and how well the electrode is cared for. Electrodes will last the longest if adhered to a plastic sheet and placed in a sealed plastic bag between uses. Once the gel coating starts to dry out, the current delivery becomes less uniform, causing uneven current density. In areas where the electrode is still conductive, the current density will be high, which can cause the skin to burn. Therefore, electrodes must be inspected regularly, and dry or discolored electrodes should be discarded.

Some patients may experience skin sensitivity to self-adhesive electrodes and may develop redness or a rash in the area where electrodes have been applied. This response generally reflects an allergy to the adhesive in the conductive gel. For these patients, "sensitive skin" electrodes may be an option. Sensitive skin electrodes usually are made with a blue

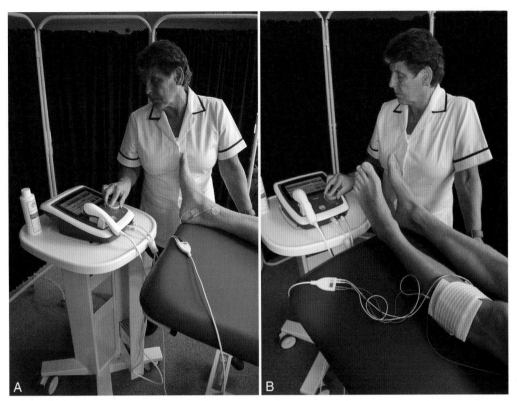

FIGURE 11.21 Electrotherapy with different electrodes. (A) With self-adhesive electrodes. (B) With carbon-impregnated silicone rubber electrodes with wet sponge conductor. (Courtesy EMS Physio, Wantage, UK.)

gel and have less adhesive and more water in the gel. Another option is to use electrodes made of carbon-impregnated silicone rubber (see Fig. 11.21). These electrodes last longer than self-adhesive electrodes and are used with a conductive gel or with a sponge soaked in tap water to promote conduction. Carbon rubber electrodes used with gel have the lowest impedance,[33] but because these types of electrodes are not self adhesive, they must be secured to the patient with tape, elastic straps, or bandages. Carbon rubber electrodes should be cleaned with warm, soapy water, not with alcohol, because alcohol can degrade the carbon rubber.

Electrodes made of conductive fabric can also be used. These electrodes are typically made from a conductive thread, such as silver, woven into another fabric in the shape of a garment, such as a glove, sock, or sleeve.[35] Garment electrodes can be used to treat an entire area that conventional gelled electrodes would not cover, and they can be fastened onto a wrap for areas that may be hard to reach, such as the lower back (Fig. 11.22). The use of this type of electrode is usually expensive because the garments themselves are

expensive, and because they are in contact with the patient's skin, they are therefore for single patient use only.

An alternative for applying electrical stimulation to the hand or foot is to immerse the area to be treated in a non-metal container of water along with the treatment electrode or lead and affix the other electrode elsewhere on the body (Fig. 11.23). Because water conducts electricity well, it serves as the electrode. Applying electrical stimulation this way is generally very comfortable to the patient because the current is delivered evenly throughout the treatment area.

The selection of electrode size, shape, and type depends on treatment goals, the area to be treated, and the amount of tissue targeted. Smaller electrodes target stimulation to a small area, whereas larger electrodes spread the stimulation over a larger area. Larger electrodes may be needed for areas with thicker subcutaneous fat tissue[17,18] and are generally more comfortable[16,36] than smaller ones, but they require a higher total current amplitude to have the same effect. Different sizes or shapes of electrodes do not generally change the overall efficacy of electrical stimulation treatments.[37]

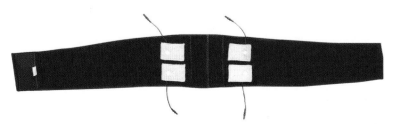

FIGURE 11.22 A garment electrode. (Courtesy BioMedical Life Systems, Carlsbad, CA.)

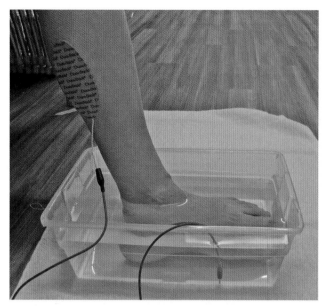

FIGURE 11.23 Application of electrical stimulation to the foot using water as the treatment electrode.

ELECTRODE PLACEMENT

To ensure even delivery of current, electrodes must lie smoothly against the skin, without wrinkles or gaps. Self-adhesive electrodes usually maintain good contact; patients with excessive hair on their arms or legs may present a challenge to proper adhesion, and hair may need to be trimmed. Flexible bandaging is generally needed with non–self-adhesive electrodes to maintain good electrode-to-skin contact. Electrodes should not be placed directly over bony prominences because the greater resistance of bone and the poor adhesion of electrodes to highly contoured surfaces reduce therapeutic effectiveness and increase the risk of discomfort and burns.

> ◎ **Clinical Pearl**
>
> Electrodes should not be placed directly over bony prominences.

The distance or spacing between electrodes affects the depth and path of the electrical current through the patient. The closer together the electrodes are placed, the more superficially the current will travel, and conversely, the greater the distance between electrodes, the deeper the current will penetrate (Fig. 11.24). The ideal electrode placement that produces the desired therapeutic effect should be documented, noting the distance from bony landmarks or anatomic structures, so that follow-up sessions can replicate the placement. Diagrams are often helpful.

> ◎ **Clinical Pearl**
>
> Document electrode placement using diagrams so that follow-up sessions can easily replicate the placement.

Documentation

The following should be documented:
- Area of the body treated
- Patient positioning
- Specific stimulation parameters
- Electrode placement
- Treatment duration
- Patient's response to treatment

Chapter Review

1. An electrical current is a flow of charged particles.
2. A therapeutic electrical current can be described by its waveform and, where relevant, the parameters of pulse duration, frequency, amplitude, on:off times, and ramp-up and ramp-down times. Appropriate parameters for particular clinical applications are summarized in tables throughout the next three chapters.
3. Most uses of electrical stimulation are based on its ability to produce APs in peripheral nerves. Once an AP is generated by an electrical current, the body responds to it in the same way as it does to an AP that is generated physiologically. An electrically stimulated AP can affect sensory nerves, producing a tingling sensation, or motor nerves, producing a muscle contraction.
4. Unbalanced electrical current waveforms can produce ionic effects independent of any APs.
5. General contraindications for electrical stimulation include demand cardiac pacemakers and implanted defibrillators, placement over carotid sinus or areas of thrombosis, and pregnancy. Precautions include cardiac disease, impaired mentation, impaired sensation, malignant tumor, skin irritation, and open wounds.
6. The reader is referred to the Evolve website for additional resources and references.

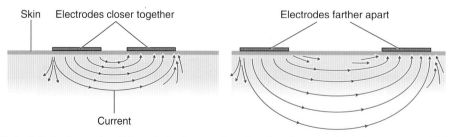

FIGURE 11.24 The effect of electrode spacing. When electrodes are closer together, the current travels more superficially. When electrodes are farther apart, the current goes deeper.

Glossary

Absolute refractory period: The period of time immediately after nerve depolarization when no action potential can be generated.

Accommodation: A transient increase in threshold to nerve excitation.

Action potential (AP): The rapid sequential depolarization and repolarization of a nerve that occurs in response to a stimulus and transmits along the axon. The AP is the message unit of the nervous system.

Alternating current (AC): A continuous sinusoidal bidirectional flow of charged particles (see Fig. 11.3). AC has equal ion flow in each direction, and thus no pulse charge remains in the tissues. With AC, when the frequency increases, the cycle duration decreases, and when the frequency decreases, the cycle duration increases (Fig. 11.25).

Amplitude: The magnitude of current or voltage (see Fig. 11.12); also called *strength* or *intensity*.

Anode: The positive electrode.

Biphasic pulsed current: A current composed of pulses, with current going in one direction and then in the opposite direction within each pulse (see Fig. 11.4B).

Bursts: Series or groups of pulses (Fig. 11.26).

Cathode: The negative electrode.

Charge: The quantity of unbalanced electricity in a body. Charge is equal to current (I) × time (t). Charge is noted as Q and is measured in coulombs (C).

Current density: The amount of current per unit area.

Depolarization: The reversal of the resting potential in excitable cell membranes, where the inside of the cell becomes positive relative to the outside.

Direct current (DC): A continuous unidirectional flow of charged particles (see Fig. 11.2).

Electrical current: The movement or flow of charged particles through a conductor in response to an applied electrical field. Current is noted as I and is measured in amperes (A).

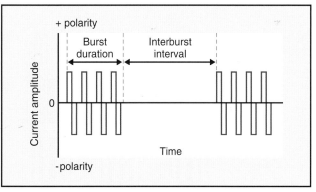

FIGURE 11.26 Burst mode.

Electrical muscle stimulation (EMS): Application of an electrical current directly to muscle to produce a muscle contraction.

Frequency: The number of cycles or pulses per second. Frequency is measured in hertz (Hz) for cycles or pulses per second (pps) for pulses (see Fig. 11.11); also called *rate*.

Impedance: The resistance to an alternating current. Impedance is noted by Z and is measured in ohms (Ω).

Interferential current: The waveform produced by the interference of two medium-frequency (1000 to 10,000 Hz) sinusoidal alternating currents (ACs) of slightly different frequencies. These two waveforms are delivered through two pairs of electrodes through separate channels in the same stimulator. Electrodes are configured on the skin so that the two ACs intersect (see Fig. 11.7A).

Interpulse interval: The time between individual pulses (see Fig. 11.10).

Iontophoresis: The delivery of ions through the skin for therapeutic purposes using an electrical current.

Medium-frequency AC: An alternating current (AC) waveform with a frequency between 1000 and 10,000 Hz (between 1 and 10 kHz). Most medium-frequency currents available on clinical units have a frequency between 2500 and 5000 Hz. Medium-frequency AC is rarely used alone therapeutically, but two medium-frequency ACs of different frequency may be applied together to produce an interferential current (see *Interferential current*).

Modulation: Any pattern of variation in one or more of the stimulation parameters. Modulation is used to limit neural adaptation to an electrical current. Modulation may be cyclic or random (Fig. 11.27).

Monophasic pulsed current: A series of pulses where the charged particles move in only one direction (see Fig. 11.4A).

Motor point: The place in a muscle where electrical stimulation will produce the greatest contraction with the least amount of electricity, generally located over the middle of the muscle belly.

Myelin: A fatty tissue that surrounds the axons of neurons, allowing electrical signals to travel more quickly (see Fig. 11.18).

Neuromuscular electrical stimulation (NMES): Application of an electrical current to motor nerves to produce contractions of the muscles they innervate.

Nodes of Ranvier: Small, unmyelinated gaps in the myelin sheath covering myelinated axons.

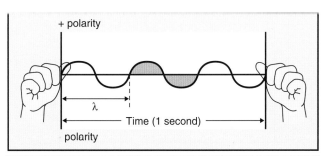

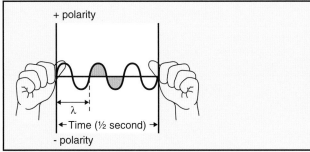

FIGURE 11.25 The inverse relationship between frequency and cycle duration for an alternating current (λ = wavelength).

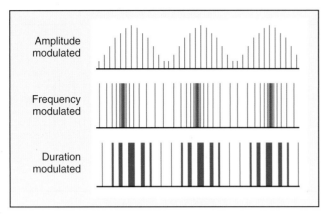

FIGURE 11.27 Modulation.

On time/off time: On time is the time during which a train of pulses occurs. Off time is the time between trains of pulses when no current flows. On and off times are usually used when the goal of electrical stimulation is to produce muscle contractions. During on time, the muscle contracts, and during off time, it relaxes. Off time is required to reduce muscle fatigue during the stimulation session (see Fig. 11.13).

Phase: In pulsed current, the period from when current starts to flow in one direction to when it stops flowing or starts to flow in the other direction. A biphasic pulsed current is made up of two phases; the first phase begins when current starts to flow in one direction and ends when the current starts to flow in the other direction, which is also the beginning of the second phase. The second phase ends when current stops flowing.

Phase duration: The duration of one phase of a pulse. Phase duration is generally expressed in microseconds (μs, 10^{-6} seconds); also called *phase width* (see Fig. 11.10).

Premodulated current: An alternating current (AC) that uses a medium-frequency sinusoidal waveform with sequentially increasing and decreasing current amplitude, produced with a single circuit using two electrodes. This current has the same waveform as an interferential current produced by the interference of two medium-frequency sinusoidal ACs requiring four electrodes (see Fig. 11.8).

Propagation: The movement of an action potential along a nerve axon; also called *conduction*.

Pulse: The period when current is flowing.

Pulse duration: Time from the beginning of the first phase of a pulse to the end of the last phase of a pulse. Pulse duration is generally expressed in microseconds (μs, 10^{-6} seconds); also called *pulse width* (see Fig. 11.10).

Pulsed current (PC): An interrupted flow of charged particles whereby the current flows in a series of pulses separated by periods when no current flows; also called *pulsatile current*.

Ramp-up time/ramp-down time: The ramp up time is the time it takes for the current amplitude to increase from zero, at the end of the off time, to its maximum amplitude during the on time. A current ramps up by having the amplitude of the first few pulses of on time gradually become sequentially higher than the amplitude of the previous pulse. The ramp-down time is the time it takes for the current amplitude to decrease from its maximum amplitude during on time back to zero (see Fig. 11.14). Ramp-up and ramp-down times are different from rise and decay times. The latter describe the time needed for the current amplitude to increase and decrease during a phase.

Relative refractory period: The period after nerve depolarization in which the nerve membrane is hyperpolarized and a greater stimulus than usual is required to produce an action potential.

Resistance: Opposition of a material to the flow of electrical current. Resistance is noted as R and is measured in ohms (Ω).

Resting membrane potential: The electrical difference between the inside of a neuron and the outside when the neuron is at rest, usually 60 to 90 mV, with the inside being negative relative to the outside.

Russian protocol: A medium-frequency burst AC with a set frequency of 2500 Hz delivered in 50 bursts/second. Each burst is 10 ms long and is separated from the next burst by a 10-ms interburst interval (see Fig. 11.9).

Saltatory conduction: The rapid propagation of an electrical signal along a myelinated nerve axon, with the signal appearing to jump from one node of Ranvier to the next (see Fig. 11.18).

Wavelength: The duration of one cycle of alternating current (AC). A cycle lasts from the time the current departs from the isoelectric line (zero current amplitude) in one direction and then crosses the isoelectric line in the opposite direction to when it returns to the isoelectric line. The wavelength of AC is similar to the pulse duration of pulsed current (Fig. 11.28).

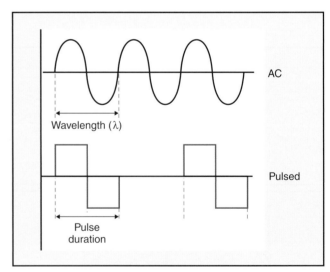

FIGURE 11.28 Wavelength.

References

1. Bussel B: History of electrical stimulation in rehabilitation medicine. *Ann Phys Rehabil Med* 58:198–200, 2015.
2. Francis J, Dingly J: Electroanaesthesia—from torpedo fish to TENS. *Anaesthesia* 70(1):93–103, 2015.
3. Duchenne G-B: *A treatise on localized electrization and its applications to pathology and therapeutics*, London, 1871, Hardwicke.
4. American Physical Therapy Association: Clinical electrophysiology. In *Electrotherapeutic terminology in physical therapy*, Alexandria, VA, 2000, APTA.
5. Baker LL, Bowman BR, McNeal DR: Effects of waveform on comfort during neuromuscular electrical stimulation. *Clin Orthop Relat Res* 233:75–85, 1988.
6. Ariel E, Ratmansky M, Levkovitz Y, et al: Efficiency of tissue penetration by currents induced by 3 electrotherapeutic techniques: a comparative study using a novel deep-tissue measuring technique. *Phys Ther* 99(5):540–548, 2019.
7. Fuentes JP, Armijo Olivo S, Magee DJ, et al: Effectiveness of interferential current therapy in the management of musculoskeletal pain: a systematic review and meta-analysis. *Phys Ther* 90:1219–1238, 2010.
8. Johnson MI, Tabasam G: An investigation into the analgesic effects of interferential currents and transcutaneous electrical nerve stimulation on experimentally induced ischemic pain in otherwise pain-free volunteers. *Phys Ther* 83:208–223, 2003.
9. Bae YH, Lee SM: Analgesic effects of transcutaneous electrical nerve stimulation and interferential current on experimental ischemic pain models: frequencies of 50 hz and 100 hz. *J Phys Ther Sci* 26:1945–1948, 2014.
10. Acedo AA, Luduvice Antunes AC, Barros dos Santos A, et al: Upper trapezius relaxation induced by TENS and interferential current in computer users with chronic nonspecific neck discomfort: an electromyographic analysis. *J Back Musculoskelet Rehabil* 28:19–24, 2015.
11. Koca I, Boyaci A, Tutoglu A, et al: Assessment of the effectiveness of interferential current therapy and TENS in the management of carpal tunnel syndrome: a randomized controlled study. *Rheumatol Int* 34:1639–1645, 2014.
12. Almeida CC, Silva VZMD, Júnior GC, et al: Transcutaneous electrical nerve stimulation and interferential current demonstrate similar effects in relieving acute and chronic pain: a systematic review with meta-analysis. *Braz J Phys Ther* 22(5):347–354, 2018.
13. Ward AR, Shkuratova N: Russian electrical stimulation: the early experiments. *Phys Ther* 82:1019–1030, 2002.
14. Hill AV: Excitation and accommodation in nerve. *Proc R Soc B* 119:305–355, 1936.
15. Nelson RM, Hunt GC: Strength-duration curve: intrarater and interrater reliability. *Phys Ther* 61:894–897, 1981.
16. Alon G, Kantor G, Ho HS: Effects of electrode size on basic excitatory responses and on selected stimulus parameters. *J Orthop Sports Phys Ther* 20:29–35, 1994.
17. Medeiros FV, Vieira A, Carregaro RL, et al: Skinfold thickness affects the isometric knee extension torque evoked by neuromuscular electrical stimulation. *Braz J Phys Ther* 19(6):466–472, 2015.
18. Doheny EP, Caulfield BM, Minogue CM, et al: Effect of subcutaneous fat thickness and surface electrode configuration during neuromuscular electrical stimulation. *Med Eng Phys* 32:468–474, 2010.
19. Baker LL, Wederich CL, McNeal DR, et al: *Neuromuscular electrical stimulation*, ed 4, Downey, CA, 2000, LAREI.
20. Petrofsky JS, Petrofsky S: A wide-pulse-width electrical stimulator for use on denervated muscles. *J Clin Eng* 17:331–338, 1992.
21. Pieber K, Herceg M, Paternostro-Sluga T, et al: Optimizing stimulation parameters in functional electrical stimulation of denervated muscles: a cross-sectional study. *J Neuroeng Rehabil* 12:51, 2015.
22. Carlson T, Andréll P, Ekre O, et al: Interference of transcutaneous electrical nerve stimulation with permanent ventricular stimulation: a new clinical problem? *Europace* 11:364–369, 2009.
23. Egger F, Hofer C, Hammerle FP, et al: Influence of electrical stimulation therapy on permanent pacemaker function. *Wien Klin Wochenschr* 131(13–14):313–320, 2019.
24. Holmgren C, Carlsson T, Mannheimer C, et al: Risk of interference from transcutaneous electrical nerve stimulation on the sensing function of implantable defibrillators. *Pacing Clin Electrophysiol* 31:151–158, 2008.
25. Badger J, Taylor P, Swain I: The safety of electrical stimulation in patients with pacemakers and implantable cardioverter defibrillators: A systematic review. *J Rehabil Assist Technol Eng* Dec 5;4, 2017.
26. Yokoyama LM, Pires LA, Ferreira EA, et al: Low- and high-frequency transcutaneous electrical nerve stimulation have no deleterious or teratogenic effects on pregnant mice. *Physiotherapy* 101:214–218, 2015.
27. Mello LF, Nóbrega LF, Lemos A: Transcutaneous electrical stimulation for pain relief during labor: a systematic review and meta-analysis [Article in English, Portuguese]. *Rev Bras Fisioter* 15:175–184, 2011.
28. Francis R: TENS (transcutaneous electrical nerve stimulation) for labour pain. *Pract Midwife* 15:20–23, 2012.
29. Báez-Suárez A, Martín-Castillo E, García-Andújar J, et al: Evaluation of different doses of transcutaneous nerve stimulation for pain relief during labour: a randomized controlled trial. *Trials* 19:652, 2018.
30. Loh J, Gulati A: The use of transcutaneous electrical nerve stimulation (TENS) in a major cancer center for the treatment of severe cancer-related pain and associated disability. *Pain Med* 16(6):1204–1210, 2015.
31. Searle RD, Bennett MI, Johnson MI, et al: Letter to editor: transcutaneous electrical nerve stimulation (TENS) for cancer bone pain. *Palliat Med* 22:878–879, 2008.
32. Satter EK: Third-degree burns incurred as a result of interferential current therapy. *Am J Dermatopathol* 30:281–283, 2008.
33. Nolan MF: Conductive differences in electrodes used with transcutaneous electrical nerve stimulation devices. *Phys Ther* 71:746–751, 1991.
34. Sha N, Kenney LP, Heller BW, et al: The effect of the impedance of a thin hydrogel electrode on sensation during functional electrical stimulation. *Med Eng Phys* 30:739–746, 2008.
35. Cowan S, McKenna J, McCrum-Gardner E, et al: An investigation of the hypoalgesic effects of TENS delivered by a glove electrode. *J Pain* 10:694–701, 2000.
36. Lyons GM, Leane GE, Clarke-Moloney M, et al: An investigation of the effect of electrode size and electrode location on comfort during stimulation of the gastrocnemius muscle. *Med Eng Phys* 26:873–878, 2004.
37. Ishimaru K, Kawakita K, Sakita M: Analgesic effects induced by TENS and electroacupuncture with different types of stimulating electrodes on deep tissues in human subjects. *Pain* 63:181–187, 1995.

Electrical Currents for Muscle Contraction

Michelle H. Cameron | Michelle Ocelnik

CHAPTER OUTLINE

CHAPTER OBJECTIVES

After reading this chapter, the reader will be able to do the following:
* Define *neuromuscular electrical stimulation.*
* Describe the physical effects of neuromuscular electrical stimulation.
* Explain the clinical indications for the use of neuromuscular electrical stimulation.
* Choose the best technique for treatment with neuromuscular electrical stimulation and list the advantages and disadvantages of each.
* Select the appropriate equipment and optimal treatment parameters for treatment with neuromuscular electrical stimulation.
* Safely and effectively apply neuromuscular electrical stimulation.
* Accurately and completely document treatment with neuromuscular electrical stimulation.

Since the late 18th century, when it was first discovered that electrical currents could cause muscle contractions, considerable research has explored the mechanisms underlying this effect and means to optimize clinical outcomes associated with electrically stimulated muscle contractions. The use of electrical currents to produce muscle contractions in innervated muscles is called **neuromuscular electrical stimulation (NMES).** NMES requires an intact and functioning peripheral nervous system, including the nerve, neuromuscular junction, and muscle. The effects of NMES have been studied in various populations, including patients with orthopedic conditions such as joint injuries or those recovering from surgery, patients with central nervous system (CNS) injury such as stroke or spinal cord injury (SCI), people with chronic or critical illness, as well as healthy adults and athletes. In addition, electrically stimulated muscle contractions can be used to help control edema caused by lack of motion, and electrical currents with appropriate parameters can stimulate contractions in denervated muscles. Electrical stimulation of contractions in denervated muscles is generally called **electrical muscle stimulation (EMS).** Although muscle contractions produced by electrical stimulation are not exactly the same as physiological contractions, both types of contractions can strengthen muscles, improve muscle endurance and cardiovascular health, retard or prevent muscle atrophy, reduce spasticity, and help restore function.

◎ Clinical Pearl

Although electrically stimulated muscle contractions are not exactly the same as physiological contractions, both physiological contractions and electrically stimulated contractions can be used to strengthen muscles, improve muscle endurance and cardiovascular health, retard or prevent muscle atrophy, reduce spasticity, and help restore function.

Effects of Electrically Stimulated Muscle Contractions

INNERVATED MUSCLE

When action potentials (APs) are propagated along motor nerves, as described in Chapter 11, the muscle fibers innervated by those nerves become depolarized and contract. Muscle contractions produced by electrically stimulated APs are similar to contractions produced by physiologically initiated APs and can therefore be used for a similarly wide range of clinical applications, including muscle strengthening, muscle education or reeducation, and edema control. However, there are differences between electrically stimulated muscle contractions and voluntary physiologically initiated muscle contractions that affect their therapeutic impact and application.

The difference between physiologically initiated muscle contractions and electrically stimulated muscle contractions that has the most clinical impact is the order of motor unit recruitment. With physiologically initiated contractions, the smaller nerve fibers, and thus the smaller, **slow-twitch type I muscle fibers,** are activated before larger nerve and muscle fibers.[1] In contrast, during electrically stimulated muscle contractions, the largest-diameter nerve fibers, which innervate the larger, **fast-twitch type II muscle fibers,** are activated first, and the smaller-diameter fibers are recruited later.[2-4] The smaller, slow-twitch muscle fibers produce lower-force contractions but are more resistant to fatigue and atrophy. The larger, fast-twitch muscle fibers produce stronger and quicker contractions but fatigue rapidly and are more prone to weakening and atrophy with disuse (Fig. 12.1). An important clinical implication of this difference in the order of motor unit recruitments is that electrically stimulated contractions, which first activate the larger type II muscle fibers, can very effectively strengthen muscle fibers atrophied and weakened by disuse. However, because these stimulated contractions are more fatiguing than physiological contractions, longer rest times are needed between them (Fig. 12.2). If possible, patients should perform physiological contractions together with electrically stimulated contractions to optimize the recruitment of all muscle fibers and the integration of strength gains.

◎ Clinical Pearl

If possible, patients should perform physiological contractions together with electrically stimulated contractions to optimize the recruitment of all muscle fibers and the functional integration of strength gains.

In addition to the difference in the order of motor unit recruitment, physiologically initiated contractions usually recruit motor units asynchronously, resulting in a gradual,

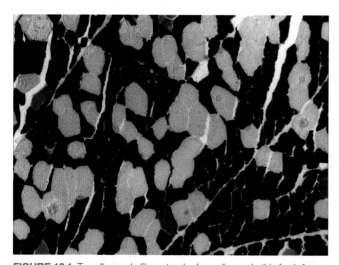

FIGURE 12.1 Type II muscle fiber atrophy from disuse. In this fresh frozen muscle biopsy specimen, the dark brown/black fibers are atrophic type II fibers, and the light beige fibers are normal-sized type I fibers. (Courtesy Sakir Gultekin, MD, Oregon Health & Science University, Portland, OR.)

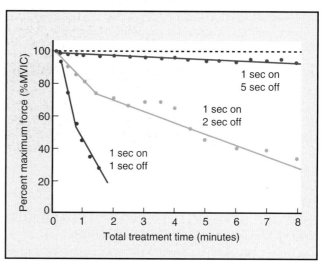

FIGURE 12.2 The effect of changing the on:off ratio on the force of contraction produced. Stronger contractions are produced when longer off times are used. *MVIC,* Maximum voluntary isometric contraction. (Adapted from Benton LA, Baker LL, Bowman BR, et al: *Functional electrical stimulation: a practical clinical guide,* Downey, CA, 1981, Rancho Los Amigos Hospital.)

smoothly graded increase in force. In contrast, electrical stimulation causes all motor units that can be recruited by the applied stimulus to fire simultaneously, when the stimulus reaches motor threshold, resulting in a rapid, often jerky, onset of the contractions.

DENERVATED MUSCLE

When a muscle becomes denervated by nerve injury or disease, it no longer contracts physiologically, and a contraction cannot be produced by the amount of charge that is effective for an innervated muscle. Electrical stimulation can generally only produce contractions in denervated muscles when a direct current (DC), or a pulsed current with a pulse duration of 10 ms or longer, is applied directly to the muscle. This stimulates APs in the muscle cells directly without input from a motor nerve. This is known as *EMS.*[5]

Although it has been suggested that EMS could delay reinnervation[6] of denervated muscles, most studies suggest that use of EMS after motor nerve injury reduces the rate of muscle atrophy and that application immediately after the injury is more effective than delaying its use.[7-11] The use of EMS has been studied most extensively in patients with Bell palsy (facial weakness caused by facial nerve dysfunction). Seven human clinical trials comparing EMS to controls for Bell palsy have been published.[12-18] Five of these trials found a weak benefit[14-18] from EMS, and two found neither benefit nor harm.[12,13] Unfortunately, the small size of these trials, poor reporting of patient factors that affect recovery, and poor reporting of outcomes, as well as variability in stimulation parameters, limit interpretation of these trial results. For example, although DC or pulses longer than 10 ms are thought to be required to produce contractions in denervated muscle, four of the seven published trials on Bell palsy used **biphasic waveforms**[12,14,17,18] with shorter pulse durations. In general, it is recommended that EMS be applied for a number of seconds for each contraction of each affected muscle, gradually increasing the current **amplitude (intensity)** to increase the strength of the contractions.

> ◎ **Clinical Pearl**
>
> Denervated muscle will not contract with the usual electrical stimulus used for NMES but will contract if DC, or a pulsed current with a pulse duration of 10 ms or longer, is applied directly to the muscle.

Clinical Applications of Electrically Stimulated Muscle Contractions
MUSCLE STRENGTHENING FOR PATIENTS WITH ORTHOPEDIC CONDITIONS

Electrical stimulation is thought to strengthen muscles by two mechanisms: overload and specificity.[19] According to the **overload principle,** the greater the load placed on a muscle and the higher-force contraction it produces, the more strength that muscle will gain. This principle applies to contractions produced by electrical stimulation and to contractions produced by physiological exercise.[20] With physiological exercise, the load can be progressively increased by increasing the resistance, usually with weights or resistance bands. With electrically stimulated contractions, the contraction force is increased by increasing the total amount of current, which can be achieved by increasing the **pulse duration,** the current amplitude, or the electrode size, all of which will recruit more muscle fibers.[21-25] An externally applied resistance will also increase the force of an electrically stimulated contraction.

According to the specificity theory, muscle contractions specifically strengthen the muscle fibers that contract. Because electrical stimulation causes fast-twitch type II muscle fibers, which produce a greater level of force, to contract before slow-twitch type I muscle fibers, electrical stimulation has more impact on strengthening fast-twitch type II muscle fibers. In patients with reduced muscle strength as a result of surgery, immobilization, or other muscle-weakening pathology, where there is primarily type II fiber atrophy, early use[26,27] of electrical stimulation, and adding electrical stimulation to physiological exercise, amplifies and accelerates strength gains.[2,28-30] After surgery, NMES has been found to have the greatest impact on strength in the early stages of rehabilitation, with waning benefits over time. By 12 months postoperatively, most studies find no difference in strength between groups that use NMES and groups that do not use NMES.[26,31,32]

> ◎ **Clinical Pearl**
>
> In patients with reduced muscle strength after surgery or immobilization, early use of electrical stimulation, and adding electrical stimulation to physiological exercise, can accelerate strength recovery.

Neuromuscular Electrical Stimulation After Anterior Cruciate Ligament Reconstruction

After joint surgery, the recovery of functional performance depends on the strength of the muscles supporting the joint, and electrical stimulation can strengthen these muscles.

Much of the early research on NMES focused on enhancing recovery from anterior cruciate ligament (ACL) reconstruction surgery. Six months after an ACL reconstruction, quadriceps strength is typically reduced by an average of 23% compared with the healthy unoperated side, and the strength of the operated side is still an average of 14% less than the unoperated side 12 months after ACL reconstruction.[33] Quadriceps strengthening is essential to functional recovery after ACL reconstruction. If quadriceps strength is restored to 90% or more than that of the unoperated side, the kinematics of the repaired knee will match an uninjured leg, but if the quadriceps strength is less than 80% of the contralateral uninjured leg, the kinematics of the repaired knee will be the same as in an ACL-deficient knee.[30]

Early studies found that NMES can retard the early decline of quadriceps strength associated with ACL reconstruction, although 9 to 12 weeks after surgery, the strength in stimulated and unstimulated muscles was equal, suggesting that applying electrical stimulation early after surgery accelerates recovery but does not alter the final outcome.[34] A 2010 systematic review of studies of NMES after ACL reconstruction found that in most studies, strength gains were significantly greater if subjects performed both NMES and exercise than if they performed exercise alone, but the impact of NMES on functional outcomes was inconsistent.[30] More recent studies, including one in soccer players who underwent ACL reconstruction, continue to support that adding NMES to standard rehabilitation enhances early recovery of muscle strength and size.[35-38]

Neuromuscular Electrical Stimulation After Total Knee Arthroplasty

Persistent quadriceps and hamstring weakness and poor activation are also common after total knee arthroplasty (TKA).[39,40] The quadriceps are generally more affected than the hamstring muscles, with quadriceps strength directly after TKA usually being between 40% and 62% of preoperative levels.[41,42] In many patients undergoing TKA, aging also contributes to type II muscle fiber atrophy, reduced number of type I and type II muscle fibers[43,44] and decreased innervation to and activation of those muscles.[11,44] Therefore, improving quadriceps strength in patients undergoing TKA is an important rehabilitation objective. Several studies have found that adding NMES to voluntary exercise after TKA improves quadriceps strength, and NMES *before* surgery is also associated with greater postoperative strength and more rapid functional improvement.[45] A 2010 Cochrane collaboration systematic review with meta-analysis based on two studies[46] and a 2016 systematic review based on four studies[31] both concluded that although patients undergoing TKA who used NMES in addition to exercise had better quadriceps activation than patients who only exercised, the evidence remained insufficient to definitively recommend NMES for patients undergoing TKA. Two subsequent reviews concluded that NMES for TKA improved outcomes compared with the standard of care. The authors attributed the better outcomes to the regular use of high-intensity NMES during the immediate postoperative phase helping to attenuate dramatic early losses in quadriceps strength and improving overall strength and function.[28,47] Studies where NMES was not associated with significant improvements in strength after TKA likely used too low of a current amplitude to produce sufficiently strong contractions or did not apply the stimulation often enough. The hypothesis that the intensity and frequency of stimulation affect the outcome is supported by a small study in 30 patients who had undergone TKA that found a significant association between NMES training intensity and change in quadriceps muscle strength and activation[48] and studies showing that stimulation needs to be performed daily to be effective.[27,47]

> ### Clinical Pearl
>
> Daily high-intensity NMES is probably most likely to help attenuate early losses in quadriceps strength and improve outcomes after TKA.

Neuromuscular Electrical Stimulation for Patients With Other Orthopedic Conditions

In addition to accelerating recovery of strength and function after knee surgery, electrical stimulation can be a helpful adjunct in nonsurgical management of patients with various other conditions affecting the knee. NMES can be as effective as exercise in decreasing pain,[49,50] increasing quadriceps strength, and improving functional performance (walking and stair climbing) in patients with osteoarthritis of the knee,[51-54] and combining exercise with NMES in these patients may be even more effective.[55-59] Similarly, electrical stimulation can improve muscle strength and endurance in patients with muscle atrophy associated with rheumatoid arthritis.[60,61] Electrically stimulated contractions may be particularly effective in these conditions because chronic inflammatory conditions also appear to disproportionately cause type II muscle fiber atrophy.[62] In patients with patellofemoral syndrome (PFS), who often have weakness of the vastus medialis oblique (VMO) muscle, NMES can selectively target the VMO, whereas voluntary contractions cannot. NMES of the VMO has been shown to increase VMO force generation and reduce patellofemoral pain during activity.[63,64] However, a 2017 Cochrane review that investigated the use of NMES for patellofemoral pain syndrome found only four randomized controlled trials, all of which they judged to be of low quality, and they therefore concluded that there was insufficient evidence to draw a conclusion[65] about the efficacy of this intervention.

Most research into NMES for orthopedic conditions has studied the effects of quadriceps stimulation. However, clinically, NMES is likely similarly effective for strengthening other muscles affected by orthopedic conditions. For example, NMES of the hand can increase strength and endurance,[60] and adding NMES of the biceps to resisted elbow flexion exercise after upper extremity immobilization is likely to accelerate and enhance strengthening and functional recovery.

CARDIORESPIRATORY AND FUNCTIONAL TRAINING FOR PATIENTS WITH CARDIAC, PULMONARY, OR CRITICAL ILLNESS

NMES has been studied in various patient populations other than those with orthopedic conditions. Many recent studies have focused on the effects of NMES in patients with serious cardiac or pulmonary conditions or with other critical illnesses because these patients cannot participate in standard exercise.

A 2016 systematic review with meta-analysis based on 13 randomized controlled trials found that the application of NMES, generally to the quadriceps, in patients with heart failure improved peak oxygen uptake, 6-minute walk test distance, muscle strength, flow-mediated dilation, depressive symptoms, and global quality of life.[66] More recent studies are mixed, with two studies[67,68] showing increased quadriceps strength and one[69] showing reduction of protein degradation with the application of NMES in patients after cardiac surgery.[69] However, two other studies[70,71] showed no difference in strength, quality of life, or walking with NMES in similar samples. Researchers have investigated the effects of NMES on mixed groups of critically ill patients and found that overall, NMES, as an adjunct to current rehabilitation practices, increases or better preserves muscle strength and possibly also muscle mass, compared with placebo or standard of care, and may also shorten the length of stay in intensive care.[72-75] Additionally, the most recent Cochrane collaboration systematic review—a meta-analysis of 18 studies with a total of 933 patients—of NMES for muscle weakness in adults with advanced disease, including chronic obstructive pulmonary disease (COPD), chronic heart failure, and thoracic cancer, found that NMES improved quadriceps strength and functional walking (6-minute walk test) in this mixed population.[76] A Cochrane review specifically focused on patients with COPD also found that NMES increased quadriceps force and endurance as well as the 6-minute walk distance (6MWD).[77] One study on COPD published since this review found that NMES was associated with improvements in quadriceps strength, 6MWD, and exercise capacity, although the effects were not greater than those achieved with resistance exercise, and the effects waned once the treatment was stopped.[78] A study on patients with chronic kidney disease on hemodialysis also found that NMES increased muscle strength and functional capacity[79] in these patients. Overall, research strongly supports that NMES improves muscle strength and functional outcomes in patients with a wide range of chronic progressive or critical illnesses associated with reduced physical activity, muscle atrophy, and loss of strength, particularly in those unable or unwilling to comply with standard resistance exercise.

> ### Clinical Pearl
>
> NMES of the quadriceps can improve muscle strength and functional outcomes in patients with reduced physical activity, muscle atrophy, and loss of strength associated with chronic, progressive, or critical illness.

MUSCLE STRENGTHENING FOR ATHLETIC PERFORMANCE

In addition to increasing strength and function in patients with disease, NMES may also further increase strength in healthy adults when added to an exercise program.[80-87] In general, strength gains in healthy muscle with contraction, whether stimulated or voluntary, depend on the force of the contraction, with contractions of at least 50% of the **maximum voluntary isometric contraction (MVIC)** force required to increase strength in healthy muscles and greater gains requiring more forceful contractions. However, most studies have found that the enhanced strength gains from adding NMES to exercise do not translate into functional performance benefits.[88] Although NMES generally improved strength in various athlete populations, including rugby players,[89] tennis players,[90] hockey players,[91] soccer players,[92] young gymnasts,[93] basketball players,[94] volleyball players,[95] and physical education students,[82] it had an inconsistent impact on their functional performance, such as squat jump height, countermovement jump, vertical jump, and sprint speed. It is likely that improving the complex, dynamic movements required for sports performance requires more than strength gains alone. Most sports require agility, coordination of agonist/antagonist muscle groups, flexibility, proprioception, and motor control and balance, which are not affected by NMES. The addition of NMES to a training program most likely assists participants in sports that rely more heavily on strength, but NMES is limited in its ability to improve overall performance in other sports that require high levels of coordination, balance, and motor control. Therefore, although incorporating NMES into an exercise program can likely improve strength, it is not a substitute for a comprehensive program of exercises that challenges performance in a more complex, functional manner.

COUNTERACT DECONDITIONING IN OLDER ADULTS

Various populations with reduced access to exercise will lose muscle strength and mass over time. Early work in astronauts used electrical stimulation of antagonist opposing muscles to provide a resistive force for exercise to prevent atrophy in a zero-gravity space environment.[96] More recent work has focused on older adults with mobility restrictions or illnesses that prevent regular, active exercise or resistance training. Loss of muscle mass and strength also occurs naturally with age, and this age-related muscle atrophy preferentially affects type II fast-twitch muscle fibers.[44] Histological studies have shown that this is at least partially due to a reduction in the number of motor units, suggesting underlying denervation of the muscle.[97] Exercise and activity are key to reducing muscle loss with aging and have both been shown to prevent and reverse age-related muscle atrophy.[11,97,98] However, not all older adults are able to participate in standard exercise programs. NMES has therefore been used to counteract progressive age-related muscle atrophy in both healthy and bedridden older adults. NMES has been shown to increase isometric strength, type II myofiber cross-sectional area, maximum torque, mobility, and function[44,99-101] in older adults, with a variety of mechanisms related to cell functioning and protein synthesis being proposed[99,100] to underlie these effects. Unfortunately, although NMES has been proven to be a safe and effective method for improving strength, function, and mobility in older adults, it has thus far had limited acceptability and implementation by clinicians, possibly because of challenges with adherence or patient-engagement concerns.[102]

IMPROVED MUSCLE COORDINATION AND MOTOR CONTROL IN PATIENTS WITH NEUROLOGICAL CONDITIONS

In addition to the traditional uses of electrical stimulation to increase strength and function in patients with weakness caused by orthopedic conditions, NMES is recommended for producing muscle contractions and thereby improving function in patients with CNS damage from stroke, SCI, or other disorders.[103] NMES can be effective in these patients because electrical stimulation only requires an intact peripheral nervous system, neuromuscular junction, and muscles and not an intact CNS. Although there is strong evidence to support these applications,[104-106] studies published as recently as 2015 indicate that few therapists use NMES for these types of patients.[107]

Neuromuscular Electrical Stimulation After Stroke

NMES can enhance functional recovery after stroke. Two systematic reviews found that NMES increased strength and improved activity after stroke and had a sustained effect on activity beyond the intervention period compared with training alone or with no intervention.[105,108] Based on these findings, the authors of these reviews suggest that "**FES [functional electrical stimulation]** should be used in stroke rehabilitation to improve the ability to perform activities."[108] In addition, two other systematic reviews and meta-analyses concluded that electrical stimulation can prevent or reduce shoulder subluxation and improve function if applied in the acute or subacute stage after stroke.[108,109] Moreover, another meta-analysis concluded that NMES combined with other interventions after stroke reduced spasticity and increased range of motion (ROM) compared with control interventions.[110]

> ◎ **Clinical Pearl**
>
> NMES can increase strength, reduce spasticity, and enhance functional recovery after stroke.

NMES may promote functional improvements in patients after stroke through peripheral and central mechanisms. Peripherally, NMES can help directly by improving muscle strength. Centrally, repetitive practice and increased general excitability of the motor neuron pool produced by motor-level and sensory-level electrical stimulation can enhance descending control of muscle activity and coordination. The motor stimulation and muscle contractions, as well as the sensory input that always accompanies motor-level stimulation, may also provide a cue for the patient to activate a muscle group or promote reflexive motor contraction.[111,112] This may in turn enhance brain plasticity and cortical motor output.[113-115] Spasticity can also be reduced by stimulating antagonist contraction, causing reciprocal inhibition of the agonist muscle. Additionally, NMES can be used to produce stationary cycling in patients with stroke, which can reduce spasticity, strengthen muscles, and increase function.[116-119] Electrically stimulated muscle contractions can also support or assist with joint positioning or movement, functioning similarly to an orthosis, in people with stroke. NMES can also be applied in conjunction with electromyographic (EMG) triggering. In this application, when the patient voluntarily contracts the agonist muscle, the device senses EMG activity, triggering NMES to assist in the contraction. EMG-triggered NMES has been found to improve upper extremity function more than NMES alone in patients with stroke.[120,121] This effect may be due to the increased force of muscle contraction, proprioceptive feedback, or increased cerebral blood flow in the sensorimotor cortex. Further details on applications of superficial EMG activity are provided in Chapter 15.

NMES can be integrated into functional activities by stimulating contractions when the muscle should contract during an activity. Electrical stimulation of muscle contractions to perform functional activities is known as *functional electrical stimulation (FES)*. FES may be delivered with transcutaneous electrodes, similar to NMES. Multichannel FES systems with implanted electrodes are also being studied but are beyond the scope of this text. For patients with stroke and footdrop, FES can initiate ankle dorsiflexion during the swing phase of gait to assist with walking, substituting for an ankle-foot orthosis (AFO) (Fig. 12.3).[122] A 2015 meta-analysis of six randomized controlled trials of footdrop stimulation in patients with stroke found this intervention to be as effective as an AFO for increasing gait speed based on the timed up-and-go and the 6-minute walk test. The footdrop stimulation was preferred to the AFO and reduced the physiological cost of walking more than the AFO.[123] NMES devices for footdrop stimulate dorsiflexion during the swing phase of gait via the peroneal nerve. The stimulation comes on when the heel contacts the ground or based on the angular velocity of the leg.[124] NMES was also found to be cost-effective for correcting footdrop in a group of patients with various CNS disorders, including stroke, multiple sclerosis (MS), SCI, cerebral palsy (CP), and others.[125]

Two hybrid orthosis/stimulation devices for the upper extremity are also available. These have an electrical stimulator inside hand and wrist splints that stimulates thumb opposition as well as wrist flexor and extensor contraction (Fig. 12.4). Patients with weakness resulting from an upper motor neuron lesion can use these devices to grasp objects with their hand—an important functional task for activities of daily living.[126]

Neuromuscular Electrical Stimulation After Spinal Cord Injury

Although NMES is not thought to reverse SCI, NMES may reduce disability and common complications of SCI and improve quality of life by strengthening affected muscles.[11,127-129] FES can also assist people with SCI with a range of body functions, including hand grasp, breathing, aerobic and cardiovascular conditioning, and bowel and bladder voiding.[130] Long-term NMES use in people with SCI may also increase epidermal thickness, providing additional protection against pressure ulcers.[129,131,132]

For FES to be effective, it must produce a contraction of sufficient force to carry out the desired activity, must not be painful, and must be controlled and repeatable. To do this, at a minimum, the lower motor neuron, the neuromuscular junction, and the muscle must be intact; the delivery method must be acceptable to the user; and the contraction must not be excessively fatiguing.[133] Many challenges have arisen in trying to achieve these minimal criteria for successful FES in people with SCI. FES was first used to help patients with SCI walk. Although FES can facilitate walking in this population, doing so requires patients to use a walker for stability and support, which necessitates substantial voluntary upper body strength and endurance. Therefore, locomotion is very slow and requires a high level of energy expenditure by the patient.[133] These limitations make FES locomotion possibly useful for short distances where a wheelchair would be cumbersome but generally impractical for community mobility, where a wheelchair is likely to be more efficient.

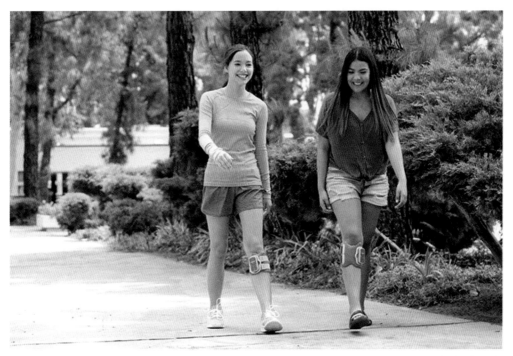

FIGURE 12.3 Functional electrical stimulation to stimulate dorsiflexion during swing phase of gait, triggered by the heel coming off the ground. (Courtesy Bioness, Santa Clarita, CA.)

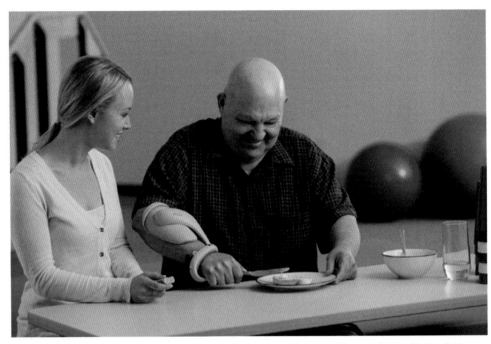

FIGURE 12.4 NESS H200 Hand Rehabilitation System. (Courtesy Bioness, Santa Clarita, CA.)

Another application of NMES in people with SCI is producing movements for exercise, such as leg cycle ergometry, arm cranking, or rowing.[134] Performing these activities when stimulated by electrical stimulation can increase muscle strength and endurance; decrease muscle atrophy; and increase energy expenditure, blood flow, oxygen uptake, stroke volume, maximal oxygen consumption, and ventilatory rate.[135-138] In addition, NMES of the gluteus muscles can increase tissue oxygenation and redistribute surface pressure in people with gluteal weakness resulting from SCI; this may reduce the risk of pressure ulcer formation.[139] Some studies have found that electrically stimulated cycling increased bone mineral density (BMD) by 10% to 30%,[140,141] thus potentially reducing the risks of osteoporosis and associated fractures in adults with SCI.[133,140,142,143] However, one study of FES cycling in children with SCI[143] and a number of similar studies in adults have not found this intervention to significantly increase BMD.[144-146] It is likely that the studies that failed to show benefit did not produce adequate loading because a load of at least 1.4 times body weight is needed to produce significant increases in BMD.[143]

Neuromuscular Electrical Stimulation in Patients With Other Central Nervous System Disorders

In addition to its use after SCI or stroke, electrically stimulated muscle contractions can be used in patients with any CNS dysfunction who have an intact peripheral nervous system, such as patients with TBI, MS, or CP. Several studies have reported improvements in activity and walking, as well as gains in muscle strength and cross-sectional area, in children with CP when NMES of the lower extremities was included in their treatment regimen.[147-153] Upper extremity function also improved when NMES of the upper extremities was included. Combining NMES and dynamic bracing in children with CP has also been found to decrease spasticity, increase function and grip strength, and improve posture.[154,155] In people with

MS, electrical stimulation of the peroneal nerve during the swing phase of gait improved walking speed and decreased the energy expenditure of walking, and FES-stimulated cycling increased the power and smoothness of movement and reduced spasticity immediately after exercise.[156-158]

Neuromuscular Electrical Stimulation for Dysphagia

Although traditionally used primarily for strengthening limb muscles, electrical stimulation can also be used for strengthening the throat muscles in patients with swallowing difficulties (dysphagia) from stroke or other disorders.[159-161] This intervention involves applying electrodes to the neck and stimulating contractions in the muscles responsible for swallowing. This approach is controversial despite several studies finding it to be more effective than other treatments for dysphagia. Early studies concluded, from the limited quantity of high-quality data available at the time, that a small but significant summary effect size supported the use of electrical stimulation to improve swallowing.[162] More recent meta-analyses also concluded that NMES was more effective than traditional therapy for improving swallowing in patients with dysphagia not due to stroke,[161] and that swallowing therapy with surface NMES was more effective than swallowing therapy alone.[159] In addition, stimulation of the pharynx directly with electrodes on a treatment catheter introduced through the nose has been found to help treat poststroke dysphagia,[163] and stimulation of the orbicularis oris muscle has been found to improve lip strength and mouth closure in patients with poststroke dysphagia.[164]

Neuromuscular Electrical Stimulation for Urinary Incontinence

Another use of electrically stimulated muscle contractions is in the treatment of **urinary incontinence (UI)**.[165-167] The urinary bladder is supposed to store urine when partially full and empty, under voluntary control, when completely full. When functioning well, the bladder stores urine by having the detrusor muscle of the bladder wall relaxed and the sphincter muscle at the entrance to the urethra contracted (Fig. 12.5A). To empty the bladder, the detrusor muscle contracts and the sphincter muscle relaxes (Fig. 12.5B). UI, which is the early involuntary leakage of urine from the bladder, can be caused either by weak sphincter muscle contraction, often called *pelvic floor weakness* or *stress incontinence* (Fig. 12.5C), or by early contraction of the detrusor muscle before the bladder is full, often called **overactive bladder (OAB)** or *urge incontinence* (Fig. 12.5D).

For UI caused by pelvic floor weakness, motor-level stimulation can be applied transcutaneously, percutaneously, or via intravaginal probes, with the goal of strengthening the pelvic floor muscles.[168–170] A 2016 systematic review with meta-analysis found that both intravaginal and superficial electrical stimulation were better than no treatment for improving quality of life and pad test in people with stress urinary incontinence.[171] A 2013 Cochrane review on electrical stimulation for urinary incontinence in men found that electrical stimulation enhanced the effect of pelvic floor muscle training in the short term but was associated with more pain and discomfort.[172] A 2017 Cochrane review on electrical stimulation for stress incontinence in women, using nonimplanted vaginal electrodes, found that electrical stimulation is better than sham treatment but may not be better than pelvic floor exercises.[173] A 2019 Cochrane review of therapies for poststroke incontinence, which can be caused by sphincter muscle weakness or OAB, found that transcutaneous stimulation may reduce the number of incontinent episodes each day and probably also improves functional ability.[174] The Agency for Healthcare Research and Quality (AHRQ) recommends the use of electrical stimulation, in conjunction with Kegel exercises, to decrease incontinence in women with stress urinary incontinence.[175]

OAB, contraction of the detrusor muscle of the bladder wall before the bladder is full, can be caused by CNS disorders, including stroke, SCI, and MS. Sensory-level electrical stimulation applied percutaneously or transcutaneously over the tibial nerve or over the sacral spine in patients with OAB can improve symptoms such as excessive urinary frequency and can also improve quality of life.[176–181] A 2016 Cochrane collaboration systematic review with meta-analysis that included studies of electrical stimulation of the bladder wall or the tibial nerve with nonimplanted electrodes to inhibit detrusor contraction found that this intervention was more effective for treating OAB in adults than either no treatment at all or treatment with medications.[182] Of children, 15% to 20%, mostly boys, have OAB.[183] Behavioral management is the primary treatment of OAB in children, with medications being used when behavioral management is insufficiently effective. Sacral and tibial transcutaneous electrical stimulation have also been explored for the treatment of OAB in children and have been found, in some studies, to reduce symptoms, including the number of wet days per week, the frequency and number of voids per day, and the number of incontinence episodes per day.[183,184] However, a 2019 Cochrane review of conservative interventions for daytime UI in children found insufficient evidence to recommend the use of electrical stimulation for daytime UI in children.[185]

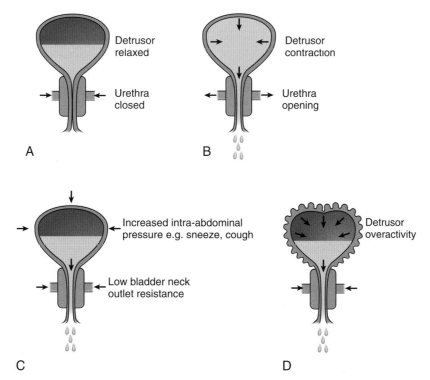

FIGURE 12.5 Causes of urinary incontinence. (A) A healthy partially full bladder storing urine by having the detrusor muscle of the bladder wall relaxed and the sphincter muscle at the entrance to the urethra contracted. (B) A healthy full bladder emptying by contraction of the detrusor muscle and relaxation of the sphincter muscle. (C) Stress urinary incontinence. Urinary leakage with a partially full bladder caused by weak sphincter contraction. (D) Urge incontinence (overactive bladder). Urinary leakage with a partially full bladder caused by early contraction of the detrusor muscle.

EDEMA CONTROL AND IMPROVED CIRCULATION

NMES can also reduce edema caused by poor peripheral circulation resulting from a lack of motion[186] but should be avoided in the presence of edema caused by inflammation because muscle contractions generally aggravate inflammation. Edema caused by inflammation can be treated using monophasic, sensory-level stimulation, as described in Chapter 14.

> ### ◎ Clinical Pearl
>
> Edema caused by poor peripheral circulation as a result of a lack of motion can be treated by electrically stimulated muscle contractions. Edema caused by inflammation can be treated using monophasic, sensory-level stimulation.

Lack of muscle contractions, particularly in a dependent limb, causes edema to form in the distal extremities because the muscles fail to pump fluid proximally through the veins and lymphatics. Contraction of the limb muscles compresses the veins and lymphatic vessels, promoting the return flow of fluid from the periphery. If the muscles do not contract, fluid accumulates in the form of edema; the area will appear pale and will feel cool. Edema of this type can be treated by applying motor-level electrical stimulation to the muscles around the main draining veins. Motor-level electrical stimulation, in conjunction with elevating the legs, has been shown to increase popliteal blood flow in healthy subjects[187,188] and in people with a history of lower limb surgery or thromboembolism[189] and to reduce the increase in foot and ankle volume produced in healthy volunteers after standing motionless for 30 minutes.[190] Motor-level stimulation alone has also been found to reduce edema in patients with chronic venous disease.[191,192] In contrast, sensory-level electrical stimulation has not been found to be effective for this application.[193] To control edema, NMES should be applied in conjunction with elevation and followed by the use of a compression garment (see Chapter 21).

The improvement in blood flow produced by NMES[194–196] can also accelerate tissue healing and help reduce the risk of deep venous thrombosis (DVT) formation.[197–199] Motor-level NMES of the calf muscles has been found to be 1.7 to 3 times more effective than intermittent pneumatic compression for promoting venous circulation, suggesting this could be a more convenient and effective way to prevent DVTs.[187,200] Even NMES of just the foot is as effective in promoting venous circulation and preventing DVTs as intermittent pneumatic compression.[201]

RETARDATION OF ATROPHY AND RETURN OF FUNCTION IN DENERVATED MUSCLE

Motor denervation causes paralysis, muscle atrophy, and fibrosis. The entire muscle and the individual muscle fibers become weaker and smaller, and fibrous tissue forms between these fibers. It has been suggested that ongoing electrical stimulation of denervated muscles may retard, or even reverse, this loss of strength, atrophy, and fibrosis.[7–11,129,200] Electrical stimulation of denervated muscles may also improve function and appearance in some patients.[202] However, studies

have found that these improvements in functional outcomes do not persist after stimulation of denervated muscles is stopped unless the muscles reinnervate. Furthermore, whether stimulation of denervated muscle facilitates reinnervation is also controversial.[12–18,203–205]

Contraindications and Precautions for Electrically Stimulated Muscle Contractions

The standard contraindications and precautions for all electrical stimulation, as described in Chapter 11, also apply to using electrical stimulation to produce muscle contractions. For more detailed information on these contraindications and precautions, refer to the section on contraindications and precautions for the application of electrical currents in Chapter 11.

In addition to the standard contraindications for all electrical stimulation, do not use electrical stimulation to contract muscle when contraction of the muscle may disrupt healing. For example, if the muscle or tendon is torn, muscle contraction may exacerbate the tear, as would a voluntary contraction. Similarly, muscle contractions in patients with tendinitis may worsen symptoms. In addition to the standard precautions for all electrical stimulation, stimulation of muscle contractions should be introduced with long off times and few contractions to assess the patient's delayed response. This is because repetitive stimulation of contractions, particularly in atrophied fibers, can result in delayed-onset muscle soreness.

CONTRAINDICATIONS FOR ELECTRICALLY STIMULATED MUSCLE CONTRACTIONS

> ### ✳ CONTRAINDICATIONS
>
> #### for Electrically Stimulated Muscle Contractions
>
> Standard contraindications for all electrical stimulation (see Chapter 11 for details):
> - Demand cardiac pacemaker, implantable cardiac defibrillator (ICD), or unstable arrhythmias
> - Placement of electrodes over carotid sinus
> - Areas where venous or arterial thrombosis or thrombophlebitis is present
> - Pregnancy—over or around the abdomen or low back (electrical stimulation may be used for pain control during labor and delivery, as discussed in Chapter 13)
>
> Additional contraindications for electrically stimulated muscle contractions:
> - When contraction of the muscle may disrupt healing (e.g., muscle or tendon tear, overuse injury)

When Contraction of the Muscle May Disrupt Healing (e.g., Muscle or Tendon Tear, Overuse Injury)

Although electrically stimulated muscle contractions differ in some ways from physiologically initiated muscle contractions, the overall forces that stimulated contractions exert on the musculotendinous unit are similar to the forces exerted by physiological contractions. Therefore, electrically stimulated contractions should be avoided when muscle contraction may disrupt healing or aggravate symptoms, such as when there is an order for no active motion or for no resisted motion or when there is a tear or inflammation in the muscle or tendon that would be aggravated by muscle contraction.

> ▪ **Ask the Patient**
> • "Do you have a torn muscle or tendon?"
> • "Do you have tendinitis?"
>
> ▪ **Assess**
> • Check for any orders for no active motion or for no resisted motion.

Although active muscle contraction is not always contra-indicated in the presence of a muscle or tendon tear or inflammation, additional caution should be applied when considering electrically stimulated contractions because the force of these contractions cannot be as finely controlled and because electrical stimulation generally produces many repetitive contractions of the same muscles.

PRECAUTIONS FOR ELECTRICALLY STIMULATED MUSCLE CONTRACTIONS

✹ PRECAUTIONS

for Electrically Stimulated Muscle Contractions

Standard precautions for all electrical stimulation (see Chapter 11 for details):
• Cardiac disease
• Impaired mentation
• Impaired sensation
• Malignant tumors
• Areas of skin irritation or open wounds
Additional precautions for electrically stimulated muscle contractions:
• May cause delayed-onset muscle soreness

Application Techniques

APPLICATION TECHNIQUE 12.1 — MUSCLE STRENGTHENING AND COORDINATION AND MOTOR CONTROL

General guidelines for applying electrical stimulation are provided in Chapter 11. The following information builds on this foundation, providing specific recommendations for techniques and parameters for electrically stimulating contractions of innervated muscles to improve muscle strength, muscle coordination, and motor control. These recommendations are summarized in Table 12.1.

Patient Positioning

When electrical stimulation is applied to strengthen muscles, contractions should generally occur with the muscle in the middle of its available length. This can be achieved by securing the limb in place to prevent motion through the range, with the joint that the stimulated

TABLE 12.1 Recommended Parameter Settings for Electrically Stimulated Muscle Contractions

Parameter Settings/ Treatment Goal	Pulse Frequency	Pulse Duration	Amplitude	On:Off Times and Ratio	Ramp Time	Treatment Time	Times per Day
Muscle strengthening	35–80 pps	125–200 μs for small muscles, 200–350 μs for large muscles	To >10% of MVIC in injured muscle, >50% MVIC in uninjured muscle	6–10 s on, 50–120 s off, ratio of 1:5, initially; may reduce off time with repeated treatments	At least 2 s	10–20 min to produce 10–20 repetitions	Every 2–3 h when awake
Muscle reeducation	35–50 pps	125–200 μs for small muscles, 200–350 μs for large muscles	Sufficient for functional activity	Depends on functional activity	At least 2 s	Depends on functional activity	NA
Muscle spasm reduction	35–50 pps	125–200 μs for small muscles, 200–350 μs for large muscles	To visible contraction	2–5 s on, 2–5 s off; equal on:off times	At least 1 s	10–30 min	Every 2–3 h until spasm relieved
Edema reduction using muscle pump	35–50 pps	125–200 μs for small muscles, 200–350 μs for large muscles	To visible contraction	2–5 s on, 2–5 s off; equal on:off times	At least 1 s	30 min	Twice a day

MVIC, Maximum voluntary isometric contraction; *NA,* not applicable; *pps,* pulses per second.

Continued

APPLICATION TECHNIQUE 12.1—*cont'd*

muscles cross in midrange (see Fig. 12.9B). This allows the patient to perform strong isometric contractions in midrange, rather than moving through the range and then applying maximum force at the end of the available ROM. The limb may be secured by placing a barrier to motion in either direction or by using cuff weights to overpower the strength of the muscle contractions. In addition, most treatment tables have positioning straps that can be used to facilitate appropriate and comfortable positioning for the patient and to maintain the joint in a single position that facilitates isometric contraction. Alternatively, when movement is not contraindicated, the muscle can be contracted isotonically during stimulation, with movement through the range consistent with that typically used for functional activities. For example, when stimulating contraction of the quadriceps, the patient may be seated with the knee bent to approximately 90 degrees and the leg secured to prevent motion during muscle contractions. Or the patient may stand in a partial squat and rise from the squat, contracting the quadriceps to extend the knee, when the quadriceps stimulation is on. Similarly, when stimulating the dorsiflexors and hip abductors, stimulation may be applied during treadmill walking.[206] When stimulating contraction of the finger flexors, a functional object, such as a plastic cup, can be used for grasping.

Electrode Type

In general, when using electrical stimulation to induce muscle contractions, self-adhesive, disposable electrodes are recommended.

Electrode Placement

When electrical stimulation is applied to produce a muscle contraction, place one electrode over the **motor point** for the muscle and the other on the muscle to be stimulated so that the current will travel between the electrodes, parallel to the direction of the muscle fibers (Fig. 12.6).[207] The electrodes should be at least 2 inches apart so that they will not be so close (less than 1 inch apart) when the muscle contracts that there is a risk the current will not penetrate deeply enough to stimulate the muscle or could arc between the electrodes.

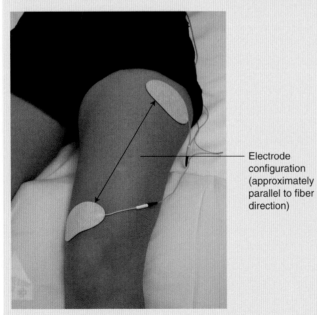

Electrode configuration (approximately parallel to fiber direction)

FIGURE 12.6 Electrodes placed over the proximal and distal ends of the quadriceps muscles for maximum efficacy.

The motor point is the place where an electrical stimulus will produce the greatest contraction with the least amount of electricity; it is the area of skin over the place where the motor nerve enters the muscle. Charts of motor points are available; however, because most motor points are over the middle of the muscle belly, it is generally easiest and most effective to start by placing electrodes there, but alternative placement may be necessary for optimal effect.

Waveform

When electrical stimulation is used to produce muscle contractions, either a **pulsed biphasic waveform** or **Russian protocol** should be used. The pulsed biphasic waveform is available on most devices and is effective for this application. The pulsed biphasic waveform is composed of two square phases in opposite directions with an adjustable pulse duration and frequency. A brief interphase interval of 100 to 250 μs between the two phases of a biphasic waveform can enhance force production and reduce fatigue with NMES without increasing discomfort.[208–211]

The Russian protocol, available on select units, was first described by Kots, who used this waveform to train Russian Olympic athletes. The Russian protocol is specifically a medium-frequency alternating current with a frequency of 2500 Hz delivered in 50 bursts per second. The burst duration and interburst interval are both 10 ms. Although it has been claimed that the Russian protocol may be more effective than pulsed biphasic waveforms for muscle strengthening, several systematic reviews with meta-analyses have concluded that medium-frequency currents such as the Russian protocol are no more or less effective or comfortable for strengthening than pulsed biphasic waveform.[212–214] When using NMES, the frequency, intensity, and pulse duration have a greater impact on efficacy and outcomes than the waveform.

Pulse Duration

When electrical stimulation is used to contract an innervated muscle, the pulse duration should be between 125 and 350 μs in order to stimulate APs in motor nerves (see Fig. 11.17). Most units with adjustable pulse duration allow a maximum duration of 300 μs, and many units intended solely for stimulating muscle contractions have a fixed pulse duration of approximately 250 to 300 μs. If the pulse duration is adjustable, shorter durations are usually more comfortable for stimulating smaller muscles, and longer durations are more comfortable for stimulating larger muscles. As the pulse duration is shortened, a higher-amplitude current will be required to achieve the same strength of muscle contraction. The selection of the ideal combination of pulse duration and current amplitude should be based on patient comfort and achievement of the desired outcome. One study, carried out in healthy volunteers, suggests that for NMES, longer pulse durations with lower amplitudes are more comfortable and less fatiguing than shorter pulse durations with higher amplitudes.[215]

Frequency

The pulse **frequency** determines the type of response that NMES will produce. When a low frequency, of under 30 pps, is used to stimulate a motor nerve, each pulse produces a separate muscle twitch contraction (Fig. 12.7). As the frequency increases to approximately 35 to 50 pps, the twitches occur so close together that they run together into a smooth tetanic contraction. Increasing the frequency further, beyond 50 to 80 pps, may produce stronger contractions, but because this requires such frequent release and recycling of acetylcholine at the neuromuscular junction, these higher frequencies also cause more rapid fatigue.[216,217] Therefore a frequency of 35 to 50 pps is generally recommended[218] for NMES. The frequency

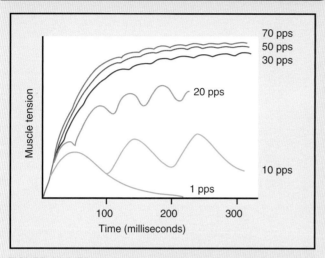

FIGURE 12.7 Effect of stimulus frequency on the type of muscle contraction produced. A frequency of at least 30 pps is needed to produce a sustained contraction.

may be increased to a maximum of 80 pps if needed for comfort. A lower frequency of 20 to 30 pps may also achieve a tetanic contraction and be better tolerated when stimulating smaller muscles, such as the muscles of the face and distal upper extremities in adults and any muscles in young children. There are some studies that also suggest that varying the pulse frequency during treatment can reduce fatigue.[219,220]

On:Off Time

When used to produce muscle contractions, an **on:off time** must be set for the muscles to contract and then relax during treatment. The relaxation is needed to limit fatigue and maintain force production[221] during the contraction.

When used for muscle strengthening, the recommended on time is between 6 and 10 seconds, and the recommended off time is between 50 and 120 seconds, with an initial on:off ratio of 1:5. The long off time is to minimize fatigue. As the patient gets stronger, the on:off ratio may be decreased with subsequent treatments to 1:4 or 1:3. When the goal of electrical stimulation is to relieve a muscle spasm, the on:off ratio is set at 1:1, with both on and off times set between 2 and 5 seconds, to produce muscle fatigue and relax the spasm. When treatment is intended to pump out edema, the on:off ratio is also set at 1:1, with both on and off times set between 2 and 5 seconds and the intensity set to produce a low force contraction.

Ramp Time

A ramp time may be needed to optimize comfort when a muscle contraction is stimulated. The ramp time allows the contraction force to gradually increase at the beginning of the on time (the ramp up) and decrease at the end of the on time (the ramp down), rather than suddenly increasing when switching on and suddenly decreasing when switching off. When stimulation is used to facilitate repetitive exercise, and when on times are in the range of 6 to 10 seconds, a **ramp-up/ramp-down time** of 1 to 4 seconds is recommended. However, for some activities, shorter or longer ramp times are preferred. For

example, when electrical stimulation is used for gait training, where muscles contract and then relax rapidly, a ramp time should not be used. In contrast, when contraction of the antagonist to a spastic muscle is stimulated in a patient with stroke, a long ramp time of 4 to 8 seconds may be necessary to avoid rapidly stretching the agonist, which would only increase the spasticity. Interestingly, one study in healthy adults found that longer ramp times were associated with greater cerebral sensorimotor activation.[222] Additional studies are needed to confirm this finding and to understand its clinical implications.

Current Amplitude

When electrical stimulation is used for muscle strengthening, the current amplitude is adjusted to produce a contraction of the desired strength. When the goal is to strengthen muscles in people without injury, the amplitude of the current must be high enough to produce a contraction that is at least 50% of MVIC strength. However, during recovery from injury or surgery, such as an ACL reconstruction, a current amplitude that produces contractions of a strength equal to or greater than 10% of the MVIC of the uninjured limb will increase strength and accelerate functional recovery better than a control intervention of strengthening without stimulation,[223] although stronger contractions are likely to be more effective. With repeated sessions, the current amplitude can be gradually increased to maximize the torque production and thus the strengthening effect.[25]

When electrical stimulation is used for motor reeducation, the goal of treatment is functional movement that may not require maximum strength. Electrical stimulation can assist functional recovery by providing sensory input, proprioceptive feedback of normal motion, and increased muscle strength. Therefore, when used for motor reeducation, the lowest current amplitude to produce the desired functional movement is probably the best. Initially, this may require strong, motor-level stimulation that makes the muscles move by stimulating the motor nerves. As the patient progresses and regains voluntary control, a lower-amplitude, sensory-level stimulus may be sufficient to cue the patient to move appropriately. Ideally, the patient will learn over time to perform the movement independently without stimulation.

When electrical stimulation is used to reduce muscle spasms or to pump out edema, the current amplitude need only be sufficient to produce a visible contraction.

Treatment Time

When electrical stimulation is used for muscle strengthening, it is generally recommended that treatment last long enough to allow for 10 to 20 contractions. This will usually take about 10 minutes. This treatment session should be repeated multiple times throughout the day if the patient has an electrical stimulation device available for home use. When treatment is provided in the clinic, electrical stimulation is generally applied once each visit for about 10 minutes; the time should be adjusted according to the number of contractions desired and the on:off times used.

When electrical stimulation is used for muscle reeducation, the treatment time will vary based on the functional activity being addressed. Although this is generally no longer than 20 minutes at a single session—less if a patient shows signs of inattentiveness or fatigue—many hours of total stimulation may be recommended in some cases.

Continued

APPLICATION TECHNIQUE 12.2   EDEMA CONTROL AND IMPROVED CIRCULATION

The following recommendations apply *only* when edema and circulatory compromise are caused by a lack of muscle activity—when the area is generally pale and cool. They do not apply to edema caused by inflammation, when the area is red and warm. Information on controlling edema caused by inflammation is presented in Chapter 14, together with other applications of electrical currents for tissue healing. The material presented here concerning control of edema caused by a lack of muscle contraction is repeated in Chapter 12 for the reader's convenience.

Patient Positioning

When electrically stimulated muscle contractions are used to control edema caused by lack of muscle activity or promote circulation. the patient should be positioned with the involved area elevated to help fluid flow from the extremity into the central circulation. In this circumstance, the electrically stimulated muscle contractions help reduce edema and improve circulation by intermittently compressing the veins and lymphatics and promoting venous and lymphatic return.

Electrode Type

Self-adhesive disposable electrodes are recommended when using electrical stimulation for muscle contractions to facilitate edema control and promote circulation.

Electrode Placement

The electrodes should be placed on the muscles around the main veins draining the area (Fig. 12.8). For example, with edema in the foot, the electrodes would be placed on the same-side calf.

Waveform

A pulsed biphasic waveform or Russian protocol is recommended.

Pulse Duration

When a pulsed biphasic waveform is used, the pulse duration should be between 125 and 350 µs—sufficient to produce a muscle contraction. When the Russian protocol is used, the cycle duration cannot be adjusted.

Frequency and On:Off Time

When using electrically stimulated muscle contractions to control edema caused by disuse, the goal is to produce short, low-force, repetitive muscle contractions to pump fluid through the vessels.

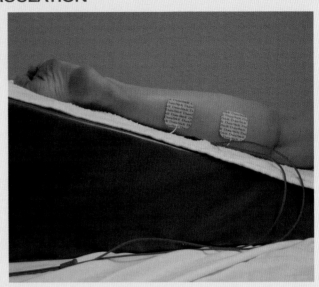

FIGURE 12.8 Electrode placement for neuromuscular electrical stimulation to control edema caused by lack of muscle activity.

There are two ways to achieve this. One option, if you have a device that allows you to set an on:off time, is to set the pulse frequency at 35 to 50 pps, as used to produce muscle contractions for other purposes. Then set the on and off times at 1 to 2 seconds. This will produce tetanic contractions lasting 1 to 2 seconds, with 1 to 2 seconds of relaxation between contractions. Alternatively, if the device does not allow you to set an on:off time, set the pulse frequency at 1 to 2 pps. This will produce one to two twitch contractions each second with relaxation between contractions.

Current Amplitude

The current amplitude should be sufficient to produce a small, visible muscle contraction.

Treatment Time

The stimulation is generally applied for 20 to 30 minutes per session but may be used more than once a day if needed to control edema.[191]

APPLICATION TECHNIQUE 12.3   STIMULATION OF DENERVATED MUSCLE

Patient Positioning

The patient should be positioned to allow easy access to the muscle or muscles to be stimulated. With denervation, there will be no active contraction without stimulation, and atrophy may limit the strength of the stimulated contractions. Therefore, in general, position the patient to allow the stimulated contractions to produce motion with minimal resistance, possibly in a gravity-neutral position.

Electrode Type

When stimulating contractions in denervated muscle, a small-diameter probe is generally used as the active electrode to focus the stimu-

lation and produce the contractions, and a larger, self-adhesive electrode is used as the inactive (dispersive) electrode to complete the electrical circuit. Alternatively, both the active and inactive electrodes can be self-adhesive.

Electrode Placement

The active electrode should be placed on the most electrically responsive point on the muscle to be stimulated. The inactive electrode, which is used only to complete the circuit and not to cause contractions, should be placed over a muscle in the same limb as the active electrode. The electrodes should be placed closer together to

APPLICATION TECHNIQUE 12.3—*cont'd*

stimulate contractions in more superficial muscles and farther apart to stimulate contractions in deeper muscles.

Waveform

A DC is recommended.

Pulse Duration

Because DC and not a pulsed waveform is used for stimulating contractions in denervated muscle, no pulse duration is set.

Frequency

With a DC, there is no frequency to be set.

On:Off Time

For treating denervated muscle, the on-time (contractions) usually lasts 5 to 10 seconds, and the off-time is 4 to 5 times longer than

the on-time to minimize fatigue. In general, there is no on:off setting available when using DC. In this device, the clinician turns the stimulation on for the desired contraction time and turns it off for the relaxation time.

Current Amplitude

When electrical stimulation is applied to denervated muscle, the goal is generally to produce as strong a contraction as possible to most effectively retard disuse atrophy and fibrosis. Therefore, the maximally tolerated current amplitude that produces the desired contraction should be used.

Treatment Time

Electrical stimulation is generally applied for 20 to 30 minutes per session but may be used for much longer and more than once a day.

Documentation

As outlined in Chapter 11, documentation of electrical stimulation is generally written in the form of a SOAP note. When using NMES, document the following:

- Area of the body treated
- Patient positioning
- Specific stimulation parameters
- Electrode placement
- Treatment duration
- Patient's response to treatment

The level of detail should be sufficient for another clinician to be able to reproduce the treatment using your notes.

EXAMPLES

When applying electrical stimulation (ES) to the right knee for quadriceps muscle reeducation after right ACL reconstruction, document the following:

S: Pt reports she is unable to independently perform the quad set exercise she was instructed to do at her last treatment.

O: **Pretreatment:** Pt unable to perform quad exercises.

Intervention: ES to R quadriceps muscles × 20 min. Pt sitting with knee extended. Electrodes placed over VMO muscle and proximal lateral anterior thigh. Pulsed biphasic waveform, pulse duration 300 μs, frequency 50 pps, on:off time 10 s:50 s, ramp up/ramp down 2 s/2 s, amplitude to produce maximum tolerated contraction. Pt instructed to attempt to contract quadriceps muscle with ES.

Posttreatment: Pt able to perform 4 visible quadriceps contractions independently after ES treatment.

A: Pt tolerated ES with increased ability to contract VMO during exercise.

P: Discontinue ES when Pt can perform quad sets × 10 independently as part of home program.

CLINICAL CASE STUDIES

The following case studies demonstrate the concepts of clinical application of electrical stimulation discussed in this chapter. Based on the scenario presented, an evaluation of the clinical findings and goals of treatment are proposed. These are followed by a discussion of the factors to be considered in the selection of electrical stimulation as an indicated intervention and in the selection of the ideal electrical stimulation parameters to promote progress toward the set goals of treatment. Electrical stimulation is not intended to be the sole component of the patient's treatment but rather should be integrated into a comprehensive plan of care.

CASE STUDY 12.1

Shortly After Total Knee Arthroplasty
Examination
History

VP is a 67-year-old woman who underwent right TKA 1 week ago and comes to the physical therapy clinic with an order from her surgeon to evaluate and treat.

Continued

CLINICAL CASE STUDIES—cont'd

Systems Review

VP is alert and cooperative. She has had difficulty straightening her right leg and bearing full weight on the right when walking and has been unable to work since surgery. VP states that right knee pain is 8/10.

Tests and Measures

On palpation, mild warmth and tenderness of the right knee are noted. The surgical sites are healing well. Girth at the level of the midpatella is 43 cm on the right and 38 cm on the left. The right knee active ROM (AROM) is 10 to 50 degrees of flexion. VP walks household distances without any assistive device but with her right knee in approximately 15 to 20 degrees of flexion during stance. She has 4–/5 quadriceps strength on the right, within the available ROM.

> Why would electrical stimulation be a good choice in this patient? Does she have any contraindications to electrical stimulation? What are some appropriate goals?

Evaluation and Goals

ICF Level	Current Status	Goals
Body structure and function	Right quadriceps weakness, knee pain, loss of motion, increased girth	Increase strength Improve ROM Control pain and edema
Activity	Limited and altered ambulation	Return to normal ambulation
Participation	Unable to work	Return to limited, then normal work hours

ICF, International Classification for Functioning, Disability and Health; *ROM,* range of motion.

◆ FIND THE EVIDENCE

PICO Terms	Natural Language Example	Sample PubMed Search
P (Population)	Patient recovering from total knee arthroplasty	("total knee arthroplasty" [text word] OR "Arthroplasty, Replacement, Knee" [MeSH])
I (Intervention)	Neuromuscular electrical stimulation (NMES)	AND ("electrically stimulated muscle contractions" [text word] OR "electrical stimulation" [text word] OR "Electric Stimulation Therapy" [MeSH])
C (Comparison)	No NMES	
O (Outcome)	Optimize functional recovery	AND ("Recovery of Function" [MeSH] OR "strength recovery" [text word] OR strength* [text word])

Key Studies or Reviews

1. Bistolfi A, Zanovello J, Ferracini R, et al: Evaluation of the effectiveness of neuromuscular electrical stimulation after total knee arthroplasty: A meta-analysis. *Am J Phys Med Rehabil* Feb;97(2):123–130, 2018.

This 2018 critical review of six randomized controlled trials of NMES for TKA compared the impact of standard rehabilitation protocols to the impact of standard rehabilitation plus NMES. Three studies showed significantly greater distance covered in the 3- or 6-minute walk test, with one also showing improvements in strength, ROM, and functional tests such as the stair-climbing test and the get-up-and-go test, with NMES as compared with without NMES. Another study showed significantly better ratings on a pain visual analog scale and improved Western Ontario and McMaster Universities Osteoarthritis Index scores in the NMES group compared with control. Of these four studies in which those who received NMES did better than those who did not, in two of the studies, the differences between groups declined over time since surgery. In addition, two studies did not find significant differences in outcomes between those who exercised and those who exercised and also used NMES. The authors of this report concluded that NMES slightly enhances early recovery after TKA, particularly in patients with a severe lack of muscular activation.

2. Volpato HB, Szego P, Lenza M, et al: Femoral quadriceps neuromuscular electrical stimulation after total knee arthroplasty: a systematic review. *Einstein (Sao Paulo)* 14:77–98, 2016.

This 2016 systematic review included four studies of NMES after TKA, three of which were the same as in the review by Kittelson et al. The authors concluded that in patients with TKA, there were no significantly greater improvements at 12 months in knee function, pain, or ROM in patients who received NMES, but the patients who received NMES achieved greater quadriceps activation early after surgery.

Prognosis

Electrical stimulation would be an appropriate treatment for this patient because it would help generate a greater level of force than the patient can generate on her own. Although the evidence supports that long-term outcomes are similar with or without NMES in this population, early NMES to optimize quadriceps activation and attenuate losses in strength accelerates early functional recovery. In this patient, NMES should help increase her quadriceps strength and may help eliminate excess fluid from around her knee, both of which would contribute to functional improvements. This patient has no contraindications for the use of electrical stimulation.

Intervention

Electrical stimulation with a pulsed biphasic waveform or the Russian protocol should be used for this patient (Fig. 12.9). With a pulsed biphasic waveform, the recommended parameters are as follows:

CLINICAL CASE STUDIES—cont'd

Type	Parameters
Patient position	Supine with knee in approximately 20° flexion, over a bolster, strapped for isometric contraction (see Fig. 12.7)
Electrode placement	One channel is set up on the quadriceps with one electrode over the VMO and the second electrode at the proximal lateral anterior thigh. Placement may need to be varied slightly, depending on the quality of contraction and the patient's comfort. A second channel could be used on additional muscle groups if needed. If stimulation is applied to the quadriceps and hamstrings, the channels should run sequentially rather than simultaneously so that the quadriceps and hamstrings contract sequentially rather than simultaneously.
Pulse duration	200–350 μs (based on patient comfort, but with longer duration if tolerated for these larger muscles)
Pulse frequency	50–80 pps to achieve a smooth tetanic contraction
On:off time	10 seconds on, 50 seconds off to initiate treatment, moving to 10 seconds on, 30 seconds off as the patient progresses
Ramp-up/ramp-down time	2–3 seconds ramp up/2 seconds ramp down for comfort
Amplitude	10%–50% of MVIC muscle contraction, as tolerated. The patient should be encouraged to actively contract with the stimulation if she is able.
Treatment time	Sufficient to produce 10–20 contractions. If available, the patient should use a portable stimulation device at home 3–4 times a day to accelerate her recovery of strength and function.

MVIC, Maximum voluntary isometric contraction; *VMO,* vastus medialis obliquus.

Documentation

S: Pt reports R knee pain, increased girth, and difficulty walking after R knee surgery.

O: Pretreatment: R quadriceps strength 4–/5 with slow activation. R knee pain 8/10. R knee girth 43 cm, L knee girth 38 cm. R knee AROM 10 to 50 degrees of flexion. R knee in about 15 to 20 degrees of flexion during stance when ambulating.

Intervention: ES with pulsed biphasic waveform, 1 channel, 1 electrode over the VMO and the other electrode over the proximal lateral anterior thigh. Pulse duration 250 μs, pulse frequency 50 pps, 10 seconds on, 50 seconds off, ramp up 3 seconds, ramp down 2 seconds, amplitude 20% of MVIC muscle contraction. Repeat for 15 contractions.

Posttreatment: Pt able to straighten knee in non–weight bearing.

A: Pt tolerated ES, with improved quadriceps control.

P: Pt given home device and demonstrated correct use. Pt to use 3 to 4 times daily at home, along with strengthening exercises.

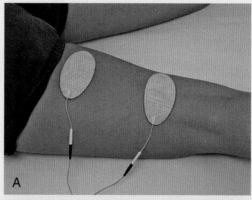
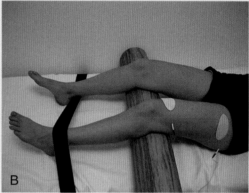

FIGURE 12.9 Electrical stimulation to increase (A) hamstring and (B) quadriceps strength.

CLINICAL CASE STUDY 12.2

Distal Radial Fracture With Weakness and Loss of Range of Motion

Examination

History

RS is a 62-year-old, right-handed housewife who fell and fractured her left distal radius 7 weeks ago. She underwent an open reduction internal fixation (ORIF), and her cast was removed 1 week ago. While her cast was on, she was able to vacuum and cook simple meals, but she could not fold laundry, cook typical meals, shop independently for all groceries, perform her usual housecleaning activities, or play golf because she could not lift with her left hand. She has not yet returned to any of these activities. Her physician's prescription for therapy says "Evaluate and treat." No limitations are prescribed.

Systems Review

RS appears in the clinic in no acute distress. She is attentive to questions and eager to begin treatment. Observation of the wrist reveals atrophy of the extensor and flexor muscles as a result of disuse because of cast immobilization. Pain severity is self-rated 0/10 at rest and 5/10 after 30 minutes of activity.

Continued

CLINICAL CASE STUDIES—*cont'd*

Tests and Measures

Wrist ROM is as follows:

	Left		Right	
	AROM	PROM	AROM	PROM
Extension	30°	45°	70°	75°
Flexion	40°	60°	80°	85°
Ulnar deviation	10°	14°	30°	30°
Radial deviation	15°	15°	20°	20°
Pronation	15°	15°	85°	85°
Supination	8°	10°	80°	80°

AROM, Active range of motion; *PROM,* passive range of motion.

Strength is 3/5 in all directions within her pain-free range. RS has no history of heart disease, cancer, or any major medical problems.

Would this patient be a good candidate for electrical stimulation? How might electrical stimulation help her condition? What parameters for electrical stimulation would be appropriate for this case?

Evaluation and Goals

ICF Level	Current Status	Goals
Body structure and function	Left wrist pain, weakness, and decreased ROM	Control pain Increase strength Increase ROM
Activity	Limited lifting capacity	Increase lifting capacity
Participation	Unable to cook, shop, clean, or play golf	Return to prior level of cooking, shopping, cleaning, and golf

ICF, International Classification for Functioning, Disability and Health; *ROM,* range of motion.

◆ FIND THE EVIDENCE

PICO Terms	Natural Language Example	Sample PubMed Search
P (Population)	Patient with weakness and decreased range of motion after distal radius fracture	"Wrist fracture" [text word] OR "broken wrist" [text word] OR "distal radius fracture" [text word] OR "Wrist" [MeSH] OR "wrist" [text word]
I (Intervention)	Neuromuscular electrical stimulation (NMES)	AND ("electrical stimulation" [text word] OR "electric stimulation therapy" [text word] OR "Electric Stimulation Therapy" [MeSH])
C (Comparison)	No NMES	
O (Outcome)	Strengthen muscle and increase range of motion in hand and wrist	AND ("strength recovery" [text word] OR strength* [text word])

Key Studies or Reviews

No published studies specifically examining the effects of NMES on muscle strength after wrist fracture were found. The many studies and reviews supporting the use of NMES for strengthening muscles after injury, surgery, or disuse and the many small studies on the use of NMES for the upper extremity after stroke support the application of NMES in this patient.

1. Rosewilliam S, Malhotra S, Roffe C, et al: Can surface neuromuscular electrical stimulation of the wrist and hand combined with routine therapy facilitate recovery of arm function in patients with stroke? *Arch Phys Med Rehabil* 93:1715–1721, 2012.

   This article describes a study in 90 patients with no upper limb function after stroke who were randomly assigned to receive NMES for 30 minutes twice a day for 6 weeks in addition to standard therapy or standard therapy only. Patients assigned to receive NMES demonstrated statistically significantly greater increases in wrist extensor and grip strength than patients receiving standard therapy alone.

Prognosis

RS has reduced muscle strength, muscle atrophy, and reduced ROM as a result of her distal radius fracture and subsequent immobilization. Electrical stimulation can help her regain strength, especially of type II muscle fibers, which have atrophied during the time her arm was immobilized in a cast, and can help increase her active ROM by stimulating repeated motion through the available passive ROM.

Intervention

Electrical stimulation, using a pulsed biphasic waveform over the flexors and/or extensors, may be applied. The two muscle groups can be worked independently or sequentially. Recommended parameters are as follows:

Type	Parameters
Patient position	Seated with forearm supported in neutral pronation/supination to allow for gravity-eliminated flexion and extension
Electrode placement	One channel is placed on the wrist extensors. The second channel is placed on the wrist flexors. Stimulation is applied alternately to the extensors and flexors, with a rest period in between. The channels should not run simultaneously because this would produce a co-contraction of the flexors and extensors.
Pulse duration	150–250 μs
Pulse frequency	20–50 pps
On:off time	10 seconds on, 50 seconds off; progressing to 10 seconds on, 30 seconds off
Ramp-up/ ramp-down time	3–4 seconds ramp up, 2 seconds ramp down

CLINICAL CASE STUDIES—cont'd

Type	Parameters
Amplitude	Intensity should be turned up so that a muscle contraction that moves the patient's wrist through the full pain-free range is achieved. RS should contract with the device as much as she is able.
Treatment time	10–20 contractions on the first day. Progress to 10–20 contractions 2 times a day on the third day and for the rest of the week, then reassess. After 1 week, resistance can probably be added to this program. A home device should be used to allow her to continue treatment in between therapy visits.

Documentation

S: Pt reports 3/10 pain, limited ROM and function following ORIF to L wrist 7 weeks ago.

O: Pretreatment: L wrist extension AROM 30 degrees, flexion 40 degrees, strength 3/5 wrist flexion and extension. L wrist pain 3/10.

Intervention: ES to wrist flexors and extensors, sequentially. Pulse duration 200 μs, frequency 30 pps, 10 seconds on, 50 seconds off, ramp up 4 seconds, ramp down 2 seconds, amplitude = muscle contraction through full range, treatment time = 10 contractions (each). During intervention, Pt picked up small objects and transferred them into a bucket.

Posttreatment: Pt was able to increase active wrist flexion and extension by 5 degrees in each direction. Pain during and after treatment 2/10.

A: Pt tolerated ES well with improved ROM and increased functional use of her hand/wrist.

P: NMES for home use to increase repetitions and sessions per day (add 1 session per day until doing 3 × /day). Encouraged Pt to sort socks and/or do other lightweight sorting activities while using NMES.

CLINICAL CASE STUDY 12.3

Critically Ill Patient in Intensive Care

Examination

History

JL is a 25-year-old, right-handed man who, 1 day ago, fell from a roof while drunk and sustained a severe TBI. At baseline, before his accident, JL was independent in all activities of daily living (ADLs), drove, was active in sports, and worked as a tree trimmer. His physician's prescription for therapy says "Evaluate and treat." No limitations are prescribed.

Systems Review

JL is intubated and sedated for airway protection and to treat seizures caused by the TBI. He is in intensive care. Review of his chart shows no history of heart conditions or cancer and no known lower extremity limb fractures or peripheral nerve injuries. He does have a right humeral fracture and a skull fracture.

Tests and Measures

On observation, there are no open wounds on his lower extremities, and on palpation, there is no warmth or edema of his thighs. He does have mild bilateral ankle edema and is wearing compression hose. Girth at the level of the midpatella is 47 cm on the right and 46.5 cm on the left. The right and left knee passive ROM (PROM) are 0 to 130 degrees of flexion. Because of the sedation, JL is not responsive to commands and is not actively moving any extremity. The physicians are hopeful that, in time, he will substantially recover.

Why would electrical stimulation be a good choice in this patient? Does he have any contraindications to electrical stimulation? What are some appropriate goals?

Evaluation and Goals

ICF Level	Current Status	Goals
Body structure and function	At risk for loss of strength and muscle mass due to prolonged immobilization	Slow loss of strength and prevent and muscle atrophy
Activity	None	Maintain strength and muscle mass in preparation for motion as sedation is reduced
Participation	Unable to participate	N/A

ICF, International Classification for Functioning, Disability and Health.

◆ FIND THE EVIDENCE

PICO Terms	Natural Language Example	Sample PubMed Search
P (Population)	Critically ill patients, traumatic brain injury	("critical illness" [text word] OR "intensive care" [MeSH]) or "critical care" [text word]
I (Intervention)	Neuromuscular electrical stimulation (NMES)	AND ("electrically stimulated muscle contractions" [text word] OR "electrical stimulation" [text word] OR "Electric Stimulation Therapy" [MeSH])
C (Comparison)	No NMES	
O (Outcome)	Optimize functional recovery	AND ("intensive care acquired weakness" [MeSH] OR "muscle wasting" [text word]

Continued

CLINICAL CASE STUDIES—cont'd

Key Studies or Reviews

1. Reid JC, Unger J, McCaskell D, et al: Physical rehabilitation interventions in the intensive care unit: a scoping review of 117 studies. *J Intensive Care* Dec 7;6:80, 2018.

   This review of 117 studies examining a wide range of rehabilitation interventions in the intensive care unit found that NMES was one of the interventions associated with better outcomes than control.

2. Silva PE, de Cássia Marqueti R, Livino-de-Carvalho K, et al: Neuromuscular electrical stimulation in critically ill traumatic brain injury patients attenuates muscle atrophy, neurophysiological disorders, and weakness: a randomized controlled trial. *J Intensive Care* Dec 12;7:59, 2019.

   This randomized controlled trial compared conventional physiotherapy plus daily NMES for 14 days to conventional physiotherapy alone in 60 critically ill patients with TBI. Those who had NMES added to their rehabilitation had preserved muscle thickness in the tibialis anterior and rectus femoris, whereas those in the control group had a significant reduction. Those in the NMES group also had a lower incidence of neuromuscular electrophysiological disorders (NEDs) and an increase in evoked peak force. The time to achieve reduction in NED and prevent weakness was 7 days.

Prognosis

Electrical stimulation would be an appropriate treatment for this patient because it would help prevent atrophy resulting from immobilization and minimize the consequences of prolonged bed rest. This patient has no contraindications for the use of electrical stimulation.

Intervention

Electrical stimulation with a biphasic pulsed waveform or the Russian protocol should be used for this patient (see Fig. 12.8). With a biphasic pulsed waveform, the recommended parameters are as follows:

Type	Parameters
Patient position	Supine with legs at ~30 degrees of flexion extended.
Electrode placement	One channel is set up on each quadriceps (right and left), with one electrode over the VMO and the second electrode at the proximal lateral anterior thigh. Placement may need to be varied slightly, depending on the quality of contraction.
Pulse duration	300–350 μs
Pulse frequency	50–80 pps to achieve a smooth tetanic contraction
On:off time	6–10 seconds on, 30-50 seconds off
Ramp-up/ramp-down time	1–2 second ramp up/1–2 second ramp down for comfort
Amplitude	Strong muscle contraction
Treatment time	Sufficient to produce 30–50 contractions.

VMO, Vastus medialis obliquus.

Documentation

S: Pt unconscious and sedated, admitted to intensive care yesterday.

O: Pretreatment: R quadriceps girth at 6″ proximal to the patella = 22″, L quadriceps girth at 6″ proximal to the patella = 23″. R and L knee PROM full, 0 to 130 degrees of flexion.

Intervention: ES with pulsed biphasic waveform, 1 channel on each quad, 1 electrode over VMO, the other electrode over proximal lateral anterior thigh. Pulse duration 300 μs, pulse frequency 50 pps, ramp up 2 s, ramp down 1 s, amplitude 20% of MVIC muscle contraction. Repeat for 40 contractions.

A: Tolerated NMES well without signs of pain or concerning changes in vital signs. No skin irritation at site of electrodes.

P: Repeat daily in intensive care 5–7 day/s week until pt can perform voluntary, active exercises.

Chapter Review

1. Electrical stimulation to produce contractions of innervated muscles is known as *NMES*.

2. NMES primarily produces contractions of type II muscle fibers, enhancing recovery from disuse atrophy but being more fatiguing than voluntary contractions.

3. NMES is primarily used to strengthen muscles according to overload and specificity principles. NMES may also increase muscle endurance, assist with joint positioning, decrease spasticity, and increase circulation.

4. NMES has been used to maintain or regain muscle strength and function in patients with orthopedic conditions, including patients recovering from ACL repair, TKA, osteoarthritis, or PFS; in patients with chronic illnesses such as heart disease and COPD; and in patients with neurological conditions such as stroke, SCI, and MS.

5. NMES should not be used if a tendon or muscle is torn because the repetitive electrical stimulation may worsen the symptoms.

Glossary

Amplitude (intensity): The magnitude of current or voltage (see Fig. 11.12).

Biphasic waveform: A current where the charged particles move first in one direction and then in the opposite direction. Biphasic currents may be pulsed or alternating.

Electrical muscle stimulation (EMS): Application of an electrical current directly to muscle to produce a muscle contraction.

Fast-twitch type II muscle fibers: Large muscle fibers that contract to produce quick, powerful movements but that fatigue quickly; also called *fast twitch*.

Frequency (rate): The number of cycles or pulses per second. Frequency is measured in Hertz (Hz) for cycles and in pulses per second (pps) for pulses (see Fig. 11.11).

Functional electrical stimulation (FES): Application of an electrical current to produce muscle contractions that are applied during a functional activity. Examples of FES include the electrical stimulation of dorsiflexion during the swing phase of gait and the stimulation of wrist extension and finger flexion during grasp activities.

Maximum voluntary isometric contraction (MVIC): The peak force produced by a muscle as it contracts while pulling against an immovable resistance.

Motor point: The place in a muscle where electrical stimulation will produce the greatest contraction with the least amount of electricity; generally located over the middle of the muscle belly.

Neuromuscular electrical stimulation (NMES): Application of an electrical current to motor nerves to produce contractions of the muscles they innervate.

On:off time: On time is the time during which a train of pulses occurs. Off time is the time between trains of pulses, when no current flows. On and off times are usually used only when electrical stimulation is used to produce muscle contractions. The muscle contracts during on time, and it relaxes during off time. Off times are needed to reduce muscle fatigue during the stimulation session.

Overactive bladder (OAB): A type of urinary incontinence where the detrusor muscle contracts before the bladder is full. Also called *urge incontinence.*

Overload principle: A principle of strengthening muscle stating that the greater the load placed on a muscle and the higher force contraction it produces, the more strength that muscle will gain.

Pulse duration (width): Time from the beginning of the first phase of a pulse to the end of the last phase of a pulse. Pulse duration is generally expressed in microseconds ($\mu s \times 10^{-6}$ seconds) (see Fig. 11.10).

Pulsed biphasic waveform: Series of pulses where the charged particles move first in one direction and then in the opposite direction (see Fig. 11.4B).

Ramp-up/ramp-down time: The ramp-up time is the time it takes for the current amplitude to increase from zero, at the end of the off time, to its maximum amplitude during the on time. A current ramps up by having the amplitude of the first few pulses of the on time gradually become sequentially higher than the amplitude of the previous pulse. The ramp-down time is the time it takes for the current amplitude to decrease from its maximum amplitude during the on time back to zero (see Fig. 11.14).

Russian protocol: A medium-frequency alternating current (AC) with a frequency of 2500 Hz delivered in 50 bursts/second. Each burst is 10 ms long and is separated from the next burst by a 10-ms interburst interval (see Fig. 11.9). This type of current is also known as *medium-frequency burst AC (MF burst AC)*; when this term is used, the frequency of the medium-frequency current or the bursts may be different from the original protocol.

Slow-twitch type I muscle fibers: Small muscle fibers that are slow to contract but do not fatigue easily; also called *slow twitch.*

Urinary incontinence (UI): Involuntary leakage of urine from the bladder that can be caused by either weak pelvic floor muscles or early contraction of the detrusor muscle.

References

1. Henneman E: Relation between size of neurons and their susceptibility to discharge. *Science* 126:1345–1347, 1957.
2. Garnett R, Stephens JA: Changes in the recruitment threshold of motor units produced by cutaneous stimulation in man. *J Physiol (London)* 311:463–473, 1981.
3. Hennings K, Kamavuako EN, Farina D: The recruitment order of electrically activated motor neurons investigated with a novel collision technique. *Clin Neurophysiol* 118:283–291, 2007.
4. Datta AK, Stephens JA: The effects of digital nerve stimulation on the firing of motor units in human first dorsal interosseous muscle. *J Physiol* 318:501–510, 1981.
5. Petrofsky JS, Petrofsky S: A wide-pulse-width electrical stimulator for use on denervated muscles. *J Clin Eng* 17:331–338, 1992.
6. Pinheiro-Dardis CM, Erbereli BT, et al: Electrical stimulation delays reinnervation in denervated rat muscle. *Muscle Nerve* 56(6):E108–E118, 2017.
7. Pieber K, Herceg M, Paternostro-Sluga T, et al: Optimizing stimulation parameters in functional electrical stimulation of denervated muscles: a cross-sectional study. *J Neuroeng Rehabil* 12:51, 2015.
8. Bueno CRS, Pereira M, Favaretto Jr IA, et al: Electrical stimulation attenuates morphological alterations and prevents atrophy of the denervated cranial tibial muscle. *Einstein (Sao Paulo)* 15(1):71–76, 2017.
9. Koh ES, Kim HC, Lim JY: The effects of electromyostimulation application timing on denervated skeletal muscle atrophy. *Muscle Nerve* 56(6):E154–E161, 2017.
10. Carraro U, Boncompagni S, Gobbo V, et al: Persistent muscle fiber regeneration in long term denervation. Past, present, future. *European Journal of Translational Myology* 25(2):77–92, 2015.
11. Carrar U, Kern H, Gava P, et al: Biology of muscle atrophy and of its recovery by FES in aging and mobility impairments: roots and by-products. *European Journal of Translational Myology* 25(4):221–230, 2015.
12. Alakram P, Puckree T: Effects of electrical stimulation on House-Brackmann scores in early Bell's palsy. *Physiother Theory Pract* 26(3):160–166, 2010.
13. Mosforth J, Taverner D: Physiotherapy for Bell's palsy. *Br Med J* 2(5097):675–677, 1958.
14. Manikandan N: Effect of facial neuromuscular re-education on facial symmetry in patients with Bell's palsy: a randomized controlled trial. *Clin Rehabil* 21(4):338–343, 2007.
15. Kim J, Choi JY: The effect of subthreshold continuous electrical stimulation on the facial function of patients with Bell's palsy. *Acta Otolaryngol* 136(1):100–105, 2016.
16. Tuncay F, et al: Role of electrical stimulation added to conventional therapy in patients with idiopathic facial (Bell) palsy. *Am J Phys Med Rehabil* 94(3):222–228, 2015.
17. Flores PF, Haro LG: Idiopathic peripheral facial paralysis treatment physic therapy versus prednisone [Tratamiento de la paralisis facial peripherica idiopatica: terapia fisica versus prednisone]. *Revista Medica del Instituto Mexicano del Seguro Social* 36(3):217–221, 1998.
18. Marotta N, et al: Neuromuscular electrical stimulation and shortwave diathermy in unrecovered Bell palsy: A randomized controlled study. *Medicine (Baltimore)* 99(8):e19152, 2020.
19. Delitto A, Snyder-Mackler L: Two theories of muscle strength augmentation using percutaneous electrical stimulation. *Phys Ther* 70:158–164, 1990.
20. DeLuca CJ, LeFever RS, McCue MP, et al: Behavior of human motor units in different muscles during linearly varying contractions. *J Physiol (London)* 329:113–128, 1982.
21. Han TR, Kim DY, Lim SJ, et al: The control of parameters within the therapeutic range in neuromuscular electrical stimulation. *Int J Neurosci* 117:107–119, 2007.
22. Dreibati B, Lavet C, Pinti A, et al: Influence of electrical stimulation frequency on skeletal muscle force and fatigue. *Ann Phys Rehabil Med* 53:266–277, 2010.
23. Gondin J, Giannesini B, Vilmen C, et al: Effects of stimulation frequency and pulse duration on fatigue and metabolic cost during a single bout of neuromuscular electrical stimulation. *Muscle Nerve* 41:667–678, 2010.
24. Gorgey AS, Dudley GA: The role of pulse duration and stimulation duration in maximizing the normalized torque during neuromuscular electrical stimulation. *J Orthop Sports Phys Ther* 38:508–516, 2008.

25. Bremner CB, Holcomb WR, Miller MG: Recommendations to increase neuromuscular electrical stimulation training intensity during quadriceps treatments for orthopedic knee conditions. *Clin J Sport Med* 31(3):330–334, 2019.

26. Bistolfi A, Zanovello J, Ferracini R, et al: Evaluation of the effectiveness of neuromuscular electrical stimulation after total knee arthroplasty: a meta-analysis. *Am J Phys Med Rehabil* 97(2):123–130, 2018.

27. Delanois R, Sodhi N, Acuna A, et al: Use of home neuromuscular electrical stimulation in the first 6 weeks improves function and reduces pain after primary total knee arthroplasty: a matched comparison. *Ann Transl Med* 7(Suppl 7):S254, 2019. doi:10.21037/atm.2019.09.150.

28. Kittelson AJ, Stackhouse SK, Stevens-Lapsley JE: Neuromuscular electrical stimulation after total joint arthroplasty: a critical review of recent controlled studies. *Eur J Phys Rehabil Med* 49:909–920, 2013.

29. Maddocks M, Gao W, Higginson IJ, et al: Neuromuscular electrical stimulation for muscle weakness in adults with advanced disease. *Cochrane Database Syst Rev* 2013(1):CD009419, 2013.

30. Kim KM, Croy T, Hertel J, et al: Effects of neuromuscular electrical stimulation after anterior cruciate ligament reconstruction on quadriceps strength, function, and patient-oriented outcomes: a systematic review. *J Orthop Sports Phys Ther* 40:383–391, 2010.

31. Volpato HB, Szego P, Lenza M, et al: Femoral quadriceps neuromuscular electrical stimulation after total knee arthroplasty: a systematic review. *Einstein (Sao Paulo)* 14(1):77–98, 2016.

32. Nussbaum EL, Houghton P, Anthony J, et al: Neuromuscular electrical stimulation for treatment of muscle impairment: critical review and recommendations for clinical practice. *Physiother Can* 69(5):1–76, 2017.

33. Lepley LK: Deficits in quadriceps strength and patient-oriented outcomes at return to activity after ACL reconstruction: a review of the current literature. *Sports Health* 7:231–238, 2015.

34. Morrissey MC, Brewster CE, Shields CL, et al: The effects of electrical stimulation on the quadriceps during postoperative knee immobilization. *Am J Sports Med* 13:40–45, 1985.

35. Taradaj J, Halski T, Kucharzewski M, et al: The effect of neuromuscular electrical stimulation on quadriceps strength and knee function in professional soccer players: return to sport after ACL reconstruction. *Biomed Res Int* 802534:2013, 2013.

36. Imoto AM, Peccin S, Almeida GJ, et al: Effectiveness of electrical stimulation on rehabilitation after ligament and meniscal injuries: a systematic review. *Sao Paulo Med J* 129:414–423, 2011.

37. Wright AR, Richardson AB, Kikuchi CK, et al: Effectiveness of accelerated recovery performance for post-ACL reconstruction rehabilitation. *Hawaii J Health Soc Welf* 78(11 Suppl 2):41–46, 2019.

38. Moran U, Gottlieb U, Gam A, et al: Functional electrical stimulation following anterior cruciate ligament reconstruction: a randomized controlled pilot study. *J Neuroeng Rehabil* 16:89, 2019.

39. Thomas AC, Stevens-Lapsley JE: Importance of attenuating quadriceps activation deficits after total knee arthroplasty. *Exerc Sport Sci Rev* 40:95–101, 2012.

40. Moon YW, Kim HJ, Ahn HS, et al: Serial changes of quadriceps and hamstring muscle strength following total knee arthroplasty: a meta-analysis. *PLoS One* 11(2):e0148193, 2016.

41. Mizner RL, Petterson SC, Stevens JE, et al: Early quadriceps strength loss after total knee arthroplasty: the contributions of muscle atrophy and failure of voluntary muscle activation. *J Bone Joint Surg Am* 87:1047–1053, 2005.

42. Mintken PE, Carpenter KJ, Eckhoff D, et al: Early neuromuscular electrical stimulation to optimize quadriceps muscle function following total knee arthroplasty: a case report. *J Orthop Sports Phys Ther* 37:364–371, 2007.

43. Lewek M, Stevens J, Snyder-Mackler L: The use of electrical stimulation to increase quadriceps femoris muscle force in an elderly patient following a total knee arthroplasty. *Phys Ther* 81:1565–1571, 2001.

44. Langeard A, Bigot L, Chastan N, et al: Does neuromuscular electrical stimulation training of the lower limb have functional effects on the elderly? A systematic review. *Exp Gerontol* 91:88–98, 2017.

45. Walls RJ, McHugh G, O'Gorman DJ, et al: Effects of preoperative neuromuscular electrical stimulation on quadriceps strength and functional recovery in total knee arthroplasty: a pilot study. *BMC Musculoskelet Disord* 11:119, 2010.

46. Monaghan B, Caulfield B, O'Mathúna DP: Surface neuromuscular electrical stimulation for quadriceps strengthening pre and post total knee replacement. *Cochrane Database Syst Rev* 2010(1):CD007177, 2010.

47. Yue C, Zhang X, Zhu Y, et al: Systematic review of three electrical stimulation techniques for rehabilitation after total knee arthroplasty. *J Arthroplasty* 33(7):2330–2337, 2018.

48. Stevens-Lapsley JE, Balter JE, Wolfe P, et al: Relationship between intensity of quadriceps muscle neuromuscular electrical stimulation and strength recovery after total knee arthroplasty. *Phys Ther* 92:1187–1196, 2012.

49. Zeng C, Li H, Yang T, et al: Electrical stimulation for pain relief in knee osteoarthritis: systematic review and network meta-analysis. *Osteoarthritis Cartilage* 23:189–202, 2015.

50. Bjordal JM, Johnson MI, Lopes-Martins RA, et al: Short-term efficacy of physical interventions in osteoarthritic knee pain. A systematic review and meta-analysis of randomised placebo-controlled trials. *BMC Musculoskelet Disord* 8:51, 2007.

51. Durmuş D, Alayli G, Cantürk F: Effects of quadriceps electrical stimulation program on clinical parameters in the patients with knee osteoarthritis. *Clin Rheumatol* 26:674–678, 2007.

52. Melo Mde O, Pompeo KD, Brodt GA, et al: Effects of neuromuscular electrical stimulation and low-level laser therapy on the muscle architecture and functional capacity in elderly patients with knee osteoarthritis: a randomized controlled trial. *Clin Rehabil* 29(6):570–580, 2015.

53. Devrimsel G, Metin Y: Serdaroglu Beyazal M: Short-term effects of neuromuscular electrical stimulation and ultrasound therapies on muscle architecture and functional capacity in knee osteoarthritis: a randomized study. *Clin Rehabil* 33(3):418–427, 2019.

54. Rabe KG, Matsuse H, Jackson A, et al: Evaluation of the combined application of neuromuscular electrical stimulation and volitional contractions on thigh muscle strength, knee pain, and physical performance in women at risk for knee osteoarthritis: a randomized controlled trial. *PM R* 10(12):1301–1310, 2018.

55. Park SH, Hwangbo G: Effects of combined application of progressive resistance training and Russian electrical stimulation on quadriceps femoris muscle strength in elderly women with knee osteoarthritis. *J Phys Ther Sci* 27:729–731, 2015.

56. Elboim-Gabyzon M, Rozen N, Laufer Y: Does neuromuscular electrical stimulation enhance the effectiveness of an exercise programme in subjects with knee osteoarthritis? A randomized controlled trial. *Clin Rehabil* 27:246–257, 2013.

57. Matsuse H, Hashida R, Takano Y, et al: Walking exercise simultaneously combined with neuromuscular electrical stimulation of antagonists resistance improved muscle strength, physical function, and knee pain in symptomatic knee osteoarthritis: a single-arm study. *J Strength Cond Res* 31:171–180, 2017.

58. Kus G, Yeldan I: Strengthening the quadriceps femoris muscle versus other knee training programs for the treatment of knee osteoarthritis. *Rheumatol Int* 39(2):203–218, 2019.

59. Novak S, Guerron G, Zou Z, et al: New guidelines for electrical stimulation parameters in adult patients with knee osteoarthritis based on a systematic review of the current literature. *Am J Phys Med Rehabil* Mar 3, 2020.

60. Brosseau LU, Pelland LU, Casimiro LY, et al: Electrical stimulation for the treatment of rheumatoid arthritis. *Cochrane Database Syst Rev* 2002(2):CD003687, 2002.

61. Almeida GJ, Khoja SS, Piva SR: Dose-response relationship between neuromuscular electrical stimulation and muscle function in people with rheumatoid arthritis. *Phys Ther* 99(9):1167–1176, 2019.

62. Piva SR, Goodnite EA, Azuma K, et al: Neuromuscular electrical stimulation and volitional exercise for individuals with rheumatoid arthritis: a multiple-patient case report. *Phys Ther* 87:1064–1077, 2007.

63. Glaviano NR, Saliba SA: Immediate effect of patterned electrical neuromuscular stimulation on pain and muscle activation in individuals with patellofemoral pain. *J Athl Train* 51(2):118–128, 2016.

64. Garcia FR, Azevedo FM, Alves N, et al: Effects of electrical stimulation of vastus medialis obliquus muscle in patients with patellofemoral pain syndrome: an electromyographic analysis. *Rev Bras Fisioter* 14:477–482, 2010.

65. Martimbianco ALC, Torloni MR, Andriolo BN, et al: Neuromuscular electrical stimulation (NMES) for patellofemoral pain syndrome. *Cochrane Database Syst Rev* 12:CD011289, 2017.

66. Gomes Neto M, Oliveira FA, Reis HF, et al: Effects of neuromuscular electrical stimulation on physiologic and functional measurements in

patients with heart failure: a systematic review with meta-analysis. *J Cardiopulm Rehabil Prev* 36:157–166, 2016.

67. Schardong J, Kuinchtner GC, Sbruzzi G, et al: Functional electrical stimulation improves muscle strength and endurance in patients after cardiac surgery: a randomized controlled trial. *Braz J Phys Ther* 21(4):268–273, 2017.

68. Fischer A, Spiegl M, Altmann K, et al: Muscle mass, strength and functional outcomes in critically ill patients after cardiothoracic surgery: does neuromuscular electrical stimulation help? The Catastim 2 randomized controlled trial. *Crit Care* 20:30, 2016.

69. Iwatsu K, Iida Y, Kono Y, et al: Neuromuscular electrical stimulation may attenuate muscle proteolysis after cardiovascular surgery: A preliminary study. *J Thorac Cardiovasc Surg* 153(2):373–379, 2017.

70. Fontes Cerqueira TC, Cerqueira Neto ML, Cacau LAP, et al: Ambulation capacity and functional outcome in patients undergoing neuromuscular electrical stimulation after cardiac valve surgery: A randomised clinical trial. *Medicine (Baltimore)* 97(46):e13012, 2018.

71. Kitamura H, Yamada S, Adachi T, et al: Effect of perioperative neuromuscular electrical stimulation in patients undergoing cardiovascular surgery: a pilot randomized controlled trial. *Semin Thorac Cardiovasc Surg* 31(3):361–367, 2019.

72. Maffiuletti NA, Roig M, Karatzanos E, et al: Neuromuscular electrical stimulation for preventing skeletal-muscle weakness and wasting in critically ill patients: a systematic review. *BMC Med* 11:137, 2013.

73. Burke D, Gorman E, Stokes D, et al: An evaluation of neuromuscular electrical stimulation in critical care using the ICF framework: a systematic review and meta-analysis. *Clin Respir J* 10:407–420, 2016.

74. Dall' Acqua AM, Sachetti A, Santos LJ, et al: Use of neuromuscular electrical stimulation to preserve the thickness of abdominal and chest muscles of critically ill patients: a randomized clinical trial. *J Rehabil Med* 49(1):40–48, 2017.

75. Silva PE, de Cássia Marqueti R, Livino-de-Carvalho K, et al: Neuromuscular electrical stimulation in critically ill traumatic brain injury patients attenuates muscle atrophy, neurophysiological disorders, and weakness: a randomized controlled trial. *J Intensive Care* 7:59, 2019.

76. Jones S, Man WD, Gao W, et al: Neuromuscular electrical stimulation for muscle weakness in adults with advanced disease. *Cochrane Database Syst Rev* 10:CD009419, 2016.

77. Hill K, Cavalheri V, Mathur S, et al: Neuromuscular electrostimulation for adults with chronic obstructive pulmonary disease. *Cochrane Database Syst Rev* 5:CD010821, 2018.

78. Latimer LE, Constantin D, Greening NJ, et al: Impact of transcutaneous neuromuscular electrical stimulation or resistance exercise on skeletal muscle mRNA expression in COPD. *Int J Chron Obstruct Pulmon Dis* 14:1355–1364, 2019.

79. Schardong J, Stein C, Della Méa Plentz R: Neuromuscular electrical stimulation in chronic kidney failure: a systematic review and meta-analysis. *Arch Phys Med Rehabil* 101(4):700–711, 2020.

80. Paillard T, Noe F, Bernard N, et al: Effects of two types of neuromuscular electrical stimulation training on vertical jump performance. *J Strength Cond Res* 22:1273–1278, 2008.

81. Paillard T: Combined application of neuromuscular electrical stimulation and voluntary muscular contractions. *Sports Med* 38:161–177, 2008.

82. Herrero AJ, Martín J, Martín T, et al: Short-term effect of plyometrics and strength training with and without superimposed electrical stimulation on muscle strength and anaerobic performance: a randomized controlled trial. Part II. *J Strength Cond Res* 24:1616–1622, 2010.

83. Herrero AJ, Martín J, Martín T, et al: Short-term effect of strength training with and without superimposed electrical stimulation on muscle strength and anaerobic performance: a randomized controlled trial. Part I. *J Strength Cond Res* 24:1609–1615, 2010.

84. Iwasaki T, Shiba N, Matsuse H, et al: Improvement in knee extension strength through training by means of combined electrical stimulation and voluntary muscle contraction. *Tohoku J Exp Med* 209:33–40, 2006.

85. Matsuse H, Iwasa C, Imaishi K, et al: Hybrid-training method increases muscle strength and mass in the forearm without adverse effect of hand function in healthy male subjects. *Kurume Med J* 57:125–132, 2011.

86. Matsuse H, Shiba N, Umezu Y, et al: Muscle training by means of combined electrical stimulation and volitional contraction. *Aviat Space Environ Med* 77:581–585, 2006.

87. Takano Y, Haneda Y, Maeda T, et al: Increasing muscle strength and mass of thigh in elderly people with the hybrid-training method of electrical stimulation and volitional contraction. *Tohoku J Exp Med* 221:77–85, 2010.

88. Gondin J, Cozzone PJ, Bendahan D: Is high-frequency neuromuscular electrical stimulation a suitable tool for muscle performance improvement in both healthy humans and athletes? *Eur J Appl Physiol* 111:2473–2487, 2011.

89. Babault N, Cometti G, Bernardin M, et al: Effects of electromyostimulation training on muscle strength and power of elite rugby players. *J Strength Cond Res* 21:431–437, 2007.

90. Maffiuletti NA, Bramanti J, Jubeau M, et al: Feasibility and efficacy of progressive electrostimulation strength training for competitive tennis players. *J Strength Cond Res* 23:677–682, 2009.

91. Brocherie F, Babault N, Cometti G, et al: Electrostimulation training effects on the physical performance of ice hockey players. *Med Sci Sports Exerc* 37:455–460, 2005.

92. Billot M, Martin A, Paizis C, et al: Effects of an electrostimulation training program on strength, jumping, and kicking capacities in soccer players. *J Strength Cond Res* 24:1407–1413, 2010.

93. Deley G, Cometti C, Fatnassi A, et al: Effects of combined electromyostimulation and gymnastics training in prepubertal girls. *J Strength Cond Res* 25:520–526, 2011.

94. Maffiuletti NA, Cometti G, Amiridis IG, et al: The effects of electromyostimulation training and basketball practice on muscle strength and jumping ability. *Int J Sports Med* 21:437–443, 2007.

95. Malatesta D, Cattaneo F, Dugnani S, et al: Effects of electromyostimulation training and volleyball practice on jumping ability. *J Strength Cond Res* 17:573–579, 2003.

96. Shiba N, Matsuse H, Takano Y, et al: Electrically stimulated antagonist muscle contraction increased muscle mass and bone mineral density of one astronaut—initial verification on the International Space Station. *PLoS ONE* 10:e0134736, 2015.

97. Carraro U, Kern H, Gava P, et al: Recovery from muscle weakness by exercise and FES: lessons from Masters, active or sedentary seniors and SCI patients. *Aging Clin Exp Res* 29(4):579–590, 2017.

98. Mosole S, Carraro U, Kern H, et al: Use it or lose it: tonic activity of slow motoneurons promotes their survival and preferentially increases slow fiber-type groupings in muscles of old lifelong recreational sportsmen. *Eur J Transl Myol* 26(4):5972, 2016.

99. Mancinelli R, Toniolo L, Di Filippo ES, et al: Neuromuscular electrical stimulation induces skeletal muscle fiber remodeling and specific gene expression profile in healthy elderly. *Front Physiol* 10:1459, 2019.

100. Di Filippo ES, Mancinelli R, Marrone M, et al: Neuromuscular electrical stimulation improves skeletal muscle regeneration through satellite cell fusion with myofibers in healthy elderly subjects. *J Appl Physiol* 123(3):501–512, 2017.

101. Nishikawa Y, Watanabe K, Kawade S, et al: The effect of a portable electrical muscle stimulation device at home on muscle strength and activation patterns in locomotive syndrome patients: A randomized control trial. *J Electromyogr Kinesiol* 45:46–52, 2019.

102. O'Connor D, Brennan L, Caulfield B: The use of neuromuscular electrical stimulation (NMES) for managing the complications of ageing related to reduced exercise participation. *Maturitas* 113:13–20, 2018.

103. Knutson JS, Fu MJ, Sheffler LR, et al: Neuromuscular electrical stimulation for motor restoration in hemiplegia. *Phys Med Rehabil Clin N Am* 26:729–745, 2015.

104. Gu P, Ran JJ, Yu L: Electrical stimulation for hemiplegic shoulder function: a systematic review and meta-analysis of 15 randomized controlled trials. *Arch Phys Med Rehabil* 97:1588–1594, 2016.

105. Howlett OA, Lannin NA, Ada L, et al: Functional electrical stimulation improves activity after stroke: a systematic review with meta-analysis. *Arch Phys Med Rehabil* 96:934–943, 2015.

106. Kafri M, Laufer Y: Therapeutic effects of functional electrical stimulation on gait in individuals post-stroke. *Ann Biomed Eng* 43:451–466, 2015.

107. Auchstaetter N, Luc J, Lukye S, et al: Physical therapists' use of functional electrical stimulation for clients with stroke: frequency, barriers, and facilitators. *Phys Ther* 96:995–1005, 2016.

108. Nascimento LR, Michaelsen SM, Ada L, et al: Cyclical electrical stimulation increases strength and improves activity after stroke: a systematic review. *J Physiother* 60:22–30, 2014.

109. Lee JH, Bakker LL, Johnson RE, et al: Effectiveness of neuromuscular electrical stimulation for management of shoulder subluxation

post-stroke: a systematic review with meta-analysis. *Clin Rehabil* 31(11):1431–1444, 2017.

110. Stein C, Fritsch CG, Robinson C, et al: Effects of electrical stimulation in spastic muscles after stroke: systematic review and meta-analysis of randomized controlled trials. *Stroke* 46:2197–2205, 2015.

111. Maenpaa H, Jaakkola R, Sandstrom M, et al: Electrostimulation at sensory level improves function of the upper extremities in children with cerebral palsy. *Dev Med Child Neurol* 46:84–90, 2004.

112. Wu M, Gordon K, Kahn JH, et al: Prolonged electrical stimulation over hip flexors increases locomotor output in human SCI. *Clin Neurophysiol* 122:1421–1428, 2011.

113. Laufer Y, Elboim-Gabyzon M: Does sensory transcutaneous electrical stimulation enhance motor recovery following a stroke? A systematic review. *Neurorehabil Neural Repair* 25:799–809, 2011.

114. Chipchase LS, Schabrun SM, Hodges PW: Peripheral electrical stimulation to induce cortical plasticity: a systematic review of stimulus parameters. *Clin Neurophysiol* 122:456–463, 2011.

115. Sullivan J, Girardi M, Hensley M, et al: Improving arm function in chronic stroke: a pilot study of sensory amplitude electrical stimulation via glove electrode during task-specific training. *Top Stroke Rehabil* 22:169–175, 2015.

116. Ferrante S, Pedrocchi A, Ferrigno G, et al: Cycling induced by functional electrical stimulation improves the muscular strength and the motor control of individuals with post-acute stroke. *Eur J Phys Rehabil Med* 44:159–167, 2008.

117. Lo HC, Tsai KH, Su FC, et al: Effects of a functional electrical stimulation-assisted leg-cycling wheelchair on reducing spasticity of patients after stroke. *J Rehabil Med* 41:242–246, 2009.

118. Bauer P, Krewer C, Golaszewski S, et al: Functional electrical stimulation-assisted active cycling—therapeutic effects in patients with hemiparesis from 7 days to 6 months after stroke: a randomized controlled pilot study. *Arch Phys Med Rehabil* 96:188–196, 2015.

119. Lo HC, Hsu YC, Hsueh YH, et al: Cycling exercise with functional electrical stimulation improves postural control in stroke patients. *Gait Posture* 35:506–510, 2012.

120. Hara Y: Neurorehabilitation with new functional electrical stimulation for hemiparetic upper extremity in stroke patients. *J Nihon Med Sch* 75:4–14, 2008.

121. de Kroon JR, IJzerman MJ: Electrical stimulation of the upper extremity in stroke: cyclic versus EMG-triggered stimulation. *Clin Rehabil* 22:690–697, 2008.

122. Bosch PR, Harris JE, Wing K, et al: Review of therapeutic electrical stimulation for dorsiflexion assist and orthotic substitution from the American Congress of Rehabilitation Medicine stroke movement interventions subcommittee. *Arch Phys Med Rehabil* 95:390–396, 2014.

123. Dunning K, O'Dell MW, Kluding P, et al: Peroneal stimulation for foot drop after stroke: a systematic review. *Am J Phys Med Rehabil* 94:649–664, 2015.

124. Melo PL, Silva MT, Martins JM, et al: Technical developments of functional electrical stimulation to correct drop foot: sensing, actuation and control strategies. *Clin Biomech (Bristol, Avon)* 30:101–113, 2015.

125. Taylor P, Humphreys L, Swain I: The long-term cost-effectiveness of the use of functional electrical stimulation for the correction of dropped foot due to upper motor neuron lesion. *J Rehabil Med* 45:154–160, 2013.

126. Meijer JW, Voerman GE, Santegoets KM, et al: Short-term effects and long-term use of a hybrid orthosis for neuromuscular electrical stimulation of the upper extremity in patients after chronic stroke. *J Rehabil Med* 41:157–161, 2009.

127. Patil S, Raza WA, Jamil F, et al: Functional electrical stimulation for the upper limb in tetraplegic spinal cord injury: a systematic review. *J Med Eng Technol* 39:419–423, 2014.

128. Lu X, Battistuzzo CR, Zoghi M, et al: Effects of training on upper limb function after cervical spinal cord injury: a systematic review. *Clin Rehabil* 29:3–13, 2015.

129. Kern H, Gargiulo P, Pond A, et al: To reverse atrophy of human muscles in complete SCI lower motor neuron denervation by home-based functional electrical stimulation. *Adv Exp Med Biol* 1088:585–591, 2018.

130. Hamid S, Hayek R: Role of electrical stimulation for rehabilitation and regeneration after spinal cord injury: an overview. *Eur Spine J* 17:1256–1269, 2008.

131. Albertin G, Kern H, Hofer C: Two years of Functional Electrical Stimulation by large surface electrodes for denervated muscles improve skin epidermis in SCI. *Eur J Transl Myol* 28(1):7373, 2018.

132. Albertin G, Hofer C, Zampieri S, et al: In complete SCI patients, long-term functional electrical stimulation of permanent denervated muscles increases epidermis thickness. *Neurol Res* 40(4):277–282, 2018.

133. Ragnarsson KT: Functional electrical stimulation after spinal cord injury: current use, therapeutic effects and future directions. *Spinal Cord* 46:255–274, 2008.

134. Wilbanks SR, Rogers R, Pool S, et al: Effects of functional electrical stimulation assisted rowing on aerobic fitness and shoulder pain in manual wheelchair users with spinal cord injury. *J Spinal Cord Med* 39:645–654, 2016.

135. Davis GM, Hamzaid NA: Fornusek C: Cardiorespiratory, metabolic, and biomechanical responses during functional electrical stimulation leg exercise: health and fitness benefits. *Artif Organs* 32:625–629, 2008.

136. Mayson TA, Harris SR: Functional electrical stimulation cycling in youth with spinal cord injury: a review of intervention studies. *J Spinal Cord Med* 37:266–277, 2014.

137. Sadowsky CL, Hammond ER, Strohl AB, et al: Lower extremity functional electrical stimulation cycling promotes physical and functional recovery in chronic spinal cord injury. *J Spinal Cord Med* 36:623–631, 2013.

138. Thrasher TA, Ward JS, Fisher S: Strength and endurance adaptations to functional electrical stimulation leg cycle ergometry in spinal cord injury. *Neurorehabilitation* 33:133–138, 2013.

139. Gyawali S, Solis L, Chong SL, et al: Intermittent electrical stimulation redistributes pressure and promotes tissue oxygenation in loaded muscles of individuals with spinal cord injury. *J Appl Physiol* 110:246–255, 2011.

140. Bélanger M, Stein RB, Wheeler GD, et al: Electrical stimulation: can it increase muscle strength and reverse osteopenia in spinal cord injured individuals? *Arch Phys Med Rehabil* 81:1090–1098, 2000.

141. Mohr T, Podenphant J, Biering-Sorensen F, et al: Increased bone mineral density after prolonged electrically induced cycle training of paralyzed limbs in spinal cord injured man. *Calcif Tissue Int* 61:22–25, 1997.

142. Gater DR, Jr Dolbow D, Tsui B, et al: Functional electrical stimulation therapies after spinal cord injury. *Neurorehabilitation* 28:231–248, 2011.

143. Lauer RT, Smith BT, Mulcahey MJ, et al: Effects of cycling and/or electrical stimulation on bone mineral density in children with spinal cord injury. *Spinal Cord* 49:917–923, 2011.

144. Rodgers MM, Glaser RM, Figoni SF, et al: Musculoskeletal responses of spinal cord injured individuals to functional neuromuscular stimulation-induced knee extension exercise training. *J Rehabil Res Dev* 28:19–26, 1991.

145. Leeds EM, Klose KJ, Ganz W, et al: Bone mineral density after bicycle ergometry training. *Arch Phys Med Rehabil* 71:207–209, 1990.

146. BeDell KK, Scremin AM, Perell KL, et al: Effects of functional electrical stimulation-induced lower extremity cycling on bone density of spinal cord-injured patients. *Am J Phys Med Rehabil* 75:29–34, 1996.

147. Cauraugh JH, Naik SK, Hsu WH, et al: Children with cerebral palsy: a systematic review and meta-analysis on gait and electrical stimulation. *Clin Rehabil* 24:963–978, 2010.

148. Merrill DR: Review of electrical stimulation in cerebral palsy and recommendations for future directions. *Dev Med Child Neurol* 51(Suppl 4):154–165, 2009.

149. Pool D, Elliott C, Bear N, et al: Neuromuscular electrical stimulation-assisted gait increases muscle strength and volume in children with unilateral spastic cerebral palsy. *Dev Med Child Neurol* 58:492–501, 2016.

150. Karabay İ, Öztürk GT, Malas FÜ, et al: Short-term effects of neuromuscular electrical stimulation on muscle architecture of the tibialis anterior and gastrocnemius in children with cerebral palsy: preliminary results of a prospective controlled study. *Am J Phys Med Rehabil* 94:728–733, 2015.

151. Pool D, Blackmore AM, Bear N, et al: Effects of short-term daily community walk aide use on children with unilateral spastic cerebral palsy. *Pediatr Phys Ther* 26:308–317, 2014.

152. Chiu HC, Ada L: Effect of functional electrical stimulation on activity in children with cerebral palsy: a systematic review. *Pediatr Phys Ther* 26:283–288, 2014.

153. Mooney JA, Rose JA: Scoping review of neuromuscular electrical stimulation to improve gait in cerebral palsy: the arc of progress and future strategies. *Front Neurol* 10:887, 2019.
154. Ozer K, Chesher SP, Scheker LR: Neuromuscular electrical stimulation and dynamic bracing for the management of upper-extremity spasticity in children with cerebral palsy. *Dev Med Child Neurol* 48:559–563, 2006.
155. Scheker LR, Chesher SP, Ramirez S: Neuromuscular electrical stimulation and dynamic bracing as a treatment for upper-extremity spasticity in children with cerebral palsy. *J Hand Surg [Br]* 24:226–232, 1999.
156. Szecsi J, Schlick C, Schiller M, et al: Functional electrical stimulation-assisted cycling of patients with multiple sclerosis: biomechanical and functional outcome—a pilot study. *J Rehabil Med* 41:674–680, 2009.
157. Taylor PN, Burridge JH, Dunkerley AL, et al: Clinical use of the Odstock dropped foot stimulator: its effect on the speed and effort of walking. *Arch Phys Med Rehabil* 80:1577–1583, 1999.
158. Ratchford JN, Shore W, Hammond ER, et al: A pilot study of functional electrical stimulation cycling in progressive multiple sclerosis. *Neurorehabilitation* 27:121–128, 2010.
159. Chen YW, Chang KH, Chen HC, et al: The effects of surface neuromuscular electrical stimulation on post-stroke dysphagia: a systemic review and meta-analysis. *Clin Rehabil* 30:24–35, 2016.
160. Poorjavad M, Talebian Moghadam S, Nakhostin Ansari N, et al: Surface electrical stimulation for treating swallowing disorders after stroke: a review of the stimulation intensity levels and the electrode placements. *Stroke Res Treat* 2014:918057, 2014.
161. Tan C, Liu Y, Li W, et al: Transcutaneous neuromuscular electrical stimulation can improve swallowing function in patients with dysphagia caused by non-stroke diseases: a meta-analysis. *J Oral Rehabil* 40:472–480, 2013.
162. Carnaby-Mann G, Crary M: Examining the evidence on neuromuscular electrical stimulation for swallowing: a meta-analysis. *Arch Otolaryngol Head Neck Surg* 133:1–8, 2007.
163. Scutt P, Lee HS, Hamdy S, et al: Pharyngeal electrical stimulation for treatment of poststroke dysphagia: individual patient data meta-analysis of randomised controlled trials. *Stroke Res Treat* 2015:429053, 2015.
164. Oh DH, Park JS, Kim WJ: Effect of neuromuscular electrical stimulation on lip strength and closure function in patients with dysphagia after stroke. *J Phys Ther Sci* 29(11):1974–1975, 2017.
165. Patidar N, Mittal V, Kumar M, et al: Transcutaneous posterior tibial nerve stimulation in pediatric overactive bladder: a preliminary report. *J Pediatr Urol* 11(6):351, 2015.
166. Borch L, Hagstroem S, Kamperis K, et al: Transcutaneous electrical nerve stimulation combined with oxybutynin is superior to monotherapy in children with urge incontinence: a randomized, placebo controlled study. *J Urol* 198(2):430–435, 2017.
167. Borch L, Rittig S, Kamperis K, et al: No immediate effect on urodynamic parameters during transcutaneous electrical nerve stimulation (TENS) in children with overactive bladder and daytime incontinence-A randomized, double-blind, placebo-controlled study. *Neurourol Urodyn* 36(7):1788–1795, 2017.
168. Govier FE, Litwiller S, Nitti V, et al: Percutaneous neuromodulation for the refractory overactive bladder: results of a multicenter study. *J Urol* 165:1193–1198, 2001.
169. van Balken MR, Vandoninck V, Gisolf KW, et al: Posterior tibial nerve stimulation as neuromodulative treatment of lower urinary tract dysfunction. *J Urol* 166:914–918, 2001.
170. Gungor Ugurlucan F, Alper N, Ayvacikli G, et al: Comparison of home-based and outpatient clinic-based intravaginal electrical stimulation for the treatment of urinary incontinence. *Minerva Ginecol* 66:347–353, 2014.
171. Moroni RM, Magnani PS, Haddad JM, et al: Conservative treatment of stress urinary incontinence: a systematic review with meta-analysis of randomized controlled trials. *Rev Bras Ginecol Obstet* 38:97–111, 2016.
172. Berghmans B, Hendriks E, Bernards A, et al: Electrical stimulation with non-implanted electrodes for urinary incontinence in men. *Cochrane Database Syst Rev* 2013(6):CD001202, 2013.
173. Stewart F, Berghmans B, Bø K, et al: Electrical stimulation with non-implanted devices for stress urinary incontinence in women. *Cochrane Database Syst Rev* 12:CD012390, 2017.
174. Thomas LH, Coupe J, Cross LD: Interventions for treating urinary incontinence after stroke in adults. *Cochrane Database Syst Rev* 2:CD004462, 2019.
175. Agency for Healthcare Research and Quality: What is urinary incontinence (UI)? http://effectivehealthcare.ahrq.gov/ehc/decisionaids/urinary-incontinence/index.cfm? Accessed April 2, 2017.
176. Booth J, Connelly L, Dickson S, et al: The effectiveness of transcutaneous tibial nerve stimulation (TTNS) for adults with overactive bladder syndrome: a systematic review. *Neurourol Urodyn* 37(2):528–541, 2018.
177. Ramírez-García I, Blanco-Ratto L, Kauffmann S, et al: Efficacy of transcutaneous stimulation of the posterior tibial nerve compared to percutaneous stimulation in idiopathic overactive bladder syndrome: randomized control trial. *Neurourol Urodyn* 38(1):261–268, 2019.
178. Jacomo RH, Alves AT, Lucio A, et al: Transcutaneous tibial nerve stimulation versus parasacral stimulation in the treatment of overactive bladder in elderly people: a triple-blinded randomized controlled trial. *Clinics (Sao Paulo)* 75:e1477, 2020.
179. Tudor KI, Seth JH, Liechti MD, et al: Outcomes following percutaneous tibial nerve stimulation (PTNS) treatment for neurogenic and idiopathic overactive bladder. *Clin Auton Res* 30(1):61–67, 2020.
180. Seth JH, Gonzales G, Haslam C, et al: Feasibility of using a novel non-invasive ambulatory tibial nerve stimulation device for the home-based treatment of overactive bladder symptoms. *Transl Androl Urol* 7(6):912–919, 2018.
181. Sharma N, Rekha K, Srinivasan KJ: Efficacy of transcutaneous electrical nerve stimulation in the treatment of overactive bladder. *J Clin Diagn Res* 10(10):QC17–QC20, 2016.
182. Stewart F, Gameiro OL, El Dib R, et al: Electrical stimulation with non-implanted electrodes for overactive bladder in adults. *Cochrane Database Syst Rev* 2016(4):CD010098, 2016.
183. Ramsay S, Bolduc S: Overactive bladder in children. *Can Urol Assoc J* 11(1–2 Suppl1):S74–S79, 2017.
184. Cui H, Yao Y, Xu Z, et al: Role of transcutaneous electrical nerve stimulation in treating children with overactive bladder from pooled analysis of 8 randomized controlled trials. *Int Neurourol J* 24(1):84–94, 2020.
185. Buckley BS, Sanders CD, Spineli L: Conservative interventions for treating functional daytime urinary incontinence in children. *Cochrane Database Syst Rev* 9(9):CD012367, 2019.
186. Man IO, Lepar GS, Morrissey MC, et al: Effect of neuromuscular electrical stimulation on foot/ankle volume during standing. *Med Sci Sports Exerc* 35:630–634, 2003.
187. Bahadori S, Immins T, Wainwright TW: The effect of calf neuromuscular electrical stimulation and intermittent pneumatic compression on thigh microcirculation. *Microvasc Res* 111:37–41, 2017.
188. Jin HK, Hwang TY, Cho SI: Effect of electrical stimulation on blood flow velocity and vessel size. *Open Med (Wars)* 12:5–11, 2017.
189. Morita H, Abe C, Tanaka K, et al: Neuromuscular electrical stimulation and an ottoman-type seat effectively improve popliteal venous flow in a sitting position. *J Physiol Sci* 56:183–186, 2006.
190. Reed BV: Effect of high voltage pulsed electrical stimulation on microvascular permeability to plasma proteins: a possible mechanism in minimizing edema. *Phys Ther* 68:491–495, 1988.
191. Burgess LC, Immins T, Swain I, et al: Effectiveness of neuromuscular electrical stimulation for reducing oedema: A systematic review. *J Rehabil Med* 51(4):237–243, 2019.
192. Williams KJ, Ravikumar R, Gaweesh AS, et al: A review of the evidence to support neuromuscular electrical stimulation in the prevention and management of venous disease. *Adv Exp Med Biol* 906, 2017:377386.
193. Man IO, Morrissey MC, Cywinski JK: Effect of neuromuscular electrical stimulation on ankle swelling in the early period after ankle sprain. *Phys Ther* 87:53–65, 2007.
194. Broderick BJ, Breathnach O, Condon F, et al: Haemodynamic performance of neuromuscular electrical stimulation (NMES) during recovery from total hip arthroplasty. *J Orthop Surg Res* 8:3, 2013.
195. Ravikumar R, Williams KJ, Babber A, et al: Randomised controlled trial: potential benefit of a footplate neuromuscular electrical stimulation device in patients with chronic venous disease. *Eur J Vasc Endovasc Surg* 53(1):114–121, 2017.
196. Ojima M, Takegawa R, Hirose T, et al: Hemodynamic effects of electrical muscle stimulation in the prophylaxis of deep vein thrombosis

for intensive care unit patients: a randomized trial. *J Intensive Care* 5:9, 2017.

197. Yilmaz S, Calbiyik M, Yilmaz BK, et al: Potential role of electrostimulation in augmentation of venous blood flow after total knee replacement: A pilot study. *Phlebology* 31(4):2516, 2016.

198. Lattimer CR, Azzam M, Papaconstandinou JA, et al: Neuromuscular electrical stimulation reduces sludge in the popliteal vein. *J Vasc Surg Venous Lymphat Disord* 6(2):154–162, 2018.

199. Wainwright TW, Burgess LC, Middleton RG: A single-centre feasibility randomised controlled trial comparing the incidence of asymptomatic and symptomatic deep vein thrombosis between a neuromuscular electrostimulation device and thromboembolism deterrent stockings in post-operative patients recovering from elective total hip replacement surgery. *Surg Technol Int* 36:sti36/1253, 2020.

200. Broderick BJ, O'Connell S, Moloney S, et al: Comparative lower limb hemodynamics using neuromuscular electrical stimulation (NMES) versus intermittent pneumatic compression (IPC). *Physiol Meas* 35:1849–1859, 2014.

201. Czyrny JJ, Kaplan RE, Wilding GE, et al: Electrical foot stimulation: a potential new method of deep venous thrombosis prophylaxis. *Vascular* 18:20–27, 2010.

202. Kern H, Carraro U, Adami N, et al: One year of home-based daily FES in complete lower motor neuron paraplegia: recovery of tetanic contractility drives the structural improvements of denervated muscle. *Neurol Res* 32:5–12, 2010.

203. Girlanda P, Dattola R, Vita G, et al: Effect of electrotherapy in denervated muscles in rabbits: an electrophysiological and morphological study. *Exp Neurol* 77:483–491, 1982.

204. Pachter BR, Eberstein A, Goodgold J: Electrical stimulation effect on denervated skeletal myofibers in rats: a light and electron microscopic study. *Arch Phys Med Rehabil* 63:427–430, 1982.

205. Johnston TE, Smith BT, Betz RR, et al: Strengthening of partially denervated knee extensors using percutaneous electric stimulation in a young man with spinal cord injury. *Arch Phys Med Rehabil* 86:1037–1042, 2005.

206. Cho MK, Kim JH, Chung Y, et al: Treadmill gait training combined with functional electrical stimulation on hip abductor and ankle dorsiflexor muscles for chronic hemiparesis. *Gait Posture* 42:73–78, 2015.

207. Gobbo M, Maffiuletti NA, Orizio C, et al: Muscle motor point identification is essential for optimizing neuromuscular electrical stimulation use. *J Neuroeng Rehabil* 11:17, 2014.

208. Laufer Y: A brief interphase interval interposed within biphasic pulses enhances the contraction force of the quadriceps femoris muscle. *Physiother Theory Pract* 29:461–468, 2013.

209. Springer S: Effects of interphase interval and stimulation form on dorsiflexors contraction force. *Technol Health Care* 23:475–483, 2015.

210. Springer S, Braun-Benyamin O, Abraham-Shitreet C, et al: The effect of electrode placement and interphase interval on force production during stimulation of the dorsiflexor muscles. *Artif Organs* 38:E142–E146, 2014.

211. Becher M, Springer S, Braun-Benyamin O, et al: The effect of an interphase interval on electrically induced dorsiflexion force and fatigue in subjects with an upper motor neuron lesion. *Artif Organs* 40:778–785, 2016.

212. da Silva VZ, Durigan JL, Arena R, et al: Current evidence demonstrates similar effects of kilohertz-frequency and low-frequency current on quadriceps evoked torque and discomfort in healthy individuals: a systematic review with meta-analysis. *Physiother Theory Pract* 31:533–539, 2015.

213. Iijima H, Takahashi M, Tashiro Y: Comparison of the effects of kilohertz- and low-frequency electric stimulations: a systematic review with meta-analysis. *PLoS One* 13(4):e0195236, 2018.

214. Aurélio Vaz M, Bortoluzzi Frasson V: Low-frequency pulsed current versus kilohertz-frequency alternating current: a scoping literature review. *Arch Phys Med Rehab* 99:792–805, 2018.

215. Jeon W, Griffin L: Effects of pulse duration on muscle fatigue during electrical stimulation inducing moderate-level contraction. *Muscle Nerve* 57(4):642–649, 2018.

216. Gorgey AS, Black CD, Elder CP, et al: Effects of electrical stimulation parameters on fatigue in skeletal muscle. *J Orthop Sports Phys Ther* 39:684–692, 2009.

217. Bickel CS, Gregory CM, Azuero A: Matching initial torque with different stimulation parameters influences skeletal muscle fatigue. *J Rehabil Res Dev* 49:323–331, 2012.

218. Glaviano NR, Saliba S: Can the use of neuromuscular electrical stimulation be improved to optimize quadriceps strengthening? *Sports Health* 8(1):79–85, 2016.

219. Deley G, Laroche D, Babault N: Effects of electrical stimulation pattern on quadriceps force production and fatigue. *Muscle Nerve* 49:760–763, 2014.

220. Deley G, Denuziller J, Babault N, et al: Effects of electrical stimulation pattern on quadriceps isometric force and fatigue in individuals with spinal cord injury. *Muscle Nerve* 52:260–264, 2015.

221. Taylor MJ, Fornusek C, Ruys AJ: Reporting for duty: The duty cycle in functional electrical stimulation research. Part I: Critical commentaries of the literature. *Eur J Transl Myol* 28(4):313–322, 2018.

222. Jiang SL, Wang Z, Yi W, et al: Current change rate influences sensorimotor cortical excitability during neuromuscular electrical stimulation. *Front Hum Neurosci* 13:152, 2019.

223. Snyder-Mackler L, Delitto A, Stralka SW, et al: Use of electrical stimulation to enhance recovery of quadriceps femoris muscle force production in patients following anterior cruciate ligament reconstruction. *Phys Ther* 74:901–907, 1994.

13

Electrical Currents for Pain Control

Michelle H. Cameron | Michelle Ocelnik

CHAPTER OBJECTIVES

After reading this chapter, the reader will be able to do the following:

- Define *transcutaneous electrical nerve stimulation* (TENS).
- Describe the physical effects of TENS.
- Explain the clinical indications for the use of TENS.
- Choose the best technique for treatment with TENS and list the advantages and disadvantages of each.
- Select the appropriate equipment and optimal treatment parameters for treatment with TENS.
- Safely and effectively apply TENS.
- Accurately and completely document treatment with TENS.

The use of transcutaneous electrical stimulation to modulate pain is usually called **transcutaneous electrical nerve stimulation (TENS).** Although *TENS* could refer to all uses of electrical stimulation that are externally applied to the skin, the term *TENS* is usually only used to refer to the use of electrical stimulation for pain control. The use of TENS started in the 1970s when portable TENS devices were used to screen patients to help determine if implanted spinal cord stimulators would help alleviate their pain; it was found that these devices provided substantial relief. TENS is thought to exert its effects on pain control via gate control and stimulation of endogenous opioid release in the midbrain, and some evidence supports that certain stimulation parameters affect the mechanism of effect.[1]

Mechanisms Underlying Electrical Current Use for Pain Control

GATE CONTROL

The **gate control theory** of pain, published by Melzac and Wall in 1965, first described how a person's perception of pain could be reduced by the application of nonnociceptive stimuli, such as mild heat, touch, or electrical stimulation, to the skin. Noxious stimuli are converted to nociception and transmitted from the periphery to the dorsal horn of the spinal cord along small, **myelinated,** A-delta nerve fibers and along small, unmyelinated, C nerve fibers. Nonnoxious stimuli activate large myelinated nonnociceptive, A-beta nerves that also terminate in the dorsal horn. When nonnociceptive input reaches sufficient intensity, it activates inhibitory interneurons in the spinal cord and thereby inhibits, or "closes the gate to," transmission of nociception from the dorsal horn to the brain (Fig. 13.1). Over the last several decades, a more detailed understanding of the mechanisms of action of TENS has been developed that encompasses central and peripheral neurons, neurotransmitters and their receptors, and the release of endogenous opioids.

Conventional TENS, also known as *high-rate or high-frequency TENS,* uses short-duration (50- to 80-μs), high-frequency (100- to 150-pps) **pulses** at a current **amplitude** sufficient to produce a comfortable sensation without muscle contractions to selectively stimulate nonnociceptor A-beta nerves and activate the gating mechanism to modulate pain (Fig. 13.2A).[2,3]

> **◎ Clinical Pearl**
>
> Sensory-level electrical stimulation (high-rate TENS) can control pain by activating nonnociceptor A-beta nerves. A-beta activity inhibits the transmission of nociceptive signals at the spinal cord level. This is known as *gate control.*

Because the primary pain-modulating effect of conventional TENS is produced by gating, which requires A-beta nerve activation by the stimulation, the effect generally lasts only while the stimulation is on. Therefore, conventional TENS should be applied when the patient has pain and may be used for up to 24 hours a day if necessary. Conventional TENS may also interrupt the pain-spasm-pain cycle. When pain is reduced by electrical stimulation, it may indirectly reduce muscle spasms, which will further reduce pain. In this case, pain relief may last after the stimulation is turned off.

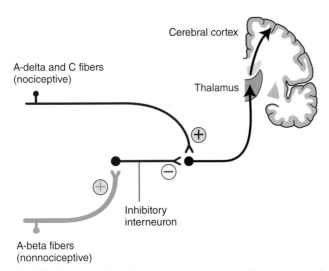

FIGURE 13.1 Simplified diagram of the gate control mechanism of pain modulation.

OPIOID RELEASE

TENS may also control pain by stimulating the production and release of endorphins and enkephalins.[4,5] These substances, which are endogenous opioids, act similarly to morphine and modulate pain perception by binding to opiate receptors in the brain and other areas, where they act as neurotransmitters and neuromodulators.[6] Opioids also activate descending inhibitory pathways that involve nonopioid (serotonin) systems.

Low-frequency pulses, at 2 to 10 pps, at an intensity high enough to produce motor contraction, known as *low-frequency* or **low-rate TENS** (Fig. 13.2B), use repetitive stimulation of motor nerves to produce brief, repetitive, muscle contractions or twitches to stimulate endogenous opioid production and release.[1,7] Further increasing the current intensity, beyond the level of muscle contraction, to produce a painful noxious stimulus through stimulation of nociceptive A-delta nerves, known as **acupuncture-like TENS,** likely also works by this mechanism. Frequencies of under 10 pps are used for low-rate TENS because this range will produce twitch muscle contractions that increase endorphin and enkephalin levels while minimizing the risk of muscle soreness.[8]

> **◎ Clinical Pearl**
>
> Motor-level electrical stimulation (low-rate TENS) can control pain by stimulating the production and release of endogenous opioids.

Early studies suggested that only low-rate TENS stimulated the production of endogenous opioids.[9] However, more recent research indicates that both high-rate TENS and low-rate TENS activate opioid receptors, although possibly different opioid receptors. For example, although low doses of naloxone, a mu-opioid receptor blocker, block the analgesia produced by low-rate TENS (4 pps) and not the analgesia produced by conventional high-rate TENS (100 pps), high doses of naloxone will block the effects of both low-rate and high-rate TENS, suggesting that high-rate TENS also stimulates some opioid production.[10] Furthermore, naltrindole, a delta opioid receptor

blocker, only blocks the analgesia produced by high-rate TENS and not the analgesia produced by low rate TENS.[4,11,12] Notably, high-rate TENS also appears to be more effective than low-rate TENS in patients taking opioids.[13]

Low-rate TENS usually controls pain for 4 to 5 hours after a 20-minute to 30-minute treatment. It is effective for this length of time because the half-life of the endogenous opioids released is approximately 4.5 hours. Low-rate TENS should not be applied for longer than 45 minutes at a time because prolonging the repetitive muscle contraction produced by the stimulus can result in delayed-onset muscle soreness.

Patients may develop tolerance to TENS-induced analgesia, particularly if low-rate TENS[14] is used. Tolerance to TENS results in higher doses of the intervention being needed to produce an effect. Patients may develop tolerance to TENS by the fourth or fifth day of stimulation.[15] TENS tolerance may be mediated by endogenous opioids as well as by cholecystokinin[12] and N-methyl-D-aspartate (NMDA).[16] **Frequency modulations,** similar to those used to prevent **adaptation,** have been shown to delay tolerance to TENS-induced analgesia.[17]

SELECTING TRANSCUTANEOUS ELECTRICAL NERVE STIMULATION APPROACHES

Although both high-rate TENS and low-rate TENS reduce pain, it is not clear which approach is more effective, and it is likely that their effectiveness depends to some degree on the patient and the source of pain. Although one study on experimentally induced cold-pressor pain found low-rate TENS to be more effective than high-rate TENS,[18] another study found that high-rate TENS controlled experimentally induced ischemic pain more effectively than low-rate TENS.[19] Consistent with their proposed mechanisms of action, low-rate TENS and high-rate TENS have been found to be equally effective at controlling pain while being applied, but low-rate TENS provided significantly more analgesia several minutes or hours after the stimulation had stopped.[20,21] Clinically, high-rate TENS is recommended when only sensation, but not muscle contraction, will be tolerated, such as after a recent injury when inflammation is present or tissues may be damaged by contraction. Low-rate TENS is recommended when a longer duration of pain control after treatment is desired and repetitive muscle contraction is likely to be tolerated. This generally occurs in the context of more chronic conditions. Selecting TENS as part of a treatment plan may also depend on the age of the patient. One study found no effect of high- or low-rate TENS in older adults,[22] whereas another showed that older adults required higher-amplitude[23] stimulation to achieve the same relief as younger users.

> **◎ Clinical Pearl**
>
> High-rate TENS is recommended when only sensation, but not muscle contraction, will be tolerated, such as after a recent injury when inflammation is present or tissues may be damaged by contraction. Low-rate TENS is recommended when a longer duration of pain control after treatment is desired and repetitive muscle contraction is likely to be tolerated.

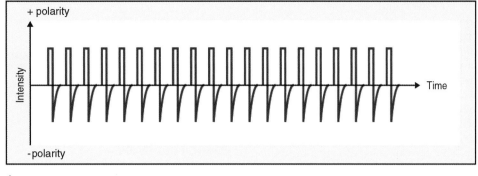

A

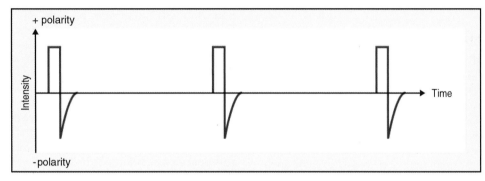

B

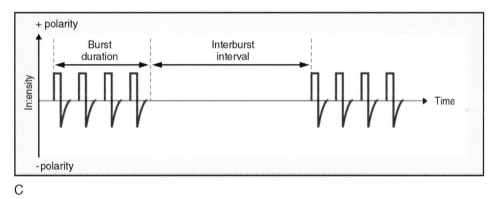

C

FIGURE 13.2 Typical waveforms for (A) conventional high-rate transcutaneous electrical nerve stimulation (TENS), (B) low-rate TENS, and (C) burst mode TENS.

Another approach to applying TENS is to use **burst mode.** For **burst mode TENS,** the stimulation is delivered in bursts, or packages, with a number of pulses in each burst (Fig. 13.2C). This mode of TENS is thought to work by the same mechanisms as low-rate TENS but may be more effective because more current is delivered, resulting in greater endorphin release, or because it combines the effects of high-rate and low-rate TENS. Some patients tolerate low-rate TENS better than burst mode, whereas others tolerate burst mode better than low-rate TENS. A study comparing the effect of burst mode TENS with the effect of high-rate TENS on experimental cold-induced pain found both forms of TENS to be more effective than placebo but neither form to be significantly more effective than the other.[24]

Electrical stimulation may also control pain when the electrodes are placed on the skin overlying acupuncture points.

This method of application is thought to stimulate energy flow along acupuncture meridians that connect acupuncture points in the body.[25,26] The application of TENS over acupuncture points has been shown to decrease myofascial pain[27] and may facilitate improvements in range of motion. Electroacupuncture has also been shown to decrease chronic neck pain when applied together with exercise and to decrease postoperative pain and analgesic use after spinal surgery and thoracic lobectomy.[28–31]

Many studies have investigated the effects of electroacupuncture, where the electrical stimulus was applied via acupuncture needles inserted into the body through the skin at the appropriate points.[32,33] Electroacupuncture has been found to reduce pain, stiffness, and disability associated with osteoarthritis of the knee.[34] It has also been found to reduce postoperative pain,[35] reduce pain and improve function in patients with frozen shoulder,[36] and reduce pain in various experimental models.[37] Recent meta-analyses found that although electroacupuncture may be effective for some applications, data were insufficient to conclude that it was effective in the treatment of pain associated with rheumatoid arthritis.[38] The mechanisms of action of electroacupuncture are uncertain but are likely similar to the mechanisms of low-rate TENS, given that the effects of electroacupuncture are reversed by naloxone, suggesting that this intervention promotes endorphin release.[34,39] Electroacupuncture has also been shown to decrease plasma cortisol, suggesting that the reduction in pain also results in a reduction in stress.[34] Electroacupuncture requires special training, as well as licensure that allows the clinician to place needles through the patient's skin.

Clinical Applications of Electrical Currents for Pain Control

The application of **electrical currents** for pain control, TENS, has been studied extensively. In recent years, a number of systematic reviews and meta-analyses have examined the efficacy of TENS for controlling pain in people with a wide range of conditions.[40–47] These[45,48–52] reviews have come to limited conclusions, largely because most studies have low-quality methodology, small sample sizes, and variable application parameters, and it is difficult to establish an appropriate placebo to control for the nonspecific effects of study participation. However, it is important to realize that the conclusions of current meta-analyses and reviews indicate a *lack* of high-quality evidence, not that there is convincing evidence that TENS is not effective. Furthermore, there is little evidence of risk of adverse effects, supporting that electrical stimulation for pain management is generally safe.

ACUTE PAIN

There is extensive research on the use of electrical currents to control acute pain. The most recent Cochrane collaboration systematic review with meta-analysis was published in 2015 and included 19 randomized controlled trials with a total of 1346 participants.[53] Many published trials were not included in this review. Eleven were excluded because all the information needed to perform a systematic review was not available, and many others were excluded because TENS was given in conjunction with other interventions or because TENS was not delivered using appropriate technique. In the reviewed trials, data were in favor of TENS compared with placebo for reducing pain on a visual analog scale and for achieving a 50% or greater reduction in pain. A systematic review and meta-analysis specifically focused on the application of TENS for acute pain in the prehospital setting found four trials of good quality. Overall, these studies found that TENS produced a clinically significant reduction in pain severity for patients with moderate to severe acute pain and reduced anxiety secondary to pain.[54] TENS has also been found to help with postoperative pain[55] following several different types of surgeries, such as total knee arthroplasty,[56,57] rotator cuff repair,[58] cardiac surgery,[59] pulmonary surgery,[60] thoracotomy, and lobectomy surgery.[61,62] Although one study[63] found no differences in postoperative pain with TENS compared with placebo, most studies showed a significant

reduction in pain and analgesic medication intake[56] in patients receiving TENS compared with those in a control group.

> ### ◉ Clinical Pearl
> TENS has been shown to reduce acute pain and significantly reduce analgesic intake after surgery.

CHRONIC PAIN

The use of electrical stimulation to control chronic pain or pain associated with chronic conditions has also been studied extensively. The most recent Cochrane collaboration publication is a 2019 overview of eight previously published Cochrane reviews of TENS for chronic pain conditions, including rheumatoid arthritis, neuropathic pain, osteoarthritic knee pain, phantom stump pain, cancer pain, fibromyalgia, and chronic low back pain.[45] This overview included 51 randomized clinical trials with a total of 2895 participants but found that the poor quality of the trials limited the authors' ability to confidently draw any conclusions.

Several studies have also evaluated the effectiveness of electrical stimulation for controlling chronic pain associated with specific conditions. Two systematic reviews have evaluated randomized controlled trials for the control of pain associated with knee osteoarthritis. They found that TENS, particularly using an interferential current, helped reduce pain intensity and pain scores in patients with this condition.[46,64] Electrical stimulation has also been found to help reduce myofascial pain and neck pain, particularly when used in combination with exercise.[65,66]

There are mixed results in studies on electrical stimulation for controlling pain associated with shoulder conditions. Two studies showed improvements in pain and function in patients with shoulder impingement and chronic tendonitis.[67,68] However, several studies found that TENS provided no significant improvements over standard treatment.[69–71] A 2016 review concluded that higher-quality, better-controlled studies were needed.[72]

TENS has also been found to reduce pain in patients with diabetic neuropathy,[73–75] temporomandibular joint disorders,[76–79] and carpal tunnel syndrome.[80] However, the effectiveness of TENS for controlling chronic low back pain remains uncertain.[81] Although some studies show a reduction in pain with TENS alone or when added to standard treatment,[82–85] others find no benefit,[86,87] especially in the long term.[48] The lack of large-scale, high-quality studies with controlled parameters prevents a definitive conclusion.

> ### ◉ Clinical Pearl
> TENS can reduce chronic pain associated with various conditions, including knee osteoarthritis and diabetic neuropathy, but its utility for chronic low back pain remains uncertain.

Lastly, there is growing use of low-rate TENS for the treatment and prevention of migraine.[88,89] Specific devices for noninvasive vagal nerve stimulation[90,91] (by applying electrodes at the neck) and supraorbital and supratrochlear nerve stimulation[92,93] (by applying stimulation to the face) for migraine therapy have been developed. The use of these devices has been shown to reduce the duration and intensity of migraine pain, reduce pain medication intake, and when used preventatively, reduce the frequency of migraines.

Contraindications and Precautions for Electrical Currents for Pain Control

The standard contraindications and precautions for all electrical stimulation, as described in detail in Chapter 11, apply to using electrical currents for pain control. For more detailed information on these contraindications and precautions, refer to Chapter 11.

In addition to the standard contraindications for all electrical stimulation, do not use motor-level electrical stimulation (i.e., that produces muscle contractions) when contraction of the muscle may disrupt or delay healing. For instance, if the muscle or tendon is torn, muscle contraction may exacerbate the tear, just like a voluntary contraction. Similarly, muscle contractions in patients with any acute injury may worsen symptoms. In addition, because the repetitive stimulation of contractions, particularly in atrophied fibers, can result in delayed-onset muscle soreness, low-rate TENS and burst, which require muscle contractions, should not be applied for longer than 30 minutes per session.

CONTRAINDICATIONS FOR ELECTRICAL CURRENTS FOR PAIN CONTROL

✷ CONTRAINDICATIONS

for the Use of Electrical Currents for Pain Control

Standard contraindications for all electrical stimulation (see Chapter 11 for details):
- Demand cardiac pacemaker, implantable cardiac defibrillator (ICD), or unstable arrhythmias
- Placement of electrodes over carotid sinus
- Areas where venous or arterial thrombosis or thrombophlebitis is present
- Pregnancy—over or around the abdomen or low back (electrical stimulation may be used for pain control during labor and delivery)

Additional contraindications for electrical currents for pain control:
- Do not use stimulated muscle contractions for pain control, as with low-rate and burst TENS, when muscle contractions may disrupt healing (e.g., muscle or tendon tear, overuse, or acute injury).

Although electrically stimulated muscle contractions differ in some ways from physiologically initiated muscle contractions, the overall forces that stimulated contractions exert on the musculotendinous unit are similar to the forces exerted by physiological contractions. Therefore electrically stimulated contractions should be avoided when muscle contraction may disrupt healing or aggravate symptoms, such as when there is an order for no active motion or for no resisted motion or when there is a tear or inflammation in the muscle or tendon or an acute injury that would be aggravated by muscle contraction.

◎ Clinical Pearl

Electrically stimulated muscle contractions should be avoided when muscle contraction may disrupt healing or aggravate symptoms.

▪ Ask the Patient
- "Do you have a torn muscle or tendon?"
- "Do you have tendinitis?"
- "How recently did your pain start?"

▪ Assess
- Check for any orders for no active motion or for no resisted motion.
- Palpate for signs of inflammation, including heat and edema.
- Observe for redness associated with inflammation.

Although active muscle contraction is not always contraindicated in the presence of a muscle or tendon tear or inflammation, low-rate TENS should generally be avoided because the repetitive contractions may aggravate the condition.

PRECAUTIONS FOR ELECTRICAL CURRENTS FOR PAIN CONTROL

✷ PRECAUTIONS

for the Use of Electrical Currents for Pain Control

Standard precautions for all electrical stimulation (see Chapter 11 for details):
- Cardiac disease
- Impaired mentation
- Impaired sensation
- Malignant tumors
- Areas of skin irritation or open wounds

Additional precautions for electrical currents for pain control:
- Because of the muscle contractions, low-rate TENS may cause delayed-onset muscle soreness.
- Because TENS can effectively reduce pain, patients may need to be instructed to avoid potentially symptom-aggravating activities while under the analgesic effects of TENS.

Adverse Effects of Transcutaneous Electrical Nerve Stimulation

Minor adverse effects have been reported in some TENS trials, including mild erythema and itching underneath the electrodes and participants disliking the TENS sensation.[53]

Application Technique

APPLICATION TECHNIQUE 13.1 PARAMETERS FOR ELECTRICAL STIMULATION FOR PAIN CONTROL

General guidelines for the application of electrical stimulation are provided in Chapter 11. The following information builds on this foundation, providing specific recommendations for application techniques and parameters for electrical stimulation for pain control. These recommendations are also summarized in Table 13.1.

Patient Positioning

When electrical stimulation is applied for acute pain control, the patient should be positioned in a position of comfort. However, in most other cases, the patient can be encouraged to move once the TENS is applied. Ideally the stimulation should allow the patient to perform more normal activity, although the patient may need to be instructed to avoid potentially symptom-aggravating activities.

Electrode Type

In general, when using electrical stimulation for pain control, self-adhesive, disposable electrodes are recommended.

Electrode Placement

When electrical stimulation is applied for pain control, a variety of electrode placements can be effective. Placement around the painful area is most common. Placement over trigger points or acupuncture points, which generally are areas of decreased skin **resistance,** has also been reported to be effective.[94] However, placing electrodes over acupuncture points has not been found to be more effective than placing electrodes around the area of pain.[96] When the electrodes cannot be placed near or over the painful area—for example, if the area is in a cast or local application of the electrodes is not tolerated—the electrodes can be placed proximal to the site of pain along the pathway of the sensory nerves supplying the area.[96] If two currents, and thus four electrodes, are used, the electrodes can also be placed to surround the area of pain. When pulsed currents are used, the electrodes may be placed in parallel, either horizontally or vertically (Fig. 13.3). Alternatively, they can be placed so that the two currents intersect, allowing the current to cross at the area of pain. However, when two pulsed currents are used, they are of the same **frequency** and therefore do not interfere with each other. If an interferential current is desired, the two **alternating currents (ACs)**, with differing frequencies, must intersect to interfere and produce the therapeutic beat frequency in the treatment area (Fig. 13.4). For all applications, the electrodes should be at least 1 inch apart.

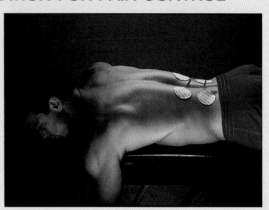

FIGURE 13.3 Electrodes placed over the low back for electrical stimulation treatment to control low back pain. (Courtesy Mettler Electronics, Anaheim, CA.)

Waveform

A **pulsed biphasic current** (also known as a *pulsed biphasic waveform*) or an **interferential current,** which is produced by two interfering ACs, is the waveform most commonly used for pain control. Most devices called "TENS" units output a pulsed **biphasic current.** This waveform, with the appropriate selection of other parameters, has been shown to reduce acute, chronic, and postoperative pain, as well as postoperative analgesic medication consumption.[55–57,59,61,62,67,68,75,76,78,85,97–99] An interferential waveform has also been shown to reduce pain associated with a wide range of conditions.[65–67,82,84,100–105] Although TENS with an interferential current may be more comfortable and penetrate to a larger, deeper area than TENS with a pulsed biphasic waveform, the evidence for either one being more effective for controlling pain is mixed.[95,106–110] For example, one study found that in patients with neck pain, an interferential current improved trapezius muscle relaxation, which increased cervical range of motion and reduced neck pain,[65,66] more effectively than a pulsed biphasic current. But in another study in patients with neck pain, when combined with ultrasound, a biphasic current with burst mode increased the pressure pain threshold and lateral cervical flexion more effectively than an interferential[111] current.

TABLE 13.1 Recommended Parameter Settings for Electrical Stimulation for Pain Control

Parameter Settings	Pulse Frequency (or Beat Frequency for Interferential)	Pulse Duration	Amplitude	Modulation (Frequency, Duration, or Amplitude)	Treatment Time	Possible Mechanism of Action
High-rate (conventional)	100–150 pps	50–80 μs	To produce tingling	Use if available	May be worn 24 h as needed for pain control	Gating at the spinal cord
Low-rate	2–10 pps	150–300 μs	To visible contraction	None or modulate	20–30 min	Endorphin release
Burst mode	Generally preset in unit at 10 bursts	Generally preset and may have maximum of 100–300 μs	To visible contraction	Generally not possible in burst mode	20–30 min	Endorphin release

APPLICATION TECHNIQUE 13.1—*cont'd*

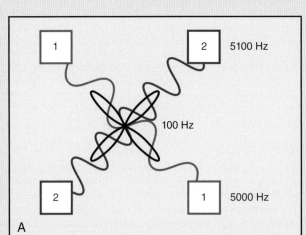

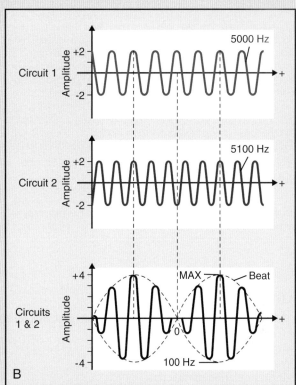

FIGURE 13.4 (A) Intersecting **medium-frequency alternating currents (ACs)** producing an interferential current between two crossed pairs of electrodes. (B) An AC with a frequency of 5000 Hz interfering with an AC with a frequency of 5100 Hz to produce an interferential current with a beat frequency of 100 Hz. (Modified from May H-U, Hansjürgens A: *Nemectrodyn Model 7 manual of Nemectron GmbH,* Karlsruhe, Germany, 1984, Nemectron GmbH.)

Premodulated current, a variation of interferential current that uses only two electrodes and delivers an AC of varying amplitude, may also be used to reduce pain, but this current probably does not provide the additional depth and distance of penetration expected from interferential current.[112,113]

Pulsed monophasic currents, such as high-volt **pulsed current,** can also be used to reduce pain.[114] Essentially, as long as the stimulus has the necessary pulse duration, amplitude, and rate of rise to stimulate the appropriate nerves, it can be effective for controlling pain.

Pulse Duration

Most clinical and portable electrical stimulation units with biphasic waveforms intended to be used for pain control have an adjustable **pulse duration.** When a pulsed biphasic waveform is used for high-rate TENS, the pulse duration should be between 50 and 80 μs to depolarize only the A-beta sensory nerves. When low-rate TENS is applied, the pulse duration should be between 200 and 300 μs to also depolarize the motor nerves and possibly the A-delta nerves.

When an interferential current is used for pain control, one cannot select the pulse duration. Interferential current is composed of alternating currents, where the **wavelength,** which is equivalent to the pulse duration of a pulsed waveform, changes inversely with the carrier frequency. If the carrier frequency is higher, the wavelength is shorter, and if the carrier frequency is lower, the wavelength is longer. When the carrier frequency is 2500 Hz, the wavelength is 400 μs; when the carrier frequency is 4000 Hz, the wavelength is 250 μs; and

when the carrier frequency is 5000 Hz, the wavelength is 200 μs. Most units that can deliver interferential current have a fixed carrier frequency of 4000 or 5000 Hz or allow the user to select from a small selection of carrier frequencies between 2500 and 10000 Hz.

Frequency

The selection of pulse frequency for pain control depends on the desired mode—high rate, low rate, or burst. For high-rate TENS, the pulse frequency is set between 100 and 150 pps, and for low-rate TENS, the pulse frequency is set below 10 pps. Portable TENS units that provide burst mode are generally preset by the manufacturer to provide 10 or fewer bursts each second, with pulses within the burst being at 100 to 150 pps (see Fig. 13.2).

On:Off Time

When applied for pain control, electrical stimulation is delivered continuously throughout the treatment time, with no off time. This is necessary because, according to the gate control theory, the current blocks the pain only when it is stimulating A-beta nerve fibers. During any off time, no A-beta nerves would be stimulated, and no reduction in pain would be felt. Similarly, endogenous opioid release is stimulated when low-rate TENS is on, not during any off time.

Current Amplitude

To control pain with electrical stimulation, the treatment should not be uncomfortable. For high-rate TENS, it is generally recommended that the amplitude be set to produce a strong tingling or vibration

Continued

APPLICATION TECHNIQUE 13.1—cont'd

sensation.[2] Because the amplitude required to achieve this effect varies between users, it is often difficult to quantify in research protocols, but higher current intensities are generally associated with greater pain reduction.[115] Therefore, some clinicians and patients increase the current amplitude during treatment when the intensity of the sensation seems to fade. Although one study using an experimental model of pain found that increasing the current amplitude during TENS application improved pain relief,[116] studies evaluating the impact of increasing the current amplitude during the treatment of painful clinical conditions have not found this to be helpful.[117,118] For low-rate and burst TENS, the current amplitude should be sufficient to produce a muscle contraction that can be seen or palpated by the clinician.

Modulation

The stimulus used for TENS is generally modulated (i.e., varied over time) to limit adaptation. Adaptation is a decrease in the frequency of **action potentials (APs)** and a decrease in the subjective sensation of stimulation when electrical stimulation is applied without variation in the applied stimulus. Adaptation is a known property of sensory receptors caused by decreased excitability of the nerve membrane with repeated stimulation. Modulations can include changes in frequency, often called "**sweep,**" changes in amplitude, often called "**scan,**" and changes in pulse duration. **Modulation** of any of the stimulation parameters is likely to equally effectively help prevent adaptation to electrical stimulation. Modulations do not increase the analgesic effects of the stimulation.[119]

Treatment Time

When electrical stimulation is used for pain control with high-rate TENS, the stimulation may be applied whenever the patient is in pain or would be expected to be in pain. Low-rate or burst mode TENS should be applied only for a maximum of 20 to 30 minutes every 2 hours. Low-rate and burst mode TENS should not be used for longer periods because the muscle contractions they produce can cause delayed-onset muscle soreness if the stimulation is applied for prolonged periods.

Documentation

When applying electrical stimulation to treat patients for pain, document the following:
- Area of the body to be treated
- Patient positioning
- Specific stimulation parameters
- Electrode placement
- Treatment duration
- Patient response to treatment

Documentation is usually provided in the SOAP note format. Ensure that the level of detail in your notes is sufficiently detailed that another clinician can reproduce the treatment. The following examples summarize only the modality component of treatment and are not intended to represent a comprehensive plan of care.

EXAMPLES

When applying TENS for relief of acute pain in bilateral (B) upper trapezius and neck resulting from a motor vehicle accident (MVA), document the following:

S: Pt reports constant B trapezius area pain after MVA 10 days ago. He awakens 6 to 10 times each night from neck pain. Pt denies pain, numbness, or tingling in his upper extremities.

O: Intervention: TENS to B upper trapezius area ×30 min, 2 channels, 4 electrodes—2 at level of cervical thoracic junction and 2 at level of proximal medial scapulae, crossed channels. Biphasic waveform, pulse duration 70 μs, frequency 120 pps, with **amplitude modulation.** Pt set amplitude to his comfort.

Posttreatment: After 20 min of treatment, Pt notes a 50% decrease in his trapezius area discomfort. Pt instructed in appropriate application and use; he then correctly demonstrated setup and operation of unit. Given written instruction for independent home use of TENS, including a drawing with electrode placement.

A: Pt tolerated stimulation, with decrease in pain.

P: Pt to use TENS independently at home up to 24 h/day for pain relief during functional activities. Pt to monitor the condition of his skin under the electrodes and discontinue TENS if irritation or redness occurs. Pt to call therapist at clinic if he has any questions or concerns about home TENS use.

CLINICAL CASE STUDIES

The following case studies demonstrate the concepts of the clinical application of electrical stimulation discussed in this chapter. Based on the scenario presented, an evaluation of the clinical findings and goals of treatment are proposed. These are followed by a discussion of the factors to be considered in the selection of electrical stimulation as an indicated intervention and in the selection of the ideal electrical stimulation parameters to promote progress toward the set goals of treatment. Electrical stimulation is not intended to be the sole component of the patient's treatment but rather should be integrated into a comprehensive plan of care.

CASE STUDY 13.1

Upper Back and Neck Pain
Examination
History

DS is a 28-year-old woman who was referred to physical therapy with a diagnosis of upper back and neck pain. DS complains of gradually increasing neck and upper trapezius pain over the past 6 weeks. She reports that her pain is worse at the end of her workday as a supermarket checker. She

CLINICAL CASE STUDIES—*cont'd*

notes that her pain has become more intense and frequent in the past month. DS states that her pain increases with lifting, carrying, and any twisting motion of her neck, and she has had to cut short some of her workdays this month because of pain.

Systems Review

DS has been evaluated by a physician, and her cervical spine x-rays were unremarkable. She has no history of cardiac arrhythmias and does not have a pacemaker. She reports no recent fatigue or dizziness but admits to worsening mood lately. DS states that her neck pain severity is 6/10.

Tests and Measures

The patient's upper extremity active range of motion (AROM) is within normal limits. Her upper extremity strength is full, although full effort exacerbates her neck pain. Her rhomboid and lower trapezius strength is 4−/5 bilaterally. Neck rotation and lateral flexion are 75% of normal in both directions, with pain on overpressure bilaterally. Forward flexion is uncomfortable in the final 30% of the range. Extension is within normal limits. On palpation, significant nodules are noted in the bilateral upper trapezius and in trigger points along the medial borders of both scapulae. The patient denies numbness or tingling in her upper extremities.

Is this patient a candidate for electrical stimulation? Why or why not? What else should be included in her treatment program? What other physical agents might be useful?

Evaluation and Goals

ICF Level	Current Status	Goals
Body structure and function	Cervical and upper back pain	Control pain
	Restricted cervical ROM	Regain normal cervical ROM
	Decreased rhomboid and lower trapezius strength	Regain normal upper body strength
Activity	Difficulty lifting and carrying	Regain usual ability to lift and carry
Participation	Decreased work hours	Perform all work-related duties and return to regular work hours
	Decreased lifting Decreased carrying	Regain ability to lift and carry objects

ICF, International Classification for Functioning, Disability and Health; *ROM,* range of motion.

◆ FIND THE EVIDENCE

PICO Terms	Natural Language Example	Sample PubMed Search
P (Population)	Patient with pain due to neck and back pain	"Neck" [title] OR "Back" [title]
I (Intervention)	Transcutaneous electric nerve stimulation (TENS)	AND ("Transcutaneous Electric Nerve Stimulation" [MeSH] OR "TENS" [title] OR "Electric Stimulation Therapy" [title] OR "electrical currents" [title])
C (Comparison)	No TENS	
O (Outcome)	Control pain	AND ("pain" [text word])

Key Studies or Reviews

1. Rodríguez-Fernández AL, Garrido-Santofimia V, Güeita-Rodríguez J, et al: Effects of burst-type transcutaneous electrical nerve stimulation on cervical range of motion and latent myofascial trigger point pain sensitivity. *Arch Phys Med Rehabil* 92(9):1353–1358, 2011.

   This study compared a single session of burst mode TENS (200-μs pulse duration, 100 pps, 2 bursts/second) for 10 minutes with sham TENS for 10 minutes in 76 people with latent myofascial trigger points in one upper trapezius muscle. Those in the active TENS group had a statistically significantly greater reduction in referred pressure point sensitivity and a statistically significantly greater increase in ipsilateral cervical rotation range of motion than the sham-treated group, but absolute differences between groups were small.

2. Martimbianco ALC, Porfírio GJ, Pacheco RL, et al: Transcutaneous electrical nerve stimulation (TENS) for chronic neck pain. *Cochrane Database Syst Rev* 12:CD011927, 2019.

   This meta-analysis included seven randomized clinical trials involving a total of 651 participants evaluating the impact of TENS on chronic neck pain. Five of the seven studies concluded that TENS was more effective than placebo. However, the overall results of this meta-analysis were inconclusive because most studies did not meet the high standards imposed by the Cochrane collaboration (sample size, randomization, adequate placebo control, etc.).

Prognosis

This patient does not appear to have a bony or neurological problem, given her normal x-ray and lack of radicular sensory

Continued

CLINICAL CASE STUDIES—cont'd

or motor signs or symptoms, such as upper extremity tingling, numbness, or weakness. The nodules in her trapezius and the scapular trigger points indicate a muscular cause of her pain. In general, TENS is an indicated treatment to reduce pain. Exercise and body mechanics training and other physical agents, such as ultrasound or ice and heat, may be used in conjunction with electrical stimulation. This patient has no contraindications for the use of electrical stimulation.

Intervention

It is proposed that electrical stimulation be used for the control of pain, with the patient using a unit at home after evaluation and instruction (Fig. 13.5). The following parameters are chosen:

Type	Parameters
Electrode placement	One pair of electrodes upper cervical, one pair lower cervical
Waveform	Pulsed biphasic (or interferential)
Frequency	100–150 pps (or 100–150 bps for interferential)
Pulse duration	50–80 µs
Modulation	Yes
Amplitude	Sensory only—to patient comfort
Treatment duration	Patient may wear unit throughout the day for pain control

The patient initially will feel a gentle humming or buzzing under the electrodes. The intensity should be turned up to a strong sensation. Once this is achieved, the patient should switch the unit to modulation mode to reduce adaptation to the stimulus. Because the patient will have a home unit, she will be able to receive treatment throughout the day to minimize her pain at all times. DS will be reevaluated weekly for revision of parameters and for an update of her home exercise program, with the frequency of visits decreasing as her problem resolves. The use of electrical stimulation is generally

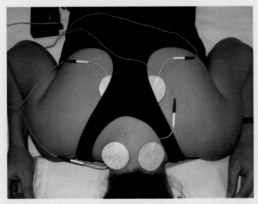

FIGURE 13.5 Treatment of upper back and neck pain with electrical stimulation.

discontinued at the patient's request on reaching tolerable resolution of pain.

If the patient is experiencing significant relief while wearing the TENS unit, she may use it at work. The lead wires can be placed under clothing, and the unit can be placed in a pocket or clipped to a waistband. With present technology, amplitude controls are covered so that they cannot be accidentally changed, thus increasing or decreasing the current.

Documentation

S: Pt reports bilateral upper back and neck pain that is worse at the end of the day.

O: Pretreatment: Overall neck pain 6/10. UE strength 4+/5 bilaterally, limited by neck pain. Rhomboid and lower trapezius strength is 4–/5 bilaterally. Neck rotation and lateral flexion 75% of normal. Forward flexion uncomfortable in final 30% of range.

Intervention: TENS home unit to bilateral cervical area × 30 min, 4 electrodes—2 upper and 2 lower cervical. Biphasic waveform, pulse duration 60 µs, frequency 130 pps, with amplitude modulation. Pt set amplitude to her comfort (sensory only).

During treatment: Approximately 50% decreased pain in neck and upper back.

A: Pt tolerated treatment with no adverse effects. Demonstrated independent setup and use of TENS.

P: Pt to use TENS at home up to 24 h/day for pain relief during functional activities and will discontinue TENS if irritation or redness occurs at the electrode site. Pt instructed in home exercises.

CASE STUDY 13.2

Chronic Low Back Pain
Examination
History

OL is a 48-year-old man who complains of chronic low back pain following a lifting injury that occurred 6 months ago at his job as a meatpacker. OL reports that his pain has progressively worsened, and he has had to take more analgesic medication to control it. He was referred to physical therapy with a diagnosis of lumbar sprain/strain and lumbago. His x-rays were normal. OL used to play tennis and go hiking but has stopped these activities because of pain with twisting during tennis and pain with lifting and carrying when hiking.

Systems Review

OL is moderately overweight and reports persistent fatigue. He has returned to work in a limited capacity, with lifting limited to 10 lb. OL has no history of heart problems, does not have a pacemaker, and does not have a cancerous tumor. His affect is positive, and he is eager to begin new treatment. OL self-reports his pain as 5/10 in severity and localized to his low back.

Tests and Measures

Lateral rotation and lateral flexion are within normal limits. Forward flexion is limited in the last 10%. Extension is 75% of normal and painful. The patient's lower extremity strength is 5/5 bilaterally. He states that the pain sometimes goes into his buttocks, but he denies any radiating pain down into his legs.

Would electrical stimulation be appropriate for this patient? What other education or interventions would be helpful to relieve his back symptoms over the long term?

Evaluation and Goals

ICF Level	Current Status	Goals
Body structure and function	Low back and buttock pain	Control pain
	Restricted lumbar ROM	Regain normal lumbar ROM
Activity	Avoids lifting, carrying, and twisting	Regain usual ability to lift, carry, and twist
Participation	Decreased lifting at work	Perform all work-related lifting duties
	Unable to play tennis or hike	Return to hobbies of tennis and hiking

ICF, International Classification for Functioning, Disability and Health; *ROM*, range of motion.

◆ FIND THE EVIDENCE

PICO Terms	Natural Language Example	Sample PubMed Search
P (Population)	Patient with lower back and buttock pain	"Back" [title]
I (Intervention)	Transcutaneous electric nerve stimulation (TENS)	AND ("Interferential Current" [title] OR "Transcutaneous Electric Nerve Stimulation" [title])
C (Comparison)	No TENS	
O (Outcome)	Reduce pain	AND ("pain" [text word])

Key Studies and Reviews

1. Gibson W, Wand BM, Meads C, et al: Transcutaneous electrical nerve stimulation (TENS) for chronic pain—an overview of Cochrane Reviews. *Cochrane Database Syst Rev* 4:CD011890, 2019.

   The most recent Cochrane publication on TENS is a 2019 overview of eight previously published Cochrane reviews of electrical stimulation for chronic pain conditions, including rheumatoid arthritis, neuropathic pain, osteoarthritis knee pain, phantom stump pain, cancer pain, fibromyalgia, and chronic low back pain. This review included 7 reviews of a total of 51 randomized clinical trials, with a total of 2895 participants, and concluded that they were "unable to confidently state whether TENS is effective in relieving pain in people with chronic pain. This is due to the very low quality of the evidence, and the overall small numbers of participants included in studies in the reviews." The authors make recommendations for future TENS study designs to meaningfully reduce this uncertainty. Unfortunately, mostly because of their small size, most studies of rehabilitation interventions do not meet the quality requirements of the Cochrane collaboration.

2. Albornoz-Cabello M, Maya-Martín J, Domínguez-Maldonado G, et al: Effect of interferential current therapy on pain perception and disability level in subjects with chronic low back pain: a randomized controlled trial. *Clin Rehabil* 31(2):242–249, 2017.

   In this randomized clinical trial, 64 individuals with chronic low back pain were treated with electrical stimulation or "usual care." Those treated with electrical stimulation had a greater decrease in pain perception and disability level than the usual-care control group.

Prognosis

Electrical stimulation could be an appropriate adjunct to help control OL's pain. His AROM is limited, but he does not have numbness, tingling, or weakness in his lower extremities, which would suggest nerve involvement. Low-rate TENS using a biphasic or interferential waveform, combined with other interventions, is most likely to be effective. Other interventions may include a home exercise program of stretching, strengthening of core musculature, and balance and coordination exercises, as well as body mechanics training and weight loss. In addition, OL may use heat or cold in conjunction with electrical stimulation to reduce muscle spasms and relieve pain.

Intervention

Electrical stimulation can be applied to reduce the patient's pain, using a pulsed biphasic current or an interferential current. The patient does not have any conditions that would be contraindications to the use of electrical stimulation. The following parameters are chosen:

Type	Parameters
Electrode placement	4 electrodes in a square on the low back, on either side of the spine
Waveform	Pulsed biphasic (or interferential)
Pulse frequency	2–10 pps (or 2–10 bps for interferential)
Pulse duration	150–300 μs
Modulation	None or modulate
Amplitude	Produces a visible muscle twitch contraction
Treatment duration	20–30 minutes, 3–4 × /day

Continued

CLINICAL CASE STUDIES—*cont'd*

Documentation

S: Pt reports continued and worsening low back pain since a lifting injury 6 months ago. Pain level 5/10.

O: Pretreatment: LE strength 5/5 throughout. Lumbar AROM: lateral flexion and rotation normal, forward flexion limited in last 10%, extension limited last 25% and painful.

Intervention: TENS using interferential current × 30 min, 4 electrodes on paraspinals with channels crossed, 5 bps, 30 min with amplitude set to visible muscle twitches.

During treatment: Approximately 40% decrease in low back pain.

A: Patient tolerated electrical stimulation with no adverse events.

P: Patient to use home interferential unit 3 to 4 times per day for 20 to 30 min for low back pain, along with hot pack and home exercise program, to maximize functional independence. Pt to discontinue use of device if irritation or redness occurs under the electrodes. Pt instructed in home exercise program.

Chapter Review

1. Electrically stimulated action potentials in sensory or motor nerves can control pain.
2. TENS is the use of transcutaneous electrical stimulation to control pain.
3. TENS appears to exert its effects through gating and stimulating the release of endogenous opioids.
4. High-rate TENS uses short-duration, high-frequency pulses to reduce the sensation of pain, primarily by gating.
5. Low-rate TENS uses long-duration, low-frequency pulses to reduce the sensation of pain, primarily by stimulating the release of endogenous opioids to mediate pain.

Glossary

Action potentials (APs): Rapid sequential depolarizations and repolarizations of a nerve that occur in response to a stimulus and transmit along the axon.

Acupuncture-like TENS: TENS with long-duration, high-amplitude pulses used to control pain; also called *low-rate TENS*.

Adaptation: A decrease in the frequency of action potentials and a decrease in the subjective sensation of stimulation that occur in response to electrical stimulation with unchanging characteristics.

Alternating current (AC): Continuous bidirectional flow of charged particles (see Fig. 11.4). AC has equal ion flow in each direction, and thus no pulse charge remains in the tissues. Most commonly, AC is delivered as a sine wave. With AC, when the frequency increases, the cycle duration decreases, and when the frequency decreases, the cycle duration increases (see Fig. 11.26).

Amplitude (intensity): The magnitude of current or voltage (see Fig. 11.12).

Amplitude modulation: Variation in peak current amplitude over time.

Biphasic current: A current where the charged particles move first in one direction and then in the opposite direction. Biphasic currents may be pulsed or alternating.

Burst mode: A current composed of a series of pulses delivered in groups (or packets) known as *bursts*. The burst is generally delivered with a preset frequency and duration. Burst duration is the time from the beginning to the end of the burst. The time between bursts is called the *interburst interval* (see Fig. 11.9).

Burst mode TENS: TENS using burst mode current.

Conventional TENS: TENS with short-duration, low-amplitude pulses used to control pain; also called *high-rate TENS*.

Electrical current: Movement or flow of charged particles through a conductor in response to an applied electrical field. Current is noted as "I" and is measured in amperes (A).

Frequency: The number of cycles or pulses per second. Frequency is measured in Hertz (Hz) for cycles and in pulses per second (pps) for pulses (see Fig. 11.11).

Frequency modulation: Variation in the number of pulses or cycles per second delivered.

Gate control theory: A theory of pain control that states that pain is modulated at the spinal cord level by inhibitory effects of nonnoxious afferent input.

Interferential current: The waveform produced by the interference of two medium-frequency (1000- to 10,000-Hz) sinusoidal alternating currents (ACs) of slightly different frequencies. These two waveforms are delivered through two sets of electrodes through separate channels in the same stimulator. The electrodes are configured on the skin so that the two ACs intersect (see Fig. 11.7).

Low-rate TENS: TENS with long-duration, high-amplitude pulses used to control pain; also called *acupuncture-like TENS*.

Medium-frequency alternating current (AC): AC with a frequency between 1000 and 10,000 Hz (between 1 and 10 kHz). Most medium-frequency currents available on clinical units have a frequency of 2500 to 5000 Hz. Medium-frequency AC is rarely used alone therapeutically, but two medium-frequency ACs of different frequency may be applied together to produce an interferential current (see *Interferential current*).

Modulation: Any pattern of variation in one or more of the stimulation parameters. Modulation is used to limit neural adaptation to an electrical current. Modulation may be cyclical or random (see Fig. 11.27).

Myelinated: Having a myelin sheath; myelin is a fatty tissue that surrounds the axons of neurons, allowing electrical signals to travel more quickly.

Premodulated current: An alternating current (AC) with a medium frequency and sequentially increasing and decreasing current amplitude that is produced with a single circuit and only two electrodes. This current has the same waveform as the interferential current resulting from the interference of two medium-frequency sinusoidal ACs that requires four electrodes (see Fig. 11.8).

Pulse duration: The time from the beginning of the first phase of a pulse to the end of the last phase of a pulse. Pulse duration is generally expressed in microseconds ($\mu s \times 10^6$ seconds) (see Fig. 11.10).

Pulsed biphasic current: A series of pulses whereby the charged particles move first in one direction and then in the opposite direction (see Fig. 11.4B).

Pulsed current (pulsatile current): An interrupted flow of charged particles whereby the current flows in a series of pulses separated by periods when no current flows.

Pulsed monophasic current: Series of pulses where the charged particles move in only one direction (see Fig. 11.5A).

Pulses: In pulsed current, periods when current is flowing in any direction.

Resistance: The opposition of a material to the flow of electrical current. Resistance is noted as "R" and is measured in ohms (Ω).

Scan: Amplitude modulation of an interferential current. Amplitude modulation of an interferential current moves the effective field of stimulation, causing the patient to feel the focus of the stimulation in a different location. This may allow the clinician to target a specific area in soft tissue.

Sweep: An alternative term for frequency modulation; usually used with interferential current.

Transcutaneous electrical nerve stimulation (TENS): The application of electrical current through the skin to modulate pain.

Voltage: The force or pressure of electricity; the difference in electrical energy between two points that produces the electrical force capable of moving charged particles through a conductor between those two points. Voltage is noted as "V" and is measured in volts (V); also called *potential difference*.

Wavelength: The duration of 1 cycle of alternating current. A cycle lasts from the time the current departs from the isoelectric line (zero current amplitude) in one direction and then crosses the isoelectric line in the opposite direction to when it returns to the isoelectric line. The wavelength of alternating current is similar to the pulse duration of pulsed current (see Fig. 11.28).

References

1. Sluka KA, Walsh D: Transcutaneous electrical nerve stimulation: basic science mechanisms and clinical effectiveness. *J Pain* 4:109–121, 2003.
2. Vance CG, Dailey DL, Rakel BA, et al: Using TENS for pain control: the state of the evidence. *Pain Manag* 4:197–209, 2014.
3. Sluka KA, Bjordal JM, Marchand S, et al: What makes transcutaneous electrical nerve stimulation work? Making sense of the mixed results in the clinical literature. *Phys Ther* 93:1397–1402, 2013.
4. Sabino GS, Santos CM, Francischi JN, et al: Release of endogenous opioids following transcutaneous electric nerve stimulation in an experimental model of acute inflammatory pain. *J Pain* 9:157–163, 2008.
5. Sjolund BH, Terenius L, Eriksson M: Increased cerebrospinal fluid levels of endorphins after electroacupuncture. *Acta Physiol Scand* 100:382–384, 1977.
6. Pert CB, Snyder SH: Opiate receptor: demonstration in nervous tissue. *Science* 179:1011–1014, 1973.
7. Xiang XH, Chen YM, Zhang JM, et al: Low- and high-frequency transcutaneous electrical acupoint stimulation induces different effects on cerebral μ-opioid receptor availability in rhesus monkeys. *J Neurosci Res* 92:555–563, 2014.
8. Mannheimer JS, Lampe GN: *Clinical transcutaneous electrical nerve stimulation*, Philadelphia, 1984, FA Davis.
9. Sjolund BH, Eriksson MBE: The influence of naloxone on analgesia produced by peripheral conditioning stimulation. *Brain Res* 173:295–301, 1979.
10. Leonard G, Goffaux P, Marchand S: Deciphering the role of endogenous opioids in high-frequency TENS using low and high doses of naloxone. *Pain* 151:215–219, 2010.
11. Kalra A, Urban MO, Sluka KA: Blockade of opioid receptors in rostral ventral medulla prevents antihyperalgesia produced by transcutaneous electrical nerve stimulation (TENS). *J Pharmacol Exp Ther* 298:257–263, 2001.
12. DeSantana JM, da Silva LF, Sluka KA: Cholecystokinin receptors mediate tolerance to the analgesic effect of TENS in arthritic rats. *Pain* 148(1):84–93, 2010.
13. Léonard G, Cloutier C, Marchand S: Reduced analgesic effect of acupuncture-like TENS but not conventional TENS in opioid-treated patients. *J Pain* 12:213–221, 2011.
14. Chandran P, Sluka KA: Development of opioid tolerance with repeated transcutaneous electrical nerve stimulation administration. *Pain* 102:195–201, 2003.
15. Liebano RE, Rakel B, Vance CG, et al: An investigation of the development of analgesic tolerance to TENS in humans. *Pain* 152:335–342, 2011.
16. Hingne PM, Sluka KA: Blockade of NMDA receptors prevents analgesic tolerance to repeated transcutaneous electrical nerve stimulation (TENS) in rats. *J Pain* 9(3):217–225, 2008.
17. Desantana JM, Santana-Filho VJ, Sluka KA: Modulation between high- and low-frequency transcutaneous electric nerve stimulation delays the development of analgesic tolerance in arthritic rats. *Arch Phys Med Rehabil* 89:754–760, 2008.
18. Chen CC, Johnson MI: A comparison of transcutaneous electrical nerve stimulation (TENS) at 3 and 80 pulses per second on cold-pressor pain in healthy human participants. *Clin Physiol Funct Imaging* 30:260–268, 2010.
19. Chen CC, Johnson MI: Differential frequency effects of strong nonpainful transcutaneous electrical nerve stimulation on experimentally induced ischemic pain in healthy human participants. *Clin J Pain* 27:434–441, 2011.
20. Francis RP, Marchant PR, Johnson MI: Comparison of post-treatment effects of conventional and acupuncture-like transcutaneous electrical nerve stimulation (TENS): a randomised placebo-controlled study using cold-induced pain and healthy human participants. *Physiother Theory Pract* 27:578–585, 2011.
21. Tousignant-Laflamme Y, Laroche C, Beaulieu C, et al: A randomized trial to determine the duration of analgesia following a 15- and a 30-minute application of acupuncture-like TENS on patients with chronic low back pain. *Physiother Theory Pract* 33(5):361–369, 2017.
22. Bergeron-Vézina K, Corriveau H, Martel M, et al: High- and low-frequency transcutaneous electrical nerve stimulation does not reduce experimental pain in elderly individuals. *Pain* 156(10):2093–2099, 2015.
23. Simon CB, Riley JL, Fillingim RB, et al: Age group comparisons of TENS response among individuals with chronic axial low back pain. *J Pain* 16(12):1268–1279, 2015.
24. Francis RP, Marchant P, Johnson MI: Conventional versus acupuncture-like transcutaneous electrical nerve stimulation on cold-induced pain in healthy human participants: effects during stimulation. *Clin Physiol Funct Imaging* 31:363–370, 2011.
25. Omura Y: Basic electrical parameters for safe and effective electro-therapeutics [electro-acupuncture, TES, TENMS (or TEMS), TENS and electro-magnetic field stimulation with or without drug field] for pain, neuromuscular skeletal problems, and circulatory disturbances. *Acupunct Electrother Res* 12:201–225, 1987.
26. Debreceni L: Chemical releases associated with acupuncture and electric stimulation: critical reviews. *Crit Rev Phys Rehabil Med* 5:247–275, 1993.
27. Aranha MFM, Müller CEE, Gavião MBD: Pain intensity and cervical range of motion in women with myofascial pain treated with acupuncture and electroacupuncture: a double-blinded, randomized clinical trial. *Braz J Phys Ther* 19(1):34–43, 2015.
28. Chiu TT, Hui-Chan CW, Chein G: A randomized clinical trial of TENS and exercise for patients with chronic neck pain. *Clin Rehabil* 19:850–860, 2005.
29. Yeh ML, Chung YC, Chen KM, et al: Pain reduction of acupoint electrical stimulation for patients with spinal surgery: a placebo-controlled study. *Int J Nurs Stud* 48:703–709, 2011.
30. Yeh ML, Chung YC, Chen KM, et al: Acupoint electrical stimulation reduces acute postoperative pain in surgical patients with patient-controlled analgesia: a randomized controlled study. *Altern Ther Health Med* 16:10–18, 2010.

31. Huang S, Peng W, Tian X, et al: Effects of transcutaneous electrical acupoint stimulation at different frequencies on perioperative anesthetic dosage, recovery, complications, and prognosis in video-assisted thoracic surgical lobectomy: a randomized, double-blinded, placebo-controlled trial. *J Anesth* 31(1):58–65, 2017.

32. Kim HW, Roh DH, Yoon SY, et al: The anti-inflammatory effects of low- and high-frequency electroacupuncture are mediated by peripheral opioids in a mouse air pouch inflammation model. *J Altern Complement Med* 12:39–44, 2006.

33. Ng MM, Leung MC, Poon DM: The effects of electro-acupuncture and transcutaneous electrical nerve stimulation on patients with painful osteoarthritis knees: a randomized controlled trial with follow-up evaluation. *J Altern Complement Med* 9:641–649, 2003.

34. Ahsin S, Saleem S, Bhatti AM, et al: Clinical and endocrinological changes after electro-acupuncture treatment in patients with osteoarthritis of the knee. *Pain* 147:60–66, 2009.

35. Lee D, Xu H, Lin JG, et al: Needle-free electroacupuncture for postoperative pain management. *Evid Based Complement Alternat Med* 696–754, 2011.

36. Cheing GL, So EM, Chao CY: Effectiveness of electroacupuncture and interferential electrotherapy in the management of frozen shoulder. *J Rehabil Med* 40:166–170, 2008.

37. Ulett GA, Han S, Han JS: Electroacupuncture: mechanisms and clinical application. *Biol Psychiatry* 44:129–138, 1998.

38. Casimiro L, Barnsley L, Brosseau L, et al: Acupuncture and electroacupuncture for the treatment of rheumatoid arthritis. *Cochrane Database Syst Rev* 2005(4):CD003788, 2005.

39. Fukazawa Y, Maeda T, Hamabe W, et al: Activation of spinal anti-analgesic system following electroacupuncture stimulation in rats. *J Pharmacol Sci* 99:408–414, 2005.

40. Kroeling P, Gross A, Graham N, et al: Electrotherapy for neck pain. *Cochrane Database Syst Rev* 2013(8):CD004251, 2013.

41. Sbruzzi G, Silveira SA, Silva DV, et al: Transcutaneous electrical nerve stimulation after thoracic surgery: systematic review and meta-analysis of 11 randomized trials. *Rev Bras Cir Cardiovasc* 27:75–87, 2012.

42. Hurlow A, Bennett MI, Robb KA, et al: Transcutaneous electric nerve stimulation (TENS) for cancer pain in adults. *Cochrane Database Syst Rev* 2012(3):CD006276, 2012.

43. Walsh DM, Howe TE, Johnson MI, et al: Transcutaneous electrical nerve stimulation for acute pain. *Cochrane Database Syst Rev* 2009(2):CD006142, 2009.

44. Rutjes AW, Nüesch E, Sterchi R, et al: Transcutaneous electrostimulation for osteoarthritis of the knee. *Cochrane Database Syst Rev* 2009(4):CD002823, 2009.

45. Gibson W, Wand BM, Meads C, et al: Transcutaneous electrical nerve stimulation (TENS) for chronic pain—an overview of Cochrane reviews. *Cochrane Database Syst Rev* 2019(4):CD011890, 2019.

46. Ferreira RM, Duarte JA, Gonçalves RS: Non-pharmacological and non-surgical interventions to manage patients with knee osteoarthritis: An umbrella review. *Acta Reumatol Port* 43(3):182–200, 2018.

47. Chen LX, Zhou ZR, Li YL, et al: Transcutaneous electrical nerve stimulation in patients with knee osteoarthritis: evidence from randomized-controlled trials. *Clin J Pain* 32(2):146–154, 2016.

48. Resende L, Merriwether E, Rampazo ÉP, et al: Meta-analysis of transcutaneous electrical nerve stimulation for relief of spinal pain. *Eur J Pain* 22(4):663–678, 2018.

49. Binny J, Joshua Wong NL, Garga S, et al: Transcutaneous electric nerve stimulation (TENS) for acute low back pain: systematic review. *Scand J Pain* 19(2):225–233, 2019.

50. Gibson W, Wand BM, O'Connell NE: Transcutaneous electrical nerve stimulation (TENS) for neuropathic pain in adults. *Cochrane Database Syst Rev* 2017(9), 2017. Sep 14.

51. Johnson MI, Claydon LS, Herbison GP, et al: Transcutaneous electrical nerve stimulation (TENS) for fibromyalgia in adults. *Cochrane Database Syst Rev* 2017(10):CD012172, 2017.

52. Page MJ, Green S, Mrocki MA, et al: Electrotherapy modalities for rotator cuff disease. *Cochrane Database Syst Rev* 2016(6):CD012225.

53. Johnson MI, Paley CA, Howe TE, et al: Transcutaneous electrical nerve stimulation for acute pain. *Cochrane Database Syst Rev* 2015(6):CD006142, 2015.

54. Simpson PM, Fouche PF, Thomas RE, et al: Transcutaneous electrical nerve stimulation for relieving acute pain in the prehospital setting: a systematic review and meta-analysis of randomized-controlled trials. *Eur J Emerg Med* 21:10–17, 2014.

55. Bjordal JM, Johnson MI, Ljunggreen AE: Transcutaneous electrical nerve stimulation (TENS) can reduce postoperative analgesic consumption. A meta-analysis with assessment of optimal treatment parameters for postoperative pain. *Eur J Pain* 7:181–188, 2003.

56. Li J, Song Y: Transcutaneous electrical nerve stimulation for postoperative pain control after total knee arthroplasty: a meta-analysis of randomized controlled trials. *Medicine (Baltimore)* 96(37):e8036, 2017.

57. Zhu Y, Feng Y, Peng L: Effect of transcutaneous electrical nerve stimulation for pain control after total knee arthroplasty: A systematic review and meta-analysis. *J Rehabil Med* 49(9):700–704, 2017.

58. Mahure SA, Rokito AS, Kwon YW: Transcutaneous electrical nerve stimulation for postoperative pain relief after arthroscopic rotator cuff repair: a prospective double-blinded randomized trial. *J Shoulder Elbow Surg* 26(9):1508–1513, 2017.

59. Ozturk NK, Baki ED, Kavakli AS, et al: Comparison of transcutaneous electrical nerve stimulation and parasternal block for postoperative pain management after cardiac surgery. *Pain Res Manag* 2016:4261949, 2016.

60. Zhou J, Dan Y, Yixian Y, et al: Efficacy of transcutaneous electronic nerve stimulation (TENS) in postoperative analgesia after pulmonary surgery: a systematic review and meta-analysis. *Am J Phys Med Rehabil* 99(3):241–249, 2020.

61. Sezen CB, Akboga SA, Celik A, et al: Transcutaneous electrical nerve stimulation effect on postoperative complications. *Asian Cardiovasc Thorac Ann* 25(4):276–280, 2017.

62. Jahangirifard A, Razavi M, Ahmadi ZH, et al: Effect of TENS on postoperative pain and pulmonary function in patients undergoing coronary artery bypass surgery. *Pain Manag Nurs* 19(4):408–414, 2018.

63. Kadı MR, Hepgüler S, Atamaz FC, et al: Is interferential current effective in the management of pain, range of motion, and edema following total knee arthroplasty surgery? A randomized double-blind controlled trial. *Clin Rehabil* 33(6):1027–1034, 2019.

64. Zeng C, Li H, Yang T, et al: Electrical stimulation for pain relief in knee osteoarthritis: systematic review and network meta-analysis. *Osteoarthritis Cartilage* 23:189–202, 2015.

65. Choi YJ, Kim HJ, Han SY, et al: Effect of interferential current therapy on forward head posture. *J Phys Ther Sci* 30(3):398–399, 2018.

66. Acedo AA, Luduvice Antunes AC, Barros dos Santos A, et al: Upper trapezius relaxation induced by TENS and interferential current in computer users with chronic nonspecific neck discomfort: An electromyographic analysis. *J Back Musculoskelet Rehabil* 28(1):19–24, 2015.

67. Gunay Ucurum S, Kaya DO, Kayali Y, et al: Comparison of different electrotherapy methods and exercise therapy in shoulder impingement syndrome: a prospective randomized controlled trial. *Acta Orthop Traumatol Turc* 52(4):249–255, 2018.

68. Lin ML, Chiu HW, Shih ZM, et al: Two transcutaneous stimulation techniques in shoulder pain: transcutaneous pulsed radiofrequency (TPRF) versus transcutaneous electrical nerve stimulation (TENS): a comparative pilot study. *Pain Res Manag* 2019:2823401, 2019.

69. Gomes CAFP, Dibai-Filho AV, Moreira WA, et al: Effect of adding interferential current in an exercise and manual therapy program for patients with unilateral shoulder impingement syndrome: a randomized clinical trial. *J Manipulative Physiol Ther* 41(3):218–226, 2018.

70. Jan F, Naeem A, Malik AN, et al: Comparison of low level laser therapy and interferential current on post stroke shoulder pain. *J Pak Med Assoc* 67(5):788–789, 2017.

71. Nazligul T, Akpinar P, Aktas I, et al: The effect of interferential current therapy on patients with subacromial impingement syndrome: a randomized, double-blind, sham-controlled study. *Eur J Phys Rehabil Med* 54(3):351–357, 2018.

72. Desmeules F, Boudreault J, Roy JS, et al: Efficacy of transcutaneous electrical nerve stimulation for rotator cuff tendinopathy: a systematic review. *Physiotherapy* 102(1):41–49, 2016.

73. Stein C, Eibel B, Sbruzzi G, et al: Electrical stimulation and electromagnetic field use in patients with diabetic neuropathy: systematic review and meta-analysis. *Braz J Phys Ther* 17:93–104, 2013.

74. Dubinsky RM, Miyasaki J: Assessment: efficacy of transcutaneous electric nerve stimulation in the treatment of pain in neurologic disorders (an evidence-based review): report of the Therapeutics and Technology Assessment Subcommittee of the. *American Academy of Neurology Neurology* 74:173–176, 2010.

75. Upton GA, Tinley P, Al-Aubaidy H, et al: The influence of transcutaneous electrical nerve stimulation parameters on the level of pain perceived by participants with painful diabetic neuropathy: A crossover study. *Diabetes Metab Syndr* 11(2):113–118, 2017.

76. Ferreira AP, Costa DR, Oliveira AI, et al: Short-term transcutaneous electrical nerve stimulation reduces pain and improves the masticatory muscle activity in temporomandibular disorder patients: a randomized controlled trial. *J Appl Oral Sci* 25(2):112–120, 2017.

77. Awan KH, Patil S: The role of transcutaneous electrical nerve stimulation in the management of temporomandibular joint disorder. *J Contemp Dent Pract* 16(12):984–986, 2015.

78. Seifi M, Ebadifar A, Kabiri S, et al: Comparative effectiveness of low level laser therapy and transcutaneous electric nerve stimulation on temporomandibular joint disorders. *J Lasers Med Sci* 8(Suppl 1):S27–S31, 2017.

79. Rezazadeh F, Hajian K, Shahidi S, et al: Comparison of the effects of transcutaneous electrical nerve stimulation and low-level laser therapy on drug-resistant temporomandibular disorders. *J Dent (Shiraz)* 18(3):187–192, 2017.

80. Huisstede BM, Hoogvliet P, Franke TP, et al: Carpal tunnel syndrome: effectiveness of physical therapy and electrophysical modalities. An updated systematic review of randomized controlled trials. *Arch Phys Med Rehabil* 99(8):1623–1634,e23; 2018.

81. Khadilkar A, Odebiyi DO, Brosseau L, et al: Transcutaneous electrical nerve stimulation (TENS) versus placebo for chronic low-back pain. *Cochrane Database Syst Rev* 2008(4):CD003008, 2008.

82. Albornoz-Cabello M, Maya-Martín J, Domínguez-Maldonado G, et al: Effect of interferential current therapy on pain perception and disability level in subjects with chronic low back pain: a randomized controlled trial. *Clin Rehabil* 31(2):242–249, 2017.

83. Sayilir S, Yildizgoren MT: The medium-term effects of diadynamic currents in chronic low back pain; TENS versus diadynamic currents: a randomised, follow-up study. *Complement Ther Clin Pract* 29:16–19, 2017.

84. Rajfur J, Pasternok M, Rajfur K, et al: Efficacy of selected electrical therapies on chronic low back pain: a comparative clinical pilot study. *Med Sci Monit* 23:85–100, 2017.

85. Jauregui JJ, Cherian JJ, Gwam CU, et al: A meta-analysis of transcutaneous electrical nerve stimulation for chronic low back pain. *Surg Technol Int* 28:296–302, 2016.

86. Franco KM, Franco YD, Oliveira NB, et al: Is interferential current before pilates exercises more effective than placebo in patients with chronic nonspecific low back pain? A randomized controlled trial. *Arch Phys Med Rehabil* 98(2):320–328, 2017.

87. Wu LC, Weng PW, Chen CH, et al: Literature review and meta-analysis of transcutaneous electrical nerve stimulation in treating chronic back pain. *Reg Anesth Pain Med* 43(4):425–433, 2018.

88. Zhu S, Marmura MJ: Non-invasive neuromodulation for headache disorders. *Curr Neurol Neurosci Rep* 16(2):11, 2016.

89. Tao H, Wang T, Dong X, et al: Effectiveness of transcutaneous electrical nerve stimulation for the treatment of migraine: a meta-analysis of randomized controlled trials. *J Headache Pain* 19(1):42, 2018.

90. Gaul C, Magis D, Liebler E, et al: Effects of non-invasive vagus nerve stimulation on attack frequency over time and expanded response rates in patients with chronic cluster headache: a post hoc analysis of the randomised, controlled PREVA study. *J Headache Pain* 18(1):22, 2017.

91. Gaul C, Diener HC, Silver N, et al: Non-invasive vagus nerve stimulation for PREVention and Acute treatment of chronic cluster headache (PREVA): A randomised controlled study, *Cephalalgia* 36(6):534–546, 2016.

92. Schoenen J, Vandersmissen B, Jeangette S, et al: Migraine prevention with a supraorbital transcutaneous stimulator: a randomized controlled trial. *Neurology* 80(8):697–704, 2013.

93. Chou DE, Shnayderman Yugrakh M, Winegarner D, et al: Acute migraine therapy with external trigeminal neurostimulation (ACME): A randomized controlled trial. *Cephalalgia* 39(1):3–14, 2019.

94. Jones DA, Bigland-Ritchie B, Edwards RH: Excitation frequency and muscle fatigue: mechanical responses during voluntary and stimulated contractions. *Exp Neurol* 64:401–413, 1979.

95. Cheing GL, Hui-Chan CW: Analgesic effects of transcutaneous electrical nerve stimulation and interferential currents on heat pain in healthy subjects. *J Rehabil Med* 35:15–19, 2003.

96. Long DM: Stimulation of the peripheral nervous system for pain control. *Clin Neurosurg* 31:323–343, 1984.

97. Machado LAC, Kamper SJ, Herbert RD, et al: Analgesic effects of treatments for non-specific low back pain: a meta-analysis of placebo-controlled randomized trials. *Rheumatology* 48:520–527, 2009.

98. Rakel B, Frantz R: Effectiveness of transcutaneous electrical nerve stimulation on postoperative pain with movement. *J Pain* 4:455–464, 2003.

99. Rushton DN: Electrical stimulation in the treatment of pain. *Disabil Rehabil* 24:407–415, 2002.

100. Jarit GJ, Mohr KJ, Waller R, et al: The effects of home interferential therapy on post-operative pain, edema, and range of motion of the knee. *Clin J Sport Med* 13:16–20, 2003.

101. Fuentes JP, Olivo SA, Magee DJ, et al: Effectiveness of interferential current therapy in the management of musculoskeletal pain: a systematic review and meta-analysis. *Phys Ther* 90:1219–1238, 2010.

102. Walker UA, Uhl M, Weiner SM, et al: Analgesic and disease modifying effects of interferential current in psoriatic arthritis. *Rheumatol Int* 26:904–907, 2006.

103. Defrin R, Ariel E, Peretz C: Segmental noxious versus innocuous electrical stimulation for chronic pain relief and the effect of fading sensation during treatment. *Pain* 115:152–160, 2005.

104. Zambito A, Bianchini D, Gatti D, et al: Interferential and horizontal therapies in chronic low back pain due to multiple vertebral fractures: a randomized, double blind, clinical study. *Osteoporos Int* 18:1541–1545, 2007.

105. Zambito A, Bianchini D, Gatti D, et al: Interferential and horizontal therapies in chronic low back pain: a randomized, double blind, clinical study. *Clin Exp Rheumatol* 24:534–539, 2006.

106. Bae YH, Lee SM: Analgesic effects of transcutaneous electrical nerve stimulation and interferential current on experimental ischemic pain models: frequencies of 50 Hz and 100 Hz. *J Phys Ther Sci* 26:1945–1948, 2014.

107. Facci LM, Nowotny JP, Tormem F, et al: Effects of transcutaneous electrical nerve stimulation (TENS) and interferential currents (IFC) in patients with nonspecific chronic low back pain: randomized clinical trial. *Sao Paulo Med J* 129:206–216, 2011.

108. Ward AR, Lucas-Toumbourou S, McCarthy B: A comparison of the analgesic efficacy of medium-frequency alternating current and TENS. *Physiotherapy* 95:280–288, 2009.

109. Yesil H, Hepguler S, Dundar U, et al: Does the use of electrotherapies increase the effectiveness of neck stabilization exercises for improving pain, disability, mood, and quality of life in chronic neck pain? A randomized, controlled, single-blind study. *Spine (Phila Pa 1976)* 43(20):E1174–E1183, 2018.

110. Albornoz-Cabello M, Pérez-Mármol JM, Barrios Quinta CJ, et al: Effect of adding interferential current stimulation to exercise on outcomes in primary care patients with chronic neck pain: a randomized controlled trial. *Clin Rehabil* 33(9):1458–1467, 2019.

111. Takla MKN: Low-frequency high-intensity versus medium-frequency low-intensity combined therapy in the management of active myofascial trigger points: a randomized controlled trial. *Physiother Res Int* 23(4):e1737, 2018.

112. Ozcan J, Ward AR, Robertson VJ: A comparison of true and premodulated interferential currents. *Arch Phys Med Rehabil* 85:409–415, 2004.

113. Beatti A, Rayner A, Chipchase L, et al: Penetration and spread of interferential current in cutaneous, subcutaneous and muscle tissues. *Physiotherapy* 97:319–326, 2011.

114. Stralka SW, Jackson JA, Lewis AR: Treatment of hand and wrist pain: a randomized clinical trial of high voltage pulsed, direct current built into a wrist splint. *AAOHN J* 46:233–236, 1998.

115. Moran F, Leonard T, Hawthorne S, et al: Hypoalgesia in response to transcutaneous electrical nerve stimulation (TENS) depends on stimulation intensity. *J Pain* 12(8):929–935, 2011.

116. Pantaleão MA, Laurino MF, Gallego NL, et al: Adjusting pulse amplitude during transcutaneous electrical nerve stimulation (TENS) application produces greater hypoalgesia. *J Pain* 12(5):581–590, 2011.

117. Elserty N, Kattabei O, Elhafez H: Effect of fixed versus adjusted transcutaneous electrical nerve stimulation amplitude on chronic mechanical low back pain. *J Altern Complement Med* 22(7):557–562, 2016.

118. Bergeron-Vézina K, Filion C, Couture C, et al: Adjusting Pulse amplitude during transcutaneous electrical nerve stimulation does not provide greater hypoalgesia. *J Altern Complement Med* 24(3):262–267, 2018.

119. Chen CC, Johnson MI: An investigation into the effects of frequency-modulated transcutaneous electrical nerve stimulation (TENS) on experimentally-induced pressure pain in healthy human participants. *J Pain* 10:1029–1037, 2009.

Electrical Currents for Soft Tissue Healing

Michelle H. Cameron | Michelle Ocelnik

CHAPTER OBJECTIVES

After reading this chapter, the reader will be able to do the following:
- Describe the effects of electrical currents on soft tissue.
- Explain the clinical indications for the use of electrical currents for soft tissue healing.
- Choose the best technique for treatment with electrical currents for soft tissue healing, and list the advantages and disadvantages of each.
- Select the appropriate equipment and optimal treatment parameters for treatment with electrical currents for soft tissue healing.
- Safely and effectively apply electrical currents for soft tissue healing.
- Accurately and completely document treatment with electrical currents for soft tissue healing.

Electricity has been used to enhance wound healing for many centuries. About 300 years ago, electrostatically charged gold leaf was found to accelerate the healing of smallpox lesions. In the mid-1800s, Du Bois-Reymond was the first to measure the naturally occurring electrical current in a wound, and since the mid-1900s, exogenous electrical currents in the form of electrical stimulation have been used to treat wounds. More recently, through research in vitro, and in animals and in humans with several different types of wounds, we have come to better understand the mechanisms underlying the effects of electrical currents on tissue healing, including the impact on cell migration, proliferation, and function.

More than 8 million Americans have chronic, nonhealing wounds. In 2012, the cost of treating chronic wounds was estimated to be $50 billion. By 2014, estimates for chronic wound care for the Medicare population alone were $30 billion per year.[1,2] Wounds may impede rehabilitation, prevent the patient from participating in usual activities, increase length of stay, and increase the overall cost of care.[3] In people with diabetes and resulting peripheral vascular disease, foot ulcers and infection are the leading causes of hospitalization, and 70% to 90% of leg amputations are caused by vascular ulcers.[4] In people with spinal cord injury, untreated pressure ulcers can lead to hypoproteinemia, malnutrition, osteomyelitis, sepsis, and death.[5] Promoting wound healing is therefore essential, potentially improving quality of life and enabling patients to participate more fully in other components of rehabilitation, optimizing functional outcomes, and decreasing overall costs.

Effective wound management requires an integrated multidisciplinary approach that includes collaboration among a team that may include nurses, physical and occupational therapists, dietitians, physicians, the patient, and the patient's family and caregivers. This chapter focuses on the role of electrical currents in promoting soft tissue healing. This chapter does not cover the use of electrical currents to promote bone (fracture) healing. This is because, although electricity, generally in the form of induced electrical fields, is used to promote fracture healing, electrical bone stimulators are almost always dispensed directly to the patient by a physician and are not used by physical therapists or occupational therapists, the primary readers of this book. This chapter also does not cover the other important aspects of wound care, such as nutrition, blood sugar control, positioning, and wound debridement and dressing. Optimizing patient nutrition, blood sugar control, and positioning can be essential to address the underlying causes or risk factors for chronic wounds. Like wound debridement and dressings, electrical stimulation can enhance healing by optimizing processes involved in tissue healing, regardless of the etiology of the wound. As with other physical agents, electrical stimulation for wound management serves as an adjunct to other aspects of care to help achieve optimal outcomes.

Electrical stimulation is an adjunct to other aspects of wound care, which include patient nutrition, blood sugar control, positioning, and wound debridement and dressing.

Mechanisms Underlying Electrical Currents for Tissue Healing

In rehabilitation, electrical stimulation is most commonly used to control pain or to produce muscle contractions by stimulating action potentials in peripheral nerves, but electrical stimulation can also promote tissue healing. Tissue healing may be aided directly by applying current to a wound or indirectly by controlling edema or promoting transdermal delivery of medications.

In chronic wounds, the endogenous healing mechanism is disrupted. Electrical stimulation is thought to promote tissue healing by imitating endogenous electrical currents to attract appropriate cell types to the area (**galvanotaxis**), activating these cells by altering cell membrane function, enhancing antimicrobial activity, reducing inflammatory cytokine production and release,[6-8] and promoting circulation and thereby reducing edema and improving tissue oxygenation.[9,10]

GALVANOTAXIS

Galvanotaxis, the directional movement of cells in response to an electrical field, is important for cells engaged in various processes, including embryogenesis, regeneration, and wound healing.[11] Galvanotaxis can cause specific cells, including neutrophils, macrophages, lymphocytes, and fibroblasts, to move to an injured healing area because these cells carry a **charge**.[12,13] Research supports that calcium ion flow from the positively charged pole (usually called the **anode**) to the negatively charged pole (usually called the **cathode**),[14] calcium and sodium channel responses,[15] and stimulation of adenosine triphosphate (ATP) release[16] may underlie galvanotaxis toward the negatively charged pole. Because the terms *anode* and *cathode* are defined differently according to the discipline, *positively charged pole* and *negatively charged pole* are used here for clarity.

Galvanotaxis is a normal healthy response to tissue injury that can be augmented with appropriate electrical stimulation.[17] When skin and cell membranes are intact, there is an electrical charge across them as a result of the action of the sodium/potassium pumps. As soon as tissue is injured, rupturing cell membranes, charged ions leak out of the cells, causing the center of the wound to become electrically charged relative to the surrounding uninjured tissue.[18,19] This charge difference is commonly termed a *skin battery,* producing an electrical current of injury that activates healing.[20] This current has been demonstrated in children with accidental finger amputations.[21] This electrical potential difference steadily declines over time, resolving after the wound closes. Electrical stimulation with a monophasic pulsed or direct current applied to the wound is thought to promote wound healing by replicating or supplementing the effects of this skin battery.

Macrophages, epidermal cells, and inactive neutrophils are attracted to the positively charged pole, whereas lymphocytes, platelets, mast cells, keratinocytes, neural progenitor cells, fibroblasts, and activated neutrophils are attracted to the negatively charged pole.[16,22,23] To attract the most appropriate cell types for the phase of tissue healing, it is generally recommended that the negative electrode be used to treat infected or inflamed wounds and the positive electrode be used if necrosis without inflammation is present and when the wound is in the proliferative stage of healing.[24]

In general, the negative electrode should be used to promote healing of inflamed or infected wounds, and the positive electrode should be used to promote healing of wounds without inflammation.

CELL ACTIVATION

Not only does electrical stimulation attract cells to an injury site, but it also activates these cells. Most of the research in this area has been carried out using fibroblasts, the cells that make collagen to close a wound. Fibroblasts and the collagen they produce are essential for the proliferation phase of tissue healing. Electrical stimulation activates fibroblasts, enhancing their replication and their synthesis of DNA and collagen, upregulating growth factor pathways, and inducing them to become myofibroblasts.[7,25-32] It is proposed that with pulsed electrical stimulation, the electrical current pulse triggers calcium channels in the fibroblast cell membrane to open. The open channels then allow calcium to flow into the cells, increasing intracellular calcium levels to induce exposure of additional insulin receptors on the cell surface. Insulin can then bind to the exposed receptors, stimulating the fibroblasts to synthesize collagen and DNA.[33,34] Electrical stimulation also modulates fibroblast gene expression. This includes genes that are active in many processes involved in tissue healing, including cell adhesion, remodeling, and spreading; cytoskeletal activity; extracellular matrix metabolism; production of cytokines, chemokines, and growth factors; and signal transduction.[35-37] Cellular responses to electrical currents are voltage dependent, with maximum calcium influx and protein and DNA synthesis occurring with high-volt **pulsed current** (HVPC) with a peak **voltage** in the range of 60 to 90 V. Both higher and lower voltages have less effect. Electrical stimulation can also promote changes in other cells involved in tissue healing, such as epidermal cell and lymphocyte migration, proliferation, and function,[38] possibly by increasing vascular endothelial growth factor (VEGF) production or release.[7,39-41] VEGF also stimulates the development of microcirculation near the wound, which enhances the delivery of oxygen and nutrients.

Although most studies using electrical stimulation for wound healing have used a monophasic pulsed current, in order specifically to have a negative and positive **polarity** electrode, there is some evidence that alternating or biphasic currents may have some benefit.[42,43] Because these currents do not have a net charge effect on the tissue, they cannot exert effects through galvanotaxis, but it is possible that **biphasic pulsed currents** activate cells through effects on the cell membrane.

ANTIMICROBIAL EFFECTS

Electrical stimulation may also promote tissue healing by having antimicrobial effects. Monophasic currents, both microampere-level **direct current (DC)** and HVPC, have been shown to kill bacteria in vitro, whereas alternating current (AC) does not appear to affect bacterial growth or survival.[24,44–46] This effect of DC and HVPC is likely due to electrolytic generation of hypochlorous acid at the negative electrode.[47] However, most research indicates that to inhibit bacterial growth, the electrical current must be applied at a much higher voltage or for much longer than used in the clinical setting.[47–52] Therefore the potential direct antimicrobial effects of electrical currents are not likely to contribute strongly to the benefits seen with standard electrical stimulation for wound management. It is more likely that electrical stimulation indirectly reduces microbial counts and activity by enhancing the body's immune response to infection and possibly by enhancing the activity of antibiotic agents against bacteria in biofilms, where they are usually resistant to antibiotics.[53–55]

ENHANCED CIRCULATION

Electrical stimulation may also facilitate tissue healing by increasing circulation during or after the stimulation.[56] This effect appears to be augmented when stimulation is applied in a warm room.[57,58] With repeated applications of electrical stimulation, there may also be some increase in circulation due to angiogenesis as a result of increased VEGF production.[59] However, it is unlikely that the sensory-level electrical stimulation typically used to promote wound healing increases circulation immediately through vessels already in the area because, in general, muscle contractions are required for electrical stimulation to increase circulation.[60–64]

Clinical Applications of Electrical Stimulation for Soft Tissue Healing

CHRONIC WOUNDS: PRESSURE ULCERS, DIABETIC ULCERS, VENOUS ULCERS

Multiple studies and systematic reviews support the benefits of electrical stimulation for enhancing the healing of chronic wounds.[24,41,64–70] In 2002, the U.S. Centers for Medicare and Medicaid Services (CMS) approved payment for electrical stimulation to treat chronic stage III or stage IV pressure ulcers, arterial ulcers, diabetic ulcers, and venous stasis ulcers that have not previously responded to standard wound treatment in 30 days.[71] The cost of electrical stimulation for wound care is only covered by CMS when it is performed by a physician or a physical therapist or incident to a physician service.

> **◎ Clinical Pearl**
>
> In 2002, the U.S. Centers for Medicare and Medicaid Services approved payment for electrical stimulation when performed by a physician or a physical therapist, or incident to a physician service, to treat chronic stage III or stage IV pressure ulcers, arterial ulcers, diabetic ulcers, and venous stasis ulcers that have not previously responded to standard wound treatment in 30 days.

Several systematic reviews on the effects of electrical stimulation on various types of wounds have been published in the last several years. Most of these concluded that electrical stimulation significantly accelerates wound healing. Three reviews[72] concluded that electrical stimulation significantly accelerates the rate of chronic wound healing compared with the standard of care or placebo.[67,73,74] A 2014 systematic review on pressure ulcers alone found moderate evidence that electrical stimulation is effective, with low risk of adverse effects and substantial savings in health care costs.[68] Two systematic reviews with meta-analysis, one published in 2014 and the other in 2015, specifically examining the impact of electrical stimulation on pressure ulcers in individuals with spinal cord injury found mixed results.[66,75] The 2014 meta-analysis came to no firm conclusion, and the 2015 meta-analysis concluded that electrical stimulation significantly decreased pressure ulcer size compared with standard wound care or sham stimulation and increased the likelihood of complete wound closure. A systematic review and a comparative effectiveness report from the Agency for Healthcare Research and Quality (AHRQ) evaluating all treatments for pressure ulcers concluded that electrical stimulation was one of the interventions that improve pressure ulcer healing but found no clear evidence to recommend one intervention, or any particular combination of interventions, over another.[76,77] More recent reviews have focused on HVPC and confirm earlier conclusions that applying electrical stimulation to chronic wounds, lower extremity wounds, and pressure ulcers accelerates healing compared with placebo or standard of care.[72,78]

Intermittent application of motor-level electrical stimulation to produce muscle contractions has also been investigated as a means to prevent deep tissue injury.[79] This type of electrical stimulation can significantly reduce pressure around the tuberosities, produce significant and long-lasting elevations in tissue oxygenation, and significantly reduce discomfort produced by prolonged sitting, performing as well as or better than both voluntary contractions and chair push-ups.

EDEMA CONTROL

Edema is a normal physiological response after tissue trauma. Edema can have protective effects, including splinting the injured area and being a component of the first stage of tissue healing, inflammation. However, edema is also associated with increased pain, decreased function, and prolonged recovery.[80] Edema management can expedite return to activities from acute injuries such as joint sprains and strains, and certain electrical stimulation can reduce inflammation-associated edema at least as well as nonsteroidal antiinflammatory medications such as ibuprofen, with fewer risks.[81]

Edema is an accumulation of fluid that produces swelling. There are several potential causes of edema, including systemic disorders, inflammation, and lack of motion. Edema caused by systemic disorders such as heart failure, liver failure, or kidney failure generally causes symmetrical swelling in the dependent distal extremities, particularly the legs, and can also cause fluid to accumulate in the lungs (pulmonary edema) and abdomen (ascites). Electrical stimulation should not be used to treat edema suspected to have a systemic cause because this intervention may drive fluid from the extremities into the central circulation, further overwhelming the failing organ system and increasing the risk of pulmonary edema. Electrical stimulation may be used to treat edema caused by inflammation or by lack of motion.

Edema Due to Inflammation

Edema can form directly after an acute injury as part of the inflammatory response. An area with this type of edema will appear red and feel warm. The application of electrical stimulation to control this type of edema was studied extensively by Fish, Mendel, and colleagues in animal models.[82–88] A 2010 systematic review concluded that HVPC may curb edema formation after acute injury, although this conclusion was based primarily on studies of intentional injury in animals.[80] This review specifically supported the use of HVPC administered using negative polarity, with a pulse frequency of 120 pulses/second and an intensity of 90% of that which produces a visible motor contraction, administered for four 30-minute sessions 4 hours apart or for one continuous 180-minute session. A 2011 review of treatments for acute edema associated with burns also supported the benefits of electrical stimulation to reduce edema formation.[88] Although studies show that applying electrical stimulation during the inflammatory response can retard the formation of edema, they have not clearly shown that this treatment reduces the amount of edema already present or accelerates return to play or activities.[89,90] Specifically, negative polarity HVPC below the threshold for motor contraction has been found to retard the formation of edema by approximately 50% compared with no treatment after acute injury in animal models.[87] The magnitude of the effect of negative polarity HVPC on the formation of acute edema is similar to that of ibuprofen[81] or cool-water immersion.[91] Positive polarity HVPC[86] has not been found to be effective for this application. Studies of biphasic currents have yielded mixed results, with one study finding no benefit[92] but another more recent pilot study suggesting that this intervention may help reduce edema following acute ankle sprains.[93]

Several mechanisms for how negative polarity HVPC retards edema formation associated with inflammation have been suggested. The negative charge can repel negatively charged serum proteins, essentially blocking their movement out of blood vessels. The current may also reduce pore size in microvessel walls, thereby preventing large plasma proteins from leaking through the pores.[94] Keeping proteins within the vessels would create osmotic pressure, keeping fluid in the vessels. In the normal histamine response to acute trauma, these pores would be enlarged. However, because both negative polarity and positive polarity HVPC decrease microvessel permeability, some other mechanism likely underlies the reduced edema formation associated only with negative polarity stimulation. The current may also decrease

blood flow by reducing microvessel diameter, although this is unlikely because negative polarity stimulation has not been shown to affect microvessel diameter.[95]

Edema Due to Lack of Muscle Contraction

The use of electrical stimulation to control edema caused by lack of muscle contraction is also discussed in Chapter 12 as one of the clinical applications of neuromuscular electrical stimulation (NMES). When edema forms because of a lack of muscle contraction, electrical stimulation is applied to produce muscle contractions in order to reduce edema caused by poor peripheral circulation due to lack of motion.[96–98]

A lack of muscle contractions, particularly in a dependent limb, causes edema to form in the distal extremities because the muscles fail to pump fluid proximally through the veins and lymphatics. Contraction of the limb muscles is needed to compress the veins and lymphatic vessels to promote the return flow of fluid from the periphery. If the muscles do not contract, fluid, in the form of edema, accumulates. An area with this type of edema will appear pale and will feel cool. Edema of this type can be treated by applying motor-level electrical stimulation to the muscles around the main draining veins. Motor-level electrical stimulation, in conjunction with elevating the legs, has been shown to increase popliteal blood flow in healthy subjects and in subjects with a history of lower limb surgery or thromboembolism[99] and to reduce the increase in foot and ankle volume produced in healthy volunteers after standing motionless for 30 minutes.[94] Motor-level stimulation alone has also been found to reduce edema in patients with chronic venous disease.[100,101] In contrast, sensory-level electrical stimulation has not been found to be effective for this application.[92] To control edema, NMES should be applied in conjunction with elevation and followed by the use of a compression garment (see Chapter 21).

The improvement in blood flow produced by NMES[98,102,103] can also accelerate tissue healing and help reduce the risk of deep venous thrombosis (DVT) formation.[104–106] Motor-level NMES of the calf muscles has been found to be 1.7 to 3 times more effective than intermittent pneumatic compression for promoting venous circulation, suggesting this could be a more convenient and effective way to prevent DVTs.[107,108] Even NMES of just the foot is as effective in promoting venous circulation[98] and preventing DVTs as intermittent pneumatic compression.[109]

TRANSDERMAL DRUG DELIVERY: IONTOPHORESIS

The use of an electrical current to promote transdermal drug delivery is known as **iontophoresis**. Iontophoresis has been used for more than 100 years to deliver therapeutic drugs while avoiding some of the side effects associated with oral, nasal, or parenteral routes of administration. When taken orally, some drugs produce gastrointestinal distress, and others are incompletely absorbed.[110] Nasal delivery allows absorption of only low-concentration drugs, and many individuals find this route of administration uncomfortable. Injections and infusions carry risks of injection-site reactions and require professional administration or monitoring. Therefore transdermal delivery is an attractive alternative if the compound can get through the skin and can be absorbed at sufficiently high rates and concentrations to be effective.

Iontophoresis is the use of low-amplitude DC to facilitate transdermal drug delivery. The use of iontophoresis was first reported in the early 1900s.[111,112] Iontophoresis works in part because like charges repel, and therefore a fixed-charge electrode on the skin can "push" the charged ions of a drug through the skin. Iontophoresis, similar to phonophoresis, may also promote transdermal drug penetration by increasing the permeability of the outermost layer of the skin, the stratum corneum, the main barrier to transdermal drug uptake. The most common use of iontophoresis in rehabilitation is to apply dexamethasone, an antiinflammatory corticosteroid.[113]

> ### ◎ Clinical Pearl
> Iontophoresis uses low-amplitude DC to facilitate the delivery of medications through the skin.

The depth to which a drug is delivered by iontophoresis is uncertain. Studies have clearly shown penetration through the skin.[114,115] Most studies support penetration to a depth of 3 to 20 mm.[116] For example, lidocaine could be detected 5 mm below the surface of the skin in humans when delivered by iontophoresis, together with epinephrine, to maintain local vasoconstriction and thus keep the drug in the local area.[117] Iontophoresis can also be used to deliver drugs systemically because once a drug crosses the skin barrier, it will enter the bloodstream, which then distributes it throughout the body.[118]

For an electrical current to facilitate transdermal drug penetration, the current must be at least sufficient to overcome the combined resistance of the skin and the electrode being used.[119] The amount of electricity used for iontophoresis is described, according to charge, in units of milliamp minutes (mA-min). A mA-min is the product of the current amplitude, measured in milliamps, and the time, measured in minutes. The number of mA-min recommended for a particular application depends on the specific electrode being used and is determined by the electrode manufacturer. At the present time, most manufacturers support using 40 or 80 mA-min for each iontophoresis treatment, with some recommending 120 mA-min for each treatment.[118,120] Historically, iontophoresis was applied by using higher-current amplitudes, in the range of 1 to 4 mA, applied by a portable device to special-purpose disposable electrodes. This current was applied for about 10 to 40 minutes during clinic visits. Today, iontophoresis is usually applied with much lower current amplitudes, in the microamp range, over longer periods of time (hours). This is done with self-powered special-purpose disposable iontophoresis electrodes applied in the clinic and that the patient wears at home for the recommended number of hours and then removes and discards.

Many drugs can be delivered by iontophoresis, as long as they can be ionized and are stable in solution, they are not altered by the application of an electrical current, and their ions are small or moderate in size. Different drugs have been administered by iontophoresis to treat different pathologies (Table 14.1). At the present time, the manufacturers of iontophoresis electrodes recommend using iontophoresis only to deliver dexamethasone. However, the use of other substances, such as acetic acid for the treatment of recalcitrant scarring, calcific tendinitis, or heel pain, has been reported.[121–123] Dexamethasone is a corticosteroid with antiinflammatory effects. Dexamethasone iontophoresis has been found to be more effective than placebo or injection in the treatment of lateral epicondylitis[124,125] and plantar fasciitis[113,126,127] and may be effective for treating other local inflammatory disorders.[128] Dexamethasone is delivered by iontophoresis using a 0.4% solution of dexamethasone sodium phosphate in the negative polarity electrode. The negative polarity electrode is used to promote penetration of the negatively charged dexamethasone phosphate ion through the skin (Fig. 14.1). The delivery of other medications by iontophoresis, such as the nonsteroidal antiinflammatory drugs naproxen and ketoprofen to control inflammation and the synthetic opiate analgesic fentanyl to control pain, has also been studied.[129,130] Iontophoretic delivery of naproxen was shown to reduce pain associated with lateral epicondylitis. An iontophoretic transdermal fentanyl delivery system was found to be as effective as morphine delivered by intravenous patient-controlled analgesia (PCA)

TABLE 14.1	Ions Used Clinically for Iontophoresis Including Ion Source, Polarity, Recommended Indications, and Concentration				
Ion	**Source**	**Polarity**	**Indications**	**Concentration (%)**	
Acetate	Acetic acid	Negative	Calcium deposits	2.5–5	
Chloride	NaCl	Negative	Sclerotic	2	
Copper	$CuSO_4$	Positive	Fungal infection	2	
Dexamethasone phosphate	$DexNa_2PO_3$	Negative	Inflammation	0.4	
Hyaluronidase	Wydase	Positive	Edema reduction	—	
Iodine	—	Negative	Scar	5	
Lidocaine	Lidocaine 1:50,000 with epinephrine	Positive	Local anesthetic	5	
Magnesium	$MgSO_4$	Positive	Muscle relaxant, vasodilator	—	
Salicylate	NaSal	Negative	Inflammation, plantar warts	2	
Tap water	—	Negative/positive	Hyperhidrosis	—	
Zinc	ZnO_2	Positive	Dermal ulcers, wounds	—	

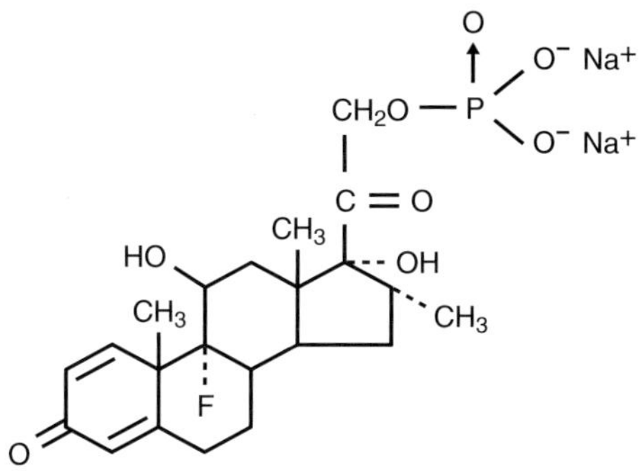

FIGURE 14.1 The molecular structure of dexamethasone sodium phosphate. The negatively charged dexamethasone phosphate ion is moved across the dermal barrier by iontophoresis using the negatively charged electrode.

for control of postoperative pain, with higher patient satisfaction, and is approved by the U.S. Food and Drug Administration for the control of postoperative pain,[131] but this device was recently withdrawn from the market in the United States and Europe.[132,133]

Much research has explored using iontophoresis to deliver a wide range of other medications, including insulin for diabetes, leuprolide for hormonal effects, calcitonin analogues for osteoporosis, cyclosporine for immunosuppression, beta blockers for hypertension, antihistamines for allergies, triptans for migraines, ondansetron for nausea and vomiting, prednisolone for bronchial asthma, zinc phthalocyanine tetrasulfonic acid for cancerous tumors, dexamethasone phosphate for dry eyes, and midazolam for pediatric sedation before surgery.[110,134–140] The primary challenges facing new applications of iontophoresis are not its ability to deliver the drug through the skin into the circulation but rather to control the precise amount of the drug that gets into the patient (bioavailability) and patient intolerance of the electrical stimulation.

Contraindications and Precautions for Electrical Currents for Tissue Healing

The standard contraindications and precautions for all electrical stimulation, as described in detail in Chapter 11, also apply to using electrical currents for tissue healing. For more detailed information on these contraindications and precautions, refer to the section on contraindications and precautions for the application of electrical currents in Chapter 11.

In addition to the standard contraindications for all electrical stimulation, do not use electrical currents for wound healing when there is concern for malignancy. Iontophoresis should also not be used after the application of any physical agent that may alter skin permeability, such as heat, ice, or ultrasound. Heat causes vasodilation and increased blood

flow that can accelerate dispersion of the drug from the treatment area. In addition, all contraindications and precautions for the drug being delivered must be observed.

CONTRAINDICATIONS FOR ELECTRICAL CURRENTS FOR TISSUE HEALING

✱ CONTRAINDICATIONS

For Electrical Currents for Tissue Healing

Standard contraindications for all electrical stimulation (see Chapter 11 for details):
- Demand cardiac pacemaker, implantable cardiac defibrillator (ICD), or unstable arrhythmias
- Placement of electrodes over carotid sinus
- Areas where venous or arterial thrombosis or thrombophlebitis is present
- Pregnancy—over or around the abdomen or low back (electrical stimulation may be used for pain control during labor and delivery, as discussed in Chapter 13)

Additional contraindications for electrical currents for tissue healing:
- Malignant tumors
- Do not apply iontophoresis after any intervention that is likely to alter skin permeability.

Malignant Tumors

The presence of malignant tumors is generally a precaution for electrical stimulation. However, when monophasic currents such as those typically used for wound healing are applied, the presence of malignancy is of even greater concern. This is because the galvanotaxis (directional movement of cells in response to an electrical field or charge) may affect metastasis (i.e., movement of cells from the primary tumor to other sites).[5,141]

▪ Ask the Patient
- "Have you ever had cancer? Do you have cancer now?"
- "Do you have fever, sweats, chills, or night pain?"
- "Do you have pain at rest?"
- "Have you had recent unexplained weight loss?"

Iontophoresis After Any Intervention That Is Likely to Alter Skin Permeability

Iontophoresis should not be administered after use of any physical agent that may alter skin permeability, such as heat, ice, or ultrasound, because this could alter the amount of drug that will penetrate the skin, resulting in a higher- or lower-than-intended amount of drug penetration. In addition, heat should be avoided before iontophoresis because heat causes vasodilation and increased blood flow, which will accelerate dispersion of the drug from the treatment area.

PRECAUTIONS FOR ELECTRICAL CURRENTS FOR TISSUE HEALING

★ PRECAUTIONS

for Electrical Currents for Tissue Healing

Standard precautions for all electrical stimulation (see Chapter 11 for details):
- Cardiac disease
- Impaired mentation
- Areas with impaired sensation
- Areas of skin irritation

Additional precautions for electrical currents for tissue healing:
- Infection control

Particular attention should be paid to the following when electrical current is used for tissue healing:
- Infection control
  - If electrodes are placed in wounds, a new electrode (typically gauze) should be used each time.

- Self-adhesive electrodes should be single-patient use only.
- Chronic open wounds should be kept clean but cannot be sterile.
- Protective covers for electrical stimulation devices and leads are available to minimize the transmission of communicable diseases, such as methicillin-resistant *Staphylococcus aureus* (MRSA). After these covers are used, they should be left in the patient's room.

Adverse Effects of Electrical Currents for Tissue Healing

Although electrical stimulation for wound healing is generally very safe, adverse effects have been reported, including excessive granulation formation, skin irritation, and burns when the stimulus intensity was set too high.[142,143]

Application Techniques

APPLICATION TECHNIQUE 14.1   WOUND HEALING

General guidelines for the application of electrical stimulation are provided in Chapter 11. The following information builds on this foundation, providing specific recommendations, techniques, and parameters for applying electrical stimulation for wound healing.[17] These recommendations are summarized in Table 14.2.

Patient Positioning

When electrical stimulation is applied for wound healing, position the patient so that the wound is readily visible and pressure on the wound is minimized.

Electrode Type

In general, when using electrical stimulation for wound healing, two or more electrodes are used: a treatment electrode, or electrodes, on or close to the wound and a dispersive electrode away from the wound. The dispersive electrode completes the electrical current circuit and is not considered a "treating" electrode.

For the dispersive electrode, use a large, self-adhesive, disposable electrode. For the treatment electrode, use a purpose-made electrode, form-fit to the shape of the wound. To do this, first place saline-soaked gauze directly in the wound and then cover it with a single-use disposable electrode, a multiuse carbon rubber electrode,

or a layer of heavy-duty aluminum foil. Then attach the electrode to the lead wire (Fig. 14.2). Alternatively, commercially available self-adhesive electrodes may be placed on either side of the wound (Fig. 14.3), but this approach is probably less effective.[144]

Electrode Placement

Treatment electrodes may be placed in or around the wound. One treatment electrode is used when it is placed directly in the wound; it should be contoured to fit the wound and kept moist[145] for optimal conduction. Two or more electrodes (of the same polarity) are used when applying stimulation to the area around the wound. Then place one large, dispersive electrode of opposite polarity to the treatment electrode on intact skin several inches away from the wound site. The dispersive electrode should be larger than the sum of the area of the treatment electrodes in or near the wounds. The large size allows the current to be dispersed over a greater area, making it more comfortable and safer while not limiting the intensity of the stimulation at the active electrode.

Waveform

When electrical stimulation is applied to promote tissue healing, a monophasic waveform—where the electrodes are of consistent

TABLE 14.2	Recommended Parameter Settings for Electrical Stimulation for Tissue Healing[10,17]					
Parameter Settings/ Goal of Treatment	**Waveform**	**Polarity**	**Pulse Frequency**	**Pulse Duration**	**Amplitude**	**Treatment Time**
Tissue healing: inflammatory phase/ infected	HVPC	Negative	100–105 pps	Usually preset for HVPC at ~100 µs	To produce comfortable tingling	45–60 min daily, 3–7 days/week
Tissue healing: proliferation phase/clean	HVPC	Positive	100–105 pps	Usually preset for HVPC at ~100 µs	To produce comfortable tingling	45–60 min daily, 3–7 days/week

HVPC, High-voltage pulsed current; *pps,* pulses per second.

APPLICATION TECHNIQUE 14.1—cont'd

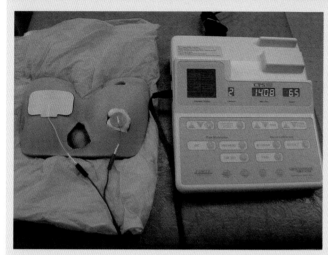

FIGURE 14.2 Electrode placement to promote tissue healing, with treatment electrode in the wound.

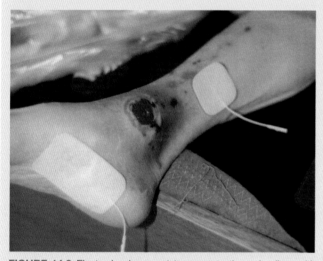

FIGURE 14.3 Electrode placement to promote tissue healing, with treatment electrodes on either side of the wound.

opposite polarity—is generally recommended. HVPC, a **monophasic pulsed current** (Fig. 14.4), was used in most studies that showed benefit for this application and is likely to be most effective.[74] Although a few studies have found low-intensity DC (LIDC), pulsed biphasic, and AC waveforms to promote wound healing, they are generally less so,[146] have a slightly higher risk of burns, and less closely mimic the endogenous current of injury.[68] Other parameter recommendations for the HVPC waveform are provided later in the chapter.

Polarity

The polarity of the electrode on or nearest to the wound is selected according to the types of cells required to advance a particular stage of wound healing and based on whether the wound is or is not infected or inflamed.[13] Although either positive or negative polarity

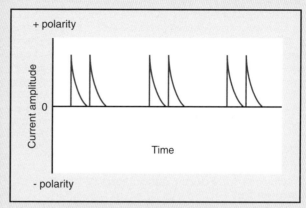

FIGURE 14.4 High-voltage pulsed current.

stimulation has been found to be more effective than placebo[64] stimulation, negative polarity is generally recommended during the early inflammatory stage of healing, whereas positive polarity is recommended for use later to facilitate epithelial cell migration across the wound bed. Kloth recommends using negative polarity for the first 3 to 7 days of treatment and changing to positive polarity thereafter.[61,62,147] Another recommendation is to use negative polarity initially and for 3 days after the wound bed becomes free of necrotic tissue and the drainage becomes serosanguineous and thereafter use positive polarity.[148,149] Consistent with many recommendations, most clinicians use negative polarity initially or when the wound shows signs of inflammation and switch polarity when there are no signs of inflammation or when wound healing plateaus.

Pulse Duration

When HVPC is used to promote wound healing, the recommended **pulse duration** is between 40 and 200 μs.[13] With most stimulators that deliver HVPC, the pulse duration for this waveform is set in the device to approximately 70 to 100 μs by the manufacturer and cannot be changed by the clinician. With other monophasic pulsed currents, the pulse duration can usually be adjusted.

Frequency

When used to promote tissue healing, the pulse **frequency** should be 60 to 125 pps.

On:Off Time

When used to promote tissue healing, the electrical stimulation is delivered continuously throughout the treatment time, with no off time.

Current Amplitude

When used to promote tissue healing, the current **amplitude** should be sufficient to produce a comfortable sensation without a motor response. If the patient has decreased or altered sensation in the treatment area, the appropriate amplitude can be determined by first applying the electrode to another area of normal, intact sensation.

Treatment Time

When used to promote tissue healing, most studies have applied the stimulation at least 5 days each week, with each treatment lasting 45 to 60 minutes.

APPLICATION TECHNIQUE 14.2   EDEMA CONTROL

When electrical stimulation is used to control edema, the therapist must determine whether the edema is caused by acute inflammation, lack of muscle contraction, or systemic causes (e.g., heart, kidney, or liver failure). Electrical stimulation can be used to treat edema associated with acute inflammation or lack of muscle contraction, but different parameters must be used for these different types of edema. Electrical stimulation should not be used to treat edema with other causes. Patients with edema with other causes should be evaluated by a medical provider. The parameters used for electrical stimulation for control of edema associated with acute inflammation or lack of muscle contraction are detailed here and are summarized in Table 14.3.

Parameters for Edema Associated With Inflammation

Electrical currents can be used to control edema associated with inflammation. Note that the following recommendations apply only when edema is caused by inflammation and not when edema and circulatory compromise are caused by a lack of muscle activity. The information presented here on application techniques to control edema caused by lack of muscle contraction is also presented in Chapter 12 for the reader's convenience.

Patient Positioning

When using electrical stimulation to inhibit the formation of edema associated with inflammation, the patient should be positioned with the involved area elevated to help promote the flow of fluid out of the extremity to the central circulation. Ice and compression may also be applied to further control inflammation and edema.

Electrode Type

In general, when using electrical stimulation to inhibit the formation of edema associated with inflammation, self-adhesive disposable electrodes are recommended.

Electrode Placement

The negative polarity treatment electrodes should be placed directly over the area of edema, with the dispersive electrode placed over another large, flat area near the area of edema (Fig. 14.5).

Waveform

HVPC is the recommended waveform.

Pulse Duration

The pulse duration for HVPC is usually fixed by the manufacturer in the range of 40 to 100 μs.

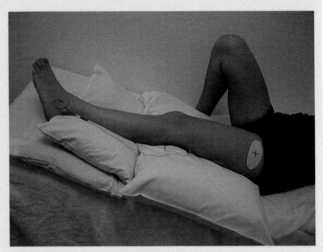

FIGURE 14.5 Electrode placement to retard acute edema formation at the ankle.

Polarity

The negative polarity electrode should be placed over the area of edema.

Frequency

The pulse frequency should be set to 120 pps.[80]

On:Off Time

Electrical stimulation is delivered continuously throughout the treatment time.

Current Amplitude

The current amplitude should be set to 90% of the visually observable motor threshold.

Treatment Time

Electrical stimulation is generally applied for 30 minutes per session and may be used more than once a day, up to every 4 hours.

Parameters for Control of Edema Associated With Lack of Muscle Contraction

Electrically stimulated muscle contractions can also be used to help control edema and improve circulation when edema and poor circulation are caused by a lack of muscle activity. Note that the following

---

TABLE 14.3	Recommended Parameter Settings for Electrical Stimulation for Edema Control					
Parameter Settings/ Goal of Treatment	Waveform	Polarity	Pulse Frequency	Pulse Duration	Amplitude	Treatment Time
Edema control: for edema associated with inflammation	HVPC	Negative	120 pps	Usually preset for HVPC at 40–100 μs	90% of visual-motor threshold	30 min
Edema control: for edema associated with lack of motion	Biphasic (can use interferential if on:off time available)	NA	35–50 pps, 2–5 s equal on:off times	150–350 μs	To visible contraction	20–30 min

HVPC, High-voltage pulsed current; *NA,* not applicable; *pps,* pulses per second.

APPLICATION TECHNIQUE 14.2—*cont'd*

recommendations apply *only* when edema and circulatory compromise are caused by a lack of muscle activity and *not* when edema is caused by inflammation. The information presented here concerning the control of edema caused by lack of muscle contraction is also presented in Chapter 12 for the reader's convenience.

Patient Positioning

When electrically stimulated muscle contractions are used to control edema or promote circulation caused by a lack of muscle activity, the patient should be positioned with the involved area elevated to help promote the flow of fluid out of the extremity to the central circulation. In this circumstance, the electrically stimulated muscle contractions facilitate edema control and promote circulation by intermittently compressing the veins and lymphatics to promote venous and lymphatic return.

Electrode Type

In general, when using electrical stimulation for muscle contractions to facilitate edema control and promote circulation, self-adhesive disposable electrodes are recommended.

Electrode Placement

The electrodes should be placed on the muscles around the main veins draining the area (Fig. 14.6). For example, with edema in the foot, the electrodes should be placed on the calf of the same side.

Waveform

A pulsed biphasic waveform or **Russian protocol** is recommended.

Pulse Duration

When a pulsed biphasic waveform is used, the pulse duration should be between 150 and 350 μs—sufficient to produce a muscle contraction. When the Russian protocol is used, the cycle duration cannot be adjusted.

Frequency and On:Off Time

When using electrically stimulated muscle contractions to control edema caused by disuse, the goal is to produce short, low-force,

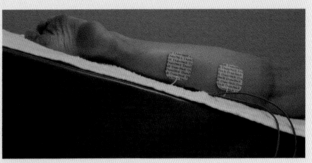

FIGURE 14.6 Electrode placement for neuromuscular electrical stimulation to control edema caused by lack of muscle activity.

repetitive muscle contractions to pump fluid through the vessels. There are two different ways to achieve this:

1. If you have a device that allows you to set an **on:off time,** set the pulse frequency at 35 to 50 pps, as used to produce muscle contractions for other purposes. Then set both the on time and the off time at 1 to 2 seconds. This will produce tetanic contractions lasting 1 to 2 seconds with 1 to 2 seconds of relaxation between contractions.
2. If you have a device that does not allow you to set an on:off time, set the pulse frequency at 1 to 2 pps. This will produce one to two twitch contractions each second with relaxation between contractions.

Current Amplitude

The current amplitude should be sufficient to produce a small, visible muscle contraction.

Treatment Time

The stimulation is generally applied for 20 to 30 minutes per session but may be used more than once a day if needed to control edema.[100]

APPLICATION TECHNIQUE 14.3   IONTOPHORESIS

The parameters used for electrical stimulation for iontophoresis are discussed in detail here and are summarized in Table 14.4.

Patient Positioning

When electrical stimulation is applied for iontophoresis, the patient should be positioned comfortably, with the locations for both electrodes clearly visible by the clinician.

Electrode Type

Two distinct types of electrodes can be used for iontophoresis. Historically, iontophoresis was delivered with a powered controller connected to two electrodes (Fig. 14.7). With this setup, the dispersive electrode is a self-adhesive transmissive electrode, and the treatment electrode is a self-adhesive electrode that can be filled with the medi-

TABLE 14.4   Recommended Parameter Settings for Electrical Stimulation for Iontophoresis

Parameter Settings/Goal of Treatment	Waveform	Pulse Frequency	Pulse Duration	Amplitude	Active Electrode Polarity	Treatment Time
Iontophoresis	DC	NA	NA	To patient tolerance, no greater than 4 mA	Same as drug ion (see Table 14.1)	Depends on amplitude, to produce a total of 40 mA-min

DC, Direct current; *NA,* not applicable.

Continued

APPLICATION TECHNIQUE 14.3—*cont'd*

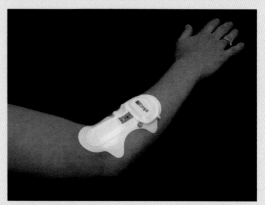

FIGURE 14.8 A 24-hour iontophoresis patch.

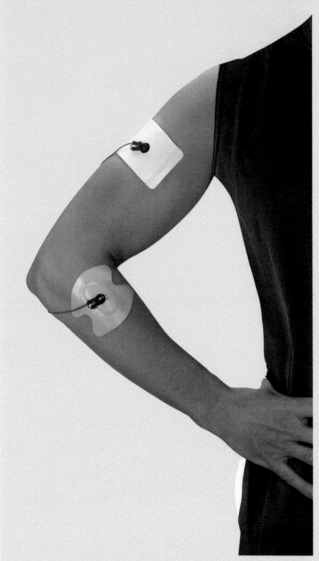

FIGURE 14.7 Electrode placement for iontophoresis with a wired unit.

over a large muscle or the belly. The electrode should be large enough that the **current density** does not exceed 0.5 mA/cm² when the negatively charged electrode is used as the delivery electrode and does not exceed 1.0 mA/cm² when the positively charged electrode is used.[61] When low-voltage patch electrodes are used, the negative and positive polarity electrodes are at either end of the same patch.

Polarity

For iontophoresis, the drug delivery electrode should have the same polarity as the active ion of the drug to be delivered.

Current Amplitude and Treatment Time

As discussed earlier, for iontophoresis, the dose of electricity is determined by the current (amperage) multiplied by the time, such as 40 mA-min. A number of combinations of current and time can be used to achieve this dose, including 1-mA current for 40 minutes, 4-mA current for 10 minutes, or 100-μA current for 400 minutes (6 hours and 40 minutes; Table 14.5). In practice, with a battery-powered controller, the current amplitude should be set to patient comfort at a maximum of 4 mA, and then the device will adjust the treatment time to produce the intended dose. It is important to check the patient's skin during this treatment because the ionic effects of

cation solution. Now, iontophoresis is more often delivered with self-powered low-voltage, low-current electrodes with no separate controller (Fig. 14.8). With this setup, a single self-adhesive patch contains both electrodes as well as the power source. When the electrode surfaces are wetted, the active polarity with the medication and the other with water, and attached to the skin, the battery activates, initiating transmission of the drug. The patch can be worn under clothing and requires no machine or external battery.

Electrode Placement

For iontophoresis, the drug delivery electrode is placed over the area of pathology. When a battery-powered controller with wired electrodes is used, the dispersive or return electrode is placed a few inches away from the treatment electrode at a site of convenience

TABLE 14.5	Examples of Different Combinations of Current Amplitude and Treatment Duration to Achieve 40- to 80-mA-min Iontophoresis Treatment Doses	
Current Amplitude	Treatment Time, min	Dose, mA-min
1 mA	40 minutes	40
4 mA	10 minutes	40
4 mA	20 minutes	80
100 μA	400 minutes (6 hours and 40 minutes)	40
100 μA	800 minutes (13 hours and 20 minutes)	80
200 μA	400 minutes	80

APPLICATION TECHNIQUE 14.3—cont'd

DC and the small electrodes used for iontophoresis produce a high current density, increasing the risk of burning the patient.

With low-voltage patch electrodes, the current amplitude is in the μA range and is preset by the manufacturer. The manufacturer will also provide instructions for the required wear time to achieve the intended mA-min treatment dose. Some research supports that with the equivalent mA-min dose, longer delivery with lower current delivers drug more effectively than shorter delivery at higher current.[120] Reducing the current amplitude also helps decrease the risk of local adverse effects, including pain, skin irritation, and chemical burns. This type of application also shortens the time spent by the patient in the clinic for this treatment.

Documentation

Documentation is generally written in the form of a SOAP note. When using electrical stimulation to reduce edema or for tissue healing, document the following:

- The area of the body to be treated
- Patient positioning
- Specific stimulation parameters
- Electrode placement
- Treatment duration
- Patient's response and response of the wound to treatment, including the condition of the skin and surrounding areas

The level of detail should be sufficient for another clinician to be able to reproduce the treatment using your notes.

EXAMPLES

When applying electrical stimulation (ES) to a full-thickness venous ulcer on the left lateral ankle, document the following:

S: Pt alert and oriented × 3. She states she has been keeping her L lower extremity elevated as much as possible because the edema in her L ankle increases with dependent positioning.

O: Intervention: Pt supine with 2 pillows under L leg for elevation. HVPC to L lower extremity × 1 h. Saline-soaked gauze treating electrode placed in wound, dispersive electrode placed on proximal posterior calf. Frequency 100 pps, negative polarity to treatment area, intensity to sensory level.

Posttreatment: Wound area decreased from 10 × 5 cm on first treatment 3 weeks ago to 8 × 3 cm today.

A: Pt tolerated treatment well. Wound size decreasing.

P: Continue HVPC to L lateral ankle area until wound closes. Change polarity if healing plateaus.

CLINICAL CASE STUDIES

The following case studies demonstrate the concepts of the clinical application of electrical stimulation discussed in this chapter. Based on the scenario presented, an evaluation of the clinical findings and goals of treatment are proposed. These are followed by a discussion of the factors to be considered in the selection of electrical stimulation as an indicated intervention and in the selection of the ideal electrical stimulation parameters to promote progress toward the set goals of treatment.

CASE STUDY 14.1

Lateral Ankle Sprain
Examination

History

MC is a 23-year-old student. He injured his left ankle during a soccer game at school earlier today. He was seen by the attending physician on the field and diagnosed with a grade II lateral ankle sprain. Ice was applied to MC's ankle, and he was sent to the locker room for immediate physical therapy follow-up. The physician instructed MC to use non–weight-bearing crutches to rest the injured ankle.

Systems Review

MC reports disappointment in his inability to finish the soccer season. Visual inspection shows MC is holding his ankle in a single position and expresses extreme hesitancy in allowing the therapist to move the joint. MC is otherwise healthy and denies a history of cancer, diabetes, or other significant health problems.

Tests and Measures

Gentle passive range of motion (PROM) reveals restrictions in all directions. Active range of motion (AROM) is minimal. The lateral talofibular joint is tender to touch, with discoloration indicating internal bleeding along the lateral surface and an inability to view the lateral malleolus because of swelling. The area is warm to the touch and slightly reddened.

What kind of process is occurring in this patient's ankle? What kind of electrical stimulation would be most useful? What aspects of the patient's injury would electrical stimulation address? What other physical agent may be used along with electrical stimulation?

Continued

CLINICAL CASE STUDIES—cont'd

Evaluation and Goals

ICF Level	Current Status	Goals
Body structure and function	Left ankle pain, edema, and decreased ROM	Control edema and pain Accelerate resolution of acute inflammatory phase of healing Increase ROM
Activity	Limited ambulation	Increase ambulation
Participation	Unable to play soccer	Return to playing soccer

ICF, International Classification for Functioning, Disability and Health; *ROM,* range of motion.

◆ FIND THE EVIDENCE

PICO Terms	Natural Language Example	Sample PubMed Search
P (Population)	Patient with pain due to sprained ankle	("sprained ankle" [text word] OR "ankle sprain" [text word] OR "Ankle Injuries" [MeSH])
I (Intervention)	Electrical stimulation	AND ("Electric Stimulation Therapy" [text word] OR "electrical currents" [text word] OR "electrical stimulation" [text word])
C (Comparison)	No electrical stimulation	
O (Outcome)	Control pain and restore function	

Key Studies or Reviews

1. Snyder AR, Perotti AL, Lam KC, et al: The influence of high-voltage electrical stimulation on edema formation after acute injury: a systematic review. *J Sport Rehabil* 19:436–451, 2010.

   This systematic review of the literature concluded that HVPC may be effective in curbing edema formation after acute injury, although this conclusion is based primarily on studies of intentional injury in animals.[80] This review specifically supported the use of HVPC administered using negative polarity, with a pulse frequency of 120 pulses/s and an intensity of 90% of the visually observed motor contraction, administered for four 30-minute sessions 4 hours apart or one continuous 180-minute session.

2. Feger MA, Goetschius J, Love H, et al: Electrical stimulation as a treatment intervention to improve function, edema or pain following acute lateral ankle sprains: a systematic review. *Phys Ther Sport* 16:361–369, 2015.

   This systematic review included four randomized controlled trials of electrical stimulation for acute ankle sprains. Overall, the authors did not find a benefit of electrical stimulation for improving function, edema, or pain following acute lateral ankle sprains. However, one

of the studies used submotor biphasic NMES,[92] which would not be expected to be effective. One of the HVPC studies used subsensory cathodal stimulation continuously for 72 hours,[89] which is likely an insufficient intensity and excessive duration. Another HVPC study found no difference in outcomes between three groups of 10 patients each, where one group used ice alone, the other used ice with negative polarity submotor stimulation at 28 pps, and the third used ice with negative polarity submotor stimulation at 80 pps.[150] The other HVPC study, with 28 subjects in three groups (control, submotor positive polarity HVPC, submotor negative polarity HVPC) with HVPC applied for 30 minutes, found that subjects who received negative polarity HVPC had greater reductions in volume and girth, had greater recovery of range of motion and gait velocity, and recovered faster than the subjects in the other two groups.[90]

Prognosis

Given the mechanism of MC's injury, an active inflammatory process is most likely occurring. Electrical stimulation using negative polarity HVPC would be an appropriate choice of treatment because it has been shown to retard the formation of edema during the inflammatory stage of healing and may specifically accelerate recovery after acute ankle sprains and help control pain. Nothing in the patient's history indicates a contraindication to using electrical stimulation.

Intervention

Electrical stimulation using HVPC waveform is chosen based on the literature indicating that it is effective in decreasing edema formation after injury (see Fig. 14.4). The following parameters are chosen:

Type	Parameter
Electrode placement	One or two treating electrodes may be used over the swollen, discolored area. (Polarity is negative for treating electrodes.) The larger dispersive electrode is placed proximally over the calf or the quadriceps. This may be based on comfort or other suspected areas of swelling. Ice may be added over the electrodes to further inhibit the formation of edema.
Pulse duration	Generally fixed at 40–100 μs for HVPC
Pulse frequency	120 pps
Mode	Continuous
Amplitude	Sensory *only.* Ask the patient to state when a tingling or vibratory sensation just begins to occur. Continue to increase the amplitude until it reaches the maximum tolerable level or a contraction is seen. Then decrease the amplitude by approximately 10%.
Treatment time	30 min, up to every 4 h for up to 72 hours after the injury

HVPC, High-voltage pulsed current.

CLINICAL CASE STUDIES—*cont'd*

Documentation

S: Pt reports severe (9/10) L ankle pain immediately after injuring himself playing soccer.

O: Pretreatment: Pt unable to bear weight. L ankle PROM limited in all directions. Edema and discoloration over lateral L ankle.

Intervention: One treating electrode, negative polarity, placed over lateral L ankle; one dispersive electrode on L calf. HVPC at 120 pps, continuous. Amplitude 90% motor threshold, sensory only, × 30 min.

Posttreatment: Pain 5/10. Mildly increased L ankle PROM. Pt unable to bear weight.

A: Pt tolerated ES well, with decreased pain and increased PROM.

P: Continue treatment two to three times daily × 30 min. Pt should remain non–weight bearing and should apply ice and elevation to L ankle.

CASE STUDY 14.2

Chronic Wound Healing
Examination
History

BT is a 72-year-old, wheelchair-bound nursing home resident who is referred to the clinic with a stage III pressure ulcer on his left buttock over his left ischial tuberosity. He recently had his right great toe amputated owing to his diabetes and has been recovering slowly. For the past month, the nursing staff has been debriding and cleaning the wound, monitoring nutrition status, frequently repositioning him, and changing the dressings on his left buttock wound following standard wound care protocols. Although the pressure ulcer has not increased in depth or size, it has not shown any signs of healing. To avoid excessive pressure on his left buttock, BT has been advised to minimize his time sitting, including in his wheelchair.

Systems Review

BT is very limited in his mobility and cannot participate in most community activities. He reports instant fatigue when attempting to practice exercises in his wheelchair and occasional shortness of breath. He acknowledges that his mood has been negatively affected in recent months but is eager to begin new treatment

Tests and Measures

BT states that his pain is 6/10. Pressure ulcer 3 × 4 cm, stage III, is present on left buttock, clean but without granulation tissue. Surrounding skin is intact but tender to palpation.

Why would electrical stimulation be beneficial for this patient? What kind of electrical stimulation should be used? What other physical agents might be used?

Evaluation and Goals

ICF Level	Current Status	Goals
Body structure and function	Left buttock stage III pressure ulcer	Control pain, reduce size of ulcer Increase ROM
Activity	Limited sitting tolerance	Increase sitting tolerance
	Limited mobility in wheelchair	Increase mobility in wheelchair
Participation	Limited participation in community activities requiring sitting (e.g., meals, games)	Return to prior level of community participation in group activities requiring sitting including meals and games

ICF, International Classification for Functioning, Disability and Health; *ROM,* range of motion.

FIND THE EVIDENCE

PICO Terms	Natural Language Example	Sample PubMed Search
P (Population)	Patient with pressure ulcer	("pressure ulcer" [text word] OR "Pressure Ulcer" [MeSH])
I (Intervention)	Electrical stimulation	AND ("Electric Stimulation Therapy" [text word] OR "electrical currents" [text word] OR "electrical stimulation" [text word])
C (Comparison)	No electrical stimulation	
O (Outcome)	Wound closure or healing	AND "treatment" [text word]

Key Studies or Reviews

1. Girgis B, Duarte JA: High voltage monophasic pulsed current (HVMPC) for stage II-IV pressure ulcer healing. A systematic review and meta-analysis. *J Tissue Viability* 27(4):274–284, 2018.

   Eleven studies examining the impact of HVPC on the reduction of wound surface area in pressure ulcers were included in this review. There were nine randomized controlled trials and two case studies. The authors concluded that HVPC plus standard wound care was better than standard wound care alone or standard wound care plus placebo HVPC in reducing wound surface area. Additionally, HVPC "increased the probability of complete healing and almost eliminated the probability of worsening of healing." The authors also concluded that HVPC was safe, based on a low incidence of adverse reactions.

Continued

CLINICAL CASE STUDIES—cont'd

2. Saha S, Smith MEB, Totten A, et al: *Pressure ulcer treatment strategies: comparative effectiveness.* Report No. 13-EHC003-EF. AHRQ Comparative Effectiveness Reviews, Rockville, MD, 2013, Agency for Healthcare Research and Quality.

   This Agency for Healthcare Research and Quality (AHRQ) review evaluated articles on the treatment of pressure ulcers published between 1985 and 2012. The review found moderate-strength evidence that electrical stimulation improves pressure ulcer healing.

Prognosis

Electrical stimulation would be an appropriate addition to the care BT is already receiving because it can accelerate healing his wound and decrease pain. BT has no contraindications for electrical stimulation. However, care should be taken when increasing amplitude to ensure adequate sensation in the area because of his diabetes.

Intervention

Electrical stimulation with HVPC can be used to reduce the size and depth of the patient's pressure ulcer, in addition to providing conventional wound care interventions. This may help to control some of the pain associated with his ulcer. Recommended parameters are as follows:

Type	Parameter
Waveform	HVPC
Electrode placement	One negative electrode in the ulcer. A larger, positively charged dispersive electrode is placed over the low back.
Pulse duration	Generally fixed at 40–100 µs for HVPC
Pulse frequency	100 pps
Mode	Continuous
Amplitude	Sensory *only*. Ask the patient to state when a tingling or vibratory sensation just begins to occur. Continue to increase the amplitude until it reaches the maximum tolerable level. If a contraction is seen, decrease the amplitude.
Treatment time	45–60 min, 5 days/week

HVPC, High-voltage pulsed current.

Documentation

S: *Pt reports pain and discomfort on left buttocks due to pressure ulcer after great toe amputation and subsequent confinement to wheelchair. Pt alert and oriented × 3. Pt states he is taking acetaminophen for pain.*

O: **Pretreatment:** *L buttock pain 6/10, full-thickness stage III wound, 3 × 4 cm, 1 cm deep, clean but without granulation tissue. Surrounding skin intact but tender to palpation.*

Intervention: *ES with HVPC waveform, 1 negative electrode in wound, 1 dispersive electrode over low back. 120 pps, sensory level 60 min.*

Posttreatment: *Pt reports decrease of pain to 4/10.*

A: *Pt tolerated ES with decreased pain.*

P: *Continue ES 5 days/week for 60 min. Monitor closely for wound changes. Change polarity if healing plateaus.*

CASE STUDY 14.3

Lateral Epicondylitis
Examination
History

TO is a 42-year-old administrative assistant who is referred to therapy with a diagnosis of right lateral epicondylitis. She usually plays golf and tennis on the weekends and reports that a significant part of her workday is spent typing on a computer. Her pain developed 1 week ago after she participated in an all-day tennis tournament. She now has trouble gripping and shaking hands. If she has to hold things for any period of time, the pain increases, especially if the objects are heavy (e.g., books). She notes that her pain is not resolving and is interfering with her ability to sleep, work, and participate in sports. She has taken the last 3 days off work. She has moderate pain with typing for longer than 10 minutes and moderate pain with gripping. She is unable to play tennis because of the pain.

Systems Review

TO reports frustration with her current inability to grip the steering wheel to drive independently. TO reports no history of previous musculoskeletal pain. She has no history of depression or anxiety and reports having a strong social support network. No radiating pain from elbow is visibly present at resting state.

Tests and Measurements

TO states that her elbow pain is consistently 5/10 but increases to 7/10 with any activity. Her grip strength in her involved hand is 15 kg, and it is 24 kg in her uninvolved hand, as measured by a dynamometer. Her wrist flexion strength is 4+/5 with pain at end-range. Her wrist extension strength is 4/5 with pain. TO is tender to palpation directly over the lateral epicondyle. Her PROM is within normal limits. Her AROM is within normal limits but with pain at end-range of both flexion and extension.

Why is this patient a candidate for electrical stimulation? What type of electrical stimulation would you select and why? What else should be included in her treatment plan? What other physical agents might be helpful?

Evaluation and Goals

ICF Level	Current Status	Goals
Body structure and function	Right elbow pain, wrist weakness, and decreased ROM	Control pain Increase strength Increase ROM
Activity	Limited gripping capacity	Increase gripping capacity

CLINICAL CASE STUDIES—*cont'd*

ICF Level	Current Status	Goals
Participation	Unable to work, hold heavy objects, grip without pain, and play tennis	Return to prior level of work activity and tennis

ICF, International Classification for Functioning, Disability and Health; *ROM,* range of motion.

◆ FIND THE EVIDENCE

PICO Terms	Natural Language Example	Sample PubMed Search
P (Population)	Patient with pain due to lateral epicondylitis	("Tennis Elbow" [MeSH] OR "tennis elbow" [text word] OR "lateral epicondylitis" [text word])
I (Intervention)	Iontophoresis	AND ("iontophoresis" [text word] OR "iontophoresis" [MeSH])
C (Comparison)	No iontophoresis	
O (Outcome)	Reduce pain and increase ROM	

Key Studies or Reviews

1. Stefanou A, Marshall N, Holdan W, et al: A randomized study comparing corticosteroid injection to corticosteroid iontophoresis for lateral epicondylitis. *J Hand Surg Am* 37:104–109, 2012.

   This study randomly assigned 82 patients with lateral epicondylitis to receive dexamethasone via iontophoresis using a self-contained patch with a 24-hour battery, a 10-mg dexamethasone injection, or a 10-mg triamcinolone injection. All patients also received the same hand therapy protocol. The patients receiving iontophoresis had statistically significant improvement in grip strength at the conclusion of hand therapy compared with baseline and were more likely to return to work without restriction. By 6-month follow-up, all groups had equivalent results for all measured outcomes. This study supports that, in combination with other therapy interventions, iontophoresis is more effective than injection at accelerating recovery from lateral epicondylitis.

2. da Luz DC, de Borba Y, Ravanello EM, et al: Iontophoresis in lateral epicondylitis: a randomized, double-blind clinical trial. *J Shoulder Elbow Surg* 28(9):1743–1749, 2019.

   This study randomly assigned 24 patients to an iontophoresis group or an electrical-stimulation-only group. The iontophoresis used a 5-mA DC for 15 minutes to deliver dexamethasone (4 mg/mL) with lidocaine, and the electrical stimulation control group had the same 5-mA DC current applied for 15 minutes with a nonmedicated current transmission medium. Both groups also received a standard program of eccentric exercises and wrist extensor stretches. Although both groups showed a reduction in pain and increased strength and function after the intervention, pain was more reduced and function was more improved in the iontophoresis group compared with the stimulation-only group. Although this study was small, it supports that iontophoresis is more effective for reducing pain and improving function than DC electrical stimulation alone in individuals with lateral epicondylitis.

3. Baktir S, Razak Ozdincler A, Kaya Mutlu E, et al: The short-term effectiveness of low-level laser, phonophoresis, and iontophoresis in patients with lateral epicondylosis. *J Hand Ther* 32(4):417–425, 2019.

   This study compared the efficacy of iontophoresis, phonophoresis, and low-level laser therapy (LLLT) in 37 individuals with lateral epicondylosis. Participants received treatment 5 times a week for 3 weeks, without any other intervention, and were evaluated for pain, function, and grip strength at the end of these 15 sessions. Both LLLT and iontophoresis were associated with significantly reduced pain, whereas phonophoresis was not. Although LLLT was associated with a slightly greater reduction in pain than iontophoresis, iontophoresis was associated with significantly improved function and grip strength, whereas LLLT was not. Although this study was small, it provides interesting data for comparing the impact of different physical agents on symptoms and function in patients with lateral epicondylitis.

Prognosis

Iontophoresis with dexamethasone, an antiinflammatory drug, would be an appropriate treatment for TO to reduce her pain and inflammation in the lateral epicondyle and improve function. This would enable her to participate in AROM exercises and passive stretching without pain, increasing her grip strength and functional ability. This patient has no contraindications for the use of electrical stimulation or dexamethasone.

Intervention

With an appropriate prescription from the referring provider, iontophoresis with dexamethasone could be used for this patient. Recommended parameters are as follows:

Type	Parameter
Iontophoresis delivery system	Low-voltage patch electrodes
Electrode placement	Negatively charged electrode loaded with dexamethasone placed on lateral epicondyle.
Polarity	Negative
Treatment time	1–24 h, depending on the design of the patch

Documentation

S: Pt reports R lateral elbow pain, increased with activity, especially gripping and playing tennis.

Continued

O: **Pretreatment:** R elbow PROM within normal limits, AROM within normal limits with pain, grip strength in R hand 20 kg (L = 24 kg), flexion strength 4+/5, extension strength 4/5.

Intervention: Iontophoresis with 0.4% dexamethasone sodium phosphate with active negative electrode over lateral epicondyle using low-voltage iontophoresis patch. Pt to keep patch on for 14 h at home and then remove.

Posttreatment: Pt able to actively flex and extend without pain. Grip strength increased in R hand to 21 kg.

A: Pt tolerated iontophoresis well with increased ROM and decreased pain. Skin under electrode sites without signs of irritation after treatment. Pt tolerated 15 min of pain-free typing posttreatment.

P: Apply ice as needed. Pt given stretching exercises to be done at home 3 or 4 times per day. Pt will monitor pain while typing, stopping before onset of pain, and will complete stretching exercises as needed during typing activity.

Chapter Review

1. Electrical stimulation promotes tissue healing by encouraging the movement and proliferation of cells.
2. Galvanotaxis is the process of attracting or repelling cells that carry a charge, and electrical stimulation facilitates this.
3. Fibroblasts are the cells that make collagen. Electrical stimulation activates fibroblasts, enhancing their replication and synthesis of DNA to accelerate wound healing.
4. Sensory-level electrical stimulation can be used to retard the formation of edema resulting from inflammation.
5. Motor-level electrical stimulation can be used to reduce edema caused by a lack of muscle contractions by improving circulation.
6. Iontophoresis is the process by which electrical current is used to promote transdermal drug delivery. It should not be applied if skin permeability has been affected by agents such as heat, ice, or ultrasound.

Glossary

Amplitude (intensity): The magnitude of current or voltage (see Fig. 11.12).

Anode: The positive electrode.

Biphasic pulsed current: A series of pulses where the charged particles move first in one direction and then in the opposite direction (see Fig. 11.4B).

Cathode: The negative electrode.

Charge: One of the basic properties of matter, which has no charge (is electrically neutral) or may be negatively (−) or positively (+) charged. Charge is noted as Q and is measured in coulombs (C). Charge is equal to current × time.

$$Q = It$$

Current density: The amount of current delivered per unit area.

Direct current (DC): A continuous, unidirectional flow of charged particles. DC is used for iontophoresis, to stimulate contractions of denervated muscle, and occasionally to facilitate wound healing (see Fig. 11.2).

Frequency: The number of cycles or pulses per second. Frequency is measured in hertz (Hz) for cycles and in pulses per second (pps) for pulses (see Fig. 11.11).

Galvanotaxis: The attraction of cells to an electrical charge.

Iontophoresis: The transcutaneous delivery of ions into the body for therapeutic purposes using an electrical current.

Monophasic pulsed current: A series of pulses where the charged particles move in only one direction (see Fig. 11.4A).

On:off time: On time is the time during which a train of pulses occurs. Off time is the time between trains of pulses when no current flows. On and off times are usually used only when electrical stimulation is used to produce muscle contractions. During on time, the muscle contracts, and during off time, it relaxes.

Polarity: The charge of an electrode that will be positive or negative with a direct or monophasic pulsed current and constantly changing with an alternating or biphasic pulsed current.

Pulse duration: The time from the beginning of the first phase of a pulse to the end of the last phase of a pulse. Pulse duration is generally expressed in microseconds ($\mu s \times 10^6$ seconds; see Fig. 11.10).

Pulsed current: An interrupted flow of charged particles where the current flows in a series of pulses separated by periods when no current flows. The current may flow in one direction only, or it may flow back and forth during each pulse; also called *pulsatile current*.

Russian protocol: A medium-frequency alternating current (AC) with a frequency of 2500 Hz delivered in 50 bursts/s. Each burst is 10 ms long and is separated from the next burst by a 10-ms interburst interval (see Fig. 11.9). This type of current is also known as *medium-frequency burst AC* (MFburstAC); when this term is used, the frequency of the medium-frequency current or of the bursts may be different from the original protocol.

Voltage: The force or pressure of electricity; the difference in electrical energy between two points that produces the electrical force capable of moving charged particles through a conductor between those two points. Voltage is noted as V and is measured in volts (V); also called *potential difference*.

References

1. Fife CE, Carter MJ, Walker D, et al: Wound care outcomes and associated cost among patients treated in US outpatient wound centers: data from the US Wound Registry. *Wounds* 24:10–17, 2012.
2. Nussbaum SR, Carter MJ, Fife CE, et al: An economic evaluation of the impact, cost, and Medicare policy implications of chronic nonhealing wounds. *Value Health* 21(1):27–32, 2018.
3. Bauer K, Rock K, Nazzal M, et al: Pressure ulcers in the United States' inpatient population from 2008 to 2012: Results of a retrospective nationwide study. *Ostomy Wound Manage* 62(11):30–38, 2016.
4. Allman RM: Pressure ulcer prevalence, incidence, risk factors, and impact. *Clin Geriatr Med* 13:421–436, 1997.
5. Mittmann N, Chan BC, Craven BC, et al: Evaluation of the cost-effectiveness of electrical stimulation therapy for pressure ulcers in spinal cord injury. *Arch Phys Med Rehabil* 92:866–872, 2011.

6. de Carmo Almeida TC, Dos Santos Figueiredo FW, Barbosa Filho VC, et al: Effects of transcutaneous electrical nerve stimulation on proinflammatory cytokines: Systematic review and meta-analysis. *Mediators Inflamm* 2018:1094352, 2018.

7. Rouabhia M, Park HJ, Atieh AD, et al: Electrical stimulation promotes the proliferation of human keratinocytes, increases the production of keratin 5 and 14, and increases the phosphorylation of ERK1/2 and p38 MAP kinases. *J Tissue Eng Regen Med* 14(7):909–919, 2020.

8. Sovak G, Budgell B: TENS-like stimulation downregulates inflammatory cytokines in a PC-12 cell line. *J Manipulative Physiol Ther* 40(6):381–386, 2017.

9. Tyler SEB: Nature's electric potential: a systematic review of the role of bioelectricity in wound healing and regenerative processes in animals, humans, and plants. *Front Physiol* 8:627, 2017.

10. Hunckler J, de Mel A: A current affair: electrotherapy in wound healing. *J Multidiscip Healthc* 10:179–194, 2017.

11. Zhao M, Penninger J, Isseroff RR: Electrical activation of wound-healing pathways. *Adv Skin Wound Care* 1:567–573, 2010.

12. Mycielska ME, Djamgoz MB: Cellular mechanisms of direct-current electric field effects: galvanotaxis and metastatic disease. *J Cell Sci* 117(Pt 9):1631–1639, 2004.

13. Uemura M, Maeshige N, Koga Y, et al: Monophasic pulsed 200-µA current promotes galvanotaxis with polarization of actin filament and integrin α2β1 in human dermal fibroblasts. *Eplasty* 16:e6, 2016.

14. Guo L, Xu C, Li D, et al: Calcium ion flow permeates cells through SOCs to promote cathode-directed galvanotaxis. *PLoS ONE* 10:e0139865, 2015.

15. Yang HY, Charles RP, Hummler E, et al: The epithelial sodium channel mediates the directionality of galvanotaxis in human keratinocytes. *J Cell Sci* 126(Pt 9):1942–1951, 2013.

16. Riding A, Pullar CE: ATP release and P2 Y receptor signaling are essential for keratinocyte galvanotaxis. *J Cell Physiol* 231:181–191, 2016.

17. Polak A, Franek A, Taradaj J: High-voltage pulsed current electrical stimulation in wound treatment. *Adv Wound Care (New Rochelle)* 3:104–117, 2014.

18. Jaffe LF, Vanable JW: Jr: Electric fields and wound healing. *Clin Dermatol* 2:34–44, 1984.

19. Borgens RB, Vanable JS, Jaffe LF: Bioelectricity and regeneration: large currents leave the stumps of regenerating newt limbs. *Proc Natl Acad Sci USA* 74:4528–4532, 1977.

20. Balakatounis KC, Angoules AG: Low-intensity electrical stimulation in wound healing: review of the efficacy of externally applied currents resembling the current of injury. *Eplasty* 8:e28, 2008.

21. Illingworth CM, Barker AT: Measurement of electrical currents emerging during the regeneration of amputated finger tips in children. *Clin Phys Physiol Meas* 1(87), 1980.

22. Babona-Pilipos R, Pritchard-Oh A, Popovic MR, et al: Biphasic monopolar electrical stimulation induces rapid and directed galvanotaxis in adult subependymal neural precursors. *Stem Cell Res Ther* 6(67), 2015.

23. Sugimoto M, Maeshige N, Honda H, et al: Optimum microcurrent stimulation intensity for galvanotaxis in human fibroblasts. *J Wound Care* 21:10–11, 2012; 5–6, 8, 10, discussion.

24. Kloth LC: Electrical stimulation for wound healing: a review of evidence from in vitro studies, animal experiments, and clinical trials. *Int J Low Extrem Wounds* 4(23), 2005.

25. Cheng N, Van Hoof H, Bock E, et al: The effects of electric currents on ATP generation, protein synthesis, and membrane transport in rat skin. *Clin Orthop Relat Res* 171:264–272, 1982.

26. Bourguignon GJ, Bourguignon LYW: Electric stimulation of protein and DNA synthesis in human fibroblasts. *FASEB J* 1:398–402, 1987.

27. Wang Y, Rouabhia M, Zhang Z: Pulsed electrical stimulation benefits wound healing by activating skin fibroblasts through the TGFβ1/ERK/NF-κB axis. *Biochim Biophys Acta* 1860:1551–1559, 2016.

28. Rouabhia M, Park H, Meng S, et al: Electrical stimulation promotes wound healing by enhancing dermal fibroblast activity and promoting myofibroblast transdifferentiation. *PLoS ONE* 8:e71660, 2013.

29. Wang Y, Rouabhia M, Lavertu D, et al: Pulsed electrical stimulation modulates fibroblasts' behaviour through the Smad signalling pathway. *J Tissue Eng Regen Med* 11(4):1110–1121, 2017.

30. Nguyen EB, Wishner J, Slowinska K: The effect of pulsed electric field on expression of ECM proteins: collagen, elastin, and MMP1 in human dermal fibroblasts. *J Electroanal Chem (Lausanne)* 812:265–272, 2018.

31. Snyder S, DeJulius C, Willits RK: Electrical stimulation increases random migration of human dermal fibroblasts. *Ann Biomed Eng* 45(9):2049–2060, 2017.

32. Tai G, Tai M, Zhao M: Electrically stimulated cell migration and its contribution to wound healing. *Burns Trauma* 6:20, 2018.

33. Ennis WJ, Lee C, Meneses P: A biochemical approach to wound healing through the use of modalities. *Clin Dermatol* 25:63–72, 2007.

34. Bourguignon GJ, Wenche JY, Bourguignon LYW: Electric stimulation of human fibroblasts causes an increase in Ca^{2+} influx and the exposure of additional insulin receptors. *J Cell Physiol* 140:379–385, 1989.

35. Park HJ, Rouabhia M, Lavertu D, et al: Electrical stimulation modulates the expression of multiple wound healing genes in primary human dermal fibroblasts. *Tissue Eng Part A* 21:1982–1990, 2015.

36. Sebastian A, Volk SW, Halai P, et al: Enhanced neurogenic biomarker expression and reinnervation in human acute skin wounds treated by electrical stimulation. *J Invest Dermatol* 137(3):737–747, 2017.

37. Chen C, Bai X, Ding Y, et al: Electrical stimulation as a novel tool for regulating cell behavior in tissue engineering. *Biomater Res* 23:25, 2019.

38. Cooper MS, Schliwa M: Electrical and ionic controls of tissue cell locomotion in DC electric fields. *J Neurosci Res* 13:223–244, 1985.

39. Asadi MR, Torkaman G, Hedayati M: Effect of sensory and motor electrical stimulation in vascular endothelial growth factor expression of muscle and skin in full-thickness wound. *J Rehabil Res Dev* 48:195–201, 2011.

40. Souza AK, Souza TR, Siqueira das Neves LM, et al: Effect of high voltage pulsed current on the integration of total skin grafts in rats submitted to nicotine action. *J Tissue Viability* 28(3):161–166, 2019.

41. Asadi MR, Torkaman G, Hedayati M, et al: Angiogenic effects of low-intensity cathodal direct current on ischemic diabetic foot ulcers: a randomized controlled trial. *Diabetes Res Clin Pract* 127:147–155, 2017.

42. Martínez-Rodríguez A, Bello O, Fraiz M, et al: The effect of alternating and biphasic currents on humans' wound healing: a literature review. *Int J Dermatol* 52:1053–1062, 2013.

43. Li Y, Gu Y, Wang H, et al: Electric pulses can influence galvanotaxis of dictyostelium discoideum. *Biomed Res Int* Aug 8, 2018:2534625, 2018.

44. Ong PC, Laatsch LJ, Kloth LC: Antibacterial effects of a silver electrode carrying microamperage direct current in vitro. *JACC Clin Electrophysiol* 6:14–18, 1994.

45. Daeschlein G, Assadian O, Kloth LC, et al: Antibacterial activity of positive and negative polarity low-voltage pulsed current (LVPC) on six typical gram-positive and gram-negative bacterial pathogens of chronic wounds. *Wound Repair Regen* 15:399–403, 2007.

46. Ibrahim ZM, Waked IS, Ibrahim O: Negative pressure wound therapy versus microcurrent electrical stimulation in wound healing in burns. *J Wound Care* 28(4):214–219, 2019.

47. Sandvik EL, McLeod BR, Parker AE, et al: Direct electric current treatment under physiologic saline conditions kills *Staphylococcus epidermidis* biofilms via electrolytic generation of hypochlorous acid. *PLoS ONE* 8:e55118, 2013.

48. Kincaid C, Lavoie K: Inhibition of bacterial growth in vitro following stimulation with high voltage, monophasic, pulsed current. *Phys Ther* 69:29–33, 1989.

49. Szuminsky NJ, Albers AC, Unger P, et al: Effect of narrow, pulsed high voltages on bacterial viability. *Phys Ther* 74:660–667, 1994.

50. Rowley BA, McKenna J, Chase GR: The influence of electrical current on an infecting microorganism in wounds. *Ann N Y Acad Sci* 238:543–551, 1974.

51. del Pozo JL, Rouse MS, Mandrekar JN, et al: The electricidal effect: reduction of *Staphylococcus* and *Pseudomonas* biofilms by prolonged exposure to low-intensity electrical current. *Antimicrob Agents Chemother* 53:41–45, 2009.

52. Ruiz-Ruigomez M, Badiola J, Schmidt-Malan SM, et al: Direct electrical current reduces bacterial and yeast biofilm formation. *Int J Bacteriol* 2016:9727810, 2016.

53. Del Pozo JL, Rouse MS, Patel R: Bioelectric effect and bacterial biofilms. A systematic review. *Int J Artif Organs* 31:786–795, 2008.

54. Freebairn D, Linton D, Harkin-Jones E, et al: Electrical methods of controlling bacterial adhesion and biofilm on device surfaces. *Expert Rev Med Devices* 10:85–103, 2013.

55. Canty MK, Hansen LA, Tobias M, et al: Antibiotics enhance prevention and eradication efficacy of cathodic-voltage-controlled

electrical stimulation against titanium-associated methicillin-resistant *Staphylococcus aureus* and *Pseudomonas aeruginosa* biofilms. *mSphere* 4(3):e00178, 2019.

56. Petrofsky J, Schwab E, Lo T, et al: Effects of electrical stimulation on skin blood flow in controls and in and around stage III and IV wounds in hairy and nonhairy skin. *Med Sci Monit* 11:CR309–CR316, 2005.

57. Lawson D, Petrofsky JS: A randomized control study on the effect of biphasic electrical stimulation in a warm room on skin blood flow and healing rates in chronic wounds of patients with and without diabetes. *Med Sci Monit* 13:CR258–CR263, 2007.

58. Malty AM, Petrofsky J: The effect of electrical stimulation on a normal skin blood flow in active young and older adults. *Med Sci Monit* 13:CR147–CR155, 2007.

59. Junger M, Zuder D, Steins A, et al: Treatment of venous ulcers with low frequency pulsed current (Dermapulse): effects on cutaneous microcirculation. *Hautarzt* 18:879–903, 1997.

60. Mohr T, Akers T, Wessman HC: Effect of high voltage stimulation on blood flow in the rat hind limb. *Phys Ther* 67:526–533, 1987.

61. Lundeberg TC, Eriksson SV, Malm M: Electrical nerve stimulation improves healing in diabetic ulcers. *Ann Plast Surg* 29:328–331, 1992.

62. Lundeberg T, Kjartansson J, Samuelsson UE: Effect of electric nerve stimulation on healing of ischemic skin flaps. *Lancet* 24:712–714, 1988.

63. Sherry JE, Oehrlein KM, Hegge KS, et al: Effect of burst-mode transcutaneous electrical nerve stimulation on peripheral vascular resistance. *Phys Ther* 81:1183–1191, 2001.

64. Polak A, Kucio C, Kloth LC, et al: A randomized, controlled clinical study to assess the effect of anodal and cathodal electrical stimulation on periwound skin blood flow and pressure ulcer size reduction in persons with neurological injuries. *Ostomy Wound Manage* 64(2):10–29, 2018.

65. Kloth LC, Feedar JA: Acceleration of wound healing with high voltage, monophasic, pulsed current. *Phys Ther* 68:503–508, 1988.

66. Lala D, Spaulding SJ, Burke SM, et al: Electrical stimulation therapy for the treatment of pressure ulcers in individuals with spinal cord injury: a systematic review and meta-analysis. *Int Wound J* 13:1214–1226, 2016.

67. Barnes R, Shahin Y, Gohil R, et al: Electrical stimulation vs. standard care for chronic ulcer healing: a systematic review and meta-analysis of randomised controlled trials. *Eur J Clin Invest* 44:429–440, 2014.

68. Kawasaki L, Mushahwar VK, Ho C, et al: The mechanisms and evidence of efficacy of electrical stimulation for healing of pressure ulcer: a systematic review. *Wound Repair Regen* 22:161–173, 2014.

69. Nair HKR: Microcurrent as an adjunct therapy to accelerate chronic wound healing and reduce patient pain. *J Wound Care* 27(5):296–306, 2018.

70. Bogie KM: The modular adaptive electrotherapy delivery system (MAEDS): an electroceutical approach for effective treatment of wound infection and promotion of healing. *Mil Med* 184(Suppl 1):92–96, 2019.

71. Centers for Medicare and Medicaid Services: Decision memo for electrostimulation for wounds (#CAG-00068R); 2002. http://www.cms.hhs.gov/mcd/viewdecisionmemo.asp?id=28. (Accessed 19 April 2007).

72. Ashrafi M, Alonso-Rasgado T, Baguneid M, et al: The efficacy of electrical stimulation in lower extremity cutaneous wound healing: a systematic review. *Exp Dermatol* 26(2):171–178, 2017.

73. Thakral G, LaFontaine J, Najafi B, et al: Electrical stimulation to accelerate wound healing. *Diabet Foot Ankle* 4, 2013.

74. Khouri C, Kotzki S, Roustit M, et al: Hierarchical evaluation of electrical stimulation protocols for chronic wound healing: An effect size meta-analysis. *Wound Repair Regen* 25(5):883–891, 2017.

75. Liu LQ, Moody J, Traynor M, et al: A systematic review of electrical stimulation for pressure ulcer prevention and treatment in people with spinal cord injuries. *J Spinal Cord Med* 37:703–718, 2014.

76. Smith ME, Totten A, Hickam DH, et al: Pressure ulcer treatment strategies: a systematic comparative effectiveness review. *Ann Intern Med* 159:39–50, 2013.

77. Saha S, Smith MEB, Totten A, et al: *Pressure ulcer treatment strategies: comparative effectiveness*, Rockville, MD, 2013, Agency for Healthcare Research and Quality. Report No. 13-EHC003-EF. AHRQ Comparative Effectiveness Reviews.

78. Girgis B, Duarte JA: High voltage monophasic pulsed current (HVMPC) for stage II-IV pressure ulcer healing. A systematic review and meta-analysis. *J Tissue Viability* 27(4):274–284, 2018.

79. Solis LR, Gyawali S, Seres P, et al: Effects of intermittent electrical stimulation on superficial pressure, tissue oxygenation, and discomfort levels for the prevention of deep tissue injury. *Ann Biomed Eng* 39:649–663, 2011.

80. Snyder AR, Perotti AL, Lam KC, et al: The influence of high-voltage electrical stimulation on edema formation after acute injury: a systematic review. *J Sport Rehabil* 19:436–451, 2010.

81. Dolan MG, Grave P, Nakazawa C, et al: Effects of ibuprofen and high-voltage electric stimulation on acute edema formation after blunt trauma to limbs of rats. *J Athl Train* 40:111–115, 2005.

82. Mendel FC, Wylegala JA, Fish DR: Influence of high voltage pulsed current on edema formation following impact injury in rats. *Phys Ther* 72:668–673, 1992.

83. Bettany JA, Fish DR, Mendel FC: The effect of high voltage pulsed direct current on edema formation following impact injury. *Phys Ther* 70:219–224, 1990.

84. Bettany JA, Fish DR, Mendel FC: The effect of high voltage pulsed direct current on edema formation following hyperflexion injury. *Arch Phys Med Rehabil* 71:677–681, 1990.

85. Bettany JA, Fish DR, Mendel FC: Influence of cathodal high voltage pulsed current on acute edema. *JACC Clin Electrophysiol* 2:724–733, 1990.

86. Fish DR, Mendel FC, Schultz AM, et al: Effect of anodal high voltage pulsed current on edema formation in frog hind limbs. *Phys Ther* 71:724–730, 1991.

87. Taylor K, Mendel FC, Fish DR, et al: Effect of high voltage pulsed current and alternating current on macromolecular leakage in hamster cheek pouch microcirculation. *Phys Ther* 71:1729–1740, 1997.

88. Edgar DW, Fish JS, Gomez M, et al: Local and systemic treatments for acute edema after burn injury: a systematic review of the literature. *J Burn Care Res* 32:334–347, 2011.

89. Mendel FC, Dolan MG, Fish DR, et al: Effect of high-voltage pulsed current on recovery after grades I and II lateral ankle sprains. *J Sport Rehabil* 19:399–410, 2010.

90. Sandoval MC, Ramirez C, Camargo DM, et al: Effect of high-voltage pulsed current plus conventional treatment on acute ankle sprain. *Rev Bras Fisioter* 14:193–199, 2010.

91. Dolan MG, Mychaskiw AM, Mendel FC: Cool-water immersion and high-voltage electric stimulation curb edema formation in rats. *J Athl Train* 38:225–230, 2003.

92. Man IO, Morrissey MC, Cywinski JK: Effect of neuromuscular electrical stimulation on ankle swelling in the early period after ankle sprain. *Phys Ther* 87:53–65, 2007.

93. Wainwright TW, Burgess LC, Middleton RG: Does neuromuscular electrical stimulation improve recovery following acute ankle sprain? A pilot. *Clin Med Insights: Arthr Musculo Disord* 12:1–6, 2019.

94. Reed BV: Effect of high voltage pulsed electrical stimulation on microvascular permeability to plasma proteins: a possible mechanism in minimizing edema. *Phys Ther* 68:491–495, 1988.

95. Karnes JL, Mendel FC, Fish DR, et al: High voltage pulsed current: its influences on diameters of histamine-dilated arterioles in hamster cheek pouches. *Arch Phys Med Rehabil* 76:381–386, 1995.

96. Man IO, Lepar GS, Morrissey MC, et al: Effect of neuromuscular electrical stimulation on foot/ankle volume during standing. *Med Sci Sports Exerc* 35:630–634, 2003.

97. Vena D, Rubianto J, Popovic MR, et al: The effect of electrical stimulation of the calf muscle on leg fluid accumulation over a long period of sitting. *Sci Rep* 7(1):6055, 2017.

98. Ravikumar R, Williams KJ, Babber A, et al: Randomised controlled trial: potential benefit of a footplate neuromuscular electrical stimulation device in patients with chronic venous disease. *Eur J Vasc Endovasc Surg* 53(1):114–121, 2017.

99. Morita H, Abe C, Tanaka K, et al: Neuromuscular electrical stimulation and an ottoman-type seat effectively improve popliteal venous flow in a sitting position. *J Physiol Sci* 56:183–186, 2006.

100. Burgess LC, Immins T, Swain I, et al: Effectiveness of neuromuscular electrical stimulation for reducing oedema: A systematic review. *J Rehabil Med* 51(4):237–243, 2019.

101. Williams KJ, Ravikumar R, Gaweesh AS, et al: A review of the evidence to support neuromuscular electrical stimulation in the prevention and management of venous disease. *Adv Exp Med Biol* 906:377386, 2017.

102. Broderick BJ, Breathnach O, Condon F, et al: Haemodynamic performance of neuromuscular electrical stimulation (NMES) during recovery from total hip arthroplasty. *J Orthop Surg Res* 8(3), 2013.

103. Ojima M, Takegawa R, Hirose T, et al: Hemodynamic effects of electrical muscle stimulation in the prophylaxis of deep vein thrombosis for intensive care unit patients: a randomized trial. *J Intensive Care* 5:9, 2017.

104. Yilmaz S, Calbiyik M, Yilmaz BK, et al: Potential role of electrostimulation in augmentation of venous blood flow after total knee replacement: a pilot study. *Phlebology* 31(4):2516, 2016.

105. Lattimer CR, Azzam M, Papaconstandinou JA, et al: Neuromuscular electrical stimulation reduces sludge in the popliteal vein. *J Vasc Surg Venous Lymphat Disord* 6(2):154–162, 2018.

106. Wainwright TW, Burgess LC, Middleton RG: A single-centre feasibility randomised controlled trial comparing the incidence of asymptomatic and symptomatic deep vein thrombosis between a neuromuscular electrostimulation device and thromboembolism deterrent stockings in post-operative patients recovering from elective total hip replacement surgery. *Surg Technol Int* 36:289–298, 2020.

107. Broderick BJ, O'Connell S, Moloney S, et al: Comparative lower limb hemodynamics using neuromuscular electrical stimulation (NMES) versus intermittent pneumatic compression (IPC). *Physiol Meas* 35:1849–1859, 2014.

108. Bahadori S, Immins T, Wainwright TW: The effect of calf neuromuscular electrical stimulation and intermittent pneumatic compression on thigh microcirculation. *Microvasc Res* 111:3741, 2017.

109. Czyrny JJ, Kaplan RE, Wilding GE, et al: Electrical foot stimulation: a potential new method of deep venous thrombosis prophylaxis. *Vascular* 18:20–27, 2010.

110. Pierce MW: Transdermal delivery of sumatriptan for the treatment of acute migraine. *Neurother* 7:159–163, 2010.

111. Leduc S: Introduction of medicinal substances into the depths of tissues by electrical current. *Ann Electrobiol* 3(545), 1900.

112. Leduc S: *Electric ions and their use in medicine*, London, 1908, Rebman.

113. Stefanou A, Marshall N, Holdan W, et al: A randomized study comparing corticosteroid injection to corticosteroid iontophoresis for lateral epicondylitis. *J Hand Surg Am* 37:104–109, 2012.

114. Manjunatha RG, Prasad R, Sharma S, et al: Iontophoretic delivery of lidocaine hydrochloride through ex-vivo human skin. *J Dermatolog Treat* 31(2):191–199, 2020.

115. Manjunatha RG, Sharma S, Narayan RP, et al: Effective permeation of 2.5 and 5% lidocaine hydrochloride in human skin using iontophoresis technique. *Int J Dermatol* 57(11):1335–1343, 2018.

116. Glass JM, Stephen RL, Jacobsen SC: The quantity and distribution of radiolabeled dexamethasone delivered to tissue by iontophoresis. *Int J Dermatol* 19:519–525, 1080.

117. Draper DO, Coglianese M, Castel C: Absorption of iontophoresis-driven 2% lidocaine with epinephrine in the tissues at 5 mm below the surface of the skin. *J Athl Train* 46:277–281, 2011.

118. Cázares-Delgadillo J, Balaguer-Fernández C, Calatayud-Pascual A, et al: Transdermal iontophoresis of dexamethasone sodium phosphate in vitro and in vivo: effect of experimental parameters and skin type on drug stability and transport kinetics. *Eur J Pharm Biopharm* 75.170 178, 2010.

119. Bertolucci LE: Introduction of anti-inflammatory drugs by iontophoresis: a double blind study. *J Orthop Sports Phys Ther* 4:103–108, 1982.

120. Anderson CR, Morris RL, Boeh SD, et al: Effects of iontophoresis current magnitude and duration on dexamethasone deposition and localized drug retention. *Phys Ther* 83:161–170, 2003.

121. Japour CJ, Vohra R, Vohra PK, et al: Management of heel pain syndrome with acetic acid iontophoresis. *J Am Podiatr Med Assoc* 09:251–257, 1999.

122. Gard K, Ebaugh D: The use of acetic acid iontophoresis in the management of a soft tissue injury. *North Am J Sports Phys Ther* 5:220–226, 2010.

123. Dardas A, Bae GH, Yule A, et al: Acetic acid iontophoresis for recalcitrant scarring in post-operative hand patients. *J Hand Ther* 27:44–48, 2014.

124. da Luz DC, de Borba Y, Ravanello EM, et al: Iontophoresis in lateral epicondylitis: a randomized, double-blind clinical trial. *J Shoulder Elbow Surg* 28(9):1743–1749, 2019.

125. Baktir S, Razak Ozdincler A, Kaya Mutlu E, et al: The short-term effectiveness of low-level laser, phonophoresis, and iontophoresis in patients with lateral epicondylosis. *J Hand Ther* 32(4):417–425, 2019.

126. Nirschl RP, Rodin DM, Ochiai DH, et al: Iontophoretic administration of dexamethasone sodium phosphate for acute epicondylitis: a randomized, double-blinded, placebo-controlled study. *Am J Sports Med* 31:189–195, 2003.

127. Gudeman SD, Eisele SA, Heidt RS Jr, et al: Treatment of plantar fasciitis by iontophoresis of 0.4% dexamethasone: a randomized, double-blind, placebo-controlled study. *Am J Sports Med* 25:312–316, 1997.

128. Mina R, Melson P, Powell S, et al: Effectiveness of dexamethasone iontophoresis for temporomandibular joint involvement in juvenile idiopathic arthritis. *Arthritis Care Res (Hoboken)* 63:1511–1516, 2011.

129. Lobo S, Yan G: Improving the direct penetration into tissues underneath the skin with iontophoresis delivery of a ketoprofen cationic prodrug. *Int J Pharm* 535(1–2):228–236, 2018.

130. Lobo S, Yan G: Evaluation iontophoretic delivery of a cationic ketoprofen prodrug for treating nociceptive symptoms in monosodium iodoacetate induced osteoarthritic rat model. *Int J Pharm* 569, 2019:118598.

131. Jorge LL, Feres CC, Teles VE: Topical preparations for pain relief: efficacy and patient adherence. *J Pain Res* 4:11–24, 2010.

132. Lindley P, Ding L, Danesi H: Meta-analysis of the ease of care from a patients' perspective comparing fentanyl iontophoretic transdermal system versus morphine intravenous patient-controlled analgesia in postoperative pain management. *J Perianesth Nurs* 32(4):320–328, 2017.

133. Pestano CR, Lindley P, Ding L, et al: Meta-analysis of the ease of care from the nurses' perspective comparing fentanyl iontophoretic transdermal system (ITS) vs morphine intravenous patient-controlled analgesia (IV PCA) in postoperative pain management. *J Perianesth Nurs* 32(4):329–340, 2017.

134. Viscusi ER, Reynolds L, Chung F, et al: Patient-controlled transdermal fentanyl hydrochloride vs intravenous morphine pump for postoperative pain: a randomized controlled trial. *JAMA* 291:1333–1341, 2004.

135. Balaguer-Fernández C, Femenía-Font A, Muedra V, et al: Combined strategies for enhancing the transdermal absorption of midazolam through human skin. *J Pharm Pharmacol* 62:1096–1102, 2010.

136. Ishii H, Suzuki T, Todo H, et al: Iontophoresis-facilitated delivery of prednisolone through throat skin to the trachea after topical application of its succinate salt. *Pharm Res* 28:839–847, 2011.

137. Souza JG, Gelfuso GM, Simão PS, et al: Iontophoretic transport of zinc phthalocyanine tetrasulfonic acid as a tool to improve drug topical delivery. *Anticancer Drugs* 22:783–793, 2011.

138. Patane MA, Cohen A, From S, et al: Ocular iontophoresis of EGP-437 (dexamethasone phosphate) in dry eye patients: results of a randomized clinical trial. *Clin Ophthalmol* 5:633–643, 2011.

139. Edwards AM, Stevens MT, Church MK: The effects of topical sodium cromoglicate on itch and flare in human skin induced by intradermal histamine: a randomised double-blind vehicle controlled intra-subject design trial. *BMC Res Notes* 4(47), 2011.

140. Zhang Y, Yu J, Kahkoska AR, et al: Advances in transdermal insulin delivery. *Adv Drug Deliv Rev* 139:51–70, 2019.

141. Zhu K, Hum NR, Reid B, et al: Electric fields at breast cancer and cancer cell collective galvanotaxis. *Sci Rep* 10(1):8712, 2020.

142. Adunsky A, Ohry A, Group DDCT: Decubitus direct current treatment (DDCT) of pressure ulcers: results of a randomized double-blinded placebo controlled study. *Arch Gerontol Geriatr* 41:261–269, 2005.

143. Houghton PE, Campbell KE, Fraser CH, et al: Electrical stimulation therapy increases rate of healing of pressure ulcers in community-dwelling people with spinal cord injury. *Arch Phys Med Rehabil* 91:669–678, 2010.

144. Karba R, Semrov D, Vodovnik L, et al: DC electrical stimulation for chronic wound healing enhancement. 1. Clinical study and determination of electrical field distribution in numerical wound model. *Bioelectrochem Bioenerg* 43:265–270, 1997.

145. Sun YS: Electrical stimulation for wound-healing: simulation on the effect of electrode configurations. *Biomed Res Int* 2017:5289041, 2017.

146. Baker LL, Ruyabi S, Villar F, et al: Effect of electrical stimulation waveform on healing of ulcers in human beings with spinal cord injury. *Wound Repair Regen* 4:21–28, 1996.

147. Griffin JW, Tooms RE, Mendius RE, et al: Efficacy of high voltage pulsed current for healing of pressure ulcers in patients with spinal cord injury. *Phys Ther* 71:433–444, 1991.

148. Unger P, Eddy J, Raimastry S: A controlled study of the effect of high voltage pulsed current (HVPC) on wound healing. *Phys Ther* 71(Suppl):S119, 1991.

149. Unger PC: A randomized clinical trial of the effect of HVPC on wound healing. *Phys Ther* 71(Suppl);S118, 1991.

150. Michlovitz SL, Smith W, Watkins M: Ice and high voltage pulsed stimulation in treatment of acute lateral ankle sprains. *J Orthop Sports Phys Ther* 9:301–304, 1988.

Electromyographic (EMG) Biofeedback

Jason E. Bennett

15

CHAPTER OUTLINE

CHAPTER OBJECTIVES

After reading this chapter, the reader will be able to do the following:
- Define *electromyographic (EMG) biofeedback*.
- Describe the physiological effects of EMG biofeedback.
- Explain the clinical indications and contraindications for the use of EMG biofeedback.
- Select appropriate equipment and optimal treatment parameters for treatment with EMG biofeedback.
- Safely and effectively apply neuromuscular electrical stimulation.
- Accurately and completely document treatment with EMG biofeedback.

Introduction
TERMINOLOGY

Readers unfamiliar with **electromyographic (EMG)** biofeedback are encouraged to review the glossary before reading this chapter; doing so will enhance the reader's understanding of the principles and application of EMG biofeedback.

HISTORY OF BIOFEEDBACK

Biofeedback refers to techniques that provide information to the user about their own physiological or biomechanical processes as a means of improving self-awareness and control of a specific, targeted process. Early biofeedback techniques were developed to address musculoskeletal conditions based on the principles of motor learning and operant conditioning and were later expanded to address psychological conditions by targeting autonomic processes. Biofeedback is usually implemented to facilitate a user's ability to self-regulate a targeted biological process to enhance performance or as part of a comprehensive treatment plan for a specific medical condition. In contrast to other modalities discussed in this text where physiological effects result from the direct transfer of energy to a targeted tissue, biofeedback requires the user to learn how to control the targeted process using attentional strategies to create a therapeutic or performance effect. Adjunctive techniques such as visualization and relaxation training, postural education, sports-specific training, and therapeutic exercise are often incorporated to improve the effectiveness of biofeedback. The use of biofeedback is increasing rapidly as a result of advances in technology, improved access to equipment, decreased cost, enhanced user interfaces, and additional evidence supporting its clinical use.

> ### ◎ Clinical Pearl
>
> Biofeedback provides information to the user about their own physiological or biomechanical processes to improve self-awareness and control of a specific, targeted process. Biofeedback is usually used to help someone self-regulate a targeted biological process.

Heart rate monitors that provide information regarding cardiovascular effort during exercise are a ubiquitous example of biofeedback in everyday use. Based on the feedback provided by the heart rate monitor, the user can increase, decrease, or maintain their effort to attain a predetermined target level (Fig. 15.1). Many types of biofeedback in addition to heart rate are used clinically to assess the performance of a specific activity or exercise, potentially to improve balance, strength, function, movement, posture, muscle tone, or cardiovascular effort. The targeted activity can be monitored using various types of equipment, including surface or needle EMG devices, electrogoniometers, force platforms, and real-time ultrasound

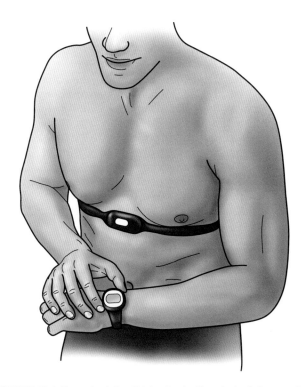

FIGURE 15.1 Example of direct biofeedback of heart rate during exercise.

imaging (Fig. 15.2). Biofeedback can be classified as direct or transformed, depending on how accurately the external information produced represents the internal biological process being recorded. For example, heart rate monitors provide **direct biofeedback** because they produce an accurate numerical representation of the user's heart rate. In contrast, EMG biofeedback is a type of **transformed biofeedback** because it provides a representative signal of electrical activity in muscle.[1] This chapter describes the principles and applications of surface EMG biofeedback in the rehabilitation of neuromusculoskeletal conditions. Unless otherwise indicated, the term *EMG biofeedback* in this book refers specifically to the use of surface electrodes—or *surface EMG* as it is commonly called—rather than invasive needle electrode applications, which require advanced training and pose additional risks to the patient.

EMG BIOFEEDBACK DEFINITION

Although EMG biofeedback does not involve the transfer of thermal, electromagnetic, or mechanical energy and therefore does not meet the strict definitions of physical agents covered in this text, EMG biofeedback is included because it is often used by rehabilitation professionals, it uses an electrical device applied to the patient, and it is generally taught along with physical agents in the same course. Understanding the principles related to EMG biofeedback will allow the

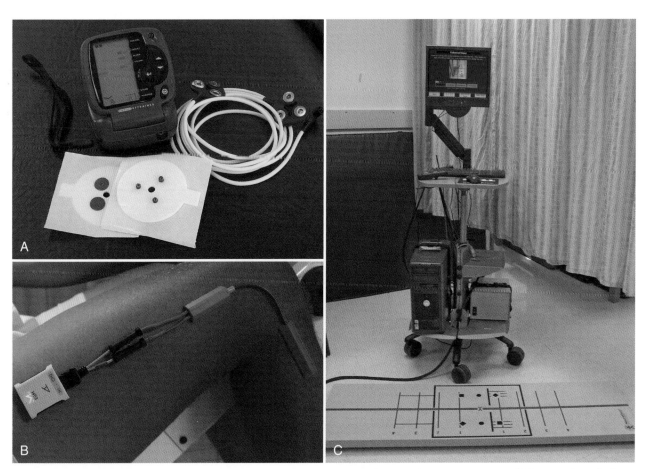

FIGURE 15.2 Example of biofeedback equipment. (A) Surface electromyography (EMG) device. (B) Electrogoniometer. (C) Force platform. (A, Courtesy Chattanooga/DJO, Vista, CA. B, Courtesy Ergotest Innovation AS, Porsgrunn, Norway.)

clinician to more effectively prescribe and monitor its use clinically.

In the most general sense, surface EMG biofeedback uses electrodes on the surface of the skin to detect the underlying intrinsic electrical activity of muscle tissue and converts this to an extrinsic auditory, visual, or haptic signal that is fed back to the user (Fig. 15.3). In this regard, electromyography functions in much the same way as a voltmeter by detecting the difference in electrical potential across two points. More advanced methods of signal delivery incorporating virtual reality and gaming technologies have been developed recently, but research is limited, and cost may be prohibitive for many users.

> ### ◎ Clinical Pearl
>
> Myoelectric (ionic) activity produced during a muscle contraction is detected by surface EMG electrodes and converted to an electrical signal, which is then amplified and processed to produce a representative auditory, visual, or haptic signal.

Surface EMG biofeedback is not a direct measure of muscle **contractility** or tension but rather a broad representation of the electrical changes occurring in the tissue underlying the electrodes. Surface electrodes detect the ionic activity of underlying muscle tissue but cannot monitor specific motor units or muscles. The spacing of electrodes during EMG biofeedback will also influence the area of muscle being targeted, similar to the impact of spacing electrodes during electrical stimulation discussed in Chapter 11. Narrow spacing will capture signal from more superficial muscles, whereas wider spacing allows for greater tissue sampling with less specificity.

Surface EMG electrodes generally consist of three silver–silver chloride (Ag-AgCl) electrodes: two active electrodes that detect changes in myoelectrical activity and one reference electrode. Some manufacturers produce a single electrode that incorporates both active and reference electrodes into a single patch (Fig. 15.4). Movement of the electrodes or poor conductivity can cause noise or artifact in the EMG signal, making it difficult for the user to successfully control the targeted process. To limit noise in the EMG signal, the skin should be cleaned thoroughly and a small amount of ultrasound gel applied between the electrode and the skin. In some cases, removing hair and denuding dead skin cells by shaving the area may be necessary to further minimize EMG signal noise. Electrodes should be oriented in parallel with the muscle fibers and secured in place with tape (Fig. 15.5). The quality of the EMG signal from skeletal muscle may also be influenced by the thickness of adipose tissue between the electrode and muscle tissue, interference from nearby electrical devices,

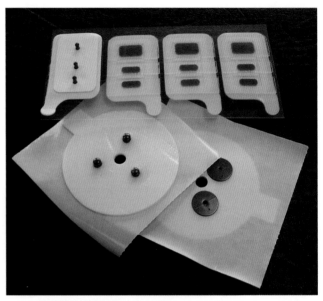

FIGURE 15.4 Surface electromyography (EMG) electrodes.

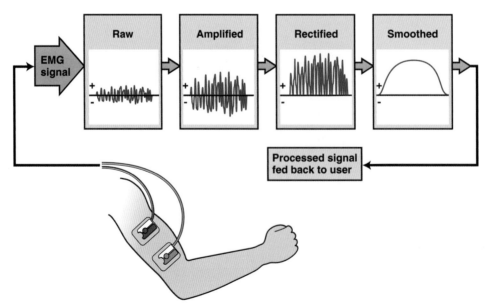

FIGURE 15.3 Example of electromyography (EMG) signal processing, from raw to amplified to rectified to smoothed, then fed back to the user.

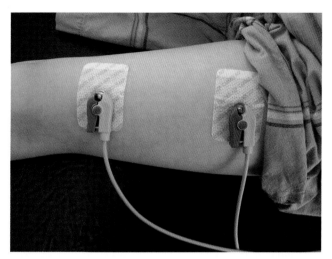

FIGURE 15.5 Electrode placement in parallel with muscle fibers.

and artifacts from the electrical activity of cardiac and respiratory muscles.

Parameters

A typical EMG biofeedback device used in rehabilitation is portable and represents the detected ionic activity in audio and visual formats. The ionic activity is measured in microvolts (µV) and then amplified and usually filtered to produce the representative signal provided to the user. EMG biofeedback devices may differ slightly based on the amplification settings allowed by the unit, but these typically range from 1 to 2000 µV. This is referred to as the **gain** setting, which determines the sensitivity of a device or its ability to reflect various levels of ionic activity (Fig. 15.6).

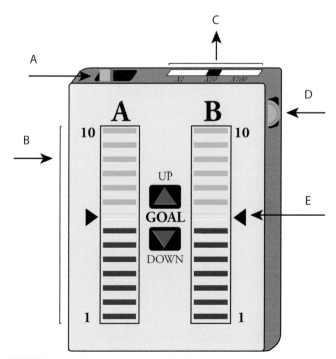

FIGURE 15.6 Electromyography (EMG) device with *arrows* marking (A) on/off, (B) amplitude (µV), (C) gain, (D) volume, and (E) threshold. (Image copyright Jodi Splinter.)

> ### ◎ Clinical Pearl
>
> The higher the gain setting, the higher the sensitivity of an EMG device; therefore small changes in electrical activity will produce an EMG signal. The inverse is true for lower gain settings.

As a general guideline, the EMG amplitude of muscle at rest is approximately 2 µV, and healthy muscle contractions have been recorded at levels greater than 20 to 30 mV. When there is a high level of ionic activity requiring less amplification, the gain (amplification) will be set lower, thereby requiring the user to contract with greater effort to change the signal output. This is often done in later stages of rehabilitation or when EMG biofeedback is used to improve performance in healthy individuals. Alternatively, when there is a low level of ionic activity, the gain must be set higher so that an EMG signal output is produced, for example, with paresis or trace muscle contractions. The gain setting should be adjusted as the user improves control of the targeted process— referred to as "shaping"—or if the user has difficulty achieving a detectable signal output.

The following EMG variables can be recorded during a typical EMG biofeedback session, allowing the clinician to establish a baseline and document changes in myoelectrical activity and muscle performance. The **peak amplitude** is the highest EMG activity (µV) recorded during a muscle contraction, and the **contraction latency** (typically approximately 0.5 second) is the time it takes to reach peak amplitude following a command to contract a muscle. The **return latency** is the time from the command to stop a muscle contraction to the point when the myoelectrical activity returns to resting or baseline levels (typically approximately 1 second). Longer return latencies reflect muscle overactivity or an inability to relax a muscle. **Hold capacity** reflects a user's ability to sustain a muscle contraction or muscle endurance by recording the time during which consistent EMG amplitude is produced. A muscle that produces an erratic EMG signal during an active contraction is considered to have poor hold capacity. The **intercontraction baseline** is the level of myoelectrical activity measured between muscle contractions when the muscle is at rest. The **threshold** is the goal level of myoelectrical activity set by the clinician based on the aforementioned therapeutic goals and measured variables. The threshold will be recorded as the level of electrical activity (µV) that must be achieved by the user to produce a signal during EMG biofeedback training. If the goal is to increase myoelectrical activity during a volitional muscle contraction (facilitation), the user will be instructed to try to reach or exceed the threshold (**above threshold**). If the goal is to reduce myoelectrical activity at rest or during functional activities (inhibition), the user will be instructed to decrease the amplitude to a level at or below the set threshold (**below threshold**).

Physiological Effects of EMG Biofeedback

As described in the introduction to this chapter, EMG biofeedback provides information to the user to allow volitional alteration of myoelectrical activity. The user must be able to interpret and learn how to modify the targeted activity based on the information provided to realize a therapeutic benefit. This is the underlying principle behind the intended neurophysiological effects of EMG biofeedback for neuromuscular **facilitation (up training), inhibition (down training),** or coordination.

NEUROMUSCULAR FACILITATION

Two primary neurophysiological mechanisms are thought to facilitate myoelectrical activity: reduced inhibition of descending motor (excitatory) signals and increased excitation of cerebromotor cortex (Fig. 15.7).[2–5] Both mechanisms increase a muscle's ability to generate force and therefore can result in muscle hypertrophy, increased strength, and improved function (performance).

Normal muscle function is inhibited in the presence of pain and swelling after injury or surgery. This may be a result of decreased excitability of the associated primary motor cortex, a phenomenon commonly referred to as **arthrogenic muscle**

inhibition (AMI).[2,6] Although AMI is protective, it can lead to muscle atrophy, weakness, and long-term disability if left untreated. Therapeutic modalities that minimize the inhibitory effects of pain and swelling or enhance the excitability of motor units, such as ice and electrical stimulation, have been described in detail in previous chapters. EMG biofeedback uses attentional strategies to disinhibit muscle activity through enhanced muscle contraction timing or increased motor unit recruitment. Reduction of AMI increases a muscle's ability to generate force, typically measured as the peak torque produced during a **maximal voluntary isometric contraction (MVIC).**

Improving muscle performance, or "up training," is often a goal after orthopedic surgery (e.g., anterior cruciate ligament [ACL] reconstruction, rotator cuff repair); in neurological conditions affecting muscle contractility (e.g., stroke, incomplete spinal cord injury, peripheral nerve injuries); in conditions affecting muscle performance related to age, trauma, or disuse (e.g., injury to the pelvic floor muscles [PFMs] after childbirth); or when trying to improve function or performance of daily,

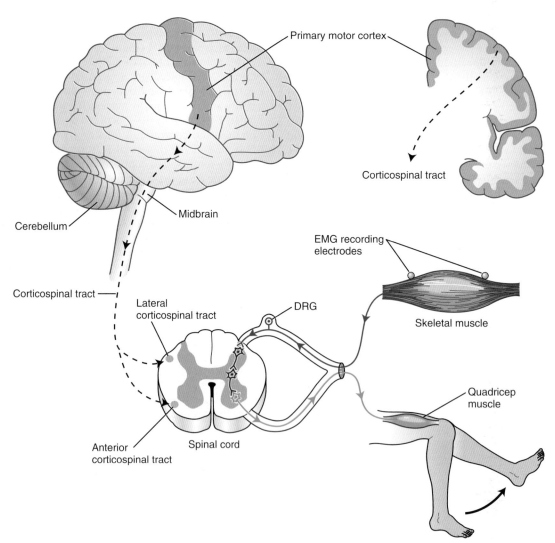

FIGURE 15.7 Neurophysiological mechanisms for facilitating myoelectrical activity. Neural information from premotor areas of the brain (involved in planning movements) is transmitted via the primary motor cortex to descending tracts in the spinal cord. These descending spinal cord tracts terminate on alpha motor neurons that then excite muscles. Two primary neurophysiological mechanisms are thought to facilitate myoelectrical activity: (1) reduced inhibition of descending excitatory motor signals or (2) increased excitation of the cerebromotor cortex. *DRG,* Dorsal root ganglion.

occupational, or sports activities. Immediate short-term effects of using EMG biofeedback to facilitate muscle contraction include greater force production during an MVIC, earlier gains in range of motion (ROM) and function following surgery, decreased latency of motor unit recruitment, and increased neural excitability and voluntary activation.[7-10] Long-term results follow the principles of therapeutic exercise and depend on the exercise dose and specificity of training.

NEUROMUSCULAR INHIBITION

To inhibit the ionic activity of a muscle ("down training"), the user must reduce the motor input to that muscle. The resulting decrease in tone is a result of activation of fewer or smaller motor units, less frequent depolarization per unit time, or a combination of these effects. As the information being fed back is received, the user attempts to reduce the signal frequency or intensity of the detected myoelectrical activity. Successful reduction of the fed-back signal reinforces the user's control over the underlying ionic activity. The neurophysiological pathways for facilitating a muscle contraction are the same pathways targeted to inhibit muscle activity; however, the intent is to increase afferent inhibition of aberrant efferent signals or decrease the excitability of the motor cortex. EMG biofeedback for muscle inhibition is commonly used in conjunction with relaxation techniques, postural training, and therapeutic exercise to decrease pain, decrease muscle tone, improve function, and increase ROM and flexibility.[11-15]

NEUROMUSCULAR COORDINATION

EMG biofeedback can also be used to improve the timing and recruitment of muscle activity to improve functional activities such as gait or the performance of higher-level activities.[16-20] The emphasis here is less on facilitation or inhibition of muscle to increase strength or decrease tone and more on the appropriate timing and intensity of motor unit firing for the specific task. EMG biofeedback to improve coordination has been used successfully in athletes, musicians, and patients with central or peripheral neurological injury.[16,17,21]

Clinical Indications for EMG Biofeedback

EMG biofeedback is typically used with other interventions to facilitate or inhibit muscle activity or to improve coordination. For example, EMG biofeedback can be used to facilitate muscle activity during the performance of an isometric contraction, with the goal of increasing strength using the principles of therapeutic exercise. In contrast, in the presence of spasticity or hypertonicity, EMG biofeedback can assist in reducing muscle activity in combination with relaxation training or neurological rehabilitation. The principles of neuromuscular reeducation and retraining are enhanced with the use EMG biofeedback for discoordination and to improve function and performance.

> ### ◎ Clinical Pearl
> EMG biofeedback up training can be used to facilitate muscle activity after stroke or for strengthening. EMG biofeedback down training can be used to inhibit muscle activity in patients with headache.

HEMIPLEGIA

EMG biofeedback may help address impairments in patients with **hemiplegia** after stroke. Examples of clinical applications in this population include decreasing footdrop, reducing shoulder subluxation, and improving hand function (Table 15.1). However, variability in measured outcomes, small sample sizes, and differing methodologies make it difficult to draw definitive conclusions regarding the overall effectiveness of EMG biofeedback in patients after stroke.

The use of EMG biofeedback for improving upper extremity function after stroke has been repeatedly supported in the literature.[22-26] A meta-analysis of eight randomized or matched-control studies concluded that EMG biofeedback is effective for neuromuscular reeducation in patients with hemiplegia after stroke.[27] The authors further identified that in most subjects in the included studies, stroke had occurred 3 or more months previously, beyond the time frame when spontaneous improvements in hemiplegia are likely to occur. However, a 2007 Cochrane Collaboration systematic review and meta-analysis comparing active physical therapy and EMG biofeedback to physical therapy alone or with sham biofeedback was less conclusive. Despite evidence from small individual studies suggesting EMG biofeedback improves gait, muscle power, and function more effectively than physical therapy alone, a combined analysis of the identified studies did not demonstrate a treatment benefit.[18] A 2009 systematic review examining all studied interventions for motor recovery after stroke found that EMG biofeedback did promote recovery of arm function, although the studies were limited by small sample sizes and the lack of blinding and allocation concealment.[24] This conclusion is supported by a 2012 randomized

TABLE 15.1	Clinical Indications for Electromyography (EMG) Biofeedback After Stroke		
Clinical Indication	**Primary Targeted Muscles**	**Neurophysiological Effect**	**Functional Goals**
Footdrop	Anterior tibialis	Facilitate	Improve gait
	Gastrocnemius	Inhibit	
Shoulder hemiparesis	Upper trapezius	Facilitate	Reduce shoulder subluxation
	Anterior deltoid	Facilitate	
Hand hemiparesis	Wrist/finger flexors	Inhibit	Improve grasp
	Wrist/finger extensors	Facilitate	

controlled trial in 40 patients with spasticity after stroke that found that combining EMG biofeedback with a traditional rehabilitation program of neurodevelopmental and conventional methods provided significantly greater improvements in spasticity and hand function than a traditional program alone.[23] The study group received 3 weeks of EMG biofeedback 5 days per week for 20 minutes, with the electrodes placed over motor points on the affected wrist flexors. Subjects were instructed to maintain a below-threshold level of myogenic activity using the audio and visual feedback provided with the forearm resting over a pillow and the wrist in 90 degrees of flexion. A recent randomized controlled trial compared the use of EMG biofeedback for serratus anterior facilitation and upper trapezius inhibition during the performance of upper extremity functional tasks with sham EMG biofeedback training. The EMG biofeedback group demonstrated significant improvements over the control group in function, active ROM (AROM), and muscle performance after 6 weeks and at 1 month after completion of the study.[26] Task-oriented retraining with EMG biofeedback of the tibialis anterior (TA) muscle has also been found to produce significant improvements in TA strength compared with task retraining without EMG biofeedback. Furthermore, the use of faded EMG biofeedback and randomized, variable TA activation at 25%, 50%, 75%, and 100% of maximum EMG signal resulted in significant improvements in anterior-posterior postural sway compared with constant TA activation at 100% EMG signal. The results of this study demonstrate the added benefit of incorporating motor learning principles when using EMG biofeedback in the treatment of patients with chronic stroke.[28]

QUADRICEPS STRENGTHENING

Quadriceps muscle inhibition, weakness, and dysfunction are commonly associated with musculoskeletal conditions presenting with knee pain.[6] Strategies to activate the quadriceps muscle to improve strength and function are fundamental in the treatment of knee pain.[8,29–33] The importance of these interventions is supported by the finding that 47% of MVIC variance in subjects following anterior cruciate ligament (ACL) reconstruction can be predicted by the level of corticospinal and spinal reflexive excitability.[7] Characteristic differences between musculoskeletal conditions associated with knee pain make it difficult to compare trials incorporating EMG biofeedback for quadriceps strengthening. For example, a significant treatment effect was reported for EMG biofeedback compared with placebo or conventional strengthening programs for quadriceps strengthening in patients with knee osteoarthritis; however, the effect on quadriceps strength was not significant when all knee conditions were evaluated together.[4] The chronicity of injury may influence the effectiveness of EMG biofeedback in the treatment of knee pain, as demonstrated in a systematic review of eight studies using EMG biofeedback of the quadriceps femoris across a number of knee conditions. Although EMG biofeedback was associated with statistically significant improvements in pain and strength after surgery, similar benefits were not realized when EMG biofeedback was used for more chronic conditions.[34] The use of EMG biofeedback to improve acute, postsurgical conditions is further supported by a randomized controlled trial with 45 subjects after knee meniscectomy. Subjects were assigned to one of three

treatment groups: (1) home exercise program (HEP), (2) HEP plus quadriceps EMG biofeedback, or (3) HEP plus quadriceps electrical stimulation. In addition to performing their HEP, subjects in the EMG biofeedback group performed isometric quadriceps contractions with EMG biofeedback 5 days per week for 2 weeks, holding each contraction above the set threshold for 10 seconds, followed by a 20-second rest, for a total treatment time of 20 minutes per day. At 2 and 6 weeks after surgery, significantly greater gains in strength and function were found in the EMG biofeedback group than in the HEP-only and electrical stimulation groups.[35]

A systematic review of all trials examining the use of therapeutic modalities for patellofemoral pain syndrome found that the addition of EMG biofeedback and taping significantly reduced pain and improved selective vastus medialis oblique (VMO) recruitment, but the addition of EMG biofeedback to exercise did not significantly enhance effects on pain or function despite increases in vastus medialis and VMO recruitment.[36] The lack of statistically significant effects may largely be attributable to the low to moderate quality of the identified studies specifically examining EMG biofeedback as a modality in the treatment of patellofemoral pain syndrome. A recent study demonstrated the benefits of adding EMG biofeedback to conventional physical therapy in the treatment of subjects with polyarticular juvenile rheumatoid arthritis (JRA).[37] Subjects aged 8 to 13 years diagnosed with JRA ($n = 36$) were randomized into one of two groups: a control group consisting of conventional physical therapy or a treatment group consisting of conventional physical therapy plus EMG biofeedback-guided isometric strengthening. All subjects were seen for 1 hour, three times per week over 12 weeks, with subjects in the treatment group performing 10-second isometric contractions assisted with above-threshold EMG biofeedback of the vastus medialis oblique and rectus femoris muscles, followed by 20 seconds of rest. At the completion of the study, subjects in the treatment group demonstrated significantly greater improvements in pain, quadriceps strength, and function, supporting the addition of EMG biofeedback-guided isometrics to conventional physical therapy in the treatment of JRA.

HEADACHE

The effectiveness of EMG biofeedback to treat migraine and tension-type headache (HA) is well established.[12,38–42] Commonly used psychophysiological strategies combine relaxation techniques and EMG biofeedback training. Although strategies may differ across age groups and HA types, the underlying intention is to improve self-efficacy and decrease muscle tension in the pericranial and upper trapezius muscles. A recent meta-analysis of 94 studies found EMG biofeedback to be effective for both migraine HA (level 4 efficacy) and tension-type HA (level 5 efficacious and specific).[40,43] EMG biofeedback for tension-type HA has traditionally targeted the frontalis muscle, but a study by Arena et al[38] found that EMG biofeedback of the upper trapezius muscle more effectively reduced tension-type HA activity (intensity and duration) than EMG biofeedback of the frontalis muscle or relaxation training. This study included 26 subjects randomly assigned to one of three treatments: (1) frontal EMG, (2) trapezius EMG, or (3) relaxation training. EMG biofeedback treatment sessions lasting approximately 50 minutes each were conducted twice weekly over a 6- to 9-week period. The authors reported significantly greater clinical success in subjects receiving trapezius EMG biofeedback, which they defined as a reduction in the HA index greater or equal to 50% of the pretreatment measure.

PELVIC FLOOR DISORDERS

EMG biofeedback targeting the PFMs is effective in treating urinary and fecal incontinence and fecal constipation. In a 2014 clinical practice guideline, the American College of Physicians recommended EMG biofeedback as a first-line intervention to manage stress urinary incontinence (SUI) in women.[44] When treating SUI, EMG biofeedback targeting the PFMs is commonly combined with Kegel exercises—isolated contraction of the PFMs—to strengthen and improve volitional muscle performance. A study of 53 women with SUI found that combining intravaginal pressure biofeedback or perineal EMG biofeedback with PFM exercise produced significantly greater improvements across all measured variables when compared with PFM exercises alone.[45] Studies involving both male and female subjects with urinary incontinence treated with EMG biofeedback and PFM training reported significant improvements in incontinence and quality-of-life measures.[46–49] The use of electrical stimulation in conjunction with EMG biofeedback and PFM exercise also has proven beneficial over EMG biofeedback and PFM exercise alone. For instance, combining transcutaneous interferential electrical stimulation of the PFMs with EMG biofeedback was found to be superior to EMG biofeedback alone when used to treat children with nonneuropathic urinary incontinence.[50] In women with multiple sclerosis, EMG biofeedback and PFM exercise combined with vaginal neuromuscular electrical stimulation produced greater improvements in lower urinary tract symptoms when compared with PFM exercise with sham neuromuscular electrical stimulation (NMES) or PFM exercise with transcutaneous tibial nerve stimulation and EMG biofeedback.[51] A systematic review of 13 studies also reported strong evidence for the use of EMG biofeedback to manage fecal incontinence.[52] EMG biofeedback can also provide information about PFM activity in patients having difficulty performing a bowel movement as a result of constipation. In a meta-analysis of studies published between 1950 and 2007 examining the treatment of fecal constipation resulting from an inability to relax the PFMs, Koh et al.[53] reported a sixfold increase in the odds of symptomatic improvement when using EMG biofeedback over other interventions, although the authors also recognized a lack of high-quality evidence. Dyssynergic defecation, a highly prevalent condition in women with chronic constipation, is characterized by incomplete defecation as a result of dysfunctional PFM contractility. Ten women with dyssynergic defecation were successfully treated with EMG biofeedback of the external anal sphincter during simulated defecation, with significant improvements in clinical symptoms, quality of life, and reduced EMG activity when compared with a control group.[54] In dyspareunia (painful intercourse), learning to control PFM overactivity decreases excessive muscle tone and pain in response to pressure.[55] Many of the techniques related to treatment of **pelvic floor disorders (PFDs)** require additional training for the appropriate evaluation and application of EMG biofeedback, especially when considering the use of intracavity devices for assessing and treating PFDs.

CHRONIC PAIN CONDITIONS

EMG biofeedback has been investigated as an intervention for reducing musculoskeletal pain across a number of conditions.[13,56–59] The physiological mechanisms underlying reductions in pain with EMG biofeedback are uncertain but are probably related to changes in muscle activation (facilitation or inhibition). Reducing muscle tone may increase blood flow to ischemic tissues, thereby clearing elevated levels of noxious (myalgic) mediators (e.g., bradykinin, substance P). Facilitation of muscle activation may reduce stress to painful tissues by restoring normal movement patterns and increasing joint stability. Angoules et al.[58] identified five studies in their systematic review of randomized controlled trials investigating the use of EMG biofeedback for the treatment of musculoskeletal pain. They found that EMG biofeedback reduced pain compared with baseline measures, but the effect was not significantly better than comparison interventions.

The use of EMG biofeedback for short-term pain relief in patients diagnosed with fibromyalgia syndrome (FMS) has also shown promise. In their systematic review of studies examining the use of **electroencephalography (EEG)** and EMG biofeedback in the treatment of FMS, EMG biofeedback significantly reduced pain, but other measured variables, such as quality of life and depression, were not significantly improved.[57] As with other areas of study, the authors identified that many of the studies included in their meta-analysis were of poor quality and that the long-term benefit of EMG biofeedback on pain has not been substantiated.[57,59–61]

TEMPOROMANDIBULAR DISORDERS

Temporomandibular disorders (TMDs) are a spectrum of conditions affecting the temporomandibular joint (TMJ). A general description of TMDs includes pain in the TMJ or masticatory muscles, joint crepitus, and limited or abnormal movement of the mandible. Summarizing the research on TMDs is challenging because of multimodal treatment designs and variations in inclusion criteria across studies. In a systematic review of 30 studies that examined physical therapy interventions for TMDs, 7 incorporated relaxation or EMG biofeedback.[14] Based on the strength of the evidence and the outcomes measured, the authors concluded that biofeedback and EMG training were effective in decreasing myofascial or muscular pain and improving opening compared with placebo or occlusional splints for the treatment of TMDs. These findings support two earlier meta-analyses and efficacy studies that found significantly greater treatment effects with EMG biofeedback compared with placebo when assessing pain and clinical examination measures.[62,63] The authors specifically identified EMG biofeedback of the muscles of mastication and relaxation training as having the most benefit in the treatment of TMDs and provided guidelines for future studies examining the use of biofeedback in the treatment of TMDs.

Contraindications and Precautions for EMG Biofeedback

As a device that detects normally occurring ionic activity of muscle tissue, the specific application of EMG biofeedback does not have any related contraindications when promoting or reducing muscle activity is indicated. However, the use of

EMG biofeedback is contraindicated in individuals with conditions that would potentially be exacerbated by promoting muscle activation, such as acute fractures or muscle strains, and in individuals with a history of allergic reaction to adhesives. The use of specialized intracavity sensors (intravaginal and intrarectal) is contraindicated during pregnancy, in the presence of bladder or vaginal infections, in the presence of genital skin conditions, following recent rectal or pelvic surgery (less than 6 weeks postoperatively), in the presence of untreated atrophic vaginitis, or when insertion of an intracavity sensor increases pain or discomfort.

✳ CONTRAINDICATIONS AND PRECAUTIONS

for EMG Biofeedback
- Acute inflammatory conditions
- Pregnancy
- Bladder or vaginal infection

CONTRAINDICATIONS AND PRECAUTIONS
Acute Inflammatory Conditions

Rest and immobilization are considered part of the immediate management of acute injuries during the inflammatory stage and after certain surgical procedures. Activities that promote muscle contraction may aggravate acutely inflamed tissue, resulting in increased pain and swelling, and may slow or disrupt the normal healing process. The use of EMG biofeedback is contraindicated during acute inflammatory conditions such as postsurgical and posttraumatic conditions, acute or unstable fractures, acutely inflamed tissue, infection, and thrombophlebitis.

■ Ask the Patient
- "When did your injury occur?"
- "When did your pain start?"
- "When was the date of your surgery?"

If injury or onset of pain occurred within the last 72 hours, the injury is likely to still be in the acute inflammatory phase, and EMG biofeedback should not be used. As inflammation resolves, EMG biofeedback may be used to promote muscle activity unless there is a risk of disrupting the normal healing of injured tissue. EMG biofeedback is contraindicated in the first 6 weeks after surgery unless otherwise directed by the surgeon and only then if no other contraindications for the use of EMG biofeedback exist.

■ Assess
- Palpate and inspect the area to detect signs of inflammation, including heat, redness, and swelling.

If signs of acute inflammation are present, it is recommended that the application of EMG biofeedback be delayed until they are resolved.

Pregnancy

Pregnant women should not use intravaginal devices because of the risk of infection. EMG biofeedback is also contraindicated in the presence of preterm labor and high-risk pregnancy, although this is primarily a result of the lack of research in this area. Pelvic floor EMG biofeedback is also contraindicated during the first 6 weeks postpartum.

■ Ask the Patient
- "Are you pregnant or is there a possibility you could be pregnant?"
- "If pregnant, how far along is your pregnancy? Is your pregnancy considered high risk?"

Bladder or Vaginal Infection

The use of an intracavity sensor may be implemented when reeducating the PFMs or perianal muscles in the presence of incontinence, dysuria (painful or difficult urination), or dyspareunia (painful or difficult sexual intercourse). Patients with known bladder or vaginal infections should not use intracavity devices as part of EMG biofeedback treatment.

■ Ask the Patient
- "Have you been diagnosed with a vaginal or bladder infection?"
- "Have you been feverish or had an increase in temperature?"
- "Have you noticed any abnormal odor or color to your urine?"
- "Have you noticed an abnormal discharge?"
- "Have you noticed pain with urination?"

Adverse Effects of EMG Biofeedback

The adverse effects of EMG biofeedback are related to potential responses when performing strengthening and cardiovascular exercise during EMG facilitation or skin reactions from the electrodes. For example, dyspnea, fatigue, angina, and other cardiac-related symptoms, as well as delayed-onset muscle soreness, may occur with excessive exercise during EMG facilitation. Increased pain may occur when EMG biofeedback is used inappropriately. A rash or other skin irritation at the site of the electrodes may be caused by an allergic reaction to the electrode adhesive.

Application Technique

APPLICATION TECHNIQUE 15.1   EMG BIOFEEDBACK

The specific application of EMG biofeedback depends on the identified impairments, the therapeutic goals, and the user's individual characteristics. The placement of the electrodes and the signal threshold are based on whether the goal is to facilitate or inhibit muscle activation, the surface area and number of targeted muscles, the type of electrodes, and the anthropometric characteristics of the patient (Fig. 15.8).

perform a strong contraction of this muscle with as much effort as possible." Record the peak amplitude.

8. Set the threshold at or just above the achieved peak amplitude and instruct the patient in performing isometric contractions with the goal of reaching and sustaining the threshold for a set amount of time with each contraction. Say, for example, "I want you to contract your muscle with enough effort to reach the

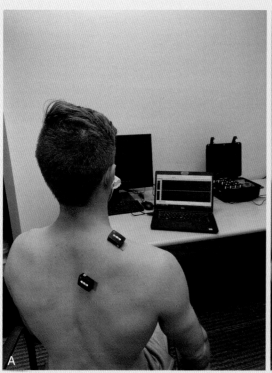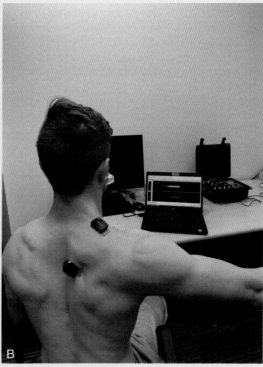

FIGURE 15.8 Patient setup for electromyography (EMG) biofeedback with wireless electrodes. (A) Upper trap and rhomboids relaxed. (B) Upper trap and rhomboids contracting.

Procedure

1. Instruct the patient in the goal of the EMG biofeedback treatment and be sure they understand and can correctly perform the prescribed activity. Say, for example, "I would like to use biofeedback to improve your ability to contract your muscles. The purpose of this intervention is to improve your strength and make it easier for you to walk and climb stairs."
2. Clean the patient's skin with alcohol, and if necessary, place a small amount of ultrasound gel on the electrode.
3. Determine the appropriate electrode location based on the specific muscles targeted.
4. Apply the electrodes, and if necessary, fix with tape to secure in place and prevent movement.
5. Attach the electrodes to the EMG biofeedback unit and turn the unit on.
6. Establish the baseline resting muscle activity over 1 to 3 minutes and record.
7. Establish the peak amplitude by asking the user to perform a maximal isometric contraction. Say, for example, "I want you to

threshold we just set. You will know you have reached the threshold when you hear the audible signal and see the display reach or surpass the set threshold. I want you to sustain the contraction above the threshold for 5 seconds and perform 15 contractions with 10 seconds of rest between each contraction."

9. Check on the patient during the treatment to determine if the threshold needs to be adjusted (i.e., the patient is easily reaching the threshold or can no longer reach the threshold because of fatigue).
10. On completion, turn off the device, remove the electrodes and discard them (do not reuse), and inspect the treatment area. Check for abnormal redness that may indicate a reaction to the electrode adhesive or signs of increased swelling or discoloration.
11. Assess the outcome of the intervention. This may include reviewing the peak amplitude achieved during the intervention, manually assessing strength, measuring AROM, and assessing functional performance and the level of pain.
12. Document the treatment.

PARAMETERS FOR EMG BIOFEEDBACK

When used to facilitate a muscle contraction, the signal threshold is set just at or above the level of the predetermined maximum volitional EMG amplitude. Instruct the patient to perform a specific activity or exercise during EMG biofeedback application with a dose that reflects the principles of strength training and neuromuscular reeducation. For example, the patient may be instructed to perform isometric quadriceps contractions at three sets of 15 repetitions twice daily, with the goal of retarding muscle atrophy and improving function after knee surgery.

When used to inhibit muscle activation, the threshold is set at or just below the lowest prerecorded amplitude that produces a signal. When the patient is able to successfully reduce muscle activation to below the threshold level, the audible feedback can be set to turn either off or on. This allows the clinician to determine whether the signal provides either positive reinforcement or negative reinforcement of the user's success in reducing muscle activity. For example, some clinicians may provide feedback to the user by setting the signal threshold to sound when the patient successfully reduces muscle activity below the set threshold. The feedback signal, possibly a pleasant signal such as music, would positively reinforce the user's success in decreasing muscle activation. EMG biofeedback for decreasing muscle activity can be set to provide continuous feedback to the user during daily living or work activities to minimize increases in muscle tension or for a set amount of time until a therapeutic benefit is achieved, as in the case of HAs or chronic pain conditions.

> ### Clinical Pearl
>
> A threshold setting requiring the user to increase muscle activity to produce an EMG signal is referred to as *above threshold*. A threshold setting requiring the user to reduce muscle activity to produce an EMG signal is referred to as *below threshold*.

Documentation

Include the following as part of your documentation as appropriate:
- Goal of treatment
- Area of the body treated
- Patient preparation
- Electrode placement
- Threshold level
- Baseline amplitude
- Peak amplitude
- Net change in amplitude
- Latency (rise/fall time)
- Treatment duration
- Exercise parameters (if appropriate)
- Patient position
- Patient's response to the treatment

Documentation is typically written in the SOAP note format. The following examples summarize only the modality component of treatment and are not intended to represent a comprehensive plan of care.

EXAMPLES

When applying EMG biofeedback to the quadriceps muscle to facilitate contraction, document the following:

S: Pt describes difficulty contracting quadriceps muscle and giving way when bearing weight.

O: EMG biofeedback to quadriceps to facilitate contraction.

Pretreatment: Trace (1/5) quadriceps contraction with knee extended in supine; EMG electrodes placed over VMO (baseline resting EMG level = 3 μV, maximum volitional EMG amplitude = 15 μV).

Intervention: Electrodes placed over VMO, signal threshold set at 17 μV. Pt instructed to perform 3 sets of 15 repetitions with 3-s hold and 60-s rest period between sets.

Posttreatment: Increased quadriceps contraction noted to palpation; maximum volitional EMG amplitude attained during treatment 23 μV (net rise = 20 μV).

A: Pt demonstrates improved quadriceps contraction, as evidenced by increase in peak amplitude after EMG biofeedback intervention.

P: Continue with EMG biofeedback for quadriceps facilitation.

When applying EMG biofeedback to the upper trapezius muscle to inhibit contraction, document the following:

S: Pt reports HA pain on verbal numeric pain rating (VNPR) scale as 4/10 located in temporal and retroorbital regions.

O: Pretreatment: Palpation of upper trapezius increases temporal pain (VNPR = 6/10). Baseline resting EMG amplitude of trapezius muscle 15 μV with erratic signal amplitude.

Intervention: Electrode placement over taut band in trapezius muscle and audible signal set using below threshold level of 12 μV for 30 min. Pt positioned in supine; instructed in relaxation techniques including diaphragmatic breathing and visual imagery.

Posttreatment: VNPR 1/10 after treatment; lowest recorded EMG amplitude during treatment 8 μV.

A: Decreased pain at rest and with palpation of upper trapezius muscle.

P: Pt instructed in use of EMG biofeedback during home activities or work for pain as needed.

CLINICAL CASE STUDIES

The following case studies summarize the concepts of applying EMG biofeedback as discussed in this chapter. Based on the scenarios presented, an evaluation of the clinical findings and goals of treatment are proposed. This is followed by a discussion of factors to be considered in the selection of EMG biofeedback as the indicated intervention modality and in the selection of the ideal treatment parameters to promote progress toward the goals.

CASE STUDY 15.1

Quadriceps Inhibition
Examination
History

MB is a 20-year-old female soccer player who underwent ACL reconstruction using a patellar bone-tendon-bone (BTB) autograft 5 days ago following a noncontact ACL tear of her right knee. MB states she injured her knee 2 weeks ago on landing single-legged from a jump during a soccer match. MB states that on landing, she felt a "pop" and sharp pain in her knee, causing her to fall to the ground. MB states she was unable to continue in the soccer match because of pain and instability and describes the onset of swelling shortly after her injury. MB states she received ice and electrical stimulation for pain and swelling before her surgery and performed isometric quadriceps strengthening and ROM exercises under the direction of the team athletic trainer. MB states that since her surgery, she has been using ice for 30 minutes every 1 to 2 hours and wearing a compression bandage. MB currently presents with knee pain and swelling and states that she is using axillary crutches to walk, weight bearing as tolerated (WBAT), and wearing a hinged knee brace set with an available range of 0 to 30 degrees of motion. MB rates her current pain as 3/10 while at rest and 7/10 at end-range when attempting to flex her knee.

Systems Review

MB is a healthy female college student with no previous history of surgery or injury involving the right knee. Before her knee injury, MB was a competitive collegiate soccer player. MB states she has 2 years of collegiate soccer eligibility and is motivated to return to competitive soccer activities. MB currently is having difficulty ambulating up and down stairs and getting to class but has access to campus assistance for transportation.

Tests and Measures

Active knee ROM measured in supine is 0/5/75. Active straight leg raise reveals a 15-degree extension lag. Quadriceps recruitment is poor with volitional contraction. Girth compared with the uninvolved limb is +1.5 cm at the joint line and +3 cm measured 7 cm proximal to the lateral joint line.

What are some reasonable goals of treatment for this patient? How would you position the patient during treatment? What therapeutic interventions could be performed in addition to EMG biofeedback?

Evaluation and Goals

ICF Level	Current Status	Goals
Body structure and function	Knee pain and swelling, decreased ROM and strength	Reduce swelling by 1 cm Increased active ROM to 0°/0°/135° Perform SLR with no extension lag
Activity	Difficulty with normal gait and ambulating stairs	Normal gait without assistive device; ambulate stairs
Participation	Unable to play collegiate soccer	Return to playing collegiate soccer

ICF, International Classification for Functioning, Disability and Health; *ROM,* range of motion; *SLR,* straight leg raise.

◆ FIND THE EVIDENCE

PICO Terms	Natural Language Example	Sample PubMed Search
P (Population)	Patient with postoperative quadriceps weakness	("Quadriceps Muscle" [MeSH] OR "quadriceps" [text word])
I (Intervention)	Surface EMG biofeedback	("Electromyography" [MeSH] OR "electromyography" [text word] OR "EMG" [text word] OR electromyographic [text word]) AND ("Biofeedback, Psychology" [MeSH] OR "Biofeedback" [text word] OR "biofeedback" [text word])
C (Comparison)	Physical therapy without EMG biofeedback	
O (Outcome)	Increased strength	AND "strength"* [text word] AND "Humans" [MeSH]

Key Studies or Reviews

1. Lepley AS, Ericksen HM, Sohn DH, et al: Contributions of neural excitability and voluntary activation to quadriceps muscle strength following anterior cruciate ligament reconstruction. *Knee* 21:736–742, 2014.

   This study demonstrated the relationship between corticospinal and spino-reflexive excitability to quadriceps MVIC strength in 29 patients who underwent unilateral ACL reconstruction, with greater activation and excitability being associated with stronger maximal contractions. Based on their findings, the authors suggest that strategies targeting neural excitation may be beneficial for strength training after ACL reconstruction.

Continued

Prognosis

MB presents with typical right knee pain and swelling after ACL reconstruction using a BTB autograft. Pain and swelling inhibit quadriceps function and result in functional deficits, including antalgic gait and difficulty with stair climbing. EMG biofeedback will allow MB to more effectively perform volitional quadriceps contractions, thereby improving strength and minimizing disuse atrophy.

Intervention

Facilitation of quadriceps contraction is indicated using single-channel EMG biofeedback with the electrodes placed over the vastus medialis approximately 50 mm superior and medial to the patella. Resting and maximal volitional quadriceps amplitudes will be recorded and the target set at 2 µV above the patient's current maximum achievable amplitude. MB will be educated on the audible and visual feedback provided and how it relates to quadriceps activity. MB will be instructed to contract her quadriceps muscle and attempt to press her posterior knee into the plinth. MB will be instructed to hold the contraction for 3 seconds, followed by a rest of 5 seconds, and to repeat this for 15 repetitions. MB will perform three sets with a 60-second rest period between sets. Maximal amplitude achieved will be recorded on completion.

Documentation

S: Pt describes difficulty contracting quadriceps muscle and giving way with weight bearing. Pt unable to walk up or down stairs and needs crutches to walk on level surfaces.

O: **Pretreatment:** Trace (1/5) muscle contraction noted with knee extended in supine; baseline resting EMG level 3 µV, maximum volitional EMG amplitude 15 µV.

Intervention: Electrodes placed over VMO, signal threshold set at 17 µV. Pt instructed to perform 3 sets of 15 repetitions with 3-s hold and 60-s rest period between sets.

Posttreatment: Increased quadriceps contraction noted to palpation; maximum volitional EMG amplitude attained during treatment 23 µV (net rise = 20 µV).

A: Pt able to demonstrate improved quadriceps contraction after EMG biofeedback treatment. Pt reports no adverse effects related to treatment.

P: Continue with home EMG biofeedback twice daily, 3 sets of 15 repetitions per session, to improve quadriceps muscle performance.

CASE STUDY 15.2

Headache
Examination
History

TB is a 43-year-old woman who presents with frequent tension-type HAs lasting up to 2 days in duration. TB states HA symptoms began insidiously approximately 6 months ago and have been progressively increasing in frequency and duration, with five to seven episodes per month. TB rates her worst HA pain as a 5/10 on the verbal numeric pain rating (VNPR) scale and localizes the pain to the suboccipital region with radiation into the temporal region. TB also describes pain in the upper shoulders, especially when performing her work activities as a certified public accountant. TB states that the specific activities that reproduce her HA pain include working at her computer and driving in her car for more than 30 minutes. TB also enjoys scrapbooking and playing the piano but admits her HA pain is disrupting her ability to enjoy these activities on a regular basis.

Systems Review

TB is a slightly overweight but otherwise healthy-appearing woman in no apparent distress and with no significant comorbidities. TB denies a history of neck or head trauma, nausea, photophobia, phonophobia, or auras preceding the onset of HA pain. Upper extremity neurological screening is normal and symmetrical for motor, sensory, and reflex testing. TB describes difficulty performing work activities related to sustained sitting postures and recreational activities, including playing the piano and scrapbooking.

Tests and Measures

TB has decreased upper cervical flexion and retraction ROM. Palpation of the upper trapezius reveals an active trigger point with palpable banding and radiation into temporal region and pain with palpation of the suboccipital and temporal muscles and hypomobility of the occipitoatlantal (OA) joint.

Evaluation and Goals

ICF Level	Current Status	Goals
Body structure and function	HA pain that refers to temporal region	Decreased HA pain
	Active trigger point in upper trapezius	Resolution of active trigger points
	Hypomobility of OA joint	Normal OA mobility
Activity	Computer activity and driving limited to 30 min	Unrestricted time performing computer work and driving
Participation	Difficulty performing scrapbooking, piano, and work activities	Unrestricted work and recreational activities

HA, Headache; *ICF,* International Classification for Functioning, Disability and Health; *OA,* occipitoatlantal.

CLINICAL CASE STUDIES—*cont'd*

◆ FIND THE EVIDENCE

PICO Terms	Natural Language Example	Sample PubMed Search
P (Population)	Patient with tension-type headache	("Headache" [MeSH] OR "headache" [text word])
I (Intervention)	Surface EMG biofeedback	("Electromyography" [MeSH] OR "electromyography" [text word] OR "EMG" [text word]) OR "electromyographic" [text word]) AND ("Biofeedback, Psychology" [MeSH] OR "Biofeedback" [text word] OR "biofeedback" [text word])
C (Comparison)	Relaxation training without biofeedback	
O (Outcome)	Decreased headache pain	

Key Studies or Reviews

1. Nestoriuc Y, Rief W, Martin A: Meta-analysis of biofeedback for tension-type headache: efficacy, specificity, and treatment moderators. *J Consult Clin Psychol* 76:379–396, 2008.

   This systematic review and meta-analysis of 32 randomized controlled trials and 21 pretest–posttest trials focused on biofeedback for tension-type HA found that EMG biofeedback provided significantly greater effect sizes in the treatment of tension-type HA compared with no treatment, placebo, or relaxation alone. EMG biofeedback with relaxation was found to be the most effective.

2. Arena JG, Bruno GM, Hannah SL, et al: A comparison of frontal electromyographic biofeedback training, trapezius electromyographic biofeedback training, and progressive muscle relaxation therapy in the treatment of tension headache. *Headache* 35:411–419, 1995.

   This early randomized controlled trial reported that upper trapezius EMG biofeedback was 100% successful in reducing tension-type HA at 3 months and provided significantly greater clinical improvement in activity than frontal EMG biofeedback or relaxation training.

Prognosis

TB meets the classification criteria for frequent tension-type HA with pericranial tenderness described by the International Headache Society.[64] Attentional strategies incorporating EMG biofeedback and relaxation training at rest, during work, and during recreational activities are likely to be beneficial. A comprehensive treatment plan should also incorporate joint mobilization techniques addressing the upper cervical mobility impairments, postural education, and ergonomic assessment of the patient's work environment.

Intervention

TB will be instructed in home use of an EMG biofeedback unit with electrode placement initially over the midportion of the upper trapezius muscle bilaterally. Baseline amplitude levels will be recorded with the patient in supine, sitting, and standing positions, and below-threshold levels will be set accordingly to promote relaxation of the upper trapezius muscle. TB will also be instructed in relaxation and breathing techniques as part of her home program and instructed in recording the frequency and duration of HA episodes in a diary to improve self-efficacy and monitor progress.

Documentation

S: Pt currently reports pain (VNPR = 4/10) located in the temporal and upper trapezius regions.

O: Pretreatment: Palpation of upper trapezius increases pain (VNPR = 6/10) with a localized taut band identified in the midportion muscle belly. Baseline resting EMG amplitude of trapezius 15 μV with erratic signal amplitude.

Intervention: Electrode placed over taut band in trapezius muscle and audible signal set using below threshold level of 12 μV for 30 min. Pt positioned in supine and instructed in relaxation techniques including diaphragmatic breathing and visual imagery.

Posttreatment: VNPR 1/10 after treatment; palpation of midportion upper trapezius produces decreased pain (VNPR = 3/10) without radiation to temporal region. Lowest recorded EMG amplitude during treatment 8 μV.

A: Decreased pain at rest and with palpation with noticeable decrease in palpable banding of upper trapezius muscle.

P: Pt instructed in use of EMG biofeedback during home or work for pain as needed.

CASE STUDY 15.3

Pelvic Floor Disorder
Examination
History

BK is a 38-year-old postpartum, primiparous woman who presents with daily episodes of stress incontinence. BK states incontinence began after the birth of her child 6 months ago. She describes a difficult labor lasting 14 hours and a vaginal birth. BK states the episodes of urinary incontinence have become more frequent as she has been returning to regular exercise and strenuous activities. BK describes episodes of incontinence with activities such as lifting her child, weight-training exercise, and jogging.

Systems Review

BK is a healthy woman in no apparent distress who recently gave birth to her first child. Before her pregnancy, BK jogged 20 to 30 miles per week and performed weight-training exercise 2 to 3 days per week. BK is anxious to return to her normal exercise routine but feels limited by the regular episodes of stress urinary incontinence. BK is a full-time mother and was active in her church before her pregnancy, but she now feels nervous about returning to church activities because of her incontinence.

Continued

CLINICAL CASE STUDIES—cont'd

Tests and Measures

Palpation of PFM contraction reveals poor recruitment. Baseline resting EMG measurement of PFMs with intravaginal electrode is 2 μV over 2-minute assessment; peak amplitude is 5 μV with erratic signal and 1- to 2-second contraction latency. Hold capacity is under 2 seconds at peak amplitude.

Evaluation and Goals

ICF Level	Current Status	Goals
Body structure and function	Decreased PFM recruitment and hold capacity	Improved PFM contraction (>10 μV) and hold capacity (>5 s)
Activity	Incontinence	Resolved urinary incontinence
Participation	Difficulty with lifting and exercise performance	Normal lifting and exercise without incontinence

ICF, International Classification for Functioning, Disability and Health; *PFM,* pelvic floor muscle.

◆ FIND THE EVIDENCE

PICO Terms	Natural Language Example	Sample PubMed Search
P (Population)	Patient with stress urinary incontinence	("Urinary Incontinence, Stress" [MeSH] OR "stress incontinence" [text word])
I (Intervention)	Surface EMG biofeedback	("Electromyography" [MeSH] OR "electromyography" [text word] OR "EMG" [text word]) OR "electromyographic" [text word]) AND ("Biofeedback, Psychology" [MeSH] OR "Biofeedback" [tw] OR "biofeedback" [text word])
C (Comparison)	Kegel exercises without biofeedback	
O (Outcome)	Decreased frequency of stress incontinence	

Key Studies or Reviews

1. Rett MT, Simoes JA, Herrmann V, et al: Management of stress urinary incontinence with surface electromyography-assisted biofeedback in women of reproductive age. *Phys Ther* 87:136–142, 2007.

   In this study, 26 women with urinary incontinence treated with EMG biofeedback–assisted PFM training demonstrated significant improvements in episodes of urine loss, nocturia, and pad use after treatment. Treatment consisted of 12 sessions lasting 40 minutes each, performed twice weekly, comprising both tonic and phasic contractions. The authors also reported significant improvements in EMG peak amplitudes and quality-of-life measures, with 88.5% of women reporting that they were "cured" or "almost cured."

2. Qaseem A, Dallas P, Forciea MA, et al: Nonsurgical management of urinary incontinence in women: a clinical practice guideline from the American College of Physicians. *Ann Intern Med* 161:429–440, 2014.

   The American College of Physicians provides six clinical recommendations for the nonsurgical management of urinary incontinence in women. PFM training as a first-line intervention for stress incontinence was given a "strong" recommendation based on the high quality of available evidence supporting the recommendation. The use of an EMG vaginal probe demonstrated weak evidence for decreasing incontinence over other nonactive interventions.

Prognosis

BK demonstrates poor coordination of PFMs during stressful activities, resulting in episodes of incontinence, following a difficult labor. BK is a good candidate for retraining of the PFMs through EMG biofeedback and exercise instruction.

Intervention

EMG biofeedback using surface electrodes over the PFMs was initially performed in a hook-lying position to facilitate muscle contraction. Treatment will also include instruction in avoiding increases in intraabdominal pressure (Valsalva) or substitution of abdominal muscles and appropriate co-contraction of the transversus abdominis muscle. Progression of EMG biofeedback will include advancement to upright postures and performance of stabilization exercises and functional activities.

Documentation

S: Pt reports frequent urinary incontinence with 8 to 10 episodes per day.

O: **Pretreatment:** External palpation of PFMs during active contraction reveals poor recruitment; palpation of rectus abdominis during contraction of PFM reveals overactivation. Baseline amplitude 2 μV; maximum amplitude 4 μV (net 2 μV) with long recruitment latency and poor hold capacity (<2 s). Normal derecruitment to baseline noted between contractions.

Intervention: Pt positioned in hook lying and electrodes placed externally at 4 o'clock and 10 o'clock perianal positions. Pt instructed to palpate rectus abdominis to avoid recruitment. Threshold set at 6 μV, and Pt instructed to perform 7-s contraction with 10-s rest. Treatment to be terminated when Pt is unable to reach threshold or maximum of 5 min.

Posttreatment: Pt demonstrated maximum amplitude of 9 μV during treatment and is able to sustain contraction for a full 10 s without fatigue.

A: Facilitation of PFM activation noted with increased amplitude and hold time during EMG biofeedback.

P: Pt instructed in home use of EMG biofeedback for 1 to 2 sessions/day for 5 min, 10-s contraction with 10-s rest. Plan to progress home use of EMG biofeedback to functional positions as PFM activation improves.

Chapter Review

1. *Biofeedback* refers to techniques that provide information to the user about their own physiological or biomechanical processes to improve self-awareness and control of a specific, targeted process (muscle or muscle groups).
2. EMG biofeedback detects changes in the electrical activity in muscle and converts it to a representative auditory or visual signal that is fed back to the patient.
3. EMG biofeedback can be used to "up train" (facilitate a muscle contraction), to "down train" (inhibit muscle activity), or to improve the timing and coordination of muscle contractions.
4. EMG biofeedback is typically combined with therapeutic exercise or relaxation training as part of a comprehensive program to increase strength, decrease pain, or decrease muscle spasm, with the goal of improving function and performance.
5. Because EMG biofeedback does not involve a transfer of energy, contraindications are relative to the specific application and individual characteristics that may pose a risk to the user (e.g., pregnancy, infection). Clinicians should always read and follow the contraindications and precautions listed for their particular EMG biofeedback unit.
6. The reader is referred to the Evolve website for additional resources and references.

Glossary

Above threshold: A threshold that requires the user to increase the level of myoelectrical activity to produce an electromyography (EMG) signal; typically used to facilitate a muscle contraction.

Arthrogenic muscle inhibition (AMI): A protective response following joint trauma that results in a decreased ability to produce a muscle contraction despite the absence of muscle or nerve injury.

Below threshold: A threshold that requires the user to decrease the level of myoelectrical activity to produce an electromyography (EMG) signal; typically used to inhibit muscle activity.

Biofeedback: Techniques that allow an individual to improve control over neuromuscular or autonomic processes through the use of devices that provide information about the targeted process using auditory, visual, or haptic stimuli.

Contractility: The capacity of muscle to contract or develop tension.

Contraction latency: The time between a command to contract a muscle and the point at which maximum amplitude is achieved during the muscle contraction (typically approximately 0.5 second).

Direct biofeedback: Biofeedback that provides accurate external information reflective of the internal biological process being monitored. A common example is a heart rate monitor.

Electroencephalography (EEG): Refers to the measurement of electrical activity occurring in brain tissue.

Electromyography (EMG): Refers to the measurement of electrical activity (μV) occurring in muscle tissue.

Facilitation (up training): Refers to increases in myoelectrical activity via reduced inhibition of descending motor signals and increased excitation of the cerebromotor cortex; the opposite of *inhibition*.

Gain: Determines the sensitivity of an electromyography (EMG) unit in detecting the electrical activity of muscle; higher gain settings are more sensitive and able to detect lower levels of electrical activity.

Hemiplegia: Paralysis of one side of the body following a cerebrovascular accident (CVA), or stroke.

Hold capacity: The ability of a muscle to maintain a contraction over time as determined by the stability of measured electromyography (EMG) activity.

Inhibition (down training): Refers to reduced myoelectrical activity as a result of increased inhibition of descending motor signals or decreased excitation of the cerebromotor cortex; the opposite of *facilitation*.

Intercontraction baseline: The level of ionic activity measured between muscle contractions.

Maximal voluntary isometric contraction (MVIC): A quantitative measure of muscle strength recorded as the greatest torque produced during a muscle contraction against an immovable object.

Peak amplitude: The maximum electromyography (EMG) activity (μV) recorded during a muscle contraction.

Pelvic floor disorders (PFDs): Conditions related to pelvic floor muscle dysfunction resulting in difficulty or pain with sexual intercourse, bowel movements, or urination or fecal or urinary incontinence.

Return latency: The time it takes for the electrical activity in muscle to return to resting levels following a command to relax (typically approximately 1 second).

Temporomandibular disorders (TMDs): Conditions resulting in orofacial pain and/or dysfunction of the temporomandibular joint, such as difficulty opening, joint locking, and crepitus.

Threshold: The level of electrical activity (μV) that must be achieved by the user to produce a signal during electromyography (EMG) biofeedback training.

Transformed biofeedback: Biofeedback that provides external processed information representative of the internal biological process being monitored. Electromyography (EMG) biofeedback is an example of transformed biofeedback.

References

1. Giggins OM, Persson UM, Caulfield B: Biofeedback in rehabilitation. *J Neuroeng Rehabil* 10:60, 2013.
2. Gabler C, Kitzman PH, Mattacola CG: Targeting quadriceps inhibition with electromyographic biofeedback: a neuroplastic approach. *Crit Rev Biomed Eng* 41:125–135, 2013.
3. Konishi Y: Tactile stimulation with kinesiology tape alleviates muscle weakness attributable to attenuation of Ia afferents. *J Sci Med Sport* 16:45–48, 2013.
4. Lepley AS, Gribble PA, Pietrosimone BG: Effects of electromyographic biofeedback on quadriceps strength: a systematic review. *J Strength Cond Res* 26:873–882, 2012.
5. Pietrosimone B, McLeod MM, Florea D, et al: Immediate increases in quadriceps corticomotor excitability during an electromyography biofeedback intervention. *J Electromyogr Kinesiol* 25:316–322, 2015.
6. Hart JM, Pietrosimone B, Hertel J, et al: Quadriceps activation following knee injuries: a systematic review. *J Athl Train* 45:87–97, 2010.
7. Lepley AS, Ericksen HM, Sohn DH, et al: Contributions of neural excitability and voluntary activation to quadriceps muscle strength following anterior cruciate ligament reconstruction. *Knee* 21:736–742, 2014.
8. Croce RV: The effects of EMG biofeedback on strength acquisition. *Biofeedback Self Regul* 11:299–310, 1986.
9. Gabriel DA, Kamen G, Frost G: Neural adaptations to resistive exercise: mechanisms and recommendations for training practices. *Sports Med* 36:133–149, 2006.

10. Takahashi R, Sano K, Kimura K, et al: Reproducibility and reliability of performance indicators to evaluate the therapeutic effectiveness of biofeedback therapy after elbow surgery: an observational case series. *Medicine* 99(34):e21889, 2020.

11. Moore A, Mannion J, Moran RW: The efficacy of surface electromyographic biofeedback assisted stretching for the treatment of chronic low back pain: a case-series. *J Bodyw Mov Ther* 19:8–16, 2015.

12. Mullally WJ, Hall K, Goldstein R: Efficacy of biofeedback in the treatment of migraine and tension type headaches. *Pain Physician* 12:1005–1011, 2009.

13. Holtermann A, Søgaard K, Christensen H, et al: The influence of biofeedback training on trapezius activity and rest during occupational computer work: a randomized controlled trial. *Eur J Appl Physiol* 104:983–989, 2008.

14. Medlicott MS, Harris SR: A systematic review of the effectiveness of exercise, manual therapy, electrotherapy, relaxation training, and biofeedback in the management of temporomandibular disorder. *Phys Ther* 86:955–973, 2006.

15. Cummings MS, Wilson VE, Bird EI: Flexibility development in sprinters using EMG biofeedback and relaxation training. *Biofeedback Self Regul* 9:395–405, 1984.

16. Aiello E, Gates DH, Patritti BL, et al: Visual EMG biofeedback to improve ankle function in hemiparetic gait. *Conf Proc IEEE Eng Med Biol Soc* 7: 7703–7706, 2005.

17. Govil K, Noohu MM: Effect of EMG biofeedback training of gluteus maximus muscle on gait parameters in incomplete spinal cord injury. *Neurorehabilitation* 33:147–152, 2013.

18. Woodford H, Price C: EMG biofeedback for the recovery of motor function after stroke. *Cochrane Database Syst Rev* 2007(2):CD004585, 2007.

19. Demircan E, Khatib O, Wheeler J, et al: Reconstruction and EMG-informed control, simulation and analysis of human movement for athletics: performance improvement and injury prevention. *Conf Proc IEEE Eng Med Biol Soc* 2009:6534–6537, 2009.

20. Larsen CM, Juul-Kristensen B, Olsen HB, et al: Selective activation of intra-muscular compartments within the trapezius muscle in subjects with subacromial impingement syndrome. A case-control study. *J Electromyogr Kinesiol* 24:58–64, 2014.

21. Markovska-Simoska S, Pop-Jordanova N, Georgiev D: Simultaneous EEG and EMG biofeedback for peak performance in musicians. *Prilozi* 29:239–252, 2008.

22. Rayegani SM, Raeissadat SA, Sedighipour L, et al: Effect of neurofeedback and electromyographic-biofeedback therapy on improving hand function in stroke patients. *Top Stroke Rehabil* 21:137–151, 2014.

23. Dogan-Aslan M, Nakipoğlu-Yüzer GF, Doğan A, et al: The effect of electromyographic biofeedback treatment in improving upper extremity functioning of patients with hemiplegic stroke. *J Stroke Cerebrovasc Dis* 21:187–192, 2012.

24. Langhorne P, Coupar F, Pollock A: Motor recovery after stroke: a systematic review. *Lancet Neurol* 8:741–754, 2009.

25. Moreland J, Thomson MA: Efficacy of electromyographic biofeedback compared with conventional physical therapy for upper-extremity function in patients following stroke: a research overview and meta-analysis. *Phys Ther* 74:534–543; discussion 544–547, 1994.

26. Lirio-Romero C, Torres-Lacomba M, Gómez-Blanco A, et al: Electromyographic biofeedback improves upper extremity function: a randomized, single-blinded, controlled trial. *Physiother* 110:54–62, 2020. doi:10.1016/j.physio.2020.02.002.

27. Schleenbaker RE, Mainous 3rd AG: Electromyographic biofeedback for neuromuscular reeducation in the hemiplegic stroke patient: a meta-analysis. *Arch Phys Med Rehabil* 74:1301–1304, 1993.

28. Tsaih PL, Chiu MJ, Luh JJ, et al: Practice variability combined with task-oriented electromyographic biofeedback enhances strength and balance in people with chronic stroke. *Behav Neurol* 26:7080218, 2018. doi:10.1155/2018/7080218.

29. Collins NJ, Bisset LM, Crossley KM, et al: Efficacy of nonsurgical interventions for anterior knee pain: systematic review and meta-analysis of randomized trials. *Sports Med* 42:31–49, 2012.

30. Draper V: Electromyographic biofeedback and recovery of quadriceps femoris muscle function following anterior cruciate ligament reconstruction. *Phys Ther* 70:11–17, 1990.

31. Krebs DE: Clinical electromyographic feedback following meniscectomy. A multiple regression experimental analysis. *Phys Ther* 61:1017–1021, 1981.

32. Oravitan M, Avram C: The effectiveness of electromyographic biofeedback as part of a meniscal repair rehabilitation programme. *J Sports Sci Med* 12:526–532, 2013.

33. Yip SL, Ng GY: Biofeedback supplementation to physiotherapy exercise programme for rehabilitation of patellofemoral pain syndrome: a randomized controlled pilot study. *Clin Rehabil* 20:1050–1057, 2006.

34. Wasielewski NJ, Parker TM, Kotsko KM: Evaluation of electromyographic biofeedback for the quadriceps femoris: a systematic review. *J Athl Train* 46:543–554, 2011.

35. Akkaya N, Ardic F, Ozgen M, et al: Efficacy of electromyographic biofeedback and electrical stimulation following arthroscopic partial meniscectomy: a randomized controlled trial. *Clin Rehabil* 26:224–236, 2012.

36. Lake DA, Wofford NH: Effect of therapeutic modalities on patients with patellofemoral pain syndrome: a systematic review. *Sports Health* 3:182–189, 2011.

37. Eid MAM, Aly SM, El-Shamy SM: Effect of electromyographic biofeedback training on pain, quadriceps muscle strength, and functional ability in juvenile rheumatoid arthritis. *Am J Phys Med Rehabil* 95(12):921–930, 2016.

38. Arena JG, Bruno GM, Hannah SL, et al: A comparison of frontal electromyographic biofeedback training, trapezius electromyographic biofeedback training, and progressive muscle relaxation therapy in the treatment of tension headache. *Headache* 35:411–419, 1995.

39. Nestoriuc Y, Martin A: Efficacy of biofeedback for migraine: a meta-analysis. *Pain* 128:111–127, 2007.

40. Nestoriuc Y, Martin A, Rief W, et al: Biofeedback treatment for headache disorders: a comprehensive efficacy review. *Appl Psychophysiol Biofeedback* 33:125–140, 2008.

41. Nestoriuc Y, Rief W, Martin A: Meta-analysis of biofeedback for tension-type headache: efficacy, specificity, and treatment moderators. *J Consult Clin Psychol* 76:379–396, 2008.

42. Rokicki LA, Holroyd KA, France CR, et al: Change mechanisms associated with combined relaxation/EMG biofeedback training for chronic tension headache. *Appl Psychophysiol Biofeedback* 22:21–41, 1997.

43. Association for Applied Psychophysiology and Biofeedback: Template for developing guidelines for the evaluation of the clinical efficacy of psychophysiological interventions. *Appl Psychophysiol Biofeedback* 27:273–281, 2002.

44. Qaseem A, Dallas P, Forciea MA, et al: Nonsurgical management of urinary incontinence in women: a clinical practice guideline from the American College of Physicians. *Ann Intern Med* 161:429–440, 2014.

45. Özlü A, Yıldız N, Öztekin Ö: Comparison of the efficacy of perineal and intravaginal biofeedback assisted pelvic floor muscle exercises in women with urodynamic stress urinary incontinence. *Neurourol Urodyn* 36(8):2132–2141, 2017. doi:10.1002/nau.23257.

46. Fernandez-Cuadros ME, Nieto-Blasco J, Geanini-Yagüez A, et al: Male urinary incontinence: associated risk factors and electromyography biofeedback results in quality of life. *Am J Mens Health* 10:NP127–NP135, 2016.

47. Huebner M, Riegel K, Hinninghofen H, et al: Pelvic floor muscle training for stress urinary incontinence: a randomized, controlled trial comparing different conservative therapies. *Physiother Res Int* 16:133–140, 2011.

48. Rett MT, Simoes JA, Herrmann V, et al: Management of stress urinary incontinence with surface electromyography-assisted biofeedback in women of reproductive age. *Phys Ther* 87:136–142, 2007.

49. Bertotto A, Schvartzman R, Uchôa S, et al: Effect of electromyographic biofeedback as an add-on to pelvic floor muscle exercises on neuromuscular outcomes and quality of life in postmenopausal women with stress urinary incontinence: a randomized controlled trial. *Neurourol Urodyn* 36(8):2142–2147, 2017. doi:10.1002/nau.23258.

50. Ladi-Seyedian SS, Sharifi-Rad L, Kajbafzadeh AM: Pelvic floor electrical stimulation and muscles training: a combined rehabilitative approach for management of non-neuropathic urinary incontinence in children. *J Pediatr Surg* 54(4):825–830, 2019. doi:10.1016/j.jpedsurg.2018.06.007.

51. Lucio A, D'ancona CAL, Perissinotto MC, et al: Pelvic floor muscle training with and without electrical stimulation in the treatment of lower urinary tract symptoms in women with multiple sclerosis. *J Wound Ostomy Continence Nurs* 43(4):414–419, 2016.

52. Vonthein R, Heimerl T, Schwandner T, et al: Electrical stimulation and biofeedback for the treatment of fecal incontinence: a systematic review. *Int J Colorectal Dis* 28:1567–1577, 2013.

53. Koh CE, Young CJ, Young JM, et al: Systematic review of randomized controlled trials of the effectiveness of biofeedback for pelvic floor dysfunction. *Br J Surg* 95:1079–1087, 2008.

54. Simon MA, Bueno AM, Otero P, et al: A randomized controlled trial on the effects of electromyographic biofeedback on quality of life and bowel symptoms in elderly women with dyssynergic defecation. *Int J Environ Res Public Health* 16:3247, 2019. doi:10.3390/ijerph16183247.

55. Gentilcore-Saulnier E, McLean L, Goldfinger C, et al: Pelvic floor muscle assessment outcomes in women with and without provoked vestibulodynia and the impact of a physical therapy program. *J Sex Med* 7(2 Pt 2):1003–1022, 2010.

56. Van Eerd D, Munhall C, Irvin E, et al: Effectiveness of workplace interventions in the prevention of upper extremity musculoskeletal disorders and symptoms: an update of the evidence. *Occup Environ Med* 73:62–70, 2016.

57. Glombiewski JA, Bernardy K, Hauser W: Efficacy of EMG- and EEG-biofeedback in fibromyalgia syndrome: a meta-analysis and a systematic review of randomized controlled trials. *Evid Based Complement Alternat Med* 2013:962741, 2013.

58. Angoules AG, Balakatounis KC, Panagiotopoulou KA, et al: Effectiveness of electromyographic biofeedback in the treatment of musculoskeletal pain. *Orthopedics* 31(10), 2008.

59. Linton SJ: Behavioral remediation of chronic pain: a status report. *Pain* 24:125–141, 1986.

60. Adams N, Sim J: Rehabilitation approaches in fibromyalgia. *Disabil Rehabil* 27:711–723, 2005.

61. Lauche R, Cramer H, Häuser W, et al: A systematic overview of reviews for complementary and alternative therapies in the treatment of the fibromyalgia syndrome. *Evid Based Complement Alternat Med* 2015:610615, 2015.

62. Crider AB, Glaros AG: A meta-analysis of EMG biofeedback treatment of temporomandibular disorders. *J Orofac Pain* 13:29–37, 1999.

63. Crider A, Glaros AG, Gevirtz RN: Efficacy of biofeedback-based treatments for temporomandibular disorders. *Appl Psychophysiol Biofeedback* 30:333–345, 2005.

64. International Headache Society: The international classification of headache disorders. http://ihs-classification.org/en/02_klassifikation/02_teil1/02.02.00_tension.html. (Accessed March 14, 2017).

Lasers, Light, and Photobiomodulation

CHAPTER OBJECTIVES

After reading this chapter, the reader will be able to do the following:

• Define *lasers, light,* and *photobiomodulation* (PBM).
• Describe the effects of PBM.
• Compare and contrast different types of laser therapy.
• Explain the adverse effects of PBM.
• Safely and effectively apply PBM.
• Choose the best technique for treatment with PBM, and list the advantages and disadvantages of each.
• Select the appropriate equipment and parameters for treatment with PBM.
• Accurately and completely document treatment with PBM.

Photobiomodulation (PBM) is the therapeutic application of **electromagnetic radiation** with wavelengths in and around visible light. Electromagnetic radiation is composed of electrical and magnetic fields that vary over time and are oriented perpendicular to one another (Fig. 16.1). All living organisms are continuously exposed to electromagnetic radiation from natural sources, such as the magnetic field of the earth and a combination of **ultraviolet (UV) radiation,** visible radiation, and infrared (IR) radiation from the sun. We are also exposed to electromagnetic radiation from manufactured sources, such as light bulbs, domestic electrical appliances, computers, and power lines.

Light is electromagnetic **energy** with **wavelengths** in or close to the visible range of the electromagnetic spectrum. Most light consists of various wavelengths of electromagnetic radiation, all within the visible range. This type of light is known as *polychromatic.* **Laser** (an acronym for *light* amplification by *stimulated* emission of *radiation*) light is also electromagnetic energy in or close to the visible range of the electromagnetic spectrum, but in contrast to other light, laser light is all of the same single wavelength. Laser light is therefore called **monochromatic** (Fig. 16.2). The waves of laser light are also all in phase with each other, known as **coherent** (Fig. 16.3), and the light is **directional** (also known as **collimated**), meaning it does not spread as it gets farther from its source (Fig. 16.4).

This chapter introduces the application of electromagnetic radiation in rehabilitation. Electromagnetic radiation in the radio-wave and microwave range of the electromagnetic spectrum is used for diathermy and is discussed in Chapter 10. Electromagnetic radiation in the UV range of the electromagnetic spectrum is discussed in Chapter 17, and because IR radiation produces superficial heating, clinical applications of IR lamps are described in Chapter 8, along with other superficial heating agents. Specific information about the therapeutic use of lasers and other light therapy is provided in this chapter. The therapeutic use of lasers and other light therapy was previously known as **low-level laser therapy (LLLT),** but to encompass the therapeutic effects of all types of light, more recently, the terms *PBM* and *photobiomodulation therapy (PBMT)* have been adopted by most experts in the field.[1] In this chapter, except when referring specifically to lasers versus other forms of light or when differentiating laser from other forms of light, the term *PBM* is used to collectively describe the therapeutic application of lasers and light in rehabilitation.

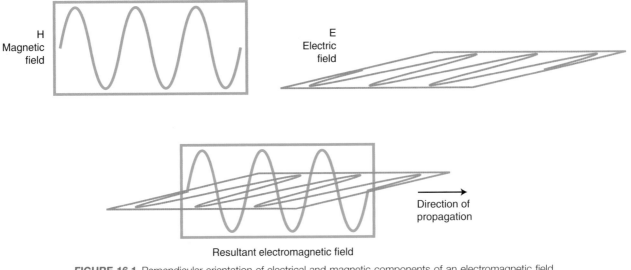

FIGURE 16.1 Perpendicular orientation of electrical and magnetic components of an electromagnetic field.

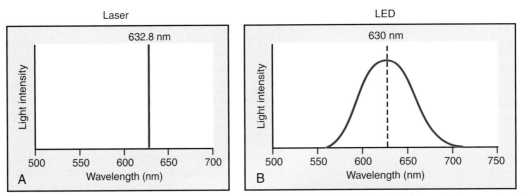

FIGURE 16.2 Wavelength distribution of different red light sources. (A) Light from a helium-neon (He-Ne) laser with a wavelength of 632.8 nm. This monochromatic light has a single wavelength. (B) Light from a red light-emitting diode (LED). This light concentrates around a wavelength of 630 nm but has a range of wavelengths.

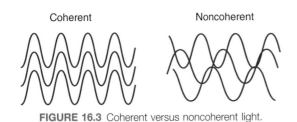

FIGURE 16.3 Coherent versus noncoherent light.

History of Electromagnetic Radiation

Electromagnetic agents have been used for therapy to varying degrees at different times. Until recently, most electromagnetic agents were used in a limited manner by therapists. However, since 2002, when the U.S. Food and Drug Administration (FDA) cleared the use of a laser device for the treatment of carpal tunnel syndrome, the use of lasers and other forms of light for therapy has gained some popularity, although limited by reimbursement in some systems.

Sunlight was the earliest form of electromagnetic energy therapy. Sunlight includes electromagnetic radiation in the UV, visible, and IR ranges of the spectrum. Prehistoric humans believed that sunlight could drive out the evil spirits

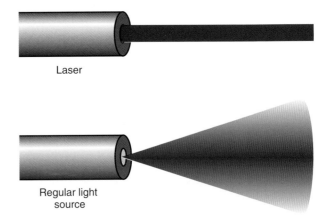

FIGURE 16.4 Directional light produced by a laser, in contrast to divergent light produced by other sources.

that caused disease. The ancient Greeks worshipped Helios, their god of light, sun, and healing. *Heliotherapy,* the term for treatment with sunlight, is derived from the word *Helios.* Although the exact purpose and effectiveness of heliotherapy as recommended by the ancient Greeks and Romans are difficult to judge, the prominent ancient physicians Celsus and Galen recommended bathing in the sun to treat many conditions, including seizures, arthritis, and asthma, as well as to prevent a wide range of medical problems and disorders.

Sunlight exposure, particularly to UV light, regained therapeutic popularity in the early 20th century. At that time, its value for preventing rickets (a bone disorder caused by vitamin D deficiency) in people rarely exposed to sunlight because of dark living and working conditions, as well as the potential effectiveness of UV in treating and preventing the transmission of tuberculosis, were recognized.[2,3] Today, although rickets and tuberculosis are rare in the developed world, UV therapy remains popular for the treatment of psoriasis and other skin disorders, and lasers and similar forms of light, generally in the red and IR range, are used clinically, particularly to treat pain and to promote tissue healing.

Other forms of treatment with electromagnetic radiation also gained popularity in the 20th century when electrically driven devices that could deliver controlled wavelengths and intensities of electromagnetic energy were produced. These included **diathermy**—devices that output energy in the shortwave or microwave wavelength range to produce heat in patients—and fluorescent and incandescent lights that output energy in the UV, visible, and IR parts of the spectrum. Today, diathermy is used for deep heating, UV light is used for the treatment of certain skin disorders, and IR lamps are sometimes used for superficial heating.

Laser and other devices delivering light in the visible or IR range are probably the most common form of electromagnetic therapy used in rehabilitation today. The idea of laser light was first proposed by Albert Einstein in 1916 when he introduced the concept of **stimulated emission** and proposed that it should be possible to make a powerful light amplifier by passing light through a substance to stimulate the emission of even more light. Einstein did not make a laser. It was not until the 1950s that research on stimulated emission devices really progressed, and in 1960, the first functioning laser was made by Theodore H. Maiman at Hughes Research Laboratories. This first laser was a ruby crystal laser. Soon thereafter, high-power lasers were adopted for a range of medical applications. Lasers were first used in medicine by ophthalmologists to "weld" detached retinas back in place and are now used for many other applications, including for finely controlled cutting and cauterization by surgeons and for treating various pigmented lesions by dermatologists. The lasers used for surgery are high-intensity "hot" lasers that destroy tissue. A **hot laser** offers a number of advantages over traditional surgical implements: the beam is sterile, it allows fine control, it cauterizes as it cuts, and it produces little scarring. In addition, because a laser has a narrow beam and because laser light is absorbed selectively by **chromophores,** it generates heat within and destroys only the more darkly colored tissue directly in the beam while avoiding damage to surrounding tissues. However, because hot lasers destroy tissue, they are not used for rehabilitation.

In the late 1960s and early 1970s, Endre Mester found that low-level (nonthermal, cold) irradiation with a helium-neon (He-Ne) gas tube laser appeared to stimulate tissue healing.[4-7] Others studied the effects of low-level (mainly He-Ne) laser irradiation, and in Eastern Europe and much of Asia, LLLT soon became the treatment of choice for a wide range of conditions.

But He-Ne gas tube lasers did not gain much popularity in the West because of their cost, bulk, and fragility and because of limitations of the evidence supporting their effectiveness. However, in the late 1980s, with the advent of relatively inexpensive semiconductor-based photodiodes to produce light, and mounting research evidence, low-intensity laser therapy, and later, other forms of light therapy, including treatment with light from **light-emitting diodes (LEDs)** and then **supraluminous diodes (SLDs)**, started to gain greater popularity in the West.[8] Light from LEDs and SLDs is not the same as laser light because neither is monochromatic, coherent, or directional. An LED is a semiconductor diode light source that produces relatively low-power light in a range of frequencies. LED light may appear to be one color (e.g., red) but is made up of a range of wavelengths and is not coherent or directional. An SLD is also a semiconductor diode light source, but it produces higher-power light than an LED in a narrower frequency range.

In June 2002, the FDA cleared the use of one laser device to treat carpal tunnel syndrome. Since then, other laser devices have received FDA clearance for the treatment of head and neck pain, knee pain, and postmastectomy lymphedema. In addition, many other light therapy devices, including **laser diodes,** LEDs, and SLDs, have been introduced to the U.S. market.

Today, many laser and light therapy devices are available in the United States and around the world. In general, these devices include one or more probes (applicators), each of which contains one or more diodes. The diodes may be laser diodes, LEDs, or SLDs, with each diode producing light in the visible or IR range of the electromagnetic spectrum. An applicator with more than one diode, called a **cluster probe,** usually contains various diodes of different types, wavelengths, and power.

The term *PBM* is generally used to describe treatment with low-power lasers and/or other low-power light devices, including LEDs, SLDs, and cluster probes. PBM is a very active area of research and publication. In contrast to other physical agents, where there is generally a dearth of research, there are multiple journals devoted entirely to PBM (e.g., *Journal of Cosmetic Laser Therapy, Laser Therapy, Lasers in Surgery and Medicine, Photomedicine and Laser Surgery, Journal of Clinical Laser Medicine and Surgery, Lasers in Medical Science, Journal of Biophotonics*), with each publishing many articles each month. Despite this immense quantity of publications, the quality of studies and clear guidance regarding the optimal use of lasers in rehabilitation remain limited. The recommendations given here are based on this author's interpretations of the current literature, which are likely to change as new discoveries about the effects of PBM are made.

Physical Properties of Electromagnetic Radiation

Electromagnetic radiation is categorized according to its **frequency** and wavelength, which are inversely related to each other (Fig. 16.5). As the frequency increases, the wavelength decreases, and as the frequency decreases, the wavelength increases. Lower-frequency, longer-wavelength electromagnetic radiation, which includes extremely low-frequency (ELF), shortwave, microwave, IR, visible light, and UV, is nonionizing. Nonionizing radiation cannot break molecular

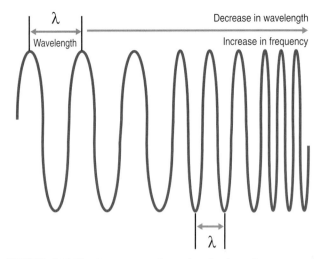

FIGURE 16.5 The frequency and wavelength of an electromagnetic wave are inversely related. As the frequency increases, the wavelength decreases.

bonds or produce ions and therefore can be used for therapeutic applications. Higher-frequency, shorter-wavelength electromagnetic radiation, such as x-ray and gamma ray, is ionizing and can break molecular bonds to form ions.[9,10] **Ionizing radiation** can also inhibit cell division, so its clinical applications are limited to low-dose exposure for imaging and higher-dose exposure to intentionally destroy tissue. Approximate frequency ranges for the different types of electromagnetic radiation are shown in Fig. 16.6 and are provided

in the sections concerning each type of radiation. Approximate ranges are given because reported values differ slightly among sources.[11]

The intensity of electromagnetic radiation reaching the patient from a radiation source is related to the energy output from the source, the inverse square of the distance of the source from the patient, and the cosine of the angle of incidence between the beam and the tissue. The intensity of energy reaching the patient is greatest when energy output is high, the radiation source is close to the patient, and the beam is perpendicular to the skin's surface. As the energy output of the device decreases, the distance of the energy source from the skin increases, or the angle with the surface decreases, the intensity of radiation reaching the skin diminishes.

> ◎ **Clinical Pearl**
>
> Because the intensity of electromagnetic radiation reaching the body is inversely proportional to the distance of the source from the patient, the impact on the patient will change a lot if the patient moves closer to or further from the radiation source.

Electromagnetic radiation can be applied to a patient to achieve a wide variety of clinical effects. The nature of these effects is determined primarily by the frequency and the wavelength range of the radiation and, to some degree, by the intensity of the radiation.

The frequencies of electromagnetic radiation used therapeutically can be in the IR, visible light, UV, shortwave, or microwave range. *Far IR* radiation, which is defined as close

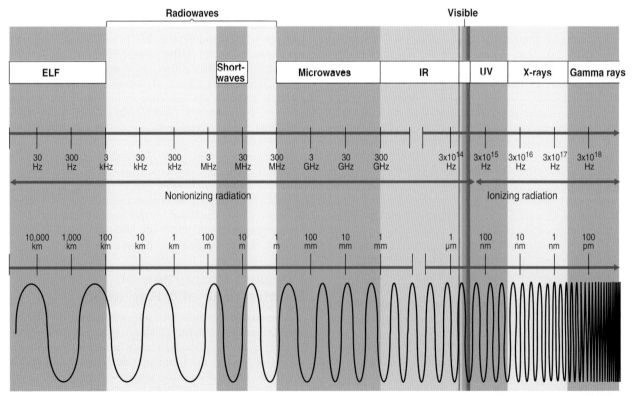

FIGURE 16.6 The electromagnetic spectrum ranges from low frequencies in the hertz range to greater than 1023 Hz, with wavelengths varying from greater than 10,000 km to less than 1 pm. *ELF,* Extremely low frequency; *IR,* infrared; *UV,* ultraviolet.

to the microwave range as opposed to *near IR,* which is close to the visible range, produces superficial heating and can be used for the same purposes as other superficial heating agents. Far IR has the advantage over other superficial heating agents of not requiring direct contact with the body. UV radiation produces skin erythema and tanning, as well as epidermal hyperplasia. Skin exposure to UV is also essential for vitamin D synthesis. UV therapy, as described in Chapter 17, is used primarily to treat psoriasis and other skin disorders. Shortwave and microwave electromagnetic energy, as described in Chapter 10, can be used to heat deep tissues. This is known as *diathermy.* When shortwave electromagnetic energy is applied at a low to average intensity using a pulsed signal, this is known as *nonthermal shortwave therapy (SWT).* SWT may decrease pain and edema and facilitate tissue healing by non-thermal mechanisms. Low-intensity lasers and other light sources in the visible and near-IR frequency ranges are generally used to promote tissue healing and to control pain and inflammation by nonthermal mechanisms.

LIGHT SOURCES

Light is electromagnetic energy in or close to the visible range of the spectrum. Light can be produced by emission from a gas-filled glass tube or a photodiode. Spontaneously emitted mixed-wavelength light, such as light from a household fluorescent tube light bulb, is generated by applying electricity to molecules of a contained gas. The electricity moves electrons in the gas molecules to a higher energy level, and when the electrons spontaneously return to their original level, they emit photons of light of various frequencies (colors), depending on the orbital they return to (Fig. 16.7). The original clinical laser devices used vacuum tube technology similar to a fluorescent tube light bulb to produce coherent, monochromatic laser light. With this type of laser, electricity is applied to molecules of specific gases contained in the tube, and the tube has mirrored ends. One end of the tube is fully mirrored, and the other end is semimirrored. When the electricity is applied, electrons in the gas jump up to a higher energy level. When these electrons return to a lower orbital, they produce photons that are reflected by the mirrored ends of the tube. As photons travel back and forth from one mirrored end of the tube to the other, they collide with other atoms of the gas, and each excited atom they encounter releases two identical photons. These two photons then travel back and forth and encounter two more atoms, causing them to release four identical photons, and so on. When the number of identical photons is sufficient, this strong single-frequency light escapes through the semimirrored end of the tube as a coherent, monochromatic, directional laser beam (Fig. 16.8).

Current therapeutic light sources generally use photodiodes instead of glass tubes to produce monochromatic or close-to-monochromatic light (Fig. 16.9). Photodiodes are composed of two layers of semiconductor: one layer of P-type material with a positive charge and the other layer of N-type material with a negative charge. When electrons fall from the N-type to the P-type layer, photons are emitted (Fig. 16.10). Laser photodiodes have mirrored ends that focus the energy

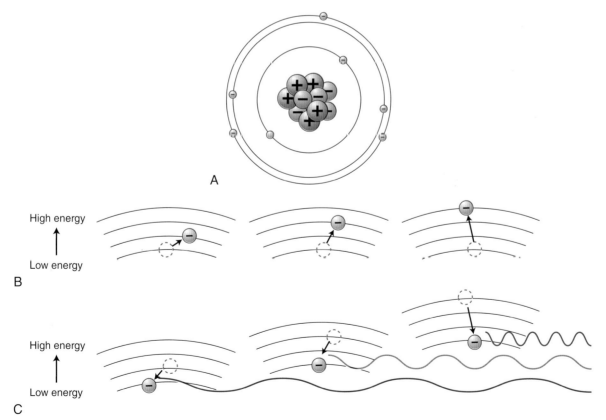

FIGURE 16.7 Spontaneous emission of light. (A) Atom with shells of electrons. (B) Electricity is applied, and electrons move up to different shells. (C) As electrons move to more inner orbitals, photons of various wavelengths are emitted.

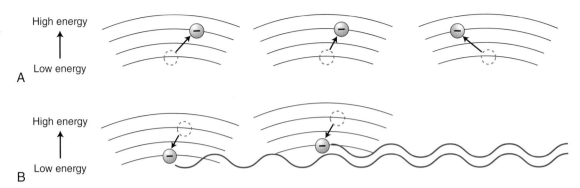

FIGURE 16.8 Stimulated emission of light. (A) Electricity is applied, and electrons all move up to the same level. (B) Electrons move to inner orbitals, and photons all with the same wavelength are emitted.

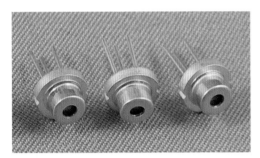

FIGURE 16.9 Photodiodes. (Courtesy LaserMate Group, Pomona, CA.)

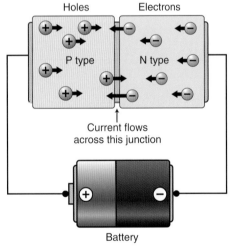

FIGURE 16.10 Light diode technology.

to produce monochromatic laser light. Photodiodes offer many advantages over tube light sources. They are small, hardy, and relatively inexpensive. Photodiodes may be laser diodes, LEDs, or SLDs.

◎ Clinical Pearl

Photodiodes can be laser diodes, LEDs, or SLDs. All of these diode types are small, sturdy, and relatively inexpensive.

Laser diodes produce light that is monochromatic, coherent, and directional, providing high-intensity light in one area. LEDs produce low-intensity light that may appear to be one color but is neither coherent nor monochromatic. LED light is not directional and spreads widely. Therapeutic applicators that use LEDs as their light source generally include 30 LEDs or more, in an array, with each LED having low-output power. Although the low power of LEDs can increase the time required for treatment, the large number of diodes and their divergence allow their light energy to be delivered to a wide area. SLDs produce high-intensity, almost monochromatic light that is not coherent but spreads less than light produced by LEDs (Fig. 16.11). Thus, SLDs require shorter application times than LEDs and deliver energy to a wider area than laser diodes. As noted previously, many clinical light therapy applicators include a few laser diodes, SLDs, and LEDs together in a cluster probe of 10 to 20 diodes or more.

WAVELENGTH

The wavelength of light most affects which chromophores absorb the light and the depth to which the light penetrates.[12,13] Light of wavelengths between 600 and 1300 nm, which is red or IR, penetrates most deeply into human tissue and therefore is used most commonly for patient treatment.[14,15] Longer-wavelength light (lower frequency) penetrates more deeply, whereas shorter-wavelength light (higher frequency) penetrates less deeply. For instance, IR light penetrates 2 to 4 cm into soft tissue, whereas red light penetrates only a few millimeters, just through and below the skin. Light may also produce physiological effects beyond its depth of penetration because the energy promotes chemical reactions that mediate processes distant from the site of application.

◎ Clinical Pearl

Light with a longer wavelength penetrates more deeply, and light with a shorter wavelength is absorbed more superficially.

POWER AND POWER DENSITY

Light intensity can be expressed in terms of **power,** usually measured in watts or milliwatts, or **power density (irradiance),** usually measured in milliwatts per centimeter squared

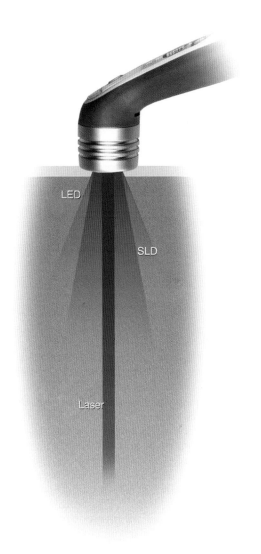

FIGURE 16.11 Comparison of the spread of laser, supraluminous diode (SLD), and light-emitting diode (LED) light. (Courtesy Chattanooga/DJO, Vista, CA.)

(mW/cm²). Power is the rate of energy flow, and power density is the amount of power per unit area. PBM applicators generally have a fixed power, although in some cases, this can be reduced by pulsing the output. If the light is pulsed, the power delivered is the average power over time, which equals the peak power multiplied by the pulse width multiplied by the pulse frequency. It is unclear if the effects of pulsed light are the same as or different from the effects of continuous light at the same average intensity.[16,17]

Because high-intensity lasers have the potential to cause harm, all lasers are assigned one of four classes, according to their power range (Table 16.1). These classes only apply to lasers, where the light energy is directional and does not spread, and not to other light sources, such as LEDs and SLDs, where the light energy spreads. The power of most laser diodes used for rehabilitation is between 5 and 500 mW. This is in the 3B class power range. When a PBM applicator includes a number of diodes, the power of the applicator is equal to the sum of the

	Power	
Class	(mW)	Effects
1	<0.5	No hazard
1M		No hazard because beam has a large diameter or is divergent
2	<1	Safe for momentary viewing; will provoke a blink reflex
3A	<5	Commonly used for laser pointers; Poses an eye hazard with prolonged exposure
3B	<500	Used for therapy; Can cause permanent eye injury with brief exposure; Direct viewing of beam should be avoided; Viewing of diffuse beam reflected from skin is safe; Can cause minor skin burns with prolonged exposure
4	>500	Surgical and industrial cutting lasers; Can cause permanent eye injury before you can react; Can cause serious skin burns; Can burn clothing; Use with extreme caution

TABLE 16.1 Laser Classifications

power of all its diodes, and the power density is equal to that total power divided by the total area, but the applicator is classified according to the power of the highest-intensity laser in it, not according to the total power of all the diodes.

Light applicators with higher power take less time to deliver a given amount of energy, but it is not known to what degree therapeutic effects differ if the same total amount of energy is delivered over a short duration with higher power compared with delivery over a longer duration with lower power.[18]

Clinical Pearl

Most laser diodes used for therapy have a power between 5 and 500 mW.

ENERGY AND ENERGY DENSITY
Energy is the power multiplied by the duration of application and is usually measured in joules:

$$\text{Energy (J)} = \text{Power (W)} \times \text{Time (s)}$$

Energy density (fluence) is the amount of power per unit area. Energy density is usually measured in joules per centimeter squared (J/cm²). Energy density is the treatment dose measure preferred by most authors and researchers in this field. This measure takes into account the power, treatment duration, and area of application.

Most PBM devices allow the user to select displaying energy or energy density. Because both energy (joules) and energy density (joules/cm²) include time, when using a PBM device, the clinician generally does not need to select the treatment time (duration).

PHYSIOLOGICAL EFFECTS OF ELECTROMAGNETIC RADIATION

When electromagnetic radiation is absorbed by tissues, it can affect them through thermal and nonthermal mechanisms. Because IR radiation and continuous shortwave and microwave diathermy delivered at sufficient intensity increase tissue temperature, these agents are thought to affect tissues primarily by thermal mechanisms. IR, having a shorter wavelength, can be used to heat superficial tissues, whereas continuous shortwave and microwave diathermy, with longer wavelengths, heat deep and superficial tissues. The physiological and clinical effects of these thermal agents are generally the same as the effects of superficial heating agents (see Chapter 8), except that the tissues affected are different.

UV radiation and low levels of pulsed diathermy or electromagnetic radiation in the visible or near-visible range do not increase tissue temperature and therefore are thought to affect tissues by nonthermal mechanisms. These types of electromagnetic energy are thought to cause changes at the cellular and subcellular levels by altering cell membrane function, permeability, and binding, as well as intracellular organelle function.[19] These changes can trigger complex sequences of cellular reactions and may cause proteins to undergo conformational changes that promote active transport across cell membranes and accelerate the synthesis and use of adenosine triphosphate (ATP).[20,21] Because these agents are thought to promote the initial steps in cellular function, this mechanism of action could explain the wide variety of effects that have been observed in response to the application of nonthermal levels of electromagnetic energy.

Many researchers have invoked the Arndt-Schulz law to explain the effects of low-level electromagnetic radiation.[22,23] According to this law, a certain minimum stimulus is needed to initiate a biological process. Although a slightly stronger stimulus may produce greater effects, beyond a certain level, stronger stimuli have a progressively less positive effect, so higher levels become inhibitory (Fig. 16.12). For example, a low level of mechanical stress during childhood promotes normal bone growth, whereas too little or too much stress can result in abnormal growth or fractures. Similarly, with some forms of electromagnetic radiation, such as shortwave or light, although too low a dose may not produce any effect, the optimal dose to achieve the desired physiological effect may be lower than that which produces heat. If even greater doses are used, they may damage tissue.

PHYSIOLOGICAL EFFECTS OF PHOTOBIOMODULATION

PBM has been studied and recommended for use in rehabilitation because, since devices were first developed, evidence suggested that this form of electromagnetic energy may facilitate healing. The clinical effects of light are thought to be related to the direct effects of light energy—photons—on chromophores

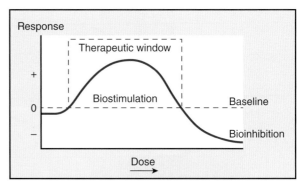

FIGURE 16.12 The Arndt–Schultz law. According to this general law of therapeutics, for many physical and pharmacological interventions, very low doses are ineffective, and low doses are effective, with increasing efficacy as the dose increases, until a maximum benefit is achieved. Beyond this dose, higher doses are less effective and then damaging.

in many different types of cells.[12,22,24–27] A chromophore is the part of a molecule that gives tissue its color by absorbing some wavelengths of light and reflecting others. Absorbed light energy can stimulate chromophores to undergo chemical reactions. To produce an effect in tissue, photons are absorbed by a target cell to promote a cascade of biochemical events that influence the tissue's function. Evidence suggests that light in the visible red and invisible near-IR spectral regions exerts a wide range of nonthermal effects at the cellular and subcellular levels as a result of its impact on cytochrome-c oxidase, also known as *Complex IV,* a chromophore with three copper atoms that is in mitochondria and affects ATP production and nitric oxide synthesis.[22,28–32] This can affect all energy- and oxygen-consuming processes in the body, including RNA production, cytokine synthesis, and collagen synthesis.[27,33,34] Laser light likely also initiates reactions at the cell membrane by affecting calcium channels[26,35,36] and intercellular communication[37,38] (Fig. 16.13).

PROMOTE ADENOSINE TRIPHOSPHATE PRODUCTION

The primary function of the mitochondrion—the powerhouse of the cell—is to generate ATP, which is used as the energy source for all other cellular reactions. Increased ATP production promoted by red and IR light is thought to be the primary contributor to many of the clinical benefits of PBM. ATP generation is a multistep process that occurs on the inner mitochondrial membrane. Red laser (632.8 nm),[39] LED (670 nm)[40] light, and IR laser (915 nm) and LED light[28] have all been shown to improve mitochondrial function and increase their production of ATP, with increases reported to be as great as 70%. It appears that light increases ATP production by enhancing electron transfer by cytochrome-c oxidase,[22,41–45] although recently, some have questioned the predominance of this mechanism[46–49] of action. The impact of PBM on ATP production is likely mediated in part by cellular or mitochondrial calcium uptake.[35,50]

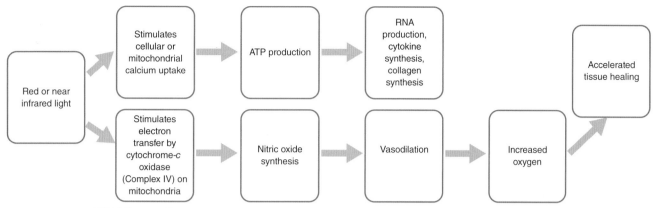

FIGURE 16.13 Proposed mechanism of action of photobiomodulation (PBM) for accelerating tissue healing.

PROMOTE COLLAGEN PRODUCTION

PBM is also thought to enhance tissue healing by promoting collagen production,[51–54] particularly the production of type I collagen, likely by stimulating the production of messenger ribonucleic acid (RNA) that codes for procollagen.[55]

MODULATE INFLAMMATION

PBM has been shown to help control inflammation in a range of animal models and clinical conditions.[22,33,34] These effects are associated with changes in cytokine levels, including prostaglandin $F_{2\alpha}$ ($PGF_{2\alpha}$),[56,57] prostaglandin E_2 (PGE_2),[55–58] interleukin-1α (IL-1α),[59,60] interleukin-6 (IL-6), interleukin-8 (IL-8), and tumor necrosis factor-α (TNF-α).[59,61] These changes in cytokine levels result in increased blood flow; enhanced keratinocyte migration and proliferation[62]; and enhanced activity of T and B lymphocytes,[63,64] mast cells,[65,66] and macrophages.[67,68] PBM can also stimulate the proliferation and activation of cells involved in tissue healing, including fibroblasts,[69–73] keratinocytes,[74,75] and endothelial cells.[76,77]

INHIBIT GROWTH OF BACTERIA

PBM can inhibit the growth of microorganisms, including bacteria and fungi. Several studies have shown that infrared, red, and blue light inhibit the growth of various bacteria, including *Staphylococcus aureus, Pseudomonas aeruginosa, Salmonella enterica,* and *Escherichia coli.*[78–84] These effects may be a result of the direct cytotoxic impact of blue light or high intensity light or the stimulation of an antibacterial immune response by red light.[29,83,85,86]

PROMOTE VASODILATION

Some authors report that PBM can induce vasodilation, particularly of the microcirculation.[87–89] This effect is likely mediated by the release of preformed nitric oxide or by increased production of nitric oxide, both of which have been found to be enhanced by irradiation with red light.[90,91] Such vasodilation could accelerate tissue healing by increasing the availability of oxygen and other nutrients and by speeding up the removal of waste products from the irradiated area.[92]

ALTER NERVE CONDUCTION VELOCITY AND REGENERATION

Research has also explored the impact of PBM on nerve function and healing.[93] The first FDA approval for PBM device was for the use of a specific low-level laser device for the treatment of carpal tunnel syndrome.[94] Some studies have also shown that PBM increases peripheral nerve conduction velocities, increases the frequency of action potentials, and decreases distal sensory latencies. In addition, mostly in animal studies, PBM has been associated with accelerated nerve regeneration and repair after injury.[93–98] These positive effects occur in response to laser irradiation over the site of nerve compression and are enhanced by irradiation of corresponding spinal cord segments.[99,100]

Clinical Indications for Photobiomodulation

SOFT TISSUE AND BONE HEALING

There are many published studies, review articles,[13,30,101–104] and meta-analyses[105–111] concerning the use of PBM to promote the healing of chronic and acute wounds in humans and animals. This area of research started with the early findings reported by Mester et al.[5] that low-level laser irradiation appeared to accelerate wound healing. Although the first meta-analyses on this topic, published in 1999[109] and 2000,[105] did not find sufficient evidence to support the use of PBM to promote venous leg ulcer healing, three more recently published meta-analyses[106,107,108] evaluating studies on wound healing in general concluded that PBM had strong (Cohen's $d = +1.81$ to $+2.22$) evidence of benefit for promoting tissue repair. Subsequently published studies continue to support this conclusion.[112–115] Furthermore, a 2014 systematic review of studies on the effects of PBM on skeletal muscle repair in animals also found that PBM reduced inflammation, modulated growth factors and myogenic regulatory factors, and increased angiogenesis after skeletal muscle injuries,[116] and other studies support that PBM can enhance oxidative energy metabolism and ATP levels and thus the aerobic potential and fatigue resistance of skeletal muscle.[117,118]

Although most of the research concerning PBM for tissue healing has focused on general soft tissue healing, as occurs with chronic wounds, local muscle trauma, or surgical incisions, some studies have examined the effects of PBM on the healing of other tissues, including tendon, ligament, and bone.[119-121] As with general soft tissue healing, most of these studies have shown positive outcomes. A 2012 systematic review of conservative management approaches for Achilles tendinopathy that included only human studies, although with fairly liberal inclusion criteria otherwise, concluded that there was moderate evidence supporting the use of PBM for this condition.[122] Similarly, a 2010 systematic review with meta-analysis of clinical trials of PBM for the treatment of tendinopathy found predominantly positive effects for both lateral epicondylitis and Achilles tendonitis,[123,124] and a more recent study suggests that PBM enhances the effect of aerobic exercise on tendon healing.[19] In comparing studies that found benefit for tendinopathy with those that did not, as with other indications, it appears that there may be an effective dose window for the treatment of tendons, although this window is likely broad in terms of all parameters.

With regard to fracture healing, several animal studies support the efficacy of PBM for accelerating fracture healing.[125,126] In addition, a systematic review and meta-analysis of randomized controlled trials (RCTs) on PBM for the treatment of fractures in human adults published in 2020 showed significantly greater pain reduction and improvement in physical function, but no difference in radiographic healing, with PBM compared with placebo.[121] Unfortunately, the certainty of these conclusions was low, and the authors recommended further research to prove the safety and effectiveness of PBM in the treatment of fractures.

Several studies have compared the effects of PBM with the effects of low-intensity pulsed ultrasound or shock wave therapy for promoting tissue healing or controlling inflammation.[66,127-130] Most of these have found both PBM and low-intensity pulsed ultrasound to be effective, without one being consistently more effective than any other.

The lack of systematic studies evaluating PBM treatment parameters for promoting tissue healing makes the selection of parameters for clinical practice challenging. Most studies and clinicians find red or IR light with an energy density of 2 to 15 J/cm^2 to be most effective, with higher levels within this range for tendon, skin, and cartilage and lower levels within this range for muscle.

ARTHRITIS

Studies have investigated the application of PBM to manage symptoms associated with joint dysfunction and arthritis.[131] A number of meta-analyses and reviews exploring the effects of PBM on patients with joint pain, rheumatoid arthritis (RA), and osteoarthritis (OA) have also been published. The most recent Cochrane collaboration reviews on PBM for RA, published in 2005, and of PBM for OA, published in 2004, found sufficient evidence to recommend consideration of PBM for short-term (up to 4 weeks) relief of pain and morning stiffness in RA, but the results were conflicting for osteoarthritis, with only five of eight studies reporting benefit.[132,133] A meta-analysis of studies on PBM for joint symptoms, published in 2012, that included 22 trials with a total of 1014 patients concluded that there was sufficient evidence to support that PBM reduces joint pain in patients and that the effect was more reliable when PBM doses were within recommended levels.[134] The researchers derived

recommended levels from a 2003 systematic review that provided dose ranges for different joints at different wavelengths.[124] These recommendations are extremely broad, including wavelengths of 632 to 1060 nm and doses between 0.5 and 2700 J. More recent systematic reviews and meta-analyses related to PBM for arthritis have focused on patients with knee OA. One in 2015 that included seven trials did not support the efficacy of PBM,[135] but the conclusions of this analysis have been questioned.[136] Furthermore, subsequent systematic reviews with meta-analyses, one in 2017 that included 14 trials[137] and another in 2019 that included 22 trials,[138] support the efficacy of PBM for reducing pain and disability in patients with knee OA, particularly if the dosages adhere to World Association for Laser Therapy (WALT) dose recommendations. There are two WALT PBM dose recommendation tables, both published in 2010, one for IR lasers at wavelengths of 780 to 860 nm and the other for IR lasers with a 904-nm wavelength. In general, they recommend, with the shorter-wavelength range, using 4 to 8 J for tendinopathies and 2 to 16 J for arthritis, and with the longer wavelength, using between 1 and 4 J for all conditions. They also recommend starting at these doses, ±50%, and reducing by 30% when inflammation is under control. Although the data supporting the efficacy of PBM for arthritis are becoming more convincing and dose recommendations are becoming narrower, there is still scant evidence to definitively recommend any particular treatment regimen or parameters for any specific condition or stage of condition.

LYMPHEDEMA

Despite concerns for promoting cancer recurrence or metastasis with any biostimulatory intervention, several studies have examined the effects of PBM on postmastectomy lymphedema. Based on findings from the first of these studies, published in 2003,[139] the FDA authorized the use of one laser device (LTU-904; RianCorp, Richmond, South Australia) as part of a therapy regimen to treat postmastectomy lymphedema. This device has a 904-nm wavelength (i.e., in the IR range), a peak pulse power of 5 W, and a fixed average power of 5 mW. In the 2003 study, laser treatment was applied at 1.5 J/cm^2 (300 mJ/0.2 cm^2 spot to 17 spots, for a total of 5.1 J) to the area of the axilla three times per week for one or two cycles of 3 weeks each. Although no significant improvement was noted immediately after any of these treatments was provided, mean affected limb volume was significantly reduced 1 and 3 months after completion of two (although not one) treatment cycles. Approximately one-third of 37 actively treated subjects had a clinically significant reduction (greater than 200 mL) in limb volume 2 to 3 months after receiving treatment with the laser.

A 2007 systematic review evaluating a range of common therapies for lymphedema concluded that, in general, more intensive, health professional–based therapies, such as laser therapy, complex physical therapy, manual lymphatic drainage, and pneumatic compression, are more effective than self-instigated approaches, such as exercise, limb elevation, and compression garments.[140] Numerous systematic reviews specifically focusing on PBM for lymphedema after breast cancer have now been published.[141-144] All of these support considering PBM in the axillary region for producing clinically meaningful reductions in limb volume and pain in women with breast cancer–related lymphedema. However, no studies have specifically evaluated the risk of cancer recurrence or metastasis in humans, and the optimal treatment parameters have yet to be elucidated.

Based on the current research and the FDA authorization, it is suggested that laser treatment to reduce limb volume associated with lymphedema after breast cancer be provided at an energy density of 1 to 2 J/cm^2 to a total area of 3 cm^2 three times per week for 3 weeks for one or two cycles.

NEUROLOGICAL CONDITIONS

Several studies have attempted to determine the impact of PBM on peripheral and central nerve conduction, regeneration, and function.[98,145–147] The first FDA clearance for laser therapy was based on a 1995 study of IR laser (830-nm) therapy in approximately 100 General Motors employees with carpal tunnel syndrome.[94] This double-blind RCT compared the effect of physical therapy combined with laser versus physical therapy alone to treat carpal tunnel syndrome. Grip and pinch strength, radial deviation range of motion (ROM), median-nerve motor conduction velocity across the wrist, and incidence of return to work were all significantly higher in the laser-treated group than in the control group. The treatment protocol was to apply 3 J (90 mW for 33 seconds) during therapy for 5 weeks. Many individual trials have since examined the efficacy of PBM for carpal tunnel syndrome, and a number of systematic reviews and meta-analyses of these trials have been published.[148–152] In general, these reports support that PBM in the infrared range with an energy density of around 8 to 12 J/cm^2 promotes recovery from carpal tunnel syndrome, but the low quality of the trials and the short duration of follow-up limits the ability to draw definitive conclusions and about benefit, duration of effect, and optimal dosing.

Laser therapy has also been investigated to treat neurological conditions other than carpal tunnel syndrome. Several studies have found that IR and red light may help reduce the pain associated with diabetic peripheral neuropathy and postherpetic neuralgia.[153–158] Some studies have also investigated the use of PBM for central nervous system (CNS) disorders, including traumatic and ischemic brain injury, stroke,[145,159] Alzheimer disease, Parkinson disease, and depression.[160–168] Studies in both animals and humans have shown promising effects, including enhanced neurogenesis, brain-derived neurotrophic factor (BDNF) synthesis, and synaptogenesis,[169] as well as altered inflammation in the lesional area, but there are few fully powered clinical RCTs in this area, and thus far, although PBM has proven safe, no study has achieved the primary outcome of statistically significant benefits.[170,171] Animal studies on the use of PBM for central nervous system conditions suggest that this intervention may be effective, but more research is needed to confirm effectiveness in humans and to delineate ideal treatment parameters.

PAIN MANAGEMENT

Many studies report that PBM reduces the pain and disability associated with a wide variety of neuromusculoskeletal conditions other than arthritis and neuropathy, including fibromyalgia,[172] acute and chronic low back and neck pain,[173–175] shoulder tendinopathy and impingement[176] syndrome, trigger points, temporomandibular disorder,[177] and delayed-onset muscle soreness.[178]

The effects of PBM on pain may be mediated by its effects on inflammation, tissue healing, nerve conduction, or endorphin release or metabolism. Analgesic effects generally are most pronounced when laser or light is applied to the skin overlying the involved nerves or nerves innervating the area of the involved dermatome. Although some studies have not found a significant difference in subjective or objective treatment outcomes when comparing treatment with PBM with alternative sham treatments, meta-analyses on the effects of laser therapy on pain described an overall positive treatment effect of PBM on pain in humans.[106,179,180]

Contraindications and Precautions for Photobiomodulation

Although the adverse effects of PBM have been reported to be no different from those reported for placebo, various authors and manufacturers list a variety of contraindications and precautions for the application of PBM. The following represents a summary of these recommendations integrated with those published from the North American Association for Laser Therapy consensus meeting in 2010.[181] To minimize risk, clinicians should also review and adhere to the recommendations provided with the specific device being used.

CONTRAINDICATIONS FOR PHOTOBIOMODULATION

> ✴ **CONTRAINDICATIONS**
>
> **for PBM**
> - Direct irradiation of the eyes
> - Malignancy
> - Low back or abdomen during pregnancy
> - Within 4 to 6 months after radiotherapy
> - Over hemorrhaging regions
> - Over the thyroid glands

Direct Irradiation of the Eyes

Because lasers can damage the eyes, throughout treatment, all patients treated with lasers and the clinician applying the laser should wear goggles opaque to the wavelength of the light emitted from the laser being used.[182] Safety goggles should be marked with the wavelength range they attenuate and their optical density within that **band (frequency band).**

> ◔ **Clinical Pearl**
>
> Both the patient and the clinician should wear protective goggles during laser treatment; the goggles should be specific to and marked with the range of wavelengths that they block.

Safety goggles suitable for one wavelength should not be assumed to be safe at any other wavelength. Particular care should be taken with IR lasers because even at high power, the radiation they produce is not visible, but it can still easily damage the retina. A laser beam should never be directed at the eyes, and one should never look directly along the axis of the laser beam.

Safety goggles are not required when nonlaser light sources, including SLDs and LEDs, are used. This is because, in contrast to lasers that produce directional light that is concentrated in one area and can damage the eye, particularly the retina, nonlaser light sources produce **divergent** light that diffuses the light energy.

Malignancy

PBM has been shown to have a range of physiological and cellular effects, including increasing blood flow and cellular energy production. These effects may benefit or harm patients with cancer. There may be benefits if the PBM damages the tumor, potentiates the cancer therapy, or stimulates the immune system. On the other hand, there may be harm if PBM accelerates the growth or metastasis rate of malignant tissue.[183-185] Given the conflicting findings, and to err on the side of safety, at this time we recommend that PBM *not* be applied in the area of a known or possible primary malignancy or secondary metastasis. Some authors do allow LLLT if the patient is undergoing chemotherapy, when PBM can be used to reduce side effects such as mucositis, and suggest consideration of PBM in terminally ill patients with cancer for palliative relief.[181]

> ### ▪ Ask the Patient
> - "Are you under the care of a physician for any major medical problem? If so, what is the problem?"
> - "Have you experienced any recent unexplained weight loss or weight gain?"
> - "Do you have constant pain that does not change?"

If the patient has experienced recent unexplained changes in body weight or has constant pain that does not change, PBM should be deferred until a physician has performed a follow-up evaluation to rule out malignancy. If the patient is known to have cancer, the following question should be asked.

> ### ▪ Assess
> - "Do you know if you have a tumor in this area?"
> - Check the patient's skin for pigment abnormalities suspicious for cancer in the treatment area.
> - Refer the patient back to their physician for evaluation of any suspicious lesions.

Low Back or Abdomen During Pregnancy

Because the effects of PBM on fetal development are unknown, this type of treatment should not be applied to the abdomen or lower back, directly over the developing fetus, during pregnancy.

> ### ▪ Ask the Patient
> - "Are you pregnant?"
> - "Do you think you may be pregnant?"
> - "Are you trying to get pregnant?"

If the patient is or may be pregnant, PBM should not be applied to the abdomen or low back.

Within 4 to 6 Months After Radiotherapy

It is recommended that PBM not be applied to areas that have recently been exposed to radiotherapy because radiotherapy increases tissue susceptibility to malignancy and burns.

> ### ▪ Ask the Patient
> - "Have you recently had radiation applied in this area (the area being considered for treatment application)?"

If the patient has recently had radiation therapy applied to an area, PBM should not be applied in that area.

Over Hemorrhaging Regions

PBM is contraindicated in hemorrhaging regions because this intervention may cause vasodilation and thus may increase bleeding.

> ### ▪ Assess
> - Check for signs of bleeding, including blood in a wound or worsening or recent bruising.

PBM should not be applied in the area of bleeding.

Over the Thyroid Glands

Studies have found that applying PBM to the area of the thyroid gland, or even the area of the mandible, can increase thyroid hormone levels in animals[186,187]; therefore, in general, irradiating the area near the thyroid gland (the midanterior neck) should be avoided. Interestingly, one group of researchers has carried out a series of small clinical trials that support the short- and long-term safety and efficacy of IR PBM for treating hypothyroidism caused by autoimmune thyroiditis.[188-190] Further research by other groups is needed to confirm this effect.

PRECAUTIONS FOR PHOTOBIOMODULATION

> ### ★ PRECAUTIONS
> **for PBM**
> - Epiphyseal plates in children
> - Impaired sensation
> - Impaired mentation
> - Photophobia, or abnormally high sensitivity to light
> - Pretreatment with photosensitizers

Epiphyseal Plates in Children

The effect of PBM on epiphyseal plate growth or closure is unknown. However, because PBM can affect cell growth, application over the epiphyseal plates before their closure is not recommended.

Impaired Sensation or Mentation

Caution is recommended when treating patients with impaired sensation or mentation because these patients may be unable to report discomfort during treatment. Although discomfort is rare during PBM, the area of the applicator in contact with the patient's skin can become warm and may burn if applied for prolonged periods or if malfunctioning.

> ■ **Ask the Patient**
> • "Do you have normal feeling in this area?"
>
> ■ **Assess**
> • Check sensation in the application area. Use test tubes containing hot and cold water or metal spoons put in hot and cold water to test thermal sensation.
> • Check alertness and orientation.

PBM should not be applied to any area where thermal sensation is impaired. PBM should not be applied if the patient is unresponsive or confused.

Photophobia or Pretreatment With Photosensitizers

Some recommend not applying PBM to any patient who has abnormally high sensitivity to light, either intrinsically or as the result of treatment with a photosensitizing medication. However, because increased skin sensitivity to light is generally limited to the UV range of the electromagnetic spectrum, only UV irradiation must be avoided in such patients. When wavelengths of light outside the UV range are being used in patients with photosensitivity, the clinician should check closely for any adverse effects and should stop treatment if adverse effects occur.

> ■ **Ask the Patient**
> • "Are you taking any medication that increases your sensitivity to light or your risk of sunburn?"
> • "Do you sunburn easily?"
>
> ■ **Assess**
> • Observe the skin for any signs of burning, including erythema or blistering.

Treatment with PBM should be stopped if the patient shows any signs of burning.

Adverse Effects of Photobiomodulation

Although most reports concerning the use of PBM devices note no adverse effects from the application of this physical agent, authors have described transient tingling, mild erythema,

Application Technique

skin rash, or a burning sensation, as well as increased pain or numbness, in response to the application of PBM.[191,192]

The primary hazards of laser irradiation are the adverse effects that can occur with irradiation of the eyes. As discussed earlier in this chapter, lasers are classified on a scale from 1 to 4 according to their power and associated risk of adverse effects on unprotected skin and eyes (see Table 16.1). The low-level lasers used in clinical rehabilitation applications are generally class 3B, which means that although they are harmless to unprotected skin, they pose a potential hazard to the eyes if viewed along the beam. Exposure of the eyes to laser light of this power can damage the retina because of the concentrated intensity of the light and the limited attenuation of the beam by the outer structures of the eye. As noted previously, this hazard does not apply to nonlaser light sources (LED and SLD), where the light is divergent and not concentrated in one particular area.

The other substantial potential hazard of applying PBM devices intended for therapy is burns. Although the mechanism of the therapeutic action of PBM is not thermal, the diodes used to apply PBM can become quite warm if they are on for a prolonged period. This is more likely to occur with lower-power LEDs because in order to deliver a therapeutic dose of energy, they need to be on for a long time, and often many diodes are used together in an array (Fig. 16.14). For this reason, take particular caution when applying laser or any other form of light therapy to patients with impaired sensation or mentation and to areas of fragile tissue such as open wounds.

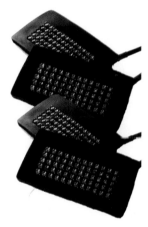

FIGURE 16.14 Light-emitting diode (LED) array light applicators. (Courtesy Anodyne Therapy, Tampa, FL.)

APPLICATION TECHNIQUE 16.1   PBM

Procedure

1. Evaluate the patient's clinical findings and set the goals of treatment.
2. Determine whether PBM is the most appropriate treatment.
3. Determine that PBM is not contraindicated for the patient or the condition. Check with the patient and check the patient's chart for contraindications regarding the application of laser or light therapy.

4. Select an applicator with the appropriate diode(s), including type (LED, SLD, and/or laser diode), wavelength, and power. See the discussion of parameters in the next section.
5. Select the appropriate energy density (fluence) (J/cm^2). Recommendations for different clinical applications are summarized in Table 16.2 and in the parameter discussion in the next section.

Continued

APPLICATION TECHNIQUE 16.1—cont'd

TABLE 16.2	Photobiomodulation Dose Suggestions Based on Tissue Type and Clinical Indication
Clinical Indication	**Suggested Treatment Dose Range**
Soft tissue healing (tendon, skin, cartilage)	$4–15$ J/cm^2
Soft tissue healing (muscle)	$2–8$ J/cm^2
Bone healing	Up to 15 J/cm^2
Arthritis	$2–15$ J/cm^2
Lymphedema	$1–2$ J/cm^2
Carpal tunnel syndrome/ neuropathy	$8–12$ J/cm^2

6. Before treating any area at risk for cross-infection, swab the face of the applicator with 0.5% alcoholic chlorhexidine or the antimicrobial approved for this use in the facility.
7. If using an applicator that includes laser diodes, the patient and the therapist should wear protective goggles that shield the eyes from the wavelength of light emitted by the laser (Fig. 16.15). *Do not* substitute sunglasses for the goggles provided with or intended for your laser device. Sunglasses do not adequately filter IR light. Never look into the beam or the laser aperture. A laser beam can damage the eyes even if the beam cannot be seen.
8. Expose the area to be treated. Remove overlying clothing, opaque dressings,[193] and any shiny jewelry from the area. Nonopaque dressings, such as thin films, do not need to be removed because most laser light can penetrate through these wound dressings.[194]
9. Apply the applicator to the skin with firm pressure, keeping the light beam perpendicular to the skin (see Fig. 16.15). If the treatment area does not have intact skin, is painful to touch, or does not tolerate contact for any reason, treatment may be applied with the applicator slightly above the tissue, without touching the skin but with the light beam kept perpendicular to the tissue surface (Fig. 16.16).
10. Start the light output and keep the applicator in place throughout the application of each dose. If the treatment area is larger than the applicator, repeat the dose to areas approximately 1 inch apart throughout the treatment area. The device will automatically stop after delivery of the set dose (J/cm^2).

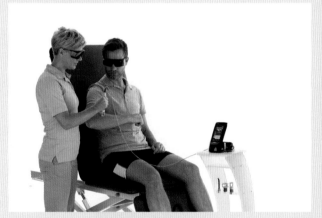

FIGURE 16.15 Patient wearing goggles during laser therapy. (Courtesy Chattanooga/DJO, Vista, CA.)

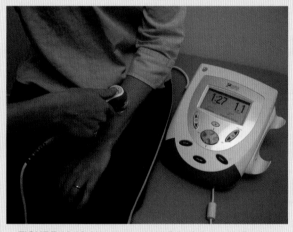

FIGURE 16.16 Noncontact laser light therapy application.

PARAMETERS FOR THE USE OF PHOTOBIOMODULATION

There is much controversy, both in the literature and among experts, about the ideal device and parameters for the therapeutic application of PBM in clinical practice.[195] Dose recommendations have been published by various authors[124] and societies,[196–198] based on their evaluation of clinical trial data and the mechanisms underlying the effects of PBM.[195] Interestingly, one author who compared the efficacy of different PBM doses concluded that tissues with more mitochondria, including muscle, brain, heart, and nerve, tend to respond to lower doses of light, whereas those with a lower number of mitochondria, such as skin, tendon, or cartilage, tend to respond to higher doses.

Type of Diode(s)

Different diodes produce light of different ranges of wavelength, coherence, and collimation, but it is not clear whether these differences have a clinical impact, and if so, what this clinical impact is. Very few studies have directly compared the effects of coherent (laser) light with the effects of noncoherent (LED and SLD) light.[199,200] In addition, there are more studies investigating the effects of laser light than studies investigating the effects of light emitted by LEDs and SLDs, largely because laser applicators were available many years earlier, but studies have shown the beneficial effects from light produced by all of these PBM devices. What remains somewhat controversial is whether the effects found with coherent laser light can be assumed to also occur in response to noncoherent LED and SLD light and thus if one device can be substituted for another or if one type of light is better than another.

LEDs provide the most diffuse light with the widest frequency range and individually are of low power. Because they output diffuse light, LEDs are therefore likely most suitable for treating larger, more superficial areas. Applicators that use LEDs as the treatment light source generally contain many LEDs in an array (see Fig. 16.14) or cluster to provide more power for the entire applicator and to treat a larger area. The power of the applicator equals the sum of the power of all of its diodes. Some cluster applicators may contain various diodes, including a small number of low-power LEDs in the visible light wavelength range primarily to indicate when the device is emitting rather than for any potential therapeutic benefit. This is common when the other diodes are higher-power SLDs or laser diodes that emit only in the invisible IR range (Fig. 16.17).

SLDs provide light that is less diffuse and of a narrower wavelength range than that provided by LEDs, and they emit higher power than LEDs (see Figs. 16.14 and 16.17). SLDs are suitable for treating superficial or moderately deep areas, depending on their wavelength.

Laser diodes provide light of a single wavelength that is very concentrated (Fig. 16.18). Laser diodes are suitable for treating small areas and, for the same wavelength and power, will deliver the most light deepest to a focused area of tissue. Because this concentrated light can damage the eyes, protective safety goggles should be worn by both the patient and the clinician when using any applicator that includes one or more laser diodes.

Wavelength

Clinically, PBM is generally provided with applicators that output light wavelengths in the near-IR ($\approx$700 to 1100 nm) and/or red ($\approx$600 to 700 nm) range, although some output blue or UV light ($\approx$450 to 500 nm). Recent research comparing the effects of different wavelength ranges generally finds stimulatory effects with PBM at wavelengths within the red to near-IR range[201] and inhibitory effects with wavelengths in the blue or UV range.[29,75,86] It is therefore recommended that PBM treatment use wavelengths in the red to IR range, and

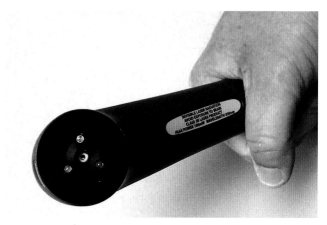

FIGURE 16.18 A laser diode applicator. This applicator includes one infrared laser diode and three blue light-emitting diodes (LEDs) that serve as indicators to show when the applicator is on. (Courtesy Mettler Electronics, Anaheim, CA.)

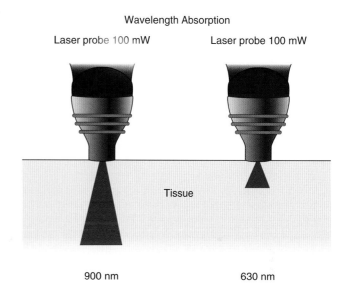

FIGURE 16.19 Depth of penetration according to wavelength.

selection within this range should be based on the desired depth of penetration. IR light, with its longer wavelengths, penetrates more deeply than red light (Fig. 16.19) and is therefore suitable for treating deeper tissues up to 30 to 40 mm deep. In contrast, red light, with its shorter wavelengths, is absorbed more superficially, at a depth of 5 to 10 mm, making it more suitable for treating superficial tissues, such as the skin and subcutaneous tissue. Blue light and UV light are likely most helpful for producing surface antimicrobial effects on the skin or exposed soft tissue.[29]

Power

PBM applicator power is measured in milliwatts (1 mW = 1/1000th of a watt). Lasers are classified by international agreement as class 1 to class 4, according to their power and associated risks (see Table 16.1). All devices with a laser in them are required to carry a label denoting their class (Fig. 16.20). Some authors also classify PBM according to the power of the device as LLLT or high-intensity laser therapy (HILT), but there are no well-accepted definitions for these terms.[202, 203]

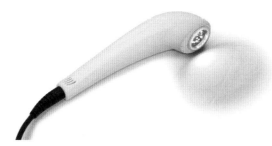

FIGURE 16.17 A cluster light applicator that includes supraluminous diodes (SLDs) of three different wavelengths, six with a wavelength of 464 nm that emit blue light, six with a wavelength of 624 nm that emit red light, and 20 with a wavelength of 850 nm that emit infrared light. (Courtesy Dynatronics, Salt Lake City, UT.)

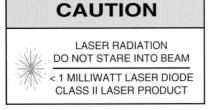

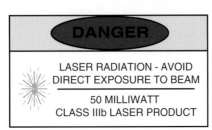

FIGURE 16.20 Labels denoting laser class.

Lasers used for rehabilitation are generally power class 3B, with the power of any individual diode being between 5 and 500 mW. When multiple laser diodes are combined in a single cluster applicator, the class is based on the power of the highest-power diode, not on the sum of the power of all the diodes. This is because the class designation was developed for safety, and safety is most dependent on the concentration of light, not the total amount of light. However, for treatment purposes, the sum of the power of all the diodes in the applicator will affect the treatment time.

The laser classification system does not apply to other PBM devices, such as LEDs and SLDs, because these diodes do not produce light that is concentrated in a small area and that therefore can injure the eyes or other tissues. The power of a single LED is generally in the range of 1 to 5 mW but can be as high as 30 to 40 mW. Numerous LEDs—often 20 to 60 but up to 200 or more—are generally placed in a pad or array applicator (see Fig. 16.14) to provide an applicator with higher total power. The power of individual SLDs is generally in the range of 5 to 35 mW but may be as high as 90 mW or more. Several SLDs—generally 3 to 10—are usually placed together in a cluster applicator to provide more total power.

As discussed earlier in this chapter, the total power of a light applicator affects the required time to deliver a given amount of energy or dose, with lower-total-power applicators taking longer than higher-total-power applicators to deliver the same amount of energy. It is not clear if, within the typical total power range of 10 to 1000 mW available for clinical use in rehabilitation, total power has any other impacts on therapeutic efficacy or outcome. Thus, at this time, the power of a PBM applicator should be selected to optimize the practicality of the treatment time.

Energy Density

The energy density (see Table 16.2) is also known as the *dose* or *fluence*. In general, very low energy densities, below 1 J/cm², are found to have minimal if any clinically relevant effects; energy densities up to around 15 J/cm² are found to be stimulatory; and too high of an energy density, much higher than 15 J/cm², can be suppressive or damaging.[72,75,97] Most authors recommend using lower doses for superficial conditions and higher doses for deeper conditions. In addition, recent analyses suggest that lower doses may be most effective for tissues with higher numbers of mitochondria, such as muscle, brain, heart, and nerve, whereas higher doses may be ineffective in these tissues but required for benefit in tissues with fewer mitochondria, such as skin, tendon, and cartilage.[195] Although most recommend using lower doses for acute conditions and for initial treatments and increasing the dose for more chronic conditions and for subsequent treatments if the prior treatment was well tolerated, WALT recommends reducing the dose by 30% as a condition becomes chronic.[196,197]

Documentation

When using laser, LED, or SLD PBM, document the following:
- Type of diode(s) (laser, LED, SLD)
- Wavelength(s) (nm)
- Total applicator power (mW)
- Area of the body treated
- Energy density (J/cm²)

The duration of treatment is not listed because this is included in the energy density parameter, and light delivery will stop automatically when the total dose (energy density) has been delivered.

EXAMPLES

When applying PBM to a pressure ulcer over the left greater trochanter in a patient with T10 level paraplegia in the second week of treatment, document the following:

S: Pt reports that his wound over the left thigh was stable for 2 months before initiating laser therapy but is now closing up.

O: Stage IV pressure ulcer over left greater trochanter, 3 cm × 4 cm, 2 cm deep.

Treatment: IR laser 904 nm, 200 mW, to area of wound, 9 J/cm² to 4 areas over wound.

A: Wound size decreased from 4 cm × 5 cm × 2.5 cm deep at initiation of laser therapy.

P: Continue current laser therapy and pressure management.

When applying PBM to a patient with lateral epicondylitis, document the following:

S: Pt reports 5/10 pain over the right lateral elbow and increased pain with gripping.

O: Tender to deep palpation over extensor carpi radialis brevis tendon.

Treatment: Red SLD, 630 nm, 500 mW cluster, 3 J/cm².

Posttreatment: Minimal tenderness, pain decreased to 2/10.

A: Reduced pain and tenderness after light therapy.

P: Continue light therapy. Modify work activities to reduce strain on wrist extensors.

CLINICAL CASE STUDIES

The following case studies summarize the concepts of PBM in rehabilitation discussed in this chapter. Based on the scenarios presented, an evaluation of the clinical findings and goals of treatment are proposed. These are followed by a discussion of the factors to be considered in the selection of PBM as an indicated intervention and in the selection of the ideal treatment parameters to promote progress toward set goals.

CASE STUDY 16.1

Open Wound

Examination

History

JM is a 78-year-old man with an open wound on his right foot. JM states that the wound has been present for 6 months and has not improved with compression bandaging, elevation, and regular dressing changes. His doctor has diagnosed his wound as being due to a combination of chronic venous insufficiency and diabetes. JM has had similar ulcers in the past that have healed slowly. JM relies on his wife to help him with daily dressing changes, and his wife notes that yellow drainage is present on the dressings when they are changed.

Systems Review

JM rates the pain from the wound as 3/10. JM has also been walking less to avoid aggravating the wound. As a result, he has not been involved in many of his usual activities, including gardening and Sunday-night bingo, and he reports mild feelings of depression. No itching or burning is present near the wound site, and both upper extremities and the left lower extremity are unaffected.

Tests and Measures

JM has mild bilateral non-pitting lower extremity edema and an ulcerated area measuring approximately 4 × 5 cm on the plantar aspect of his right foot with purulent drainage and no evidence of granulation tissue or bleeding. Light touch and sharp/dull sensation in both feet and around the wound are moderately impaired. His left lower extremity does not have any wounds and has normal sensation.

> *Why might the clinician need to use caution when applying laser or light to this patient? Should the patient continue compression? How will you know whether this patient is or is not improving?*

Evaluation and Goals

ICF Level	Current Status	Goals
Body structure and function	Chronic right foot ulcer Bilateral lower extremity edema	Closure of right foot ulcer Control lower extremity edema
Activity	Decreased ambulation	Restore ambulation tolerance and activity to prewound distances
Participation	Decreased participation in hobbies such as gardening and bingo	Return to gardening and bingo

ICF, International Classification for Functioning, Disability and Health.

◆ FIND THE EVIDENCE

PICO Terms	Natural Language Example	Sample PubMed Search
P (Population)	Patients with right foot ulcer	("ulcer" [text word] OR "varicose ulcer" [MeSH])
I (Intervention)	Laser and light therapy	AND "Low-Level Light Therapy/Therapeutic Use" [MeSH] OR "Low-Level Light Therapy/Therapy" [MeSH] OR "low-level light therapy" [text word]
C (Comparison)	No laser and light therapy	
O (Outcome)	Reduction of ulcer pain; healing of wound	

Key Studies or Reviews

1. Tchanque-Fossuo CN, Ho D, Dahle SE, et al: A systematic review of low-level light therapy for treatment of diabetic foot ulcer. *Wound Repair Regen* 24:418–426, 2016.

   This systematic review of four RCTs with 131 participants concluded that despite limitations of all studies, including small sample size, unclear allocation concealment, lack of screening phases to exclude rapid healers, unclear inclusion/exclusion criteria, short follow-up, and unclear treatment settings, all RCTs reviewed demonstrated positive therapeutic outcomes with no adverse events with the use of PBM for treating diabetic foot ulcers.

2. Li S, Wang C, Wang B, et al: Efficacy of low-level light therapy for treatment of diabetic foot ulcer: a systematic review and meta-analysis of randomized controlled trials. *Diabetes Res Clin Pract* 143:215–224, 2018.

   This systematic review and meta-analysis of seven RCTs with 194 participants found that PBM reduced diabetic ulcer area, improved complete healing rate, accelerated granulation tissue formation, and shortened closure time while also alleviating ulcer-related pain.

Continued

Prognosis

This patient presents with a chronic ulcer of the foot that is likely a result of chronic venous insufficiency and diabetes. The wound has not healed over several months despite compression bandaging, elevation, and regular dressing changes. At this point, it is reasonable to try adding a new modality to promote tissue healing. PBM, electrical stimulation, and ultrasound might be options for this patient. PBM offers the advantage of short treatment time and the ability to be applied without touching the wound, thus minimizing the risk of cross-infection. There is support from the literature for PBM promoting healing of diabetic foot ulcers but not for promoting healing of ulcers caused by venous insufficiency. It will be important to closely evaluate progress to assess if in this case, the addition of PBM helps promote healing of this patient's wound.

Intervention

PBM was selected as an adjunctive treatment modality to promote tissue healing. PBM has been shown in various studies and meta-analyses to accelerate wound healing, with stronger evidence for diabetic ulcers than for venous ulcers.

A cluster probe that included laser diodes and SLDs was selected because it provides both focal and broad coverage with light. Red light with approximately 600-nm wavelength was selected because it has shallow penetration, consistent with the depth of tissue involved with this wound. A cluster probe with a total power of 500 mW was selected so that treatment time could be fairly short.

The dose for the first treatment was 4 J/cm^2, which was increased by 2 J/cm^2 at each subsequent treatment up to 14 J/cm^2. Treatment was provided twice a week for 8 weeks.

Documentation

S: Pt reports right foot ulcer present for 6 months.
O: Pretreatment: 4 x 5 cm ulcer on plantar surface of right foot.
Intervention: Laser SLD cluster, 630 to 650 nm, 500 mW, 4 J/cm^2, applied to right foot ulcer **without** contact.
A: Pt tolerated intervention with no signs of discomfort.
P: Continue PBM treatment 2 x /week, increasing by 2 J/cm^2 at each subsequent treatment up to 14 J/cm^2 until wound has healed. Educate pt to keep his lower extremities elevated and in the proper use of compression bandages or stockings.

CASE STUDY 16.2

Rheumatoid Arthritis
Examination

History

RM is a 42-year-old electrical engineer with RA. She has been referred to therapy for stiffness and pain, particularly in the joints of her hands. In the past, when RM received therapy, she was taught ROM exercises that she now performs three times a week. The patient's work involves using her hands on the computer and troubleshooting projects involving fine wires. RM finds that she has become slower at these fine

motor tasks and is unable to do some of the finest work. RM is worried that this will affect her ability to continue her current job or to maintain other types of employment.

The patient's medications include methotrexate and ibuprofen. These provide some relief of hand pain and stiffness.

Systems Review

RM appears to be generally healthy, although she walks somewhat stiffly. She reports hand pain that varies from 4/10 at rest to 7/10 with motion. She reports that her hands are particularly stiff for the first 1 to 1½ hours each morning. RM complains of fatigue, which she attributes to the longer hours spent at work to stay on top of her responsibilities.

Tests and Measures

ROM appears to be generally decreased in all joints of both hands, and mild ulnar drift is noted at the metacarpophalangeal joints. Measurements of passive ROM (PROM) in various finger joints follow:

Joint	Right	Left
Thumb IP flexion	80°	80°
Thumb IP extension	−20°	−20°
Index finger PIP joint flexion	90°	90°
Index finger PIP joint extension	−20°	−25°
Middle finger PIP flexion	100°	90°
Middle finger PIP extension	−20°	−30°

IP, Interphalangeal; *PIP,* proximal interphalangeal.

Grip strength is 4/5 bilaterally and is limited by pain and stiffness.

What would be reasonable goals for therapy with laser or light therapy? What other interventions would you consider in addition to laser or light therapy? What are the advantages and disadvantages for this patient of laser or light therapy compared with other interventions?

Evaluation and Goals

ICF Level	Current Status	Goals
Body structure and function	Bilateral hand joint pain, stiffness, and decreased ROM	Decrease pain by 50%, shorten duration of morning stiffness to 30 min, and increase ROM by ≥5° in measured joints in both hands
Activity	Decreased fine motor skill and speed	Improve fine motor skill and speed Be aware of adaptive tools and other methods to perform certain fine motor skills

CLINICAL CASE STUDIES—*cont'd*

ICF Level	Current Status	Goals
Participation	Slowed and limited work performance	Continue working at current job at an acceptable level

ICF, International Classification for Functioning, Disability and Health; *ROM,* range of motion.

◆ FIND THE EVIDENCE

PICO Terms	Natural Language Example	Sample PubMed Search
P (Population)	Patients with rheumatoid arthritis	("Rheumatoid Arthritis" [text word] OR "Arthritis, Rheumatoid" [MeSH])
I (Intervention)	Laser and light therapy	AND "Low-Level Light Therapy/Therapeutic Use" [MeSH] OR "Low-Level Light Therapy/Therapy" [MeSH] OR "low-level light therapy" [text word]
C (Comparison)	No laser and light therapy	
O (Outcome)	Reduction of joint pain and stiffness	

Key Studies or Reviews

1. Brosseau L, Robinson V, Wells G, et al: Low level laser therapy (classes I, II and III) for treating rheumatoid arthritis. *Cochrane Database Syst Rev* 2005(4):CD002049, 2005. This systematic review of five RCTs with 130 patients randomly assigned to PBM concluded that PBM should be considered for the short-term treatment for relief of pain and morning stiffness for patients with RA. Clinicians should consistently report the characteristics of the PBM device and the application techniques used.

Prognosis

This patient presents with reduced functional abilities and participation as a result of pain and stiffness in her fingers and reduced ROM from RA. PBM has been found in individual studies and in a meta-analysis of current studies to reduce pain and morning stiffness in patients with RA. This form of therapy would be a good choice for RM because laser light could be delivered quickly and easily to many of her joints with the appropriate applicator. Given the chronic and progressive

nature of RA, treatment should be provided in conjunction with medications, body mechanics, and adaptive equipment evaluation and intervention to optimize function and participation over the long term.

Intervention

PBM was selected as an adjunctive treatment modality to modify inflammation. A cluster probe that included laser diodes and SLDs was selected because this provides both focal and broad coverage with light and could be used to treat several involved joints at once. Alternatively, a single diode could be used and applied to individual joints separately, or an array of LEDs could be applied to most or all of each hand, although this likely would require a longer application time because these arrays output light with a low-energy density. IR light with approximately 800- to 900-nm wavelength was selected because its deep penetration may reach involved joint structures. A cluster probe with a total power of 200 to 500 mW would be ideal so that treatment time could be fairly short.

The dose for the first treatment was 2 J/cm^2. This low dose is used at first because higher doses have been found by some clinicians to exacerbate inflammation. If this dose is well tolerated, the dose may be increased to 4 or possibly 8 J/cm^2. Treatment was provided two times a week for 4 weeks.

Documentation

S: *Pt reports stiffness of her hands that is worst for the first 60 to 90 min each morning and that interferes with fine motor tasks at work.*

O: *Pretreatment PROM:*

Joint	Right	Left
Thumb IP flexion	80°	80°
Thumb IP extension	−20°	−20°
Index finger PIP joint flexion	90°	90°
Index finger PIP joint extension	−20°	−25°
Middle finger PIP flexion	100°	90°
Middle finger PIP extension	−20°	−30°

Intervention: *Laser SLD cluster, 800 to 900 nm, 500 mW, 2 J/cm^2 applied to both hands, 2 different areas to focus on IP joints.*

A: *Pt tolerated laser with no signs of discomfort.*

P: *Continue laser treatment 2 × /week. Recheck ROM in 1 week; if improved and Pt tolerating treatment well, increase dose to 4 to 8 J/cm^2. Educate patient in joint protection techniques.*

Chapter Review

1. Electromagnetic radiation is composed of electrical and magnetic fields that vary over time and are oriented perpendicular to each other.
2. Different frequencies of electromagnetic radiation have different names, different properties, and different applications. Shortwave, microwave, IR, visible light, and UV radiation all have clinical therapeutic applications.
3. Laser light has the unique features of being monochromatic (one frequency), coherent, and directional; light produced by LEDs and SLDs has a range of frequencies, is noncoherent, and spreads. Low-intensity laser or noncoherent light may be used as physical agents in rehabilitation.
4. Lasers and light affect cells via their interaction with intracellular chromophores. This interaction leads to a range of cellular effects, including increased ATP and RNA synthesis.

These effects can promote tissue healing, reduce pain, and improve function in patients with a range of conditions, including arthritis, neuropathy, and lymphedema.

5. Contraindications to the use of lasers include direct irradiation of the eyes, malignancy, within 4 to 6 months after radiotherapy, hemorrhaging regions, and application to the endocrine glands. Precautions include application to the low back or abdomen during pregnancy, epiphyseal plates in children, impaired sensation and mentation, photophobia or abnormally high sensitivity to light, and pretreatment with one or more photosensitizers. Clinicians should always read and follow the contraindications and precautions listed for a particular unit.

6. When selecting a device for PBM, the clinician should first consider whether PBM will be effective for the patient's condition. After deciding on the type of diode (laser, LED, or SLD), the clinician should set the appropriate parameters, including wavelength, power, and energy density.

Glossary

Band (frequency band): A range of wavelengths within the electromagnetic spectrum; for example, the band for UVA radiation is 320 to 400 nm.

Chromophores: The parts of a molecule that give it color by absorbing certain wavelengths and reflecting others.

Cluster probe: A light therapy applicator with multiple diodes that may consist of any combination of laser diodes, light-emitting diodes, or supraluminous diodes. The use of multiple diodes allows coverage of a larger treatment area, takes advantage of the properties of different types of diodes and may reduce treatment time.

Coherent: Light in which all waves are in phase with each other; lasers produce coherent light.

Diathermy: The application of shortwave or microwave electromagnetic energy to produce heat within tissues, particularly deep tissues.

Directional (collimated): Light with parallel waves.

Divergent: Light that spreads; the opposite of collimated.

Electromagnetic radiation: Radiation composed of electrical and magnetic fields that vary over time and are oriented perpendicular to each other. This type of radiation does not need a medium to propagate.

Energy: The total amount of electromagnetic energy delivered over the entire treatment time. Energy is usually measured in joules (J). Energy is equal to power multiplied by time.

$$1\,J = 1\,W \times 1\,s$$

Energy density (fluence): The total amount of electromagnetic energy delivered per unit area over the entire treatment time. Energy density is generally measured in joules per centimeter squared (J/cm^2). Most authors agree that this should be the standard dosage measure for laser light therapy.

Frequency: The number of waves per unit time, generally measured in hertz (Hz), which indicates waves per second.

Hot laser: A laser that heats and destroys tissue directly in beam and is used for surgery; also called *high-intensity laser*.

Ionizing radiation: Electromagnetic radiation that can penetrate cells and displace electrons from atoms or molecules to create ions. Ionizing radiation includes x-rays and gamma rays. Ionizing radiation can damage the internal structures of living cells.

Laser: Acronym for *l*ight *a*mplification by *s*timulated *e*mission of *r*adiation. Laser light has the unique properties of being monochromatic, coherent, and directional.

Laser diode: A light source that uses semiconductor diode technology and optics to produce laser light.

Light-emitting diode (LED): A semiconductor diode light source that produces relatively low-power light in a range of frequencies. LED light may appear to be one color (e.g., red) but that has a range of wavelengths and is not coherent or directional.

Low-level laser therapy (LLLT): Application of laser light for therapeutic purposes. LLLT generally uses laser light diodes that have less than 500-mW power per diode. LLLT cluster probes may contain a number of diodes with a total combined power greater than 500 mW; also known as *cold laser, low-intensity, low-power,* or *soft laser.*

Monochromatic: Light of single frequency, wavelength, and color. Laser light is monochromatic. Other light sources produce light with a range of wavelengths.

Photobiomodulation (PBM): Therapeutic application of lasers or other forms of light, including light from light-emitting diodes, supraluminous diodes, or broadband sources.

Power: Rate of energy production, generally measured in milliwatts (mW) for laser light.

Power density (irradiance): The concentration of power per unit area, measured in watts per centimeter squared (W/cm^2).

Stimulated emission: Occurs when a photon hits an atom that is already excited (i.e., electrons are at a higher energy level than usual). The atom being hit releases a new photon that is identical to the incoming photon—the same color, traveling in the same direction.

Supraluminous diode (SLD): A light source that uses semiconductor diode technology to produce high-power light in a narrow frequency range.

Ultraviolet (UV) radiation: Electromagnetic radiation with wavelength from less than 290 to 400 nm, which lies between x-ray and visible light.

Wavelength: The length of a wave of light from peak to peak determines frequency and color. Longer wavelengths are associated with deeper penetration.

References

1. American Society for Laser Medicine and Surgery. Home page. https://www.aslms.org. (Accessed August 1, 2020).
2. Rajakumar K, Greenspan SL, Thomas SB, et al: Solar ultraviolet radiation and vitamin D: a historical perspective [published correction appears in *Am J Public Health* 97(12):2121, 2007. doi:10.2105/AJPH.2006.091736.] *Am J Public Health* 97(10):1746–1754, 2007.
3. Mester E, Spiry T, Szende B, et al: Effects of laser rays on wound healing. *Am J Surg* 122:532–535, 1971.
4. Mester E, Ludany G, Sellyei M, et al: The stimulating effects of low power laser rays on biological systems. *Laser Rev* 1:3, 1968.
5. Mester AF, Mester A: Wound healing. *Laser Ther* 1:7–15, 1989.
6. Mester AF, Mester A: Clinical data of laser biostimulation in wound healing. *Lasers Surg Med* 7:78, 1987.
7. Beckerman H, de Bie RA, Bouter LM, et al: The efficacy of laser therapy for musculoskeletal and skin disorders: a criteria-based meta-analysis of randomized clinical trials. *Phys Ther* 72:483–491, 1992.
8. Sears FW, Zemansky MW, Young HD: *College physics*, Reading, MA, 1987, Addison-Wesley.
9. Hitchcock RT, Patterson RM: *Radio-frequency and ELF electromagnetic energies: a handbook for health professionals*, New York, 1995, Van Nostrand Reinhold.
10. Thomas CL: *Taber's cyclopedic medical dictionary*, Philadelphia, 1993, FA Davis.

11. Hawkins D, Houreld N, Abrahamse H: Low level laser therapy (LLLT) as an effective therapeutic modality for delayed wound healing. *Ann N Y Acad Sci* 1056:486–493, 2005.
12. Chaves ME, Araüjo AR, Piancastelli AC, et al: Effects of low-power light therapy on wound healing: laser x LED. *An Bras Dermatol* 89(4):616–623, 2014. doi:10.1590/abd1806-4841.20142519.
13. Ash C, Dubec M, Donne K, et al: Effect of wavelength and beam width on penetration in light-tissue interaction using computational methods. *Lasers Med Sci* 32(8):1909–1918, 2017.
14. Gupta A, Dai T, Hamblin MR: Effect of red and near-infrared wavelengths on low-level laser (light) therapy-induced healing of partial-thickness dermal abrasion in mice. *Lasers Med Sci* 29(1):257–265, 2014.
15. Hashmi JT, Huang YY, Sharma SK, et al: Effect of pulsing in low-level light therapy. *Lasers Surg Med* 42:450–466, 2010.
16. Barolet D, Duplay P, Jacomy H, et al: Importance of pulsing illumination parameters in low-level-light therapy. *J Biomed Opt* 15(4), 2010:048005. doi:10.1117/1.3477186.
17. Trelles MA, Mayayo E, Miro L: The action of low reactive laser therapy on mast cells. *Laser Ther* 1:27–30, 1989.
18. de Oliveira AR, da Silva FS, Bortolin RH, et al: Effect of photobiomodulation and exercise on early remodeling of the Achilles tendon in streptozotocin-induced diabetic rats. *PLoS One* 14(2): e0211643, 2019.
19. Tsong TY: Deciphering the language of cells. *TIBS* 14:89–92, 1989.
20. Escoffre JM, Dean DS, Hubert M, et al: Membrane perturbation by an external electric field: a mechanism to permit molecular uptake. *Eur Biophys J* 36(8):973–983, 2007. doi:10.1007/s00249-007-0194-7.
21. Hamblin MR: Mechanisms and applications of the anti-inflammatory effects of photobiomodulation. *AIMS Biophys* 4(3):337–361, 2017. doi:10.3934/biophy.2017.3.337.
22. Huang YY, Sharma SK, Carroll J, et al: Biphasic dose response in low level light therapy - an update. *Dose Response* 9(4):602–618, 2011. doi:10.2203/dose-response.11-009.
23. Belkin M, Schwartz M: New biological phenomena associated with laser radiation. *Health Phys* 56:687–690, 1989.
24. Karu T: Photobiology of low-power laser effects. *Health Phys* 56:691–704, 1989.
25. Ferrando S, Agas D, Mirata S, et al: The 808 nm and 980 nm infrared laser irradiation affects spore germination and stored calcium homeostasis: a comparative study using delivery hand-pieces with standard (Gaussian) or flat-top profile. *J Photochem Photobiol B* 199, 2019:111627. doi:10.1016/j.jphotobiol.2019.111627.
26. de Freitas LF, Hamblin MR: Proposed mechanisms of photobiomodulation or low-level light therapy. *IEEE J* 22(3):7000417, 2016. doi:10.1109/JSTQE.2016.2561201.
27. Belletti S, Uggeri J, Mergoni G, et al: Effects of 915 nm gaAs diode laser on mitochondria of human dermal fibroblasts: analysis with confocal microscopy. *Lasers Med Sci* 30:375–381, 2015.
28. Lunova M, Smolková B, Uzhytchak M, et al: Light-induced modulation of the mitochondrial respiratory chain activity: possibilities and limitations. *Cell Mol Life Sci*, 2019. [published online ahead of print, 2019 Oct 3]. doi:10.1007/s00018-019-03321-z.
29. Amaroli A, Ravera S, Baldini F, et al: Photobiomodulation with 808-nm diode laser light promotes wound healing of human endothelial cells through increased reactive oxygen species production stimulating mitochondrial oxidative phosphorylation. *Lasers Med Sci* 34(3):495–504, 2019. doi:10.1007/s10103-018-2623-5.
30. Ahamed BA, Mathangi DC, Shyamala R: Effect of LED photobiomodulation on fluorescent light induced changes in cellular ATPases and Cytochrome c oxidase activity in Wistar rat. *Lasers Med Sci* 31(9):1803–1809, 2016. doi:10.1007/s10103-016-2054-0.
31. Poyton RO, Ball KA: Therapeutic photobiomodulation: nitric oxide and a novel function of mitochondrial cytochrome c oxidase. *Discov Med* 11(57):154–159, 2011.
32. Marcos RL, Leal Junior EC, Messias FM, et al: Infrared (810 nm) low-level laser therapy in rat achilles tendinitis: a consistent alternative to drugs. *Photochem Photobiol* 87(6):1447–1452, 2011.
33. Torres-Silva R, Lopes-Martins RA, Bjordal JM, et al: The low level laser therapy (LLLT) operating in 660 nm reduce gene expression of inflammatory mediators in the experimental model of collagenase-induced rat tendinitis. *Lasers Med Sci* 30(7):1985–1990, 2015.
34. Smith KC: The photobiological basis of low level laser radiation therapy. *Laser Ther* 3:19–24, 1991.
35. Pall ML: Electromagnetic fields act via activation of voltage-gated calcium channels to produce beneficial or adverse effects. *J Cell Mol Med* 17(8):958–965, 2013.
36. Baxter D: Low intensity laser therapy. In Kitchen S, Bazin S, editors: *Clayton's electrotherapy*, ed 10, London, 1996, WB Saunders.
37. Kitchen SS, Partridge CJ: A review of low level laser therapy. *Physiotherapy* 77:161–168, 1991.
38. Passarella S, Casamassima E, Molinari S, et al: Increase of proton electrochemical potential and ATP synthesis in rat liver mitochondria irradiated in vitro by helium-neon laser. *FEBS Lett* 175:95–99, 1984.
39. Eells JT, Henry MM, Summerfelt MTT, et al: Therapeutic photobiomodulation for methanol-induced retinal toxicity. *Proc Natl Acad Sci USA* 100:3439–3444, 2003.
40. Eells JT, Wong-Riley MT, VerHoeve J, et al: Mitochondrial signal transduction in accelerated wound and retinal healing by near-infrared light therapy. *Mitochondrion* 4:559–567, 2004.
41. Winterle JS, Einarsdottir O: Photoreactions of cytochrome C oxidase. *J Photochem Photobiol* 82:711–719, 2006.
42. Silveira PC, Streck EL, Pinho RA: Evaluation of mitochondrial respiratory chain activity in wound healing by low-level laser therapy. *J Photochem Photobiol* 86:279–282, 2006.
43. Benedicenti S, Pepe IM, Angiero F, et al: Intracellular ATP level increases in lymphocytes irradiated with infrared laser light of wavelength 904 nm. *Photomed Laser Surg* 26:451–453, 2008.
44. Hamblin MR: Mechanisms and mitochondrial redox signaling in photobiomodulation. *Photochem Photobiol* 94(2):199–212, 2018. doi:10.1111/php.12864.
45. Sommer AP, Schemmer P, Pavláth AE, et al: Quantum biology in low level light therapy: death of a dogma. *Ann Transl Med* 8(7):440, 2020. doi:10.21037/atm.2020.03.159.
46. Sommer AP: Revisiting the photon/cell interaction mechanism in low-level light therapy. *Photobiomodul Photomed Laser Surg* 37(6):336–341, 2019. doi:10.1089/photob.2018.4606.
47. Lima PLV, Pereira CV, Nissanka N, et al: Photobiomodulation enhancement of cell proliferation at 660 nm does not require cytochrome c oxidase. *J Photochem Photobiol B* 194:71–75, 2019. doi:10.1016/j.jphotobiol.2019.03.015.
48. Sommer AP: Mitochondrial cytochrome c oxidase is not the primary acceptor for near infrared light—it is mitochondrial bound water: the principles of low-level light therapy. *Ann Transl Med* 7(Suppl 1):S13, 2019. doi:10.21037/atm.2019.01.43.
49. Greco M, Vacca R, Moro L, et al: Helium-neon laser irradiation of hepatocytes can trigger increase of the mitochondrial membrane potential and can stimulate c-fos expression in a Ca[2+]-dependent manner. *Lasers Surg Med* 29:433–441, 2001.
50. Carney SA, Lawrence JC, Ricketts CR: The effect of light from a ruby laser on the metabolism of skin tissue culture. *Biochem Biophys Acta* 148:525–530, 1967.
51. Chen MH, Huang YC, Sun JS, et al: Second messengers mediating the proliferation and collagen synthesis of tenocytes induced by low-level laser irradiation. *Lasers Med Sci* 30:263–272, 2015.
52. De Jesus JF, Spadacci-Morena DD, Rabelo ND, et al: Low-level laser therapy on tissue repair of partially injured Achilles tendon in rats. *Photomed Laser Surg* 32:345–350, 2014.
53. Lam TS, Abergel RP, Castel JC, et al: Laser stimulation of collagen synthesis in human skin fibroblast cultures. *Laser Life Sci* 1:61–77, 1986.
54. Anders JJ, Geuna S, Rochkind S: Phototherapy promotes regeneration and functional recovery of injured peripheral nerve. *Neurol Res* 26:234–240, 2004.
55. Mester E, Mester AF, Mester A: The biomedical effects of laser application. *Lasers Surg Med* 5:31–39, 1985.
56. Bjordal JM, Lopes-Martins RA, Iversen VV: A randomised, placebo controlled trial of low level laser therapy for activated Achilles tendinitis with microdialysis measurement of peritendinous prostaglandin E2 concentrations. *Br J Sports Med* 40:76–80; discussion 76–80, 2006.
57. Dos Santos LS, Saltorato JC, Monte MG, et al: PBMT and topical diclofenac as single and combined treatment on skeletal muscle injury in diabetic rats: effects on biochemical and functional aspects. *Lasers Med Sci* 34(2):255–262, 2019. doi:10.1007/s10103-018-2580-z.
58. Hwang MH, Shin JH, Kim KS, et al: Low level light therapy modulates inflammatory mediators secreted by human annulus fibrosus cells

during intervertebral disc degeneration in vitro. *Photochem Photobiol* 91:403–410, 2015.

59. Mantineo M, Pinheiro JP, Morgado AM: Low-level laser therapy on skeletal muscle inflammation: evaluation of irradiation parameters. *J Biomed Opt* 19:98002, 2014.

60. Gupta A, Keshri GK, Yadav A, et al: Superpulsed (ga-as, 904 nm) low-level laser therapy (LLLT) attenuates inflammatory response and enhances healing of burn wounds. *J Biophotonics* 8:489–501, 2015.

61. Yu HS, Chang KL, Yu CL, et al: Low-energy helium-neon laser irradiation stimulates interleukin-1 alpha and interleukin-8 release from cultured human keratinocytes. *J Invest Dermatol* 107:593–596, 1996.

62. Kupin IV, Bykov VS, Ivanov AV, et al: Potentiating effects of laser radiation on some immunologic traits. *Neoplasma* 29:403–406, 1982.

63. Passarella S, Casamassima E, Quagliariello E, et al: Quantitative analysis of lymphocyte-Salmonella interaction and the effects of lymphocyte irradiation by He-Ne laser. *Biochem Biophys Res Commun* 130:546–552, 1985.

64. Wang L, Zhang D, Schwarz W: TRPV channels in mast cells as a target for low-level-laser therapy. *Cells* 3(3):662–673, 2014. doi:10.3390/cells3030662.

65. Kouhkheil R, Fridoni M, Abdollhifar MA, et al: Impact of photobiomodulation and condition medium on mast cell counts, degranulation, and wound strength in infected skin wound healing of diabetic rats. *Photobiomodul Photomed Laser Surg* 37(11):706–714, 2019. doi:10.1089/photob.2019.4691.

66. Zhang J, Sun J, Zheng Q, et al: Low-level laser therapy 810-nm up-regulates macrophage secretion of neurotrophic factors via PKA-CREB and promotes neuronal axon regeneration in vitro. *J Cell Mol Med* 24(1):476–487, 2020. doi:10.1111/jcmm.14756.

67. de Brito Sousa K, Rodrigues MFSD, de Souza Santos D, et al: Differential expression of inflammatory and anti-inflammatory mediators by M1 and M2 macrophages after photobiomodulation with red or infrared lasers. *Lasers Med Sci* 35(2):337–343, 2020. doi:10.1007/s10103-019-02817-1.

68. Vinck EM, Cagnie BJ, Cornelissen MJ, et al: Increased fibroblast proliferation induced by light emitting diode and low power laser irradiation. *Laser Med Sci* 18:95–99, 2003.

69. Pereira AN, Eduardo Cde P, Matson E, et al: Effect of low-power laser irradiation on cell growth and procollagen synthesis of cultured fibroblasts. *Lasers Surg Med* 31:263–267, 2002.

70. Webb C, Dyson M, Lewis WHP: Stimulatory effect of 660 nm low level laser energy on hypertrophic scar-derived fibroblasts: possible mechanisms for increase in cell counts. *Lasers Surg Med* 22:294–301, 1998.

71. Ren C, McGrath C, Jin L, et al: Effect of diode low-level lasers on fibroblasts derived from human periodontal tissue: a systematic review of in vitro studies. *Lasers Med Sci* 31(7):1493–1510, 2016. doi:10.1007/s10103-016-2026-4.

72. Martignago CC, Oliveira RF, Pires-Oliveira DA, et al: Effect of low-level laser therapy on the gene expression of collagen and vascular endothelial growth factor in a culture of fibroblast cells in mice. *Lasers Med Sci* 30(1):203–208, 2015. doi:10.1007/s10103-014-1644-y.

73. Grossman N, Schneid N, Reuveni H, et al: 780 nm low power diode laser irradiation stimulates proliferation of keratinocyte cultures: involvement of reactive oxygen species. *Lasers Surg Med* 29:105–106, 2001.

74. de Abreu PTR, de Arruda JAA, Mesquita RA, et al: Photobiomodulation effects on keratinocytes cultured in vitro: a critical review. *Lasers Med Sci* 34(9):1725–1734, 2019. doi:10.1007/s10103-019-02813-5.

75. Schindl A, Merwald H, Schindl L, et al: Direct stimulatory effect of low-intensity 670 nm laser irradiation on human endothelial cell proliferation. *Br J Dermatol* 148:334–336, 2003.

76. Bagheri HS, Mousavi M, Rezabakhsh A, et al: Low-level laser irradiation at a high power intensity increased human endothelial cell exosome secretion via Wnt signaling [published correction appears in *Lasers Med Sci* (1):295–296, 2020]. *Lasers Med Sci* 33(5):1131–1145, 2018. doi:10.1007/s10103-018-2495-8.

77. de Simone NA, Christiansen C, Dore D: Bactericidal effect of 0.95mW helium-neon and 5-mW indium-gallium-aluminum-phosphate laser irradiation at exposure times of 30, 60 and 120 seconds on photosensitized *Staphylococcus aureus* and *Pseudomonas aeruginosa* in vitro. *Phys Ther* 79:839–846, 1999.

78. Nussbaum EL, Lilge L, Mazzuli T: Effects of 630-, 660-, 810- and 905-nm laser irradiation delivering radiant exposure of 1-50 J/cm2 on three species of bacteria in vitro. *J Clin Laser Med Surg* 20:325–333, 2002.

79. Guffey SJ, Wilborn J: Effect of combined 405-nm and 880-nm light on *Staphylococcus aureus* and *Pseudomonas aeruginosa* in vitro. *Photomed Laser Surg* 24:680–683, 2006.

80. Guffey JS, Wilborn J: In vitro bactericidal effects of 405 nm and 470 nm blue light. *Photomed Laser Surg* 24:684–688, 2006.

81. Silva DC, Plapler H, Costa MM, et al: Low level laser therapy (AlGaInP) applied at 5j/cm2 reduces the proliferation of *Staphylococcus aureus* MRSA in infected wounds and intact skin of rats. *An Bras Dermatol* 88:50–55, 2013.

82. de Sousa NT, Gomes RC, Santos MF, et al: Red and infrared laser therapy inhibits in vitro growth of major bacterial species that commonly colonize skin ulcers. *Lasers Med Sci* 31(3):549–556, 2016. doi:10.1007/s10103-016-1907-x.

83. Bumah VV, Masson-Meyers DS, Enwemeka CS: Blue 470nm light suppresses the growth of Salmonella enterica and methicillin-resistant *Staphylococcus aureus* (MRSA) in vitro. *Lasers Surg Med* 47(7):595–601, 2015. doi:10.1002/lsm.22385.

84. Lee SY, Seong IW, Kim JS, et al: Enhancement of cutaneous immune response to bacterial infection after low-level light therapy with 1072 nm infrared light: a preliminary study. *J Photochem Photobiol B* 105:175–182, 2011.

85. Mignon C, Uzunbajakava NE, Castellano-Pellicena I, et al: Differential response of human dermal fibroblast subpopulations to visible and near-infrared light: Potential of photobiomodulation for addressing cutaneous conditions. *Lasers Surg Med* 50(8):859–882, 2018. doi:10.1002/lsm.22823.

86. Schindl A, Heinze G, Schindl M, et al: Systemic effects of low-intensity laser irradiation on skin microcirculation in patients with diabetic microangiopathy. *Microvasc Res* 64:240–246, 2002.

87. Pereira MC, de Pinho CB, Medrado AR, et al: Influence of 670 nm low-level laser therapy on mast cells and vascular response of cutaneous injuries. *J Photochem Photobiol B* 98:188–192, 2010.

88. Plass CA, Loew HG, Podesser BK, et al: Light-induced vasodilation of coronary arteries and its possible clinical implication. *Ann Thorac Surg* 93(4):1181–1186, 2012. doi:10.1016/j.athoracsur.2011.12.062.

89. Chennoufi R, Cabrié A, Nguyen NH, et al: Light-induced formation of NO in endothelial cells by photoactivatable NADPH analogues targeting nitric-oxide synthase. *Biochim Biophys Acta Gen Subj* 1863(6):1127–1137, 2019.

90. Lingard A, Hulten LM, Svensson L, et al: Irradiation at 634 nm releases nitric oxide from human monocytes. *Laser Med Sci* 22:30–36, 2007.

91. Linares SN, Beltrame T, Ferraresi C, et al: Photobiomodulation effect on local hemoglobin concentration assessed by near-infrared spectroscopy in humans. *Lasers Med Sci* 35(3):641–649, 2020. doi:10.1007/s10103-019-02861-x.

92. Tezcan S, Ulu Ozturk F, Uslu N, et al: Carpal tunnel syndrome: evaluation of the effects of low-level laser therapy with ultrasound strain imaging. *J Ultrasound Med* 38(1):113–122, 2019. doi:10.1002/jum.14669.

93. Anderson TE, Good WT, Kerr HH, et al: *Low level laser therapy in the treatment of carpal tunnel syndrome*, 1995, Microlight Corporation. http://www.laserhealthproducts.com/gmstudy.pdf. (Accessed June 13, 2012).

94. de Oliveira RF, De Andrade Salgado DM, Trevelin LT, et al: Benefits of laser phototherapy on nerve repair. *Lasers Med Sci* 30:1395–1406, 2015.

95. Rochkind S: Phototherapy in peripheral nerve regeneration: from basic science to clinical study. *Neurosurg Focus* 26:E8, 2009.

96. Andreo L, Soldera CB, Ribeiro BG, et al: Effects of photobiomodulation on experimental models of peripheral nerve injury. *Lasers Med Sci* 32(9):2155–2165, 2017. doi:10.1007/s10103-017-2359-7.

97. Wang CZ, Chen YJ, Wang YH, et al: Low-level laser irradiation improves functional recovery and nerve regeneration in sciatic nerve crush rat injury model. *PLoS One* 9(8):e103348, 2014. doi:10.1371/journal.pone.0103348.

98. Shamir MH, Rochkind S, Sandbank J, et al: Double-blind randomized study evaluating regeneration of the rat transected sciatic nerve after suturing and postoperative low-power laser treatment. *J Reconstr Microsurg* 17:133–137, 2001.

99. Rochkind S, Nissan M, Alon M, et al: Effects of laser irradiation on the spinal cord for the regeneration of crushed peripheral nerve in rats. *Lasers Surg Med* 28:216–219, 2001.

100. Walker JB, Akhanjee LK, Cooney MM, et al: Laser therapy for pain of rheumatoid arthritis. *Clin J Pain* 3:54–59, 1987.

101. Matic M, Lazetic B, Poljacki C, et al: Low level laser irradiation and its effect on repair processes in the skin. *Med Pregl* 56:137–141, 2003. [in Croatian].

102. Enwemeka CS: Laser biostimulation of healing wounds: specific effects and mechanisms of action. *J Orthop Sports Phys Ther* 9:333–338, 1988.

103. Lucas C, Criens-Poublon LJ, Cockrell CT, et al: Wound healing in cell studies and animal model experiments by low level laser therapy: were clinical studies justified? A systematic review. *Lasers Med Sci* 17:110–134, 2002.

104. Flemming K, Cullum N: Laser therapy for venous leg ulcers. *Cochrane Database Syst Rev* 2000(2):CD001182, 2000.

105. Enwemeka CS, Parker JC, Dowdy DS, et al: The efficacy of low-power lasers in tissue repair and pain control: a meta-analysis study. *Photomed Laser Surg* 22:323–329, 2004.

106. Woodruff LD, Bounkeo JM, Brannon WM, et al: The efficacy of laser therapy in wound repair: a meta-analysis of the literature. *Photomed Laser Surg* 22:241–247, 2004.

107. Fulop AM, Dhimmer S, Deluca JR, et al: A meta-analysis of the efficacy of phototherapy in tissue repair. *Photomed Laser Surg* 27:695–702, 2009.

108. Flemming KA, Cullum NA, Nelson EA: A systematic review of laser therapy for venous leg ulcers. *J Wound Care* 8:111–114, 1999.

109. Machado RS, Viana S, Sbruzzi G: Low-level laser therapy in the treatment of pressure ulcers: systematic review. *Lasers Med Sci* 32(4):937–944, 2017. doi:10.1007/s10103-017-2150-9.

110. Tchanque-Fossuo CN, Ho D, Dahle SE, et al: A systematic review of low-level light therapy for treatment of diabetic foot ulcer. *Wound Repair Regen* 24(2):418–426, 2016. doi:10.1111/wrr.12399.

111. Frangež I, Nizič-Kos T, Frangež HB: Phototherapy with LED shows promising results in healing chronic wounds in diabetes mellitus patients: a prospective randomized double-blind study. *Photomed Laser Surg* 36(7):377–382, 2018. doi:10.1089/pho.2017.4382.

112. Langella LG, Casalechi HL, Tomazoni SS, et al: Photobiomodulation therapy (PBMT) on acute pain and inflammation in patients who underwent total hip arthroplasty-a randomized, triple-blind, placebo-controlled clinical trial. *Lasers Med Sci* 33(9):1933–1940, 2018. doi:10.1007/s10103-018-2558-x.

113. de Alencar Fonseca Santos J, Campelo MBD, de Oliveira RA, et al: Effects of low-power light therapy on the tissue repair process of chronic wounds in diabetic feet. *Photomed Laser Surg* 36(6):298–304, 2018. doi:10.1089/pho.2018.4455.

114. Mathur RK, Sahu K, Saraf S, et al: Low-level laser therapy as an adjunct to conventional therapy in the treatment of diabetic foot ulcers. *Lasers Med Sci* 32(2):275–282, 2017. doi:10.1007/s10103-016-2109-2.

115. Alves AN, Fernandes KP, Deana AM, et al: Effects of low-level laser therapy on skeletal muscle repair: a systematic review. *Am J Phys Med Rehabil* 93:1073–1085, 2014.

116. Hayworth CR, Rojas JC, Padilla E, et al: In vivo low-level light therapy increases cytochrome oxidase in skeletal muscle. *Photochem Photobiol* 86(3):673–680, 2010. doi:10.1111/j.1751-1097.2010.00732.x.

117. Ferraresi C, de Sousa MV, Huang YY, et al: Time response of increases in ATP and muscle resistance to fatigue after low-level laser (light) therapy (LLLT) in mice. *Lasers Med Sci* 30(4):1259–1267, 2015. doi:10.1007/s10103-015-1723-8.

118. Tsai WC, Hsu CC, Pang JH, et al: Low-level laser irradiation stimulates tenocyte migration with up-regulation of dynamin II expression. *PLoS One* 7(5):e38235, 2012.

119. Martimbianco ALC, Ferreira RES, Latorraca COC, et al: Photobiomodulation with low-level laser therapy for treating Achilles tendinopathy: a systematic review and meta-analysis. *Clin Rehabil* 34(6):713–722, 2020. doi:10.1177/0269215520912820.

120. Neto FCJ, Martimbianco ALC, de Andrade RP, et al: Effects of photobiomodulation in the treatment of fractures: a systematic review and meta-analysis of randomized clinical trials. *Lasers Med Sci* 35(3):513–522, 2020. doi:10.1007/s10103-019-02779-4.

121. Rowe V, Hemmings S, Barton C, et al: Conservative management of midportion Achilles tendinopathy: a mixed methods study, integrating systematic review and clinical reasoning. *Sports Med* 42:941–967, 2012.

122. Tumilty S, Munn J, McDonough S, et al: Low level laser treatment of tendinopathy: a systematic review with meta-analysis. *Photomed Laser Surg* 28(1):3–16, 2010. doi:10.1089/pho.2008.2470.

123. Bjordal JM, Couppé C, Chow RT, et al: A systematic review of low level laser therapy with location-specific doses for pain from chronic joint disorders. *Aust J Physiother* 49:107–116, 2003.

124. Pinheiro ALB, Soares LGP, da Silva ACP, et al: Laser/LED phototherapy on the repair of tibial fracture treated with wire osteosynthesis evaluated by Raman spectroscopy. *Lasers Med Sci* 33(8):1657–1666, 2018. doi:10.1007/s10103-018-2508-7.

125. Pinheiro ALB, Soares LGP, da Silva ACP, et al: Raman spectroscopic study of the effect of the use of laser/LED phototherapy on the repair of complete tibial fracture treated with internal rigid fixation [published online ahead of print, Apr 18, 2020]. *Photodiagnosis Photodyn Ther* 101773, 2020. doi:10.1016/j.pdpdt.2020.101773.

126. Coradini JG, Mattjie TF, Bernardino GR, et al: Comparison of low level laser, ultrasonic therapy and association in joint pain in Wistar rats. *Rev Bras Reumatol* 54(1):7–12, 2014.

127. Li X, Zhang L, Gu S, et al: Comparative effectiveness of extracorporeal shock wave, ultrasound, low-level laser therapy, noninvasive interactive neurostimulation, and pulsed radiofrequency treatment for treating plantar fasciitis: a systematic review and network meta-analysis. *Medicine (Baltimore)* 97(43):e12819, 2018. doi:10.1097/MD.0000000000012819.

128. Tantawy SA, Abdelbasset WK, Kamel DM, et al: Laser photobiomodulation is more effective than ultrasound therapy in patients with chronic nonspecific low back pain: a comparative study. *Lasers Med Sci* 34(4):793–800, 2019. doi:10.1007/s10103-018-2665-8.

129. Bayat M, Virdi A, Rezaei F, Chien S: Comparison of the in vitro effects of low-level laser therapy and low-intensity pulsed ultrasound therapy on bony cells and stem cells. *Prog Biophys Mol Biol* 133:36–48, 2018. doi:10.1016/j.pbiomolbio.2017.11.001.

130. Herpich CM, Amaral AP, Leal-Junior EC, et al: Analysis of laser therapy and assessment methods in the rehabilitation of temporomandibular disorder: a systematic review of the literature. *J Phys Ther Sci* 27(1):295–301, 2015.

131. Brosseau L, Welch V, Wells G, et al: Low level laser therapy (classes I, II and III) in the treatment of rheumatoid arthritis. *Cochrane Database Syst Rev* 2005(2):CD002049, 2005.

132. Brosseau L, Welch V, Wells G, et al: Low level laser therapy (classes I, II and III) for treating osteoarthritis. *Cochrane Database Syst Rev* 2004(3):CD002046, 2004.

133. Jang H, Lee H: Meta-analysis of pain relief effects by laser irradiation on joint areas. *Photomed Laser Surg* 30:405–417, 2012.

134. Huang Z, Chen J, Ma J, et al: Effectiveness of low-level laser therapy in patients with knee osteoarthritis: a systematic review and meta-analysis. *Osteoarthritis Cartilage* 23(9):1437–1444, 2015. doi:10.1016/j.joca.2015.04.005.

135. Stausholm MB, Bjordal JM, Lopes-Martins RAB: Methodological flaws in meta-analysis of low-level laser therapy in knee osteoarthritis: a letter to the editor. *Osteoarthritis Cartilage* 25(4):e9–e10, 2017. doi:10.1016/j.joca.2016.09.022.

136. Rayegani SM, Raeissadat SA, Heidari S, et al: Safety and effectiveness of low-level laser therapy in patients with knee osteoarthritis: a systematic review and meta-analysis. *J Lasers Med Sci* 8(Suppl 1):S12–S19, 2017. doi:10.15171/jlms.2017.s3.

137. Stausholm MB, Naterstad IF, Joensen J, et al: Efficacy of low-level laser therapy on pain and disability in knee osteoarthritis: systematic review and meta-analysis of randomised placebo-controlled trials. *BMJ Open* 9(10), 2019:e031142. doi:10.1136/bmjopen-2019-031142.

138. Carati CJ, Anderson SN, Gannon BJ, et al: Treatment of post-mastectomy lymphedema with low-level laser therapy: a double blind, placebo controlled trial. *Cancer* 98:1114–1122, 2003.

139. Moseley AL, Carati CJ, Piller NB: A systematic review of common conservative therapies for arm lymphoedema secondary to breast cancer treatment. *Ann Oncol* 18:639–640, 2007.

140. Omar MT, Shaheen AA, Zafar H: A systematic review of the effect of low-level laser therapy in the management of breast cancer-related lymphedema. *Support Care Cancer* 20:2977–2984, 2012.

141. E Lima MT, E Lima JG, de Andrade MF, et al: Low-level laser therapy in secondary lymphedema after breast cancer: systematic review. *Lasers Med Sci* 29:1289–1295, 2014.

142. Smoot B, Chiavola-Larson L, Lee J, et al: Effect of low-level laser therapy on pain and swelling in women with breast cancer-related lymphedema: a systematic review and meta-analysis. *J Cancer Surviv* 9(2):287–304, 2015. doi:10.1007/s11764-014-0411-1.

143. Baxter GD, Liu L, Petrich S, et al: Low level laser therapy (photobiomodulation therapy) for breast cancer-related lymphedema: a systematic review. *BMC Cancer* 17(1):833, 2017. doi:10.1186/s12885-017-3852-x.

144. Hennessy M, Hamblin MR: Photobiomodulation and the brain: a new paradigm. *J Opt* 19(1), 2017:013003. doi:10.1088/2040-8986/19/1/013003.

145. Chen YJ, Wang YH, Wang CZ, et al: Effect of low level laser therapy on chronic compression of the dorsal root ganglion. *PLoS One* 9(3):e89894, 2014. doi:10.1371/journal.pone.0089894.

146. Fallah A, Mirzaei A, Gutknecht N, et al: Clinical effectiveness of low-level laser treatment on peripheral somatosensory neuropathy. *Lasers Med Sci* 32(3):721–728, 2017. doi:10.1007/s10103-016-2137-y.

147. Naeser MA: Photobiomodulation of pain in carpal tunnel syndrome: review of seven laser therapy studies. *Photomed Laser Surg* 24:101–110, 2006.

148. Bekhet AH, Ragab B, Abushouk AI, et al: Efficacy of low-level laser therapy in carpal tunnel syndrome management: a systematic review and meta-analysis. *Lasers Med Sci* 32(6):1439–1448, 2017. doi:10.1007/s10103-017-2234-6.

149. Burger M, Kriel R, Damon A, et al: The effectiveness of low-level laser therapy on pain, self-reported hand function, and grip strength compared to placebo or "sham" treatment for adults with carpal tunnel syndrome: a systematic review. *Physiother Theory Pract* 33(3):184–197, 2017. doi:10.1080/09593985.2017.1282999.

150. Franke TP, Koes BW, Geelen SJ, et al: Do patients with carpal tunnel syndrome benefit from low-level laser therapy? A systematic review of randomized controlled trials. *Arch Phys Med Rehabil* 99(8):1650–1659.e15, 2018. doi:10.1016/j.apmr.2017.06.002.

151. Rayegani SM, Moradi-Joo M, Raeissadat SA, et al: Effectiveness of low-level laser therapy compared to ultrasound in patients with carpal tunnel syndrome: a systematic review and meta-analysis. *J Lasers Med Sci* 10(Suppl 1):S82–S89, 2019. doi:10.15171/jlms.2019.S15.

152. Leonard DR, Farooqi MH, Myers S: Restoration of sensation, reduced pain, and improved balance in subjects with diabetic peripheral neuropathy: a double-blind, randomized, placebo-controlled study with monochromatic near-infrared treatment. *Diabetes Care* 27:168–172, 2004.

153. Zinman LH, Ngo M, Ng ET, et al: Low-intensity laser therapy for painful symptom diabetic sensorimotor polyneuropathy: a controlled trial. *Diabetes Care* 27:921–924, 2004.

154. Kemmotsu O, Sato K, Furumido H, et al: Efficacy of low reactive-level laser therapy for pain attenuation of postherpetic neuralgia. *Laser Ther* 3:71–75, 1991.

155. Iijima K, Shimoyama M, Shimoyama N, et al: Effect of repeated irradiation of low-power He-Ne laser in pain relief from postherpetic neuralgia. *Clin J Pain* 5:271–274, 1989.

156. Anju M, Ummer V S, Maiya AG, et al: Low level laser therapy for the patients with painful diabetic peripheral neuropathy - a systematic review. *Diabetes Metab Syndr* 13(4):2667–2670, 2019. doi:10.1016/j.dsx.2019.07.035.

157. Chen YT, Wang HH, Wang TJ, et al: Early application of low-level laser may reduce the incidence of postherpetic neuralgia (PHN). *J Am Acad Dermatol* 75(3):572–577, 2016. doi:10.1016/j.jaad.2016.03.050.

158. Sanderson TH, Wider JM, Lee I, et al: Inhibitory modulation of cytochrome c oxidase activity with specific near-infrared light wavelengths attenuates brain ischemia/reperfusion injury. [published correction appears in Sci Rep Apr 25;8[1]:6729, 2018]. *Sci Rep* 8(1):3481, 2018. doi:10.1038/s41598-018-21869-x.

159. Naeser MA, Martin PI, Ho MD, et al: Transcranial, red/near-infrared light-emitting diode therapy to improve cognition in chronic traumatic brain injury. *Photomed Laser Surg* 34(12):610–626, 2016. doi:10.1089/pho.2015.4037.

160. Wang R, Dong Y, Lu Y, et al: Photobiomodulation for global cerebral ischemia: targeting mitochondrial dynamics and functions. *Mol Neurobiol* 56(3):1852–1869, 2019. doi:10.1007/s12035-018-1191-9.

161. Lampl Y, Zivin JA, Fisher M, et al: Infrared laser therapy for ischemic stroke: a new treatment strategy: results of the NeuroThera Effectiveness and Safety Trial-1 (NEST-1). *Stroke* 38:1843–1849, 2007.

162. Stemer AB, Huisa BN, Zivin JA: The evolution of transcranial laser therapy for acute ischemic stroke, including a pooled analysis of NEST-1 and NEST-2. *Curr Cardiol Rep* 12:29–33, 2010.

163. Lu Y, Wang R, Dong Y, et al: Low-level laser therapy for beta amyloid toxicity in rat hippocampus. *Neurobiol Aging* 49:165–182, 2017. doi:10.1016/j.neurobiolaging.2016.10.003.

164. Foo ASC, Soong TW, Yeo TT, et al: Mitochondrial dysfunction and Parkinson's disease-near-infrared photobiomodulation as a potential therapeutic strategy. *Front Aging Neurosci* 12:89, 2020.

165. Salehpour F, Hamblin MR: Photobiomodulation for Parkinson's disease in animal models: a systematic review. *Biomolecules* 10(4):610, 2020. doi:10.3390/biom10040610.

166. Caldieraro MA, Cassano P: Transcranial and systemic photobiomodulation for major depressive disorder: A systematic review of efficacy, tolerability and biological mechanisms. *J Affect Disord* 243:262–273, 2019. doi:10.1016/j.jad.2018.09.048.

167. Askalsky P, Iosifescu DV: Transcranial photobiomodulation for the management of depression: current perspectives. *Neuropsychiatr Dis Treat* 15:3255–3272, 2019.

168. Yang L, Tucker D, Dong Y, et al: Photobiomodulation therapy promotes neurogenesis by improving post-stroke local microenvironment and stimulating neuroprogenitor cells. *Exp Neurol* 299(Pt A):86–96, 2018. doi:10.1016/j.expneurol.2017.10.013.

169. Zivin JA, Albers GW, Bornstein N, et al: Effectiveness and safety of transcranial laser therapy for acute ischemic stroke. *Stroke* 40:1359–1364, 2009.

170. Huisa BN, Stemer AB, Walker MG, et al: Transcranial laser therapy for acute ischemic stroke: a pooled analysis of NEST-1 and NEST-2. *Int J Stroke* 8(5):315–320, 2013. doi:10.1111/j.1747-4949.2011.00754.x.

171. Yeh SW, Hong CH, Shih MC, et al: Low-level laser therapy for fibromyalgia: a systematic review and meta-analysis. *Pain Physician* 22(3):241–254, 2019.

172. Huang Z, Ma J, Chen J, et al: The effectiveness of low-level laser therapy for nonspecific chronic low back pain: a systematic review and meta-analysis. *Arthritis Res Ther* 17:360, 2015. doi:10.1186/s13075-015-0882-0.

173. Glazov G, Yelland M, Emery J: Low-level laser therapy for chronic non-specific low back pain: a meta-analysis of randomised controlled trials. *Acupunct Med* 34(5):328–341, 2016. doi:10.1136/acupmed-2015-011036.

174. Chow RT, Johnson MI, Lopes-Martins RA, et al: Efficacy of low-level laser therapy in the management of neck pain: a systematic review and meta-analysis of randomized placebo or active-treatment controlled trials. [published correction appears in Lancet 375[9718]:894, 2010]. *Lancet* 374(9705):1897–1908, 2009. doi:10.1016/S0140-6736(09)61522-1.

175. Yavuz F, Duman I, Taskaynatan MA, et al: Low-level laser therapy versus ultrasound therapy in the treatment of subacromial impingement syndrome: a randomized clinical trial. *J Back Musculoskelet Rehabil* 27(3):315–320, 2014. doi:10.3233/BMR-130450.

176. Xu GZ, Jia J, Jin L, et al: Low-level laser therapy for temporomandibular disorders: a systematic review with meta-analysis. *Pain Res Manag* 4230583, 2018. Published 2018 May 10. doi:10.1155/2018/4230583.

177. Fisher SR, Rigby JH, Mettler JA, et al: The effectiveness of photobiomodulation therapy versus cryotherapy for skeletal muscle recovery: a critically appraised topic. *J Sport Rehabil* 28(5):526–531, 2019. doi:10.1123/jsr.2017-0359.

178. Fulop AM, Dhimmer S, Deluca JR, et al: A meta-analysis of the efficacy of laser phototherapy on pain relief. *Clin J Pain* 26:729–736, 2010.

179. Ezzati K, Fekrazad R, Raoufi Z: The effects of photobiomodulation therapy on post-surgical pain. *J Lasers Med Sci* 10(2):79–85, 2019. doi:10.15171/jlms.2019.13.

180. Cotler HB, Chow RT, Hamblin MR, et al: The use of low level laser therapy (LLLT) for musculoskeletal pain. *MOJ Orthop Rheumatol* 2(5):00068, 2015. doi:10.15406/mojor.2015.02.00068.

181. Goldman L, Michaelson SM, Rockwell RJ, et al: Optical radiation with particular reference to lasers. In Suess M, Benwell-Morrison D, editors: *Nonionizing radiation protection*, ed 2, Geneva, 1989, World Health Organization. European Series No. 25.

182. Frigo L, Luppi JS, Favero GM, et al: The effect of low-level laser irradiation (In-Ga-Al-Asp—660 nm) on melanoma in vitro and in vivo. *BMC Cancer* 9:404, 2009.

183. Myakishev-Rempel M, Stadler I, Brondon P, et al: A preliminary study of the safety of red light phototherapy of tissues harboring cancer. *Photomed Laser Surg* 30:551–558, 2012.

184. Hamblin MR, Nelson ST, Strahan JR: Photobiomodulation and cancer: what is the truth? *Photomed Laser Surg* 36(5):241–245, 2018. doi:10.1089/pho.2017.4401.

185. Azevedo LH, Correaaranha AC, Stolf SF, et al: Evaluation of low intensity laser effects on the thyroid gland of male mice. *Photomed Laser Surg* 23:567–570, 2005.
186. Weber JB, Mayer L, Cenci RA, et al: Effect of three different protocols of low-level laser therapy on thyroid hormone production after dental implant placement in an experimental rabbit model. *Photomed Laser Surg* 32(11):612–617, 2014. doi:10.1089/pho.2014.3756.
187. Höfling DB, Chavantes MC, Juliano AG, et al: Low-level laser therapy in chronic autoimmune thyroiditis: a pilot study. *Lasers Surg Med* 42(6):589–596, 2010. doi:10.1002/lsm.20941.
188. Höfling DB, Chavantes MC, Juliano AG, et al: Low-level laser in the treatment of patients with hypothyroidism induced by chronic autoimmune thyroiditis: a randomized, placebo-controlled clinical trial. *Lasers Med Sci* 28(3):743–753, 2013. doi:10.1007/s10103-012-1129-9.
189. Höfling DB, Chavantes MC, Buchpiguel CA, et al: Safety and efficacy of low-level laser therapy in autoimmune thyroiditis: long-term follow-up study. *Int J Endocrinol* 8387530, 2018. Published 2018 Nov 4. doi:10.1155/2018/8387530.
190. Chartered Society of Physiotherapy, Safety of Electrotherapy Equipment Working Group: *Guidelines for the safe use of lasers in physiotherapy*, London, 1991, Chartered Society of Physiotherapy.
191. Moholkar R, Zukowski S, Turbill H, et al: The safety and efficacy of low level laser therapy in soft tissue injuries: a double-blind randomized study. *Phys Ther* 81:A49, 2001.
192. de Jesus Guirro RR, de Oliveira Guirro EC, Martins CC, et al: Analysis of low-level laser radiation transmission in occlusive dressings. *Photomed Laser Surg* 28(4):459–463, 2010. doi:10.1089/pho.2009.2524.
193. Lilge L, Tierney K, Nussbaum E: Low-level laser therapy for wound healing: feasibility of wound dressing transillumination. *J Clin Laser Med Surg* 18:235–240, 2000.
194. Zein R, Selting W, Hamblin MR: Review of light parameters and photobiomodulation efficacy: dive into complexity. *J Biomed Opt* 23(12):1–17, 2018. doi:10.1117/1.JBO.23.12.120901.
195. World Association for Laser Therapy: Recommended treatment doses for low level laser therapy: laser class 3 B, 780 - 860nm GaAlAs lasers. https://waltza.co.za/wp-content/uploads/2012/08/Dose_table_780-860nm_for_Low_Level_Laser_Therapy_WALT-2010.pdf. (Accessed June 14, 2020).
196. World Association for Laser Therapy: Recommended treatment doses for low level laser therapy: laser class 3B, 904 nm GaAs lasers. https://waltza.co.za/wp-content/uploads/2012/08/Dose_table_904nm_for_Low_Level_Laser_Therapy_WALT-2010.pdf. (Accessed June 14, 2020).
197. Swedish Laser Medical Society: The laser therapy—LLLT internet guide. http://laser.nu/. (Accessed June 14, 2020).
198. Klebanov GI, Shuraeva NI, Chichuk TV, et al: A comparative study of the effects of laser and light-emitting diode irradiation on the wound healing and functional activity of wound exudate leukocytes. *Biofizika* 50:1137–1144, 2005.
199. Osipov AN, Rudenko TG, Shekhter AB, et al: A comparison of the effects of laser and light-emitting diodes on superoxide dismutase activity and nitric oxide production in rat wound fluid. *Biofizika* 51:116–122, 2006.
200. Albuquerque-Pontes GM, Vieira RP, Tomazoni SS, et al: Effect of pre-irradiation with different doses, wavelengths, and application intervals of low-level laser therapy on cytochrome c oxidase activity in intact skeletal muscle of rats. *Lasers Med Sci* 30(1):59–66, 2015. doi:10.1007/s10103-014-1616-2.
201. Song HJ, Seo HJ, Lee Y, et al: Effectiveness of high-intensity laser therapy in the treatment of musculoskeletal disorders. *Medicine* 97(51):e13126, 2018. doi:10.1097/MD.0000000000013126.
202. Kheshie AR, Alayat MS, Ali MM: High-intensity versus low-level laser therapy in the treatment of patients with knee osteoarthritis: a randomized controlled trial. *Lasers Med Sci* 29(4):1371–1376, 2014. doi:10.1007/s10103-014-1529-0.Di atum ut moluptatecum ipiendiciis ab iduntia tquodis et fugiatquibus ipsunt ut rehent es

Ultraviolet Therapy

CHAPTER OBJECTIVES

After reading this chapter, the reader will be able to do the following:
- Define *ultraviolet (UV) radiation*.
- Describe the physical effects of UV therapy.
- Explain the clinical indications for the use of UV therapy.
- Choose the best technique for treatment with UV therapy, and list the advantages and disadvantages of each.
- Select the appropriate equipment and optimal treatment parameters for treatment with UV therapy.
- Safely and effectively apply UV therapy.
- Accurately and completely document treatment with UV therapy.

Physical Properties of Ultraviolet Radiation

Ultraviolet (UV) radiation is electromagnetic radiation with a frequency range of between 7.5×10^{14} and over 10^{15} Hz and a wavelength range of between 400 nm and under 290 nm. The frequency of UV radiation lies between that of x-rays and visible light (see Fig. 16.6). UV radiation is divided into three bands—UVA, UVB, and UVC—with wavelengths of 320 to 400 nm (UVA), 290 to 320 nm (UVB), and under 290 nm (UVC) (Fig. 17.1). UVA, also known as *long-wave UV*, can also be divided into UVA1, with a wavelength of 340 to 400 nm, and UVA2, with a wavelength of 320 to 340 nm. UVB can also be subcategorized as narrowband, with a wavelength of 311 to 313 nm, or broadband, with a wavelength of 270 to 390 nm, with a peak at 313 nm. UVA produces fluorescence in many substances. UVB, or middle-wave UV, produces the most skin **erythema.** UVC, or short-wave UV, is germicidal. Because UV radiation does not produce heat, it is thought to produce physiological effects by nonthermal mechanisms. The most significant source of UV radiation is the sun, which emits a broad spectrum of UV radiation, including UVA, UVB, and UVC. Both UVA and UVB reach the earth from the sun; however, UVC is filtered out by the ozone layer. Patients can be treated with UV radiation of specific wavelength ranges using a UV lamp.

The physiological effects of UV radiation are influenced by the wavelength of the radiation, the intensity of radiation reaching the skin, the depth of penetration, and the concurrent use of certain systemic or topical medications. The intensity of UV radiation reaching the patient's skin is proportional to the power output of the lamp, the inverse square of the distance of the lamp from the patient, and the cosine of the angle of incidence of the radiation beam with the tissue (Fig. 17.2). Thus the intensity reaching the skin is greatest when a high-power lamp is used, when the lamp is close to the patient, and when the radiation beam is perpendicular to the surface of the skin.

The depth that UV penetrates the skin is most affected by the wavelength of the radiation, with the longest wavelength penetrating the deepest. Thus UVA penetrates farthest, with UVA1 penetrating further than UVA2, and penetrates through the dermis, whereas UVB and UVC penetrate less deeply and are almost entirely absorbed in the superficial epidermal layers. Penetration is also affected by the intensity of radiation

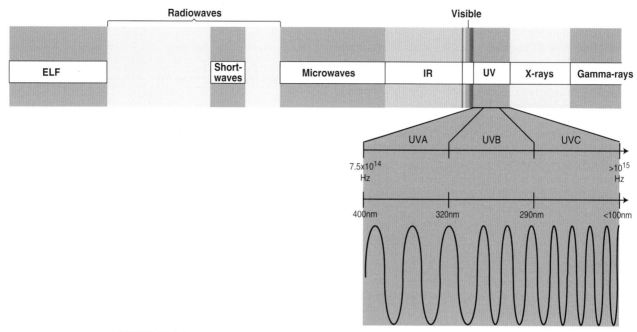

FIGURE 17.1 Bands of ultraviolet (UV) radiation. *ELF,* Extremely low frequency; *IR,* infrared.

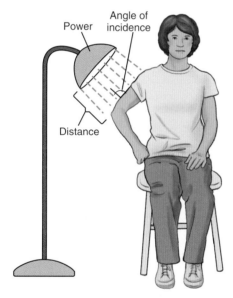

FIGURE 17.2 Factors affecting the intensity of ultraviolet radiation reaching the patient's skin: inverse square of the distance of the lamp from the patient, power output of the lamp, and cosine of the angle of incidence of the beam with the tissue.

reaching the skin, the power of the radiation source, the size of the area being treated, the thickness and pigmentation of the skin, and the duration of treatment. Penetration is deeper when the intensity of the radiation reaching the skin is higher and the skin is thinner and more lightly colored.[1]

> **◎ Clinical Pearl**
>
> To maximize the intensity of UV radiation reaching the skin, use a high-power lamp positioned close to the patient with the radiation beam perpendicular to the skin surface.

Effects of Ultraviolet Radiation

UV radiation exposure produces skin erythema, tanning, **epidermal hyperplasia,** and vitamin D synthesis while also being bactericidal and leading to skin aging and carcinogenesis.[2] These effects are the result of absorption of electromagnetic energy by the cells of exposed skin, inducing apoptotic cell death and immune suppression.[3]

ERYTHEMA PRODUCTION

Erythema (Fig. 17.3), or redness of the skin resulting from dilation of superficial blood vessels caused by the release of histamines, is one of the most common and obvious effects of exposure to UV radiation.[4] Erythema is produced primarily in response to UVB exposure or in response to UVA exposure after drug sensitization. Without drug sensitization,

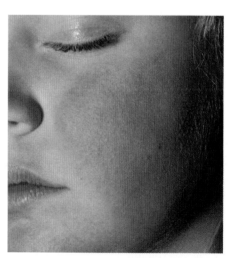

FIGURE 17.3 Erythema. (From Habif TP: *Clinical dermatology,* ed 4, Edinburgh, 2004, Mosby.)

UVA is 100 to 1000 times less potent in inducing erythema than UVB. With sensitization, the erythemal efficacy of UVA is similar to that of UVB alone, with less risk of overexposure or burning. The precise mechanism of UV-induced erythema is unknown; however, it is known that this effect is mediated by prostaglandin release from the epidermis and that it may be related to the DNA-damaging effects of UV radiation. The severity of erythema, which can produce blistering, tissue burning, and pain, and the risk of cell damage are the primary factors limiting the intensity and duration of UV exposure that can be used clinically. Because patients vary in their degree of erythemal response to UV, a **minimal erythemal dose (MED)** is determined for each patient before treatment with UV radiation is initiated. How to determine the MED and the treatment dose are detailed later in this chapter.

TANNING

Tanning, a delayed pigmentation of the skin, occurs in response to UV radiation exposure. This effect is the result of increased production and upward migration of melanin granules and oxidation of premelanin in the skin.[5] Because the darkening of skin pigmentation that occurs with tanning reduces the penetration of UV to deeper tissue layers, despite its many risks, tanning is thought to be a protective response of the body.[6]

EPIDERMAL HYPERPLASIA

Epidermal hyperplasia, thickening of the superficial layer of the skin, occurs approximately 72 hours after exposure to UV radiation and increases with repeated exposure, eventually resulting in thickening of the epidermis and the stratum corneum that persists for several weeks. This effect is thought to be caused in part by epidermal growth factor (EGFR) activation[7] and the release of prostaglandin precursors, leading to increased DNA synthesis by epidermal cells, increased epithelial cell turnover, and cellular hyperplasia.[8] Epidermal hyperplasia is most pronounced in response to UVB exposure and is thought to be a protective response to UV exposure. Because tanning and epidermal hyperplasia impair UV penetration, progressively higher doses of UV radiation are generally required during a course of clinical treatment with UV radiation.

> ◎ **Clinical Pearl**
>
> Because UV causes tanning and skin thickening, progressively higher doses of UV are generally needed during a course of UV treatment.

VITAMIN D SYNTHESIS

UV irradiation of the skin is necessary to convert ingested provitamin D to active vitamin D (Fig. 17.4).[9,10] Although exposure to UV light in sunlight is sufficient for many individuals to maintain adequate blood levels of vitamin D production, UV exposure may be inadequate in certain populations and in certain areas of the world. Risk factors for inadequate blood vitamin D levels include covering all exposed skin or using sunscreen whenever outdoors, dark skin, aging, institutionalization, exclusively breast-fed infants,

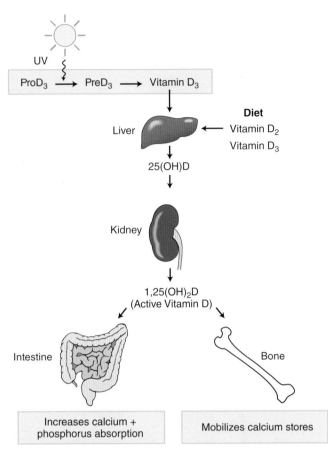

FIGURE 17.4 Conversion of provitamin D to active vitamin D and some of the physiological roles of vitamin D. *UV,* Ultraviolet (radiation).

fat malabsorption syndromes, inflammatory bowel disease, obesity, and living far from the equator.[11]

Vitamin D controls calcium absorption and exchange and is therefore essential for bone formation. Vitamin D deficiency can result in poor intestinal absorption of calcium, which can lead to rickets, a disease characterized by failure of bone mineralization. Although the importance of vitamin D for calcium absorption and bone health is not disputed, research has uncovered subtler associations of low vitamin D levels with a wide range of diseases, including multiple sclerosis, cancer, diabetes, and infections.[12,13] This has generated strong interest in the effects of vitamin D supplements to prevent or contribute to the treatment of these disorders. For example, some studies have found that increased levels of vitamin D and vitamin D supplementation are associated with prevention of preeclampsia, improved blood glucose levels in people with diabetes, and improved symptoms of rheumatoid arthritis and multiple sclerosis, but in general, the evidence for these effects continues to be conflicting and inconclusive.[14,15]

The connection between vitamin D and skin disease dates back to the 1980s, when vitamin D was found to be an effective treatment for patients with psoriasis,[16,17] who tended to have decreased levels of vitamin D and its metabolites compared with disease-free control subjects.[18] Furthermore, treatment with broadband UVB induces an increase in the level of active vitamin D in patients with psoriasis and in control subjects.[16] Thus restoration of vitamin D levels by UV phototherapy may account in part for its beneficial response in psoriasis.

BACTERICIDAL EFFECTS

In the laboratory setting, UV, particularly UVC with a 265-nm wavelength, can be bactericidal.[19-21] UVC radiation is used to kill bacteria in food; in one small study, UVC was found to be as effective as standard hospital cleaners in removing pathogens from hospital surfaces.[22] UVC radiation may also help reduce bacterial load in open wounds and may improve wound healing, but this benefit must be weighed against the potential damage to host cells.[23,24]

OTHER EFFECTS

UVB radiation affects the immune system, reducing contact sensitivity, changing the distribution of circulating lymphocytes, and suppressing mast cell–mediated whealing.[25-27] It is proposed that these effects are dose dependent: With low doses, the immune response is suppressed, and with higher doses, the immune response is activated. UVA has also been shown to inhibit cyclooxygenase 2 expression and prostaglandin E_2 production.[28] This mechanism is thought to underlie the beneficial effects of **psoralen with UVA (PUVA)** and, more recently, UVA1, which is high-intensity, long-wavelength UVA (340 to 400 nm[29]), in the treatment of scleroderma.[28,30] In patients with **vitiligo**, PUVA is thought to act by creating a favorable milieu for the growth of melanocytes, whereas UVB directly stimulates the proliferation and migration of melanocytes.[31,32]

Clinical Indications for Ultraviolet Radiation

The earliest modern clinical use of UV radiation, for which Niels Finsen was awarded the Nobel Prize in 1903, was for the treatment of cutaneous tuberculosis. In the 1920s and 1930s, the use of UV radiation for the treatment of skin disorders, including **psoriasis,** acne, and alopecia, became very popular; however, with the advent of antibiotics and other medications, the role of UV radiation in dermatological medicine decreased. At the present time, UV radiation is used primarily to treat psoriasis[33] and other dermatological conditions, including scleroderma, eczema, atopic dermatitis, cutaneous T-cell lymphoma (mycosis fungoides), vitiligo, and palmoplantar pustulosis.[28,34-37] These treatments may be applied in conjunction with a range of topical medications.[38] UV radiation is also used occasionally as a component of treatment for chronic open wounds.[24,34] Although the clinical application of UV radiation in the treatment of skin disorders is within the scope of physical therapy, such treatments are generally provided by dermatologists or their assistants. However, the treatment of chronic wounds with UV radiation is often provided by a physical therapist.

Various forms of UV, including UVB alone or with a range of topical medications,[38,39] and PUVA, are the current gold-standard intervention for psoriasis phototherapy.[40] More recently, UVA1, UV laser diodes, and UV light-emitting diodes have also been introduced as phototherapy options for psoriasis,[41,42] particularly for the treatment of more focused areas, but clinical trial

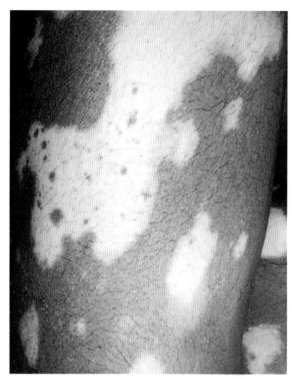

FIGURE 17.5 Vitiligo. (From Kumar V, Abbas AK, Fausto N: *Robbins and Cotran pathologic basis of disease,* ed 7, Philadelphia, 2005, Saunders.)

data for these approaches are still limited. In addition, UV phototherapy is sometimes used for a variety of other photosensitive disorders, including eczema, acne, pityriasis lichenoides, vitiligo (Fig. 17.5), pruritus, and scleroderma.[29,30,32] Clinical recommendations for using UV in the treatment of psoriasis are provided in the next section. Recommendations for using UV for other skin disorders are available in the literature,[32,41] and specific individual clinical protocols should be developed and agreed on in collaboration with the referring physician.

PSORIASIS

Psoriasis is a common benign, acute or chronic, inflammatory skin disease that appears to be based on genetic predisposition. Psoriasis is characterized by bright red plaques with silvery scales, usually on the knees, elbows, and scalp, and is associated with mild itching (Fig. 17.6). These dermatological manifestations may be associated with joint changes known as **psoriatic arthritis.**

Numerous reports have described successful treatment of psoriasis with UV radiation alone or in conjunction with sensitizing drugs.[40] **Phototherapy** of psoriasis with UV light has been provided for almost 100 years: in 1921, Goeckerman at the Mayo Clinic developed a therapy combining topical crude coal tar and subsequent UV irradiation, known as *Goeckerman therapy,* as a treatment for psoriasis. This treatment is still an option for the treatment of moderate to severe psoriasis but is rarely used because the tar application is messy and cumbersome, and other highly effective and easier-to-apply therapies are available. Psoriasis causes hyperproliferation of keratinocytes. UV phototherapy inhibits keratinocyte division, inhibits

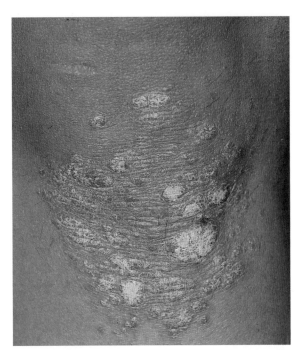

FIGURE 17.6 Psoriatic plaques. (From Habif TP: *Clinical dermatology,* ed 4, Edinburgh, 2004, Mosby.)

DNA synthesis and mitosis of hyperproliferating keratinocytes, induces keratinocyte apoptosis, and inhibits proinflammatory cytokine pathways.

Several systematic reviews clearly demonstrate that psoriasis is responsive to UV therapy, and the American Academy of Dermatology in conjunction with the National Psoriasis Foundation published guidelines of care for the management and treatment of psoriasis with phototherapy in 2019.[40,43–45] These guidelines are used as the basis for recommendations for UV therapy for psoriasis that follow here and should be consulted for a more detailed current review of this topic.

Although topical and/or systemic medications can often adequately control psoriasis with acceptable risk, topical therapies are not effective enough, and systemic medications are associated with too much risk for many patients to find them acceptable. Phototherapy serves as a reasonably safe and effective alternative or adjunctive therapy for these patients.

Psoriasis is most responsive to UVA administered in conjunction with oral or topical **psoralen** sensitization (PUVA). Although not very responsive to broadband UVB, psoriasis is almost as responsive to narrowband (NB) UVB as it is to PUVA, with less associated risk. The lower risk profile, cost, and convenience make NB-UVB the current preferred form of phototherapy for psoriasis. NB-UVB is associated with less frequent symptomatic erythema and blistering than PUVA (7.8% vs. 17%) but is slightly less effective at clearing psoriasis plaques (70% vs. 80%) and requires more treatment sessions (25 vs. 17).[46] The widespread availability and ease of administering NB-UVB combined with the expense of psoralens and the relative scarcity of UVA units have also contributed to PUVA not being as widely used.

NB-UVB is usually administered in the clinic, but home-based NB-UVB units are available. Despite most dermatologists having the impression that clinic-based therapy is more effective and safer, studies, including one with 196 patients, found similar efficacy and side-effect rates with home-based treatment, with lower patient burden and greater patient satisfaction.[47,48]

UVB therapy can be targeted to specific lesions using a laser or targeted UVB light, sparing unaffected skin and allowing higher doses, and thus greater efficacy with fewer sessions, at targeted lesions,[49] but there is less evidence for this approach than for NB-UVB lamp treatment. The use of UV sensitizers in conjunction with UV radiation to treat psoriasis has been studied extensively. Previously, the most commonly used sensitizers were tar-based topicals and psoralen-derived drugs. However, studies on the use of tar-based derivatives in conjunction with UV radiation to manage psoriasis have yielded mixed results, with some reporting that these products are valuable adjuncts to treatment and others reporting that tar-based products are no more effective than simple oil-based ointments. These findings, in addition to the fact that tar-based products are messy and expensive, have reduced the use of tar-based products and increased the use of other topical medications for this application. In contrast, the combination of psoralens with UVA, known as *PUVA*, is still used today for some patients with psoriasis. This treatment combination was first described by Tronnier and Schule[50] in 1972 and has since been shown by numerous other researchers to be effective. Psoralens can be administered topically as a cream or in bathwater, or they may be ingested orally. Psoralens reduce the appearance of psoriatic plaques by causing cross-links to form between adjacent strands of DNA when activated by UVA, interfering with cell replication and preventing the excessive cell proliferation characteristic of psoriasis. They also facilitate the production of reactive oxygen species, which damage cell membranes and result in cell death. The benefits of psoralens with UVA led to the evaluation of the addition of topical psoralens to NB-UVB treatment. One study found that this made the treatment more effective and quicker but also increased side effects, and given the lack of subsequent studies, this is therefore not currently recommended.[51] The addition of various systemic medications has been found to enhance the efficacy of UV therapy but is beyond the scope of this text.

WOUND HEALING

UV radiation is used occasionally as a component of the treatment of chronic wounds despite limited high-quality research on the effectiveness of this intervention.[52] When UV radiation is used for wound treatment, UVC is the **frequency band** most commonly chosen[53,54] because it may help the wound to heal while causing little erythema or tanning. UVC also has a low carcinogenic effect and is absorbed almost equally by all skin colors. UV radiation is thought to facilitate wound healing by increasing the turnover of epithelial cells,[23] causing epidermal cell hyperplasia,[35] accelerating granulation tissue formation, increasing blood flow,[55] killing bacteria,[23] increasing vitamin D production by the skin, and promoting sloughing of necrotic tissue.[56] Although data on the efficacy of UVC for this application are limited and mixed, with some studies reporting faster or more complete healing with the addition of UVC to the treatment protocol for wounds and others reporting no significant benefit, this physical agent has proved beneficial in some cases[52]; thus it may be appropriate to consider adding UVC to the treatment of wounds that have not responded to or are inappropriate for other types of treatment.

Contraindications and Precautions for Ultraviolet Radiation

UV phototherapy used in a controlled fashion not only is effective but also is generally safe in both children[57] and adults.[40] However, important contraindications and precautions for practitioners should be considered to administer this therapy while minimizing risk to the patient. In the event of an adverse effect, therapy should be stopped, and the patient should be evaluated by a physician.

CONTRAINDICATIONS FOR ULTRAVIOLET RADIATION

> **✱ CONTRAINDICATIONS**
>
> **for Ultraviolet Radiation**
>
> - Irradiation of the eyes or genitals
> - Skin cancer
> - Pulmonary tuberculosis
> - Cardiac, kidney, or liver disease
> - Systemic lupus erythematosus
> - Fever
> - Recent x-ray therapy

Irradiation of the Eyes or Genitals

UV irradiation of the eyes should be avoided because UV radiation can damage the cornea, the eyelids, or the lens. UV irradiation of the genitals should be avoided because UV radiation increases the risk of genital skin cancers. Exposure of the eyes can be avoided by having the patient wear UV-opaque goggles throughout treatment, as well as having the therapist wear UV-opaque goggles when at risk of irradiation while turning the UV lamp on or off. These goggles or glasses should wrap around to optimize eye protection and must be proven to block the wavelength range of the delivered therapy. Patients taking UV-sensitizing drugs, such as psoralens, with UVA treatment should continue to wear UVA-opaque eye protection on the day of treatment and the following day.[58] UV irradiation of the genitals can be avoided by keeping them covered during UV therapy.

Certain Systemic Conditions

UV radiation should not be applied to areas in which skin cancer is present because UV exposure may be carcinogenic.[59] Details of the carcinogenic effects of UV radiation can be found in the section on adverse effects. It is generally recommended that UV radiation not be used in patients with pulmonary tuberculosis; cardiac, kidney, or liver disease; systemic lupus erythematosus; or fever because these conditions may be exacerbated by exposure to UV radiation.

Recent X-Ray Therapy

It is recommended that UV radiation not be applied to areas that have had recent x-ray radiation exposure because the skin in these areas may be more likely to develop malignancies.

PRECAUTIONS FOR ULTRAVIOLET RADIATION

> **✱ PRECAUTIONS**
>
> **for Ultraviolet Radiation**
>
> - Photosensitizing medications and dietary supplements
> - Photosensitivity
> - Recurrent oral herpes simplex virus infection
> - No dose of UV radiation should be repeated until the effects of the previous dose have disappeared.

Photosensitizing Medications and Dietary Supplements

Care should be taken when applying UVA to patients who are taking photosensitizing medications or supplements because almost all photosensitizing medications have an action spectrum in the UVA range. Photosensitizing oral medications include sulfonamide, tetracycline, and quinolone antibiotics; gold-based medications used to treat rheumatoid arthritis; amiodarone hydrochloride and quinidines for cardiac arrhythmias; phenothiazines for anxiety and psychosis; and psoralens for psoriasis. Certain dietary supplements, including St. John's wort, are also known to be photosensitizing.[60] Topical preparations, including topical psoralen or calcipotriol, can also enhance UV photosensitivity.[61] While patients are taking these medications or supplements, their sensitivity to UV radiation increases, resulting in a decrease in the MED and increased risk of adverse effects. A patient's minimal erythemal dose must be remeasured if the patient starts to take a photosensitizing medication or supplement during a course of UV treatment.

Photosensitivity

Some individuals, particularly individuals with fair skin and hair color and individuals with red hair, have greater sensitivity to UV exposure, and some have photosensitive disorders, such as xeroderma pigmentosa. Because these individuals have an accelerated and exaggerated skin response to UV radiation, either UV should be avoided or only low levels of UV radiation should be used both when determining the MED and for treatment.

Recurrent Oral Herpes Simplex Virus Infection

UV therapy should be used with caution in people with recurrent oral herpes simplex virus infection because UV may trigger a recurrence.

Erythema From Prior Ultraviolet Dose

To minimize the risk of burns or an excessive erythemal response, UV irradiation should not be repeated until the erythemal effects of the previous dose have resolved.

Adverse Effects of Ultraviolet Radiation[62]

BURNING

Burning[63] by UV radiation will occur if the dose used is too high. Burning usually can be avoided by carefully assessing the MED before starting treatment, by appropriately using the

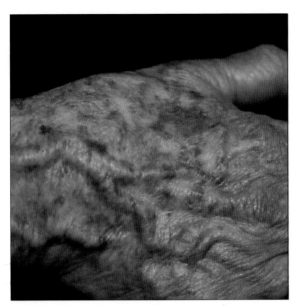

FIGURE 17.7 Actinic skin damage. (From Marks JG, Miller JJ: *Lookingbill and Marks' principles of dermatology,* ed 4, Philadelphia, 2008, Saunders.)

treatment lamp, and by avoiding further exposure if signs of erythema from a prior dose are present.

PREMATURE AGING OF SKIN

Chronic exposure to UV radiation, including sunlight, is associated with premature aging of the skin. This effect, known as **actinic damage,** causes the skin to have a dry, coarse, leathery appearance, with wrinkling and pigment abnormalities (Fig. 17.7). It is thought that these changes are primarily the result of the collagen degeneration that accompanies long-term exposure to UV radiation.

CARCINOGENESIS

Most of the data available regarding the carcinogenic effect of UV radiation concerns the effect of prolonged or intense sunlight exposure. Prolonged exposure to UV radiation, as occurs with excessive exposure to sunlight, is considered to be a major risk factor for developing basal cell carcinoma, squamous cell carcinoma, and malignant melanoma. A review of the literature published in 2012 on the carcinogenicity of UV phototherapy, with and without psoralens, concluded that there is a definite cutaneous carcinogenic risk associated with PUVA treatment when oral systemic psoralens are used.[64] An earlier study, published in 2008, with almost 4000 patients, found no association between NB-UVB treatment and skin cancers,[65] and in 2014, a study specifically evaluating the risk of skin cancer in patients treated with UVB therapy also found no greater risk in these patients than in the general population; however, caution is recommended when prescribing UVB for patients with a history of melanoma, multiple nonmelanoma skin cancers, arsenic intake, or exposure to ionizing radiation.[59] The increased cancer risk with PUVA may be a result of the carcinogenicity of the psoralens or may be a response specific to the wavelength of UV radiation used for this treatment application. PUVA treatments may also exacerbate the effects of previous exposure to carcinogens.[66]

Because of the potential cumulative adverse effects of repeated, low-level exposure to UV radiation, it is recommended that clinicians avoid frequent or excessive exposure during patient treatment. This can be achieved by wearing UV-opaque goggles and UV-opaque clothing.

EYE DAMAGE

UV irradiation of the eyes can cause various eye problems, including **photokeratitis, conjunctivitis,** and **cataracts.**[67,68] Photokeratitis and conjunctivitis can occur acutely after exposure to UVB or UVC. Symptoms of photokeratitis, an inflammation of the cornea that can be extremely painful, generally appear 6 to 12 hours after UV exposure and resolve fully within 2 days, without permanent or long-term damage. Conjunctivitis, an inflammation of the insides of the eyelids and the membrane that covers the cornea, results in a sensation of gritty eyes and varying degrees of photophobia, tearing, and blepharospasm. Chronic UVA and UVB exposures have been associated with the development of cataracts, characterized by the loss of transparency of the lens or lens capsule of the eye. Although theoretically this association would be expected to be even stronger for PUVA because psoralens are deposited in the lens of the eye, no association between increasing exposure to PUVA and cataract risk was found in a 24-year longitudinal observational study of more than 1200 adults treated with PUVA who were instructed to use eye protection.[69]

Because of risks of eye irritation or damage, UV-opaque eye protection for the appropriate UV band should always be worn by the patient and the clinician during UV treatment. Patients should also wear UV-opaque eye protection for the day after psoralen administration to protect their eyes from sunlight exposure.

ADVERSE EFFECTS OF PSORALEN WITH ULTRAVIOLET A

PUVA is associated with all the adverse effects of UV radiation, as described previously. In addition, oral psoralens are associated with nausea and vomiting that can last for 1 to 4 hours after ingestion. Prolonged high-dose PUVA therapy can cause skin damage, including small hyperpigmented nonmalignant lesions, keratotic lesions that may have premalignant histological characteristics, and squamous cell carcinomas.[70,71]

Application Techniques

When applying UV radiation for therapeutic purposes, first determine the individual patient's sensitivity to UV radiation.[72] This varies widely among individuals and can be affected by skin pigmentation, age, prior exposure to UV radiation, type of UV radiation, and use of sensitizing medications.[73] For example, even for Caucasians, a fourfold to sixfold variation in MED can occur.[74] Sensitivity to UV radiation is assessed using the dosimetry procedure described in the next section.

Because the response to UV radiation can vary significantly with even slightly different frequencies of radiation, the same lamp must be used to assess an individual's sensitivity and for all subsequent treatments. For example, the skin is 100 times more sensitive to UV radiation with a wavelength of 300 nm than to UV radiation with a wavelength of 320 nm.

If the lamp must be changed, the individual's response to the new lamp must be assessed before it is used for treatment. Reassessment is also necessary if there is a long gap between treatments because lamp output intensity decreases with prolonged use and skin tanning, and hyperplasia decreases over prolonged periods. Once the individual's responsiveness to a particular UV lamp has been determined, the treatment dose can be selected to produce the desired erythemal response.

> ### ◎ Clinical Pearl
>
> The same lamp that will be used for treatment should be used to assess a person's UV sensitivity.

DOSE-RESPONSE ASSESSMENT

The UV dose is graded according to the individual's erythemal response and is categorized as follows[75]:

- **Suberythemal dose (SED):** Dose that produces no change in skin redness in the 24 hours after UV radiation exposure.
- **Minimal erythemal dose (MED):** Smallest dose producing erythema within 8 hours after exposure that disappears within 24 hours after exposure.
- **First-degree erythema (E_1):** Definite redness with some mild desquamation appears within 6 hours after exposure and lasts for 1 to 3 days; dose is generally about 2½ times the MED.
- **Second-degree erythema (E_2):** Intense erythema with edema, peeling, and pigmentation appears within 2 hours after treatment and is similar to a severe sunburn; dose is generally about 5 times the MED.

- **Third-degree erythema (E_3):** Erythema with severe blistering, peeling, and exudation; dose is generally about 10 times the MED.

In general, the skin response is assessed visually; however, a spectrophotometer may also be used. Spectrophotometers provide measures of darkness, hue, and redness. For patients receiving PUVA therapy, the MED should be determined after they have taken psoralen. When using an oral psoralen, the MED should be determined 2 hours after ingestion. When using a topical psoralen, the MED should be determined immediately after bathing in the psoralen. For UVB, the maximal erythemal response generally occurs within 12 to 15 hours, whereas for PUVA, the erythemal response may be delayed, typically first appearing 24 to 48 hours after exposure and peaking after 100 or more hours.[75]

> ### ◎ Clinical Pearl
>
> The MED for patients receiving PUVA therapy should be determined after the patient has taken psoralen orally or has bathed in psoralen.

Once an individual's MED for a particular lamp has been determined, the treatment dose is set according to the disease being treated and the protocol being used. Guidelines for the treatment of psoriasis with UVB or with PUVA are given in the next section. Guidelines for using UV radiation to treat other problems can be obtained from UV lamp manufacturers or from texts focusing on the particular problem or disease.

APPLICATION TECHNIQUE 17.1

DETERMINING AN INDIVIDUAL'S MINIMAL ERYTHEMAL DOSE OF ULTRAVIOLET RADIATION[75]

Procedure

1. Place UV-opaque goggles on the patient and the clinician.
2. Remove all clothing and jewelry from and wash an area of the body least exposed to natural sunlight. The areas usually used are the volar forearm, the abdomen, hips, or buttocks.
3. Cover all other areas of the skin.
4. Take a piece of cardboard approximately 4 × 20 cm, and cut four square holes of 2 × 2 cm in it. Alternatively, a premade patch with appropriate holes can be purchased (e.g., from www.Daavlin.com or www.rchabmart.com).
5. Place the cardboard on the test area, and drape the area around the cardboard so that the surrounding skin will not be exposed to UV radiation.
6. Place the lamp 60 to 80 cm away from, and perpendicular to, the area to be exposed. Measure and record the exact distance of the lamp from the area to be exposed.
7. Cover all but one of the holes in the cardboard.
8. Turn on the lamp. If using an **arc lamp,** allow the lamp to warm up for 5 to 10 minutes to reach full power before turning it toward the patient. A **fluorescent lamp** will reach full power and can be used within 1 minute of being turned on.

9. Once the lamp has reached full power, direct the beam directly toward the area to be exposed.
10. Depending on the lamp being used, the dose of UV may be controlled using a timer or by mJ/cm^2 dose. For all lamps, start delivery with all testing areas open, then cover one more area after a given time or dose.
11. If using time as a guide, after 120 seconds, cover one hole; after another 60 seconds, cover the next hole; after another 30 seconds, cover the next hole; and after another 30 seconds, turn off the lamp.

According to this protocol, the first window will have been exposed for 240 seconds, the second for 120 seconds, the third for 60 seconds, and the fourth for 30 seconds (Fig. 17.8). This protocol can be adjusted according to the individual's self-reported tanning and burning response to sunlight. For individuals who tan and never or rarely burn, longer exposures can be used; shorter exposures are recommended for individuals who burn easily but do not tan and individuals taking photosensitizing drugs. More holes with shorter time differences between exposures can be used to increase the accuracy of the dose sensitivity assessment. For example, there could be eight holes in the cardboard, and one hole could be covered every 10 seconds.

Continued

APPLICATION TECHNIQUE 17.1—cont'd

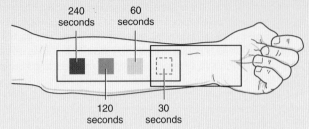

240 seconds   60 seconds

120 seconds   30 seconds

FIGURE 17.8 Setup for ultraviolet sensitivity assessment.

Fair Skin; Red or Blond Hair; Blue, Hazel, or Green Eyes	Fair Skin With Other Eye Colors; Brown or Typical Mediterranean White Skin
250	350
400	500
550	650
700	800
850	950
1000	1100
1150	1250
1300	1400

MED testing should not be performed in patients with dark brown or black skin. These patients should be started at an initial NB-UVB dose of 800 mJ/cm² and increased as tolerated per the protocol.

12. If using mJ/cm² dose as a guide, the following are recommended sequential exposures for NB-UVB. If using UVA, PUVA, or BB-UVB, please refer to an alternative text focused on this topic.[40]

13. The patient should observe the area for up to 4 days after exposure. The area that shows mild reddening of the skin within 8 hours that disappears within 24 hours is treated as the MED.

DOSIMETRY FOR THE TREATMENT OF PSORIASIS WITH ULTRAVIOLET RADIATION

In general, treatment time is selected as a proportion of the MED. The MED for an individual is determined in the manner described earlier. Because repeated exposure to UV radiation generally decreases sensitivity to UV radiation, prior exposure should be taken into account when UV treatment dosage parameters are determined.

When people build up a tolerance to UV radiation with repeated exposure as a result of darkening of their skin by tanning and thickening of their skin by epidermal hyperplasia, their MED will also increase. Thus to maintain effective treatment with a consistent proportion of the MED, exposure time should be increased, or the distance of the lamp from the skin should be decreased with repeated treatments. For UVB, if there was minimal erythema lasting less than 24 hours following the previous treatment, the dose should be increased by 20%. If erythema lasted 24 to 48 hours after the previous treatment, stay at the same dose. If erythema lasted more than 48 hours, skip the treatment, and at the next scheduled treatment, return to one dose lower than the previous dose. If the patient misses treatments, the dose may also need to be decreased, starting back at the initial dose if they miss 4 or more weeks.

Using Ultraviolet B

Initial dose recommendations of NB-UVB to treat psoriasis vary from 50% of the MED to an E_1 dose (approximately 2½ times the MED), with increases of 10% to 40% at each treatment, depending on the skin response.[62,76] It is recommended that a thin layer of emollient, such as petrolatum, be applied before NB-UVB treatment to improve effectiveness and reduce erythema. Do not apply a thick layer of emollient because this can decrease UVB transmission. Treatment is initially given two to three times each week. Treatment two or three times a week is equally likely to achieve plaque clearance, but treatment three times a week works about 1.5 times faster, achieving clearance in a mean of 58 days rather than 88 days.[77] Maintenance treatment can then be applied less frequently, usually once a week. Recent meta-analyses indicate that around 60% to 70% of patients will achieve at least 75% plaque clearance with this therapy and that the average clearance rate is about 70%.

Using Psoralen With Ultraviolet A (PUVA)

Psoralens for PUVA treatment can be delivered orally or topically. When PUVA treatments are provided using oral psoralens for the treatment of psoriasis, UV irradiation is usually applied 2 hours after taking the drug. When the psoralen is delivered topically, UV exposure is provided either immediately after the patient has soaked in a bath of weak psoralen solution for 15 to 30 minutes or, for local application, immediately after the affected area has been covered with psoralen in an emollient applied for 20 minutes. Topical delivery of psoralens is less common than oral administration, although this route of drug delivery is associated with fewer acute side effects.

Erythema in response to PUVA has a delayed onset compared with UVB-induced erythema and at first usually appears 24 to 48 hours after exposure, peaking 72 hours after exposure. PUVA-induced erythema also differs from erythema induced by UV radiation alone in that even two to three times the MED causes only a slightly greater effect. PUVA treatments are usually given two or three times a week to allow time for the erythema of one treatment to resolve before applying the next treatment. Treatment dose is determined by assessing the MED after the patient has taken the psoralen. Treatment is generally applied to the whole body and is usually started at 40% to 70% of the MED and is increased by 10% to 40% each week to maintain the response. Complete clearance usually takes approximately 6 weeks, although there is much variation among individuals.

APPLICATION TECHNIQUE 17.2   ULTRAVIOLET THERAPY

Procedure

The setups for UVB and PUVA application are the same, except that for PUVA, radiation is applied after psoralen sensitization.

1. Warm up the lamp if necessary. If using an arc lamp, it can take several minutes for the lamp to reach full power. If there is a glass filter on the lamp, the lamp should be run for approximately 20 minutes so that the filter reaches thermal equilibrium before the lamp is used for treatment. A fluorescent lamp requires only a brief warm-up period (about 1 minute after being switched on) but will also need to be run for 20 minutes before it is used for treatment if there is a glass filter on the lamp. During the warm-up period, cover the lamp beam with a UV-opaque card or direct the lamp away from the patient or other people or toward a wall or the floor.
2. Place UV-opaque goggles on the patient and the clinician.
3. Remove clothing and jewelry from the area to be treated.
4. Wash and dry the area to be treated.
5. Cover all areas not needing treatment that may otherwise be exposed to radiation with a UV-opaque material, such as a cloth or paper towel.
6. Position the area to be exposed comfortably. When psoriatic plaques are treated with UVB, a non–UVB-absorbing lubricant, such as mineral oil, may be applied to the plaques to decrease reflectance by the scale on the plaques. Do not apply agents containing salicylic acid, which absorbs UVB light.
7. Adjust the position of the lamp or the patient so that the distance between the lamp and the area to be exposed is the same as it was when the MED was determined. Also, place the lamp so that the UV beam will be as perpendicular to the treatment area as possible. Measure and record the distance of the lamp from the patient.
8. Stay close to the patient, or give the patient a call bell and a means to turn off the lamp. Also, provide the patient with a means to open the cabinet if a whole-body treatment is being given.
9. Direct the beam at the treatment area, and start the timer. Select the treatment time according to the recommendations for dosimetry.
10. When treatment is complete, observe the treated area; document the treatment given and any observable response to the treatment.

Documentation

The following should be documented:

- If and how psoralen was given
- Area of the body treated
- Type of UV radiation used
- Serial number of the lamp
- Distance of the lamp from the patient
- Treatment duration
- Response to treatment

EXAMPLE

S: Pt reports itching of the psoriatic plaque on R dorsal elbow.

O: **Pretreatment:** Well-demarcated scaling plaque approximately 3 × 4 cm on R dorsal elbow area.

Intervention: UVB to R dorsal elbow, lamp No. 6555, 60 cm from Pt, 4 min.

Posttreatment: Mild erythema 6 h after exposure; lasted for 24 h. Psoriatic plaque 50% resolved since initial treatment 3 weeks ago.

A: Pt tolerated treatment well, with appropriate erythema response and excellent plaque clearance.

P: Continue treatment every other day until plaque resolves. Increase dose by 10% of MED for next treatment.

Ultraviolet Lamps
SELECTING A LAMP

Numerous lamps with output of UV radiation at different ranges in the UV spectrum and that use different technology to produce radiation are currently available in the United States (Fig. 17.9). Output ranges include broad-spectrum UVA, BB-UVB, NB-UVB, and broad-spectrum UVC with wavelengths of 200 to 290 nm and a peak at 250 nm. The lamps can be of the arc or fluorescent type. An **arc lamp** is generally small and emits radiation of a consistent intensity, whereas a **fluorescent lamp** is long and emits higher-intensity radiation in the middle than at the ends.[78] Single-arc lamps are recommended for treating small areas such as the hand, whereas units incorporating an array of arc lamps are recommended for treatment of larger body areas. Fluorescent tubes generally are not recommended because of the variability of intensity along their length. The ideal lamp is one that produces a narrow band of radiation and uniform treatment of the area within a reasonable amount of time.

LAMP MAINTENANCE

Lamp surfaces should be cleaned regularly to remove dust or oils, which will attenuate the radiation. Lamps should be replaced when their intensity decreases to the point where treatment times become unacceptably long. The useful lifetime of most UV lamps is 500 to 1000 hours. Beyond this time, lamp output decreases by approximately 20% compared with the initial output.

> **⊚ Clinical Pearl**
>
> Most UV lamps last 500 to 1000 hours.

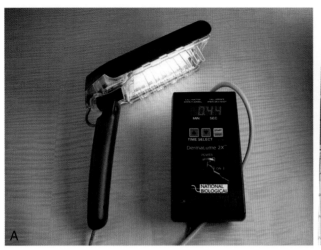
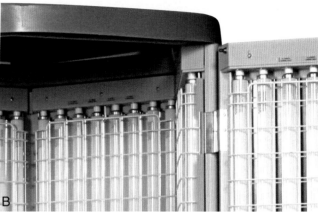

FIGURE 17.9 Ultraviolet (UV) lamps. (A) Handheld narrowband UVB lamp for treatment of small areas. Comes with a distance comb for treatment of scalp psoriasis. (B) UV cabinet for whole-body therapy that can be fit with narrowband UVB bulbs, UVA bulbs, or a combination. (Courtesy National Biological Corporation, Twinsburg, OH.)

CLINICAL CASE STUDY

The following case study summarizes some of the concepts of the clinical use of UV therapy discussed in this chapter. Based on the scenario presented, an evaluation of the clinical findings and goals of treatment are proposed. These are followed by a discussion of the factors to be considered in treatment selection.

CASE STUDY 17.1

Psoriasis

Examination

History

FR is a 25-year-old woman with psoriasis. She has had this disease for about 8 years and has been successfully treated with PUVA in the past. Prior courses of treatment generally have taken about 6 weeks and have cleared her plaques for 6 months, but they gradually recurred thereafter. Her last course of PUVA treatments was completed 1 year ago.

Systems Review

FR is alert and cooperative. She has plaques on the dorsal aspects of both elbows and on the anterior aspects of both knees. She complains that these areas itch and are unsightly, and she always wears clothing that covers her elbows and knees when in public. She has not been participating in her local soccer league because she is embarrassed to have other people see her arms and legs. She has no atrophy and no self-reported weakness, range-of-motion restrictions, or sensory changes in the upper or lower extremities.

Tests and Measures

The patient has plaques approximately 4 × 8 cm on both dorsal elbows and approximately 5 × 7 cm on both anterior knees.

What types of UV therapy would you consider for this patient? What history do you need to obtain from this patient? How do you determine the appropriate dose?

Evaluation and Goals

ICF Level	Current Status	Goals
Body structure and function	Itchiness Impaired skin integrity	Complete clearing of psoriatic plaques in 6 weeks
Activity	Avoids wearing clothes that expose unsightly psoriatic plaques	Return to feeling of comfort when wearing clothes that expose the elbows or knees
Participation	Stopped playing soccer	Return to playing in local soccer league

ICF, International Classification for Functioning, Disability and Health.

◆ FIND THE EVIDENCE

PICO Terms	Natural Language Example	Sample PubMed Search
P (Population)	Patient with psoriasis	("Psoriasis" [MeSH] OR "Psoriasis" [text word])
I (Intervention)	Ultraviolet therapy	AND ("Ultraviolet Therapy" [MeSH] OR "Ultraviolet" [text word])
C (Comparison)	No PUVA	
O (Outcome)	Clearance of plaques	AND "Plaque" [text word] AND English [lang] AND "Humans" [MeSH]

CLINICAL CASE STUDY—cont'd

Key Studies or Reviews

1. Elmets CA, Lim HW, Stoff B, et al: Joint American Academy of Dermatology–National Psoriasis Foundation guidelines of care for the management and treatment of psoriasis with phototherapy. *J Am Acad Dermatol* 81(3):775–804, 2019. This clinical guideline includes a thorough overview of the evidence concerning the use of UV therapy in its various forms, including narrowband and broadband UVB, UVA with photosensitizing agents, and UV laser, for the treatment of psoriasis. The authors provide an evidence-based discussion of the efficacy and safety of each modality and provide detailed recommendations and guidance for the use of these therapies. They conclude that, based on relative risk and benefit, NB-UVB is the phototherapy treatment of choice for plaque psoriasis.

2. Unrue EL, Cline A, Collins A, et al: A novel ultraviolet B home phototherapy system: Efficacy, tolerability, adherence, and satisfaction. *Dermatol Online J* 25(2), pii: 13030/qt3vn1z0s2, 2019.

   This article describes a study in which eight patients with plaque psoriasis used a home narrowband UVB device on some of their lesions. At 10 weeks, all patients experienced improvement in the treated lesions, and there was excellent treatment adherence. This study supports that home narrowband UVB therapy is safe, feasible, and effective.

Prognosis

UVA in conjunction with psoralen sensitization and NB-UVB are effective interventions for psoriasis, having been shown to temporarily clear psoriatic plaques. Although this patient used PUVA in the past, NB-UVB is now recommended for this patient because evidence supports that this treatment is almost as likely

to be effective and is safer and more cost-effective. If NB-UVB is not effective for her, return to PUVA should be considered.

Intervention

To provide treatment with NB-UVB, the patient's skin sensitivity to NB-UVB radiation should first be assessed by determining her MED. Because FR has several areas with plaques, treatment should be provided in a UV cabinet, and the areas without plaques should be covered. Alternatively, a single lamp, a UVB laser, or a home NB-UVB phototherapy system could be used to treat each of the four involved areas sequentially. Once FR's sensitivity to UV radiation from the selected device has been determined, treatment with 50% of her MED to E_1, increasing by 10% to 40% each week, applied two or three times per week, is recommended. This treatment regimen should be continued until her skin has cleared completely, and remission may then be maintained with ongoing weekly treatments.

Documentation

S: Pt reports itchy, scaly psoriatic plaques on both knees and elbows that have been successfully treated with PUVA in the past.

O: Pretreatment: Well-demarcated, scaling plaques approximately 4 × 8 cm on bilateral dorsal elbows and 5 × 7 cm on bilateral anterior knees.

Intervention: Pt's MED to NB-UVB determined before treatment: Pt placed in UV cabinet, lamp No. 9624, NB-UVB to bilateral knees and elbows for 4 min.

Posttreatment: No change in appearance of plaques. No erythema.

A: Pt tolerated NB-UVB well, with no adverse effects.

P: Continue NB-UVB therapy three times per week, increasing dose by 10% to 40% of MED each week, depending on Pt's response.

Chapter Review

1. UV radiation is electromagnetic radiation with a wavelength from under 290 nm to up to 400 nm, lying between x-ray and visible light. UV is emitted by the sun and by UV lamps. UV radiation is divided into three categories defined by wavelength. UVA has the longest wavelength (320 to 400 nm), UVB is in the middle (290 to 320 nm), and UVC has the shortest wavelength (less than 290 nm). UVA has the greatest depth of skin penetration, whereas UVC affects the most superficial exposed layers.

2. Effects of UV radiation include erythema, tanning, epidermal hyperplasia, and vitamin D synthesis. UVC may be bactericidal, whereas UVA and UVB can affect immune activity and inflammation, depending on the dose applied.

3. UV radiation is used primarily to treat psoriasis and other skin disorders. For this application, narrowband (311 to 313 nm) UVB is preferred. UVA in combination with oral psoralen (PUVA) is most effective, but UVB is usually recommended because it has fewer and less severe side effects, is easier and less expensive to apply, and is almost as effective.

UVC is occasionally used to augment standard wound care interventions in patients with chronic wounds.

4. Contraindications to the use of UV radiation include irradiation of the eyes and skin of the gonads; skin cancer; pulmonary tuberculosis; cardiac, kidney, or liver disease; systemic lupus erythematosus; fever; and recent x-ray therapy. Precautions include photosensitizing medication use and photosensitivity. No dose of UV radiation should be repeated until the effects of the previous dose have disappeared.

5. The MED is the smallest dose of UV radiation needed to produce erythema that appears within 8 hours of exposure and that disappears within 24 hours after exposure. Dosing of UV radiation is determined by the MED. If a patient is undergoing PUVA therapy, the MED should be determined after the patient has taken psoralen. For skin conditions, a series of treatments over the course of weeks is typically needed. The patient should be closely monitored for erythema and therapeutic response, with the dose generally being increased as treatment proceeds.

Glossary

Actinic damage: Skin damage caused by chronic exposure to ultraviolet radiation. The skin becomes dry, coarse, and leathery, with wrinkling and pigment abnormalities.

Arc lamp: A lamp that produces light when electrical current flows across the gap between two electrodes.

Cataracts: Loss of transparency of the lens of the eye that causes blurry, hazy, or distorted vision and is caused by aging and by chronic ultraviolet radiation exposure.

Conjunctivitis: Inflammation of the insides of the eyelids and the membrane covering the cornea that causes light sensitivity, tearing, eyelid twitching, and a sensation of gritty eyes.

Epidermal hyperplasia: Thickening of the superficial layer of the skin.

Erythema: Redness of the skin.

First-degree erythema (E_1): Definite redness with some mild desquamation that appears within 6 hours after exposure to ultraviolet radiation and lasts for 1 to 3 days.

Fluorescent lamp: A lamp that uses electricity to excite mercury vapor in argon or neon gas and that can produce ultraviolet light.

Frequency band: A range within the electromagnetic spectrum defined by frequency or wavelength. For example, the band for UVA radiation is 320 to 400 nm wavelength; also called *band*.

Minimal erythemal dose (MED): The smallest dose of ultraviolet radiation to produce erythema, which appears within 8 hours of exposure and disappears within 24 hours after exposure.

Photokeratitis: Temporary inflammation of the cornea that occurs after ultraviolet radiation exposure, causing discomfort, blurred vision, and light sensitivity.

Phototherapy: The therapeutic use of light.

Psoralen: A photosensitizing chemical administered orally or topically to increase the skin's reaction to light for a therapeutic effect.

Psoralen with UVA (PUVA): A combination of psoralen and UVA radiation that is used to treat some skin conditions.

Psoriasis: A chronic skin disorder marked by itchy, scaly red patches.

Psoriatic arthritis: Arthritis that may accompany the skin manifestations of psoriasis.

Second-degree erythema (E_2): Intense erythema with edema, peeling, and pigmentation appearing within 2 hours after exposure to ultraviolet radiation.

Suberythemal dose (SED): A dose of ultraviolet radiation that produces no change in skin redness in the 24 hours after exposure.

Third-degree erythema (E_3): Erythema with severe blistering, peeling, and exudation.

Ultraviolet (UV) radiation: Electromagnetic radiation with a frequency range of 7.5×10^{14} to more than 10^{15} Hz and wavelengths from 400 nm to less than 290 nm; lies between x-ray and visible light.

Vitiligo: A chronic skin condition that causes loss of pigmentation, resulting in patches of pale skin; also called *leukoderma*.

References

1. Battie C, Jitsukawa S, Bernerd F, et al: New insights in photoaging, UVA induced damage and skin types. *Exp Dermatol* 23(Suppl 1):7–12, 2014. doi:10.1111/exd.12388.
2. Christensen L, Suggs A, Baron E: Ultraviolet Photobiology in Dermatology. *Adv Exp Med Biol* 996:89–104, 2017. doi:10.1007/978-3-319-56017-5_8.
3. Matos TR, Sheth V: The symbiosis of phototherapy and photoimmunology. *Clin Dermatol* 34(5):538–547, 2016. doi:10.1016/j.clindermatol.2016.05.003.
4. Sklar LR, Almutawa F, Lim HW, et al: Effects of ultraviolet radiation, visible light, and infrared radiation on erythema and pigmentation: a review. *Photochem Photobiol Sci* 12(1):54–64, 2013. doi:10.1039/c2pp25152c.
5. O'Leary RE, Diehl J, Levins PC: Update on tanning: More risks, fewer benefits. *J Am Acad Dermatol* 70(3):562–568, 2014. doi:10.1016/j.jaad.2013.11.004.
6. Mohania D, Chandel S, Kumar P, et al: Ultraviolet radiations: skin defense-damage mechanism. *Adv Exp Med Biol* 996:71–87, 2017. doi:10.1007/978-3-319-56017-5_7.
7. El-Abaseri TB, Putta S, Hansen LA: Ultraviolet irradiation induces keratinocyte proliferation and epidermal hyperplasia through the activation of the epidermal growth factor receptor. *Carcinogenesis* 27(2):225–231, 2006.
8. Eaglestein W, Weinstein G: Prostaglandin and DNA synthesis in human skin: possible relationship to ultraviolet light effects. *J Invest Dermatol* 64:386–396, 1975.
9. Barrett KE, Barman SM, Brooks HL, et al: *Ganong's review of medical physiology*, ed 26, New York, NY, 2019, McGraw-Hill Education.
10. Holick MF: Ultraviolet B radiation: The vitamin D connection. *Adv Exp Med Biol* 996:137–154, 2017. doi:10.1007/978-3-319-56017-5_12.
11. Holick MF: Vitamin D deficiency. *N Engl J Med* 357:266–281, 2007.
12. Laursen JH, Søndergaard HB, Sørensen PS, et al: Association between age at onset of multiple sclerosis and vitamin D level-related factors. *Neurology* 86:88–93, 2016.
13. Korf H, Decallonne B, Mathieu C: Vitamin D for infections. *Curr Opin Endocrinol Diabetes Obes* 21:431–436, 2014.
14. Arain N, Mirza WA, Aslam M: Vitamin D and the prevention of preeclampsia: a systematic review. *Pak J Pharm Sci* 28:1015–1021, 2015.
15. Jorde R, Grimnes G: Vitamin D and health: the need for more randomized controlled trials. *J Steroid Biochem Mol Biol* 148:269–274, 2015.
16. Sage RJ, Lim HW: UV-based therapy and vitamin D. *Dermatol Ther* 23:72–81, 2010.
17. Holick MF, Smith E, Pincus S: Skin as the site of vitamin D synthesis and target tissue for 1,25-dihydroxyvitamin D3: use of calcitriol (1,25-dihydroxyvitamin D3) for treatment of psoriasis. *Arch Dermatol* 123:1677–1683a, 1987.
18. Staberg B, Oxholm A, Klemp P, et al: Is the effect of phototherapy in psoriasis partly due to an impact on vitamin D metabolism? *Acta Derm Venereol* 68:436–439, 1988.
19. Sullivan PK, Conner-Kerr TA: A comparative study of the effects of UVC irradiation on select procaryotic and eucaryotic wound pathogens. *Ostomy Wound Manage* 46:28–34, 2000.
20. Coohill TP, Sagripanti JL: Overview of the inactivation by 254 nm ultraviolet radiation of bacteria with particular relevance to biodefense. *Photochem Photobiol* 84(5):1084–1090, 2008.
21. Vermeulen N, Keeler WJ, Nandakumar K, et al: The bactericidal effect of ultraviolet and visible light on *Escherichia coli*. *Biotechnol Bioeng* 99(3):550–556, 2008.
22. Anderson BM, Banrud H, Boe E, et al: Comparison of UV C light and chemicals for disinfection of surfaces in hospital isolation units. *Infect Control Hosp Epidemiol* 27:729–734, 2006.
23. Thai TP, Keast DH, Campbell KE, et al: Effect of ultraviolet light C on bacterial colonization in chronic wounds. *Ostomy Wound Manage* 51:32–45, 2005.
24. Gupta A, Avci P, Dai T, et al: Ultraviolet radiation in wound care: sterilization and stimulation. *Adv Wound Care (New Rochelle)* 2:422–437, 2013.
25. Rasanen L, Reunala T, Lehto M, et al: Immediate decrease in antigen-presenting function and delayed enhancement of interleukin-I production in human epidermal cells after in vivo UV-B irradiation. *Br J Dermatol* 120:589–596, 1989.
26. Horkay I, Bodolay E, Koda A: Immunologic aspects of prophylactic UV-B and PUVA therapy in polymorphic light eruption. *Photodermatol* 3:47–49, 1986.
27. Gollhausen R, Kaidbey K, Schechter N: UV suppression of mast cell mediated whealing in human skin. *Photodermatol* 2:58–67, 1985.
28. Kanekura T, Higashi Y, Kanzaki T: Cyclooxygenase-2 expression and prostaglandin E2 biosynthesis are enhanced in scleroderma fibroblasts and inhibited by UVA irradiation. *J Rheumatol* 28:1568–1572, 2001.
29. Zandi S, Kalia S, Lui H: UVA1 phototherapy: a concise and practical review. *Skin Therapy Lett* 17(1):1–4, 2012.

30. Keyal U, Bhatta AK, Wang XK: UVA1 a promising approach for scleroderma. *Am J Transl Res* 9(9):4280–4287, 2017. PMC5622270. PMID: 28979701.

31. Wu CS, Lan CC, Wang LF, et al: Effects of psoralen plus ultraviolet A irradiation on cultured epidermal cells in vitro and patients with vitiligo in vivo. *Br J Dermatol* 156:122–129, 2007.

32. Grimes PE: New insights and new therapies in vitiligo. *JAMA* 293:730–735, 2005.

33. Racz E, Prens EP: Phototherapy and photochemotherapy for psoriasis. *Dermatol Clin* 33:79–89, 2015.

34. Reynolds NJ, Franklin V, Gray JC, et al: Narrow-band ultraviolet B and broad-band ultraviolet A phototherapy in adult atopic eczema: a randomised controlled trial. *Lancet* 357:2012–2016, 2001.

35. Marsland AM, Chalmers RJ, Hollis S, et al: Interventions for chronic palmoplantar pustulosis. *Cochrane Database Syst Rev* 2006(1):CD001433, 2006.

36. Pothiawala SZ, Baldwin BT, Cherpelis BS, et al: The role of phototherapy in cutaneous T-cell lymphoma. *J Drugs Dermatol* 9:764–772, 2010.

37. Hart PH, Norval M, Byrne SN, et al: Exposure to ultraviolet radiation in the modulation of human diseases. *Annu Rev Pathol* 14:55–81, 2019. doi:10.1146/annurev-pathmechdis-012418-012809.

38. Lotti T, Buggiani G, Troiano M, et al: Targeted and combination treatments for vitiligo: comparative evaluation of different current modalities in 458 subjects. *Dermatol Ther* 21(Suppl 1):S20–S26, 2008.

39. Valkova S: UVB phototherapeutic modalities: comparison of two treatments for chronic plaque psoriasis. *Acta Derm Venereol* 16:26–30, 2007.

40. Elmets CA, Lim HW, Stoff B, et al: Joint American Academy of Dermatology–National Psoriasis Foundation guidelines of care for the management and treatment of psoriasis with phototherapy. *J Am Acad Dermatol* 81(3):775–804, 2019. doi:10.1016/j.jaad.2019.04.042.

41. Zhang P, Wu MX: A clinical review of phototherapy for psoriasis. *Lasers Med Sci* 33(1):173–180, 2018. doi:10.1007/s10103-017-2360-1.

42. Kemény L, Varga E, Novak Z: Advances in phototherapy for psoriasis and atopic dermatitis. *Expert Rev Clin Immunol* 1: 1–10, 2019. doi:10.1080/1744666X.2020.1672537.

43. Almutawa F, Thalib L, Hekman D, et al: Efficacy of localized phototherapy and photodynamic therapy for psoriasis: a systematic review and meta-analysis. *Photodermatol Photoimmunol Photomed* 31:5–14, 2015.

44. Chen X, Yang M, Cheng Y, et al: Narrow-band ultraviolet B phototherapy versus broad-band ultraviolet B or psoralen-ultraviolet A photochemotherapy for psoriasis. *Cochrane Database Syst Rev* 2013(10):CD009481, 2013.

45. Almutawa F, Alnomair N, Wang Y, et al: Systematic review of UV-based therapy for psoriasis. *Am J Clin Dermatol* 14:87–109, 2013.

46. Archier E, Devaux S, Castela E, et al: Efficacy of psoralen UV-Atherapy vs. narrowband UV-B therapy in chronic plaquepsoriasis: a systematic literature review. *J Eur Acad DermatolVenereol* 26(Suppl 3):11–21, 2012.

47. Koek MB, Buskens E, van Weelden H, et al: Home versus outpatient ultraviolet B phototherapy for mild to severe psoriasis: pragmatic multicentre randomised controlled non-inferiority trial (PLUTO study). *BMJ* 338:b1542, 2009.

48. Unrue EL, Cline A, Collins A, et al: A novel ultraviolet B home phototherapy system: Efficacy, tolerability, adherence, and satisfaction. *Dermatol Online J* 25(2):13030/qt3vn1z0s2, 2019.

49. Mudigonda T, Dabade TS, Feldman SR: A review of targeted ultraviolet B phototherapy for psoriasis. *J Am Acad Dermatol* 66(4):664–672, 2012.

50. Tronnier H, Schule D: First results of therapy with long wave UV-A after photosensitization of the skin. In *Abstracts of the sixth international congress of photobiology*, Bochum, Germany. August 21–25, 1972.

51. Jain VK, Jangra S, Aggarwal K: Comparative efficacy of narrow-band ultraviolet B phototherapy alone and its combination with topical 8-methoxypsoralen in psoriasis. *Indian J Dermatol Venereol Leprol* 76(6):666–670, 2010.

52. Chen C, Hou WH, Chan ES, et al: Phototherapy for treating pressure ulcers. *Cochrane Database Syst Rev* 2014(7):CD009224, 2014.

53. Freytes H, Fernandez B, Fleming W: Ultraviolet light in the treatment of indolent ulcers. *South Med J* 58:223–226, 1965.

54. Nussbaum EL, Flett H, Hitzig SL, et al: Ultraviolet-C irradiation in the management of pressure ulcers in people with spinal cord injury: a randomized, placebo-controlled trial. *Arch Phys Med Rehabil* 94:650–659, 2013.

55. Ramsay C, Challoner A: Vascular changes in human skin after ultraviolet irradiation. *Br J Dermatol* 94:487–493, 1976.

56. Kloth LC: Physical modalities in wound management: UVC, therapeutic heating and electrical stimulation. *Ostomy Wound Manage* 41:18–20, 22–24, 26–27, 1995.

57. Ersoy-Evans S, Altaykan A, Sahin S, et al: Phototherapy in childhood. *Pediatr Dermatol* 25:599–605, 2008.

58. Leow YH, Tham SN: UV-protective sunglasses for UVA irradiation protection. *Int J Dermatol* 34:808–810, 1995.

59. Osmancevic A, Gillstedt M, Wennberg AM, et al: The risk of skin cancer in psoriasis patients treated with UVB therapy. *Acta Derm Venereol* 94:425–430, 2014.

60. Beattie PE, Dawe RS, Traynor NJ, et al: Can St John's wort (hypericin) ingestion enhance the erythemal response during high-dose ultraviolet A1 therapy? *Br J Dermatol* 153:1187–1191, 2005.

61. Ozkan I, Köse O, Ozmen I, et al: Efficacy and safety of non-laser, targeted UVB phototherapy alone and in combination with psoralen gel or calcipotriol ointment in the treatment of localized, chronic, plaque-type psoriasis. *Int J Dermatol* 51:609–613, 2012.

62. Epstein JH: Phototherapy and photochemotherapy. *N Engl J Med* 322:1149–1151, 1990.

63. Tilkorn DJ, Schaffran A, Al-Benna S, et al: Severe burn injuries induced by PUVA chemotherapy. *J Burn Care Res* 34:e195–e200, 2013.

64. Archier E, Devaux S, Castela E, et al: Carcinogenic risks of psoralen UV-A therapy and narrowband UV-B therapy in chronic plaque psoriasis: a systematic literature review. *J Eur Acad Dermatol Venereol* 26(Suppl 3):22–31, 2012.

65. Hearn RM, Kerr AC, Rahim KF, et al: Incidence of skin cancers in 3867 patients treated with narrow-band ultraviolet B phototherapy. *Br J Dermatol* 159:931–935, 2008.

66. Burns F: Cancer risks associated with therapeutic irradiation of the skin. *Arch Dermatol* 125:979–981, 1989.

67. Taylor HR: The biological effects of ultraviolet-B on the eye. *Photochem Photobiol* 50:489–492, 1989.

68. See JA, Weller P: Ocular complications of PUVA therapy. *Australas J Dermatol* 34:1–4, 1993.

69. Malanos D, Stern RS: Psoralen plus ultraviolet A does not increase the risk of cataracts: a 25-year prospective study. *J Am Acad Dermatol* 57:231–237, 2007.

70. Stern RS, Liebman EJ, Vakeva L: Oral psoralen and ultraviolet-A light (PUVA) treatment of psoriasis and persistent risk of nonmelanoma skin cancer: PUVA follow-up study. *J Natl Cancer Inst* 90:1278–1284, 1998.

71. Hirose-Matsuda H, Okamoto O, Sakai I, et al: Multiple malignant changes and recurrent infections in the skin associated with long-term exposure to ultraviolet light and topical psoralen plus ultraviolet A therapy. *J Dermatol* 42:536–537, 2015.

72. Tromovitch TA, Thompson LR, Jacobs PH: Testing for photosensitivity. *J Am Phys Ther Assoc* 143:348–349, 1963.

73. Man I, Dawe RS, Ferguson J: An intraindividual study of the characteristics of erythema induced by bath and oral methoxsalen photochemotherapy and narrowband ultraviolet B. *Photochem Photobiol* 78:55–60, 2003.

74. Kaidbey K, Agin P, Sayre R, et al: Photoprotection by melanin: a comparison of black and Caucasian skin. *J Am Acad Dermatol* 1:249–260, 1979.

75. Heckman CJ, Chandler R, Kloss JD, et al: Minimal erythema dose (MED) testing. *J Vis Exp* 75:50175, 2013.

76. Levine M, Parrish JA: Out-patient phototherapy of psoriasis. *Arch Dermatol* 116:552–554, 1980.

77. Cameron H, Dawe RS, Yule S, et al: A randomized, observer-blinded trial of twice vs. three times weekly narrowband ultraviolet B phototherapy for chronic plaque psoriasis. *Br J Dermatol* 147(5):973–978, 2002.

78. Chue B, Borok M, Lowe NJ: Phototherapy units: comparison of fluorescent ultraviolet B and ultraviolet A units with high-pressure mercury system. *J Am Acad Dermatol* 18:641–645, 1998.

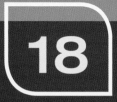

Shock Wave Therapy

OBJECTIVES

After reading this chapter, the reader will be able to do the following:
- Define *extracorporeal shock wave therapy (ESWT)*.
- Describe effects and clinical applications of ESWT.
- Safely and effectively apply ESWT.
- Choose the best technique for treatment with ESWT, and list the advantages and disadvantages of each.
- Select the appropriate equipment and parameters for treatment with ESWT.
- Accurately and completely document treatment with ESWT.

Shock wave therapy, also known as *pressure wave therapy, acoustic compression therapy,* or **extracorporeal shock wave therapy (ESWT),** is the most recently introduced physical agent to rehabilitation practice. Shock wave therapy was first used in medical practice in the 1970s and 1980s when focused shock waves were introduced for treating kidney stones,

known as *lithotripsy.* In this application, the shock waves are focused on larger kidney stones and break them into smaller fragments that can then be passed with the urine. When applying this intervention, providers noticed that this treatment affected bone and soft tissue healing in the area exposed to the shock waves. Although they first appreciated the destruction of bony tissue, through animal and then human studies involving multiple tissue types, researchers were able to optimize the treatment parameters, generally reducing the energy levels, to promote tissue healing and achieve other therapeutic benefits.

Since the 1990s, numerous papers have reported the benefits of ESWT for soft tissue problems, most commonly calcific tendonitis and other chronic tendinopathies and localized inflammation such as plantar fasciitis and bursitis. In addition, ESWT has been found to promote soft tissue healing after sprains and strains and in chronic wounds and to promote healing of nonunion, delayed union, and acute fractures. These benefits are ascribed to both the promotion of healing by the stimulation of growth factors and collagen production and by controlling inflammation and pain. This chapter focuses on the application of ESWT for the treatment of musculoskeletal conditions.

Physical Properties of Shock Waves

Shock waves are high-amplitude, short-duration sound waves. Although shock waves and ultrasound waves are both sound waves, they have some features that differ from ultrasound and that may underlie differences in effects. Shock waves are asymmetrical; last a total of under 10 microseconds; and start with a brief, rapidly rising (~10-nanosecond), high-intensity compressive phase, followed by a much longer, low-intensity tensile phase. In contrast, therapeutic ultrasound waves are symmetrical, with a sinusoidal rise and fall, with each wave lasting 0.33 or 1 microsecond for 3- or 1-MHz ultrasound, respectively (Fig. 18.1).

TYPES OF SHOCK WAVES

Two types of ESWT are currently used in therapy, **focused ESWT** (fESWT) and **radial ESWT**[1] (rESWT; Fig. 18.2 and Table 18.1), with rESWT devices being less expensive and more widely available than fESWT devices. There is substantial controversy about whether rESWT is true shock wave therapy and also whether fESWT or rESWT is more effective than the other. There is little research comparing these directly.

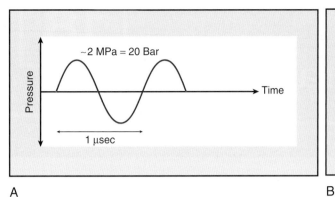
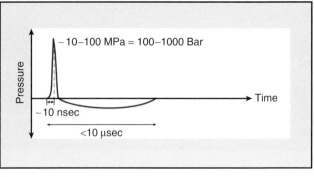

A   B

FIGURE 18.1 Comparison of therapeutic ultrasound and focused extracorporeal shock wave therapy (ESWT) waves. (A) Ultrasound is a sinusoidal compression rarefaction wave with a wavelength of 0.33 microseconds (for 3-MHz ultrasound) to 1.0 microseconds (for 1-MHz ultrasound). (B) Shock waves are also compression rarefaction waves but with a very short compression phase (~10 nanoseconds to peak pressure) and much longer rarefaction phases, with an overall wavelength of <10 microseconds.

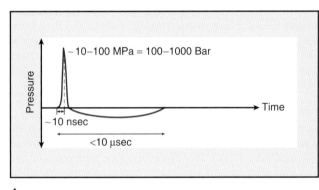
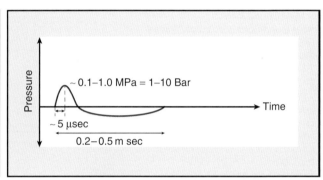

A   B

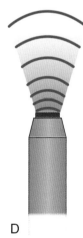

FIGURE 18.2 Comparison of focused and radial shock waves. (A) Focused shock waves have a very rapid rise, and each entire wave lasts under 10 microseconds. (B) Focused shock waves are diffuse at the applicator and focus within the tissue at a depth of ~2 to 4 inches. (C) Radial shock waves, also known as pressure waves, have a slower rise, and each entire wave lasts around 0.2–0.5 milliseconds. (D) Radial shock waves are concentrated at the applicator and diffuse within the tissue as they get farther from the applicator.

C   D

 Clinical Pearl

There are two types of shock wave therapy, focused and radial. There is substantial controversy and little agreement about whether one of these is more effective than the other, and few studies directly compare one to the other.

Focused ESWT waves are very short-duration waves with a high peak pressure, taking about 10 nanoseconds to reach their peak pressure of 10 to 100 megapascals (MPa = 10^6 pascals,

100 to 1000 bar) and lasting a total of under 10 microseconds (see Fig. 18.2A). These waves are dispersed at the applicator and focus within the tissue to apply the greatest energy density to a target about 2 to 4 inches (5 to 10 cm) deep over an area of about 1/8 to 1 inch (2 to 30 mm) in diameter (see Fig. 18.2B). The original ESWT devices used to treat kidney stones are fESWT devices and are designed to produce the greatest intensity at the kidney stone. Focused ESWT devices can also be used to treat musculoskeletal conditions and, in this case, are focused on the target tissue identified clinically or by imaging. In general, fESWT is less uncomfortable than rESWT. Focused ESWT, like most other physical agents, such as therapeutic

TABLE 18.1	Focused Versus Radial Shock Waves	
	Focused	**Radial**
Shock wave duration	<10 microseconds	0.2–0.5 milliseconds
Time to peak pressure (rise time)	~10 nanoseconds	5 microseconds
Peak pressure	10–100 megapascals (MPa) 100–1000 bar	–1 MPa 1–10 bar
Energy	150–200 mJ	20–35 mJ
Energy flux density	0–3 mJ/mm²	0–0.3 mJ/mm²
Distribution	Focused in ⅛- to 1-inch area at about 2–4 inches deep (5–10 cm), can make more superficial with standoff	Dispersing with distance from the applicator, depth 1½ inches (3–4 cm max), superficial
U.S. Food and Drug Administration class	II	I

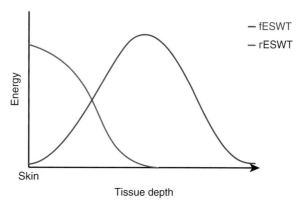

FIGURE 18.3 Distribution of focused and radial shock waves within the tissue. Focused extracorporeal shock wave therapy (fESWT; shown in red) produces the highest-intensity energy at a focal area about 2 to 4 inches deep in the tissue. The focal depth and area vary among applicators, and the focal depth within the tissue can also be modified using a standoff attached to the applicator. The energy from radial extracorporeal shock wave therapy (rESWT; shown in blue) is most concentrated at the skin surface and dissipates with increasing tissue depth.

ultrasound and neuromuscular electrical stimulation devices, is classified by the U.S. Food and Drug Administration (FDA) as a Class II medical device. Class II devices are those with a moderate potential risk of harm for which special controls combined with general controls are necessary to provide a reasonable assurance of safety and effectiveness. Examples of other medical devices with this Class II classification are syringes and powered wheelchairs.

Radial ESWT devices were introduced to the market more recently and are technologically less expensive to produce. Radial ESWT waves last longer and have a lower peak pressure than fESWT waves, taking about 5 microseconds to reach their peak pressure of 0.1 to 1 MPa (1 to 10 bar) and lasting a total of about 0.2 to 0.5 milliseconds (see Fig. 18.2C). This is about 1000 times longer than an fESWT wave. Because rESWT waves do not have the rapid rate of pressure rise or the high peak pressure of fESWT waves, some authors consider rESWT waves not to be true shock waves and therefore call them *pressure waves*. Radial ESWT waves are most concentrated at the applicator and disperse eccentrically from the applicator tip, resulting in higher concentrations superficially and lower concentrations in the tissue at depth (Fig. 18.3; see also Fig. 18.2D). In general, rESWT is more uncomfortable than fESWT. Radial ESWT devices are classified by the FDA as a Class I medical device. This means they "present minimal potential for harm to the user."[2] Examples of other devices with this Class I classification are sunglasses and adhesive or elastic bandages. The greater safety and lower cost of radial ESWT devices allow for their use by a wider range of clinicians.

GENERATION OF SHOCK WAVES

Shock waves may be generated in a number of ways. Focused shock waves are usually generated using piezoelectric, electrohydraulic, or electromagnetic devices. Piezoelectric devices apply an electrical current to a piezoelectric crystal to produce a mechanical pressure wave, as is done to produce therapeutic or diagnostic ultrasound. Piezoelectric devices produce shock

waves with the smallest **focal area.** Electrohydraulic devices use an electrical spark to rapidly create a water-vapor-filled gas bubble. The creation of the bubble causes the compressive phase of the shock wave, and its implosion causes the tensile phase. Electrohydraulic devices produce shock waves with the largest focal area. Electromagnetic devices use an electromagnetic coil to produce a rapidly changing electromagnetic field that moves a metal membrane to produce the shock wave. Radial shock waves are usually produced by pneumatic compression, where compressed air accelerates a ballistic projectile in the handpiece of the device. The ballistic projectile then abruptly slows down when it hits the transmitter of the handpiece. When the elastically suspended transmitter is touching the patient's skin, with a coupling medium to ensure good contact, it exerts a rapid compressive force on the tissue, followed by a slower distractive rarefaction force as it recoils (Fig. 18.4).

SHOCK WAVE PROPAGATION

Being sound waves, shock waves propagate to and through human tissue very similarly to ultrasound waves. To be transmitted from the applicator to the tissues, gel or water must be used as a coupling or transmission agent as air does not transmit shock waves well. When propagating through soft tissue, which has similar viscoelasticity to gel or water, the waves transmit in a fairly linear manner. When the waves reach a soft tissue bone interface, where the tissues have very differing viscoelasticity, there is substantial reflection of the energy, and the energy that does go into the bone is quickly absorbed in the first couple of millimeters and is not transmitted onwards.

SHOCK WAVE PARAMETERS

ESWT is delivered to the body by the machine's transducer. The ESWT may be focused or radial, as described previously.

When delivering fESWT, the provider generally selects the total energy delivered at the focal point in a single session. This is described in terms of **total energy flux** (also known as **energy flux density [EFD]**), measured in mJ/mm². Total energy flux may be categorized as low, medium, or high. Although ranges for these vary among publications, it is

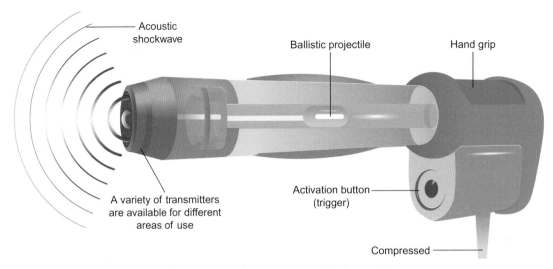

Acoustic shockwave

Ballistic projectile

Hand grip

A variety of transmitters are available for different areas of use

Activation button (trigger)

Compressed

FIGURE 18.4 Electrohydraulic method of generation.

common for low energy to be classified as up to around 0.1 mJ/mm^2, medium energy to be classified as around 0.1 to 0.25 mJ/mm^2, and high energy to be classified as around 0.25 to over 0.6 mJ/mm^2.[2,3,4]

When delivering rESWT, the provider selects the peak pressure. The peak pressure is measured in **bars** or **megapascals** (MPa). One bar is defined as equal to 0.1 MPa (10 bar = 1MPa) and is approximately equal to the atmospheric pressure on Earth at an altitude of 111 meters at 15°C. ESWT is delivered as a series of shocks.

Both fESWT and rESWT allow the user to select the **shock frequency** and **total shock number** produced by the transmitter. The shock frequency is usually measured in hertz (Hz), which is the number of shocks per second, and is generally in the range of around 1 to 10 Hz. Some devices report the shock frequency in shocks/minute. The total shock number is the total number of shocks delivered in a single session and is usually in the range of 500 to 2000 per session. The treatment duration is how long the entire treatment lasts and is usually a few minutes.

> ### ◎ Clinical Pearl
>
> When delivering fESWT, the selected treatment parameters are the energy flux density (in mJ/mm^2), the shock frequency, and the total shock number. When delivering rESWT, the selected treatment parameters are the peak pressure (in bars), the shock frequency, and the total shock number.

Although, as clinicians, we would like to be able to apply findings and treatment parameters from studies of fESWT to the application of rESWT, this is difficult to do because the dose measures of one do not translate directly into the dose measure of the other. EFD, the dose measure of fESWT, is an estimate of the energy/session at the location in the tissue where the fESWT is focused. In contrast, peak pressure, the dose measure of rESWT, is a measure of the pneumatic compression produced by the projectile inside the handpiece of an rESWT device. At

this time, the author of this chapter therefore recommends looking to studies of either type of ESWT to evaluate if ESWT is effective for a given problem and to then seek out studies using the type of ESWT clinically available to select the optimal treatment parameters. The recommended parameters provided in the Application Techniques section of this chapter were derived using this approach.

Effects of Shock Waves

Shock waves produced by an ESWT device are transmitted through and absorbed by soft tissues and are reflected at tissue interfaces. As they pass through soft tissues, they have a variety of effects on biological processes. These effects likely underlie the clinical benefits of ESWT. Although the evidence base for fESWT is larger than that for rESWT because it has been available for longer, overall, studies tend to show similar effects for both forms of ESWT.[5] When shock waves move through soft tissues, they cause **cavitation**—the formation of small, vapor-filled low-pressure cavities or bubbles. Cavitation increases cell membrane permeability and can also break up calcifications.[5,6] The increase in cell membrane permeability then acts as a trigger to activate a series of cellular events involved in cellular repair and tissue healing, including an increase in microcirculation, which increases local blood flow, and also an increase in cellular metabolic rate that contributes to regulating the inflammatory response. ESWT can promote the transition of tissues from a chronic inflammatory to an acute inflammatory state, which can then reactivate stalled tissue repair and induce cell migration, differentiation, and proliferation.[7,8] Increased release of various cytokines in response to ESWT, including substance P, prostaglandin E2 (PGE2), nitric oxide (NO), transforming growth factor beta (TGF-beta), and vascular endothelial growth factor (VEGF), are associated with these processes. The mechanical stimulation of ESWT likely also helps break down calcific deposits in tendons and remodel fibrotic tissue and scars. Furthermore, the mechanical stimulus can serve as a counterirritant, with overstimulation of mechanoreceptors at the treated site resulting in reduced nociceptive signal transmission to the brainstem.

ESWT is thought to exert therapeutic effects by cavitation, which breaks up calcifications and increases cell membrane permeability to trigger cellular repair and tissue healing. ESWT can also gate pain transmission.

Clinical Indications for Shock Waves

Although ESWT has only been introduced to the rehabilitation field fairly recently, there are many reports of studies evaluating the efficacy of this intervention. Unfortunately, the results of these studies are difficult to translate into clearly evidence-based recommendations for clinical practice. The studies vary considerably in quality, with most being small and poorly controlled; the ESWT type and parameters differ; and results are mixed, although they are overall more supportive than not. The influence of publication bias toward positive results is also uncertain. The resulting challenge in clinical practice is that although many studies suggest that ESWT may help patients with a range of musculoskeletal conditions, there is no clear consensus regarding the optimal approach to treatment. This includes the selection of the ideal patient; the selection of focused versus radial ESWT; definitions and selection of low- and high-energy ESWT; and determination of optimal dose and frequency of treatment, whether the treatment should be targeted with imaging, and whether local anesthetic should be used to control treatment-related pain.[9]

Overall, it seems reasonable to consider ESWT as another adjunctive option for treating recalcitrant chronic inflammatory conditions such as tendinopathies and calcific tendonitis, as well as plantar fasciitis and trochanteric bursitis. ESWT may also help promote healing of chronic wounds and delayed union and nonunion fractures. The FDA-approved uses for rESWT are for reducing muscle pain and aches, temporarily increasing blood flow, and activating connective tissue, and the FDA-approved uses for fESWT include treatment of kidney stones, plantar fasciitis,[10,11] lateral epicondylitis, and most recently, diabetic foot ulcers. The most common and well-supported clinical uses of ESWT are for plantar fasciitis, calcific rotator cuff tendonitis and other tendinopathies (e.g., Achilles; patellar, medial, and lateral epicondylitis; biceps; supraspinatus/rotator cuff), and trochanteric bursitis. The evidence regarding these clinical applications, and some others with modest evidence, is reviewed here.

The most common and well-supported clinical uses of ESWT are for plantar fasciitis, calcific rotator cuff tendonitis and other tendinopathies, and trochanteric bursitis.

PLANTAR FASCIITIS

Plantar fasciitis (Fig. 18.5), a foot disorder associated with pain originating from the insertion of the plantar fascia on the calcaneus, is the most common cause of heel pain. Widely ranging conservative interventions, including rest or immobilization, orthotics, ice, exercise, nonsteroidal antiinflamma-

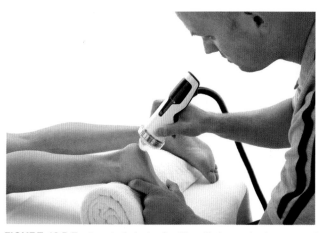

FIGURE 18.5 Treatment of plantar fasciitis with focused extracorporeal shock wave therapy (fESWT). (Courtesy Chattanooga, Lewisville, TX.)

tory drugs (NSAIDs), corticosteroid injections, taping, and soft tissue mobilization techniques, are used to treat plantar fasciitis. ESWT is FDA cleared for the treatment of plantar fasciitis based on a randomized controlled trial (RCT) with 172 patients with chronic plantar fasciitis who had not responded to at least two prior conservative interventions.[12] Systematic reviews with meta-analyses of RCTs of ESWT for managing plantar fasciitis have also concluded that ESWT is effective for the treatment of plantar fasciitis,[4,9,13–17] with effectiveness ranging from around 35% to 90%. Some analyses compared different forms and intensities of ESWT, and these concluded that the higher end of the medium-intensity range (low EFD is ≤0.08 mJ/mm^2, medium is 0.08 to 0.28 mJ/mm^2, and high is ≥0.28 mJ/mm^2) of fESWT is the ideal option, and one concluded that rESWT is an appropriate alternative because of its lower price and likely better effectiveness.[4,15,17]

The evidence for the effectiveness of ESWT relative to corticosteroid injection for plantar fasciitis has been evaluated in both a 2018 meta-analysis based on comparing studies of each[18] and in a 2019 meta-analysis of directly comparative studies.[19] The authors of the earlier meta-analysis concluded that high-intensity ESWT is likely more effective than corticosteroid injection but that corticosteroid injection is likely more effective than low-intensity ESWT. The latter meta-analysis did not evaluate the impact of different intensities of ESWT and concluded that both injection and ESWT were effective for improving function and pain, with ESWT being more effective for relieving pain. One study also supports that rESWT has a longer duration of effect[20] than corticosteroid injection, and at least one more study directly comparing these interventions in patients with plantar fasciitis is planned.[21]

Overall, current research supports that ESWT is effective for improving symptoms and reducing disability associated with plantar fasciitis. It appears that medium-intensity ESWT, although likely at the high end of this range, is most effective. Most studies have evaluated fESWT, but there is also some support for the effectiveness of rESWT, and this therapy has the advantages of lower cost and risk.

CALCIFIC ROTATOR CUFF TENDONITIS

Rotator cuff tendonitis (Fig. 18.6) is one of the most common causes of shoulder pain. Rotator cuff tendonitis may be associated with calcium deposits in the tendons, most commonly

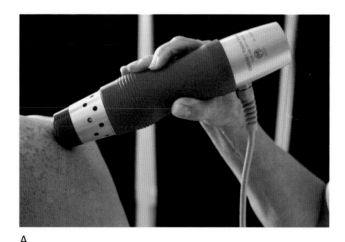

A

Original Calcification   After 4 Weeks

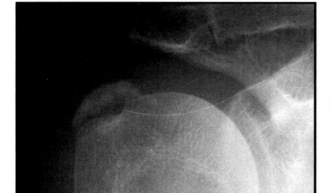

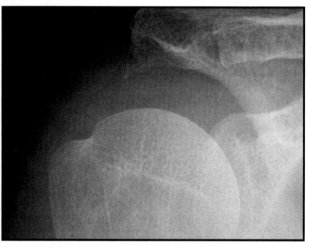

B

FIGURE 18.6 (A) Treatment of calcific rotator cuff tendonitis with radial extracorporeal shock wave therapy (rESWT). (B) Resolution of subacromial rotator cuff calcification after 4 weeks of treatment with rESWT. (A, Courtesy EMS Physio, Wantage, UK. B, From Cacchio A, Paoloni M, Barile A: Effectiveness of radial shock-wave therapy for calcific tendinitis of the shoulder: single-blind, randomized clinical study. *Phys Ther* 86(5):672–682, 2006. doi:10.1093/ptj/86.5.672.)

the supraspinatus tendon near its insertion. This is known as *calcific rotator cuff tendonitis.* The presence of calcium deposits cannot be ascertained by history or physical examination but can be identified by x-ray. As with plantar fasciitis, wide-ranging interventions, including rest, ice, exercise, NSAIDs, taping, and soft tissue mobilization techniques, are used to treat rotator cuff tendonitis, but treatment resistance is not uncommon, and calcific rotator cuff tendonitis tends to be more treatment resistant than noncalcific rotator cuff tendonitis and may require surgery.

Several studies and systematic reviews have evaluated the impact of ESWT on chronic shoulder tendonitis.[6,22–28] In general, these have concluded that although most studies are of low quality, ESWT tended to improve shoulder pain, function, and calcifications in patients with calcific tendonitis but not in those with noncalcific tendonitis. Results more consistently support the effectiveness of high-energy (≥ 0.28 mJ/mm^2) ESWT than medium- or low-energy (< 0.28 mJ/mm^2) ESWT, suggesting some dose dependence of effect. Very few studies have compared

the effects of ESWT with other interventions, and most, but not all,[29] studies have used fESWT and not rESWT.

TROCHANTERIC BURSITIS

Trochanteric bursitis, inflammation of the bursa overlying the greater trochanter, is associated with lateral hip pain. Because it can be difficult to ascertain the exact structure involved or the exact nature of the pathology associated with lateral hip pain, this syndrome is also sometimes called *greater trochanteric pain syndrome.* Trochanteric bursitis is commonly treated with activity modification, NSAIDs, use of a cane, steroid injections, stretching, and strengthening. Studies have also examined the impact of ESWT in the treatment of trochanteric bursitis. A systematic review published in 2018 examining the effect of ESWT on common lower limb conditions, including greater trochanteric pain syndrome, concluded that rESWT was more effective than control treatments in the short and long term, less effective than corticosteroid injection in the short term, but more effective than corticosteroid injection in the mid- and long term.[30]

TENDINOPATHIES—LATERAL EPICONDYLITIS, ACHILLES TENDINOPATHY, PATELLAR TENDINOPATHY

In addition to being effective for calcific rotator cuff tendonitis, some evidence supports that ESWT is effective for other chronic tendinopathies, including lateral epicondylitis, Achilles tendonitis, and patellar tendonitis. The benefits of ESWT for chronic tendinopathy appear to be related primarily to the stimulatory effect of this modality on tissue healing. It is likely that in patients with symptoms lasting over 6 months that do not respond to steroids, NSAIDs, ice, or other antiinflammatory interventions, chronic tendinopathy may reflect tissue weakness and failure to heal rather than inflammation. ESWT may be particularly effective in these patients because it can promote the transition to an acute inflammatory response and thus trigger resumption of tissue healing after it has stalled.

Lateral Epicondylitis

Lateral epicondylitis (tennis elbow), the most common overuse syndrome of the elbow, is a tendinopathy of the extensor muscles of the forearm and is often slow to resolve. Studies have evaluated the effect of ESWT on lateral epicondylitis. Although a 2005 meta-analysis of RCTs of ESWT in patients with lateral epicondylitis (tennis elbow[31]) concluded, based on the evidence available at that time, that ESWT provides little or no benefit in terms of pain and function, a 2020 meta-analysis of RCTs of ESWT in patients with lateral epicondylitis concluded, based on nine studies, that although ESWT did not significantly reduce average pain scores, it was associated with significantly more patients achieving at least 50% pain reduction and also with significant improvements in grip strength.[32] A meta-analysis of four studies specifically comparing the effects of ESWT with corticosteroid injection for lateral epicondylitis also concluded that ESWT was more effective than corticosteroid injection for reducing pain intensity and increasing grip strength.[33] It is likely that the differences in results may be related to the stage of tissue healing, with acute tendonitis being more responsive to antiinflammatory interventions and chronic tendinopathy being more responsive to stimulatory interventions like ESWT.

Achilles Tendinopathy

Several RCTs have investigated the effectiveness of ESWT for the treatments of Achilles tendinopathy. An early systematic review of these studies published in 2013 found four RCTs at that time.[34] These studies consistently found low-energy ESWT to be associated with superior outcomes at 3 months compared with control, although combining ESWT with eccentric loading was associated with even better results. Unfortunately, in these studies, participants and clinicians were not well blinded to intervention versus control. The 2018 systematic review examining the effect of ESWT on common lower limb conditions discussed earlier in this chapter also included an evaluation of studies on Achilles tendinopathy.[30] The authors concluded that rESWT is better than a wait-and-see approach and comparable to eccentric training for mid-portion Achilles tendinopathy and that combining rESWT with eccentric training is most effective. These authors also specifically recommended a protocol for rESWT of 3 bars pressure (EFD 0.1 mJ/mm^2) at a frequency of 8 Hz and a total of 2000 shocks/session for three sessions 1 week apart. They had slightly different findings for insertional Achilles tendinopathy, where rESWT was found to be superior to eccentric training, and the recommended protocol was 2.5 bars pressure (EFD 0.12), also at a frequency of 8 Hz and a total of 2000 shocks/session for three sessions 1 week apart. Studies of mixed, nonspecific Achilles tendinopathy also suggested ESWT was superior to placebo but were too heterogeneous to derive a specific suggested treatment protocol.

Patellar Tendinopathy

The 2018 systematic review examining the effect of ESWT on common lower limb conditions also included studies on patellar tendinopathy (Fig. 18.7).[30] The authors concluded that fESWT was no more effective than placebo but was more effective than control conservative treatment and that fESWT and rESWT combined with eccentric exercises produced comparable results.

DIABETIC FOOT ULCERS

The use of ESWT for the treatment of chronic wounds is one of the most recent applications. A 2018 systematic review and meta-analysis examining studies of ESWT for diabetic foot ulcers found five relevant RCTs, three comparing ESWT to standard wound care and the other two comparing ESWT to hyperbaric oxygen.[35] Despite the high risk of bias, in these studies, ESWT was associated with a higher odds ratio (OR 2.66) of complete wound healing and shorter time to healing (64.5 ± 8.06 days vs. 81.17 ± 4.35 days) than standard wound care ESWT, and healing improved more with ESWT than with hyperbaric oxygen. More recently published case studies also support this benefit, although up to 12 sessions were required to see benefit in some patients.[36] An electrohydraulic fESWT device was also recently FDA cleared specifically for the treatment of chronic diabetic foot ulcers based on the results of two phase III RCTs.[37,38] Combined, these trials included 336 patients with diabetic foot ulcers, 172 treated with ESWT and 164 treated with sham ESWT. At 24 weeks, those treated with usual care plus ESWT had a 37.8% wound closure rate, whereas those treated with usual care plus sham ESWT had a 26.2% closure rate ($p = 0.023$) in the same time period. In addition, wound area reduction (48.6% vs. 10.7%) and perimeter reduction (46.4% vs. 25.0%) were significantly greater in the ESWT-treated group than the sham-treated group,[39] whereas time to wound closure was shorter and amputation number was also

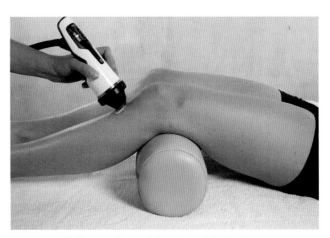

FIGURE 18.7 Treatment of patellar tendonitis with focused extracorporeal shock wave therapy (fESWT). (Courtesy Venn Healthcare, Liverpool, UK.)

lower in the ESWT-treated group. Although with regard to chronic wounds, the evidence, and thus far FDA clearance, has focused on ESWT for chronic diabetic foot ulcers, the proposed mechanisms underlying these effects suggest that ESWT may have similar benefits for other chronic wounds, but further research is needed to evaluate this.

FRACTURES

The therapeutic challenge of delayed and nonunion fractures, the efficacy found in many studies for low-intensity pulsed ultrasound (LIPUS) enhancing fracture healing, and the similarity of LIPUS and ESWT has led a number of investigators to explore the efficacy of ESWT for fracture healing. To date, most of the studies of ESWT for fracture healing have been performed in animals,[40,41] but a recent systematic review published in 2019 found 2 RCTs and 28 nonrandomized studies examining the impact of ESWT on delayed union and nonunion fractures in humans.[42] Although there is a substantial risk of bias in many of these studies because of the absence of a control group, the fact that the average union rate of delayed union fractures after ESWT was 86% and that for nonunion fractures was 73% is encouraging. It has been suggested that improved capillary blood flow in response to ESWT underlies this effect.[43] Further well-designed RCTs are needed to fully elucidate the impact of ESWT on fracture healing.

Contraindications and Precautions for Shock Waves

ESWT is generally safe. However, important contraindications and precautions should be considered to administer this therapy while minimizing risk. There is some general agreement in the literature regarding recommended contraindications and precautions for the clinical application of ESWT, although all sources vary to some degree, and most express more concern for the use of high-energy fESWT than for low-energy fESWT or rESWT.[44,45] In the event of an adverse effect, therapy should be stopped, and the patient should be evaluated by a physician.

CONTRAINDICATIONS FOR SHOCK WAVES

> ### ✴ CONTRAINDICATIONS
>
> **for Shock Waves**
> - Malignancy in the treatment area
> - Pregnancy
> - Lung tissue
> - Bleeding in the treatment area or increased bleeding risk (e.g., hemophilia, use of anticoagulants)
> - Epiphyseal plates
> - Central nervous system (brain and spinal cord)
> - Infection or skin abrasion at the treatment site
> - Pacemaker or implanted cardiac defibrillator in the treatment area
> - Cemented prostheses

Malignancy

Malignancy in the treatment area is considered by all sources as a contraindication to the use of ESWT because of the concern that the therapy may accelerate growth of the malignant tissue and/or promote metastasis. However, cancer itself is not a contraindication for the use of ESWT, and the use of this physical agent is allowed and may be helpful for known indications when the malignant tumor is not in the treatment area.[45]

> ### ▪ Ask the Patient
> - "Have you ever had cancer? Do you have cancer now?"
> - "Do you have fevers, chills, sweats, or night pain?"
> - "Do you have pain at rest?"
> - "Have you had recent unexplained weight loss?"

If the patient presently has cancer, ESWT should not be used in any area where the waves may reach the tumor. If the patient has a history of cancer or signs of cancer, such as fevers, chills, sweats, night pain, pain at rest, or recent unexplained weight loss, the therapist should consult with the referring physician to rule out the presence of malignancy before applying ESWT.

Pregnancy

Concerns have been raised regarding potential harm by ESWT to the embryo or fetus during pregnancy.[46] Therefore, ESWT should not be applied to the low back, trunk, or abdomen of a woman who is or might be pregnant.

> ### ▪ Ask the Patient
> - "Are you pregnant, might you be pregnant, or are you trying to become pregnant?"

The patient may not know if she is pregnant, particularly in the first few days or weeks after conception; however, because damage may occur at any time during fetal development, ESWT should not be applied in any area where the beam may reach the fetus of a patient who is or might be pregnant.

Lung Tissue

Lung tissue can be damaged by shock waves. Therefore, ESWT should not be applied where the waves may reach the lungs.

Bleeding and Bleeding Disorders (Coagulopathy or Use of Anticoagulant Medication)

ESWT can damage blood vessels and cause bleeding and bruising. Therefore, ESWT should not be used in patients at increased risk for bleeding, including those with bleeding disorders (e.g., hemophilia) and those taking anticoagulant medications (e.g., warfarin, apixaban, rivaroxaban).

> ### ▪ Ask the Patient
> - "Do you have any condition that puts you at increased risk for bleeding?"
> - "Are you taking blood thinner medications such as warfarin or another anticoagulant?"
>
> ### ▪ Assess
> - Check the treatment area for any signs of bleeding or bruising.

Epiphyseal Plates Until Bone Growth Is Complete

As with other physical agents, the effects of ESWT on epiphyseal plate growth and closure is not completely clear. Early studies, particularly with high-energy fESWT, suggested that this intervention could damage bones. There is also concern that because ESWT can stimulate tissue growth, it may promote bone growth or closure at unclosed epiphyseal plates.[47] However, rESWT has been reported to be safe in case series of children with Osgood–Schlatter disease (patellar ligament apophysitis) and those with Sever disease (calcaneal apophysitis[48]). Today, most authors recommend against the use of ESWT in the area of epiphyseal plates until bone growth is complete. Because the age of epiphyseal closure varies, radiographic evaluation rather than age should be used to determine whether epiphyseal closure is complete.

Central Nervous System (Brain and Spinal Cord)

Most authors currently recommend not applying ESWT to the brain or spinal cord, although some animal studies have specifically examined the impact of ESWT, particularly rESWT, on improving recovery after stroke and on Alzheimer disease.[49,50]

Infection or Skin Abrasion at the Treatment Site

Although ESWT may promote tissue healing and immune reaction to infection, ESWT is generally not recommended at sites of superficial infection or skin abrasion because of the concern that application of the device to the skin may transmit infection or mechanically disrupt healing.

Pacemaker or Implanted Cardiac Defibrillator in the Treatment Area

ESWT should generally not be applied if the focus point is less than 6 inches from an implanted cardiac pacemaker or defibrillator because ESWT can alter the functioning of some of these devices, particularly when the device is programmed to sensitive settings.[51] If ESWT is considered the ideal treatment for a patient with a pacemaker, some pacemakers may allow their settings to be altered to make this safe.[52]

> ■ **Ask the Patient**
> • "Do you have a pacemaker?"

Cemented Prostheses

Some recommend against using ESWT in the area of cemented prostheses because shock waves can be used intraoperatively to loosen cemented prostheses if they need replacement.

> ■ **Ask the Patient**
> • "Do you have a joint replacement in this area?"
> • "Was cement used to hold it in place?"

PRECAUTIONS FOR SHOCK WAVES

> ✱ **PRECAUTIONS**
>
> **for Shock Waves**
> • Unexplained calf pain (deep vein thrombosis [DVT])
> • Bony prominences
> • Stop for significant or unexpected pain

Unexplained Calf Pain

ESWT should be used with caution over the calf when there is unexplained calf pain because of the concern that this may be caused by a DVT and that the ESWT may dislodge the thrombosis.

Bony Prominences

It is generally recommended that ESWT not be applied directly over bony prominences because local reflection may result in discomfort.

Stop for Significant or Unexpected Pain

Stop ESWT if the patient reports significant or unexpected pain at the treatment site.

Adverse Effects of Shock Waves

• Bruising, hematomas, petechiae
• Reddening/skin irritation
• Swelling
• Pain during treatment and/or for the following 1 to 2 days

The most common adverse effects of ESWT reported in clinical studies are petechiae, small bruises and hematomas, local erythema, and acute pain, with more adverse events being reported with high-energy compared with low-energy ESWT.

> ◎ **Clinical Pearl**
>
> The most common adverse effects of ESWT are petechiae or bruises at the treatment site after the treatment and discomfort during the treatment. Patients should be advised that bruising or redness after the treatment is normal and to be expected. Discomfort during the treatment can be minimized by starting at a lower-than-goal pressure and gradually increasing this to goal during the session.

BRUISING, HEMATOMAS, PETECHIAE

Bruising, hematomas, and petechiae are all signs of local bleeding. ESWT can cause small amounts of local bleeding at the site of application because the cavitation produced by ESWT can cause microtrauma to small blood vessels. These signs of local bleeding generally resolve in 1 to 2 days.

REDDENING/SKIN IRRITATION, LOCAL SWELLING, AND PAIN DURING OR AFTER TREATMENT

Reddening or irritation of the skin, swelling at the site of ESWT application, and pain during and/or for the following 1 or 2 days are also signs of microtrauma and an inflammatory response.

Application Techniques

This section provides guidelines for the sequence of procedures required for safe and effective application of ESWT.

APPLICATION TECHNIQUE 18.1   EXTRACORPOREAL SHOCK WAVE THERAPY

Equipment Required

- ESWT device (Fig. 18.8)
- Transmission gel (This may be the same as ultrasound gel.)
- Antimicrobial agent for cleaning the device
- Cloth or paper towel for wiping the gel off the patient

Procedure

1. Evaluate the patient's clinical findings and set the goals of treatment.
2. Determine whether ESWT is the most appropriate intervention.
3. Confirm that ESWT is not contraindicated for the patient or the condition. Check with the patient, and check the patient's chart for contraindications or precautions regarding the application of ESWT.
4. Remove all clothing and jewelry from the treatment area.
5. Apply an ESWT transmission gel, which is the same as ultrasound gel, to the treatment area. Apply enough gel to eliminate any air between the applicator head and the treatment area. Select a gel that does not stain, is not allergenic, is not rapidly absorbed by the skin, and is inexpensive. Gels or lotions meeting these criteria have been specifically formulated for use with ESWT.
6. Select the optimal treatment parameters, including EFD for fESWT, peak pressure and total shock number for rESWT, and shock frequency for either form of ESWT, as well as the number

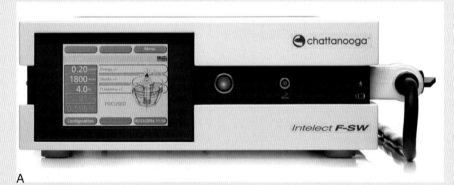

A

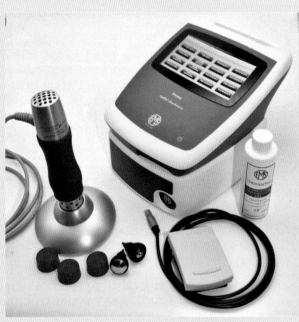

B

FIGURE 18.8 (A) Focused extracorporeal shock wave therapy (fESWT) machine. (B) Radial extracorporeal shock wave therapy (rESWT) machine. (A, Courtesy Chattanooga, Lewisville, TX. B, Courtesy EMS Physio, Wantage, UK.)

APPLICATION TECHNIQUE 18.1—cont'd

and frequency of treatments. See the next section for a general discussion of parameter selection. Some detailed information on parameters for specific conditions is also included in the previous section.

7. Place the applicator head on the skin overlying the treatment area (Figs. 18.9 and 18.10).

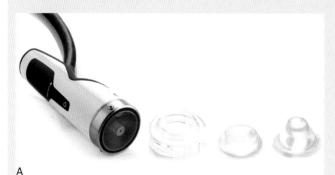

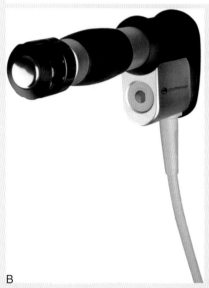

8. Start the shock wave delivery. With focused ESWT, keep the applicator stationary and directed at the target. The target can be localized using ultrasound imaging or initially by slightly moving or tilting the applicator to find the painful area. With rESWT, the applicator should always be moved over the treatment area during ESWT application. Failure to move the applicator may increase the risk of local bruising.

9. Check with the patient that they are not feeling pain from the treatment. They should expect about a 5/10 level of discomfort and no more than 7/10. For rESWT, the treatment can be made more comfortable by starting with a lower bar pressure and, during the treatment, gradually increasing as tolerated. In general, fESWT is more comfortable than rESWT, especially in areas with more reflection, such as near superficial bone.

10. Take the applicator off the skin and return it to its holder on the machine. Wipe the transmission gel off the patient with a cloth or paper towel.

11. When treatment is complete, assess the treated area.

12. Document the treatment and any response to the treatment.

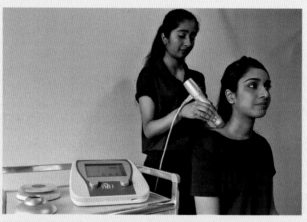

FIGURE 18.9 (A) Focused extracorporeal shock wave therapy (fESWT) applicator and standoffs to modify the depth of the focal point in the tissue. (B) Radiant extracorporeal shock wave therapy (rESWT) applicator. (Courtesy Chattanooga, Lewisville, TX.)

FIGURE 18.10 Extracorporeal shock wave therapy (ESWT) applicator head in contact with the skin overlying the treatment area. (Courtesy V2U Healthcare, Midview City, Singapore.)

○ Clinical Pearl

Always use transmission gel for ESWT treatment. For fESWT, keep the applicator stationary and directed at the target tissue. For rESWT, move the applicator continuously over the treatment area.

ESWT TREATMENT PARAMETERS

In general, a range of ESWT parameters can be used successfully for various pathologies, without any specific ones being recommended uniquely based on the pathology.

Focused or Radial Device

As discussed previously in this chapter, there is no clear evidence unequivocally supporting that either fESWT or rESWT is more effective overall or for any specific pathology. However, in general, if both options are available, because fESWT penetrates more deeply than rESWT, it is recommended that fESWT be used to treat deeper pathologies, such as trochanteric bursitis in a heavier patient, whereas rESWT be used to treat more superficial pathologies, such as lateral epicondylitis.

Energy Flux Density

The EFD for ESWT is generally in the range of 0.08 to 0.6 mJ/mm^2 and is often classified as low, medium, or high, with slightly different ranges for these in different publications. Low energy is generally below 0.1 mJ/mm^2, medium energy is generally around 0.1 to 0.25 mJ/mm^2, and high energy is around 0.25 to over 0.6 mJ/mm^2.[3,4]

Peak Pressure

The peak pressure is usually set between 2 and 4 bar.

Frequency

The frequency is usually set between 8 and 15 Hz.

Total Pulse Number

The total pulse number is usually set between 2000 and 2500 shocks/session, with some sources recommending limiting to a maximum of 6000 shocks/session.

Number of Sessions

A course of rESWT treatment is usually two to five sessions, and occasionally up to seven sessions, usually administered once or twice each week, after waiting for any reaction from the prior session to subside before the next session. However, if there has been no improvement with three sessions, consider if you are using the ideal parameters or if this is the ideal intervention. A course of fESWT, particularly with a higher EFD, may be shorter, often requiring only one or two sessions.

Documentation

The following should be documented:
- Area of the body treated
- Type of device (focused or radial)
- Treatment parameters
  - EFD for fESWT
  - Peak pressure for rESWT
  - Total shock number for rESWT
  - Frequency for fESWT or rESWT
- Response to treatment

EXAMPLE

S: Pt reports right lateral elbow pain that increases with resisted wrist extension and limits her work as a carpenter. This has been ongoing for 4 to 6 months.

O: Pretreatment: 4/10 tenderness with palpation of right extensor carp radialis brevis tendon and 4/10 pain with resisted wrist extension.

Intervention: rESWT, 3 bar, 10Hz, 2000 total shock number.

Posttreatment: Mild erythema at treatment site. 2/10 tenderness with palpation of right extensor carp radialis brevis tendon and 2/10 pain with resisted wrist extension.

A: Pt tolerated treatment well, with expected mild erythema and good reduction in pain.

P: Repeat treatment weekly for 3 to 5 sessions.

CLINICAL CASE STUDIES

The following case studies summarize some of the concepts of the clinical use of ESWT discussed in this chapter. Based on the scenario presented, an evaluation of the clinical findings and goals of treatment are proposed. These are followed by a discussion of the factors to be considered in treatment selection.

CASE STUDY 18.1

Plantar Fasciitis
Examination
History

FR is a 25-year-old woman with left plantar fasciitis. She has had left heel pain on and off for the last 12 to 18 months. This pain started after she went for a 6-mile walk with a new pair of shoes without any arch support. She got rid of those shoes, got orthotics for her other shoes, has been stretching her Achilles tendon, and has had one corticosteroid injection. All of these interventions have been helpful, but the pain has not fully resolved. She always has pain when she first steps out of bed in the morning, and this is worse, and lasts longer, if she has walked more than a couple of miles the day before. She can walk fairly comfortably in sneakers with orthotics for her usual activities of daily living (ADLs) but is not able to walk in pumps with heels as she used to do at work and is not able to go on walks that are longer than 2 miles.

Systems Review

FR is alert and cooperative. She is sitting comfortably and wearing sneakers. She reports that she is not able to walk in heels because of pain in the sole and heel of her left foot.

Tests and Measures

In standing barefoot, FR is noted to have bilateral rear foot pronation, greater on the left than the right. She has tenderness on palpation at the origin of the plantar fascia on the left and reduced dorsiflexion (DF) range of motion (ROM), as follows:
- Left: DF active ROM (AROM) −10°, passive ROM (PROM) 0°
- Right: DF AROM 0°, PROM 5°

  What types of ESWT therapy would you consider for this patient? What history do you need to obtain from this patient? How do you determine the appropriate dose?

Evaluation and Goals

ICF Level	Current Status	Goals
Body structure and function	Reduced active and passive DF ROM, left more restricted than right. Tenderness left plantar fascia insertion. Heel pain, worst with first steps after awakening.	Normalize DF ROM Resolve plantar fascia tenderness and heel pain

CLINICAL CASE STUDIES—*cont'd*

ICF Level	Current Status	Goals
Activity	Limited ambulation	Return to normal ambulation
Participation	Unable to walk more than 2 miles. Unable to walk in heeled pumps.	Able to walk at least 6 miles and able to wear heeled pumps at work

ICF, International Classification for Functioning, Disability and Health.

◆ FIND THE EVIDENCE

PICO Terms	Natural Language Example	Sample PubMed Search
P (Population)	Patient with plantar fasciitis	("Plantar fasciitis" [MeSH] OR "Plantar fasciitis" [text word])
I (Intervention)	ESWT	AND "Extracorporeal shock wave therapy" [MeSH]
C (Comparison)	No ESWT	
O (Outcome)	Reduced of pain, improved function	AND English [lang] AND "Humans" [MeSH]

Key Studies or Reviews

1. Chang KV, Chen SY, Chen WS, et al: Comparative effectiveness of focused shock wave therapy of different intensity levels and radial shock wave therapy for treating plantar fasciitis: a systematic review and network meta-analysis. *Arch Phys Med Rehabil* 93(7):1259–1268, 2012.

   This is one of the few analyses that not only examined the effectiveness of ESWT in general on plantar fasciitis but that also specifically compared the effectiveness of fESWT and rESWT. The authors concluded that both fESWT and rESWT were more effective in reducing pain and improving function than placebo and that medium-intensity fESWT or rESWT was most likely to be effective.

2. Canadian Agency for Drugs and Technologies in Health: Shockwave therapy for pain associated with lower extremity orthopedic disorders: a review of the clinical and cost-effectiveness [Internet], Ottawa, 2016, Canadian Agency for Drugs and Technologies in Health.

   This review of systematic reviews of ESWT for pain associated with lower extremity orthopedic disorders included five systematic reviews related to foot- and ankle-related disorders, four of which were focused on plantar fasciitis and heel pain. The authors concluded that overall, ESWT is an effective treatment option for plantar fasciitis compared with placebo, with rare and mild adverse events.

Prognosis

ESWT is an indicated treatment for plantar fasciitis and has been shown to reduce pain and improve function in patients with plantar fasciitis. ESWT is recommended for this patient because although her symptoms have improved with the use of an orthotic, stretching, and a corticosteroid injection, she still has pain and has not been able to return to her prior level of function.

Intervention

fESWT or rESWT may be used for this patient. If fESWT is used, an EFD in the high end of the medium range, around 0.25 mJ/mm^2, at a frequency of around 10 Hz is recommended, with a total of two sessions 1 week apart. If rESWT is used, a pressure of 2.0 to 3.0 bar, a total shock number of 2000 at 10 Hz, with a total of three to six treatments about 1 week apart is recommended.

Documentation

S: Pt reports left heel pain that is worst when she first steps out of bed in the morning, particularly if she has walked a lot the day before.

O: Pretreatment: 4/10 tenderness with palpation of left plantar fascia insertion and left DF AROM −10°, PROM 0°.

Intervention: rESWT, 3 bar, 10Hz, 2000 total shock number.

Posttreatment: Mild erythema at treatment site. 2/10 tenderness with palpation of left plantar fascia insertion.

A: Pt tolerated treatment well, with expected mild erythema and good reduction in pain.

P: Repeat treatment weekly for 3 to 5 sessions.

CASE STUDY 18.2

Calcific Rotator Cuff Tendonitis
Examination
History

JW is a 59-year-old man who has been struggling with recurrent right rotator cuff tendonitis on and off for the last 4 years. He has had prior courses of physical therapy that have included stretching, strengthening, and stabilization exercises; body mechanics training; and LIPUS. He is adherent to his exercise program, but each time he has physical therapy, his symptoms improve about 50% and then worsen again within a few months. He recently had an x-ray of his shoulder that revealed he has calcific rotator cuff tendonitis. He is wondering if physical therapy can help him or if he should have surgery. His shoulder pain limits his ability to lie on his right side to sleep and also bothers him with lifting more than 20 lb, in midrange as he reaches out to the side or overhead, and in keeping his arm overhead for more than a few moments. For example, he has pain if he tries to screw a light bulb into a ceiling fixture. He also has pain when he tries to serve when playing tennis.

Systems Review

JW is alert and cooperative. He is sitting comfortably with his arms at his sides. He reports that he has followed through with all of the interventions recommended by his physical therapists, including exercises and gradual return to activity, but his pain keeps recurring. He finds that this pain disturbs his sleep when he tries to turn over in bed and also particularly limits overhead activities such as lifting or tennis serves.

Continued

Tests and Measures

JW has full AROM and PROM of both shoulders, but he has a painful arc at 70° to 110° of active abduction on the right. He has tenderness on palpation of the right supraspinatus tendon and pain with right shoulder resisted external rotation.

What types of ESWT therapy would you consider for this patient? What history do you need to obtain from this patient? How do you determine the appropriate dose?

Evaluation and Goals

ICF Level	Current Status	Goals
Body structure and function	Painful arc at 70°–110° of right shoulder active abduction Tenderness of right supraspinatus tendon Pain with resisted shoulder external rotation Rotator cuff calcification on x-ray of right shoulder	Full pain-free AROM of right shoulder Pain-free palpation of right supraspinatus tendon Pain-free resisted motion of right shoulder Resolution of rotator cuff calcification on x-ray
Activity	Pain limiting overhead reaching	Able to reach overhead without pain
Participation	Sleep disturbed by right shoulder pain Tennis serve and other overhead reaching limited by pain	Sleep through the night Able to tennis serve and perform other overhead activities without pain

ICF, International Classification for Functioning, Disability and Health.

◆ FIND THE EVIDENCE

PICO Terms	Natural Language Example	Sample PubMed Search
P (Population)	Patient with calcific rotator cuff tendonitis	("Rotator cuff tendinitis" [MeSH] OR "Rotator cuff tendinosis" [MeSH])
I (Intervention)	ESWT	AND "Extracorporeal shock wave therapy" [MeSH]
C (Comparison)	No ESWT	
O (Outcome)	Reduced pain, improved function	AND English [lang] AND "Humans" [MeSH]

Key Studies or Reviews

1. Canadian Agency for Drugs and Technologies in Health: Shockwave therapy for pain associated with upper extremity orthopedic disorders: a review of the clinical and cost-effectiveness [Internet], Ottawa, 2016, Canadian Agency for Drugs and Technologies in Health.

This review of systematic reviews of ESWT for pain associated with upper extremity orthopedic disorders included four systematic reviews on ESWT for chronic shoulder tendonitis. The authors concluded that ESWT is an effective treatment option compared with placebo, and compared with transcutaneous electrical nerve stimulation (TENS), for reducing pain in calcific shoulder tendonitis but not in noncalcific shoulder tendonitis, with rare and mild adverse events. The results more consistently support the effectiveness of high-energy ($\geq$0.28 mJ/mm^2) ESWT than medium- or low-energy (<0.28 mJ/mm^2) ESWT, suggesting some dose dependence of effect.

2. Duymaz T, Sindel D: Comparison of radial extracorporeal shock wave therapy and traditional physiotherapy in rotator cuff calcific tendinitis treatment. *Arch Rheumatol* 34(3):281–287, 2019.

This recent paper describes an RCT comparing standard physical therapy with standard physical therapy plus rESWT with a total pulse number of 1500 shocks and frequency of 150 shocks/minute (2.5 Hz). Unfortunately, although the device used in this study does allow control of the pressure from 0.3 to 5 bar, the authors describe the output in terms of EFD, with the first treatment starting at 0.03 mJ/mm^2 for the first 5 minutes and then progressively increasing to 0.28 mJ/mm^2 and subsequent treatments being at 0.28 mJ/mm^2 for the entire treatment. rESWT was applied once a week for a total of 4 weeks. Although patients in both groups had better improved pain, ROM, and QuickDASH (a shortened version of the Disabilities of the Arm, Shoulder and Hand questionnaire) scores after treatment, the patients in the rESWT group had statistically significant improvements in these measures, whereas those in the control group did not.

Prognosis

ESWT is an indicated treatment for rotator cuff tendonitis and has been shown to reduce pain and increase ROM and function in patients with calcific, but not noncalcific, rotator cuff tendonitis. ESWT is recommended for this patient because he has calcific rotator cuff tendonitis with functional impacts. Furthermore, he has failed other therapeutic interventions.

Intervention

fESWT or rESWT may be used for this patient. If fESWT is used, a high EFD is recommended, at around 0.30 mJ/mm^2, at a frequency of around 10 Hz, with a total of two sessions 1 week apart. If rESWT is used, a pressure of 2.0 to 3.0 bar, a total shock number of 1500 at 2.5 Hz, and a total of three to six treatments about 1 week apart is recommended.

Documentation

S: Pt reports right shoulder pain when he lies on his right side, in midrange when raising his arm to the side, and if he keeps his arm overhead.

O: Pretreatment: 4/10 tenderness with palpation of right supraspinatus tendon and 4/10 pain with resisted shoulder

CLINICAL CASE STUDIES—cont'd

ER. Painful arc at 70° to 110° of shoulder abduction.

Intervention: rESWT, 2.5 bar, 2.5 Hz, 1500 total shock number.

Posttreatment: Mild erythema at treatment site. 2/10 tenderness with palpation of right supraspinatus tendon and 2/10 pain with resisted ER. Painful arc at 90° to 100° of shoulder abduction.

A: Pt tolerated treatment well, with expected mild erythema and good reduction in pain.

P: Repeat treatment weekly for 3 to 5 sessions.

CASE STUDY 18.3

Achilles Tendinopathy
Examination
History

AT is a 19-year-old college student with a basketball scholarship who reports struggling with chronic left Achilles tendonitis for the last year. She has pain at the middle of the left Achilles tendon that worsens when she does a lot of jumping drills and improves with rest and stretching; the pain is limiting her basketball playing and threatening her scholarship.

Systems Review

AT is an athletic-appearing, slender, tall young woman. She is eager to engage in therapy and to try something new for her Achilles tendon pain. She reports that prior physical therapy has been modestly helpful but her pain always comes back when she goes back to her usual activities, including lots of jumping during basketball. She reports that she usually pushes off on the left when she jumps. She reports consistently stretching before games and practice and icing afterward.

Tests and Measures

Pain ranges from 1 to 2 out of 10 at rest to 6 to 7 out of 10 with and after activity. Ankle dorsiflexion AROM is +5 degrees bilaterally, and PROM is +10 degrees bilaterally. There is tenderness and swelling consistent with edema and possible scarring at the middle of the Achilles tendon on the left and pain with unilateral active heel raises on the left.

What types of ESWT therapy would you consider for this patient? What history do you need to obtain from this patient? How do you determine the appropriate dose?

Evaluation and Goals

ICF Level	Current Status	Goals
Body structure and function	Reduced active and passive DF ROM bilaterally Tenderness left mid Achilles tendon with swelling Left Achilles tendon pain with jumping or body-weight-resisted activity	Normalize DF ROM Resolve Achilles tendon tenderness and swelling Able to jump and heel raise on left without pain
Activity	Limited jumping	Return to normal jumping

ICF Level	Current Status	Goals
Participation	Unable to fully participate in basketball and thus at risk for losing her college scholarship	Able to fully participate in competitive basketball

ICF, International Classification for Functioning, Disability and Health.

◆ FIND THE EVIDENCE

PICO Terms	Natural Language Example	Sample PubMed Search
P (Population)	Patient with Achilles tendinopathy	("Achilles tendon" [MeSH] OR "Achilles tendonitis" [text word] OR "Achilles tendinitis" [text word] OR "Achilles tendinopathy" [text word])
I (Intervention)	ESWT	AND "Extracorporeal shock wave therapy" [MeSH]
C (Comparison)	No ESWT	
O (Outcome)	Reduced pain, improved function	AND English [lang] AND "Humans" [MeSH]

Key Studies or Reviews

1. Korakakis V, Whiteley R, Tzavara A, et al: The effectiveness of extracorporeal shockwave therapy in common lower limb conditions: a systematic review including quantification of patient-rated pain reduction. *Br J Sports Med* 52(6):387–407, 2018.

   This 2018 systematic review that examined the effect of ESWT on a variety of common lower limb conditions concluded that rESWT is better than a wait-and-see approach and comparable to eccentric training for mid-portion Achilles tendinopathy and that combined rESWT with eccentric training is most effective. The researchers also specifically recommended a protocol of rESWT at 3 bars (EFD 0.1 mJ/mm^2) at a frequency of 8 Hz and a total of 2000 shocks/session for three sessions 1 week apart.

Prognosis

ESWT is an indicated treatment for Achilles tendinopathy and has been shown to reduce pain and increase ROM and function in patients with Achilles tendinopathy. ESWT is recommended for this patient because she has Achilles tendinopathy with functional impacts. Furthermore, she has failed other therapeutic interventions.

Intervention

Radial ESWT will be applied to the tender, swollen area of AT's left Achilles tendon. The treatment parameters will be 3 bars pressure at a frequency of 8 Hz and a total of 2000 shocks/session for three sessions 1 week apart.

Continued

CLINICAL CASE STUDIES—cont'd

Documentation

S: Pt reports left heel pain that is worst when she jumps or after jumping, such as after a basketball game.

O: Pretreatment: 2/10 tenderness with palpation of mid-portion of left Achilles tendon.

Intervention: rESWT, 3 bar, 8 Hz, 2000 total shock number.

Posttreatment: Mild erythema at treatment site. No tenderness with palpation of mid-portion of left Achilles tendon.

A: Pt tolerated treatment well, with expected mild erythema and good reduction in pain.

P: Repeat treatment weekly for 3 sessions. Continue combined with eccentric strengthening program.

Chapter Review

1. ESWT is the use of shock waves to promote tissue healing and control inflammation and pain.

2. Effects of ESWT include cavitation when moving through soft tissues, increasing cell membrane permeability, activating a series of cellular events involved in cellular repair and tissue healing, and breaking up calcifications.

3. ESWT has clinical benefits in part because it stimulates the production of growth factor and collagen.

4. ESWT is used primarily for conditions associated with chronic inflammation, including plantar fasciitis, calcific rotator cuff tendonitis, other tendinopathies, and trochanteric bursitis.

5. rESWT is FDA cleared for treating muscle pain and aches, temporarily increasing blood flow, and activating connective tissue. fESWT is FDA cleared to treat kidney stones, plantar fasciitis, lateral epicondylitis, and diabetic foot ulcers.

6. Contraindications to the use of ESWT include malignancy in the treatment area, pregnancy, lung tissue, bleeding in the treatment area, increased bleeding risk, use of anticoagulants, epiphyseal plates, central nervous system impairment, infection or skin abrasion at the treatment site, pacemaker or implanted cardiac defibrillator in the treatment area, or cemented prostheses. Precautions include unexplained calf pain, bony prominences, or significant or unexpected pain.

7. Dose summary: For ESWT, low energy is below 0.1 mJ/mm², medium energy is generally around 0.1 to 0.25 mJ/mm², and high energy is around 0.25 to over 0.6 mJ/mm²; peak pressure is usually set between 2 and 4 bar; frequency is usually set between 8 and 15 Hz; the total pulse number is usually set between 2000 and 2500 shocks/session; and a course of rESWT treatment is usually two to five sessions, administered once or twice each week, whereas a course of fESWT often requires only one or two sessions.

Glossary

Bar: A measure of pressure; 1 bar is equal to 100,000 pascals and is approximately equal to the atmospheric pressure on Earth at an altitude of 111 m at 15°C.

Cavitation: The formation of small, vapor-filled low-pressure cavities or bubbles

Extracorporeal shock wave therapy (ESWT): Delivery of shock waves to musculoskeletal tissues with the goal of reducing pain and promoting tissue healing.

Focal area: The area in which the pressure is ≥50% of the peak pressure.

Focused ESWT (fESWT): Focused ESWT waves are dispersed at the applicator and focus within the tissue to apply the greatest energy density to a target about 2 to 4 inches deep and about ¼ to ½ inch in diameter.

Megapascal: (MPa) A measure of pressure; 1 MPa = 10 Bar.

Radial ESWT (rESWT): Radial ESWT waves, also known as *radial pressure waves* (RPWs), are most concentrated at the applicator and disperse eccentrically from the applicator tip, resulting in a lower concentration in the tissue at depth.

Shock frequency: Number of shock waves/second, generally measured in Hz.

Shock wave: Pulsed high-amplitude, short-duration sound wave.

Total energy flux (energy flux density [EFD]): The energy per unit area, generally measured in mJ/mm².

Total shock number: Total number of shock waves in a treatment session.

References

1. Schmitz C, Császár NB, Milz S, et al: Efficacy and safety of extracorporeal shock wave therapy for orthopedic conditions: a systematic review on studies listed in the PEDro database. *Br Med Bull* 116:115–138, 2015.

2. U.S. Food and Drug Administration: Learn if a medical device has been cleared by FDA for marketing. https://www.fda.gov/medical-devices/consumers-medical-devices/learn-if-medical-device-has-been-cleared-fda-marketing. (Accessed August 10, 2020).

3. Rompe JD, Kirkpatrick CJ, Küllmer K, et al: Dose-related effects of shock waves on rabbit tendo Achillis. A sonographic and histological study. *J Bone Joint Surg Br* 80(3):546–552, 1998.

4. Chang KV, Chen SY, Chen WS, et al: Comparative effectiveness of focused shock wave therapy of different intensity levels and radial shock wave therapy for treating plantar fasciitis: a systematic review and network meta-analysis. *Arch Phys Med Rehabil* 93(7):1259–1268, 2012.

5. Rogoveanu OC, Muşetescu AE, Gofiţă CE, et al: The effectiveness of shockwave therapy in patients with lateral epicondylitis. *Curr Health Sci J* 44(4):368–373, 2018.

6. Canadian Agency for Drugs and Technologies in Health: Shockwave therapy for pain associated with upper extremity orthopedic disorders: a review of the clinical and cost-effectiveness [Internet], Ottawa (ON), 2016, Canadian Agency for Drugs and Technologies in Health. PMID: 27831675.

7. Zhang J, Kang N, Yu X: Radial extracorporeal shock wave therapy enhances the proliferation and differentiation of neural stem cells by notch, PI3K/AKT, and Wnt/β-catenin signaling. *Sci Rep* 7:15321, 2017.

8. Aschermann I, Noor S, Venturelli S, et al: Extracorporeal shock waves activate migration, proliferation and inflammatory pathways in fibroblasts and keratinocytes, and improve wound healing in an open-label, single-arm study in patients with therapy-refractory chronic leg ulcers. *Int J Experimental Cellular Physiol Biochem Pharmacol* 41:890–906, 2017.

9. Canadian Agency for Drugs and Technologies in Health: Shockwave Therapy for pain associated with lower extremity orthopedic disorders: a review of the clinical and cost-effectiveness [Internet]. Ottawa (ON): Canadian Agency for Drugs and Technologies in Health; 2016 Sep 16.

10. U.S. Food and Drug Administration: Premarket approval (PMA). https://www.accessdata.fda.gov/scripts/cdrh/cfdocs/cfPMA/pma.cfm?id=P040026. (Accessed October 4, 2020).

11. U.S. Food and Drug Administration: Summary of safety and effectiveness. https://www.accessdata.fda.gov/cdrh_docs/pdf/P010039b.pdf. (Accessed October 31, 2020).

12. U.S. Food and Drug Administration: Summary of safety and effectiveness data. https://www.accessdata.fda.gov/cdrh_docs/pdf4/P040026B.pdf. (Accessed October 5, 2020).

13. Aqil A, Siddiqui MR, Solan M, et al: Extracorporeal shock wave therapy is effective in treating chronic plantar fasciitis: a meta-analysis of RCTs. Clin Orthop Relat Res 471(11):3645—3652, 2013.

14. Sun J, Gao F, Wang Y, et al: Extracorporeal shock wave therapy is effective in treating chronic plantar fasciitis: A meta-analysis of RCTs. Medicine (Baltimore) 96(15):e6621, 2017.

15. Dizon JN, Gonzalez-Suarez C, Zamora MT, et al: Effectiveness of extracorporeal shock wave therapy in chronic plantar fasciitis: a meta-analysis. Am J Phys Med Rehabil 92(7):606–620, 2013.

16. Lou J, Wang S, Liu S, et al: Effectiveness of extracorporeal shock wave therapy without local anesthesia in patients with recalcitrant plantar fasciitis: a meta-analysis of randomized controlled trials. Am J Phys Med Rehabil 96(8):529–534, 2017.

17. Wang YC, Chen SJ, Huang PJ, et al: Efficacy of different energy levels used in focused and radial extracorporeal shockwave therapy in the treatment of plantar fasciitis: a meta-analysis of randomized placebo-controlled trials. J Clin Med 8(9):1497, 2019.

18. Li S, Wang K, Sun H, et al: Clinical effects of extracorporeal shock-wave therapy and ultrasound-guided local corticosteroid injections for plantar fasciitis in adults: a meta-analysis of randomized controlled trials. Medicine (Baltimore) 97(50):e13687, 2018.

19. Xiong Y, Wu Q, Mi B, et al: Comparison of efficacy of shock-wave therapy versus corticosteroids in plantar fasciitis: a meta-analysis of randomized controlled trials. Arch Orthop Trauma Surg 139(4):529–536, 2019.

20. Hocaoglu S, Vurdem UE, Cebicci MA, et al: Comparative effectiveness of radial extracorporeal shockwave therapy and ultrasound-guided local corticosteroid injection treatment for plantar fasciitis. J Am Podiatr Med Assoc 107(3):192–199, 2017.

21. Zhao J, Luo WM, Li T: Extracorporeal shock wave therapy versus corticosteroid injection for chronic plantar fasciitis: A protocol of randomized controlled trial. Medicine (Baltimore) 99(19):e19920, 2020.

22. Bannuru RR, Flavin NE, Vaysbrot E, et al: High-energy extracorporeal shock-wave therapy for treating chronic calcific tendinitis of the shoulder: a systematic review. Ann Intern Med 160(8):542–549, 2014.

23. Louwerens JK, Veltman ES, van Noort A, et al: The effectiveness of high-energy extracorporeal shockwave therapy versus ultrasound-guided needling versus arthroscopic surgery in the management of chronic calcific rotator cuff tendinopathy: a systematic review. Arthroscopy 32(1):165–175, 2016.

24. Speed C: A systematic review of shockwave therapies in soft tissue conditions: focusing on the evidence. Br J Sports Med 48(21):1538–1542, 2014.

25. Huisstede BM, Gebremariam L, van der Sande R, et al: Evidence for effectiveness of extracorporal shock-wave therapy (ESWT) to treat calcific and non-calcific rotator cuff tendinosis—a systematic review. Man Ther 16(5):419–433, 2011. [Internet].

26. Harmiman EC, Carette S, Kennedy C, et al: Extracorporeal shock wave therapy for calcific and noncalcific tendinitis of the rotator cuff: a systematic review. J Hand Ther 17:132–151, 2004.

27. Duymaz T, Sindel D: Comparison of radial extracorporeal shock wave therapy and traditional physiotherapy in rotator cuff calcific tendinitis treatment. Arch Rheumatol 34(3):281–287, 2019.

28. Surace SJ, Deitch J, Johnston RV, et al: Shock wave therapy for rotator cuff disease with or without calcification. Cochrane Database Syst Rev 3(3):CD008962, 2020.

29. Cacchio A, Paoloni M, Barile A, et al: Effectiveness of radial shock-wave therapy for calcific tendinitis of the shoulder: single-blind, randomized clinical study. Phys Ther 86:672–682, 2006.

30. Korakakis V, Whiteley R, Tzavara A, et al: The effectiveness of extracorporeal shockwave therapy in common lower limb conditions: a systematic review including quantification of patient-rated pain reduction. Br J Sports Med 52:387–407, 2018.

31. Buchbinder R, Green SE, Youd JM, et al: Shock wave therapy for lateral elbow pain. Cochrane Database Syst Rev (4):CD003524, 2005.

32. Zheng C, Zeng D, Chen J, et al: Effectiveness of extracorporeal shock wave therapy in patients with tennis elbow: a meta-analysis of randomized controlled trials. Medicine (Baltimore) 99(30):e21189, 2020.

33. Xiong Y, Xue H, Zhou W, et al: Shock-wave therapy versus corticosteroid injection on lateral epicondylitis: a meta-analysis of randomized controlled trials. Phys Sportsmed 47(3):284–289, 2019.

34. Al-Abbad H, Simon JV: The effectiveness of extracorporeal shock wave therapy on chronic achilles tendinopathy: a systematic review. Foot Ankle Int 34(1):33–41, 2013.

35. Hitchman LH, Totty JP, Raza A, et al: Extracorporeal shockwave therapy for diabetic foot ulcers: a systematic review and meta-analysis. Ann Vasc Surg 56:330–339, 2019.

36. Chou WY, Wang CJ, Cheng JH: Extended extracorporeal shockwave therapy for chronic diabetic foot ulcers: a case series. Wounds 31(5):132–136, 2019.

37. U.S. Food and Drug Administration. FDA permits marketing of device to treat diabetic foot ulcers. https://www.fda.gov/news-events/press-announcements/fda-permits-marketing-device-treat-diabetic-foot-ulcers. (Accessed October 31, 2020).

38. Snyder R, Galiano R, Mayer P, et al: Diabetic foot ulcer treatment with focused shockwave therapy: two multicentre, prospective, controlled, double-blinded, randomised phase III clinical trials. J Wound Care 27(12):822–836, 2018.

39. Galiano R, Snyder R, Mayer P, et al: Focused shockwave therapy in diabetic foot ulcers: secondary endpoints of two multicentre randomised controlled trials. J Wound Care 28(6):383–395, 2019.

40. Mackert GA, Schulte M, Hirche C, et al: Low-energy extracorporeal shockwave therapy (ESWT) improves metaphyseal fracture healing in an osteoporotic rat model. PLoS One 12(12), 2017:e0189356.

41. Kobayashi M, Chijimatsu R, Yoshikawa H, et al: Extracorporeal shock wave therapy accelerates endochondral ossification and fracture healing in a rat femur delayed-union model. Biochem Biophys Res Commun 530(4):632–637, 2020.

42. Willems A, van der Jagt OP, Meuffels DE: Extracorporeal shock wave treatment for delayed union and nonunion fractures: a systematic review. J Orthop Trauma 33(2):97–103, 2019.

43. Schleusser S, Song J, Stang FH, et al: Blood flow in the scaphoid is improved by focused extracorporeal shock wave therapy. Clin Orthop Relat Res 478(1):127–135, 2020.

44. International Society for Medical Shockwave Treatment: Consensus statement on ESWT indications and contraindications. 2016. https://www.shockwavetherapy.org/fileadmin/user_upload/dokumente/PDFs/Formulare/ISMST_consensus_statement_on_indications_and_contraindications_20161012_final.pdf. (Accessed October 24, 2020).

45. Crevenna R, Mickel M, Keilani M: Extracorporeal shock wave therapy in the supportive care and rehabilitation of cancer patients. Support Care Cancer 27(11):4039–4041, 2019.

46. Kiessling MC, Milz S, Frank HG, et al: Radial extracorporeal shock wave treatment harms developing chicken embryos. Sci Rep 5:8281, 2015.

47. Ramesh S, Zaman F, Madhuri V, et al: Radial extracorporeal shock wave treatment promotes bone growth and chondrogenesis in cultured fetal rat metatarsal bones. Clin Orthop Relat Res 478(3):668–678, 2020.

48. Lohrer H, Nauck T, Korakakis V, et al: Historical ESWT paradigms are overcome: A narrative review. Biomed Res Int 3850461:2016, 2016.

49. Kang N, Zhang J, Yu X, et al: Radial extracorporeal shock wave therapy improves cerebral blood flow and neurological function in a rat model of cerebral ischemia. Am J Transl Res 9(4):2000–2012, 2017.

50. Beisteiner R, Matt E, Fan C, et al: Transcranial pulse stimulation with ultrasound in Alzheimer's disease—a new navigated focal brain therapy. Adv Sci (Weinh) 7(3), 2019:1902583.

51. Cooper D, Wilkoff B, Masterson M, et al: Effects of extracorporeal shock wave lithotripsy on cardiac pacemakers and its safety in patients with implanted cardiac pacemakers. Pacing Clin Electrophysiol 11(11 Pt 1):1607–1616, 1988.

52. Fetter J, Patterson D, Aram G, et al: Effects of extracorporeal shock wave lithotripsy on single chamber rate response and dual chamber pacemakers. Pacing Clin Electrophysiol 12(9):1494–1501, 1989.

Hydrotherapy and Negative Pressure Wound Therapy

CHAPTER OBJECTIVES

After reading this chapter, the reader will be able to do the following:
- Define *hydrotherapy* and *negative pressure wound therapy*.
- Describe effects of hydrotherapy and negative pressure wound therapy.
- Compare and contrast the different techniques for hydrotherapy and negative pressure wound therapy.
- Safely and effectively apply hydrotherapy and negative pressure wound therapy.
- Choose the best technique for treatment with hydrotherapy and negative pressure wound therapy, and list the advantages and disadvantages of each.
- Select the appropriate equipment and parameters for treatment with hydrotherapy and negative pressure wound therapy.
- Accurately and completely document treatment with hydrotherapy and negative pressure wound therapy.

Hydrotherapy, derived from the Greek words *hydro,* meaning "water," and *therapeia,* meaning "healing," is the application of water, internally or externally, for the treatment of physical or psychological dysfunction. This chapter concerns the external application of water when used as a component of physical rehabilitation. Hydrotherapy can be applied externally by immersing the whole body or parts of the body in water, or without immersion by spraying or pouring water onto the body. The effects and applications of immersion and nonimmersion hydrotherapy are discussed here. Although not a form of hydrotherapy, **negative pressure wound therapy (NPWT)** is also included in this chapter because NPWT is often used in conjunction with nonimmersion hydrotherapy as a component of wound care.

◎ Clinical Pearl

Although not a form of hydrotherapy, negative pressure wound therapy (NPWT) is often used in conjunction with nonimmersion hydrotherapy as a component of wound care.

Bathing in water has been considered healing since the beginning of recorded time and across many cultures, from

Hippocrates in the 4th and 5th centuries BCE, who used hot and cold water to treat a variety of diseases; to the Romans at the beginning of the 1st century CE, who constructed therapeutic baths across their empire; to the Japanese, who have used ritual baths from ancient times to the modern day.[1] Therapeutic use of water gained particular popularity in Europe in the late 19th century, with the development of health spas in areas of natural springs, such as Baden-Baden and Bad Ragaz, and shortly thereafter in the United States in similar areas of natural hot springs. At that time, hydrotherapy was used for its effects on both the mind and the body: "It is readily shown that no remedy for lunacy exists which is at all comparable to the bath, owing to its purifying action on the blood."[2] The transition of hydrotherapy from a preventive and recreational role to a curative or rehabilitative role for diseases and their sequelae occurred during the polio epidemic of the 1940s and 1950s, when Sister Kenny included activities in water as a component of her treatment of patients recovering from polio. She found that the unique properties of the water environment, including **buoyancy, resistance,** and support, allowed these weakened patients to perform a wide range of therapeutic activities with greater ease and safety than was possible on dry land.[3] Although hydrotherapy has been shown to have wide-ranging therapeutic effects and benefits, it is used today primarily as a component of the treatment of wounds and to provide an enhanced environment for therapeutic exercise.

Physical Properties of Water

Water has a number of physical properties that make it well suited to specific rehabilitation applications. Water is a solvent and can apply **hydrostatic pressure,** resistance, and buoyancy to the body. Water also has a relatively high **specific heat** and **thermal conductivity.**

SOLVENT

Water is a universal solvent that can dissolve many chemical compounds while not reacting with them. Therefore, water running over the body or over an open wound will remove some contaminants or necrotic material by dissolving them. Although adding a surfactant such as a detergent will make a solution that dissolves fatty material that is hydrophobic,

and adding water-soluble antimicrobials will make a solution that inactivates certain microbes, surfactants and antimicrobials are generally not used to clean wounds because they can also damage healthy exposed cells. Other additives, such as salt, may be dissolved in water used for wound cleansing.

RESISTANCE

The **viscosity** of water produces pressure that provides resistance. This resistance occurs against the relative direction of the motion of the water and the body and increases in proportion to the relative speed of the motion and the frontal area of the body parts in contact with the water (Fig. 19.1).[4] When water is used for debriding and cleansing wounds, the speed of the water is adjusted to vary the pressure against the wound bed. When water is used as an environment for exercise, either the speed of the water or the speed of the patient can be changed to vary the resistance of water. When there is no water flow or body motion, water provides no resistance. As the speed of water flow increases, the speed of the body's motion through the water increases, or the frontal area of the body part in contact with the water increases, the resistance provided by the water increases. The frontal area of the body in contact with the water can be increased by the patient using paddles or fins and can be decreased by the patient keeping their limbs more parallel to the direction of movement (Fig. 19.2). The velocity-dependent resistance of water makes it a particularly safe and effective strengthening and conditioning medium for a wide range of patients.

HYDROSTATIC PRESSURE

Hydrostatic pressure is the **pressure** exerted by a fluid on a body immersed in it. According to Pascal's law, a fluid exerts equal and inward pressure on all surfaces of a body at rest in proportion to the depth of the body in the fluid (Fig. 19.3). Water exerts 0.73 mm Hg of pressure per centimeter of depth (22.4 mm Hg/ft). Because hydrostatic pressure increases as the depth of immersion increases, the pressure exerted on the distal extremities of an upright immersed patient is greater than that exerted on the more proximal or cranial parts of the body. For example, when a patient's feet are immersed under 4 feet of water, the pressure exerted by the water will be approximately 88.9 mm Hg, which is slightly

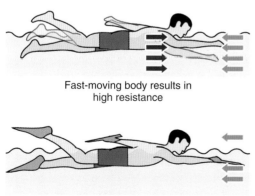

Fast-moving body results in high resistance

Paddles and fins increase frontal area and increase resistance

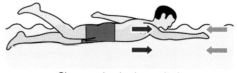

Slow-moving body results in moderate resistance

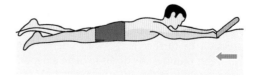

Limbs straight in front decrease frontal area and decrease resistance

FIGURE 19.1 Resistance.

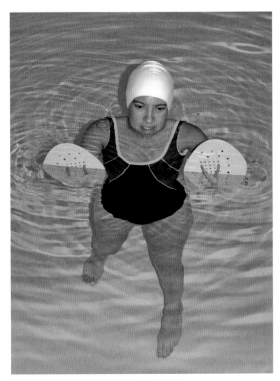

FIGURE 19.2 Patient exercising in water using handheld devices to increase the frontal area and thus increase the resistance of the water.

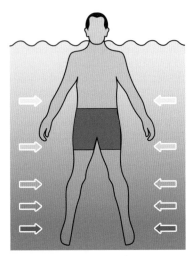

FIGURE 19.3 Hydrostatic pressure.

above normal diastolic blood pressure. This external pressure can have the same effects as the pressure exerted by compression devices, such as elastic garments or bandages, including promoting circulation or alleviating peripheral **edema** caused by venous or lymphatic insufficiency, as described in detail in Chapter 21. However, in contrast to most other external compression devices that allow the limbs to be elevated during compression to further assist with edema control, compression in water requires the limbs to be in a dependent position. This means some of the potential benefits of immersion compression are counteracted by the increase in circulatory hydrostatic pressure produced by placing a limb in this dependent position.

Because hydrostatic pressure increases with the depth of immersion, the physiological and clinical benefits of the hydrostatic pressure of water will vary with the patient's positioning. The greatest effects will occur with vertical positioning, with the feet immersed most deeply. The effects will be much less pronounced if the patient is swimming or performing other activities in more horizontal positions close to the water's surface with the limbs at lower depths of immersion. There are no therapeutic hydrostatic pressure effects when nonimmersion hydrotherapy techniques are used.

BUOYANCY

Buoyancy is a force experienced as an upward thrust on the body in the opposite direction to the force of gravity. According to Archimedes' principle, when a body at rest is entirely or partially immersed in fluid, it experiences an upward thrust equal to the weight of the fluid it displaces. If the density of the immersed body is less than that of the fluid, it will displace less than the body's total volume of fluid and will float. Conversely, if the density of the body is greater than the density of the fluid, it will displace a volume of fluid equal to its own volume, but because the body weighs more, it will sink. Because the human body is less dense than water (having a **specific gravity** of approximately 0.974 compared with that of water), it floats (Table 19.1). If the relative density of the body compared with the water is further decreased by adding salt to the water or by attaching air-filled objects such as a belt, vest, or armbands to the patient, the body will float even higher in the water (Fig. 19.4). This occurs when a person swims in sea water or uses a life jacket.

Exercising in water takes advantage of the buoyancy of the human body in water. Submersion of most of the body decreases stress and gravitational compression on weight-bearing joints, muscles, and connective tissue (Fig. 19.5). Submersion may also be used to help raise weakened body parts against gravity or to assist the therapist in supporting the weight of the patient's body during therapeutic activities.

> ### ◎ Clinical Pearl
>
> Water is a particularly safe and effective strengthening medium because its resistance depends on the speed of the person's movement, and it unloads weight-bearing structures.

TABLE 19.1	Specific Gravity of Different Substances
Substance	Specific Gravity
Pure water	1
Salt water	1.024
Ice	0.917
Air	1.21×10^{-3}
Average human body	0.974
Subcutaneous fat	0.85

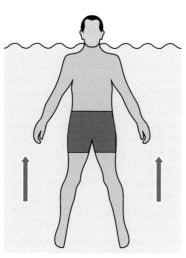
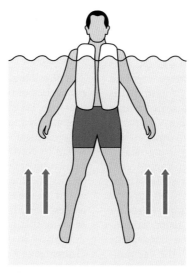
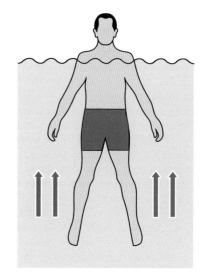

Person in water, floating head above water

Person with air-filled vest in water, floating head and shoulders above water

Person in water, with a high concentration of dissolved salt, floating head and shoulders above water

FIGURE 19.4 Buoyancy.

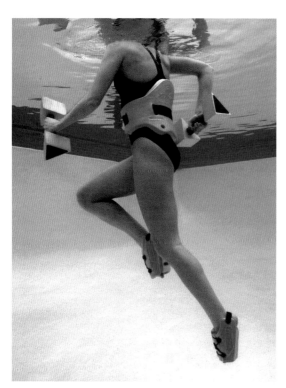

FIGURE 19.5 Patient exercising in water while wearing a foam vest to increase buoyancy. (© 2020 BD. Used with permission.)

SPECIFIC HEAT AND THERMAL CONDUCTIVITY

Water can transfer heat by conduction and convection and therefore can be used as a superficial heating or cooling agent. Stationary water transfers heat by conduction; moving water transfers heat by convection. The rate of heat transfer by convection increases as the rate of fluid flow relative to the body increases. Water is particularly effective for these applications because it has high specific heat and thermal conductivity. The specific heat of water is approximately 4 times that of air, and its thermal conductivity is approximately 25 times that of air (Table 19.2). Thus, water retains 4 times as much thermal energy as an equivalent mass of air at the same temperature, and it transfers this thermal energy 25 times faster than air at the same temperature.

The ability of water to transfer heat rapidly and efficiently is one of the advantages of using moist hot packs rather than dry hot packs and also of performing exercises in a cool swimming pool. A moist hot pack transfers more heat more quickly than a dry hot pack at the same temperature. Similarly, exercising in cool water helps dissipate the heat generated by the patient through exertion and counteracts the heat of a hotter climate more effectively than exercising in cool air. Because heat transfer by convection is quicker than heat transfer by conduction, heat transfer is faster with a whirlpool than with a hot pack at the same temperature, and the cooling of a patient in a cold swimming pool is accelerated if the patient moves quickly through the water. Additional details regarding the effects of specific heat and thermal conductivity on heat transfer and on the principles of heat transfer by conduction and convection are provided in Chapter 7 in the section on modes of heat transfer.

TABLE 19.2	Comparison of Specific Heat and Thermal Conductivity of Water and Air	
	Specific Heat, J/g/°C	Thermal Conductivity (cal/s)/(cm² × °C/cm)
Water	4.19	0.0014
Air	1.01	0.000057
Water:air ratio	4.14	24.56

Physical Properties of Negative Pressure Wound Therapy

NPWT, also known as *vacuum-assisted wound therapy,* uses a pump that applies a subatmospheric pressure to a wound bed via tubing that goes into the wound. The wound bed is filled with a foam dressing that is covered and sealed with a film dressing (Fig. 19.6). NPWT is not new. Early forms of negative pressure were used by the Chinese and others when they created static, negative pressure suction using heated glass bowls placed on the skin. Early Western nonpowered techniques used a syringe and catheter or water-sealed drainage bottles; these were followed by dressings with surgical drains connected to wall or portable suction. Purpose-designed, electrical NPWT devices using a foam wound-filling dressing covered with a thin film and a stand-alone suction device were first described in 1997.[5,6] The vacuum-assisted closure (VAC) device was the first dedicated NPWT device, and a number of others have entered this market since.

SUCTION/ASPIRATION

NPWT applies a controlled suction force to the wound through a filling dressing covered with an impermeable membrane that seals the wound. The suction force pulls toward the dressing in the wound bed, drawing fluid from the circulation into the wound and drawing fluid out of the wound and into a collection canister.

FLUID INSTILLATION

In addition to applying suction, the newer NPWT devices also allow **instillation** of a user-selected fluid into the wound and allow this fluid to stay on the wound for a predetermined amount of time, known as the **dwell time.** NPWT resumes after the dwell time. NPWT has also been modified successfully to promote the healing of infected wounds by combining it with a closed-suction irrigation system that allows for fluid instillation and removal.[7]

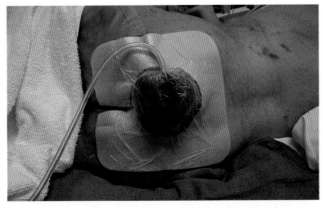

FIGURE 19.6 Vacuum-assisted wound therapy for a sacral pressure ulcer. (From Cameron MH, Monore LG: *Physical rehabilitation: evidence-based examination, evaluation, and intervention,* St Louis, 2007, Saunders.)

Physiological Effects of Hydrotherapy and Negative Pressure Wound Therapy

The physiological effects of water are the result of its physical properties of being a solvent; being able to apply hydrostatic pressure, resistance, and buoyancy to the body; and having a relatively high specific heat and thermal conductivity. The physiological effects of superficial heating or cooling by warm or cold water are the same as the physiological effects of heating or cooling with other superficial heating or cooling agents and include hemodynamic, neuromuscular, and metabolic changes and modification of soft tissue extensibility, as described in detail in Chapter 8. The physiological effects of water distinct from those of superficial thermal agents are described in the following section. These effects include cleansing as well as musculoskeletal, cardiovascular, respiratory, renal, and psychological changes (Box 19.1).

The physiological effects of NPWT are the result of its physical properties of suction and fluid instillation.

CLEANSING

Water can be used as a cleanser because it can dissolve and soften materials and exert pressure. Water is used most commonly, with or without a surfactant or antimicrobial, for cleansing intact skin. In rehabilitation, the cleansing properties of water are most often used to treat open wounds where the skin is not intact and subcutaneous tissue is exposed. In this circumstance, the solvent and resistance properties of water soften and remove debris lodged in the wound or

---

Box 19.1　Physiological Effects of Hydrotherapy

Cleansing Effects
- Pressure to remove debris
- Dissolved surfactants and antimicrobials to assist with cleaning

Musculoskeletal Effects
- Decreased weight bearing
- Strengthening
- Effects on bone density loss
- Less fat loss than with other forms of exercise

Cardiovascular Effects
- Increased venous circulation
- Increased cardiac volume
- Increased cardiac output
- Decreased heart rate, systolic blood pressure, and rate of oxygen uptake ($\dot{V}O_2$) response to exercise

Respiratory Effects
- Decreased vital capacity
- Increased work of breathing
- Decreased exercise-induced asthma

Renal Effects
- Diuresis
- Increased sodium and potassium excretion

Psychological Effects
- Relaxing or invigorating, depending on temperature

adhered to the tissue. This debris may be exogenous waste, such as gravel or adhered dressing materials, or endogenous debris, such as wound **exudate** or **necrotic tissue.** Excessive bacterial burden in a wound may also be reduced by hydrotherapy. Wounds should be cleansed because exogenous debris, necrotic tissue, and high concentrations or multiple types of microorganisms delay wound healing.[8] Water is well suited to wound cleansing because it can dissolve some wound debris, and the force exerted by water can be controlled by adjusting its rate of flow. In addition, water can quickly and easily get into and out of the contoured areas of open wounds.

> ### Clinical Pearl
> Water is well suited to wound cleansing. It is important to cleanse wounds because necrotic tissue and high concentrations of microorganisms delay wound healing.

NPWT with instillation is also effective for wound cleansing. The repeated instillation of fluid followed by its removal by suction disrupts bacterial attachment to tissues and removes bacteria. This reduces bacterial load in wounds with virulent pathogens, which can then allow spontaneous wound healing or prepare the wound for successful graft uptake.

Various water-soluble products, such as surfactants and antimicrobials, can be added to hydrotherapy water or NPWT instillation fluid to increase its cleansing effectiveness. Surfactants, such as soap or detergents, reduce surface tension and thereby reduce the adhesion of debris to the tissue. Antimicrobials, such as Dakin's solution, reduce microbial count in the water and on the wound surface. Several clinical benefits and risks are associated with putting additives in the water used for treating open wounds. These benefits and risks are discussed in detail in the sections on clinical indications for hydrotherapy later in the chapter.

TISSUE HEALING

Hydrotherapy is thought to aid wound healing by maintaining a moist wound bed and removing exogenous and endogenous waste and microorganisms. Warm water, as well as the physical stimulus of water pressure, may also promote tissue healing by enhancing local circulation and thus the delivery of oxygen and nutrients to wounds.

NPWT is also thought to aid wound healing by maintaining a moist wound environment, removing interstitial fluid and exudate, and decreasing edema.[9] NPWT promotes granulation tissue formation, angiogenesis, and tissue perfusion while also reducing wound contamination and has been used successfully to promote the healing of a wide variety of acute and chronic wounds.[10] NPWT is recommended by the Association for the Advancement of Wound Care and by the Wound, Ostomy and Continence Nurses Society for the treatment of venous ulcers and stage III and IV pressure ulcers that have failed to heal with standard wound care.[11,12]

NPWT with instillation and dwell time is intended to provide the benefits of NPWT in wound management while also cleansing the wound by instilling a cleansing fluid and then removing it.[13,14] This intervention can also have antimicrobial effects if the instillation fluid includes an antimicrobial (Fig. 19.7).[15,16] NPWT with instillation is intended to help prevent or eradicate infection and can be more effective at

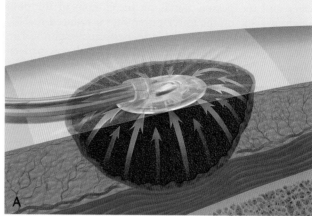

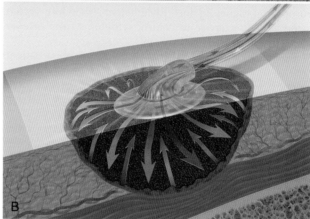

FIGURE 19.7 (A) Negative pressure (vacuum-assisted) wound therapy, applying a suction force to the wound. (B) Negative pressure wound therapy with instillation, instilling fluid to irrigate the wound and applying suction. (Used with Permission. Courtesy of 3M.)

promoting wound healing or preparing wounds for surgical closure, particularly in high-risk patients, than either hydrotherapy or NPWT alone.[10,17–20]

> ### Clinical Pearl
> NPWT applies controlled suction to the wound through a dressing covered with an impermeable membrane that seals the wound. NPWT with instillation adds instillation and removal of a fluid to the wound to NPWT, and NPWT with instillation and dwell time allows the fluid to stay in the wound for a controlled amount of time. NPWT is recommended for treating deep wounds that have failed to heal with standard care.

Additional Physiological Effects of Hydrotherapy
MUSCULOSKELETAL

The buoyancy of water allows it to unload weight-bearing anatomical structures. This can allow patients with load-sensitive joints to perform exercises with less trauma and pain.[21–23] For example, when 75% of the body is immersed in water and the person stands on the bottom of the pool, weight bearing on the lower extremities is reduced by 75%. The patient may then be able to perform weight-bearing exercises or walk unassisted with a normal gait pattern, whereas they can only perform these activities on dry land with the support of crutches. In addition, weight bearing on the lower extremities can be completely eliminated in a pool if the patient wears a floatation swim vest. The load-reducing effect of water buoyancy can help patients with arthritis, ligamentous instability, cartilage breakdown, or other degenerative or traumatic conditions of the articular or periarticular structures of the weight-bearing joints perform and progress more comfortably and rapidly with rehabilitation activities.[24] Many organizations, including the Osteoarthritis Research Society, the American College of Rheumatology, and the European League Against Rheumatism, therefore recommend aquatic exercise to control symptoms from osteoarthritis of the weight-bearing joints.

Buoyancy can also be particularly helpful for obese patients because excess body weight can place excessive stress on weight-bearing joints. In addition, because obese individuals have more low-density, subcutaneous fat than average-weight people, they are more buoyant in water (see Table 19.1), making water-based activities even more effective for reducing joint loading. Therefore, water-based exercises may be used to restore fitness in obese adults and children who have difficulty with other forms of exercise.[25–27] Earlier research suggested that exercise in water produced less weight loss and fat loss than exercise of similar intensity and duration on dry land,[28–30] but more recent research has found that weight loss in obese people is similar, or even greater, when exercise is performed in water rather than on dry land.[31,32] Therefore water-based exercise is now recommended both for improving fitness and function of obese patients and for safer and more comfortable weight loss.

The velocity-dependent resistance provided by water can be used to provide a force against which muscles can work to gain or maintain strength and cardiovascular fitness. If the direction of water flow is adjusted to be in the same direction as the patient's motion, the resistance of the water can also be used to aid the patient's motion. Water-based exercise can increase extremity strength in patients with musculoskeletal, cardiovascular, and neurological diseases such as fibromyalgia, arthritis, heart failure, and multiple sclerosis, as well as in healthy individuals.[33–41]

Exercise in water also has some limitations. The kinematics of weight-bearing activities such as running and walking will be altered by performing the activities in water rather than on dry land.[42,43] In addition, the reduced weight bearing may result in less improvement in bone health than would occur with land-based exercise.[24]

CARDIOVASCULAR

The cardiovascular effects of hydrotherapy include the fitness benefits of aerobic exercise as well as circulatory changes that result from hydrostatic pressure with immersion. Hydrostatic pressure exerted on the distal extremities when the person is upright and immersed in water displaces venous blood proximally from the extremities. This enhances venous return by shifting blood from the periphery to the trunk vessels and then to the thorax and the heart. Central venous pressure increases with immersion to the chest and continues to increase until the body is fully immersed.[44,45] With immersion to the neck, central blood volume increases by approximately 60%, and cardiac volume increases by nearly 30%.[45,46] This increase in cardiac volume increases right atrial pressure by 14 to 18 mm Hg, to which the heart responds, according to Starling's law, with an increase in contraction force and stroke volume.[47] This results in approximately 30% increased cardiac output over baseline in response to upright immersion up to the neck (Fig. 19.8).[47] In addition, water immersion is associated with a reduced heart rate response to exercise.[45,48] This reduced heart rate response results in a lower rate of oxygen consumption ($\dot{V}O_2$) when exercise is performed in water compared with when exercise at the same level of perceived exertion is performed on dry land. For example, the maximum rate of oxygen consumption ($\dot{V}O_{2max}$) is slightly lower with maximal running in deep water than with maximal running on dry land.[42,49–51] Because of these altered physiological responses, exercise in water has often been considered to be less effective for cardiac conditioning than similar exercise on dry land. However, because the reduction in heart rate and $\dot{V}O_{2max}$ are accompanied by an increase in stroke volume and cardiac output, which may

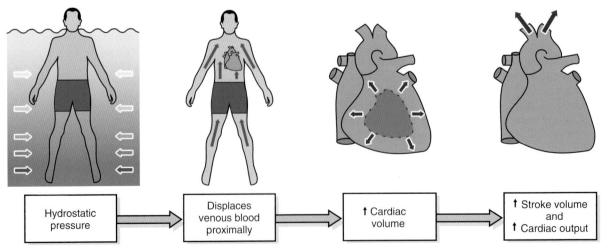

| Hydrostatic pressure | → | Displaces venous blood proximally | → | ↑ Cardiac volume | → | ↑ Stroke volume and ↑ Cardiac output |

FIGURE 19.8 Cardiovascular effects of immersion.

increase myocardial efficiency, exercise in water can be effective for cardiac conditioning in healthy adults and for rehabilitation in those with cardiovascular disease.[40,51,52]

In patients with heart failure, there is some concern that the increase in cardiac volume that occurs during immersion (as a result of hydrostatic pressure) may overwhelm the pumping ability of the heart. However, when immersed in warm water, these patients have reduced afterload as a result of peripheral vasodilation,[44] increased early diastolic filling, and a decreased heart rate, leading to an increase in stroke volume and ejection fraction.[53] These responses are similar to responses in healthy control subjects.[54] A number of studies have shown that patients with stable heart failure can safely and effectively improve their exercise capacity, muscle strength, and quality of life with aquatic-based exercise.[39,55] However, because of the changes in cardiac demand with exercise, including water-based exercise, clinicians should carefully monitor responses to these activities in patients with heart failure. In addition, because the heart rate response to exercise is blunted in water, when patients with or without heart failure exercise in water, the level of perceived exertion, rather than the heart rate response, should be used to guide exercise intensity.[56]

> ### ◎ Clinical Pearl
>
> When a person exercises in water, the heart rate response is blunted. Therefore, perceived exertion rather than heart rate should be used to guide exercise intensity.

In addition to immersion blunting the heart rate response to exercise, when an activity is performed at the same speed in water as it is on dry land, the water's velocity-dependent resistance to motion increases the metabolic rate and energy expenditure about threefold.[57] Therefore, to achieve the same level of exertion and metabolic demand as with exercise performed on dry land, exercise performed in water should be performed at about one-third the speed of similar exercise on dry land.[58] This can allow individuals with conditions that limit their speed of movement to perform exercise in water to maintain or improve their cardiovascular fitness.

RESPIRATORY

Immersion of the whole body in water increases the work of breathing because the shift of venous blood from the peripheral to the central circulation increases the circulation in the chest cavity and because hydrostatic pressure on the chest wall increases resistance to lung expansion (Fig. 19.9).[34,47] Immersion in water up to the neck decreases expiratory reserve volume by approximately 50% and decreases vital capacity by 6% to 12%. These effects increase the total work of breathing by approximately 60%.[59–61] Thus the workload challenge on the respiratory system with exercise in water can improve the efficiency and strength of the respiratory system. However, because this additional respiratory demand may overload patients with respiratory or cardiovascular impairments that prevent or limit adaptation to the additional workload, such patients should always be carefully monitored during water-based exercise.[62]

Water-based exercise is often recommended for people with asthma because studies have shown that it is less likely to trigger exercise-induced bronchospasm in these individuals than exercising on dry land.[63,64] Various factors,[65] including the absence of pollen over the water, hydrostatic pressure on the chest, hypoventilation, hypercapnia, peripheral vasoconstriction, and the high humidity of the inspired air in the pool environment, have been proposed as mechanisms for this effect.[66] Although most of these factors have not been studied experimentally, it appears that the high humidity of the air inspired during water exercise, which prevents drying or cooling of the respiratory mucosa, is the most important.

RENAL

Immersion of an individual up to the neck in water has been shown to increase urine production and the excretion of urinary sodium and potassium (Fig. 19.10).[66–69] It is proposed that these effects are the result of increased renal blood flow and decreased production of antidiuretic hormone (ADH) and aldosterone. Water immersion is thought to cause these circulatory and hormonal changes in response to the redistribution of blood volume and the relative central hypervolemia that result from the hydrostatic pressure that water exerts on the periphery. These renal effects can be taken advantage of when treating patients with hypervolemia, hypertension, or peripheral edema. In patients with chronic kidney disease, compared with no exercise, low-intensity water exercise twice weekly for 12 weeks has been found to improve kidney and cardiorespiratory function and to decrease resting blood pressure.[70]

PSYCHOLOGICAL

As is well known to people who bathe or exercise in water, water immersion can be invigorating or relaxing. Variations in these psychological effects appear to depend primarily on the temperature of the water. Soaking in warm water is generally relaxing, whereas most people find immersion in cold water to be invigorating and energizing. The neutral stimulation and support of warm water can be used clinically to provide a comforting and calming environment for over-stimulated or agitated patients, and the invigorating effects of cold water can be used to facilitate more active exercise participation by patients who are generally less active or responsive. Water-based exercise has also been found to improve quality of life in many patient populations, including older adults, patients with osteoarthritis and other musculoskeletal conditions, and patients with heart failure.[39,71–73] The clinically observed psychological effects of water immersion are thought to be mediated by a central process within the reticular activating system.

Clinical Indications for Hydrotherapy and Negative Pressure Wound Therapy

WOUND CARE

Hydrotherapy may accelerate the healing of chronic open wounds, including those caused by diabetes mellitus, pressure, vascular insufficiency, or burns. Hydrotherapy may also be used in the care of wounds from trauma, surgery, abscesses, dehisced incisions, necrotizing fasciitis, or cellulitis. Hydrotherapy is used

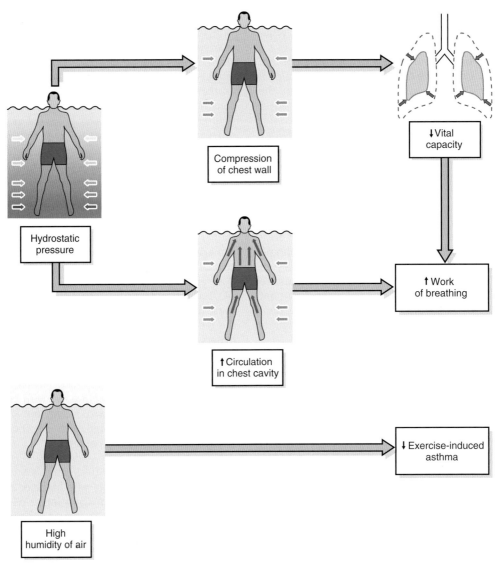

FIGURE 19.9 Respiratory effects of immersion.

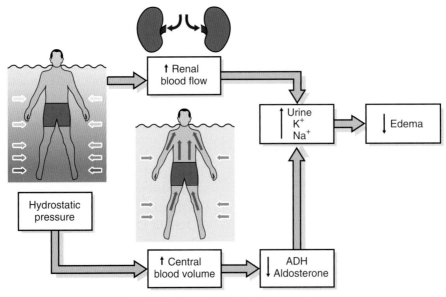

FIGURE 19.10 Renal effects of immersion.

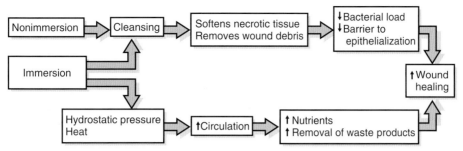

FIGURE 19.11 Effects of hydrotherapy for wound care.

for wound care because its cleansing properties facilitate rehydration, softening, and **debridement** of necrotic tissue and removal of exogenous wound debris and excessive microbial burden, and the hydrostatic pressure of water immersion and the heat of warm water improve circulation (Fig. 19.11). The use of hydrotherapy is also consistent with the current understanding that wounds heal better and more quickly when kept moist rather than dry.[12]

The use of hydrotherapy for wound care is not new. In 1734, a German physician, Dr. Johann Hahn, recommended prolonged immersion in water to treat leg sores.[74] Immersion hydrotherapy using whirlpools remained the most common method of applying wound hydrotherapy for many years. But immersion hydrotherapy has fallen out of favor and has largely been replaced by nonimmersion hydrotherapy techniques because of concerns about the pressure exerted by water agitated by a whirlpool turbine damaging regenerating tissue in wounds and driving bacteria into the wound, with[75] contaminated tanks and tank water increasing **infection** transmission. Whirlpool tank water may become contaminated by microorganisms from the patient being treated at that time or by microorganisms that become lodged in the crevices of the tank from prior treatments or between treatments.

Outbreaks of wound infections, most commonly caused by *Pseudomonas aeruginosa* but occasionally caused by *Staphylococcus aureus, Acinetobacter baumannii, Klebsiella pneumonia,* or *Candida albicans,* have been reported after immersion hydrotherapy.[76–81] Although immersion hydrotherapy–associated infections are rare, the fact that wound infections can be associated with significant morbidity and mortality, and that there are alternative cleaner and safer ways to apply hydrotherapy, have made whirlpools fall out of favor.[79,82,83] At the present time, if wounds are treated in a whirlpool, a whirlpool liner is generally used to reduce the risk of contamination and infection. The American Physical Therapy Association specifically recommends against using whirlpools for wound management because "whirlpools are a nonselective form of mechanical debridement. Utilizing whirlpool to treat wounds predisposes the patient to risks of bacterial cross-contamination, damage to fragile tissue from high turbine forces, and complications in extremity edema when arms and legs are treated in a dependent position."[84] Therefore, the use of whirlpools for wound care is not covered further in this book.

A variety of devices can be used to apply hydrotherapy to wounds without immersion. These devices must deliver fluid at pressure between 4 and 15 pounds per square inch (psi) because bacteria and debris are not effectively removed below

this level, and at higher pressures, wound trauma may occur, or bacteria may be driven into the tissue.[85–87]

◎ Clinical Pearl

When used for wound care, nonimmersion irrigation devices should deliver fluid at 4 to 15 psi pressure to remove debris without damaging tissue.

A number of devices deliver fluid within the safe and effective pressure range for wound care (Table 19.3). These include a saline squeeze bottle with an irrigation cap and a 35-mL syringe with a 19-gauge needle. Fluid can also be poured over the wound bed, although the low pressure of this approach may make it less effective. Electrically **pulsed lavage** devices can also deliver pressure within this range. These devices spray water onto the wound and then use suction or negative pressure to remove contaminated water from the area. These devices also allow fine adjustment of the water pressure. However, because pulsed lavage can aerosolize the bacteria in a wound, as demonstrated by the presence of bacteria from wounds in the noses of the therapist and the patient after pulsed lavage,[88] the U.S. Food and Drug Administration (FDA) has devised specific guidelines for using pulsed lavage. These include using a private single-patient room, allowing only essential equipment in the treatment room, covering surfaces at greatest risk for aerosol contamination, and thoroughly cleaning and disinfecting surfaces touched by hand after each patient treatment (see Fig. 19.16). During the treatment, anyone in the room must wear full personal protective equipment, including a fluid-proof gown, gloves, mask/goggles or face shield, and hair cover. The patient should also wear a surgical mask, and all patient lines, ports, and wounds that are not being treated should be covered with a drape or a towel.[89] The considerable time and resources needed to implement these precautions have reduced the popularity of this intervention.

NPWT with instillation is a means of applying nonimmersion hydrotherapy that does not aerosolize bacteria and therefore does not require the complex precautions associated with the use of pulsed lavage.[14] NPWT with instillation can cleanse wounds by applying and then removing fluid, but it does not apply the fluid with pressure to enhance the removal of debris and microorganisms. However, NPWT with installation has been found to reduce bioburden in wounds and to be superior for promoting wound healing to either hydrotherapy or NPWT alone.[16,20]

Various fluids can be used for wound hydrotherapy by immersion or nonimmersion approaches. Because open wounds

TABLE 19.3 Irrigation Pressure Delivered by Various Devices		
Device	Irrigation Pressure, psi	psi Level for Safe and Effective Wound Cleansing
Spray bottle—Ultra Klenz[a] (Carrington Laboratories Inc., Dallas, TX)	1.2	Too little
Bulb syringe[a] (Davol Inc., Cranston, RI)	2.0	Too little
Piston Irrigation Syringe, 60 mL, with catheter tip[b] (Premium Plastics Inc., Chicago, IL)	4.2	Appropriate
Saline Squeeze Bottle, 250 mL, with irrigation cap[b] (Baxter Healthcare Corp., Deerfield, IL)	4.5	Appropriate
Water Pik at lowest setting[b] (Teledyne Water Pik, Fort Collins, CO)	6.0	Appropriate
Irrijet DS Syringe with tip[b] (Ackrad Laboratories, Inc., Cranford, NJ)	7.6	Appropriate
35-mL syringe with 19-gauge needle or angiocatheter[b]	8.0	Appropriate
Water Pik at middle setting[c] (Teledyne Water Pik, Fort Collins, CO)	42	Too much
Water Pik at highest setting[c] (Teledyne Water Pik, Fort Collins, CO)	50	Too much
Pressurized Cannister Dey Wash[c] (Dey Laboratories, Napa, CA)	50	Too much

[a]Too little pressure for effective wound cleansing at less than 4 psi.
[b]Appropriate pressure for safe and effective wound cleansing at 4 to 15 psi.
[c]Too much pressure for safe wound cleansing at greater than 15 psi.
From U.S. Department of Health and Human Services (USDHHS): *Treatment of pressure ulcers: clinical practice guidelines,* Rockville, MD, 1994, USDHHS.

are not sterile, sterile fluid is not required to clean them. Using sterile fluids rather than drinkable tap water to clean wounds has also not been found to be associated with improvements in infection or healing rates.[90,91] A systematic review found no strong evidence for recommending any particular solution for cleaning pressure ulcers, and current guidelines generally recommend using lukewarm drinkable tap water, or possibly distilled water, cooled boiled water, or saline, for wound cleaning.[12,90,92,93]

Generally, nonimmersion hydrotherapy is recommended for cleaning wounds containing necrotic, nonviable tissue or debris. This type of treatment can help remove necrotic tissue, promote healing, and increase patient comfort.[94] Nonimmersion hydrotherapy should be continued until all necrotic, nonviable material has been removed and a full granulation bed is present. When applying hydrotherapy to wounds, it is important to balance its potential benefits to the wound with the potential that its mechanical disruption will damage regenerating **granulation tissue** in the wound bed or that **maceration** as a result of excessive moisture will damage the intact skin surrounding the wound. Therefore, hydrotherapy should be discontinued when the wound base is fully covered with granulation tissue, and the intact skin surrounding a wound should always be thoroughly, although gently, dried immediately after completing hydrotherapy treatment.

Clinical Pearl

Hydrotherapy should be discontinued when the wound base is fully covered with granulation tissue. The skin surrounding the wound should be dried immediately after hydrotherapy to avoid maceration.

Special Concerns Regarding the Use of Hydrotherapy in the Treatment of Burns

Most burn centers consider hydrotherapy an important component of the treatment of acute burn injury, but there is considerable variation in specific practice.[81,95,96] The purposes and uses of hydrotherapy for burn care are generally the same as for other types of wounds, except for a few noteworthy differences. As with other types of wounds, hydrotherapy is used early during treatment to cleanse, soften, and loosen necrotic tissue before debridement and to reduce bacterial load. However, unlike most other types of wounds where such debridement is relatively painless, debridement of burn wounds is frequently extremely painful because the wounds are less deep and many of the sensory nerves are still intact. Therefore high-dose analgesics, sometimes with other distracting interventions, such as virtual reality, computer tablet use, or music, are generally used during this procedure, necessitating closer monitoring of the patient during treatment.[97–99]

Because burn wounds are often extensive, covering a large area of the body, special nonimmersion techniques, or immersion hydrotherapy combined with nonimmersion techniques, may be used.[78,100] When immersion hydrotherapy is used, most centers use disposable whirlpool liners[96] to reduce the risk of cross-infection among patients.[81] Nonimmersion hydrotherapy is generally provided by showering the patient while they lie on a surface such as a mesh net stretcher or a trauma table, which allows the water to drain.[101] Although this hydrotherapy approach is associated with a low risk of infection, wound infections have occurred.[102]

In addition to using hydrotherapy during the early treatment of burn wounds when necrotic tissue is present, hydrotherapy may also be used in the later stages of wound healing, such as recovery after reepithelialization has occurred. At this stage there is little risk of wound infection, and water is used to provide a comfortable environment for exercise and range-of-motion (ROM) activities to help prevent the development of contractures and to facilitate increased ROM in scarred areas.

Additional Clinical Indications for Hydrotherapy
EDEMA CONTROL

Water immersion can reduce peripheral edema, likely because of the effect of the hydrostatic pressure of water on circulation and renal function. Water immersion has therefore been recommended for the treatment of peripheral edema with a variety of causes, including venous or lymphatic insufficiency, renal dysfunction, and postoperative inflammation.[103,104] In addition to the effects of hydrostatic pressure on postoperative edema, the cooling effects of cold water may further reduce edema by causing vasoconstriction and reducing vascular permeability. Therefore, immersion of a limb, or part of a limb, in cold water is frequently included in the treatment of edema resulting from recent trauma when other signs of acute inflammation are present. Immersion in warm or hot water is not recommended in such circumstances because heating the area and placing it in a dependent position can increase tissue temperature and intravascular pressure. This will increase inflammation and peripheral arterial flow and thus increase, rather than decrease, edema.[105] The higher the temperature of the water, the greater the amount of edema.[105] However, **contrast baths,** where the hand or foot is alternately submerged in hot and cold water, are frequently used clinically when the treatment goal is to achieve the benefits of heat, including decreased pain and increased flexibility, while avoiding increased edema. This application is discussed in detail, along with other superficial thermal agents, in Chapter 8.

WATER EXERCISE
Types of Water Exercise

Various types of exercise, including swimming, running with or without a vest or belt, walking, cycle ergometry, and other forms of upright exercise can be performed in water (Fig. 19.12). In general, for water exercise, patients are free to move about the pool while exercising, although they may be tethered to the side, as during in-place water running. The tether allows the therapist to monitor the exercise, to increase resistance, and to control a range of activities, particularly in a small pool. The principles, mechanisms of action, and rationales for performing exercise in water are discussed later in this chapter; however, specific water exercise programs are not covered because they are described in detail in other texts devoted to aquatic therapy.[106]

General Uses of Water Exercise

Exercise in water can increase circulation and muscle strength as well as joint viscoelasticity, flexibility, and ROM. Water exercise may also improve ambulation, coordination, and

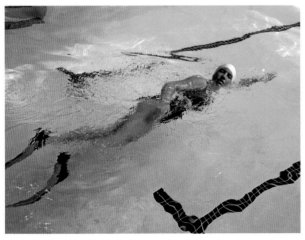

FIGURE 19.12 Water exercise in a swimming pool.

cardiovascular and respiratory conditioning as well as psychological well-being. Furthermore, water exercise can decrease pain, muscle spasm, and stiffness.

The resistance provided by water during movement can serve as a force against which muscles can work to develop strength or, when applied in the direction of patient movement, can be used to assist weakened muscles in the production of movement. Because the buoyancy of water decreases the gravitational forces placed on weight-bearing structures, patients with weakened limbs or load-sensitive joints can often perform strengthening, conditioning, and coordination exercises in water that they would be unable to perform on dry land. This can contribute to improved functional mobility and strength.

Because the hydrostatic pressure provided by immersion in water can facilitate venous return from the extremities, circulation may be enhanced during exercise in water compared with similar exercise performed on dry land. As described previously, the circulatory changes produced by the hydrostatic pressure of water on the extremities during water-based exercise can facilitate cardiovascular and respiratory conditioning and can help reverse and control the formation of peripheral edema.

The ability of water to retain and conduct heat is used clinically when a patient or a part of a patient exercises while immersed in warm water. The combination of heat transfer and exercise is particularly effective because increasing the temperature of soft tissue can augment the vasodilation, increased circulation, decreased joint stiffness, increased joint ROM, and enhanced functional abilities that result from exercise.[107,108] The relaxing effects of immersion in warm water may also improve the psychological well-being of the patient during and after water-based exercise.

Specific Uses of Water Exercise (Box 19.2)
Orthopedic Rehabilitation. The water environment provides graded weight bearing and patient-controlled resistance that can help individuals with spinal or peripheral musculoskeletal dysfunction perform exercises they would have difficulty performing on dry land.[73] This can allow for earlier exercise participation after injury, surgery, or immobilization and for greater exercise participation by patients with load-sensitive conditions such as osteoarthritis or spinal disc disorders.[109] Such exercise participation may help these patients recover earlier and achieve greater functional mobility.

Several studies and meta-analyses have examined the effects of water exercise on people with hip and knee osteoarthritis. Overall, these conclude that aquatic exercise is safe, has greater benefits than no exercise, and has similar or greater benefits than land-based exercise.[21,110–112] In addition, aquatic exercise is associated with greater adherence and satisfaction than land-based exercise.

Several studies and meta-analyses have also examined the effects of water immersion or water exercise on people with fibromyalgia. The two most recent systematic reviews and meta-analyses, both published in 2014, concluded that although the quality of the evidence is not high, compared with control interventions, aquatic training improves wellness, symptoms, and fitness in people with fibromyalgia without serious adverse effects,[113] and aquatic exercise of suitable intensity improves the functional aerobic capacity of

Box 19.2 Benefits of Water Exercise for Specific Conditions

Orthopedic Rehabilitation
- Decreased weight bearing on joints
- Velocity-dependent resistance
- Closed-chain or open-chain exercises
- Effects on bone density loss
- Fibromyalgia

Neurological Rehabilitation
- Proprioceptive input
- Increased safety
- Improved balance

Cardiovascular Fitness
- Cardiac conditioning in patients with poor tolerance for land-based exercise

Pregnancy
- Decreased weight bearing
- Less elevation of heart rate with exercise
- Decreased risk of maternal hyperthermia

Exercise-Induced Asthma
- Less exercise-induced asthma than with other forms of exercise

Age-Related Deficits
- Improved balance
- Improved strength
- Improved cardiorespiratory fitness
- Improved functional mobility

adults with fibromyalgia.[114] In addition, a 2014 systematic review of 24 studies of hydrotherapy (immersion in plain water) or balneotherapy (immersion in mineral water or natural therapeutic gas or spa treatment) in patients with fibromyalgia concluded that these interventions reduced tender-point count and significantly improved pain and health-related quality of life.[115] Based on the current literature, experts recommend water therapy as a nonpharmacological approach for improving pain, fatigue, and quality of life in patients with fibromyalgia.[116]

Exercising in water allows weight bearing to easily be graded to suit individual patient needs. The depth of immersion in water can be varied, or flotation devices such as belts, armbands, or handheld floats can be used to grade weight bearing. Deeper immersion or adding flotation devices increases unloading and reduces weight bearing. Flotation devices also allow greater muscular relaxation in the water by eliminating or reducing the amount of work required by the patient to stay afloat. Therefore, flotation devices are particularly helpful for patients who can benefit from both decreased joint loading and decreased muscular activity. For example, patients with load-sensitive spinal conditions such as disc bulges or herniations or nerve root compression, or with load-sensitive knees or hips, may benefit from relaxed vertical floating in water, supported by a flotation belt, to unload the intraarticular structures and relax the surrounding muscles.

Varying the resistance during water exercise, by altering the water's speed or direction of flow or the patient's movement speed through the water, can alter the clinical effects of the exercise. The faster the relative flow of water against the patient's movement, created by faster water flow or faster patient movement, the greater the resistance to the patient's movement and thus the greater the strengthening or endurance-building effect of the activity. Conversely, by directing the water's flow so that it is in the same direction as the patient's motion, the water can assist with motion when the patient's muscles are weak, allowing strengthening through greater ROM.

Hydrotherapy is often also recommended to control pain. Studies on water exercise in patients with osteoarthritis, fibromyalgia, or ankylosing spondylitis show that along with other benefits, patients experience decreased pain with water exercise.[110,111,116–118] Hydrotherapy is thought to control pain by providing a high level of sensory stimulation to peripheral mechanoreceptors, thereby gating the transmission of pain sensations at the spinal cord. Such a mechanism is consistent with reports by many clinicians that forms of hydrotherapy that provide the greatest sensory stimulation, such as water at a high temperature with a high level of agitation, are particularly effective in reducing pain. Water immersion may also aid pain control by decreasing weight-bearing stress and increasing the ease of movement, and cold water may reduce acute inflammation.

The types of exercises performed in water must be carefully designed and selected to address different conditions and to avoid exacerbating existing problems or causing new ones. The patient can perform closed-chain or open-chain exercises in water. **Closed-chain exercises** can be performed in shallow water using the bottom of the pool to fix the patient's distal extremity (Fig. 19.13) or using the side of the pool to fix the distal extremity when the patient is in deeper water. **Open-chain exercises** can be performed in either deep or shallow water, depending on the area of the body involved and the type of exercise to be performed (Fig. 19.14). It is important to select the appropriate exercise for a particular problem and to be aware of the changes in biomechanics that

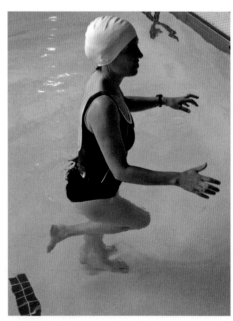

FIGURE 19.13 Closed-chain exercise in water.

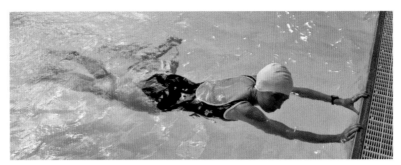

FIGURE 19.14 Open-chain exercise in water.

may occur if an exercise that is usually performed on dry land is transferred to a water environment.[119]

> ◎ **Clinical Pearl**
>
> Biomechanics are likely to be altered when an exercise typically performed on land is performed in the water.

For example, running on dry land is primarily a closed-chain activity, whereas running in deep water using a flotation vest is entirely an open-chain activity. This change may reduce pain from tibiofemoral joint compression by decreasing weight bearing on this joint, but it may increase patellofemoral joint pain by increasing compression at this joint during open-chain knee extension. When designing rehabilitation programs that involve swimming, it is particularly important to guard against adverse effects of compensatory motions because such motions can cause problems in other areas.[120]

> ◎ **Clinical Pearl**
>
> Water rehabilitation programs should be designed so that compensatory motions do not cause problems in other areas.

For example, if the patient has limited shoulder ROM and increases lumbar or cervical motion to bring the shoulder out of the water during freestyle swimming, problems in these spinal areas may result. Similarly, if a patient with hypomobility of the thoracic spine overuses their shoulder during freestyle or breaststroke swimming, they may increase subacromial compression on their rotator cuff, causing the tendon to break down.

Because exercise in water reduces weight bearing on the bones, it was assumed that exercise in this environment did not promote the maintenance of bone density in postmenopausal women. However, observational and experimental studies indicate that aquatic exercise can slow the loss of bone mineral density while enhancing bone formation in this population[121-123] and may be as effective as resistance training.[124] This is likely because of the compressive forces exerted on bones by muscle contraction during water-based exercise. Water exercise can also positively affect the health of women with osteoporosis in other ways while being a safe way to exercise for individuals at high risk for falls.

Neurological Rehabilitation. In recent years there has been a substantial increase in the research on aquatic exercise to address the impairments, disabilities, and handicaps resulting

from neurological dysfunction. A 2015 systematic review on the effects of aquatic therapy on the mobility of individuals with neurological diseases concluded, based on 20 studies, that there was fair evidence for aquatic therapy improving dynamic balance and gait speed in people with stroke or multiple sclerosis.[119] More recent systematic reviews of research in patients with specific neurological conditions have come to similar conclusions. They have concluded that aquatic therapy had a greater impact on multiple measures of mobility and balance than land-based therapy in people with stroke,[125] improved quality of life in people with multiple sclerosis,[126] and improved disability in people with Parkinson disease.[127] In addition, individual small studies have shown that water exercise can increase fitness after brain injury,[128] can reduce spasticity and improve functional independence after spinal cord injury,[129] can improve gait efficiency in adolescents with cerebral palsy,[130] and can increase walking speed and step length in patients with hereditary spastic paraparesis.[131] However, overall, the studies of aquatic therapy in people with neurological conditions are criticized for having small numbers of subjects, aquatic exercise not showing consistently better outcomes than land-based exercise, not having standardized outcome measures, not documenting safety measures or adverse effects, and for often underdosing the exercise in both intensity and duration[132,133] for optimal outcomes.

Water-based exercise is often recommended for patients with neurological dysfunction because it provides proprioceptive input, weight relief, and a safe environment for movement. The proprioceptive input may be particularly beneficial for patients with central sensory deficits resulting in weakness or impaired motor control, such as those that occur after a stroke or traumatic brain injury; the weight relief can ease movement and reduce the risk of falling, thereby facilitating greater movement exploration, functional activity training, and strengthening. It has also been proposed that the greater movement exploration and the increased production of movement errors that occur in water-based exercise are responsible for the balance enhancement associated with water-based exercise.[134] Reduced loading as a result of buoyancy and increased abdominal support from the hydrostatic pressure of water may also help improve breathing for patients with diaphragmatic weakness, which can occur after a spinal cord injury or with amyotrophic lateral sclerosis (ALS), although this must be balanced against the increased breathing workload produced by the shift of fluids to the central circulation. Decreased weight bearing because of the buoyancy of the patient's body when in water and the support provided by buoyancy and the hydrostatic pressure may also contribute by allowing the therapist to more easily handle the patient.

Exercise in water using a variety of specific approaches, such as neurodevelopmental training (NDT) or the Bad Ragaz method, has been recommended for improving stability and motor control in patients with neurological problems.[135,136] These methods use verbal instructions and tactile cues to guide the patient to practice normal movement progression and sequencing. The challenge of the activities can then be modified by varying the depth of the water or by using the support of one or more flotation devices.

Cardiorespiratory Fitness. Because water-based exercise programs have been shown to maintain and increase aerobic conditioning, exercise in water can be used to provide general conditioning for deconditioned patients or for patients who wish to increase their cardiovascular and respiratory fitness. This form of exercise can be particularly beneficial for cardiac conditioning in patients with conditions such as osteoarthritis or joint instability, which are aggravated by joint loading and thus limit land-based exercise.[137] Water exercise has also been found to benefit patients with chronic obstructive pulmonary disease (COPD).[30,46] A 2013 systematic review and meta-analysis that included five studies with 176 participants with COPD, 71 of whom participated in water-based exercise, found that water-based exercise improved walking endurance and quality of life,[62] and more recent research supports that water-based exercise has greater benefits than land-based exercise for respiratory and skeletal muscle function in patients with COPD.[138]

Increased cardiac output resulting from the hydrostatic pressure of water immersion, as described previously, has led some authors to investigate the effects of exercise in water for cardiac rehabilitation, particularly for patients with musculoskeletal comorbidities that limit land-based exercise.[139] A meta-analysis of studies of aquatic exercise in patients with stable heart failure found aquatic exercise to be more effective for improving walking endurance and peak power than land-based exercise while providing similar benefits for $\dot{V}O_{2max}$, muscle strength, and quality of life.[39] Aquatic exercise has also been recommended as a safe and effective method for high-intensity interval training to improve cardiometabolic health for both clinical and athletic populations.[40]

Exercise in Water During Pregnancy. Exercise in water may be particularly appropriate for pregnant women because this form of exercise unloads the weight-bearing joints; controls peripheral edema; and causes less elevation of heart rate, blood pressure, and body temperature than similar exercise performed on dry land.[67,140-142] Pregnant women who participated in a 1-hour water exercise program three times weekly for 6 weeks had less physical discomfort, greater mobility, and improved body image and health-promoting behaviors than control subjects who did not exercise.[143] The American College of Obstetricians and Gynecologists recommends that women continue to exercise during pregnancy and states that "the principles of exercise prescription for pregnant women do not differ from those for the general population," with a goal of 20 to 30 minutes per day of moderate-intensity exercise on most or all days of the week.[144] Aquatic exercise has also been shown to help prevent excessive maternal weight gain during pregnancy, preserve birth weight, and lower the risk of postpartum depression.[145,146]

Immersion in water, and thus upright exercise or even immersion in an upright position in water, places hydrostatic pressure on the immersed areas and can help reduce peripheral edema in pregnant patients. This effect is the result of improved venous and lymphatic flow and renal-influenced diuresis caused by the hydrostatic pressure of water on the lower extremities. Because hydrostatic pressure increases at increasing depths of water, control of peripheral edema is most marked when the patient exercises in an upright position to produce the greatest pressure on the distal lower extremities.

> **Clinical Pearl**
>
> Water-based exercise is particularly appropriate during pregnancy because it unloads the weight-bearing joints; controls peripheral edema; and causes less elevation of heart rate, blood pressure, and body temperature than similar exercise on dry land.

Exercise-Induced Asthma. Water-based exercise, including swimming, is well suited to patients with exercise-induced asthma, particularly children, because the water environment may reduce the incidence of asthma in these individuals while increasing their fitness.[63,64,147-149]

Age-Related Deficits. Although exercise in general can benefit older adults, aquatic exercise is thought to be particularly helpful for this population for improving strength, functional mobility, balance, and quality of life, with less risk than other forms of exercise.[150-153] The buoyancy of water helps alleviate pressure on degenerated intraarticular structures during exercise and helps support people who have poor balance. Working against the resistance of water can provide finely adjustable resistance to help increase strength.

SUPERFICIAL HEATING OR COOLING

Warm or cold water can be used clinically to heat or cool superficial tissues. Warm water and cold water transfer heat primarily by conduction, whereas warm and cold whirlpools transfer heat by convection. The effects and clinical applications of heating or cooling superficial tissues with water are the same as those of other superficial heating or cooling agents, as described in detail in Chapter 8. However, water has certain advantages over most other superficial thermal agents: it provides perfect contact with the skin, even in very contoured areas; it does not need to be fastened to the body; it has high thermal conductivity and specific heat; and it allows movement during heating or cooling. Its primary disadvantage is that when applied to the extremities only, the distal extremity must be in a dependent position, which may aggravate edema. However, the edema-producing effect of the dependent position is somewhat counteracted during immersion by the compression produced by the water's hydrostatic pressure.

Contraindications and Precautions for Hydrotherapy and Negative Pressure Wound Therapy

Although hydrotherapy is a relatively safe treatment modality, its use is contraindicated in some circumstances, and it should be applied with caution in others. When hot or cold water is applied to a patient, all the contraindications and precautions that apply to the use of other superficial heating or cooling agents, as described in Chapter 8, also apply. In addition, certain contraindications and precautions apply specifically to the application of hydrotherapy by nonimmersion methods, to the application of NPWT, and to full-body immersion hydrotherapy in a pool. These are listed in the following boxes and are discussed in detail in the text.

NONIMMERSION HYDROTHERAPY

✱ PRECAUTIONS

for Nonimmersion Hydrotherapy

- Maceration
- Recent skin grafts
- May not be effective

Maceration Around a Wound

Caution should be taken to minimize the wetting of intact skin surrounding a wound because this can cause or aggravate maceration of this skin. Intact skin around a wound should also be gently and thoroughly dried after any type of hydrotherapy to minimize the risk of maceration.

Recent Skin Grafts

Extra care should be taken when treating recent skin grafts with hydrotherapy because a graft may not tolerate high levels of mechanical agitation or may not have a sufficient vascular response to compensate for extremes of heat or cold. Therefore, near a graft, the water pressure should be kept at a minimum while still being effective, and water with neutral warmth (33°C to 35.5°C [92°F to 96°F]) or mild warmth (35.5°C to 37°C [96°F to 98°F]) should be used.

May Not Be Effective

Because nonimmersion hydrotherapy does not provide buoyancy or hydrostatic pressure, it is effective for only a limited number of problems that can be addressed by hydrotherapy. Nonimmersion hydrotherapy can be used for cleansing but should not be used when cardiovascular, respiratory, musculoskeletal, or renal effects of immersion are desired. Nonimmersion hydrotherapy also produces little heat transfer because water contact with the tissue is so brief.

NEGATIVE PRESSURE WOUND THERAPY

✱ CONTRAINDICATIONS

for Negative Pressure Wound Therapy[154]

- Necrotic tissue with eschar present
- Untreated osteomyelitis
- Malignancy in the wound
- Untreated malnutrition
- Exposed blood vessels, nerves, anastomotic sites, or organs
- Nonenteric and unexplored fistulas

Necrotic Tissue with Eschar Present

NPWT will not debride necrotic tissue and therefore should be applied only after a wound has been cleansed and is free of necrotic tissue and **eschar**. NPWT can then promote the healing of potentially viable tissue.

> ▪ **Assess**
> • Examine the wound bed for necrotic tissue, and debride as much as possible before applying NPWT.

Untreated Osteomyelitis

NPWT should not be applied in an area of untreated osteomyelitis because this treatment may promote soft tissue growth over infected bone or promote the spread of infection.

> ▪ **Assess**
> • Examine all wounds for exposed bone.

If exposed bone is noted, the physician should complete an evaluation for osteonecrosis before applying NPWT.

Malignancy

Because NPWT may promote the growth of any tissue, including malignant tissue, it should not be applied in an area of malignancy.

Untreated Malnutrition

Wounds require adequate nutrition to obtain the energy and substrates needed for healing. Therefore, malnutrition should be treated before NPWT is initiated.

> ▪ **Assess**
> • Request evaluation by a nutritionist before initiating NPWT.

Exposed Blood Vessels, Nerves, Anastomotic Sites, or Organs

Because of concerns that the force of NPWT may damage exposed blood vessels, nerves, anastomotic sites, or organs, this intervention should be avoided in such areas.

Nonenteric and Unexplored Fistulas

Application of NPWT over a fistula may cause excessive fluid loss and damage. Careful exploration of the fistula should be performed by a physician to determine whether the application of NPWT is appropriate. Occasionally, NPWT may be applied to enteric (bowel) fistulas.

> ▪ **Assess**
> • Examine the wound bed for exposed arteries, veins, or organs.

for Negative Pressure Wound Therapy
- High risk of bleeding (e.g., anticoagulant therapy, difficult hemostasis)
- Confusion or disorientation

High Risk of Bleeding (e.g., Anticoagulant Therapy, Difficult Hemostasis)

NPWT should be applied with caution to patients with a high risk of bleeding, such as those taking anticoagulant therapy, including warfarin (Coumadin) and heparin, or where there may be difficulty with hemostasis. Patients with a high risk of bleeding are at risk for excessive blood loss with NPWT, and this can be fatal.

■ **Ask the Patient**
- "Are you taking an anticoagulant or blood thinner? Which?"

■ **Assess**
- If the patient is taking an anticoagulant, check with their physician before initiating NPWT. If NPWT is initiated, carefully check the area for signs of bleeding, and discontinue treatment if bleeding occurs.

Confusion or Disorientation

NPWT should be used with caution in patients who are confused or disoriented because such patients may inadvertently disrupt the operation of the dressing or the negative pressure suction device.

IMMERSION FORMS OF HYDROTHERAPY

★ **CONTRAINDICATIONS**

for Immersion Forms of Hydrotherapy
- Cardiac instability
- Confusion or impaired cognition
- Maceration around a wound
- Bleeding
- Infection in the area to be immersed
- Bowel incontinence
- Severe epilepsy
- Suicidal patients

Cardiac Instability

Full-body immersion is contraindicated in patients with cardiac instability, such as uncontrolled hypertension or heart failure, because the heart in such circumstances may be unable to adapt sufficiently in response to the changes in circulation produced by hydrotherapy to maintain cardiac homeostasis.

■ **Assess**
- Check with the patient's physician and review the patient's chart to determine whether any cardiac instability is present.

Heart rate and blood pressure should be monitored during and after immersion in all patients with a history of cardiac problems.

Confusion or Impaired Cognition

When patients are confused or have impaired cognition, immersion hydrotherapy in a pool should be applied only with the direct supervision of the therapist in the pool because of the risk of drowning.

■ **Assess**
- Check the patient's level of cognition and alertness. Check whether the patient can effectively communicate discomfort.

When a patient is confused or is unable to effectively report discomfort or other problems for any reason, immersion hydrotherapy in a pool should be applied only if the therapist can be in the pool directly supervising the patient.

Maceration Around a Wound

Immersion hydrotherapy is contraindicated when maceration of intact skin is present around a wound because treatment is likely to increase the maceration and thus increase the size of the wound.

■ **Assess**
- Inspect the skin around the wound for signs of maceration, including pallor and other early indications of breakdown.

When maceration around a wound is noted, prolonged immersion should be avoided. If the cleansing benefits of hydrotherapy are desired, nonimmersion techniques should be used.

Bleeding

Immersion hydrotherapy in warm or hot water should not be applied if bleeding is noted in or near an area being considered for treatment because immersion hydrotherapy may increase bleeding by promoting venous circulation through hydrostatic pressure and may increase arterial circulation as a result of vasodilation.

■ **Assess**
- Check for bleeding in or near the area being considered for treatment.
- If bleeding is mild and has been determined not to be dangerous to the patient, nonimmersion hydrotherapy may be used.

Infection in the Area to Be Immersed

Immersion hydrotherapy is no longer recommended for the treatment of wounds. Patients with infectious conditions that may be spread by water should avoid any type of hydrotherapy in which the water is not changed between uses. Therefore, patients with open wounds should not immerse the wounds in a pool.

> ▪ **Assess**
> • Check the skin for open wounds.

Bowel Incontinence

Patients with bowel incontinence may not be immersed in water that will be used by other patients. In a patient with both bowel incontinence and open wounds, care should be taken to avoid contaminating the water and thus the wound with bacteria from the patient's own feces.

> ▪ **Assess**
> • Check the patient's chart for any notation regarding bowel incontinence.

Nonimmersion forms of hydrotherapy can be used to treat open wounds in patients with bowel incontinence.

Severe Epilepsy

Full-body immersion hydrotherapy should not be applied to patients with poorly controlled epilepsy because such patients are at increased risk of drowning.

Suicidal Patients

Full-body immersion hydrotherapy should not be applied to suicidal patients because they are at increased risk of drowning.

★ PRECAUTIONS

for Immersion Forms of Hydrotherapy

• Impaired thermal sensation in the area to be immersed
• Alcohol ingestion by the patient
• Limited strength, endurance, balance, or ROM
• Medications
• Urinary incontinence
• Fear of water
• Respiratory problems

Impaired Thermal Sensation in the Area to Be Immersed

Areas with impaired thermal sensation have an increased risk for burns. To minimize this, always use a thermometer and your hand to check the temperature of the water to be used for hydrotherapy before the patient enters.

> ▪ **Ask the Patient**
> • "Can you feel heat and cold in this area?"
>
> ▪ **Assess**
> • Test thermal sensation by applying test tubes filled with cold or warm water to the area and asking the patient to report the sensation of the stimulus.

If the patient has impaired thermal sensation, only water close to body temperature should be used for applying hydrotherapy.

Alcohol Ingestion

Full-body water immersion should be avoided if the patient has ingested alcohol because the impairment of judgment and cognitive functions that occurs with intoxication and the hypotensive effects of alcohol ingestion can increase the risk of drowning.

> ▪ **Ask the Patient**
> • "Have you had a drink of alcohol in the last few hours?" (Ask if you suspect that a patient has recently been drinking alcohol—for example, if you smell alcohol on the patient's breath.)

Limited Strength, Endurance, Balance, or Range of Motion

Although hydrotherapy is frequently used to treat limitations of strength, endurance, balance, or ROM, extreme limitations in any of these pose a safety hazard for full-body immersion hydrotherapy. Therefore, for full-body immersion treatment, a patient must have the ability to hold their head above water or, if unable to do so, must be well and safely secured with their head above water. Direct, hands-on assistance, with the therapist in the water, can be provided for patients who have difficulty doing this.

> ▪ **Assess**
> • Check strength, balance, and ROM before the patient enters the water.

If any of these are significantly limited, secure the patient so that their head cannot enter the water, or accompany the patient into the water, at least for the first treatment, to assess the patient's safety.

Medications

Some medications, particularly medications used to treat cardiovascular disease, alter the cardiovascular response to exercise. Therefore, for any patient taking medications, it is recommended that a physician be consulted to establish safe limits of the patient's cardiovascular response before an aquatic exercise program is begun.

Urinary Incontinence

A patient with urinary incontinence may be catheterized to allow full-body immersion hydrotherapy; however, this is generally not recommended because immersion may increase the risk of urinary tract infection in a catheterized patient.

Fear of Water

Patients having a fear of water will generally refuse to participate in immersion hydrotherapy. Alternative treatments, such as immersing only the area requiring treatment, using nonimmersion hydrotherapy, or using an intervention such as exercise on dry land, should be considered.

Respiratory Problems

Although water-based exercise can provide respiratory and general conditioning for patients with exercise-induced asthma or other breathing problems, water immersion increases the work of breathing, so patients with respiratory problems should be carefully monitored for signs of respiratory distress throughout their immersion. Some patients with asthma may be sensitive to chlorine and other agents used to decontaminate exercise pools and whirlpools; these patients should be closely monitored.

★ PRECAUTIONS

for Full-Body Immersion in Hot or Very Warm Water
- Pregnancy
- Multiple sclerosis
- Poor thermal regulation

Pregnancy

Maternal hyperthermia has been found to be teratogenic and is associated with a variety of central nervous system abnormalities in the child. Therefore full-body immersion in a hot pool should be avoided during pregnancy to minimize the possibility of maternal hyperthermia, particularly during the first trimester, when the effects of heat are most hazardous to the fetus.[140,155]

> ■ **Ask the Patient**
> - "Are you pregnant?"
> - "Do you think you might be pregnant?"

Multiple Sclerosis

Patients with multiple sclerosis should not be placed in a hot or warm pool because increasing their body temperature can increase their fatigue and other symptoms.[156]

Poor Thermal Regulation

Thermal regulation in response to body heating is generally accomplished by a combination of conduction, convection, radiation, and evaporation. If a small area of the body is immersed in hot water, a patient with impaired thermal regulation may still be able to dissipate heat by conduction to areas in direct contact with the heated area and by direct radiation of heat from the skin; however, the production of sweat and the dissipation of heat through convection by blood circulating from other areas that have not been heated may be impaired. Because all these mechanisms are impaired when large areas of the body are heated, such as occurs with full-body immersion in hot or warm water, a patient with poor thermal regulation may be at risk for thermal shock if large areas of their body are immersed in hot water.

> ■ **Assess**
> - Check for any history of thermal shock or any other signs of poor thermal regulation.

Because thermal regulation is frequently impaired in elderly adults and in infants, warm or hot water hydrotherapy should be limited to small areas in these individuals.

Adverse Effects of Hydrotherapy

HYPONATREMIA

Immersion hydrotherapy has been associated with hyponatremia in patients with extensive burn wounds.[155] Hyponatremia occurs because these patients can lose salt from open wounds into the water if the water's salinity is less than that of tissue fluids. To minimize the possibility of this occurring, salt should be added to the water when treating these patients.[157]

INFECTION

A number of reports have documented the association of both immersion hydrotherapy and NPWT with wound infections.[76–78,158] This is thought to occur because bacteria from one patient can lodge in a whirlpool and be transmitted to others and because these interventions can trap bacteria in the wound. This risk can be reduced by using nonimmersion hydrotherapy techniques or, when using immersion, by installing a whirlpool liner and strictly adhering to cleaning protocols. However, nonimmersion hydrotherapy with pulsed lavage to clean wounds can aerosolize wound bacteria, which then contaminates exposed surfaces and is inhaled by both the clinician and the patient.[88] Special precautions, as described subsequently, must therefore be taken to protect both the patient being treated and others from infection by wound bacteria.

DROWNING

The most severe potential adverse effect of hydrotherapy is death by drowning, and it is imperative that adequate precautions be taken to minimize this risk. The American Red Cross has identified the three most common causes of drowning to be (1) failure to recognize hazardous conditions and practices, (2) inability to get out of dangerous situations, and (3) lack of knowledge of the safest ways to aid a drowning person.[159] Specific recommendations for safety precautions to be taken to minimize the risk of drowning are provided in the "Safety Issues Regarding Hydrotherapy" section.

BURNS, FAINTING, AND BLEEDING

Treatment by immersion in warm or hot water has the risks associated with other forms of superficial thermotherapy, including burning, fainting, and bleeding. To minimize the possibility of any of these occurring, the water temperature should be kept within the appropriate range and should always be checked with a thermometer and the therapist's hand before the patient touches the water. The use of hot water should be avoided when treating elderly patients, very young patients, and patients with impaired sensation or other neurological deficits because they are at increased risk of burns.[160]

The risk of fainting as a result of hypotension is greatest when large areas of the patient's body are immersed in warm or hot water. This risk is further increased in patients taking antihypertensive medications. Therefore, to minimize the possibility of fainting, only the parts of the body requiring treatment in warm water should be immersed, and all patients taking antihypertensive medications should be closely monitored. All patients should be well supported during warm water immersion to prevent falling should they faint.

AGGRAVATION OF EDEMA

Immersion in hot or warm water has been shown to increase edema in the hands of patients with upper extremity disorders[159]; this effect becomes more pronounced as the temperature of the water increases.[105] Therefore to avoid aggravating edema, use only cool water, and avoid having the extremity in a dependent position in the water when signs of acute inflammation are present.

ASTHMA EXACERBATION

The humidity around exercise pools and whirlpools may help alleviate the symptoms of exercise-induced asthma, but exposure to chlorinated pools can reduce forced expiratory volume in patients with asthma, even if they have no symptoms.[161] Additionally, some research suggests that children exposed to swimming pools with chlorinated water may be at increased risk of developing asthma, but the evidence for this association is only suggestive and not conclusive.[162] In addition, various studies suggest that swimming pool workers are at increased risk for respiratory symptoms, likely related to exposure to trichloramine and reduced ventilation around the pool.[163-165] Patients with asthma using chlorinated exercise pools or whirlpools should be closely monitored for asthma symptoms.

Adverse Effects of Negative Pressure Wound Therapy

The U.S. FDA has issued a warning that a number of adverse events, including some deaths from bleeding, have been reported with the use of NPWT when used for certain wound types that are contraindications (see box, " Contraindications for the Use of Negative Pressure Wound Therapy").[158] Specifically, there have been reports of retention of foam or liner dressings in the wound, blood vessel perforation, and cardiac rupture. Patients should be selected carefully for NPWT based on their individual risk factors and wound types.

Application Techniques

This section provides guidelines on the sequence of procedures required for safe and effective application of hydrotherapy and NPWT.

GENERAL HYDROTHERAPY

Hydrotherapy may be applied in several circumstances, but it must first be determined whether this is the best intervention for the patient. Following is a list of steps for the use of hydrotherapy in general.

APPLICATION TECHNIQUE 19.1   GENERAL HYDROTHERAPY

Procedure

1. Evaluate the patient and set the goals of treatment.
2. Determine whether hydrotherapy is the most appropriate intervention.

    Hydrotherapy may be an appropriate intervention when progress toward the goals of treatment can be achieved through wound cleansing and debridement, controlling edema, or exercise in a water environment. Hydrotherapy is the ideal intervention for wound cleansing and debridement when a moderate amount of debris or necrotic tissue is present. When a large amount of necrotic tissue is present, more aggressive treatment, such as surgical debridement, may be required. If a wound is clean, hydrotherapy is not indicated, although NPWT may be appropriate. Exercise in water is indicated for patients with load-sensitive conditions or when the benefits of resistance or hydrostatic pressure of water can promote progress toward the goals of treatment.

3. Determine that hydrotherapy is not contraindicated for this patient or this condition.

    The treatment area should be inspected for the presence of open wounds, rash, or other signs of infection, and sensation in the area should be assessed. The patient's chart should be checked for previous adverse responses to hydrotherapy, and the patient should be asked pertinent questions regarding contraindications. It is recommended that heart rate and blood pressure be measured and recorded if a large area of the body will be immersed.

4. Select the appropriate form of hydrotherapy according to the condition to be treated and the desired treatment effects. Select from the following list (see specific application recommendations for each hydrotherapy agent):
    • Nonimmersion irrigation device
    • Pool

    The form of hydrotherapy selected should produce the desired treatment effects, be appropriate for the size of the area to be treated, allow for adequate safety and control of infection, and be cost-effective. Advantages and disadvantages of the different forms of hydrotherapy, based on treatment goals, are provided here, together with directions for their application. Detailed information on safety and infection control is provided in the section on safety issues. Because adequate infection control is very difficult if not impossible to achieve when using a whirlpool sequentially for different patients, some of whom may have open wounds, the use of whirlpools is generally no longer recommended.[84] Therefore their use is not discussed here. Readers needing detailed information on the use and cleaning of whirlpools are referred to earlier editions of this book.

    Explain to the patient the procedure, the reason for applying hydrotherapy, and the sensations the patient can expect to feel.

    During the application of hydrotherapy, the patient may feel a sensation of warmth or cold, depending on the temperature of the water used. The patient will also feel gentle pressure if the water is being agitated. The patient should not feel either excessive hot or cold or excessive pressure, and the patient should not feel faint. In general, hydrotherapy is not painful unless it is being used in conjunction with debridement for burns or other sensate wounds. Pain associated with this procedure can usually be reduced by administering high-dose analgesics before beginning hydrotherapy.

5. Apply the appropriate form of hydrotherapy.
6. When hydrotherapy is completed, assess the outcome of treatment. Remeasure and assess progress relative to the initial patient evaluation and the goals of treatment.
7. Document the treatment.

NONIMMERSION IRRIGATION AND PULSED LAVAGE

A variety of devices, including handheld showers, syringes, and purpose-designed pulsatile irrigation units, can apply hydrotherapy without immersing the area to be treated, by spraying water onto the treatment area.[78,101] Nonimmersion irrigation devices are particularly well suited for applying hydrotherapy to open wounds because they involve less risk of infection than whirlpools and because some of these devices can spray fluid onto an open wound within the safe yet effective pressure limits of 4 to 15 psi (see Table 19.3). Without immersion, water does not produce buoyancy or hydrostatic pressure and therefore does not reduce weight bearing or edema or increase circulation. Therefore, nonimmersion hydrotherapy should only be used for patients who do not need reduced weight bearing or edema or increased circulation to achieve their treatment goals.

Because electrical pulsatile irrigation devices deliver fluid at a controlled pressure and provide suction to remove contaminated fluid, they are ideally suited to the treatment of open wounds.[166,167] This type of treatment is known as *pulsed lavage* (Fig. 19.15).

Pulsed lavage devices pump an intermittent stream of fluid from an irrigation bag or bottle through tubing to a handpiece that directs the flow of fluid onto the wound (Fig. 19.16). The contaminated fluid is then removed from the treatment area back through the handpiece through other tubing into a collection canister. The handpiece has a trigger to control the flow of fluid and can be fitted with a variety of tips to vary

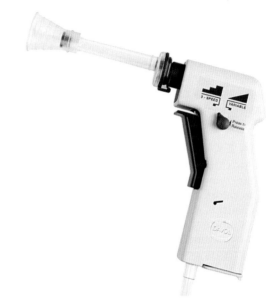

FIGURE 19.15 Pulsed lavage with suction handpiece with tip used to deliver water to the wound bed and to suction contaminated wound. (© 2020 BD. Used with permission.)

the fluid dispersion. On most of these devices, the tubing, handpiece, and tips are discarded after each treatment to minimize the risk of cross-infection. Electrical pulsatile irrigation devices are available in portable and clinical models.

APPLICATION TECHNIQUE 19.2   NONIMMERSION IRRIGATION DEVICE

Equipment Required

- Nonimmersion irrigation (pulsed lavage) device
- Irrigation fluid
- Towels
- Personal protective equipment for the clinician including gloves, waterproof gown, mask/goggles or face shield, and hair cover
- Personal protective equipment for the patient, including surgical mask

Procedure

When applying nonimmersion irrigation, the following guidelines should be used. Because pulsed lavage can spray contaminated fluid, the FDA recommends the use of a private, single-patient room containing only essential equipment. Surfaces at risk for aerosol contamination should be covered. During treatment, the clinician and anyone else in the room must wear full personal protective equipment, including a fluid-proof gown, gloves, mask/goggles or face shield, and hair cover (see Fig. 19.16). The patient should also wear a surgical mask, and all patient lines, ports, and wounds that are not being treated should be covered with a drape or towel. After the treatment of each patient, all surfaces touched by hands must be thoroughly cleaned and disinfected.

To maximize patient comfort and optimize wound healing, clean, warm fluid should always be used for irrigation. Clean, warm water can be used for this procedure, although sterile normal saline is often recommended when irrigation is provided by pulsed lavage. It is recommended that treatment be applied daily for long enough to hydrate hard eschar or loosen debris. The appropriate frequency and

duration of treatment will depend primarily on the size of the wound and the amount of necrotic tissue, exudate, or other debris present. In addition, when an electrical pulsatile irrigation device is used, the following treatment guidelines should be followed. Further specific directions for the use of different brands and models of these devices are provided by the device manufacturers.

1. Although patients may be treated at the bedside with this type of device, all irrigation treatments should be performed in a private room to reduce the risk of transmitting infection.
2. Position patient comfortably to allow access to wound, and pad area with towels or other absorbent materials.
3. Sterile normal saline in 1000-mL bags is generally used as the irrigation fluid. Multiple bags may be needed. In cases of wound infection, antimicrobials may be added. It is recommended that the saline be warmed to 102°F to 106°F by placing it in a basin of hot tap water. Hang the bags of fluid on the device or on an intravenous (IV) pole.
4. Attach tubing, suction canister, handpiece, and irrigation tip to the device.
5. Turn on the pump.
6. Select the treatment pressure. Most devices can spray fluid at pressures of between 0 and 60 psi and have a half-switch to limit the maximum pressure to 30 psi. Pressures of 4 to 15 psi are generally sufficient to clean or debride most wounds; however, the pressure can be adjusted according to the nature of the wound, the tip used, and the sensitivity of the patient. It is recommended that the lowest pressure that effectively loosens and removes debris be used and that the pressure be

APPLICATION TECHNIQUE 19.2—*cont'd*

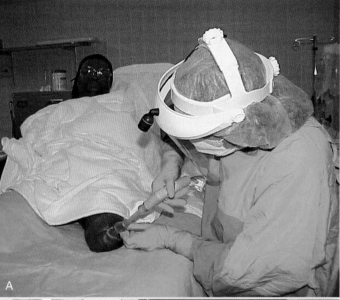

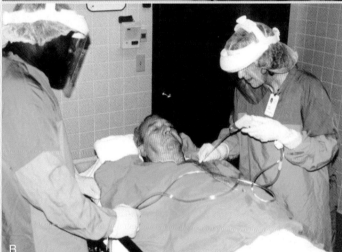

FIGURE 19.16 Using a nonimmersion hydrotherapy device to cleanse and debride a wound. (Courtesy Harriett Loehne, PT, DPT, CWS, FACCWS.)

decreased if the patient complains of pain, if bleeding occurs, or if the tip is near a major or exposed vessel. The pressure may need to be increased in the presence of tough eschar or when a large amount of necrotic tissue is present.

7. Apply the treatment until adequate hydration or debridement is achieved. This typically takes 15 to 30 minutes.

8. This form of treatment may be followed by sharp debridement if necessary to remove adhered necrotic tissue.

9. Dry intact skin with towel and pat open areas gently with sterile gauze to absorb irrigant.

10. Reapply the appropriate wound dressing.

11. Pulsed lavage is generally applied once a day but may be applied more frequently to wounds that have greater than 50% necrotic, nonviable tissue with purulent drainage or a foul odor and less frequently to other wounds. Treatment with this type of device should result in a decrease in necrotic tissue and an increase in granulation within 1 week of treatment initiation. If this does not occur, the treatment approach should be reevaluated.

Advantages

- Control of fluid pressure to stay within a safe and effective range for application to open wounds
- Ability to direct jet of fluid to stay within wound bed
- Does not require filling, draining, and cleaning a whirlpool
- Does not require the patient to be transferred to the whirlpool area
- Uses less fluid than a whirlpool
- Can be used where whirlpool treatment is not recommended, such as with an unresponsive or incontinent patient

Disadvantages

- Requires extensive precautions to minimize risks associated with aerosolization of wound bacteria
- Additional expense of using new tubing, handpiece, and tip for each application
- Does not provide the therapeutic benefits associated with buoyancy and hydrostatic pressure of immersion hydrotherapy

NEGATIVE PRESSURE WOUND THERAPY

NPWT may be used in conjunction with nonimmersion irrigation of wounds to promote wound healing, with the irrigation specifically intended for wound cleansing. NPWT may promote the healing of chronic wounds of various causes, including pressure ulcers, diabetic foot wounds, and large surgical wounds. NPWT involves applying a continuous or intermittent negative (subatmospheric) pressure over a wound bed and using a filler dressing, a covering dressing, and a pump (Fig. 19.17). As discussed earlier, current NPWT devices can also instill topical antimicrobial or antiseptic and remove the waste fluid during NPWT. This is known as *negative pressure wound therapy with instillation* (NPWTi). The most recent development in NPWT is NPWT with instillation and dwell time (NPWTi-d). NPWTi-d combines NPWTi with intermittent, automated, volumetrically controlled instillation of topical wound solutions that stay on the wound for a fixed period, called the *dwell time,* rather being continuously fed and removed. Further research is needed to fully evaluate the potential additional benefits of NPWTi-d.[168]

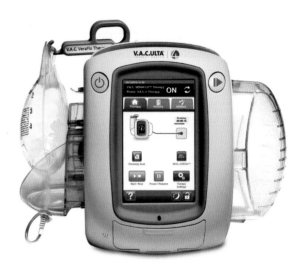

FIGURE 19.17 Negative pressure wound therapy unit. (Used with Permission. Courtesy 3M.)

APPLICATION TECHNIQUE 19.3   NEGATIVE PRESSURE WOUND THERAPY[14]

Note: These are general instructions for NPWT, including recommendations for instillation with or without dwell time. Because devices from different manufacturers vary, the clinician must check for specific instructions for the device being used.

Equipment Required

- NPWT pump
  Pumps of different sizes and made by different manufacturers are available. Smaller devices, often intended for surgical wounds, are generally single-use disposable units.
- Canister
  Traditional, full-size NPWT devices usually come with canisters that hold 250 to 1000 mL. Smaller, portable, disposable NPWT devices have small canisters or may not have any, relying on the fluid to absorb and evaporate through the wound dressing.
- Dressings
  In general, dressings for NPWT consist of an optional nonadherent layer placed directly on the wound bed, an absorbent wound filling, and a transparent layer that seals over the top of the wound. Different devices may have specific-purpose-designed dressings. In addition, some of the small, portable NPWT devices are intended to be used with premade complete layered dressings.
- A nonadherent dressing may be placed directly on the wound before the dressing that fills the wound to prevent dressings from adhering to the wound.
- A dressing that fills the wound is generally a foam or saline-moistened gauze. This is intended to absorb fluid and to prevent the transparent film from being pressed against the wound bed when suction is applied. The selection of a filler generally depends on the specific device being used. Gauze fillers have been found to be as effective as foam fillers, tend to adhere less to the wound bed, and are less expensive.[169]
- A transparent film dressing seals over the wound bed to keep the periwound skin dry and to allow the suction to be effective.
- Drain tubing
- Irrigation fluid
  Irrigation fluid may be used to cleanse the wound using pulsed lavage before applying the NPWT dressings or may be instilled into

the dressing of NPWTi or NPWTi-d devices. Various instillation fluids have been used, including water, saline, antibiotics, and other antimicrobials, but[14] normal saline is the preferred solution, except in special situations.[19]

- Gloves

Procedure

1. Prepare the wound for NPWT.
   a. Remove old wound dressings and clean the wound bed using an irrigation device and normal saline.
   b. Clean and dry the periwound area.
   c. Inspect the wound bed for any contraindications, including necrotic tissue; untreated osteomyelitis; bleeding; malignancy in the wound; exposed arteries, veins, nerves, anastomotic sites, or organs; or nonenteric and unexplored fistulas. If any of these are found, do not use this type of treatment.
2. Apply contact layer and filling dressing.
   a. If the previous dressing adheres to the wound, consider placing a nonadherent mesh dressing contact layer directly on the wound before placing the filling dressing in the wound. Cover superficial or retention sutures with a single layer of nonadherent dressing.
   b. Assess wound size and shape. Cut or select a filling dressing of a size that can be gently placed into the wound without overlapping intact, periwound skin. Gently place the filling dressing into the wound bed, ensuring contact with all wound surfaces and avoiding contact with the periwound skin. Do not pack or force the dressing into any part of the wound. Do not place the dressing into blind or unexplored tunnels where the distal aspect is not visible.
3. Apply the transparent film dressing. *Note:* Depending on the specific device, the drain tube (step 4 in these directions) will be placed *before* or *after* the transparent film dressing.
   a. Select, trim, and place the transparent film to cover the dressing inside the wound and an additional 3 to 5 cm of intact periwound skin. The dressing may be cut into multiple pieces if necessary. Do not discard excess transparent film; this may be needed later to patch difficult areas.

APPLICATION TECHNIQUE 19.3—*cont'd*

b. Place the transparent film, adhesive side down, over the filling dressing in the wound and over the intact periwound skin. Do not pull or stretch the transparent film over the filling dressing. Minimize wrinkles to avoid pressure leaks.

c. Pat the transparent film around its margins to ensure a good seal.

4. Place the drain tube, and if using NPWTi-d, place the instillation tube. *Note:* Depending on the specific device, the tube(s) will be placed *before* or *after* the transparent film dressing.

   a. Choose the tube application site, taking into consideration fluid flow and tubing position to allow for optimal drainage; avoid placing over bony prominences or within tissue creases.

   b. If the tubing is applied before the transparent film dressing, the tubing should generally be placed on top of the first layer of wound filling dressing.

   c. If the tubing is applied after the transparent film dressing, pinch the transparent film and cut a 2-cm hole through it large enough to allow for removal of fluid or exudate. Cut a hole rather than a slit because a slit may self-seal during therapy. Apply the tubing directly over the hole in the transparent film. Apply gentle pressure on the tubing and skirt to ensure complete adhesion.

5. Connect the drain tubing and, if using NPWTi-d, the instillation tube to the NPWT unit.

   a. Place the canister in the NPWT unit.

   b. Connect the drain and canister tubing, and ensure that the clamps on each tube are open. Some devices have additional connection tubing to attach to the drain tubing and the NPWT unit.

6. If using NPWTi-d, hang instillation solution and connect instillation tubing to the solution. Instillation solution is usually normal saline.

7. Turn on and set the NPWT unit.

   a. Turn on the NPWT unit. Most units have a rechargeable battery; check that the unit powers up. Select the appropriate settings, including the amount and timing (continuous or intermittent) of the pressure and, with NPWTi-d, the dwell time. Target pressures generally are between −50 and −200 mm Hg and vary according to the device, manufacturers' instructions, filler dressing, and patient's comfort. Dwell times are typically 10 to 20 minutes but can be anywhere from 1 to 30 minutes depending on solution and the size and location of wound.

   b. Assess the transparent film dressing to ensure it seals properly. If so, the dressing will contract and collapse, and there

should be no hissing sounds. Secure excess tubing to prevent interference with the patient's mobility.

8. Treatment time and ongoing management

   a. It is recommended that NPWT be on for 22 out of 24 hours for best results.

   b. Check the dressing every 2 or 3 hours to ensure that the seal is still intact, no bleeding is occurring, and the device is running. Leaks may be patched with an additional piece of transparent film dressing. The unit may be disconnected for shorter periods of time without replacing the dressing. If treatment is stopped for longer than 2 hours, the dressings should be removed, the wound irrigated, and the dressings replaced.

   c. An alarm will sound when the canister is full. Change the canister when it becomes full or at least once a week to control odor. Large (1000-mL) canisters should not be used for patients at risk of bleeding or for elderly patients or children, who cannot tolerate a large loss of fluid volume.

   d. The dressing should be changed two to four times per week, depending on the filler dressing, the amount of exudates, and specific manufacturer instructions. More frequent dressing changes, up to every 12 to 24 hours, may be needed if the wound is infected. Before a new dressing is applied, be sure that all of the old dressing, including any nonadhesive dressing, filler, and film, is removed.

   e. If using NPWTi-d, this is typically performed in 2- to 4-hour therapy cycles.

   f. The wound should be reassessed at 2 weeks for signs of healing. The average length of treatment is 4 to 6 weeks.

Advantages

- Enhances wound healing
- Provides continuous coverage to large wounds, reducing wound contamination and infection risk
- Can allow instillation of wound-cleansing solution
- Comfortable
- Maintains optimally moist wound environment while keeping surrounding skin dry
- Infrequent dressing changes reduce mechanical disruption and cooling of healing tissues.

Disadvantages

- More expensive in the short run than standard dressing changes
- Patient is tethered to suction unit.
- Potential for skin irritation from the adhesive dressing
- More time-consuming to set up than standard dressing changes

EXERCISE POOL

To optimize the cardiovascular, respiratory, renal, and psychological benefits of hydrotherapy, an exercise pool that allows full-body immersion and exercise is recommended, unless immersing the patient in water that will be used by other individuals is contraindicated. An exercise pool is generally the optimal way to apply hydrotherapy to achieve the musculoskeletal benefits associated with water immersion, although a whirlpool may be used when only the extremities require immersion.

Swimming pools and specialized hydrotherapy pools can be used for hydrotherapy. Most swimming pools are at least 100 feet

long and 25 feet wide, have a maximum depth of 8 feet, and have a sloping bottom allowing gradual descent. Most specialized hydrotherapy pools are smaller than a swimming pool and position the patient in the middle or at the edge of the pool to perform specific types of exercises. Some hydrotherapy pools are equipped with an underwater treadmill, an adjustable water flow rate, adjustable depths, and movable floors to provide graded exercise activity (Fig. 19.18).[170,171] An exercise pool may be available in the clinic, or the patient may have access to a public or private swimming pool. Depending on its size, either type of pool may be used for individual or group treatment with a therapist present or for independent home exercise.

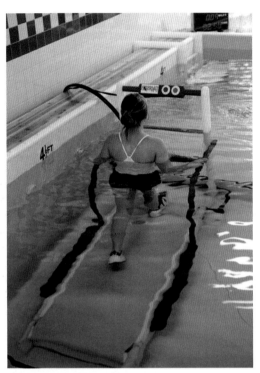

FIGURE 19.18 Purpose-designed exercise pool with treadmill. (Courtesy Hudson Aquatics, Angola, IN.)

Pool Temperature

The water temperature in an exercise pool should be kept at 26°C to 36°C (79°F to 97°F). The amount of movement performed by the patient should be used to determine the optimal temperature within this range. The warmer end of the range, 34°C to 36°C (93°F to 97°F), should be used for low-intensity activities, such as light exercise by deconditioned patients or patients with arthritis. Warmer temperatures are more comfortable and help patients who move less to conserve body heat while in the water. The cooler end of the range, 26°C to 28°C (79°F to 82°F), is recommended for recreational pools or when more intense exercise will be performed because the cooler temperature dissipates heat produced by patients, thereby allowing them to perform more exercise or more vigorous exercise with less fatigue. The water temperature should not be allowed to be below 18.5°C (65°F) because such low temperatures can impair the ability of muscles to contract.

> ### ◎ Clinical Pearl
>
> The temperature of an exercise pool should be kept at 26°C to 36°C (79°F to 97°F), with the warmer end of the range being used for low-intensity activities and the cooler end of the range being used for vigorous exercise.

APPLICATION TECHNIQUE 19.4   POOL EXERCISE

Equipment Required

- Appropriate space for pool—adequate size, support, ventilation, and heating
- Space to store auxiliary equipment, including chemicals and mechanical systems
- Space for patients to shower and change clothes
- Water supply
- Nonslip area around the pool
- Safety equipment
- Infection control equipment, including pump and filter, chemicals, and testing kit
- Towels
- Thermometer

Procedure

1. The patient and the therapist should wear bathing suits for pool exercise. The therapist may wear light clothing over the bathing suit if not planning to enter the water except in the case of an emergency.
2. The therapist should help the patient enter the pool if necessary. Provide ramps, stairs, a ladder, or a lift when needed.
3. The patient may perform activities to improve strength, cardiovascular fitness, endurance, or functional activities, as determined by the evaluation and plan of care. Activities may include upright exercise, walking in the pool, swimming, or other forms of exercise. The patient may use flotation devices, a tether, or other objects to alter resistance or the buoyancy effects of the water. Water-based exercise programs can be progressed by increasing the number of repetitions of an activity, increasing the speed of the activity, changing the length of the lever arm,

decreasing the degree of stabilization provided, or using larger floats to increase resistance. More detailed descriptions of water exercise programs are beyond the scope of this text and can be found in books devoted to aquatic therapy.
4. The therapist should stay with the patient throughout treatment and should monitor vital signs during exercise if the patient has risk factors or any history indicating that this may be necessary. For example, heart rate and blood pressure should be monitored in patients recovering from myocardial infarction, and heart rate should be monitored in pregnant patients.
5. After completion of water activities, the therapist should help the patient to get out of the pool if necessary. The patient should dry their body and immediately wrap up to avoid chilling.

Advantages

- Patient can move freely during exercises, with less risk of falling.
- Decreases weight bearing on joints—with immersion in water 60 inches deep, weight bearing on lower extremities is reduced by 88% to 95%.
- Buoyancy may assist weak muscles, allowing increased performance of more active exercise.

Disadvantages

- Risk of falling when patient gets into and out of the water because water around pool can make the floor slippery
- Risk of infection from other individuals who have been in the water
- Difficulty stabilizing or isolating body parts during exercise
- Risk of drowning
- Fear among some patients of water immersion

Safety Issues Regarding Hydrotherapy

To optimize safety and infection control during hydrotherapy, the following general guidelines should be followed.[172,173] A facility hydrotherapy safety and infection control program that addresses the specific needs of the facility should be developed in collaboration with an infection control specialist or with the facility's infection control committee. This program should take into account the specific safety hazards associated with this type of treatment and the types of microorganisms most commonly encountered at that time and place. The program must comply with the guidelines, rules, and regulations of the local public health department. Infection control experts should be consulted if a problem with infection control arises, such as frequent patient infections after the use of hydrotherapy.

SAFETY PRECAUTIONS AND INFECTION CONTROL FOR EXERCISE POOLS
Safety

Personnel Training. Individuals responsible for cleaning, disinfecting, and maintaining an exercise pool must be trained in the use and hazards of the chemicals used. They should also be provided with the appropriate protective clothing and equipment for handling these substances.

Staff working with individuals in the pool should have lifesaving and rescue training and knowledge of personal water safety techniques. At a minimum, they should be certified to perform cardiopulmonary resuscitation (CPR) and to provide advanced first aid. Ideally, a certified lifeguard should be present whenever anyone is in the pool. Staff should be trained in emergency evacuation procedures and should know the emergency action plan.

Safety in and Around the Pool. To ensure safety around an exercise pool and to minimize the risk of a patient slipping and falling, the area surrounding the pool should have nonslip surfaces. Pool regulations, water depth, emergency procedures, and phone numbers should be clearly posted in the pool area. Means of entering the pool should be appropriate for the ambulatory ability of the patients and may include stairs, ramps, ladders, or lifts for nonambulatory or impaired patients. For safety in the pool, the depth of the water should be clearly marked at intervals around the pool edge, and handgrip bars should be provided all the way around the edge of the pool.

The pool should be evacuated during power outages and floods, and outdoor pools should not be used during electrical storms. Emergency equipment should be kept near the pool at all times, and all such equipment should be inspected regularly. Emergency equipment should include a shepherd's crook, a life ring, a rescue tube, resuscitation equipment, a spine board, a blanket, scissors, and a first aid kit.

All chemicals for use in the pool should be kept in their original containers, off the floor, and in a locked cabinet. Material Safety Data Sheets for all chemicals must be maintained and filed in compliance with Occupational Safety and Health Administration (OSHA) and Environmental Protection Agency (EPA) regulations. Electrical shocks can be avoided by keeping electrical equipment such as hair dryers, electrotherapy devices, and heaters out of the wet environment of the pool and poolside.

Infection Control

Because water is not drained from an exercise pool between uses, the pool water must be continuously filtered and chemically treated to prevent infection transmission. Coliform bacteria, *Giardia lamblia*, *Pseudomonas aeruginosa*, and various types of staphylococcal bacteria, which can cause intestinal, skin, or ear infection in exposed individuals, are commonly found in water; the risk of excessive bacterial growth is elevated if the water is warm. Airborne endotoxins around a pool may cause respiratory problems in susceptible individuals.

Adequate infection control can be achieved in a pool through continuous filtering and chemical disinfection of the pool water with chlorine or bromine. The pH and chlorine or bromine residual levels appropriate for a pool are set by local and state health agencies and should be tested at the beginning of each day and at least two additional times during the day. The total alkalinity and calcium hardness of the water should be checked twice a month. Chemical testing kits designed for this application indicate safe levels for these tests. To minimize the risk of high bacterial levels in a pool, it is essential that patients with conditions that may be a source of infection not be allowed to use an exercise pool that would be reused by themselves or by others, as previously detailed in the section on contraindications.

Documentation

Documentation of hydrotherapy should include the following:
- Type of hydrotherapy used
- Patient position and/or activities
- Water temperature
- Duration of treatment
- Outcome of or response to treatment
- Fluid pressure, if applicable
- Water additives, if applicable

Documentation is typically written in the SOAP note format. The following examples summarize only the modality component of treatment and are not intended to represent a comprehensive plan of care.

EXAMPLES

When applying NPWT to a sacral pressure ulcer, document the following:

S: Pt oriented to name but not to date or place.

O: Intervention: NPWT. Removed prior dressing. Cleaned wound with water spray. Filled wound with moist gauze, covered with thin film. Negative pressure 100 mm Hg.

A: Pt appeared to tolerate dressing change well, with wound improvement.

P: Check every 2 h. Change dressing in 2 to 3 days.

When using pool exercise (exer) to increase the fitness of a patient with exercise-induced asthma and obesity, document the following:

S: Pt reports that ambulation continues to be limited by asthma.

O: **Intervention:** Pool exer, pool at 30°C, forward and backward walking across pool, 20 min at slow pace with 1 min rest at each end of the pool.

Posttreatment: Functional ambulation tolerance increased from 30 min to 1 h over the last month.

A: Pt tolerated exer without onset of asthma.

P: Continue pool exer program as above, increasing time from 20 min to 25 min next session.

CLINICAL CASE STUDIES

The following case studies summarize the concepts of hydrotherapy discussed in this chapter. Based on the scenarios presented, an evaluation of the clinical findings and goals of treatment are proposed. These are followed by a discussion of factors to be considered in the selection of hydrotherapy as an intervention and guidelines for selection of the appropriate hydrotherapy device and application technique.

CASE STUDY 19.1

Pressure Ulcers

Examination

History

ST is an 85-year-old woman with stage IV pressure ulcers near both femoral greater trochanters and a stage II pressure ulcer over the sacrum. She has a history of two strokes, one 3 years ago and the other 8 years ago. She has hypertension controlled by medication that generally keeps her blood pressure at or below 145/100 mm Hg. The pressure ulcers place her at risk for sepsis and limit safe positioning because lying on either side should be avoided in the presence of pressure ulcers over both greater trochanters.

Systems Review

ST is bedridden, oriented to name and place. Although not combative, ST is not cooperative during formal strength testing. She has atrophy of all four extremities but is able to move both arms through partial ROM against gravity and move both legs but not against gravity. She has increased tone of all four extremities that is moderately severe.

Tests and Measures

The ulcer near the right greater trochanter is approximately 8 cm long, 8 cm wide, and 2 cm deep and has no undermining. The ulcer near the left greater trochanter is approximately 9 cm long, 10 cm wide, and 1 cm deep and has approximately 1 cm of undermining along the proximal border. Both of these wounds have yellow necrotic tissue and a heavy, thick exudate; no granulation tissue is visible. The ulcer over the sacrum measures approximately 5 cm × 10 cm and is very shallow, with no necrotic tissue. No tunnels or sinus tracts are apparent in any of these wounds.

Hydrotherapy should be used for which of this patient's wounds? What type of hydrotherapy should be used and why? What precaution should be taken when using warm water for this patient?

Evaluation and Goals

Hydrotherapy is indicated for this patient because this intervention can soften and debride necrotic tissue, cleanse wound debris,

and improve circulation by immersion in warm water. Removing necrotic tissue from a wound bed and improving the local circulation can accelerate the healing and closure of the wounds. For the best outcome, other interventions, such as pressure relief, electrical stimulation, exercise, appropriate wound dressings, and possibly other forms of debridement, should also be applied.

Examination of this patient does not indicate that hydrotherapy would be contraindicated, but hydrotherapy is indicated only for the trochanteric wounds, where necrotic tissue is present, not for the sacral wound, where no necrotic tissue is apparent. Care should be taken to ascertain that the patient can feel and report heat in areas to be treated before warm or hot water is used. Because it is most likely that this patient has impaired sensation and circulation in the areas of the pressure ulcers, water temperature should be no higher than 35.5°C (96°F).

ICF Level	Current Status	Goals
Body structure and function	Impaired soft tissue integrity	Soften and remove necrotic tissue in trochanteric wounds
	Abnormal muscle tone	Facilitate wound closure
	Reduced functional mobility	Reduce risk of infection and further tissue breakdown
	At risk for developing further pressure ulcers and systemic infection	Improve circulation to wound areas
Activity	Unsafe to lie on either side	Safe lying in any position
Participation	Dependent	Dependent—no change expected

ICF, International Classification for Functioning, Disability and Health.

◆ FIND THE EVIDENCE

PICO Terms	Natural Language Example	Sample PubMed Search
P (Population)	Patient with pressure ulcers and history of stroke	("ulcer" [text word] OR "wound" [text word])
I (Intervention)	Hydrotherapy	AND "hydrotherapy" [text word]
C (Comparison)	No hydrotherapy	
O (Outcome)	Wound healing	(AND English [lang] AND "humans" [MeSH terms])

Key Studies or Reviews

1. Moore ZE, Cowman S: Wound cleansing for pressure ulcers. *Cochrane Database Syst Rev* 2013(3):CD004983, 2013.

   The objective of this systematic review was to compare the effect of different wound cleansing solutions and different wound cleansing techniques on the rate of healing of pressure ulcers. A total of three studies met the inclusion criteria for this review. Overall, these studies found that cleansing with water was as effective as saline, although a saline solution that also included aloe vera, silver chloride, and decyl glucoside may be more effective than saline, and also that use of pulsatile lavage is more effective than sham lavage.

2. Fernandez R, Griffiths R: Water for wound cleansing. *Cochrane Database Syst Rev* 2012(2):CD003861, 2012.

   The objective of this systematic review was to assess the effects of water compared with other solutions for wound cleansing. The review included 11 trials, but only 2 of these reported on wound healing, and both were related to postoperative, not chronic, wounds.

Prognosis

It is predicted that the necrotic tissue will be removed and the amount of granulation tissue in the wound will increase within 1 week of initiating treatment. If other factors, including positioning, turning, and nutrition, can be optimized, ST may achieve full wound closure of the trochanteric wounds over many months. Alternatively, once the wound beds are clean and fully granulated, ST may undergo skin grafting to achieve or accelerate wound closure.

Intervention

Nonimmersion techniques should be used to apply hydrotherapy to this patient. Nonimmersion hydrotherapy can be provided with a mechanical or electrical device, with a mechanical device such as a 60-mL piston irrigation syringe with a catheter tip being less expensive but likely taking longer than an electrical pulsed lavage device. Warm tap water will be used with either device selected. The addition of antimicrobials to the fluid is not recommended because this has not been shown to improve outcomes. It is recommended that the selected hydrotherapy treatment be applied once each day until the wound bed is fully granulated and be discontinued if bleeding occurs, if the amount of necrotic tissue does not decrease, or if the amount of granulation does not increase within 1 week. If sharp debridement of necrotic tissue is indicated, it is recommended that this be performed after hydrotherapy, when the necrotic tissue is likely to be softer and easier to remove.

Documentation

S: Bedbound Pt oriented to person and place.

O: Pretreatment: R greater trochanter ulcer 8 cm diameter, 2 cm deep, no undermining. L greater trochanter ulcer 9 cm × 10 cm, 1 cm deep, with 1 cm of proximal border undermining. Both wounds have yellow necrotic tissue, thick exudate with no granulation tissue. Sacral ulcer 5 cm × 10 cm, with no necrotic tissue.

Intervention: Wound cleansing with warm water applied with 60-mL piston irrigation syringe with catheter tip to R and L trochanteric pressure ulcers. Pt on gurney on L side for R ulcer treatment and on R side for L ulcer treatment.

Posttreatment: Both ulcers free of necrotic debris and exudate.

A: Pt tolerated irrigation without discomfort or bleeding.

P: Continue as above once daily until granulation tissue appears. Consider use of NPWT if wound healing does not progress. Discuss optimization of pressure distribution and nutrition with team.

CASE STUDY 19.2

Bilateral Knee Pain

Examination

History

FR is a 65-year-old woman with osteoarthritis of both knees. FR reports bilateral knee pain that is worse on the right (6/10) than on the left (4/10) and that worsens with standing or walking for longer than 5 minutes. She does not tolerate antiinflammatory medications because of gastric side effects. The pain in her right knee started about 5 years ago, with no known initiating event, and has gradually worsened since that time. The pain in her left knee started about 2 years ago, also with no known initiating event. She has had no prior treatment for her knee pain. As the patient's pain has worsened over the years, she has limited her activities, spending most of her time in her home or at work, where she is usually sitting. She cannot enjoy walks with friends and has not gone to church in 6 months because her knees hurt so much after walking from the parking lot to her seat. She used to attend church once or twice a week.

Systems Review

FR is alert and engaged. She uses a cane in her left hand to control her knee pain and to assist with balance during community and most household ambulation. She is able to walk at a moderate pace approximately one-half block on a flat, level surface with her cane. She reports restricted ROM in her left lower extremity but no atrophy and no self-reported weakness, ROM restrictions, or sensory changes in the right lower extremity or either upper extremity.

Tests and Measures

The patient is obese (265 lb) and has bilateral genu valgum, bilateral foot pronation, and weakness and shortness of the quadriceps and hamstring muscles. Knee passive ROM is −5 degrees extension to 95 degrees flexion on the right and 0 degrees extension to 120 degrees flexion on the left. FR uses a step-to gait for ascending and descending stairs.

What kind of hydrotherapy is appropriate for this patient, and why? What are some reasonable short-term and long-term goals for her?

Continued

CLINICAL CASE STUDIES—*cont'd*

Evaluation and Goals

Although many forms of exercise could be used to increase this patient's lower extremity strength and knee ROM, the best option is exercise with limited weight bearing. This will help avoid aggravating the patient's symptoms, given her body weight and the reported degeneration of her knee joints. Non–weight-bearing exercises such as straight leg raises or reduced weight-bearing exercises such as stationary cycling could be used. However, water-based exercises are recommended because they offer a number of advantages over non–weight-bearing, land-based exercises, including (1) allowing the patient to perform normal functional activities such as walking without an assistive device to train the muscles and to develop the balance skills required for normal function, (2) providing some pain control during the exercise, (3) allowing fine grading of joint loading by varying the depth of the water, and (4) allowing fine grading of resistance by varying the speed of patient movement. Should the patient have lower extremity edema, as is common in inactive obese individuals, the hydrostatic pressure of immersion may reduce it.

From the examination, it does not appear that hydrotherapy would be contraindicated for this patient. However, before beginning hydrotherapy, the clinician should ascertain whether the patient is afraid of being in water, if she has any infections that may be spread by water, or if she has any medical conditions that would contraindicate the treatment.

ICF Level	Current Status	Goals
Body structure and function	Bilateral knee pain	Minimal knee pain (<2/10 bilaterally)
	Weak quadriceps and hamstrings	Normal quadriceps and hamstring strength
	Reduced knee PROM	0° extension to 120° flexion PROM of both knees
	Obesity	10-lb weight loss and active involvement in a home exercise program to lose further weight and improve fitness
Activity	Limited ability to stand (≈5 min) and walk (≈½ block)	*Short term (4 weeks)*
		Increase standing tolerance to 20 min
		Increase walking tolerance to 2 blocks
		Discontinue use of a cane
		Long term (3 months)
		Involvement in a home exercise program to

ICF Level	Current Status	Goals
		lose further weight and improve fitness
Participation	Not attending church because of knee pain	Able to attend church once a week without pain

ICF, International Classification for Functioning, Disability and Health; *PROM,* passive range of motion.

◆ FIND THE EVIDENCE

PICO Terms	Natural Language Example	Sample PubMed Search
P (Population)	Adult with knee osteoarthritis	("Osteoarthritis" [MeSH] OR "osteoarthritis" [text word])
I (Intervention)	Hydrotherapy	AND "hydrotherapy" [text word]
C (Comparison)	No hydrotherapy	
O (Outcome)	Reduction of knee pain; enhanced quality of life	(AND English [lang] AND "humans" [MeSH term])

Key Studies or Reviews

1. Bartels EM, Juhl CB, Christensen R, et al: Aquatic exercise for the treatment of knee and hip osteoarthritis. *Cochrane Database Syst Rev* 2016(3):CD005523, 2016.

   This systematic review included 13 trials in 1190 participants, of whom 75% were female, with an average age of 68 and an average body mass index (BMI) of 29.4 (BMI of 25 to 29.9 = overweight, BMI ≥30 = obese). This review concluded that there is moderate-quality evidence that aquatic exercise may have small, short-term, and clinically relevant effects on patient-reported pain, disability, and quality of life in people with knee and hip osteoarthritis.

2. Dong R, Wu Y, Zhang L, et al: Is aquatic exercise more effective than land-based exercise for knee osteoarthritis? *Medicine* 97(52):e13823, 2018.

   This systematic review included eight trials involving a total of 579 patients with knee osteoarthritis. The meta-analysis found no significant difference in pain relief, physical function, or improvement in quality of life between land-based and aquatic exercise, but adherence and satisfaction were higher for the aquatic exercise than for the land-based exercise.

Prognosis

It is expected that this patient will be able to participate comfortably in aquatic exercise to increase her lower extremity strength, to lose weight, and to improve her general fitness. It is predicted that within 1 month, she will perform supervised

CLINICAL CASE STUDIES—*cont'd*

aquatic exercise for 30 minutes two times a week, and she will be able to stand on land for 20 minutes and walk on land for two blocks. She will have also lost 3 to 5 lb of body weight and be seeking a pool in which to independently perform aquatic exercises.

Intervention

Pool exercise is the only form of hydrotherapy that would address all the proposed goals of intervention for this patient. For her treatment, the pool water should be kept slightly warmer than generally used for recreation, at 34°C to 36°C (93°F to 95°F), to allow FR to exercise comfortably at the slow pace to which she will probably be limited. A pool exercise program may include forward and backward walking while holding on to the hand rail if necessary for balance, partial squats, kicking, and a variety of other closed-chain and open-chain lower extremity activities. This program is likely to be most effective if provided in conjunction with land-based exercises, active and passive stretching, joint mobilization, and a home exercise plan.

Documentation

S: Pt reports ambulation and standing limited by knee pain.

O: Pretreatment: Standing and ambulation tolerance 5 min. Knee passive ROM −5 degrees, extension to 95 degrees flexion on right and 0 degrees extension to 120 degrees flexion on left.

Intervention: Pool exer, pool at 30°C, forward and backward walking across pool, 15 min at slow pace with 1 min rest at each end of the pool, 10 partial squats.

Posttreatment (after 2 weeks): Standing and ambulation tolerance 15 min. Knee ROM −5 degrees extension to 110 degrees flexion on right and −5 degrees extension to 130 degrees flexion on left.

A: Tolerated exercise without pain.

P: Continue pool exer program as above, increasing time to 20 min next session. Pt was taught land-based exercises, active and passive stretching, and joint mobilization to incorporate into home routine. Next sessions to include home exercise plans.

Chapter Review

1. Hydrotherapy is the application of water for therapeutic purposes. The unique physical properties of water, including its high specific heat and thermal conductivity, buoyancy, resistance, and hydrostatic pressure, contribute to its therapeutic efficacy.
2. Water can be used therapeutically through immersion or nonimmersion techniques. Immersion in water can produce cardiovascular, respiratory, musculoskeletal, renal, and psychological changes. Nonimmersion hydrotherapy is used to reduce bacterial load and remove debris during wound care. Nonimmersion hydrotherapy can be applied with a shower or a specialized irrigation device and is recommended when only the cleansing effects of hydrotherapy are desired. Immersion hydrotherapy is rarely used for wound care because of the risk of infection.
3. NPWT, which involves applying vacuum suction to the wound, in conjunction with nonimmersion hydrotherapy or with instillation with or without dwell time, is often used to promote wound healing.
4. Immersion hydrotherapy is generally used for aquatic exercise in a pool. Clinical benefits include controlling pain, modifying musculoskeletal demands, and reducing edema. Contraindications and precautions for immersion hydrotherapy include open wounds, bleeding, impaired cognition or thermal sensation, infection, cardiac instability, and pregnancy. Contraindications and precautions for nonimmersion hydrotherapy and NPWT include wound maceration, exposed vessels, malignancy in the wound bed, and bleeding.
5. To optimize the outcome of hydrotherapy treatment, the treatment plan and equipment selection should take into account the risks and benefits associated with different means of applying hydrotherapy, and all appropriate precautions should be taken to provide a safe environment for treatment.

Glossary

GENERAL TERMS

Buoyancy: An upward force on an object immersed in a fluid that is equal to the weight of the fluid it displaces, enabling it to float or to appear lighter.

Closed-chain exercises: Exercises where the distal extremity is stationary on a stable support. When closed-chain exercises are performed in a pool, the distal extremity is supported on the bottom or side of the pool.

Contrast baths: Alternating immersion in hot and cold water.

Edema: Swelling that results from accumulation of fluid in the interstitial space.

Hydrostatic pressure: The pressure exerted by a fluid on a body immersed in the fluid. Hydrostatic pressure increases with increased depth of immersion.

Hydrotherapy: Therapeutic use of water.

Open-chain exercises: Exercises where the distal extremity is free to move. Open-chain exercises can be performed in a pool if the distal extremity is not touching the side or bottom of the pool.

Pressure: Force per unit area, generally measured in pounds per square inch (psi).

Resistance: A force counter to the direction of movement. Resistance to a body's movement in water is proportional to the relative speed of body and water motion and to the frontal areas of body parts in contact with the water.

Specific gravity: Ratio of the density of a material to the density of water.

Specific heat: The amount of energy required to raise the temperature of a given weight of a material by a given number of degrees, usually expressed in J/g/°C.

Thermal conductivity: The rate at which a material transfers heat by conduction, usually expressed in (cal/s)/(cm² × °C/cm).

Viscosity: Resistance to flow of a liquid, caused by friction between molecules of the liquid. Water, a liquid with low viscosity, pours quickly and easily; a more viscous liquid is thick and pours slowly.

WOUND-RELATED TERMS

Debridement: Removal of foreign material or dead, damaged, or infected tissue from a wound to expose healthy tissue.

Dwell time: The amount of time instillation fluid stays in a wound during negative pressure wound therapy (NPWT) with instillation.

Eschar: Dead tissue or a scab that forms on a wound.

Exudate: Wound fluid composed of serum, fibrin, and white blood cells.

Granulation tissue: Tissue composed of new blood vessels, connective tissue, fibroblasts, and inflammatory cells that fills an open wound when it starts to heal; tissue typically appears deep pink or red, with an irregular, berry-like surface.

Infection: Establishment and growth of microorganisms causing disease. With infection, more microorganisms or more pathological microorganisms are seen than with colonization.

Instillation: Delivery of fluid to a wound during negative pressure wound therapy (NPWT).

Maceration: Softening of tissues from excessive soaking in liquid.

Necrotic tissue: Dead tissue.

Negative pressure wound therapy (NPWT): The application of continuous or intermittent subatmospheric pressure vacuum suction to an open wound to promote wound healing; also known as *vacuum-assisted wound closure*.

Pulsed lavage: Nonimmersion pulsatile irrigation, often used to clean and debride wounds, thereby promoting wound healing.

References

1. Bettmann OL: City life: beware of contagion. In Bettmann OL, Hench PC, editors: *A pictorial history of medicine*, Springfield, IL, 1956, Charles C Thomas.
2. Shepard CH: Insanity and the Turkish bath. *JAMA* 34:604–606, 1900.
3. Kenney E, Ostenso M: *And they shall walk*, New York, 1943, Dodd, Mead & Company.
4. Roberts P: Hydrotherapy: its history, theory and practice. *Occup Health Safe* 33:235–244, 1982.
5. Argenta LC, Morykwas MJ: Vacuum-assisted closure: a new method for wound control and treatment: clinical experience. *Ann Plast Surg* 38:563–576, 1997.
6. Morykwas MJ, Argenta LC, Shelton-Brown EI, et al: Vacuum-assisted closure: a new method for wound control and treatment: animal studies and basic foundation. *Ann Plast Surg* 38:553–562, 1997.
7. Chen K, Lin JT, Sun SB, et al: Vacuum-assisted closure combined with a closed suction irrigation system for treating postoperative wound infections following posterior spinal internal fixation. *J Orthop Surg Res* 13(1):321, 2018. doi:10.1186/s13018-018-1024-6.
8. Edwards R, Harding KG: Bacteria and wound healing. *Curr Opin Infect Dis* 17(2):91–96, 2004.
9. Mouës CM, Heule F, Hovius SER: A review of topical negative pressure therapy in wound healing: sufficient? *Am J Surg* 201:544–556, 2011.
10. Ge S, Orbay H, Silverman RP, et al: Negative pressure wound therapy with instillation and dwell time in the surgical management of severe hidradenitis suppurativa. *Cureus* 10(9):e3319, 2018.
11. Association for the Advancement of Wound Care (AAWC): AAWC venous ulcer guideline. 2011. http://aawconline.org/wp-content/uploads/2011/04/AAWC-VU_Guideline.pdf. (Accessed January 1, 2020).
12. Wound, Ostomy and Continence Nurses Society-Wound Guidelines Task Force: WOCN 2016 guideline for prevention and management of pressure injuries (ulcers): an executive summary. *J Wound Ostomy Continence Nurs* 44(3):241–246, 2017. doi:10.1097/WON.0000000000000321.
13. Omar M, Gathen M, Liodakis E, et al: A comparative study of negative pressure wound therapy with and without instillation of saline on wound healing. *J Wound Care* 25(8):475–478, 2016. doi:10.12968/jowc.2016.25.8.475.
14. Kim PJ, Attinger CE, Crist BD, et al: Negative pressure wound therapy with instillation: review of evidence and recommendations. *Wounds* 27(12):S2–S19, 2015.
15. Allen D, LaBarbera LA, Bondre IL, et al: Comparison of tissue damage, cleansing and cross-contamination potential during wound cleansing via two methods: lavage and negative pressure wound therapy with instillation. *Int Wound J* 11:198–209, 2014.
16. Yang C, Goss SG, Alcantara S, et al: Effect of negative pressure wound therapy with instillation on bioburden in chronically infected wounds. *Wounds* 29(8):240–246, 2017.
17. Wolvos T: The evolution of negative pressure wound therapy: negative pressure wound therapy with instillation. *J Wound Care* 24(4 Suppl):15–20, 2015.
18. Kim PJ, Attinger CE, Steinberg JS, et al: The impact of negative-pressure wound therapy with instillation compared with standard negative-pressure wound therapy: a retrospective, historical, cohort, controlled study. *Plast Reconstr Surg* 133:709–716, 2014.
19. Kim PJ, Attinger CE, Steinberg JS, et al: Negative-pressure wound therapy with instillation: international consensus guidelines. *Plast Reconstr Surg* 132:1569–1579, 2013.
20. Fernández L, Ellman C, Jackson P: Use of negative pressure wound therapy with instillation in the management of complex wounds in critically ill patients. *Wounds* 31(1):E1–E4, 2019.
21. Bartels EM, Juhl CB, Christensen R, et al: Aquatic exercise for the treatment of knee and hip osteoarthritis. *Cochrane Database Syst Rev* 3:CD005523, 2016. doi:10.1002/14651858.CD005523.pub3.
22. Rahmann AE, Brauer SG, Nitz JC: A specific inpatient aquatic physiotherapy program improves strength after total hip or knee replacement surgery: a randomized controlled trial. *Arch Phys Med Rehabil* 90:745–755, 2009.
23. Quintrec JL, Verlhac B, Cadet C, et al: Physical exercise and weight loss for hip and knee osteoarthritis in very old patients: a systematic review of the literature. *Open Rheumatol J* 8:89–95, 2014.
24. Simas V, Hing W, Pope R, et al: Effects of water-based exercise on bone health of middle-aged and older adults: a systematic review and meta-analysis. *Open Access J Sports Med* 8:39–60, 2017. doi:10.2147/OAJSM.S129182.
25. Wouters EJ, Van Nunen AM, Geenen R, et al: Effects of aquajogging in obese adults: a pilot study. *J Obes* 2010:231074. pii.
26. Kittichaikarn C, Kuptniratsaikul V: Design of an underwater treadmill system for rehabilitation of older obese adults: a pre-post study. *BMC Geriatr* 19(1):310, 2019. doi:10.1186/s12877-019-1334-5.
27. Yaghoubi M, Fink PW, Page WH, et al: Kinematic comparison of aquatic- and land-based stationary exercises in overweight and normal weight children. *Pediatr Exerc Sci* 31(3):314–321, 2019. doi:10.1123/pes.2018-0188.
28. Gwinup G: Weight loss without dietary restriction: efficacy of different forms of aerobic exercise. *Am J Sport Med* 15:275–279, 1987.
29. Kieres J, Plowman S: Effect of swimming and land exercises on body composition of college students. *J Sport Med Phys Fitness* 31:192–193, 1991.
30. Ruoti RG, Troup JT, Berger RA: The effects of nonswimming water exercises on older adults. *J Orthop Sports Phys Ther* 19:140–145, 1994.
31. Gappmaier E, Lake W, Nelson AG, et al: Aerobic exercise in water versus walking on land: effects on indices of fat reduction and weight loss of obese women. *J Sports Med Phys Fitness* 46:564–569, 2006.
32. Cox KL, Burke V, Beilin LJ, Puddey IB: A comparison of the effects of swimming and walking on body weight, fat distribution, lipids, glucose, and insulin in older women—the Sedentary Women Exercise Adherence Trial 2. *Metabolism* 59(11):1562–1573, 2010. doi:10.1016/j.metabol.2010.02.001.
33. Pariser G, Madras D, Weiss E: Outcomes of an aquatic exercise program including aerobic capacity, lactate threshold, and fatigue in two individuals with multiple sclerosis. *J Neurol Phys Ther* 30:82–90, 2006.
34. Henker L, Provast-Craig M, Sestili P, et al: Water running and the maintenance of maximum oxygen consumption and leg strength in runners. *Med Sci Sport Exerc* 24:3–5, 1991.

35. Gusi N, Tomas-Carus P, Hakkinen A, et al: Exercise in waist-high warm water decreases pain and improves health-related quality of life and strength in the lower extremities in women with fibromyalgia. *Arthritis Rheum* 55:66–73, 2006.

36. Epps H, Ginnelly L, Utley M, et al: Is hydrotherapy cost-effective? A randomised controlled trial of combined hydrotherapy programmes compared with physiotherapy land techniques in children with juvenile idiopathic arthritis. *Health Technol Assess* 9:1–59, 2005. iii–iv, ix–x.

37. Latorre Román PÁ, Santos E, Campos MA, García-Pinillos F: Effects of functional training on pain, leg strength, and balance in women with fibromyalgia. *Mod Rheumatol* 25:943–947, 2015.

38. Assis MR, Silva LE, Alves AM, et al: A randomized controlled trial of deep water running: clinical effectiveness of aquatic exercise to treat fibromyalgia. *Arthritis Rheum* 55:57–65, 2006.

39. Adsett JA, Mudge AM, Morris N, et al: Aquatic exercise training and stable heart failure: a systematic review and meta-analysis. *Int J Cardiol* 186:22–28, 2015.

40. Nagle EF, Sanders ME, Franklin BA: Aquatic high intensity interval training for cardiometabolic health: benefits and training design. *Am J Lifestyle Med* 11(1):64–76, 2016. doi:10.1177/1559827615583640.

41. Marinho-Buzelli AR, Masani K, Rouhani H, et al: The influence of the aquatic environment on the center of pressure, impulses and upper and lower trunk accelerations during gait initiation. *Gait Posture* 58:469–475, 2017. doi:10.1016/j.gaitpost.2017.09.008.

42. Killgore GL: Deep-water running: a practical review of the literature with an emphasis on biomechanics. *Phys Sportsmed* 40:116–126, 2012.

43. Killgore GL, Wilcox AR, Caster BL, et al: A lower-extremities kinematic comparison of deep-water running styles and treadmill running. *J Strength Cond Res* 20:919–927, 2006.

44. Meyer K, Leblanc MC: Aquatic therapies in patients with compromised left ventricular function and heart failure. *Clin Invest Med* 31:E90–E97, 2008.

45. Risch WD, Koubenec HJ, Beckmann U, et al: The effect of graded immersion on heart volume, central venous pressure, pulmonary blood distribution and heart rate in man. *Pfleugers Arch* 374:115–118, 1978.

46. Haffor AA, Mohler JG, Harrison AAC: Effects of water immersion on cardiac output of lean and fat male subjects at rest and during exercise. *Aviat Space Environ Med* 62:123–127, 1991.

47. Arborelius M, Balldin UI, Lilja B, et al: Hemodynamic changes in man during immersion with the head above water. *Aerospace Med* 43:593–599, 1972.

48. Reilly T, Dowzer CN, Cable NT: The physiology of deep-water running. *J Sports Sci* 21:959–972, 2003.

49. Butts NK, Tucker M, Smith R: Maximal responses to treadmill and deep water running in high school female cross country runners. *Res Q Exerc Sports* 62:236–239, 1991.

50. Butts NK, Tucker M, Greening C: Physiologic responses to maximal treadmill and deep water running in men and women. *Am J Sports Med* 19:612–614, 1991.

51. Michaud T, Brennan D, Wilder R, et al: Aquarun training and changes in treadmill running maximal oxygen consumption. *Med Sci Sports Exerc* 24:5–7, 1991.

52. Hamer TW, Morton AR: Water-running: training effects and specificity of aerobic, anaerobic and muscular parameters following an eight week interval training programme. *Aust J Sci Med Sport* 22:13–22, 1990.

53. Cider A, Svealv BG, Tang MS, et al: Immersion in warm water induces improvement in cardiac function in patients with chronic heart failure. *Eur J Heart Fail* 8:308–313, 2006.

54. Cider A, Sunnerhagen KS, Schaufelberger M, et al: Cardiorespiratory effects of warm water immersion in elderly patients with chronic heart failure. *Clin Physiol Funct Imaging* 25:313–317, 2005.

55. Neto MG, Conceição CS, de Jesus FL, et al: Hydrotherapy on exercise capacity, muscle strength and quality of life in patients with heart failure: a meta-analysis. *Int J Cardiol* 198:216–219, 2015. doi:10.1016/j.ijcard.2014.10.132.

56. Carvalho VO, Bocchi EA, Guimarães GV: The Borg scale as an important tool of self-monitoring and self-regulation of exercise prescription in heart failure patients during hydrotherapy. A randomized blinded controlled trial. *Circ J* 73:1871–1876, 2009.

57. Gleim GW, Nicholas JA: Metabolic costs and heart rate responses to treadmill walking in water at different depths and temperatures. *Am J Sports Med* 17:248–252, 1989.

58. Evans BW, Cureton KJ, Purvis JW: Metabolic and circulatory responses to walking and jogging in water. *Res Q* 49:442–449, 1978.

59. Hong SK, Cerretelli P, Cruz JC, et al: Mechanics of respiration during submersion in water. *J Appl Physiol* 27:535–536, 1969.

60. Perk J, Perk L, Boden C: Adaptation of COPD patients to physical training on land and in water. *Eur Respir J* 9:248–252, 1996.

61. Agostoni E, Gurtner G, Torri G, et al: Respiratory mechanics during submersion and negative pressure breathing. *J Appl Physiol* 21:251–258, 1966.

62. McNamara RJ, McKeough ZJ, McKenzie DK, et al: Water-based exercise training for chronic obstructive pulmonary disease. *Cochrane Database Syst Rev* 2013(12):CD008290, 2013. doi:10.1002/14651858.CD008290.pub2.

63. Bar-Yishay E, Gur I, Inbar O, et al: Differences between swimming and running as stimuli for exercise-induced asthma. *Eur J Appl Physiol* 48:387–397, 1982.

64. Fitch KD, Morton AR: Specificity of exercise in exercise-induced asthma. *Br Med J* 4:577–581, 1971.

65. Philpott J, Houghton K, Luke A: Physical activity recommendations for children with specific chronic health conditions: Juvenile idiopathic arthritis, hemophilia, asthma and cystic fibrosis. *Paediatr Child Health* 15(4):213–225, 2010.

66. Bar-Or O, Inbar I: Swimming and asthma benefits and deleterious effects. *Sports Med* 14:397–405, 1992.

67. Katz VL, McMurray R, Goodwin WE, et al: Nonweight-bearing exercise during pregnancy on land and during immersion; a comparative study. *Am J Perinatol* 7:281–284, 1990.

68. Murray E: Renal effects of head-out water immersion in humans: a 15-year update. *Physiologic Rev* 72(3):563–570, 1992.

69. Katz VL, McMurray R, Berry MJ, et al: Renal responses to immersion and exercise in pregnancy. *Am J Perinatol* 7:118–121, 1990.

70. Pechter U, Ots M, Mesikepp S, et al: Beneficial effects of water-based exercise in patients with chronic kidney disease. *Int J Rehabil Res* 26:153–156, 2003.

71. Oh S, Lim JM, Kim Y, et al: Comparison of the effects of water- and land-based exercises on the physical function and quality of life in community-dwelling elderly people with history of falling: a single-blind, randomized controlled trial. *Arch Gerontol Geriatr* 60:288–293, 2015.

72. Waller B, Ogonowska-Slodownik A, Vitor M, et al: Effect of therapeutic aquatic exercise on symptoms and function associated with lower limb osteoarthritis: systematic review with meta-analysis. *Phys Ther* 94:1383–1395, 2014.

73. Barker AL, Talevski J, Morello RT, et al: Effectiveness of aquatic exercise for musculoskeletal conditions: a meta-analysis. *Arch Phys Med Rehabil* 95:1776–1786, 2014.

74. Hahn JS: *Lecture on the power and effect of fresh water on the human body*, 1734, Germany.

75. Wheeler CB, Rodeheaver GT, Thacker JG, et al: Side effects of high-pressure irrigation. *Surg Gynecol Obstet* 143:775–778, 1976.

76. McGuckin M, Thorpe R, Abrutyn E: Hydrotherapy: an outbreak of *Pseudomonas aeruginosa* wound infections related to Hubbard tank treatments. *Arch Phys Med Rehabil* 62:283–285, 1981.

77. Tredget EE, Shankowsky HA, Joffe AAM, et al: Epidemiology of infections with *Pseudomonas aeruginosa* in burn patients: the role of hydrotherapy. *Clin Infect Dis* 15:641–649, 1992.

78. Shankowsky HA, Callioux LS, Tredget EE: North American survey of hydrotherapy in modern burn care. *J Burn Care Rehabil* 15:143–146, 1994.

79. Richard P, LeFoch R, Chamoux C, et al: *Pseudomonas aeruginosa* outbreak in a burn unit: role of antimicrobials in the emergence of multiply resistant strains. *J Infect Dis* 170:377–383, 1994.

80. Wisplinghoff H, Perbix W, Seifert H: Risk factors for nosocomial bloodstream infections due to *Acinetobacter baumannii*: a case-control study of adult burn patients. *Clin Infect Dis* 28:59–66, 1999.

81. Ziwa M, Jovic G, Ngwisha CLT, et al: Common hydrotherapy practices and the prevalence of burn wound bacterial colonisation at the University Teaching Hospital in Lusaka, Zambia. *Burns* 45(4):983–989, 2019. doi:10.1016/j.burns.2018.11.019.

82. Braslow JT: Punishment or therapy: patients, doctors, and somatic remedies in the early twentieth century. *Psychiatr Clin North Am* 17:493–513, 1994.

83. Stanwood W, Pinzur MS: Risk of contamination of the wound in a hydrotherapeutic tank. *Foot Ankle Int* 19:173–176, 1998.

84. White NT, Delitto A, Manal TJ, et al: The American Physical Therapy Association's top five Choosing Wisely recommendations. *Phys Ther* 95:9–24, 2015.

85. Winter GD: Formation of scab and the rate of epithelialization in superficial wounds of the domestic pig. *Nature* 193:293–294, 1962.

86. Bhaskar SN, Cutright DE, Gross A: Effect of water lavage on infected wounds in the rat. *J Periodontol* 40:671–672, 1969.

87. Brown LL, Shelton HT, Bornside GH, et al: Evaluation of wound irrigation by pulsatile jet and conventional methods. *Ann Surg* 187:170–173, 1978.

88. Maragakis LL, Cosgrove SE, Song X, et al: An outbreak of multidrug-resistant *Acinetobacter baumannii* associated with pulsatile lavage wound treatment. *JAMA* 292:3006–3011, 2004.

89. Fuller J: Cover up and clean up to prevent deadly infections. *Nursing* 35:31, 2005.

90. Fernandez R, Griffiths R: Water for wound cleansing. *Cochrane Database Syst Rev* 2012(2):CD003861, 2012.

91. Chan MC, Cheung K, Leung P: Tap water versus sterile normal saline in wound swabbing: a double-blind randomized controlled trial. *J Wound Ostomy Continence Nurs* 43(2):140–147, 2016. doi:10.1097/WON.0000000000000213.

92. Moore ZE, Cowman S: Wound cleansing for pressure ulcers. *Cochrane Database Syst Rev* 2013(3):CD004983, 2013.

93. Ubbink DT, Brölmann FE, Go PM, et al: Evidence-based care of acute wounds: a perspective. *Adv Wound Care (New Rochelle)* 4:286–294, 2015.

94. Morgan D, Hoelscher J: Pulsed lavage: promoting comfort and healing in home care. *Ostomy Wound Manage* 46:44–49, 2000.

95. Langschmidt J, Caine PL, Wearn CM, et al: Hydrotherapy in burn care: a survey of hydrotherapy practices in the UK and Ireland and literature review. *Burns* 40:860–864, 2014.

96. Davison PG, Loiselle FB, Nickerson D: Survey on current hydrotherapy use among North American burn centers. *J Burn Care Res* 31:393–399, 2010.

97. Protacio J: Patient-directed music therapy as an adjunct during burn wound care. *Crit Care Nurse* 30:74–76, 2010.

98. Hoffman HG, Patterson DR, Magula J, et al: Water-friendly virtual reality pain control during wound care. *J Clin Psychol* 60:189–195, 2004.

99. Burns-Nader S, Joe L, Pinion K: Computer tablet distraction reduces pain and anxiety in pediatric burn patients undergoing hydrotherapy: a randomized trial. *Burns* 43(6):1203–1211, 2017. doi:10.1016/j.burns.2017.02.015.

100. Hoffman HG, Patterson DR, Seibel E, et al: Virtual reality pain control during burn wound debridement in the hydrotank. *Clin J Pain* 24:299–304, 2008.

101. Neville C, Dimick AR: The trauma table as an alternative to the Hubbard tank in burn care. *J Burn Care Rehabil* 8:574–575, 1987.

102. Embil JM, McLoed JA, Al-Barak AM, et al: An outbreak of methicillin resistant *Staphylococcus aureus* on a burn unit: potential role of contaminated hydrotherapy equipment. *Burns* 27:681–688, 2001.

103. Becker BE: The biological aspects of hydrotherapy. *J Back Musculoskel Rehabil* 4:255–264, 1994.

104. Tovin BJ, Wolf SL, Greenfield BH, et al: Comparison of the effects of exercise in water and on land on the rehabilitation of patients with intraarticular anterior cruciate ligament reconstructions. *Phys Ther* 74:710–719, 1994.

105. Magnes J, Garret T, Erickson D: Swelling of the upper extremity during whirlpool baths. *Arch Phys Med Rehabil* 51:297–299, 1970.

106. Brody LT, Geigle PR: *Aquatic exercise for rehabilitation and training*, Champaign, IL, 2009, Human Kinetics.

107. Hoyrup G, Kjorvel L: Comparison of whirlpool and wax treatments for hand therapy. *Physiother Can* 38:79–82, 1986.

108. Templeton MS, Booth DL, O'Kelly WD: Effects of aquatic therapy on joint flexibility and functional ability in subjects with rheumatic disease. *J Orthop Sport Phys Ther* 23:376–381, 1996.

109. Konlian C: Aquatic therapy: making a wave in the treatment of low back injuries. *Orthop Nurs* 18:11–18, 1999.

110. Lu M, Su Y, Zhang Y, et al: Effectiveness of aquatic exercise for treatment of knee osteoarthritis: systematic review and meta-analysis. *Z Rheumatol* 74:543–552, 2015.

111. Batterham SI, Heywood S, Keating JL: Systematic review and meta-analysis comparing land and aquatic exercise for people with hip or knee arthritis on function, mobility and other health outcomes. *BMC Musculoskelet Disord* 12:123, 2011.

112. Dong R, Wu Y, Xu S, et al: Is aquatic exercise more effective than land-based exercise for knee osteoarthritis? *Medicine (Baltimore)* 97(52):e13823, 2018. doi:10.1097/MD.0000000000013823.

113. Bidonde J, Busch AJ, Webber SC, et al: Aquatic exercise training for fibromyalgia. *Cochrane Database Syst Rev* 2014(10):CD011336, 2014.

114. García-Hermoso A, Saavedra JM, Escalante Y: Effects of exercise on functional aerobic capacity in adults with fibromyalgia syndrome: a systematic review of randomized controlled trials. *J Back Musculoskelet Rehabil* 28:609–619, 2015.

115. Naumann J, Sadaghiani C: Therapeutic benefit of balneotherapy and hydrotherapy in the management of fibromyalgia syndrome: a qualitative systematic review and meta-analysis of randomized controlled trials. *Arthritis Res Ther* 16:R141, 2014.

116. Zamunér AR, Andrade CP, Arca EA, et al: Impact of water therapy on pain management in patients with fibromyalgia: current perspectives. *J Pain Res* 12:1971–2007, 2019. doi:10.2147/JPR.S161494.

117. Zhao Q, Dong C, Liu Z, Li M, Wang J, Yin Y, Wang R: The effectiveness of aquatic physical therapy intervention on disease activity and function of ankylosing spondylitis patients: a meta-analysis. *Psychol Health Med* 2:1–12, 2019. doi:10.1080/13548506.2019.1659984.

118. Liang Z, Fu C, Zhang Q, Xiong F, Peng L, Chen L, He C, Wei Q: Effects of water therapy on disease activity, functional capacity, spinal mobility and severity of pain in patients with ankylosing spondylitis: a systematic review and meta-analysis. *Disabil Rehabil* 29:1–8, 2019. doi:10.1080/09638288.2019.1645218.

119. Marinho-Buzelli AR, Barela AMF, Craven BC, et al: Effects of water immersion on gait initiation: part II of a case series after incomplete spinal cord injury. *Spinal Cord Ser Cases* 16(5):84, 2019. doi:10.1038/s41394-019-0231-7.

120. Cole AJ, Eagleston RE, Moschetti M, et al: Spine rehabilitation aquatic rehabilitation strategies. *J Back Musculoskel Rehabil* 4:273–286, 1994.

121. Tsukahara N, Toda A, Goto J, et al: Cross-sectional and longitudinal studies on the effect of water exercise in controlling bone loss in Japanese postmenopausal women. *J Nutr Sci Vitaminol (Tokyo)* 40:37–47, 1994.

122. Ay A, Yurtkuran M: Influence of aquatic and weight-bearing exercises on quantitative ultrasound variables in postmenopausal women. *Am J Phys Med Rehabil* 84:52–61, 2005.

123. Moreira LD, Fronza FC, Dos Santos RN, et al: The benefits of a high-intensity aquatic exercise program (HydrOS) for bone metabolism and bone mass of postmenopausal women. *J Bone Miner Metab* 32:411–419, 2014.

124. Balsamo S, Mota LM, Santana FS, et al: Resistance training versus weight-bearing aquatic exercise: a cross sectional analysis of bone mineral density in postmenopausal women [article in English, Portuguese]. *Rev Bras Reumatol* 53:193–198, 2013.

125. Iliescu AM, McIntyre A, Wiener J, et al: Evaluating the effectiveness of aquatic therapy on mobility, balance, and level of functional independence in stroke rehabilitation: a systematic review and meta-analysis. *Clin Rehabil* 18:269215519880955, 2019. doi: 10.1177/0269215519880955.

126. Corvillo I, Varela E, Armijo F, et al: Efficacy of aquatic therapy for multiple sclerosis: a systematic review. *Eur J Phys Rehabil Med* 53(6):944–952, 2017. doi:10.23736/S1973-9087.17.04570-1.

127. Carroll LM, Volpe D, Morris ME, et al: Aquatic exercise therapy for people with Parkinson disease: a randomized controlled trial. *Arch Phys Med Rehabil* 98(4):631–638, 2017. doi:10.1016/j.apmr.2016.12.006.

128. Driver S, O'Connor J, Lox C, et al: Evaluation of an aquatics programme on fitness parameters of individuals with a brain injury. *Brain Inj* 18:847–859, 2004.

129. Kesiktas N, Paker N, Erdogan N, et al: The use of hydrotherapy for the management of spasticity. *Neurorehabil Neur Repair* 18:268–273, 2004.

130. Ballaz L, Plamondon S, Lemay M: Group aquatic training improves gait efficiency in adolescents with cerebral palsy. *Disabil Rehabil* 33:1616–1624, 2011.

131. Zhang Y, Roxburgh R, Huang L, et al: The effect of hydrotherapy treatment on gait characteristics of hereditary spastic paraparesis patients. *Gait Posture* 39:1074–1079, 2014.

132. Carroll LM, Morris ME, O'Connor WT, et al: Is aquatic therapy optimally prescribed for Parkinson's disease? A systematic review and meta-analysis. *J Parkinsons Dis*, Dec 6, 2019. doi:10.3233/JPD-191784. [Epub ahead of print].

133. Terrens AF, Soh SE, Morgan PE: The efficacy and feasibility of aquatic physiotherapy for people with Parkinson's disease: a systematic review. *Disabil Rehabil* 40(24):2847–2856, 2018. doi:10.1080/09638288.2017.1362710.

134. Simmons V, Hansen PD: Effectiveness of water exercise on postural mobility in the well elderly: an experimental study on balance enhancement. *J Gerontol A Biol Sci Med Sci* 51:M233–M238, 1996.

135. Harris SR: Neurodevelopmental treatment approach for teaching swimming to cerebral palsied children. *Phys Ther* 58:979–983, 1978.

136. Boyle AM: The Bad Ragaz ring method. *Physiotherapy* 67:265–268, 1981.

137. Ha GC, Yoon JR, Yoo CG, et al: Effects of 12-week aquatic exercise on cardiorespiratory fitness, knee isokinetic function, and Western Ontario and McMaster University osteoarthritis index in patients with knee osteoarthritis women. *J Exerc Rehabil* 14(5):870–876, 2018. doi:10.12965/jer.1836308.154.

138. Wu W, Liu X, Liu J, et al: Effectiveness of water-based Liuzijue exercise on respiratory muscle strength and peripheral skeletal muscle function in patients with COPD. *Int J Chron Obstruct Pulmon Dis* 13:1713–1726, 2018. doi:10.2147/COPD.S165593.

139. Lee JY, Joo KC, Brubaker PH: Aqua walking as an alternative exercise modality during cardiac rehabilitation for coronary artery disease in older patients with lower extremity osteoarthritis. *BMC Cardiovasc Disord* 17(1):252, 2017. doi:10.1186/s12872-017-0681-4.

140. McMurray RG, Katz VL: Thermoregulation in pregnancy: implications for exercise. *Sports Med* 10:146–158, 1990.

141. Watson WJ, Katz VL, Hackney AC, et al: Fetal response to maximal swimming and cycling exercise during pregnancy. *Obstet Gynecol* 77:382–386, 1991.

142. Ward EJ, McIntyre A, van Kessel G, et al: Immediate blood pressure changes and aquatic physiotherapy. *Hypertens Pregnancy* 24:93–102, 2005.

143. Smith SA, Michel Y: A pilot study on the effects of aquatic exercises on discomforts of pregnancy. *J Obstet Gynecol Neonatal Nurs* 35:315–323, 2006.

144. American College of Obstetricians and Gynecologists: Physical activity and exercise during pregnancy and the postpartum period. https://www.acog.org/Clinical-Guidance-and-Publications/Committee-Opinions/Committee-on-Obstetric-Practice/Physical-Activity-and-Exercise-During-Pregnancy-and-the-Postpartum-Period. (Accessed January 22, 2020).

145. Bacchi M, Mottola MF, Perales M, et al: Aquatic activities during pregnancy prevent excessive maternal weight gain and preserve birth weight: a randomized clinical trial. *Am J Health Promot* 32(3):729–735, 2018. doi:10.1177/0890117117697520.

146. Aguilar-Cordero MJ, Sánchez-García JC, Rodriguez-Blanque R, et al: Moderate physical activity in an aquatic environment during pregnancy (SWEP Study) and its influence in preventing postpartum depression. *J Am Psychiatr Nurses Assoc* 25(2):112–121, 2019. doi:10.1177/1078390317753675.

147. Huang SW, Veiga R, Sila U, et al: The effect of swimming in asthmatic children participants in a swimming program in the city of Baltimore. *J Asthma* 26:117–121, 1989.

148. Beggs S, Foong YC, Le HC, et al: Swimming training for asthma in children and adolescents aged 18 years and under. *Cochrane Database Syst Rev* 30(4):CD009607, 2013. doi:10.1002/14651858.CD009607.pub2.

149. Lahart IM, Metsios GS: Chronic physiological effects of swim training interventions in non-elite swimmers: a systematic review and meta-analysis. *Sports Med* 48(2):337–359, 2018. doi:10.1007/s40279-017-0805-0.

150. Tsourlou T, Benik A, Dipla K, et al: The effects of a twenty-four-week aquatic training program on muscular strength performance in healthy elderly women. *J Strength Cond Res* 20:811–818, 2006.

151. Devereux K, Robertson D, Briffa NK: Effects of a water-based program on women 65 years and over: a randomised controlled trial. *Austral J Physiother* 51:102–108, 2005.

152. Takeshima N, Rogers ME, Watanabe E, et al: Water-based exercise improves health-related aspects of fitness in older women. *Med Sci Sports Exerc* 34:544–551, 2002.

153. Broman G, Quintana M, Engardt M, et al: Older women's cardiovascular responses to deep-water running. *J Aging Phys Act* 14(1):29–40, 2006.

154. U.S. Food and Drug Administration: UPDATE on serious complications associated with negative pressure wound therapy systems: FDA safety communication. http://wayback.archive-it.org/7993/20170722215801/https://www.fda.gov/MedicalDevices/Safety/AlertsandNotices/ucm244211.htm. (Accessed January 26, 2020).

155. Said RA, Hussein MM: Severe hyponatremia in burn patients secondary to hydrotherapy. *Burns Incl Therm Inj* 13:327–329, 1987.

156. Christogianni A, Bibb R, Davis SL, et al: Temperature sensitivity in multiple sclerosis: an overview of its impact on sensory and cognitive symptoms. *Temperature (Austin)* 5(3):208–223, 2018. doi:10.1080/23328940.2018.1475831.

157. Headley BJ, Robson MC, Krizek TJ: Methods of reducing environmental stress for the acute burn patient. *Phys Ther* 55:5–9, 1975.

158. U.S. Food and Drug Administration: 2011 safety communications. http://wayback.archive-it.org/7993/20170722043347/https://www.fda.gov/MedicalDevices/Safety/AlertsandNotices/ucm559435.htm. (Accessed January 26, 2020).

159. American National Red Cross: *Lifesaving rescue and water safety*, Washington, DC, 1989, Water Safety Program.

160. Hwang JCF, Himel HN, Edlich RF: Bilateral amputations following hydrotherapy tank burns in a paraplegic patient. *Burns* 21:70–71, 1995.

161. Stav D, Stav M: Asthma and whirlpool baths. *N Engl J Med* 353:1635–1636, 2005.

162. Weisel CP, Richardson SD, Nemery B, et al: Childhood asthma and environmental exposures at swimming pools: state of the science and research recommendations. *Environ Health Perspect* 117(4):500–507, 2009. doi:10.1289/ehp.11513.

163. Thickett KM, McCoach JS, Gerber JM, et al: Occupational asthma caused by chloramines in indoor swimming pool air. *Eur Respir J* 19:827–832, 2002.

164. Jacobs JH, Spaan S, van Rooy GB, et al: Exposure to trichloramine and respiratory symptoms in indoor swimming pool workers. *Eur Respir J* 29(4):690–698, 2007.

165. Lévesque B, Vézina L, Gauvin D, et al: Investigation of air quality problems in an indoor swimming pool: a case study. *Ann Occup Hyg* 59(8):1085–1089, 2015. doi:10.1093/annhyg/mev038.

166. Luedtke-Hoffmann KA, Schafer DS: Pulsed lavage in wound cleansing. *Phys Ther* 80.292–300, 2000.

167. Bastawros DS: 5 things you need to know about: pulsed lavage. *Adv Skin Wound Care* 16(6):282, 2003.

168. Gupta S, Gabriel A, Lantis J, et al: Clinical recommendations and practical guide for negative pressure wound therapy with instillation. *Int Wound J* 13(2):159–174, 2016. doi:10.1111/iwj.12452.

169. Birke-Sorensen H, Malmsjo M, Rome P: Evidence-based recommendations for negative pressure wound therapy: treatment variables (pressure levels, wound filler and contact layer). Steps towards an international consensus. *J Plast Reconstr Aesthet Surg* 64:S1–S16, 2011.

170. Conners RT, Caputo JL, Coons JM, et al: Impact of underwater treadmill training on glycemic control, blood lipids, and health-related fitness in adults with type 2 diabetes. *Clin Diabetes* 37(1):36–43, 2019. doi:10.2337/cd17-0066.

171. Stevens SL, Caputo JL, Fuller DK, et al: Effects of underwater treadmill training on leg strength, balance, and walking performance in adults with incomplete spinal cord injury. *J Spinal Cord Med* 38(1):91–101, 2015. doi:10.1179/2045772314Y.0000000217.

172. American Physical Therapy Association: *Hydrotherapy/therapeutic pool infection control guidelines*, Alexandria, VA, 1994, APTA.

173. Centers for Disease Control and Prevention: Water use in hydrotherapy tanks. https://www.cdc.gov/healthywater/other/medical/hydrotherapy.html. (Accessed January 27, 2020).

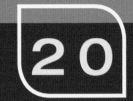

Traction

Michelle H. Cameron | Tony Rocklin

CHAPTER OUTLINE

CHAPTER OBJECTIVES

After reading this chapter, the reader will be able to do the following:
- Define traction.
- Describe the physical effects of traction.
- Explain the clinical indications for the use of traction.
- Choose the best technique for treatment with traction, and list the advantages and disadvantages of each.
- Select the appropriate equipment and optimal treatment parameters for treatment with traction.
- Safely and effectively apply traction.
- Accurately and completely document treatment with traction.

Traction is a tensional mechanical force applied to the body in a way that separates the joint surfaces and elongates surrounding soft tissues. Traction can be applied manually by the clinician or mechanically by a machine or by the patient using body weight and gravity. Traction is most often applied to the spinal or peripheral joints. This chapter focuses on the application of **mechanical traction (electrical mechanical traction)** to the cervical and lumbar spine. Brief discussions of applying traction to the spine by other means and applying mechanical traction to the hip are also provided. Information on applying traction to the other peripheral joints is not provided in this chapter because such traction is generally provided manually by the therapist and therefore is considered to be manual therapy rather than a physical agent. For information on the application of **manual traction** to peripheral joints, the reader should consult a manual therapy text.[1-3]

Spinal traction gained popularity in the 1950s and 1960s in response to recommendations by James Cyriax[4] regarding the efficacy of this technique to treat back and leg pain caused by disc protrusions. A number of early studies also suggested that spinal traction was more effective for reducing back pain and returning patients to activity than other conservative measures, such as heat, rest, and massage.[5-7] The use of spinal traction varies around the world,[8-10] likely in part because of differing interpretations and applications of current evidence.

Traction has been reported to improve symptoms and function in patients with lumbosacral radiculopathy; however, the most recent Cochrane Collaboration systematic review of traction for low back pain with or without sciatica, published in 2013 and based on 32 randomized controlled trials (RCTs) with a total of 2762 participants, concluded that "traction, either alone or in combination with other treatments, has little or no impact on pain intensity, functional status, global improvement and return to work among people with low-back pain."[11] Although the studies leading to this conclusion were of limited quality, given the preponderance of evidence, the authors recommended "little priority should be given to new studies on the effect of traction treatment alone or as part of a package." Other reviews have similarly concluded that traction is not effective for back pain or sciatica.[12,13] Ongoing clinical trials of varying quality continue to fuel this controversy. For example, a study published in 2018 found that in 47 patients with back pain, average pain, anxiety, and depression scores were improved after traction, but there was no group to control for potential placebo effects[14] in this study. Similarly, another small study published in 2018 carried out with 30 patients with chronic back pain found that both manual spinal traction and intermittent mechanical spinal traction were associated with decreases in pain and disability, but again, there was no non-traction control group included to control for placebo effects.[15] In both of these recent studies, all patients also received superficial heat and a range of other interventions. In addition, a study published in 2016 of 120 patients with low back pain with nerve root symptoms, who were specifically selected because of the expectation that traction would be beneficial, found no difference in outcomes between patients treated with extension-oriented treatment alone compared with patients treated with extension-oriented treatment and the addition of mechanical traction.[16] Despite the lack of clear supportive evidence from RCTs, lumbar traction continues to be used and recommended for some patients with symptoms attributable to lumbar spine disorders. A survey of 4,000 orthopedic physical therapists published in 2015 found that over 75% of respondents reported using lumbar traction, including both manual and mechanical traction.[17] Because of this ongoing wide use, the existence of some favorable evidence for lumbar traction, and the improvement noted by many patients with lumbar spine–related symptoms after traction, traction is therefore covered in this text.

In contrast to the lack of evidence in support of lumbar traction, recent studies on cervical spine traction have been more positive. The most recent Cochrane Collaboration systematic review on this topic, published in 2008, found that the literature at that time was insufficient to support or refute the efficacy of cervical traction for patients with neck pain with or without radiculopathy and that large RCTs were needed, but subsequent studies have provided more supportive evidence.[18] For example, a 2014 study of 86 patients with neck pain and cervical radiculopathy found that adding mechanical cervical traction to exercise resulted in lower disability and pain, particularly at long-term follow-up evaluations.[19] A 2013 systematic review of physical modalities for neck pain and associated disorders found intermittent traction to be better than placebo for chronic neck pain, although static traction was no better than placebo.[20] Two systematic reviews, one published in 2017 and one in 2018, with meta-analysis of RCTs both concluded that cervical traction may have benefits for relieving neck pain, although additional high-quality RCTs are still needed to clarify the long-term effects[21,22] and the effects on function and disability.

◎ Clinical Pearl

Studies on lumbar traction have not clearly demonstrated a benefit of this intervention, but studies on cervical traction are more positive. This may be because much more force is needed to distract the joints of the lumbar spine than to distract the joints of the cervical spine.

This chapter presents the basic principles underlying the application of lumbar and cervical spinal traction, provides suggestions for specific clinical applications of spinal traction, and makes recommendations for safe and effective spinal traction techniques. Some information on mechanical hip traction is also included because a mechanical hip traction device has recently become available. This device was developed to provide long-axis hip traction, as usually provided manually by a clinician, in order to provide symptomatic relief for patients with hip pain as a result of osteoarthritis.[23,24] There is evidence that long-axis manual hip traction is associated with significantly improved hip function and reduced pain and disability, with higher forces being more effective.[25,26] There are currently no published controlled trials on the effects of mechanical hip traction.

Effects of Traction

Spinal traction can distract joint surfaces, reduce protrusions of nuclear discal material, stretch soft tissue, relax muscles, and mobilize joints. These effects may reduce the pain associated with spinal dysfunction. Stimulation of sensory mechanoreceptors by traction may also gate the transmission of pain along afferent neural pain pathways.

A basic understanding of spinal anatomy is helpful in thinking about how traction may work and in identifying its effects on the joints of the spine. The spine consists of 24 vertebrae, stacked one on top of the other, connected by ligaments. Between the bodies of the vertebrae are discs that connect one vertebra to the adjacent vertebra and that also serve as shock absorbers (Fig. 20.1A). These discs have a soft center called the **nucleus pulposus** surrounded by the tough, fibrous **annulus fibrosus** (see Fig. 20.1B). The spinal cord is posterior to the discs and the spinal bodies and runs through the spinal canal. The primary joints of the spine are the facet joints, also known as *spinal apophyseal* or *zygapophyseal joints,* which connect the posterior elements of the vertebrae. Foramina, or holes between the posterior elements of the vertebrae, serve as exit points for spinal nerve roots coming off the spinal cord. Spinal traction pulls longitudinally on the spine, potentially reducing pressure on the discs and facet joints; enlarging the intervertebral foramina; and stretching the ligaments, tendons, and muscles running along the spine.

JOINT DISTRACTION

Joint distraction is defined as "the separation of two articular surfaces perpendicular to the plane of the articulation."[27] Distraction of the spinal apophyseal joints can help patients with signs and symptoms related to the loading of these joints or compression of spinal nerve roots as they pass through the intervertebral foramina. Joint distraction reduces compression on the joint surfaces and widens the intervertebral foramina, potentially reducing pressure on articular surfaces, intraarticular structures, or spinal nerve roots.[28] Thus joint distraction may reduce pain originating from spinal joint injury or inflammation or from nerve root compression.

It has been proposed that applying a traction force to the spine can cause distraction of the spinal apophyseal joints.[4] One study showed approximately 3 mm of joint distraction between the L2 to S1 intervertebral joints using gravitational traction in healthy subjects and patients with low back pain.[29] For distraction to occur, the force applied must be enough to cause sufficient elongation of soft tissues surrounding the joint to allow the joint surfaces to separate. Smaller amounts of force may elongate the soft tissues of the spine without separating the joint surfaces. For example, a force equal to 25% of the patient's body weight has been shown to be sufficient to increase the length of the lumbar spine; however, a force equal to 50% of the patient's body weight is needed to distract the lumbar apophyseal joints.[30,31] The amount of force required to distract the spinal joints varies with the location and the health of the joints. In general, larger lumbar joints, which have more and tougher surrounding soft tissues, require

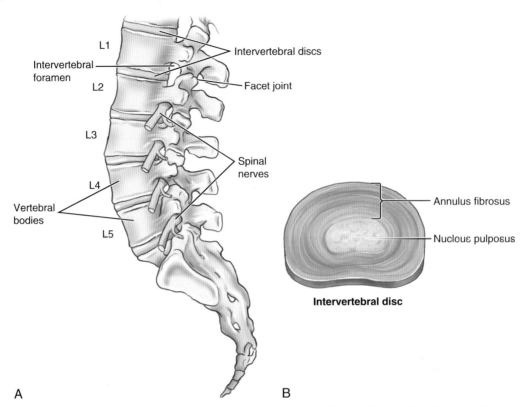

FIGURE 20.1 Spinal anatomy. (A) Left lateral view of lumbar vertebrae showing vertebral bodies, intervertebral discs, facet joints, and intervertebral foramen and spinal nerves. (B) Cross section of an intervertebral disc (showing annulus fibrosus and nucleus pulposus).

more force to achieve joint distraction than is required for smaller cervical joints. As mentioned, distraction of the lumbar apophyseal joints has been demonstrated with a force equal to 50% of total body weight; in contrast, a force equal to approximately 7% of total body weight has been reported to be sufficient to distract the cervical vertebrae.[32] It has also been shown that the same magnitude of force produces greater vertebral separation in healthy spines than in spines with signs of disc degeneration.[33]

Long-axis traction of the hip of sufficient force can also produce hip joint distraction. Vacuum phenomena appear at 90 to 135 lb (400 to 600 N) of traction, varying with joint position.[34,35] Similar amounts of force can also improve pain, mobility, and function in patients with hip-related disability.[25] Low-force hip traction of 22 to 56 lb (100 to 250 N) is probably not enough to produce joint distraction and has only minor effects on range of motion (ROM), pain, stiffness, and function in individuals with hip osteoarthritis.[36,37]

REDUCTION OF SPINAL DISC PROTRUSION

In 1982, Cyriax[4] wrote, "Traction is the treatment of choice for small nuclear protrusions." Proposed mechanisms for disc realignment included clicking back of a disc fragment; suction caused by decreased intradiscal pressure pulling displaced parts of the disc back toward the center; and tensing of the posterior longitudinal ligament at the posterior aspect of the disc, thereby pushing any posteriorly displaced discal material anteriorly toward its original position (Fig. 20.2).[4,38]

Spinal traction can increase disc height and reduce spinal discal protrusions, and it has been proposed that relief of back pain and related symptoms with the application of traction is the result of reduced protrusions of nuclear discal material.[39,40] Studies using a variety of diagnostic imaging techniques, including discography, epidurography, computed tomography (CT), and magnetic resonance imaging (MRI), have demonstrated that lumbar traction using a force of 27 to 55 kg (60 to 120 lb) can reduce a lumbar disc prolapse, cause retraction of **herniated disc** material, reduce the size of a disc herniation, increase disc height, increase space within the spinal canal, widen the neural foramina, and result in clinical improvement in patients whose discal defects are reduced.[38,41–45] Various imaging techniques have also demonstrated reduction of cervical disc herniations with cervical spine traction forces of approximately 7 to 13 kg (15 to 30 lb).[46,47] Symptoms

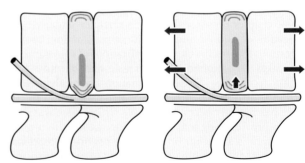

FIGURE 20.2 Suction caused by traction leading to realignment of nuclear discal material.

generally do not improve when traction force is too low[40,48-50] or when traction is applied to patients with large discal herniations that fill the spinal canal or calcification of the disc protrusion.[38]

Although spinal traction does not always reduce discal protrusions, it appears that with sufficient traction force of at least 27 kg (60 lb) to the lumbar spine or 7 to 13 kg (15 to 30 lb) to the cervical spine, some disc protrusions are reduced. Spinal traction may also reduce symptoms in some patients with local back or neck pain or radicular spinal symptoms caused by a disc protrusion if the protrusion is reduced. These symptomatic improvements may be the result of reduced discal protrusion or may be caused by concurrent changes in other associated structures, such as increased size of the neural foramina, changes in tension on soft tissues or nerves, or modification of the tone of paraspinal muscles.

> ### ◎ Clinical Pearl
>
> Lumbar disc protrusions may be reduced with traction force of at least 60 lb, and cervical disc protrusions may be reduced with traction force of at least 15 to 30 lb.

SOFT TISSUE STRETCHING

Traction has been reported to elongate the spine and increase the distance between vertebral bodies and facet joint surfaces.[51-54] It is proposed that these effects are a result of an increase in the length of soft tissues in the area, including muscles, tendons, ligaments, and discs. Soft tissue stretching using a moderate-load, prolonged force, such as that provided by spinal traction, has been shown to increase the length of tendons and to increase joint mobility.[55-57] Increasing the length of soft tissues of the spine may provide clinical benefit by contributing to spinal joint distraction or reduction of disc protrusion, as described previously, or by increasing spinal ROM and decreasing pressure on facet joint surfaces, discs, and intervertebral nerve roots, even when complete joint surface separation is not achieved.

MUSCLE RELAXATION

Spinal traction may facilitate relaxation of the paraspinal muscles.[58-60] This effect may be attributable to a decrease in pain caused by reduced pressure on pain-sensitive structures or gating of pain transmission by stimulation of mechanoreceptors by oscillatory movements produced by **intermittent traction.**[61] Reducing pain by any means can allow muscles to relax, which then decreases muscle spasms by interrupting the pain–spasm–pain cycle. **Static traction** may cause muscle relaxation as a result of a depression in monosynaptic response caused by stretching the muscles for several seconds, whereas intermittent traction may cause small changes in muscle tension that produce muscle relaxation by stimulating the Golgi tendon organs (GTOs) to inhibit alpha motor neuron firing.[62]

JOINT MOBILIZATION

Traction has been recommended as a means of mobilizing spinal and peripheral joints to increase joint mobility or to decrease joint-related pain.[23,24,63,64] Joint mobility is thought to be increased by high-force traction stretching surrounding soft tissue structures. When lower levels of force are applied, the repetitive oscillatory motion of intermittent traction may move the joints sufficiently to stimulate the mechanoreceptors, thus decreasing joint-related pain by gating the afferent transmission of pain stimuli. In this manner, the effects of mechanical traction may be similar to effects produced by manual joint mobilization techniques, except that a number of joints are mobilized at one time with most mechanical traction techniques, whereas the mobilizing force can be more localized with manual techniques.

Clinical Indications for Traction

Substantial evidence demonstrates that spinal traction has mechanical effects on the spine that could be therapeutic. Spinal traction may be helpful for some patients with spinal pain with or without radiating symptoms when caused by a disc bulge or herniation, nerve root impingement, joint hypomobility, subacute joint inflammation, and paraspinal muscle spasm. Hip traction may be helpful for patients with hip-related pain and disability.

Indications and suggestions for selecting traction as a treatment modality, which are provided in the following section, along with guidelines for selecting treatment parameters, are based on the pathophysiology of the pathologies that can cause signs and symptoms in patients. If a patient's signs and symptoms are known to be caused by a disc bulge or herniation, nerve root impingement, subacute joint inflammation, or muscle spasm, and if they are aggravated by joint loading and eased by distraction or reduction of joint loading, then traction may help reduce or control symptoms. Traction is less likely to be effective when a large disc herniation protrudes into the spinal canal or when herniated or protruding discal material has become calcified. Current evidence also suggests that cervical traction is more likely to be effective than lumbar traction.

> ### ◎ Clinical Pearl
>
> Traction may help reduce or control symptoms in patients with signs and symptoms caused by a disc bulge or herniation, nerve root impingement, subacute joint inflammation, or muscle spasm and in whom symptoms are aggravated by joint loading and eased by distraction or reduction of joint loading.

SPINAL DISC BULGE OR HERNIATION

Spinal traction is often used to treat patients with spinal disc bulges or herniations because traction may decrease the size of the herniated disc material and thus reduce compression on spinal nerve roots. The lack of overall significant clinical benefit in response to the application of lumbar traction to patients with lumbar disc injuries may be related to the severity of disc protrusions among subjects studied or sample sizes that were too small to allow a treatment effect to be detected. Given the positive outcomes with cervical traction, where the structures are smaller and lower forces are needed to affect changes, it also seems likely that lumbar traction has been less successful than cervical traction because insufficient traction force may have been used. The ongoing use of lumbar spinal traction is likely a result of the logically appealing rationale for its effectiveness, its tolerability and simplicity, and the limited alternative conservative interventions clearly proven effective for patients with signs and symptoms caused by lumbar spinal disc disease.

SPINAL NERVE ROOT IMPINGEMENT

Traction may help alleviate signs and symptoms associated with spinal nerve root impingement, particularly if it is applied shortly after the onset of such symptoms[5] and if the impingement is of the cervical nerve root. Such impingement may be caused by bulging or herniation of discal material, as described previously, or by ligament encroachment, narrowing of the intervertebral foramen as a result of loss of disc height or osteophyte encroachment, spinal nerve root swelling, or **spondylolisthesis** (Fig. 20.3). In the latter cases, if sufficient traction force is applied, the size of the neural foramen may be increased temporarily, thus reducing pressure on the spinal nerve root.[44,45] For example, when cervical lateral flexion and rotation to the same side, both of which narrow the intervertebral foramina, are markedly limited by arm pain on the same side, indicating impingement of cervical nerve roots, applying traction may reduce arm pain by increasing the size of the neural foramina and decreasing pressure on involved nerves.

Although available data do not readily indicate which patients will benefit from spinal traction in general, patients who report aggravation of symptoms with increased spinal loading and easing of symptoms with decreased spinal loading are most likely to respond well to treatment with traction.

JOINT HYPOMOBILITY

Because longitudinal spinal traction can glide and distract the spinal facet joints and stretch the soft tissues surrounding these joints, spinal traction may improve symptoms caused by spinal joint hypomobility. Similarly, because long-axis hip traction can distract the hip joint and stretch the surrounding soft tissues, hip traction may improve symptoms and function in patients with hip joint hypomobility. However, because spinal traction applies a mobilizing force to multiple rather than single spinal levels, spinal traction is not generally the optimal treatment if only individual segments are hypomobile. Such nonspecific mobilization could exacerbate symptoms in a patient with hypomobility of one segment and hypermobility of adjoining segments because the general mobilizing force of spinal traction would most probably cause the greatest increase in motion in the most extensible areas—the hypermobile segments—resulting in joint laxity while having no effect on the mobility of the less mobile segments that need to be mobilized. Adjusting the degree of spinal flexion during the application of traction localizes the mobilizing effect of the force to some degree and thus may help to alleviate this problem.[65] For example, positioning the lumbar spine in more flexion localizes the force to the upper lumbar and lower thoracic spine, whereas positioning it in neutral or extension localizes the force to the lower lumbar area. Similarly, for the cervical spine, a flexed position focuses the forces on the lower cervical area, and a neutral or slightly extended position focuses the forces on the upper cervical area.[65] More detailed recommendations for patient positioning are provided in the section on application techniques.

SUBACUTE JOINT INFLAMMATION

Traction has been recommended for reducing the pain and limitations of function associated with subacute joint inflammation. However, there is limited research in this area. The force of traction can be used to reduce the pressure on inflamed spinal and peripheral joint surfaces, whereas small movements of intermittent traction may control pain by gating transmission at the spinal cord level. These movements may also help maintain normal fluid exchange in the joints to relieve edema caused by chronic inflammation of the joints. Traction can be used safely in the subacute or chronic stages of joint inflammation; however, intermittent traction should be avoided immediately after an injury, during the acute inflammatory phase, and when repetitive motion may cause further injury or may amplify the inflammatory response. Static traction may be used at this time.

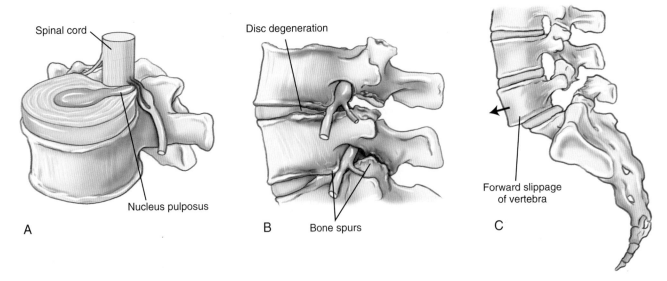

FIGURE 20.3 Causes of spinal nerve root compression. (A) Disc herniation. (B) Osteophyte encroachment and disc degeneration causing narrowing of the intervertebral foramen. (C) Spondylolisthesis.

MUSCLE SPASM

The maintained stretch of static traction or the repetitive motion of low-load, intermittent traction may help to reduce muscle spasm around joints. This effect may be because traction reduces pain, and this interrupts the pain–spasm–pain cycle, or traction may inhibit alpha motor neuron firing by depression of the monosynaptic response or stimulation of the GTOs. Higher-load traction may also alleviate protective muscle spasms by reducing the underlying cause of pain, such as a disc protrusion or herniation, nerve root impingement, or excessive joint compression, thus interrupting the pain–spasm–pain cycle.

Contraindications and Precautions for Traction

The application of spinal traction is contraindicated in some circumstances, and it should be applied with extra caution in other circumstances.[66,67] In all cases, to minimize the risk of adverse consequences, traction should first be applied using a small amount of force while monitoring the patient's response to treatment.

Clinical Pearl

To minimize the risk of adverse consequences, traction should be applied with a low force at first while monitoring the patient's response. If the response is positive, traction force can then be gradually increased until maximum benefit is obtained.

If the patient's condition worsens in response to traction, with symptoms becoming more severe, peripheralizing, increasing in distribution, or progressing to other domains (e.g., from pain to numbness or weakness), the treatment approach should be reevaluated and changed. If the patient's signs or symptoms do not improve within two or three treatments, the treatment approach should be reevaluated and changed, or the patient should be referred for further evaluation.

The patient should be instructed to try to avoid sneezing or coughing while on full traction because these activities increase intraabdominal pressure and thus can increase intradiscal pressure. It is recommended that patients empty their bladder and not have a heavy meal before lumbar traction because constriction of the pelvic belts may cause discomfort on a full bladder or stomach.

CONTRAINDICATIONS FOR TRACTION

✱ CONTRAINDICATIONS

for Traction

- Where motion is contraindicated
- Acute injury or inflammation
- Joint hypermobility or instability
- Peripheralization of symptoms with traction
- Uncontrolled hypertension

Where Motion Is Contraindicated

Traction should not be used if motion is contraindicated in the area to be affected. Examples include an unstable fracture, cord compression, and immediately after spinal surgery.

▪ Ask the Patient
- "Have you been instructed not to move your neck or back? If so, by whom?"
- If wearing a brace or corset: "Have you been instructed not to remove your brace at any time?"
- "How recent was your injury or surgery?"

No form of traction should be used if motion in the area is contraindicated. Treatment with other traction in other areas where motion is allowed can be considered.

Acute Injury or Inflammation

Acute inflammation may occur immediately after trauma or surgery or as the result of an inflammatory disease such as rheumatoid arthritis (RA) or osteoarthritis. Because intermittent or static traction may aggravate acute inflammation or may interfere with the healing of an acute injury, traction should not be applied under these conditions.

▪ Ask the Patient
- "When did your injury occur?"
- "When did your pain start?"

If injury or onset of pain occurred within the last 72 hours, the injury is likely to still be in the acute inflammatory phase, and traction should not be used. As inflammation resolves, static traction may be used initially, with progression to intermittent traction as the area tolerates greater motion.

▪ Assess
- Palpate and inspect the area to detect signs of inflammation, including heat, redness, and swelling.

If signs of acute inflammation are present, the application of traction should be delayed until they are resolved.

Hypermobile or Unstable Joint

High-force traction should not be used in areas of joint hypermobility or instability because it may further increase the mobility of the area. Therefore, the mobility of joints in the area where one is considering applying traction should be assessed before traction is applied. Joint hypermobility may be the result of recent fracture, joint dislocation, or surgery, or it can be caused by an old injury, high relaxin levels during pregnancy and lactation, poor posture, or congenital ligament laxity. Joint hypermobility and instability, particularly of the C1 to C2 articulations, are also associated with RA, Down syndrome, and Marfan syndrome as a result of degeneration of the transverse atlantal ligament. Therefore, cervical traction should not be applied to patients with these diagnoses until the integrity of the transverse atlantal ligament and the stability of the C1 to C2 articulations have been ascertained.

> **▪ Ask the Patient**
> • "Have you dislocated a joint in this area?"
> • "Do you have rheumatoid arthritis, Down syndrome, or Marfan syndrome?"
> • "Are you pregnant?"

> **▪ Assess**
> • Assess joint mobility in the area that will be affected by the traction. All levels of the cervical or lumbar spine should be assessed, not just the symptomatic ones, because traction can affect the mobility of multiple levels.
> • Check the patient's chart for a diagnosis of RA, Down syndrome, or Marfan syndrome, and if they have one of these, request radiographic studies to rule out C1 to C2 instability before applying traction.

Traction should not be applied in areas where joint hypermobility is detected on manual or radiographic examination or in areas where dislocation has previously occurred. When some segments are hypomobile and adjacent segments are hypermobile, it is recommended that hypomobile segments be treated with manual techniques rather than mechanical traction because manual techniques can mobilize individual spinal segments more specifically.

Peripheralization of Symptoms

Traction should be discontinued or modified immediately if it causes peripheralization of symptoms because, in general, progression of spinal symptoms from a central area to a more peripheral area indicates worsening nerve function and increasing compression. Continuing treatment when symptom peripheralization occurs may aggravate the initial injury and prolong the worsening of signs and symptoms.

> **▪ Tell the Patient**
> • "Let me know immediately if you notice increased pain or other symptoms farther down your arms or legs." (Stop the traction if this occurs.)

> **▪ Assess**
> • Recheck sensation, motor function, and reflexes in the appropriate extremity if patient complains of peripheralization of symptoms.

Traction should be discontinued or modified if signs or symptoms peripheralize. Traction may be modified by decreasing the load or changing the patient's position. Modified traction may be continued if peripheralization of symptoms no

longer occurs. Mild aggravation of central symptoms alone in a patient with prior central and peripheral symptoms should not be a cause for discontinuation of treatment.

Uncontrolled Hypertension

Inversion traction should be avoided in patients with uncontrolled hypertension because inversion has been found to significantly increase blood pressure.[68] In addition, in patients with no history of hypertension, cervical traction can transiently increase blood pressure when traction forces are only 10% of body weight, with greater increases at higher forces.[69,70] Although this increase in blood pressure is generally mild and may not be problematic in healthy individuals, to avoid exacerbating poorly controlled hypertension in some patients, clinicians should assess a patient's cardiovascular status before applying cervical traction and avoid cervical traction forces greater than 30% of body weight.

> **▪ Ask the Patient**
> • "Do you have high blood pressure? If so, is it well controlled with medications?"

> **▪ Assess**
> • Take the patient's blood pressure.

In a patient with a resting blood pressure greater than 140/90 mm Hg, blood pressure and heart rate should be checked during and after application of cervical traction, and treatment should be discontinued if systolic or diastolic blood pressure increases by more than 10 mm Hg or if heart rate increases by more than 10 beats/min.

PRECAUTIONS FOR TRACTION

> **★ PRECAUTIONS**
>
> **for Traction**
> • Structural diseases or conditions affecting the tissues in the area being treated (e.g., tumor, infection, rheumatoid arthritis, osteoporosis, prolonged systemic corticosteroid use, local radiation therapy)
> • When pressure of the belts may be hazardous (e.g., with pregnancy, hiatal hernia, vascular compromise, osteoporosis)
> • Displaced annular fragment
> • Medial disc protrusion
> • When severe pain fully resolves with traction
> • Claustrophobia or other psychological aversion to traction
> • Inability to tolerate prone or supine position
> • Disorientation

In cases where traction should be applied with caution, the referring physician may be consulted before traction is initiated. First, a low level of force should be applied, and then progress should be made slowly while closely monitoring the patient's response to treatment.

Structural Diseases or Conditions Affecting the Tissues in the Area Being Treated

Traction should be applied with caution when the structural integrity of the tissues in the area may be compromised. Such structural compromise can occur with a tumor, infection, RA, osteoporosis, prolonged systemic corticosteroid use, or local radiation therapy. In these circumstances, the tissues may not be strong enough to sustain strong traction forces, and injury may result. Radiographic reports and other studies that may indicate the nature and severity of the structural compromise should be checked before a decision is made on whether to apply traction to patients with these conditions.

> ■ **Ask the Patient**
> • "Do you have any disease affecting your bones or joints?"
> • "Do you have cancer, an infection in your bones, rheumatoid arthritis, or osteoporosis?"
> • "Do you take steroid medications? If so, how long have you taken them?"
> • "Have you had radiation therapy? If so, where was the radiation?"

Only low-force traction should be applied to patients with structural compromise of the local tissues. For these patients, manual traction, which allows more direct monitoring of patient response, may be more appropriate.

When Pressure From the Belts May Be Hazardous

Pelvic belts used to apply mechanical lumbar traction may exert excessive abdominal pressure to pregnant patients or to patients with hiatal hernia and may place excessive pressure on the inguinal region in individuals with compromised femoral arteries. Because of their positioning, the belts used for hip traction are not likely to compress vessels in the lower extremity or inguinal region. Compression of the inguinal vessels by the pelvic belt used for hip traction can be avoided by positioning the lower edge of the belt superior to the femoral triangle and by tightly securing the belt and keeping it in direct contact with the skin to prevent it from slipping down during treatment. Concern has arisen that pelvic or thoracic belts may apply excessive pressure to the pelvis or the ribs of patients with osteoporosis. Because the thoracic belts used for fixation of the patient during application of lumbar traction may constrict respiration, lumbar traction should be applied with caution to patients with cardiac or pulmonary disorders.[71]

Cervical traction should be applied with caution to patients with cerebrovascular compromise, as indicated by a positive vertebral artery test, because poor placement of the halter may further compromise circulation to the brain. The halter should be positioned away from the carotid arteries in patients with compromise of these arteries. This is most easily achieved by using a halter that distracts via the occiput rather than one that applies force to both the occiput and the mandible (see Figs. 20.7A and 20.13).

> ■ **Ask the Patient**
> • "Are you pregnant?"
> • "Do you have a hiatal hernia?"
> • "Have you had any trouble with blocked arteries?"
> • "Do you have pain in your calves when walking a short distance?" (This is a sign of intermittent claudication, indicating possible arterial insufficiency to the lower extremities.)
> • "Do you have osteoporosis?"
> • "Do you have problems with your breathing?"
> • "Have you had a stroke?"
> • "Do you get dizzy when you put your head back?"

If compression by the belts used for mechanical traction could be hazardous to the patient, consider using other forms of traction, such as **self-traction** or manual traction, which do not require these belts. Fastening the belts less tightly is generally not recommended because they can slip during treatment, rendering treatment ineffective or increasing pressure in the inguinal region. If the patient's responses indicate possible compromise of the cervical or lower extremity vessels, the halter or belts used for traction must be positioned so that they do not compress these vessels.

Displaced Annular Fragment

Once a fragment of annulus has become displaced and is no longer connected to the body of the disc, traction is not likely to change the position of the disc fragment; therefore, treatment with traction is not likely to improve the patient's symptoms.

> ■ **Ask the Patient**
> • "Has an MRI or CT scan of your spine been performed? Please bring me the reports from these tests."

Traction should not be used to treat symptoms resulting from a displaced disc fragment that is no longer attached to the body of the disc.

Medial Disc Protrusion

Traction may aggravate symptoms caused by a medial disc protrusion because medial movement of the nerve root caused by traction force may increase impingement of the disc on the nerve root in such circumstances (Fig. 20.4).[72]

> ■ **Ask the Patient**
> • "Has an MRI or CT scan of your spine been performed? Please bring me the reports from these tests."

When Severe Pain Resolves Fully With Traction

If severe pain resolves fully with traction, this may indicate that the traction has increased rather than decreased compression on a nerve root, causing a complete nerve block.

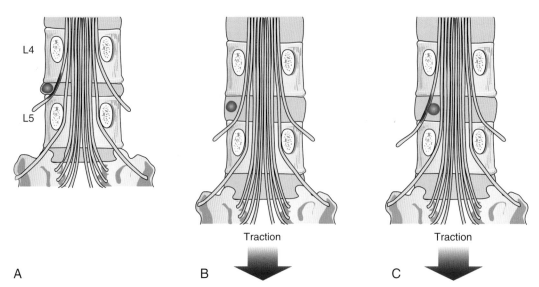

FIGURE 20.4 (A) Lateral disc protrusion compressing the L4 nerve root. (B) L4 nerve root compression by lateral disc protrusion relieved by traction caused by elongation of the lumbar spine and a consequent medial movement of the nerve root. (C) L4 nerve root compression by medial disc protrusion aggravated by traction caused by medial movement of the nerve root.

▪ **Ask the Patient**
• After a few minutes of traction: "Have your symptoms changed?"
• If the patient had severe pain and reports that the pain has decreased: "Has the pain completely gone away, or is it just less severe?"

▪ **Assess**
• Test sensation, reflexes, and strength before treatment. If the patient reports complete resolution of severe pain during treatment, check these again, and assess for any changes.
• If severe pain is fully relieved by traction, it is recommended that the clinician immediately recheck other indicators of nerve conduction, including sensation, reflexes, and strength, to rule out increasing nerve compression. If these are worse, traction should be stopped immediately. If these are not worse, the force of traction may be reduced by 50% or the direction of the traction force modified, and traction may be continued. If traction is maintained at a level that causes a nerve block, the patient may sustain a severe nerve injury as a result of treatment.

Claustrophobia or Other Psychological Aversion to Traction

Some patients are psychologically averse to the use of traction because this procedure generally involves considerable restriction of movement and loss of control. In particular, patients with claustrophobia may not tolerate the restriction of movement required for mechanical lumbar traction. In such cases, other forms of traction that do not require immobilization with belts, such as manual or **positional traction,** may be better tolerated.

Inability to Tolerate the Prone or Supine Position

Some patients cannot tolerate the prone or supine position for the period of time necessary to apply traction because of their spinal condition or other medical problems, such as reflux esophagitis. In such cases, the use of a support such as a lumbar roll may allow the patient to tolerate the position. Cervical traction may be applied in the sitting position; for lumbar traction, some self-traction techniques may be effective.

▪ **Ask the Patient**
• "Does lying on your back with your knees bent for 15 to 20 minutes cause any problems for you?"
• "Does lying on your stomach for 15 to 20 minutes cause any problems for you?"

Disorientation

Mechanical traction should not be applied to disoriented patients because they may move in the halter or belts, becoming entangled or altering the amount of force they receive. Only manual traction techniques should be used to treat disoriented patients.

ADDITIONAL PRECAUTIONS FOR CERVICAL TRACTION

★ **PRECAUTIONS**

for Cervical Traction
• Temporomandibular joint (TMJ) problems
• Dentures

Temporomandibular Joint Problems

In patients with TMJ problems or a history of TMJ problems, a halter that applies pressure only through the occiput should be used rather than one that applies pressure through both the mandible and the occiput because the latter may place pressure on the TMJs and preexisting joint pathology. Many clinicians use an occipital halter with all patients to avoid the possibility of causing TMJ problems in patients who did not have such problems previously.

> ■ **Ask the Patient**
> • "Do you have problems with your jaw?"

Dentures

Patients who wear dentures should be instructed to keep the dentures in place during cervical traction treatment because their removal can alter the alignment of the TMJs and may cause problems if pressure is applied to these joints through the mandible. An occipital halter should be used to protect dentures and teeth as well as the TMJ.

> ■ **Ask the Patient**
> • "Do you wear dentures?"
> • "Do you have them in now?"

Adverse Effects of Spinal Traction

Although no systematic research has been performed on the adverse effects of spinal traction, case reports suggest that prior signs and/or symptoms may increase after the application of traction, particularly when stronger forces are used.[64] Because a rebound increase in pain can occur after the initial application of high-force traction, it is generally recommended that traction force be kept low for the initial treatment and then be gradually increased until maximum benefit is obtained. Specific recommendations for the amount of traction force to be used for different regions of the spine and different spinal conditions are given in the section on application techniques.

It has also been reported that some patients experience lumbar radicular discomfort after receiving treatment with intermittent cervical traction for cervical radicular symptoms.[73,74] Of patients who were reported to experience this adverse effect, 33% had transitional lumbar vertebrae evident on radiographs, and 83% had evidence of spinal osteoarthritis. The onset of lumbar radiculopathy after cervical traction suggests that axial tension induced in the dural covering of the spinal cord was transmitted from the cervical spine to the lumbar nerve roots and that limitations in nerve root excursion caused by structural abnormalities and degenerative changes in these patients probably resulted in excessive tension on the nerve roots, provoking lumbar radicular symptoms. In addition, there is one published case report of unilateral facial nerve paralysis associated with slowing of facial nerve electrical conduction velocity after 4 weeks of intermittent cervical traction.[75] Signs and symptoms fully resolved after treatment with corticosteroids and cessation of traction. Although this presentation may have been caused by compression of the facial nerve or of the blood supply to the facial nerve by the traction harness, it is also possible that this was a coincidental occurrence of Bell palsy.

There is also the potential for discomfort if the belts irritate the skin or cause local pressure. Other adverse effects of spinal traction have been described in detail in the section describing contraindications and precautions.

Application Techniques

Traction can be applied in many ways. At the present time, traction is applied using electrical and weighted mechanical devices, self-traction, positional traction, inversion traction, and manual traction. In the past, spinal traction used very low-load, prolonged static force applied for hours to days.[31] This was thought to relieve symptoms aggravated by spinal motion by limiting mobility and enforcing bed rest.[76] This approach has fallen out of favor because of its high cost and the growing awareness that most patients with back pain do not benefit from prolonged bed rest and inactivity.[77]

When the type of traction, patient position, traction force, and duration and frequency of treatment to be used are selected, the effects of these different parameters of treatment, the nature of the patient's problem, and the patient's response to prior treatments should be considered. Guidelines for the standard application technique for each of these types of traction and advantages and disadvantages of each are provided in the next sections. However, if the clinician understands the principles underlying the application of this type of treatment, many of these techniques can be modified or adapted to suit individual clinical situations, such as when a patient does not tolerate the standard positions used for treatment or when preferred equipment is unavailable.

For all forms of traction, the clinician should first determine whether presenting symptoms and problems are likely to respond to treatment with traction. The clinician should confirm that traction is not contraindicated for this patient or condition.

MECHANICAL TRACTION

Mechanical traction can be applied to the lumbar or cervical spine or the hip. A variety of belts and halters, as well as different patient treatment positions, can be used to apply traction to particular areas of the body and to focus the effect on different segments or structures. Types of mechanical traction devices include motorized traction units, **over-the-door cervical traction** devices, hip traction, and other home devices. Traction can be applied continuously (static traction) or intermittently. With static traction, the same amount of force is applied throughout the treatment session. With intermittent traction, the traction force is varied between set values during the treatment session. The force is held at a maximum for a number of seconds—the hold period—and then is usually reduced by approximately 50% for the following relaxation period. Some motorized traction devices also allow control of the rate of force application, enabling finer control of the force to more closely mimic forces applied during manually applied traction or other manual joint mobilization techniques. Although the manufacturers of these newer devices claim that these features improve outcomes, and clinicians report that lower speeds of force are generally more comfortable and better tolerated, as yet, no published studies have clearly proven specific benefits to be associated with these features.[78] Weighted mechanical traction units apply static traction only, with the amount of force being determined by the amount of weight used.

Advantages of Mechanical Traction

- Force and time well controlled, readily graded, and replicable
- Once applied, does not require the clinician to be with the patient throughout treatment
- Allows the application of static or intermittent traction
- Static weighted devices, such as over-the-door cervical traction, are inexpensive and convenient for independent use by the patient at home.

Disadvantages of Mechanical Traction

- Electrical motorized devices are expensive.
- Time-consuming to set up
- Lack of patient control or participation
- Restriction by belts or halter poorly tolerated by some patients
- Mobilizes broad regions of the spine rather than individual spinal segments, potentially promoting hypermobility in normal or hypermobile joints

Motorized Mechanical Traction Units

Motorized mechanical traction units use an electrically powered motor to apply traction forces to the lumbar or cervical spine statically or intermittently and can generally be used to apply forces up to 70 kg (154 lb). These units offer the advantage of being able to apply static or intermittent traction to the lumbar or cervical spine, and they allow fine, accurate control of the forces being applied.

These units also allow considerable variation in patient position. Newer computerized models can finely control the speed of traction application, store a number of clinician-specific or patient-specific protocols, and track each patient's pain severity and location over time. The most significant limitations of electrical mechanical traction devices are their high cost and large size (Fig. 20.5).

Over-the-Door Cervical Traction Devices

Over-the-door cervical traction units can be used for the application of static cervical traction only. The limited treatment flexibility of these devices makes them appropriate primarily for home use. In this setting, they have the additional advantages of being inexpensive, easy to set up, and compact (Fig. 20.6). Before using this device at home, the patient should be educated on positioning and the amount and duration of force that should be used.

Other Home Spinal Traction Devices

Various other spinal traction devices are available for home application of static or intermittent lumbar or cervical traction (Fig. 20.7). These devices offer more treatment options but are more expensive than over-the-door devices, are more complex to use, and take up more space in the home.

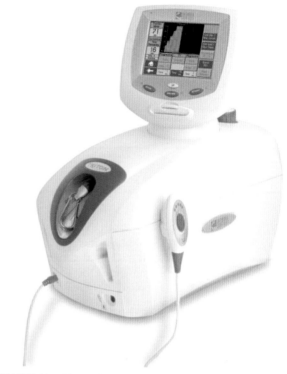

FIGURE 20.5 Mechanical traction unit. (Courtesy Chattanooga/DJO, Vista, CA.)

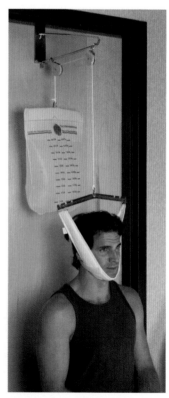

FIGURE 20.6 Over-the-door traction device. (Courtesy Chattanooga/DJO, Vista, CA.)

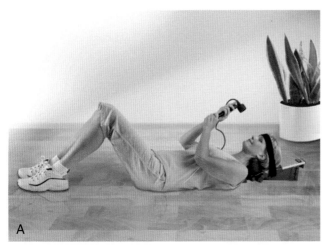
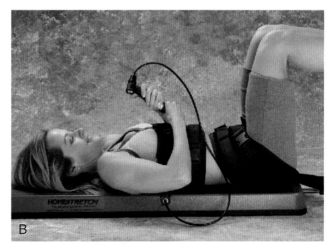

FIGURE 20.7 Examples of home traction devices. (A) Home cervical traction device. (B) Home lumbar traction device. (A, Courtesy Chattanooga/DJO, Vista, CA. B, Courtesy Glacier Cross, Inc., Kalispell, MT.)

MECHANICAL LUMBAR TRACTION

APPLICATION TECHNIQUE 20.1 — MECHANICAL LUMBAR TRACTION

Equipment Required for Electrical Mechanical Traction

- Traction unit
- Thoracic and pelvic belts
- Spreader bar
- Extension rope
- Split traction table (optional)

Equipment Required for Weighted Mechanical Traction

- Traction device (ropes, pulley, weights)
- Thoracic and pelvic belts
- Spreader bar
- Weight bag for water, weights, or sand

Procedure for Mechanical Lumbar Traction

1. Select the appropriate mechanical traction device.

   Various devices are available for applying mechanical traction to the lumbar spine in the clinic or home setting. The choice depends on the amount of force to be applied, whether static or intermittent traction is desired, and the setting in which the treatment will be applied.

2. Determine optimal patient position.

   When positioning the patient, try to achieve a comfortable position that allows muscle relaxation while maximizing the separation between involved structures. The relative degree of flexion or extension of the spine during traction determines which surfaces are most effectively separated.[79-82] The flexed position generally results in greater separation of posterior structures, including the facet joints and intervertebral foramina, whereas the neutral or extended position results in greater separation of anterior structures, including the disc spaces (Fig. 20.8). In most cases, a symmetrical central force is used, with the direction of force in line with the central sagittal axis of the patient (Fig. 20.9); however, if the patient presents with unilateral symptoms, a unilateral traction force that applies more force to one side of the spine than to the other may prove more effective.[83] A unilateral force can be applied

by offsetting the axis of traction in the direction that best reduces the patient's symptoms. For example, if the patient presents with right low back and lower extremity pain that is aggravated by right side bending but is relieved by left side bending, traction should be offset to apply a left side bending force.

For the application of traction to the lumbar spine, the patient may be positioned prone or supine (Fig. 20.10). Although supine positioning is most commonly used, prone positioning may be advantageous if the patient does not tolerate flexion or the supine position or if symptoms are reduced by extension or by being in the prone position. Greater lumbar paraspinal muscle relaxation and less electromyographic (EMG) activity have been reported during traction in the prone rather than the supine position,[84] and overall, traction in the prone position has been found to be more effective than in the supine position when applied to patients with chronic low back pain and lumbosacral nerve root involvement.[85] This may be because clinically, such symptoms are often caused by spinal disc dysfunction, and symptoms of discal origin are usually most reduced in the prone position,

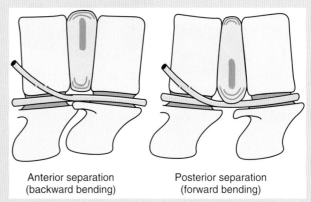

Anterior separation
(backward bending)   Posterior separation
(forward bending)

FIGURE 20.8 Effects of anterior and posterior separation on the spinal disc.

Continued

APPLICATION TECHNIQUE 20.1—*cont'd*

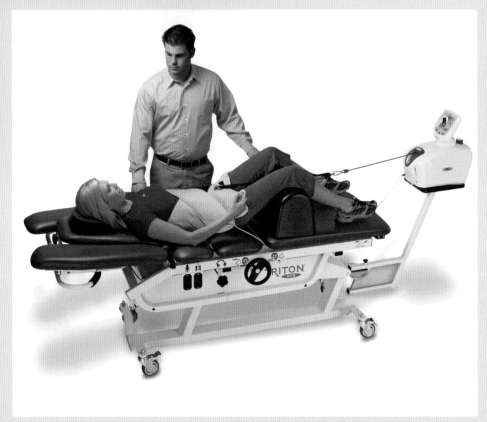

FIGURE 20.9 Central axis lumbar traction. (Courtesy Chattanooga/DJO, Vista, CA.)

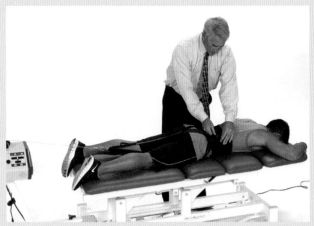

FIGURE 20.10 Prone lumbar traction with spine in neutral or slight extension. (Courtesy Mettler Electronics, Anaheim, CA.)

when the lumbar spine is in neutral or extension and the disc space is most separated (see Fig. 20.8). In contrast, symptoms caused by facet joint dysfunction are most reduced when the patient is positioned supine with the hips flexed, the lumbar spine is flexed, and the facet joints are most separated.[64] Prone neutral positioning of the lumbar spine localizes the force of the traction to the lower lumbar segments, whereas supine flexed positioning localizes the traction force to the upper lumbar and lower thoracic segments.

3. The patient should lie on a split traction table, with the area of the spine to be distracted positioned over the split and, if supine, with the lower extremities supported on a stool that does not interfere with the motion of the traction rope. A split traction table separates into two sections: one section slides away from the other when the sections are unlocked and traction is applied (Fig. 20.11). This type of table reduces the amount of traction force lost to friction between the patient and the table because the lower half of the patient's body moves with the lower section of the table. Thus less traction force is needed when a split table is used than when a one-piece table is used to provide the same amount of distractive force to the lumbar spine.[86] Initially, the patient should be positioned with the sections of the table locked together so that the table does not move as the patient moves into the treatment position. Apply appropriate belts or halter.

   Heavy-duty, nonslip thoracic and pelvic belts should be used to secure the patient during the application of mechanical lumbar traction (Fig. 20.12A). These belts must be placed with the nonslip surface directly in contact with the patient's skin and not over the clothing. Both belts must be securely tightened to prevent slipping when the traction force is applied.

APPLICATION TECHNIQUE 20.1—cont'd

◎ Clinical Pearl

The nonslip surface of the traction belt should be placed directly in contact with the patient's skin and not over clothing.

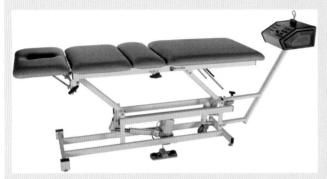

FIGURE 20.11 Split traction table. (Courtesy Mettler Electronics, Anaheim, CA.)

The belts can be placed on the table at the appropriate level and then adjusted when the patient lies down on them, or they can be secured around the patient first and secured to the table after the patient lies down. The thoracic belt is used to stabilize the upper body above the level at which traction force is desired, to prevent the patient from being pulled down the table by the force on the pelvic belt and to isolate the traction force to appropriate spinal segments. The thoracic belt should be placed so that its lower edge aligns with the superior limit at which the traction force is desired, which will generally result in its upper edge being aligned approximately with the xiphoid immediately below the greatest diameter of the thorax. The pelvic belt should be placed so that its superior edge aligns with the inferior limit

at which traction force is desired, generally just superior to the iliac crests (or superior to the superior edge of the sacrum if the patient is prone; see Fig. 20.9).

Newer belts are shaped to be more comfortable than older models and have Velcro attachments (see Fig. 20.12B). Because their placement differs slightly from that of the older belts, it is best to follow the manufacturer's instructions when applying them. Instructions for applying the type of belt shown in Fig. 20.12B are included on the Evolve website.

When the patient is supine with the lumbar spine in slight flexion, as recommended to maximize distraction of the posterior spinal structures, the pelvic belt should be placed with the fastening anteriorly and the rope posteriorly so that the pull is primarily from the posterior aspect of the pelvis (see Fig. 20.9). When the patient is prone, with the lumbar spine in neutral or slight extension, as recommended to maximize distraction of anterior spinal structures, the pelvic belt may be placed with the fastening posteriorly and the rope anteriorly so that the pull is primarily from the anterior aspect of the pelvis.[87]

4. Connect the belts or the halter to the traction device. Fasten the thoracic belt to the table above the patient's head, and connect the pelvic belt to the traction unit using a rope and a spreader bar.
5. Set the appropriate traction parameters (Table 20.1). See also the discussion of parameters in the next section. Select static or intermittent traction, and then, for static traction, set the maximum traction force and the total traction duration, or for intermittent traction, set the maximum and minimum traction force, hold and relax times, and total traction duration.
6. Start the traction.

When applying traction to the lumbar spine using a split table, first allow the traction to pull for one hold cycle to take up the slack in the belt and rope, and then, during the following relaxation of the traction, slowly release the sections of the table. The sections should be released slowly to gradually apply the initial traction force. If static traction is being used, the table's sections may be released slowly after the traction force is applied. The therapist should manually control the rate of separation of the sections to prevent sudden motion of the patient and the lower section of the table. If a split table

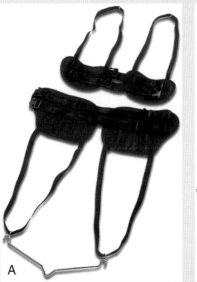

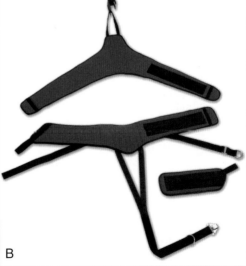

A   B

FIGURE 20.12 Traction belts: (A) old and (B) new styles. (Courtesy Chattanooga/DJO, Vista, CA.)

Continued

APPLICATION TECHNIQUE 20.1—cont'd

is not available, the traction device will take up the slack in the belt and rope during the first hold cycle. When a split table is used, once the sections are released, the force of the traction pulls the patient and the lower section of the table simultaneously and so does not have to overcome the friction between the patient and the surface of the table. For this to occur, it is essential that the lower section of the table actually move back and forth during hold and relax cycles, rather than being stationary at its position of maximal excursion, where it will act as a static surface. The clinician should observe the traction being applied and movement of the table for a few cycles and then should make any necessary adjustments to ensure that the traction is producing the desired effect.

7. Assess the patient's response.

It is recommended that the clinician assess the patient's initial response to the application of traction within the first 5 minutes of treatment so that any needed adjustments can be made then. Give the patient a means to call you and to stop the traction.

Most electrical mechanical traction units are equipped with a patient safety cutoff switch that turns off the unit and rings a bell when activated. Instruct the patient to use this switch if they experience any increase in or peripheralization of pain or other symptoms.

8. Release traction and assess the patient's response.

When the traction time is completed, lock the split sections of the table, release the tension on the traction ropes, and allow the patient to rest briefly before getting up and recompressing the joints. Then reexamine the patient.

TABLE 20.1	Recommended Parameters for the Application of Lumbar Spinal Traction		
Area of Spine and Goals of Treatment	Force	Hold/Relax Times (s)	Total Traction Time (min)
Initial/acute phase	13–20 kg (29–44 lb)	Static	5–10
Joint distraction	22.5 kg (50 lb); 50% of body weight	15/15	20–30
Decreased muscle spasm	25% of body weight	5/5	20–30
Disc problems or stretch of soft tissue	25% of body weight	60/20	20–30

Parameters for Mechanical Lumbar Traction

Static Versus Intermittent Traction. Mechanical traction may be administered statically, with the same force throughout treatment, or intermittently, with the force varying every few seconds throughout treatment. Some authors recommend that only static traction should be applied to avoid a stretch reflex of the muscles[28]; however, others report that static traction and intermittent traction are equally effective but that higher forces can be used with intermittent traction.[88] No differences in lumbar sacrospinalis EMG activity or vertebral separation have been found when static traction and intermittent traction of the same force have been compared.[89,90] It is generally recommended that static traction be used if the area being treated is inflamed, if the patient's symptoms are easily aggravated by motion, or if the patient's symptoms are related to a disc protrusion.[28] Intermittent traction with long hold times may be effective to treat symptoms related to disc protrusion, whereas shorter hold and relax times are recommended for symptoms related to joint dysfunction.

Clinical Pearl

Static traction can help relieve symptoms associated with inflammation or a disc protrusion, as well as symptoms aggravated by motion. Intermittent traction can also help relieve symptoms associated with a disc protrusion or joint dysfunction.

Hold and Relax Times. If intermittent traction is selected, the maximum traction force is applied during the hold time, and a lower traction force is applied during the relax time. The recommended ratio and duration of hold and relax times depend on the patient's condition and tolerance. In general, if intermittent traction is used to treat a disc problem, longer hold times of approximately 60 seconds and shorter relax times of approximately 20 seconds are recommended. If intermittent traction is used to treat a spinal joint problem, shorter hold and relax times of approximately 15 seconds each are recommended.[30] Symptom severity should also be used to guide hold and relax times. When the patient's symptoms are severe, long hold times and long relax times are recommended to limit the amount of movement. As symptoms become less severe, the relax time can gradually be decreased, and when discomfort has decreased to a local ache rather than a pain, the hold time can also be reduced so that when the symptoms are mild, traction produces an oscillatory motion with very short hold and relax times of approximately 3 to 5 seconds each.

Force. Recommendations for the amount of force to use for traction vary; however, most agree that the optimal amount of force depends on the patient's clinical presentation, the goals of treatment, and the patient's position during treatment.[28,40] For all applications, the force should be kept low during the initial traction session to reduce the risk of reactive muscle guarding and spasms and to determine whether traction is likely to aggravate the patient's symptoms. The traction force can be increased gradually in subsequent sessions as the patient becomes used to the procedure. It is recommended for all applications that the traction force to the lumbar spine start at 30 to 45 lb (13 to 20 kg).

The traction force to the lumbar spine should start at 30 to 45 lb (13 to 20 kg) and may increase gradually as needed up to approximately 60% of the patient's body weight.

When the goal is to decrease compression on a spinal nerve root or facet joint, sufficient force must be used to separate the facet joints in the area being treated. In the lumbar spine, this requires a force of between 50 lb (22.5 kg) and approximately 60% of the patient's body weight.[30,39,48,89]

When the goal is to decrease muscle spasm, stretch soft tissue, or exert a centripetal force on the disc by spinal elongation without joint surface separation, lower forces of 25% of total body weight for the lumbar spine are generally effective. When this is the goal, applying a hot pack in conjunction with traction may result in greater spinal elongation and thus more effective relief of symptoms.

Higher traction forces are needed when patient positioning or the harness requires the traction force to overcome gravity or friction between the patient and the table. For example, when lumbar traction is applied without a split table, the traction has to overcome the friction between the patient's body and the surface of the table, so higher traction forces are necessary, whereas when a split table is used, gravity and friction are reduced, so lower traction forces may be sufficient.

The force of traction can be adjusted during or between treatments. The force should be decreased during treatment if any peripheralization of signs or symptoms occurs or, as mentioned in the section on precautions, if complete relief of severe pain is attained. If the patient's symptoms are moderately decreased by traction, the force can be increased by 2 to 5 kg (5 to 15 lb) for lumbar traction at each subsequent treatment session until optimal relief of symptoms is achieved.

When intermittent traction is used, the relaxed force should be approximately 50% of the maximum force or less. Total release of the force during the relaxed phase of intermittent traction is not recommended because this can cause rebound aggravation of the patient's symptoms.

Total Treatment Duration. Studies have not compared the effects of different traction treatment durations; however, most authors recommend that to assess the patient's response, the duration of a patient's first treatment with traction should be brief (i.e., about 5 minutes if initial symptoms are severe and 10 minutes if initial symptoms are moderate).[30,91] If severe symptoms are significantly relieved by brief, low-force traction, the duration of treatment should be kept short; otherwise, exacerbation of symptoms after treatment is likely. If the patient's symptoms are partially relieved after 10 minutes of traction, it is recommended that the duration of the initial treatment not be extended; if symptoms are unchanged after 10 minutes, the hold force may be increased slightly or the angle of pull modified, and treatment may be continued for an additional 10 minutes. Recommendations for the duration of subsequent treatments vary from 8 to 10 minutes for treatment of a disc protrusion[30] to 20 to 40 minutes for this and other indications.[92] Treatment for longer than 40 minutes is generally thought to provide no additional benefit.

Treatment Frequency. Some authors state that spinal traction must be administered daily to be effective, although the outcomes of different treatment frequencies have not been systematically evaluated.[30,92]

MECHANICAL CERVICAL TRACTION

MECHANICAL CERVICAL TRACTION

Equipment Required for Motorized Mechanical Traction

- Traction unit
- Cervical traction halter
- Spreader bar
- Extension rope

Equipment Required for Weighted Mechanical Traction

- Traction device (ropes, pulley, weights)
- Cervical traction halter
- Weight bag for water, weights, or sand

Procedure for Mechanical Cervical Traction[93]

1. Select the appropriate mechanical traction device.
   Various devices are available for applying mechanical traction to the cervical spine in the clinic or home setting. The choice depends on the region of the body to be treated, the amount of force to be applied, whether static or intermittent traction is desired, and the setting in which the treatment will be applied.
2. Determine optimal patient position.

When positioning the patient, try to achieve a comfortable position that allows muscle relaxation while maximizing the separation between involved structures. The relative degree of flexion or extension of the spine during traction determines which surfaces are most effectively separated. The flexed position results in greater separation of posterior structures, including the facet joints and intervertebral foramina, whereas the neutral or extended position results in greater separation of anterior structures, including the disc spaces (see Fig. 20.8). In most cases, a symmetrical central force is used, in which the direction of force is in line with the central sagittal axis of the patient; however, if the patient presents with unilateral symptoms, a unilateral traction force that applies more force to one side of the spine than to the other may prove more effective.[83] A unilateral force can be applied by offsetting the axis of the traction in the direction that best reduces the patient's symptoms. For example, if the patient presents with right neck or arm pain that is aggravated by right side bending and is relieved by left side bending, the traction should be offset so that it applies a left side bending force.

To apply traction to the cervical spine, the patient may be in the supine or the sitting position, but the impact on the cervical spine is less predictable in sitting because the patient's hip joint stiffness can alter the effects (Fig. 20.13; see Fig. 20.6).[94] Certain cervical traction

Continued

APPLICATION TECHNIQUE 20.2—cont'd

devices can be used in only one of these positions, whereas others can be used in either position. For example, over-the-door cervical traction units must be applied while the patient is sitting, whereas the Saunders occipital cervical traction halter can be used only with the patient supine. In the supine position, the cervical spine is supported and non–weight bearing, resulting in increased patient comfort and muscle relaxation and greater separation between cervical segments than when the same amount of traction force is applied with the patient in the sitting position.[32] When the patient is supine, cervical flexion, rotation, and side bending can be adjusted for patient comfort and to focus the traction force on the involved area. When cervical traction is applied in the sitting position, cervical flexion and extension can be controlled to a limited degree by placing the patient facing toward (more flexion) or away from (neutral or more extension) the traction force, although cervical side bending and rotation are difficult to adjust in the sitting position. Placing the cervical spine in a neutral or slightly extended position focuses the traction forces on the upper cervical spine, whereas placing the cervical spine in a flexed position focuses the traction forces on the lower cervical spine.[68,95] Maximum posterior elongation of the cervical spine is achieved when the neck and the angle of pull are at approximately 25 to 35 degrees of flexion, as shown in Fig. 20.13.[68]

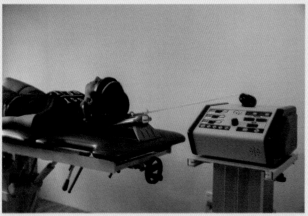

FIGURE 20.13 Supine cervical traction with soft occipital halter with approximately 20- to 30-degree angle of pull to maximize separation of the intervertebral foramina and disc spaces. (Courtesy V2U Healthcare, MidView City, Singapore.)

3. Apply the appropriate halter.

Different cervical halters have been developed to maximize patient comfort and avoid excessive pressure on the TMJs during the application of cervical traction (see Figs. 20.7A and 20.13). Some soft fabric halters apply pressure through both the mandibles and the occiput, whereas others, such as the Saunders frictionless halter, apply pressure only through the occiput. The adjustability of the halter, the patient position, and the status of the TMJs should be considered in selecting the most appropriate cervical halter for a particular patient. The halter should be adjustable to accommodate variations in the shape and size of patients' heads and necks and to allow for different angles of traction pull. A halter that applies force through the mandibles and the occiput should allow adjustment of the distance between the occiput and the spreader bar, the chin and the spreader bar, and the mandibles and the occiput. Tension on the straps should be adjusted so that the pull is comfortably and evenly applied to both the occiput and the mandibles. A halter that applies pressure only through the occiput

should adjust to fit snugly enough to stay on during the application of traction. Soft halters can be used in the sitting or supine position, whereas the Saunders halter can be used only in the supine position. Soft halters that apply pressure through the occiput tend to slip off the patient's head when traction is applied, even when appropriately adjusted for size, whereas the Saunders halter, which also avoids pressure on the TMJs, generally remains securely in place when traction is applied. The Saunders halter is designed with a low-friction sliding component for the patient's head so that the traction force does not have to overcome the friction between the patient's head and the table. Therefore, slightly less force should be applied when this type of halter rather than a soft fabric halter is used.

4. Connect the belts or the halter to the traction device.

For cervical traction, all types of soft fabric halters are connected to the traction device by a rope and a spreader bar. The Saunders halter is connected directly to the traction device by a rope.

5. Set the appropriate traction parameters (Table 20.2; see parameter discussion in the next section).

Select static or intermittent traction; then, for static traction, set the maximum traction force and the total traction duration, or for intermittent traction, set the maximum and minimum traction force, hold and relax times, and total traction duration.

6. Start the traction.

The patient should be observed for the first few cycles of cervical traction to ensure that the halter is staying in place and is exerting force through appropriate areas and to ensure that the patient is comfortable and is not experiencing any adverse effects from the treatment.

7. Assess the patient's response.

Assess the patient's initial response to the application of traction within the first 5 minutes of treatment and make any needed adjustments. Give the patient a means to call you and to stop the traction.

Most electrical mechanical traction units are equipped with a patient safety cutoff switch that turns off the unit and rings a bell when activated. Instruct the patient to use this switch if they experience any increase in or peripheralization of pain or other symptoms.

8. Release traction and assess the patient's response.

When the traction time is completed, release tension on the traction ropes, and allow the patient to rest briefly before getting up and recompressing the joints. Then reexamine the patient.

TABLE 20.2	Recommended Parameters for the Application of Cervical Spine Traction		
Area of the Spine and Goals of Treatment	Total Traction Force	Hold/Relax Times (s)	Total Traction (min)
Initial/acute phase	3–4 kg (7–9 lb)	Static	5–10
Joint distraction	9–13 kg (20–29 lb); 7% of body weight	15/15	20–30
Decreased muscle spasm	5–7 kg (11–15 lb)	5/5	20–30
Disc problems or stretch of soft tissue	5–7 kg (11–15 lb)	60/20	20–30

Parameters for Mechanical Cervical Traction

The principles for selecting parameters for mechanical cervical traction are similar to the principles used for lumbar traction, with a few exceptions mentioned in the next section. For a detailed discussion of the principles used for selecting treatment parameters for mechanical cervical traction, see the previous section on mechanical lumbar traction. It should be noted that far less force is used for cervical traction than for lumbar traction.

Intermittent traction may be most effective for reducing pain and increasing cervical ROM in a variety of cervical conditions[96] and may be particularly helpful for reducing symptoms associated with mechanical neck disorders.[97]

Force. The greatest difference between parameters used for lumbar and cervical traction is the amount of force. For all cervical traction applications, the traction force should start at 8 to 10 lb (3 to 4 kg).

> ### Clinical Pearl
>
> The traction force to the cervical spine should start at 8 to 10 lb (3 and 4 kg) and may increase gradually as needed up to approximately 7% of the patient's body weight.

When the goal is to decrease compression on a spinal nerve root or facet joint, sufficient force must be used to separate facet joints in the area being treated. In the cervical spine, 20 to 30 lb (9 to 13 kg), or approximately 7% of the patient's body weight, is generally sufficient to achieve this outcome.[30,48,89] When the goal is to decrease muscle spasm, stretch soft tissue, or exert a centripetal force on the disc by spinal elongation without joint surface separation, 12 to 15 lb (5 to 7 kg) of force will generally be effective. An alternative approach to selecting the traction force is to set the maximum at the minimum amount required to reduce radicular symptoms and to set the minimum at the least value before radicular symptoms recur.[98]

Applying a hot pack in conjunction with traction may result in greater spinal elongation and thus more effectively relieve symptoms.

Higher traction forces are needed when patient positioning, the harness, or the table requires the traction force to overcome gravity or friction. For cervical traction, higher forces are needed when the patient is sitting and traction has to overcome the force of gravity on the patient's head. In contrast, when the patient is supine, gravity is not opposing the force of the traction, and if the Saunders frictionless halter is used, there is little friction, so lower traction forces may be sufficient.

The force of traction can be adjusted during or between treatments. Force should be decreased during treatment if any peripheralization of signs or symptoms occurs or, as mentioned in the section on precautions, if complete relief of severe pain is attained. If the patient's symptoms are moderately decreased by mechanical cervical traction, the traction force can be increased by 3 to 5 lb (1.5 to 2 kg) at each subsequent treatment session until maximal relief of symptoms is achieved. Traction force to the cervical spine generally should not exceed 30 lb (15 kg).

HIP TRACTION WITH TRACTION DEVICE OR RESISTANCE BAND

Mechanical hip traction can also be performed by the patient securing a resistance band on the lower extremity, with a figure-eight loop above the malleoli, and anchoring the other end around a strong, stable structure. These bands, sometimes called SuperBands or CrossFit Bands, are not the typical exercise bands that are used traditionally in physical therapy for exercise. They are able to create hundreds of pounds of tension without breaking. The patient then lies supine or on their side and carefully moves their body away from the anchor, placing the desired amount of tension through the band. The patient can then relax and allow the band to exert the traction force (Fig. 20.14). The patient may secure the band at various heights on the stable structure for

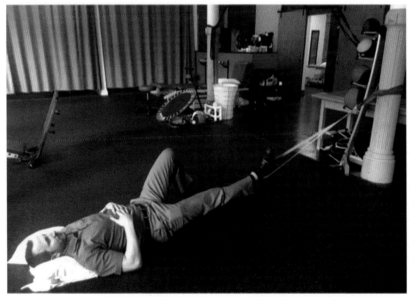

FIGURE 20.14 Hip traction with a resistance band.

traction in varying degrees of flexion. The patient can also position their body so that their hip is in varying degrees of abduction. Resistance bands are relatively inexpensive and can be used in situations when strong hip traction is not needed or desired.

Alternatively, the HipTrac (MedRock, Inc., Portland, OR, www.medrock.com) may be used when the patient is seeking both pain relief and strong joint capsule mobilization, such as in the case of hip osteoarthritis. HipTrac is a lightweight, portable, and pneumatic long-axis hip traction device that simulates manual traction that is usually applied by a health care provider (Fig. 20.15). This device may be used in the clinic or at home. It can position the hip between 0 and 30 degrees of flexion and any degree of abduction, rotation, and extension. It produces forces of more than 180 lb (0 to 800 N) and is

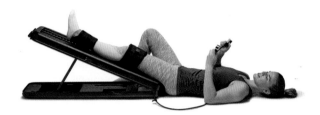

FIGURE 20.15 Hip traction with the HipTrac device. (Courtesy HipTrac, Portland, OR.)

designed to apply traction to the hip joint specifically in isolation, limiting force through the lumbar spine or in combination with the lumbar spine unilaterally.

APPLICATION TECHNIQUE 20.3   MECHANICAL HIP TRACTION

Equipment Required for Mechanical Hip Traction

- HipTrac device
- HipTrac bindings

Procedure for Mechanical Hip Traction

1. Place the HipTrac on a firm, flat, nonslippery surface. Make sure there is enough space for the patient to lie down fully and that the device is not resting on top of the air pump hose.
2. Offer a pillow for the patient's head for comfort.
3. While seated, wrap the ankle binding around the lower leg with its lower edge just above the malleoli, and center the back hook on the Achilles tendon. The position of the hook medial or lateral to the Achilles will offer more internal or external rotation during use as desired. If the goal is available and comfortable external rotation, then rotate so that hook is centered on Achilles tendon. After securing tightly, stretch and secure the two elastic Velcro bands around the ankle tightly enough to prevent the binding from slipping during use but not so tightly that they cause discomfort.
4. Wrap the thigh binding around the thigh directly above the patella. Stretch and tightly secure the two elastic Velcro bands around the binding.
5. Connect the hook on the adjustable strap of the thigh binding to the plastic D-ring at the top of the ankle binding. With the patient's leg straight (knee extended), tighten this adjustable strap.
6. Open the HipTrac and set the flexion angle by placing its support legs into one of the four available positions; three positions are placed into the "shark teeth," whereas the fourth is used when the unit is closed all the way. These different positions support different amounts of hip flexion (0 to 30 degrees) and should be selected per Table 20.3 according to the goals of treatment.
7. Have the patient lie down and place their leg, with bindings attached on the solid plastic part of the HipTrac, next to the metal slide carriage, ready to insert the metal hook into one of the holes on the HipTrac face. The patient should then use the Pull Strap to pull the HipTrac into their involved buttocks (ischial tuberosity), with pad in between, as tightly as possible while reaching for the highest hook opening they can insert into. Ensure that the patient is securely connected to the slide carriage and that the foam pad is still between their buttocks and the HipTrac.

8. Adjust the degree of hip abduction by rotating the rest of the body opposite the HipTrac while keeping the involved leg still to achieve the desired goals of treatment, per Table 20.3. Individuals may differ in their response to different positions. Therefore, each person's position should be adjusted to achieve the greatest benefits.
9. Select the treatment parameters, including maximum traction force, hold time, and total treatment time, according to the recommendations in Table 20.4. The HipTrac manufacturer also provides specific protocol recommendations for different patient presentations.
10. Gradually pump air into the cylinder to achieve the desired amount of traction force (see Table 20.4). The HipTrac can apply a force of up to 180 lb. Because individuals differ in their response to different amounts of traction force, adjust the force so that it achieves the greatest benefit for the patient.
11. Stop pumping when the desired maximum amount of traction force has been attained. The hand pump will hold the pressure automatically.
12. After adjusting to achieve the maximum traction force, sustain this force for the hold time (see Table 20.4). Then release approximately 50% of the force for 5 to 10 seconds, and then return to the full maximum force. Continue to progress through the treatment protocol with the hold and release duty cycle selected. In general, the patient can be instructed to do this independently. As per Table 20.4, hold times can be gradually increased with subsequent treatments.
13. Assess the patient's response.
    It is recommended that the clinician assess the patient's initial response to the application of traction during the first few hold periods and then again within the first 5 minutes of treatment so that any needed adjustments can be made.
14. Give the patient a means to call you and to stop the traction.
    Instruct the patient to alert you if they experience any increase in symptoms.
15. After the recommended treatment time (see Table 20.4), release traction and assess the patient's response.
    When the traction time is completed, press the release button to release the traction. While holding the release button depressed, gently assist the slide carriage back to its original position by pulling heel toward buttocks.

APPLICATION TECHNIQUE 20.3—cont'd

16. Have the patient relax for a couple of minutes before removing their leg from the HipTrac.
17. To disconnect the ankle binding from the slide carriage, first remove the foam pad from between the patient's buttocks and the HipTrac. The patient can then use the Pull Strap to pull the HipTrac toward their buttocks while bending their knee slightly. If the patient maintains pressure of the HipTrac toward their buttocks with the Pull Strap while they simply straighten their knee, the hook should easily lift out of the HipTrac. Once the hook is removed, the patient can rest their heel on the solid part of the HipTrac next to the metal slide carriage for a few minutes if needed and then roll away from the HipTrac.
18. Reassess the patient's response at the end of the intervention.

TABLE 20.3	Suggested Positioning for the Application of Mechanical Hip Traction		
Goal	Degrees of Hip Flexion	Degrees of Hip Abduction	Hip Rotation
Pain relief	20–30	15–30	Maximum external rotation
Increase ROM	Extension as tolerated	Abduction as tolerated	Maximum internal rotation

ROM, Range of motion.

TABLE 20.4	Suggested Hold Times, Maximum Traction Force, and Total Treatment Times for Mechanical Hip Traction[a]		
Days of Treatment	Hold Time (min)	Maximum Traction Force (psi)	Total Treatment Time (min)
1–7	2	30–40	10–12
8–21	2–4	40–50	12–15
≥22	3–10	Progress gradually to 50 to 100	15–30

[a]Traction force should be released about halfway for 5–10 seconds between hold times.

SELF-TRACTION

Self-traction uses gravity and the weight of the patient's body or force exerted by the patient to exert a distractive force on the spine. Self-traction can be used for the lumbar spine but not the cervical spine.

Self-traction of the lumbar spine is appropriate for home use when symptoms are relieved by low loads of mechanical traction or are associated with mild to moderate compression of spinal structures. Because the amount and duration of force that can be applied by self-traction are limited by the upper body strength of the patient and the weight of the lower body, self-traction is not generally effective when high forces are required to relieve symptoms with mechanical traction or when distraction of the spinal joints is necessary. Self-traction can be applied in several ways, a few of which are described in Application Technique 20.4. All methods of self-traction attempt to fix the patient's upper body by using the body weight or the force of the arms to pull on the lumbar spine. Positions and ways to apply self-traction other than those described can be developed by the clinician or the patient familiar with the principles of self-traction.

APPLICATION TECHNIQUE 20.4   SELF-TRACTION

Procedure for Self-Traction: Sitting

The patient should do the following:
1. Sit in a sturdy armchair, keeping both feet on the floor at all times to control lumbopelvic position.
2. Hold on to the arms of the chair and push down, lifting your trunk to reduce the weight on the spine (Fig. 20.16). Grade the force of the traction by varying the force of downward pressure on the arms of the chair and thus the degree of unweighting of the spine.

Procedure for Self-Traction: Between Corner Counters

The patient should do the following:
1. Stand in a corner that has solid counter surfaces behind you.
2. Place your forearms on the counter and push down to decrease the weight on the spine by unweighting your feet (Fig. 20.17), but leave your feet on the ground to control lumbopelvic position.

Procedure for Self-Traction: Overhead Bar

The patient should do the following:
1. Stand in a partial squat under a horizontal bar.
2. Hold on to the bar and pull to reduce the weight on the spine (Fig. 20.18); leave your feet on the ground to control lumbopelvic position.

Advantages

- Minimal or no equipment needed
- Easy for patient to perform
- Easy for patient to control
- Can be performed in many environments and thus many times during the day

Continued

APPLICATION TECHNIQUE 20.4—cont'd

Disadvantages

- Low maximum force and so may not be effective
- Requires strong, injury-free upper extremities
- Cannot be used for the cervical spine

- No research data to support the efficacy of this form of traction
- Patient must have adequate postural awareness and control to position the body appropriately for maximum benefit.

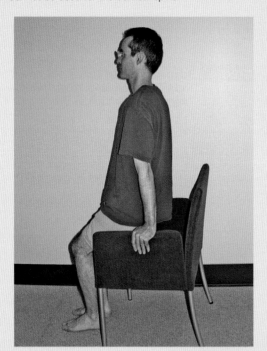

FIGURE 20.16 Sitting self-traction for the lumbar spine.

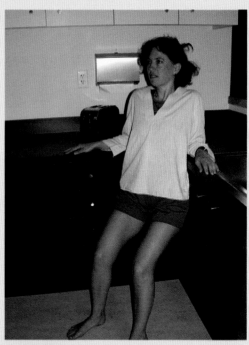

FIGURE 20.17 Self-traction between corner counters.

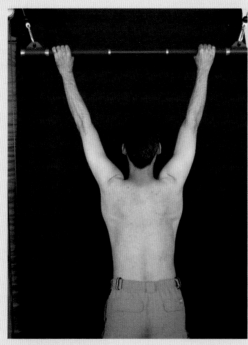

FIGURE 20.18 Self-traction with overhead bar.

POSITIONAL TRACTION

Positional traction involves prolonged placement of the patient in a position that places tension on only one side of the lumbar spine (Fig. 20.19). This type of traction gently stretches the lumbar spine by applying a prolonged low-load longitudinal force to one side of the spine. Although the low force associated with this form of traction is unlikely to cause joint distraction, it may decrease muscle spasm, stretch soft tissue, or exert a centripetal force on the disc by spinal elongation without joint surface separation. Positional traction may be used to treat unilateral symptoms originating from the lumbar spine and can be a valuable component of a patient's home program during the early stages of recovery when symptoms are severe and irritable.

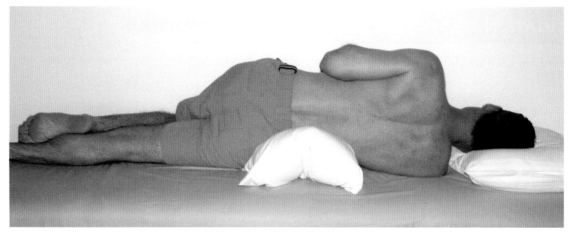

FIGURE 20.19 Positional traction to stretch and distract the left lumbar area.

APPLICATION TECHNIQUE 20.5   POSITIONAL LUMBAR TRACTION

Equipment Required

- Pillow(s)

Procedure

The patient should do the following:
1. Lie on their side with the involved side up and a pillow under the waist at approximately the level of the dysfunction. The pillow side bends the lumbar spine away from the involved side, opening the joints and disc spaces on the involved side.
2. Rotate toward the involved side by moving the lower shoulder forward and the upper shoulder back.
3. Rotate further toward the involved side by straightening the inferior lower extremity, bending the superior lower extremity, and hooking the superior foot behind the inferior leg. Rotation toward the involved side further stretches and opens the involved area.

4. Adjust flexion/extension to the position of greatest comfort and symptom relief.
5. Maintain the position for 10 to 20 minutes.

Advantages

- Requires no equipment or assistance
- Inexpensive
- Can be applied by the patient at home
- Low force and so not likely to aggravate an irritable condition
- Position readily adjustable

Disadvantages

- Low force and so not likely to be effective where joint distraction is required
- Requires agility and skill by the patient to perform correctly
- No research data to support the efficacy of this form of traction

INVERSION TRACTION

Inversion traction, which is applied by placing the patient in a device that requires a head-down position, uses the weight of the patient's upper body to apply traction to the lumbar spine. Although inversion traction devices are rarely used in the clinical setting, individuals can easily purchase them for home use. Despite evidence for effectiveness, the popularity of this form of traction has varied because of concerns for adverse effects. One study found that the addition of inversion traction to standard physical therapy allowed 10 of 13 (76.9%) patients with symptoms associated with single-level lumbar disc disease to have sufficient symptom reduction to avoid surgery compared with 2 of 11 receiving physical therapy without inversion traction, but patients with significant cardiorespiratory disorders were excluded from this study.[99] Another study also found that inversion traction provided similar clinical effectiveness as conventional mechanical spinal traction in patients with low back pain and sciatica resulting from lumbar disc herniation.[100] However, the implications of this are unclear because, as discussed earlier in this chapter, most studies have not found conventional mechanical traction to be effective for low back pain with sciatica. Small, although statistically significant, increases in systolic and diastolic blood pressure and ophthalmic artery pressure have been documented in subjects without cardiovascular disease or a history of hypertension in response to the application of inversion traction.[68,101,102] This has generated concern about stroke or myocardial infarction in patients with uncontrolled hypertension. Given the potential benefits and risks of spinal inversion traction, this form of traction should be used only with carefully selected patients.

> ### ◎ Clinical Pearl
>
> Because inversion traction can increase systolic and diastolic blood pressure and ophthalmic artery pressure, it should be used only with carefully selected patients.

APPLICATION TECHNIQUE 20.6   INVERSION TRACTION

Procedure for Lumbar Spine Inversion Traction (Fig. 20.20)

1. Adjust the inversion traction device to the patient's height.
2. Ensure that the safety strap limiting the maximum degree of inversion is connected.
3. Set the angle of inversion to be comfortable and reduce symptoms. Most patients find partial inversion to be most comfortable and effective.
4. Place securing devices on feet or ankles if necessary. Different devices use different ways to secure the feet, such as ankle cuffs or straps. If used, put these on the patient before they step into the table.
5. Have the patient step into the inversion traction device so that their back lies directly on the table.
6. Secure the patient's feet.
7. Instruct the patient to gradually raise their hands above their head, tilting and inverting the table head down to the desired degree of inversion (Fig. 20.21).
8. Sustain this inversion for up to 2 minutes.
9. Have the patient lower their arms to return to the head-up position for 1 to 2 minutes.
10. Repeat the inversion up to six times, to patient tolerance and comfort.

11. Have the patient return to the head-up position and step out of the device.
12. Remove any securing devices from the feet or ankles.

Advantages

- The equipment has a small "footprint" and may be used in the clinic or at home.
- The equipment is inexpensive.
- Easy for patient to perform
- Easy for patient to control

Disadvantages

- Inversion may elevate systemic and intraocular blood pressure.
- Cannot be used for cervical spine
- Limited research to support efficacy

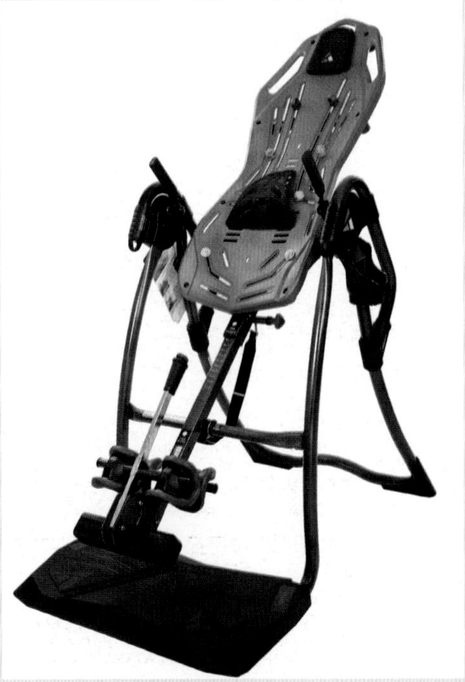

FIGURE 20.20 Inversion traction device. (Courtesy Teeter.)

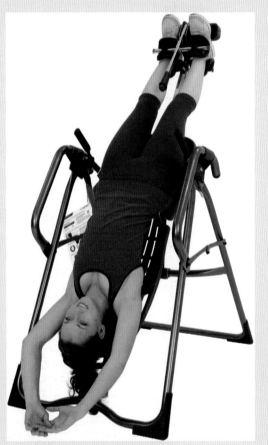

FIGURE 20.21 Using the weight of the patient's upper body to apply traction to the lumbar spine. (Courtesy Teeter.)

MANUAL TRACTION

Manual traction is the application of force by the therapist in the direction of distracting the joints. Manual traction can be used for the cervical and lumbar spine as well as for the peripheral joints. Many techniques can be used to apply manual traction; however, because manual traction is generally classified as manual therapy rather than as a physical agent, only a few basic techniques for applying manual traction to the spine are described here. For more detailed descriptions of these and other techniques for applying manual traction to the spine or to the peripheral joints, please consult a manual therapy text.[1-3]

APPLICATION TECHNIQUE 20.7   MANUAL TRACTION

Procedure for Manual Lumbar Traction (Fig. 20.22)

1. Position the patient in the position of least pain. This is usually supine, with the hips and knees flexed.
2. Position yourself. Kneel at the patient's feet, facing the patient.
3. Place your hands in the appropriate position, behind the patient's proximal legs, over the muscle belly of the triceps surae.
4. Apply traction force to the patient's spine by leaning your body back and away from the patient, keeping your spine in a neutral position.
5. Maintain this force for at least 15 seconds. Apply the force for 5 minutes or longer for static traction for patients whose symptoms are relieved by traction and are aggravated by motion. Apply the force for 15 to 30 seconds, then release for 15 to 30 seconds for intermittent traction for patients whose symptoms are relieved by traction and motion.

Adjust the force of the traction according to the desired outcome and the patient's report.

Procedure for Manual Cervical Traction: Patient Supine (Fig. 20.23)

1. Position the patient supine.
2. Position yourself. Stand at the head of the patient, facing the patient.
3. Place your hands in the appropriate position. Supinate your forearms so that your hands are facing up; place the lateral border of your second finger in contact with the patient's occiput and your thumbs behind the patient's ears.
4. Apply traction. Apply force through the occiput by leaning back, keeping your spine in a neutral position.

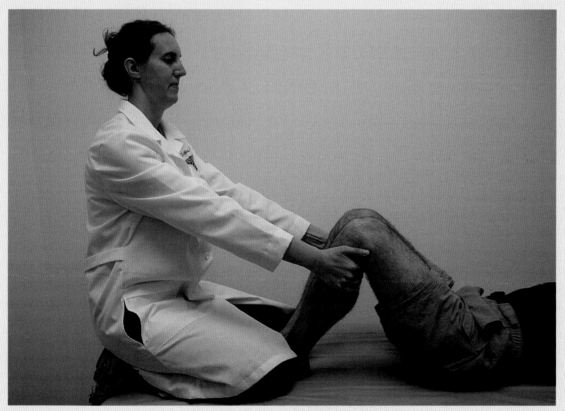

FIGURE 20.22 Manual lumbar traction.

Continued

APPLICATION TECHNIQUE 20.7—*cont'd*

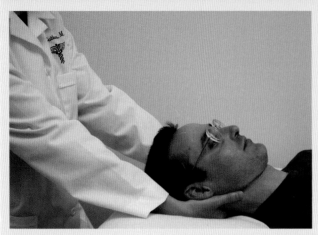

FIGURE 20.23 Manual cervical traction—supine.

Procedure for Manual Cervical Traction: Patient Sitting (Fig. 20.24)

1. Position the patient in the sitting position.
2. Stand behind the patient.
3. Place your hands in the appropriate position. With your arms in a neutral position, place your thumbs under the patient's occiput and the rest of your hands along the side of the patient's face.
4. Apply traction through the patient's occiput by lifting up.

Adjust the force of the traction according to the desired outcome and the patient's report. Manual traction to the cervical spine may be static or intermittent.

Advantages

- No equipment required
- Short setup time
- Force can be finely graded.
- The clinician is present throughout treatment to monitor and assess the patient's response.
- Can be applied briefly, before setting up mechanical traction, to help determine whether longer application of traction would be beneficial
- Can be used with patients who do not tolerate being placed in halters or belts

Disadvantages

- Limited maximum traction force, probably not sufficient to distract the lumbar facet joints
- The amount of traction force cannot be easily replicated or specifically recorded.
- Cannot be applied for a prolonged period of time
- Requires a skilled clinician to apply

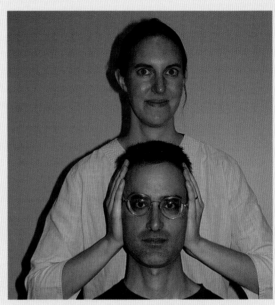

FIGURE 20.24 Manual cervical traction—sitting.

Documentation

When applying traction, document the following:
- Type of traction
- Area of the body where traction is applied
- Patient position
- Type of halter if one is used
- Maximum force
- Total treatment time
- Response to treatment
- With intermittent traction, also document the following:
  - Hold time
  - Relax time
  - Force during the relax time

Documentation is typically written in the SOAP note format. The following examples summarize only the modality component of treatment and are not intended to represent a comprehensive plan of care.

EXAMPLES

When applying intermittent (int) mechanical (mech) cervical (cerv) traction (txn) to a right upper extremity (UE), document the following:

S: Pt reports R UE pain from shoulder to wrist aggravated by turning his neck to the right or bending his neck backward.

O: Pretreatment: R UE pain 6/10 from shoulder to wrist. Cervical ROM 20% backward bend, 20% R side bend, aggravating R UE pain.

Intervention: Int mech cerv txn, Pt supine, soft occipital halter. 10 kg/5 kg, 60 s/20 s, 15 min.

Posttreatment: R UE pain 4/10 from shoulder to elbow. Cervical ROM 40% backward bend, 50% R side bend.

A: Pt tolerated cerv txn well, with decreased pain and increased cervical ROM.

P: Continue int mech cerv txn, Pt supine, soft occipital halter. Increase force to 12 kg/7 kg next treatment.

When instructing a patient in the application of self-traction to a lower extremity, document the following:

S: Pt reports low back and L LE pain that increases with sitting.
O: **Pretreatment:** Pt unable to sit × 30 min without low back and L LE pain increasing to 8/10.
Intervention: Pt instructed in self traction in chair with arms. Pt unweighted approximately 50% of body weight, 30-s hold/relax × 3.
Posttreatment: Low back and L LE pain decreased 50% for 2 to 3 h after self-traction. Pt able to continue working in sitting position for 2 h without getting out of his chair.
A: Pt able to perform self-traction appropriately and symptoms improved.

P: Pt advised to perform self-traction as above every 20 min at work.

When applying lumbar positional traction, document the following:

S: Pt reports low back pain that awakens her 3 to 5 times per night.
O: **Pretreatment:** Low back pain 5/10 when lying in bed at night.
Intervention: Lumbar positional txn, R side lying with pillow at waist, R side bend, L rotation × 20 min.
Posttreatment: Pain decreased to 2/10.
A: Pt had successful trial of positional txn with decreased pain.
P: Pt to perform traction as above at home 2 to 3 times per day, including immediately before sleeping.

CLINICAL CASE STUDIES

The following case studies summarize the concepts of spinal traction discussed in this chapter. Based on the scenario presented, an evaluation of the clinical findings and goals of treatment are proposed. These are followed by a discussion of the factors to be considered in selection of spinal traction as the indicated intervention and in selection of the ideal patient position, traction technique, and traction parameters to promote progress toward the goals.

CASE STUDY 20.1

Osteoarthritis With Facet Joint Degeneration and Cervical Radiculopathy
Examination
History

AW is a 75-year-old woman referred to physical therapy with a diagnosis of osteoarthritis with moderately severe facet joint degeneration at C4 through C6. She reports neck pain and stiffness that make her feel unsafe while driving. When the pain is severe, she is also unable to participate in her sewing class at the local senior center. AW has had similar but gradually worsening symptoms intermittently for the past 20 years. Her symptoms are always worse during the winter. In the past, AW has been referred to physical therapy for treatment of these symptoms, and her treatment has included traction, heat, massage, and a few exercises. Within four to six visits, this combination of interventions helps relieve her symptoms for about a year until the following winter.

Systems Review

AW is accompanied to the clinic by her granddaughter. She complains of bilateral neck pain that is worse on the right than on the left. She also reports that her neck is stiff first thing in the morning, loosening up throughout the day but becoming stiff and sore late in the afternoon and for the rest of the evening. She reports right upper extremity pain when she extends her neck or looks far to the right. Today, she rates the pain in the right side of her neck at 7/10, the pain in the left side of her neck at 4/10, and also 4/10 pain into her right arm when she turns to look to the far right. This pain negatively affects AW's mood when it prevents her from partaking in activities that she enjoys. She reports no pain, numbness, tingling, or weakness of the lower extremities.

Tests and Measures

The objective examination reveals a kyphotic thoracic posture with a forward head position. Cervical ROM is restricted by approximately 50% in all planes. There is moderate hypertonicity of the cervical paraspinal muscles and stiffness of all cervical facet joints on passive intervertebral motion testing, with the lower cervical joints being stiffer than the upper cervical joints. Right arm pain is reproduced at end-range cervical extension and right rotation. Shoulder flexion and abduction are limited to 140 degrees bilaterally, and all other objective tests, including upper extremity sensation, strength, and reflexes, are within normal limits for this patient's age.

What are the indications for spinal traction in this patient? What other physical agent could be useful for this patient in conjunction with traction? How would you improve her long-term benefits? What should you examine (including elements of the history, as well as tests and measures) before applying traction to this patient?

Evaluation and Goals

ICF Level	Current Status	Goals
Body function and structure	Neck pain and stiffness	Decrease neck pain by 50%
	Kyphotic thoracic posture	Improve posture
	Loss of neck movement in all planes	Increase active and passive cervical ROM to 75% of normal
	Right upper extremity pain with cervical extension and right rotation	Resolve upper extremity pain
	Hypertonic paraspinal cervical muscles	Normalize cervical muscle tone
	Limited bilateral shoulder flexion and abduction	Improve shoulder ROM

Continued

CLINICAL CASE STUDIES—cont'd

ICF Level	Current Status	Goals
Activity	Unable to turn head to see far to the side or behind	Improve ability to turn head so patient can see all the way to the side
	Unable to look down to write or sew for >10 min	Increase tolerance for looking down to 30 min
Participation	Able to drive but feels unsafe	Improve ability to drive safely within 2 weeks
	Unable to participate in sewing class	Return to full participation in sewing class within 2 weeks

ICF, International Classification for Functioning, Disability and Health; *ROM,* range of motion.

◆ FIND THE EVIDENCE

PICO Terms	Natural Language Example	Sample PubMed Search
P (Population)	Patients with symptoms due to cervical nerve root impingement	("Spinal Nerve Roots*" [MeSH]) OR "radiculopathy" [MeSH])
I (Intervention)	Spinal traction	AND ("Traction*" [MeSH] AND English [lang] AND "Humans" [MeSH])
C (Comparison)	No traction	
O (Outcome)	Symptom relief	

Key Studies or Reviews

1. Romeo A, Vanti C, Boldrini V, et al: Cervical radiculopathy: effectiveness of adding traction to physical therapy—a systematic review and meta-analysis of randomized controlled trials. *Phys Ther* 98(4):231–242, 2018.

   This systematic review and meta-analysis of RCTs on the effects of cervical traction combined with other physical therapy procedures versus physical therapy alone on pain and disability, which included five studies, found that mechanical traction had significant effects on pain and disability and that manual traction had significant effects on pain.

2. Kjaer P, Kngsted A, Hartvigsen J, et al: National clinical guidelines for non-surgical treatment of patients with recent onset neck pain or cervical radiculopathy. *Eur Spine J* 26(9):2242–2257, 2017.

   This Danish evidence-based national clinical guideline includes cervical traction as a recommended treatment for recent-onset (<12 weeks) cervical radiculopathy.

Prognosis

Cervical spinal traction is indicated for the treatment of joint hypomobility, cervical radiculopathy, and symptoms caused by subacute joint inflammation, particularly when multiple spinal segments are involved. Spinal traction may also help alleviate this patient's spinal pain by gating its transmission at the spinal cord or by reducing joint compression and inflammation. Intermittent traction may help to reduce symptoms resulting from inflammation by facilitating normal fluid exchange in the joints to relieve edema caused by chronic inflammation. This change, combined with stretching of periarticular soft tissue structures, may increase spinal joint and soft tissue mobility and cervical active ROM. Applying a deep or superficial heating agent to the patient's neck before or during the application of traction may optimize the benefits of treatment by increasing soft tissue extensibility to facilitate greater increases in soft tissue length. As in previous years, traction and other passive modalities alone are likely to result in temporary control of this patient's symptoms. More long-lasting benefits may be achieved by additionally addressing her posture and thoracic mobility and by modifying her home activities.

At the age of 75, this patient should be cleared for impairment of vertebral or carotid artery circulation and for osteoporosis before cervical traction is applied. If she normally wears dentures, she should wear them during treatment. It is important to not assume that because this patient has tolerated traction well in the past, she will tolerate it equally well at this time, particularly if she has experienced any medical events, such as a cerebrovascular accident, since she was last treated with traction.

Intervention

Once this patient is cleared for application of traction, a trial of manual traction is recommended to assess her response to traction and to help determine the ideal position before considering other forms of traction. If manual traction provides her some relief of symptoms, electrical mechanical traction should be used in the clinic to provide optimal efficiency and consistency of treatment. An occipital halter should be used to avoid compression on the TMJs, and the patient should be positioned supine, with her cervical spine in approximately 24 degrees of flexion to achieve maximum separation of the lower cervical joints and elongation of the posterior spinal structures.

As with all traction treatments, for the first session, the force of traction should initially be low, at approximately 4 kg (10 lb). The amount of force may then be increased by 1.5 to 2 kg (3 to 5 lb) at each subsequent session until optimal symptom control is achieved. A low force of 5 to 7 kg (12 to 15 lb), which can elongate the cervical spine without distracting the joints, will probably be sufficient to alleviate this patient's symptoms, and applying more force probably will not provide greater benefit. Traction force should never exceed 13 kg (30 lb). Intermittent traction should employ short hold and relax times of approximately 15 seconds each because this ratio is generally effective at reducing symptoms associated with the joints. The total duration of the traction treatment should be between 10 and 40 minutes, depending on the patient's response.

CLINICAL CASE STUDIES—cont'd

Because this patient presents with recurrent symptoms that probably are a result of progressive and chronic osteoarthritis, it is recommended that she obtain and be instructed in the use of a simple mechanical traction device, such as an over-the-door cervical traction unit, for use at home. She may then use this device to treat aggravation of similar symptoms that she may experience in the future.

Documentation

S: Pt reports neck stiffness and pain that is worse in the morning and evening and right arm pain with cervical extension and right rotation.

O: Pretreatment: Pain 7/10. Kyphotic thoracic posture. Cervical ROM restricted by 50% in all planes. Moderate hypertonic cervical paraspinal muscles. Stiff cervical facet joints on passive intervertebral motion testing. Bilateral shoulder flexion and abduction active ROM 140 degrees.

Intervention: Hot pack to neck before txn. After trial of manual txn, int mech cerv txn applied, Pt supine, soft occipital halter, cervical spine approximately 24 degrees flexion. 4 kg/2 kg (10 lb/5 lb), 15 s/15 s, 10 min.

Posttreatment: Pain 3/10. Cervical ROM restricted by 40% in all planes. Cervical paraspinal muscles mildly hypertonic. Shoulder flexion and abduction unchanged.

A: Pt tolerated txn well with some improvement in symptoms.

P: Continue int mech txn 3 × week for the next week, gradually increasing weight or length of time txn is applied. Give Pt exercises to improve posture, suggest use of home txn device.

CASE STUDY 20.2

Neck Pain in a Patient With Rheumatoid Arthritis

Examination

History

MS is a 30-year-old female high school teacher. MS was diagnosed with RA at age 22 and has been referred to physical therapy for treatment of neck pain. She complains of constant and severe pain in her neck that is aggravated by all neck movement, and she reports intermittent dizziness that is brought on by moving from sitting to standing or by looking up. The neck pain started about 3 or 4 years ago and has gradually become more severe; the dizziness started only a few weeks ago.

Systems Review

MS is a pleasant-appearing woman who is eager to receive therapy. She reports that at this time, pain keeps her awake at night, and dizziness interferes with her ability to write on the chalkboard when she is at work. MS has no numbness or tingling of her extremities and reports that no x-ray films have been taken of her neck in the past 3 years.

Tests and Measures

Her objective examination reveals postural abnormalities, including standing with approximately 20 degrees of hip and knee flexion bilaterally, bilateral genu valgum, a moderately increased lumbar lordosis, a flat thoracic spine, and a forward head position. The flat thoracic spine and forward head position are maintained in sitting. Cervical ROM testing was deferred at the initial evaluation because of the severity of the patient's reports of pain with motion. Her upper extremity strength was 4+/5 throughout within the available ROM, and her upper extremity sensation and reflexes were within normal limits.

What part of this patient's history needs further evaluation before the use of traction? Would you expect complete relief of symptoms in this patient?

Evaluation and Goals

ICF Level	Current Status	Goals
Body function and structure	Neck pain and stiffness	Ascertain ligamentous stability and bony integrity of her upper cervical spine
	Dizziness	Relieve pain and dizziness
	Abnormal posture	Improve cervical ROM
	Limited cervical ROM	
Activity	Unable to sleep	Improve sleep until patient able to sleep through night
	Unable to write on chalkboard	Improve chalkboard writing to 100% of normal in 1 month
Participation	Decreased ability to teach	Return to full-time teaching without restrictions in 1 month

ICF, International Classification for Functioning, Disability and Health; *ROM*, range of motion.

◆ FIND THE EVIDENCE

PICO Terms	Natural Language Example	Sample PubMed Search
P (Population)	30-year-old woman with rheumatoid arthritis	("Arthritis, Rheumatoid" [MeSH])
I (Intervention)	Spinal traction	(AND "Traction*" [MeSH] AND English [lang] AND "Humans" [MeSH])
C (Comparison)	No traction	
O (Outcome)	Symptom relief	(AND "Treatment outcome" [MeSH] OR Range of Motion, Articular [MeSH])

Findings From Search Results

Although this search yielded a few results, none was directly relevant to conservative treatment of this patient. However,

Continued

CLINICAL CASE STUDIES—cont'd

many of the articles discussed surgical approaches to address atlantoaxial subluxation in patients with RA, drawing attention to the importance of ruling out this complication of RA before providing physical therapy interventions.

Prognosis

Although treatment goals could include resolving any of the aforementioned impairments or functional limitations, this patient's reports of dizziness associated with neck pain and the diagnosis of RA should alert the clinician to the possibility that this patient may have an unstable C1 to C2 articulation as a result of ligamentous instability, or she may have osteoporosis as a result of prolonged systemic steroid use. Because instability at C1 to C2 poses a significant risk to the patient, and because the presence of osteoporosis requires special caution with the application of traction, the initial goal, before traction or any other treatment is applied, should be to ascertain the ligamentous stability and bony integrity of her upper cervical spine. Because these both require radiographic studies that generally must be ordered by a physician, the patient should be referred back to her physician for further evaluation.

If all radiographic reports indicate that her upper cervical spine is stable and that she does not have osteoporosis, she may return to physical therapy for treatment of her complaints, with goals as listed in the previous table. Because this patient has a systemic disease that affects the joints and that appears to have caused permanent changes in other joints, including her hips and knees, complete relief of symptoms or return of ROM probably will not occur. If all tests indicate that spinal traction is not contraindicated, traction may improve this patient's cervical mobility and decrease her neck pain. Distraction or mobilization of the cervical joints or relaxation of the cervical paraspinal muscles can achieve these effects. Cervical traction may also help alleviate the patient's dizziness because she associates this symptom with neck motion; however, her dizziness may be the result of an inner ear or vestibular dysfunction, which would also be affected by head position, in which case this symptom probably would not respond to treatment with traction. Although traction may reduce this patient's symptoms sufficiently to allow her to write on a chalkboard, it is recommended that job site adaptations, such as the use of an overhead projector, be instituted to reduce the stress on her cervical spine.

Intervention

To constantly monitor this patient's severe symptoms and to allow adjustment of the traction force and direction during treatment, manual traction should be used initially. If the patient reports moderate relief of her pain with manual traction, optimal cervical positioning for traction should be determined, and static mechanical traction may be substituted if it is thought that a longer duration of treatment would be beneficial. Static cervical traction may be provided by an electrical or weighted device, but in either case, it is recommended that the patient be treated supine rather than sitting to achieve

maximum muscle relaxation, and low forces should be used initially because of the severity of the patient's symptoms.

As treatment progresses, the force of traction may be increased up to a maximum of 13 kg (30 lb) to achieve joint distraction if necessary, and intermittent traction may be used if this is more comfortable as the patient tolerates more motion. Treatment with spinal traction should occur in conjunction with postural education and recommendations for home or work-site modifications to minimize the risk of symptom reaggravation or progression.

Documentation

S: Pt reports neck pain worsening over the past 4 years and dizziness that began 3 weeks ago, which is worse when looking up and moving from sitting to standing.

O: Pretreatment: Neck pain 8/10. 20-degree hip and knee flexion bilaterally, bilateral genu valgum, lumbar lordosis, flat thoracic spine, and forward head position when standing. Flat thoracic spine and forward head position when sitting. Cervical ROM testing deferred. UE strength 4+/5 throughout.

Intervention: Manual txn applied initially. Static cerv mech txn, Pt supine, soft occipital halter. 4 kg (10 lb), 10 min.

Posttreatment: Neck pain 6/10. Continued exacerbation of neck pain with neck movement.

A: Pt tolerated txn well, with mildly reduced neck pain.

P: Continue static cervical mech txn and increase weight gradually as tolerated for further symptom reduction. Postural education. Discuss home and work-site modifications with Pt.

CASE STUDY 20.3

Low Back Pain With Radiculopathy

Examination

History

TR is a 45-year-old man who has been referred to physical therapy with a diagnosis of a right L5, S1 radiculopathy. The pain started about 6 weeks ago, the morning after TR spent a day stacking firewood, at which time he woke up with severe low back pain and right lower extremity pain down to his lateral calf; he also had difficulty standing up straight. He has had similar problems in the past, but these have always resolved fully after a couple of days of bed rest and a few aspirin. TR first saw his doctor regarding his present problem 5 weeks ago. At that time, he was prescribed a nonsteroidal antiinflammatory drug (NSAID) and a muscle relaxant and was told to rest. His symptoms improved to their current level over the next 2 weeks but have not changed since that time. TR has been unable to return to his job as a telephone installer since the onset of symptoms 6 weeks ago. An MRI scan last week showed a mild posterolateral disc bulge at L5 to S1 on the right. TR has had no previous physical therapy for his back problem.

Systems Review

TR is a pleasant man accompanied to the clinic by his longtime girlfriend. He reports constant mild to moderately severe

CLINICAL CASE STUDIES—*cont'd*

(4/10 to 7/10) right low back pain that radiates to his right buttock and lateral thigh after sitting for longer than 20 minutes that is relieved to some degree by walking or lying down. He reports no numbness, tingling, or weakness of the lower extremities. No signs of discomfort or weakness are visibly present.

Tests and Measures

The patient's weight is 91 kg (200 lb). The objective examination is significant for a 50% restriction of lumbar ROM in forward bending and right side bending, both of which cause increased right low back and lower extremity pain. Left side bending decreases the patient's pain. Passive straight leg raising is 35 degrees on the right, limited by right lower extremity pain, and 60 degrees on the left, limited by hamstring tightness. Palpation reveals stiffness and tenderness to right unilateral posterior-anterior pressure at L5 to S1 and no notable areas of hypermobility. All other tests, including lower extremity sensation, strength, and reflexes, are within normal limits.

What is the likely cause of this patient's problem? What symptoms point to this as the cause?

Evaluation and Goals

ICF Level	Current Status	Goals
Body function and structure	Right low back pain with radiation to right buttock and lateral thigh	Decrease pain to <3/10 in 1 week
		Eliminate pain completely in 3 weeks
	Restricted lumbar ROM	
	Restricted lumbar nerve root mobility on the right (limited right SLR)	Return lumbar ROM and SLR to normal
	Bulging L5–S1 disc	
Activity	Decreased sitting tolerance	Increase sitting tolerance to 1 h in 1 week
	Unable to stand straight or lift	Stand straight in 1 week
		Lift 20 lb in 2 weeks
Participation	Unable to work	Return to limited work duties within 2 weeks
		Return to full work duties within 1 month

ICF, International Classification for Functioning, Disability and Health; *ROM,* range of motion; *SLR,* straight leg raise.

◆ FIND THE EVIDENCE

PICO Terms	Natural Language Example	Sample PubMed Search
P (Population)	Patients with symptoms due to lumbar disc bulge or herniation	("Intervertebral Disc Displacement" [MeSH] OR "herniation" [all fields])

PICO Terms	Natural Language Example	Sample PubMed Search
I (Intervention)	Spinal traction	(AND "Traction*" [MeSH] AND English [lang] AND "Humans" [MeSH])
C (Comparison)	No traction	
O (Outcome)	Symptom relief	

Key Studies or Reviews

1. Moustafa IM, Diab AA: Extension traction treatment for patients with discogenic lumbosacral radiculopathy: a randomized controlled trial. *Clin Rehabil* 27:51–62, 2013.

   This study of 64 patients with confirmed unilateral lumbosacral radiculopathy resulting from L5 to S1 disc herniation found that patients who received mechanical lumbar traction in addition to hot packs and interferential therapy had significantly less disability and significantly less back and leg pain at 10 weeks after treatment compared with the control group, who received only hot packs and interferential therapy.

2. Hahne AJ, Ford JJ, McMeeken JM: Conservative management of lumbar disc herniation with associated radiculopathy: a systematic review. *Spine (Phila Pa 1976)* 35:E488–504, 2010.

   This systematic review included 18 controlled trials of conservative management of referred leg symptoms and radiological confirmation of lumbar disc herniation in 1,671 participants. Seven trials included spinal traction as an intervention. The authors concluded that one trial showed some additional benefit from adding mechanical traction to medication and electrotherapy, but traction was also associated with adverse effects of pain, anxiety, lower limb weakness, and fainting.

3. Biligilsoy FM, Kilic Z, Uckun A, et al: Mechanical traction for lumbar radicular pain: Supine or prone? A randomized controlled trial. *Am J Phys Med Rehabil* 97(6):433–439, 2018.

   This RCT compared the effects of adding traction in prone or supine to 15 sessions of physical therapy in 125 people with lumbar radiculopathy. Although both groups showed significant improvements in disability, pain severity, and lumbar flexion ROM, there was significantly greater improvement in disability and pain in those treated with prone traction than in those treated with supine traction.

Prognosis

The distribution of this patient's pain and its response to changes in loading indicate that his symptoms probably are related to the mild posterolateral disc bulge at L5 to S1 on the right, as noted on his MRI scan. Traction is an indicated intervention for reducing symptoms associated with a disc bulge or lumbar nerve root compression and therefore should

Continued

be considered for this patient. Studies have shown that lumbar traction can reduce disc protrusions and may also enhance relief of symptoms related to low back pain and sciatica. Traction may provide additional benefit for this patient if it is applied in conjunction with other physical therapy treatment techniques, including strengthening, stabilization, and stretching exercises; joint mobilization; and body mechanics training. Treatment in the clinic should be integrated with a complete home program. Spinal traction is not contraindicated in this patient because there is no displaced fragment of annulus or areas of hypermobility, and there are no indications of a hiatal hernia or a cardiac or pulmonary condition that may be aggravated by use of the belts for mechanical traction.

Intervention

Electrical mechanical traction is the best option for this patient because this type of traction allows the greatest control of lumbar traction force and the application of sufficient force to distract the lumbar vertebrae. Prone positioning, if tolerated, will place the spine in a neutral or slightly extended position and thus will provide greater separation of the disc spaces anteriorly and localization of the force to the lower lumbar segments, and it has been shown to be more effective than supine positioning.

A traction force of 25% of the patient's body weight may be sufficient to help this patient reach the set goals of treatment because this amount of traction force can produce a centripetal force on the lumbar disc and can reduce a disc displacement. However, traction force as great as 50% of the patient's body weight may be needed if joint distraction is required to alleviate this patient's symptoms. Initial treatment should use a low force of approximately 25% of the patient's body weight, or 13 to 20 kg (25 to 50 lb), to allow assessment of the patient's response to the intervention and to minimize the risk of protective muscle spasms. The traction force may then be increased for subsequent treatments, if necessary, until a level is reached at which the patient responds with

approximately a 50% reduction in symptom severity after treatment. The application of a hot pack in conjunction with traction may improve the patient's response to the intervention by increasing superficial tissue extensibility and decreasing pain.[56,57]

Intermittent traction with a long hold time, approximately 60 seconds, and a short relax time, approximately 20 seconds, is likely to have the greatest effect on the discs. Static traction may also be effective. The initial treatment should be limited to 10 minutes if the patient reports some reduction of symptoms in this time. If this does not reduce the patient's symptoms, the treatment time may be extended to 20 to 40 minutes for subsequent treatments.

If application of mechanical traction in the manner described relieves this patient's symptoms, and particularly if lower forces and shorter durations of treatment are effective, the use of self-traction or positional traction at home, with the patient lying on the left side with the left side bent and in right rotation, may help this patient progress toward his treatment goals.

Documentation

S: Pt reports constant 4/10 to 7/10 R low back pain radiating to R buttock and lateral thigh after sitting for longer than 20 min, relieved somewhat by walking or lying down.

O: Pretreatment: 50% restricted lumbar ROM with forward bend and R side bend, limited by R low back and R LE pain 7/10. L side bend decreases pain. Passive SLR 35 degrees on R, limited by R LE pain, and 60 degrees on L, limited by hamstring tightness. Tenderness to palpation R posterior-anterior pressure at L5-S1.

Intervention: Int mech lumbar txn, Pt prone. 22 kg/11 kg (48 lb/24 lb), 60 s/20 s, 10 min.

Posttreatment: 30% restricted lumbar ROM with R forward and side bend. Pain 4/10 with R side bend.

A: Pt tolerated txn well, and symptoms improved.

P: Continue int mech txn at these parameters once daily. Teach patient positional lumbar txn.

Chapter Review

1. Traction is a mechanical force applied to the body to distract joints, stretch soft tissue, relax muscles, or mobilize joints. Types of traction include electrical mechanical traction, weighted mechanical traction, over-the-door cervical traction, various home traction devices, self-traction, positional traction, and manual traction.

2. Traction may be static (continuous force) or intermittent (varying force). Static traction is recommended when the area being treated is inflamed, when the patient's symptoms are aggravated by motion, or when the patient's symptoms are related to a disc protrusion. All types of spinal traction discussed in this chapter can be used to apply static traction. Intermittent traction is used for symptoms related to disc protrusion and joint dysfunction. Electrical mechanical traction units and manual techniques can be used to apply intermittent traction.

3. Spinal traction can be used to relieve signs, symptoms, and functional limitations associated with disc bulge or herniation, nerve root impingement, joint hypomobility, subacute joint inflammation, and paraspinal muscle spasm. The effects and clinical benefits of spinal traction depend on the amount of force used, the direction of the force, and the status of the area to which the traction is applied.

4. Hip traction can help relieve signs, symptoms, and functional limitations in patients with hip-related disability.

5. Selection of a traction technique depends on the nature of the problem being treated, specific contraindications, and whether the treatment is to be applied in the clinic or at home.

6. Traction is contraindicated where motion is contraindicated, with an acute injury or inflammation, with joint hypermobility or instability, with peripheralization of symptoms with traction, and with uncontrolled hypertension. Precautions for the application of spinal traction

include structural diseases or conditions affecting the spine, when the pressure of the belts may be hazardous, displacement of an annular fragment, medial disc protrusion, severe pain fully relieved by traction, claustrophobia, intolerance of the prone or supine position, disorientation, TMJ problems, and dentures.

Glossary

Annulus fibrosus: A ring of fibrocartilage that forms the outer layer of the **intervertebral disc.**

Herniated disc: Bulging of the intervertebral disc into the spinal canal.

Intermittent traction: Traction in which the force varies every few seconds.

Intervertebral disc: Structure located between the vertebrae that acts as a shock absorber for the spine.

Joint distraction: The separation of two articular surfaces perpendicular to the plane of articulation; the widening of a joint space.

Manual traction: Application of force by the therapist in the direction of distracting the joints.

Mechanical traction (electrical mechanical traction): Application of static or intermittent force by an electrical motor, through belts or a halter, in the direction of distracting the joints of the spine.

Nucleus pulposus: Elastic, pulpy substance found at the center of an intervertebral disc.

Over-the-door cervical traction: Application of static force to the neck, through a halter, using a device hung on a door that can be adjusted to provide differing amounts of distractive force.

Positional traction: Prolonged specific positioning to place tension on one side of the lumbar spine.

Self-traction: A form of traction that uses gravity and the weight of the patient's body, or force exerted by the patient, to exert a distractive force on the spine.

Spondylolisthesis: Forward displacement of one vertebra on another that can cause nerve root compression and pain.

Static traction: Traction in which the same force is applied throughout treatment.

Traction: A mechanical force applied to the body in a way that separates, or attempts to separate, joint surfaces and elongates soft tissues surrounding a joint.

References

1. Edmond SL: *Joint mobilization/manipulation: extremity and spinal techniques*, St Louis, MO, 2016, Elsevier.
2. Manske RC, Lehecka B, Reiman MP, et al: *Orthopedic joint mobilization and manipulation: An evidence-based approach*, Champaign, IL, 2018, Human Kinetics.
3. Hengeveld E, Banks K: *Maitland's peripheral manipulation: management of neuromusculoskeletal disorders*, ed 5, London, 2013, Churchill Livingstone.
4. Cyriax J: *Textbook of orthopedic medicine: diagnosis of soft tissue lesions*, London, 1982, Bailliere Tindall.
5. Mathews JA, Mills SB, Jenkins YM, et al: Back pain and sciatica: Controlled trials of manipulation, traction, sclerosant and epidural injections. *Br J Rheumatol* 26:416–423, 1987.
6. Larsson U, Choler U, Lindstrom A, et al: Auto-traction for treatment of lumbago-sciatica. *Acta Orthop Scand* 51:791–798, 1980.
7. Lidstrom A, Zachrisson M: Physical therapy on low back pain and sciatica. *Scand J Rehabil Med* 2:37–42, 1970.
8. Freburger JK, Carey TS, Holmes GM: Physical therapy for chronic low back pain in North Carolina: overuse, underuse, or misuse? *Phys Ther* 91:484–495, 2011.
9. Pensri P, Foster NE, Srisuk S, et al: Physiotherapy management of low back pain in Thailand: a study of practice. *Physiother Res Int* 10:201–212, 2005.
10. Harte AA, Gracey JH, Baxter GD: Current use of lumbar traction in the management of low back pain: results of a survey of physiotherapists in the United Kingdom. *Arch Phys Med Rehabil* 86:1164–1169, 2005.
11. Wegner I, Widyahening IS, van Tulder MW, et al: Traction for low-back pain with or without sciatica. *Cochrane Database Syst Rev* 2013(8):CD003010, 2013.
12. Lewis RA, Williams NH, Sutton AJ, et al: Comparative clinical effectiveness of management strategies for sciatica: systematic review and network meta-analyses. *Spine J* 15:1461–1477, 2015.
13. Casazza BA: Diagnosis and treatment of acute low back pain. *Am Fam Physician* 85:343–350, 2012.
14. Shalaby AS, El-Sharaki DR, Salem GM: Anxiety, depression, and quality of life in backache patients before and after spinal traction. *Egypt J Neurol Psychiatr Neurosurg* 54(1):44, 2018.
15. Oh H, Choi S, Lee S, et al: The impact of manual spinal traction therapy on the pain and Oswestry disability index of patients with chronic back pain. *J Phys Ther Sci* 30(12):1455–1457, 2018. doi:10.1589/jpts.30.1455.
16. Thackeray A, Fritz JM, Childs JD, et al: The effectiveness of mechanical traction among subgroups of patients with low back pain and leg pain: a randomized trial. *J Orthop Sports Phys Ther* 46(3):144–154, 2016.
17. Madson TJ, Hollman JH: Lumbar traction for managing low back pain: A survey of physical therapists in the United States. *J Orthop Sports Phys Ther* 45(8):586–595, 2015.
18. Graham N, Gross A, Goldsmith CH, et al: Mechanical traction for neck pain with or without radiculopathy. *Cochrane Database Syst Rev* 2008(3):CD006408, 2008 doi:10.1002/14651858.CD006408.pub2.
19. Fritz JM, Thackeray A, Brennan GP, et al: Exercise only, exercise with mechanical traction, or exercise with over-door traction for patients with cervical radiculopathy, with or without consideration of status on a previously described subgrouping rule: a randomized clinical trial. *J Orthop Sports Phys Ther* 44:45–57, 2014.
20. Graham N, Gross AR, Carlesso LC, et al: An ICON overview on physical modalities for neck pain and associated disorders. *Open Orthop J* 7:440–460, 2013.
21. Yang JD, Tam KW, Huang TW, et al: Intermittent cervical traction for treating neck pain: a meta-analysis of randomized controlled trials. *Spine (Phila Pa 1976)* 42(13):959–965, 2017. doi:10.1097/BRS.0000000000001948.
22. Romeo A, Vanti C, Boldrini V, et al: Cervical radiculopathy: effectiveness of adding traction to physical therapy—a systematic review and meta-analysis of randomized controlled trials. *Phys Ther* 98(4):231–242, 2018. doi:10.1093/physth/pzy001.
23. Maitland GD:Peripheral manipulation, Oxford, 1991, Butterworth-Heinemann.
24. Kaltenborn F: *Mobilization of the extremity joints: Examination and basic treatment techniques*, Oslo, 1980, Olaf Norlis Bokhandel.
25. Vaarbakken K, Ljunggren AE: Superior effect of forceful compared with standard traction mobilization in hip disability? *Adv Physiother* 9:117–128, 2007.
26. Wright AA, Abbott JH, Baxter D, et al: The ability of a sustained with-in session finding of pain reduction during traction to dictate improved outcomes from a manual therapy approach on patients with osteoarthritis of the hip. *J Man Manip Ther* 18:166–172, 2010.
27. Paris SV, Loubert PV: *Foundations of clinical orthopedics*, St Augustine, FL, 1999, Institute Press.
28. Hengeveld E, Banks K: *Maitland's vertebral manipulation*, ed 8, London, 2013, Churchill Livingstone.
29. Tekeoglu I, Adak B, Bozkurt M, et al: Distraction of lumbar vertebrae in gravitational traction. *Spine* 23:1061–1063, 1998.
30. Judovich B, Nobel GR: Traction therapy: A study of resistance forces. *Am J Surg* 93:108–114, 1957.
31. Judovich B: Lumbar traction therapy. *JAMA* 159:549, 1955.
32. Deets D, Hands KL, Hopp SS: Cervical traction: a comparison of sitting and supine positions. *Phys Ther* 57:255–261, 1977.
33. Twomey LT: Sustained lumbar traction: An experimental study of long spine segments. *Spine* 10:146–149, 1985.
34. Samuelsen G, Høiseth A: X-ray examination: Manual physical traction treatment of painful hip conditions. *Fysioterapeuten* 57:20–23, 1990.
35. Arvidsson I: The hip joint: forces needed for distraction and appearance of the vacuum phenomenon. *Scand J Rehabil Med* 22:157–161, 1990.

36. Nyfos L: Traction therapy of osteoarthrosis of the hip. A controlled study. *Ugeskr Laeger* 145:2837–2840, 1983.

37. Marques B, Toldbod M, Ostrup EL, et al: The effect of naproxen compared with that of traction in patients with osteoarthrosis of the hip. A single-blind controlled study. *Ugeskr Laeger* 145:2840–2844, 1983.

38. Onel D, Tuzlaci M, Sari H, et al: Computed tomographic investigation of the effect of traction on lumbar disc herniations. *Spine* 14:82–90, 1989.

39. Chow DHK, Yuen EMK, Xiao L, et al: Mechanical effects of traction on lumbar intervertebral discs: A magnetic resonance imaging study. *Musculoskelet Sci Pract* 29:78–83, 2017. doi:10.1016/j.msksp.2017.03.007.

40. Cyriax J: *Textbook of orthopaedic medicine*, ed 11, Eastbourne, UK, 1984, Balliere Tindall.

41. Apfel CC, Cakmakkaya OS, Martin W, et al: Restoration of disk height through non-surgical spinal decompression is associated with decreased discogenic low back pain: a retrospective cohort study. *BMC Musculoskelet Disord* 11:155,2010.

42. Sari H, Akarimak U, Karacan I, et al: Computed tomographic evaluation of lumbar spinal structures during traction. *Physiother Theory Pract* 21:3–11, 2005.

43. Chung TS, Yang HE, Ahn SJ, et al: Herniated lumbar disks: real-time MR imaging evaluation during continuous traction. *Radiology* 275:755–762, 2015.

44. Mitchell UH, Helgeson K, Mintken P: Physiological effects of physical therapy interventions on lumbar intervertebral discs: A systematic review. *Physiother Theory Pract* 33(9):695–705, 2017. doi:10.1080/09593985.2017.1345026.

45. Liu J, Ebraheim NA, Sanford Jr CG, et al: Quantitative changes in the cervical neural foramen resulting from axial traction: In vivo imaging study. *Spine J* 8(4):619–623, 2008.

46. Chung T, Lee Y, Kang S, et al: Reducibility of cervical disc herniation: evaluation at MR imaging during cervical traction with nonmagnetic traction device. *Radiology* 225(3), 2002.

47. Saal JS, Saal JA, Yurth EF: Nonoperative management of herniated cervical intervertebral disc with radiculopathy. *Spine* 21:1877–1883, 1996.

48. Meszaros TF, Olson R, Kulig K, et al: Effect of 10%, 30%, and 60% body weight traction on the straight leg raise test of symptomatic patients with low back pain. *J Orthop Sports Phys Ther* 30:595–601, 2000.

49. Andersson GBJ, Schultz AB, Nachemson AL: Intervertebral disc pressures during traction. *Scand J Rehabil Med* 9:88–91, 1983.

50. Lundgren AE, Eldevik OP: Auto-traction in lumbar disc herniation with CT examination before and after treatment, showing no change in appearance of the herniated tissue. *J Oslo City Hosp* 36:87–91, 1986.

51. Basmajian JV: *Manipulation, traction and massage*, ed 3, Baltimore, 1985, Williams & Wilkins.

52. Coalchis SC, Strohm BR: Cervical traction relationship of time to varied tractive force with constant angle of pull. *Arch Phys Med Rehabil* 46:815–819, 1965.

53. Worden RE, Humphrey TL: Effect of spinal traction on the length of the body. *Arch Phys Med Rehabil* 45:319–320, 1964.

54. Janke AW, Kerkow TA, Griffiths HJ, et al: The biomechanics of gravity-dependent traction of the lumbar spine. *Spine (Phila Pa 1976)* 22(3):253–260, 1997.

55. LaBan MM: Collagen tissue: implications of its response to stress in vitro. *Arch Phys Med Rehabil* 43:461–466, 1962.

56. Lehmann J, Masock A, Warren C, et al: Effect of therapeutic temperatures on tendon extensibility. *Arch Phys Med Rehabil* 51:481–487, 1970.

57. Lentall G, Hetherington T, Eagan J, et al: The use of thermal agents to influence the effectiveness of a low-load prolonged stretch. *J Orthop Sports Phys Ther* 16:200–207, 1992.

58. Grieve GP: *Mobilization of the spine*, New York, 1984, Churchill Livingstone.

59. Mathews JA: The effects of spinal traction. *Physiotherapy* 58:64–66, 1972.

60. Falkenberg J, Podein RJ, Pardo X, et al: Surface EMG activity of the back musculature during axial spinal unloading using an LTX 3000 Lumbar Rehabilitation System. *Electromyogr Clin Neurophysiol* 41(7):419–427, 2001.

61. Wall PD: The mechanisms of pain associated with cervical vertebral disease. In Hirsch C, Zollerman Y, editors: *Cervical pain: proceedings of the International Symposium in Wenner-Gren Center*, Oxford, 1972, Pergamon.

62. Seliger V, Dolejs L, Karas V: A dynamometric comparison of maximum eccentric, concentric and isometric contractions using EMG and energy expenditure measurements. *Eur J Appl Physiol* 45:235–244, 1980.

63. Swezey RL: The modern thrust of manipulation and traction therapy. *Semin Arthritis Rheum* 12:322–331, 1983.

64. Saunders HD: Use of spinal traction in the treatment of neck and back conditions. *Clin Orthop Relat Res* 179:31–38, 1983.

65. Coalchis SC, Strohm BR: A study of tractive forces and angle of pull on vertebral interspaces in the cervical spine. *Arch Phys Med Rehabil* 46:820–824, 1965.

66. Saunders HD: Lumbar traction. *J Orthop Sports Phys Ther* 1:36–46, 1979.

67. Gay RE, Brault JS: Traction. In Dagenais S, Haldeman S, editors: *Evidence-based management of low back pain*, St Louis, MO, 2012, Elsevier.

68. Haskvitz EM, Hanten WP: Blood pressure response to inversion traction. *Phys Ther* 66:1361–1364, 1986.

69. Utti VA, Ege S, Lukman O: Blood pressure and pulse rate changes associated with cervical traction. *Niger J Med* 15:141–143, 2006.

70. Tsai CT, Chang WD, Kao MJ, et al: Changes in blood pressure and related autonomic function during cervical traction in healthy women. *Orthopedics* 34:e295–e301, 2011.

71. Quain MB, Tecklin JS: Lumbar traction: Its effect on respiration. *Phys Ther* 65:1343–1346, 1985.

72. Frymoyer JW, Moskowitz RW: Spinal degeneration: pathogenesis and medical management. In Frymoyer JW, editor: *The adult spine: principles and practice*, New York, 1991, Raven Press.

73. LaBan MM, Macy JA, Meerschaert JR: Intermittent cervical traction: A progenitor of lumbar radicular pain. *Arch Phys Med Rehabil* 73:295–296, 1992.

74. Laban MM, Mahal BS: Intraspinal dural distraction inciting spinal radiculopathy: Cranial to caudal and caudal to cranial. *Am J Phys Med Rehabil* 84:141–144, 2005.

75. So EC: Facial nerve paralysis after cervical traction. *Am J Phys Med Rehabil* 89:849–853, 2010.

76. Cheatle MD, Esterhai JL: Pelvic traction as treatment for acute back pain. *Spine* 16:1379–1381, 1991.

77. Pal B, Mangion P, Hossain MA, et al: A controlled trial of continuous lumbar traction in the treatment of back pain and sciatica. *Br J Rheumatol* 25:181–183, 1986.

78. Tadano S, Tanabe H, Arai S, et al: Lumbar mechanical traction: a biomechanical assessment of change at the lumbar spine. *BMC Musculoskelet Disord* 20(1):155, 2019. doi:10.1186/s12891-019-2545-9.

79. Wong AM, Leong CP, Chen CM: The traction angle and cervical intervertebral separation. *Spine (Phila Pa 1976)* 17(2):136–138, 1992.

80. Moustafa IM, Diab AA: Extension traction treatment for patients with discogenic lumbosacral radiculopathy: a randomized controlled trial. *Clin Rehabil* 27(1):51–62, 2013. doi:10.1177/0269215512446093.

81. Farajpour H, Jamshidi N: Effects of different angles of the traction table on lumbar spine ligaments: a finite element study. *Clin Orthop Surg* 9(4):480–488, 2017. doi:10.4055/cios.2017.9.4.480.

82. Vaughn HT, Having KM, Rogers JL: Radiographic analysis of intervertebral separation with a 0 degrees and 30 degrees rope angle using the Saunders cervical traction device. *Spine (Phila Pa 1976)* 31(2):E39–E43, 2006.

83. Saunders HD: Unilateral lumbar traction. *Phys Ther* 61:221–225, 1981.

84. Weatherell VF: Comparison of electromyographic activity in normal lumbar sacrospinalis musculature during static pelvic traction in two different positions. *J Orthop Sports Phys Ther* 8:382–390, 1987.

85. Bilgilisoy Filiz M, Kiliç Z, Uçkun A, et al: Mechanical traction for lumbar radicular pain: supine or prone? A randomized controlled trial. *Am J Phys Med Rehabil* 97(6):433–439, 2018. doi:10.1097/PHM.0000000000000892.

86. Goldish GD: A study of mechanical efficiency of split table traction. *Spine* 15:218–219, 1989.

87. Saunders HD: Lumbar traction. *J Orthop Sports Phys Ther* 1:36–41, 1979.

88. Rogoff JB: Motorized intermittent traction. In Basmajian JV, editor: *Manipulation, traction, and massage*, Baltimore, 1985, Williams & Wilkins.

89. Coalchis SC, Strohm BR: Effects of intermittent traction on separation of lumbar vertebrae. *Arch Phys Med Rehabil* 50:251–253, 1969.

90. Hood CJ, Hart DL, Smith HG, et al: Comparison of electromyographic activity in normal lumbar sacrospinalis musculature during continuous and intermittent pelvic traction. *J Orthop Sports Phys Ther* 2:137–141, 1981.

91. Hickling J: Spinal traction technique. *Physiotherapy* 58:58–63, 1972.

92. Weber H: Traction therapy in sciatica due to disc prolapse. *J Oslo City Hosp* 23:167–176, 1973.

93. Harris PR: Cervical traction: review of literature and treatment guidelines. *Phys Ther* 57:910–914, 1977.

94. Wong LKF, Luo Z, Kurusu N, et al: A multi-body model for comparative study of cervical traction simulation - comparison between inclined and sitting traction. *Comput Methods Biomech Biomed Engin* 22(8):861–868, 2019. doi:10.1080/10255842.2019.1600684.

95. Daugherty RJ, Erhard RE: Segmentalized cervical traction. In Kent BE, editor: *International Federation of Orthopaedic Manipulative Therapists Proceedings*, Vail, CO.

96. Zylbergold RS, Piper MC: Cervical spine disorders: a comparison of three types of traction. *Spine* 10:867–871, 1985.

97. Graham N, Gross AR, Goldsmith C, et al: Mechanical traction for mechanical neck disorders: a systematic review. *J Rehabil Med* 38:145–152, 2006.

98. Erhard RE: *Manual therapy in the cervical spine. HSC 96 –1. The cervical spine*, La Crosse, WI, 1996, APTA, Inc.

99. Prasad KS, Gregson BA, Hargreaves G, et al: Inversion therapy in patients with pure single level lumbar discogenic disease: a pilot randomized trial. *Disabil Rehabil* 34(17):1473–1480, 2012. doi:10.3109/09638288.2011.647231.

100. Guevenol K, Tuzun C, Peke O: A comparison of inverted spinal traction and conventional traction in the treatment of lumbar disc herniations. *Physiother Theory Pract* 16:151–160, 2009.

101. Giankopoulos G, Waylonis GW, Grant PA, et al: Inversion devices: their role in producing lumbar distraction. *Arch Phys Med Rehabil* 66:100–102, 1985.

102. Zito M: Effect of two gravity inversion methods on heart rate, systolic brachial pressure, and ophthalmic artery pressure. *Phys Ther* 68:20–25, 1988.

Compression

CHAPTER OBJECTIVES

After reading this chapter, the reader will be able to do the following:
- Define *compression*.
- Describe the physical effects of compression.
- Explain the clinical indications for the use of compression.
- Choose the best technique for treatment with compression, and list the advantages and disadvantages of each.
- Select the appropriate equipment and optimal treatment parameters for treatment with compression.
- Safely and effectively apply compression.
- Accurately and completely document treatment with compression.

Compression is an inward-directed mechanical force that increases external pressure on the body or a body part. Compression is generally used to improve fluid balance and circulation or to modify the formation of scar tissue. Fluid balance is improved by increasing **hydrostatic pressure** in the interstitial space so that the pressure becomes greater in the interstitial space than in the vessels. This can limit or reverse fluid outflow from blood vessels and lymphatics. Keeping fluid in, or returning it to, the vessels allows the fluid to circulate rather

than accumulate in the periphery. Compression can be static—exerting a constant force, or intermittent—with the force varying over time. With **intermittent pneumatic compression (IPC),** pressure may be applied to the entire limb at the same time, or it may be applied sequentially, starting distally and progressing proximally.

The primary clinical application for compression is to control peripheral **edema** caused by vascular or lymphatic dysfunction. There has also been recent interest in the use of compression to control edema formation after flying, trauma, or exercise.[1-3] Compression can also be applied to help prevent the formation of **deep venous thromboses (DVTs)** and to facilitate residual limb shaping after amputation, and it is the first-line, gold-standard approach for the treatment of venous leg ulcers.[4,5]

⊙ Clinical Pearl

Compression is usually used to control peripheral edema but can also be applied to prevent the formation of deep vein thromboses, to facilitate residual limb shaping after amputation, to facilitate the healing of venous ulcers, and to control scar formation.

Effects of External Compression
IMPROVES VENOUS AND LYMPHATIC CIRCULATION

The controlled application of external compression has a range of effects on the body that vary with the pressure applied and the nature of the device used. Both static and intermittent compression devices can increase circulation by increasing hydrostatic pressure in the interstitial space outside the blood and lymphatic vessels. This increase in extravascular pressure can limit the outflow of fluid from the vessels into the interstitial space, where it tends to pool, keeping fluid in the circulatory system, where it can circulate. Intermittent compression may improve circulation more effectively than **static compression** because the varying amount of pressure may milk fluids from the distal to the proximal vessels. When venous and lymphatic vessels are compressed, the fluid within them is pushed proximally. When compression is then reduced, the vessels open and refill with new fluid from the interstitial space, ready to be pushed proximally at the next compression cycle. Sequential multichamber compression is thought to provide more effective milking than single-chamber, intermittent compression because sequential multichamber compression can cause a wave of vessel constriction moving in a proximal direction, ensuring that fluid is pushed along the vessels toward the heart rather than in a distal direction. Improving circulation can benefit patients with edema, may help prevent DVT formation in high-risk patients, and may facilitate healing of ulcers caused by venous stasis.

LIMITS SHAPE AND SIZE OF TISSUE

Static compression garments or bandaging can act as a form that, having an elastic compression element or being less extensible than natural skin, limits the shape and size of new tissue growth. This effect is exploited when compression bandaging or garments are applied over residual limbs after amputation, over skin damaged by burns, and to edematous limbs.

INCREASES TISSUE TEMPERATURE

Most compression devices, except those with built-in cooling mechanisms, increase the temperature of superficial tissue because the devices insulate the area to which they are applied. Although this temperature increase is not a direct effect of compressive forces, it is possible that this warmth increases the activity of temperature-sensitive enzymes such as collagenase, thereby controlling scar formation by breaking down excessive collagen formation.

Clinical Indications for External Compression

EDEMA
Causes of Edema

Edema is caused by increased fluid in the interstitial spaces of the body. Fluid equilibrium in the tissues is maintained by the balance between hydrostatic pressure and **oncotic pressure** inside and outside the blood vessels. Hydrostatic pressure is the mechanical force pushing fluid out of the capillaries and is primarily influenced by blood pressure and the effects of gravity. Oncotic pressure is the osmotic pressure pulling fluid into the capillaries because of the higher concentration of proteins inside the vessels (Fig. 21.1).

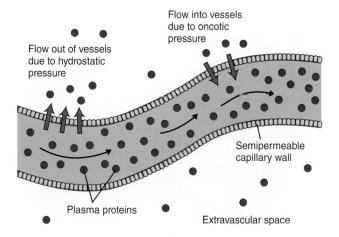

FIGURE 21.1 Effects of hydrostatic and osmotic pressure on tissue fluid balance.

> ### ◎ Clinical Pearl
>
> In a healthy body, the hydrostatic pressure pushing fluid out of the blood vessels is slightly higher than the oncotic pressure keeping fluid inside the blood vessels, and the lymphatics return the resulting fluid pushed out of the vessels back to the venous circulation.

Under normal circumstances, the hydrostatic pressure pushing fluid out of the veins is slightly higher than the osmotic pressure keeping fluid in, resulting in a slight loss of fluid into the interstitial space. The fluid that is pushed out of the veins and into the interstitial space is then taken up by the lymphatic capillaries to be returned to the venous circulation at the subclavian veins. This fluid, known as **lymphatic fluid (lymph),** is rich in protein, water, and macrophages.

A healthy diet, vascular system, and **lymphatic system**, combined with muscle contraction, will ensure that the appropriate amount of fluid exits the veins and flows back toward the heart. Dysfunction in any of these mechanisms can increase the movement of fluid from the vessels into the extravascular space or reduce the flow of venous blood or lymph back toward the heart, thus forming edema.

Major causes of edema include systemic illnesses such as kidney, liver, or heart failure, as well as venous or lymphatic insufficiency or dysfunction. Edema caused by venous or lymphatic insufficiency or dysfunction can be helped by compression; thus, these forms of edema are discussed in detail in the following sections. Treatment of edema caused by systemic illnesses with compression should only be undertaken with the guidance of the medical provider addressing the systemic illness because although compression may reduce the edema, it will likely do so by placing further load on the failing organ system and thus could worsen the patient's underlying condition and overall health.

Edema may also occur after exercise, trauma, surgery, burns, or infection because of the increase in blood flow and vascular capillary permeability that occurs with the acute inflammation associated with these events. Increased vascular capillary permeability increases the fluid flow out of the capillaries, causing an accumulation of fluid at the site of trauma or infection. More details about the formation of edema in association with acute inflammation are provided in Chapter 3.

Airline travel can also cause edema, probably because prolonged sitting and reduced external air pressure can impair lower extremity circulation. A Cochrane database systematic review first published in 2006 and then updated in 2016 concluded from studies in over 2500 subjects that wearing compression stockings for flights of at least 5 to 7 hours was associated with reduced edema formation and that these stockings were well tolerated.[1,6] In general, the stockings were below-knee length and provided either 10 to 20 mm Hg or 20 to 30 mm Hg of compression. A more recent 2019 randomized controlled trial (RCT) also found that compression stockings reduced edema formation associated with flights lasting as little as 3 hours, with no additional discomfort or adverse events, supporting that passengers may benefit from wearing compression stockings for short-haul as well as long-haul flights.[7] Pregnancy is also associated with edema formation, particularly in the legs. Contributors include increased blood volume, altered venous smooth muscle tone, and increased pressure within the veins caused by the gravid uterus reducing venous return from the lower body, leading to **venous insufficiency** and leg edema. Compression may help to control lower extremity edema during pregnancy, although this edema may also signal preeclampsia, which needs careful monitoring by a physician.[8]

Edema Caused by Venous Insufficiency. Peripheral veins carry deoxygenated blood from the periphery back to the heart. In a healthy vascular system, the resting hydrostatic venous pressure at the entrance to the right atrium of the heart averages 4.6 millimeters of mercury (mm Hg); this pressure increases by 0.77 mm Hg for each centimeter below the right atrium to reach an average of 90 mm Hg at the ankle.[9] When the calf muscles contract, they exert a pressure of approximately 200 mm Hg on the outside of the veins, which pushes the blood proximally through the veins. After the contraction, pressure on the veins falls to about 10 to 30 mm Hg, allowing the veins to refill. A healthy amount of skeletal muscle activity, as occurs during walking, running, or with any rhythmical muscle contraction, exerts a milking action that propels the blood in the veins from the periphery back toward the heart. Muscle contraction is the primary force propelling venous flow back to the heart. Valves within the vessels prevent backflow of the fluid, ensuring that the fluid moves proximally toward the heart rather than being pushed toward the distal extremities (Fig. 21.2).

Lack of physical activity, dysfunction of the venous valves caused by degeneration, or mechanical obstruction of the veins by a tumor or inflammation can result in venous insufficiency and accumulation of fluid in the periphery.

> ⊚ **Clinical Pearl**
>
> Lack of physical activity, venous or lymphatic valve dysfunction, or venous obstruction can result in peripheral edema.

The most common cause of venous insufficiency is inflammation of the veins, known as **phlebitis.** Phlebitis thickens the vessel walls, makes them less elastic, and also damages the valves. Thickening and loss of elasticity of the vessel walls elevate the hydrostatic pressure in the venous system, and damage to the valves allows blood to flow in both proximal (i.e., anterograde) and distal (i.e., retrograde) directions, rather than just proximally through the veins when the muscles contract (see Fig. 21.2). The retrograde flow reduces the circulation of deoxygenated blood out of the veins, thus increasing pressure in the venous system if fluid inflow from the arterial system is unchanged. This elevated venous pressure pushes fluid into the extravascular space, causing edema. If the limbs are in a dependent position, the edema will worsen further because of increased hydrostatic pressure from gravity.

Lymphedema. As explained previously, the hydrostatic pressure that pushes fluid out of the veins normally exceeds the oncotic pressure keeping fluid inside them. This causes fluids and proteins to flow into the interstitial space, producing a fluid called *lymph.* To prevent this lymph from accumulating, the lymphatic system acts as an accessory channel to return this fluid to the blood circulation. The lymphatic system consists of a large network of vessels and nodes through which the lymphatic fluid flows. Lymphatic vessels are found in

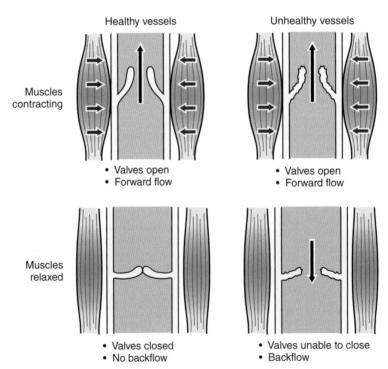

Healthy vessels   Unhealthy vessels

Muscles contracting
• Valves open
• Forward flow

Muscles relaxed
• Valves closed
• No backflow

• Valves open
• Forward flow

• Valves unable to close
• Backflow

FIGURE 21.2 Normal and abnormal valves in venous and lymphatic vessels and their relation to backflow.

almost every area where there are blood vessels. Lymph flows along the lymphatic vessels, passing through numerous lymph nodes, to empty into the subclavian veins (Fig. 21.3). Lymph nodes are concentrated in the axillary, throat, groin, and para-aortic areas, where they filter the lymph, removing bacteria and other foreign particles. The lymphatic vessels of the right arm terminate in the right lymphatic duct and empty into the right subclavian vein. The lymphatic vessels from all other areas terminate in the thoracic duct and empty into the left subclavian vein. Once lymphatic fluid reenters the circulatory system, it is processed by the kidneys, along with other fluids, waste products, and electrolytes, and then eliminated.

Fluid flows into the lymphatic system because the concentration of proteins inside the lymphatic vessels is generally higher than in the interstitial space. This oncotic pressure draws fluid out of the interstitial space into the lymphatic vessels. As with the veins, flow along the lymphatic vessels in a proximal direction depends on muscle activity, such as walking or running, to compress the vessels and their valves and prevent backflow. Decreased levels of plasma proteins, particularly albumin; mechanical obstruction of the lymphatics; abnormal distribution

of lymphatic vessels or lymph nodes; and reduced activity can all reduce lymphatic flow and cause **lymphedema.**

> ### ◎ Clinical Pearl
>
> Low serum albumin, lymphatic obstruction, abnormal lymphatic vessel distribution, and reduced activity can all cause lymphedema.

Decreased levels of plasma proteins cause fluid to accumulate in the extravascular space because the oncotic pressure that normally keeps fluid in the lymphatic vessels and the veins is reduced. If the total level of plasma protein decreases below the normal range of 6 to 8 g/dL, or if the level of plasma albumin falls below 3.3 g/dL, lymphedema is likely to result. A healthy diet and adequate protein absorption are required to keep plasma protein at an appropriate level. When lymphedema is caused by hypoproteinemia, this underlying problem should be addressed first to prevent further edema formation and other adverse consequences.

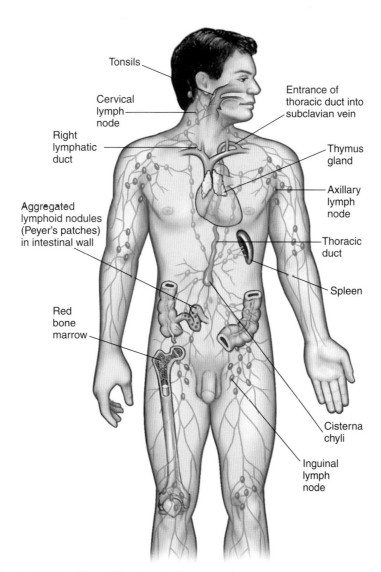

FIGURE 21.3 Lymphatic circulation. (From Thibodeau GA, Patton KT: *Anatomy and physiology,* ed 6, St Louis, 2006, Mosby.)

Lymphedema can be primary or secondary, although it is usually secondary. Primary lymphedema is caused by a congenital disorder of the lymphatic vessels, whereas secondary lymphedema is caused by some other disease or dysfunction. An example of primary lymphedema is Milroy disease, in which a person has hypoplastic, aplastic, or varicose and incompetent lymphatic vessels. Patients with primary lymphedema often have backflow in the lymphatic vessels, and the rate of protein reabsorption across the vessel walls is usually slowed. In secondary lymphedema, lymphatic flow is impaired by blockage or insufficiency of the lymphatics.

The most common cause of secondary lymphedema worldwide is filariasis, a disease characterized by infestation of the lymphatics and obstruction of the lymph vessels and nodes by microscopic filarial worms. Although this disease is common in the tropics and subtropics of Africa, the Caribbean, South America, and Asia, it is rare in the United States, Australia, and Europe. In these parts of the world, infection, neoplasm, radiation therapy, trauma, surgery, arthritis, chronic venous insufficiency, and lipedema are the main causes of secondary lymphatic obstruction, with cancer treatment with lymph node removal or radiation being most common.[10] Other causes of lymphedema in the United States include mechanical obstruction of the vessels by a tumor or inflammation, dysfunction of the valves caused by degeneration, and accidental damage to the lymphatics during non–cancer-related surgery. Most research has been done on breast cancer–related upper extremity lymphedema, but there is a growing interest and body of work on cancer-related lower extremity lymphedema.[11,12]

Compression can be applied to control lymphedema of the upper or lower extremities using various approaches, including bandaging, garments, and IPC. Compression bandaging and garments are widely recommended for the treatment of lymphedema.[13] Compression bandaging is usually used early in the treatment of lymphedema because despite being associated with greater impairment of upper extremity functional status than a garment, bandaging provides more effective edema reduction than a garment.[14] Garments are generally then used to maintain the reduction achieved with multilayer bandaging. However, recent studies support that in patients with breast cancer, the use of a light (15 to 21 mm Hg) compression sleeve immediately after lymph node surgical interventions, with ongoing use for the following 2 years, can help prevent the formation of edema and improve quality of life. This suggests that early use of light garment compression may prevent lymphedema formation after lymph node dissection and thus prevent later need for higher-level compression with multilayer bandages.[15,16] Lower extremity lymphedema can also be treated effectively with compression bandaging. A 2018 study found compression bandaging to be as or more effective for reducing lower extremity lymphedema while requiring less time, expertise, and cost compared with complex decongestive therapy, which generally includes manual lymphatic drainage, exercise, and skin care as well as compression.[17] A recent introduction to the field of bandaging for lymphedema control is taping.[18] In support of this approach, a small study in 30 women with breast cancer–related lymphedema found that kinesiotaping was associated with greater reductions in volume, greater shoulder range of motion (ROM), and greater comfort compared with compression garments.[19] However, it is not clear that the addition of kinesiotaping to complex decongestive therapy provides additional benefit,[20] and it is unlikely that taping can substitute for multilayer bandaging.

IPC is also widely used for the treatment of lymphedema, despite ongoing controversy in the literature regarding this therapy.[21] There are concerns that IPC may increase the risk for edema recurrence because of residual proteins remaining in the interstitial space, and there is also concern of risk for lymphatic structure damage and increased risk of fibrosis with high pressures. When IPC is used, it is generally as a component of a complete lymphedema management program that also includes skin care, manual lymphatic drainage, and compression bandaging or garments. However, a recent study found that IPC alone was as effective as manual lymphatic drainage alone for controlling edema and other signs and symptoms associated with breast cancer lymphedema.[22] In addition, a 2012 systematic review of IPC for lymphedema concluded that IPC may provide additional benefits beyond those associated with only wearing compression garments.[23] More recent studies also suggest that IPC, particularly high-pressure IPC to 120 mm Hg,[24] can promote the reduction of lymphedema as well as improve quality of life while also reducing overall costs.[25]

Adverse Consequences of Edema

Edema of any origin can impair ROM, limit function, and cause pain. Persistent chronic edema, particularly lymphedema, can cause collagen to be laid down in the area, leading to subcutaneous tissue fibrosis and hard induration of the skin. This edema may eventually cause disfiguring and disabling contractures and deformities (Fig. 21.4). Chronic edema also increases the risk of infection because it is often associated with skin breakdown and reduction of tissue oxygenation; this risk is further elevated with lymphedema because of the presence of a protein-rich environment for bacterial growth.[10] Advanced chronic lymphatic or venous obstruction may result in cellulitis, ulceration, and if unmanaged, partial limb amputation. These more serious sequelae are more likely to occur if pressure from excess fluid accumulated in the interstitial extravascular spaces causes arterial obstruction. Chronic venous insufficiency also often causes itching as a result of stasis dermatitis and brown pigmentation of the skin resulting from hemosiderin deposition. These signs are commonly seen on the medial lower leg (Fig. 21.5). Early edema control can help prevent the progression and development of signs and symptoms of chronic edema and its associated complications.

> ◎ **Clinical Pearl**
>
> Edema can lead to restricted ROM, pain, disfigurement, infection, ulceration, amputation, itching, brown skin pigmentation, and functional impairment. Effective edema control can help minimize these sequelae.

How Compression Reduces Edema

Compression is thought to control edema by increasing extravascular hydrostatic pressure and promoting circulation.[26,27] Underlying causes of edema, such as infection, malnutrition, inadequate physical activity, or organ dysfunction, must also

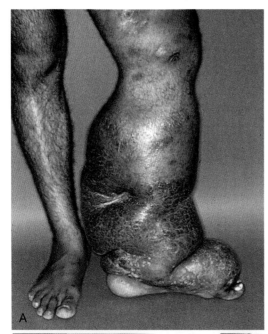

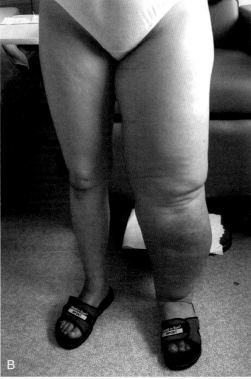

FIGURE 21.4 (A) Lymphedema caused by elephantiasis. (B) Lymphedema affecting function. (A, From Goldstein B, editor: *Practical dermatology,* ed 2, St Louis, 1997, Mosby. B, From Walsh D, Caraceni AT, Fainsinger R, et al: *Palliative medicine,* Philadelphia, 2008, Saunders.)

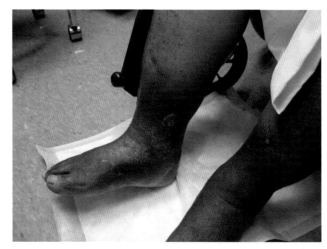

FIGURE 21.5 Venous stasis ulcer. Note the areas of darkened skin around the ulcer caused by hemosiderin deposits. (From Cameron MH, Monroe LG: *Physical rehabilitation: evidence-based examination, evaluation, and intervention,* St Louis, 2007, Saunders.)

be addressed to achieve an optimal outcome and to prevent recurrence of the edema.

Compression of a limb with a static or intermittent device increases the pressure surrounding the extremity to counterbalance any increased oncotic or hydrostatic pressure causing fluid to flow out of the vessels and into the extravascular space. If sufficient compression is applied, the hydrostatic pressure in the interstitial spaces becomes greater than the pressure in the veins and lymphatic vessels, reducing outflow from the vessels and potentially driving fluid in the interstitial spaces back into the vessels. Once fluid is in the vessels, it can be circulated out of the periphery, preventing or reversing edema formation. Intermittent sequential compression may also help to move the fluid proximally through the vessels.

PREVENTION OF DEEP VENOUS THROMBOSIS

A DVT is a blood clot (thrombus) in the deep veins. The risk for DVT formation increases when local circulation is reduced because slowly flowing blood can coagulate and form a thrombus. Therefore, any intervention that increases the circulatory rate may reduce this risk. Note, however, that although interventions that increase the circulatory rate can help prevent DVT formation, these interventions do not break down DVTs that are already present. In fact, increasing circulation where a DVT is present can increase the risk of the thrombus moving to a site where it can cause more damage, such as the lungs, where it can cause pulmonary emboli. Therefore, although compression is indicated for DVT prophylaxis, it is not indicated for the treatment of DVTs that are already present. Risk factors for DVT formation include reduced mobility and factors associated with increased blood coagulation. Reduced mobility is often associated with advanced age, surgery, trauma, hospital or nursing home confinement, or paralysis. Increased blood coagulation is associated with cancer, central vein catheterization, transvenous pacemaker, prior superficial vein thrombosis, varicose veins, the use of oral contraceptives, pregnancy, and hormone therapy.[28] DVT formation is most common in immobilized patients, and more than 50% of all DVTs occur in hospitalized patients and patients in nursing homes. Other known risk factors account for 25% of DVTs, and 25% are of unknown cause.[29]

DVTs can cause a post-thrombotic syndrome, characterized by pain, swelling, and skin changes in the area of the thrombus, but a more significant health risk occurs if the thrombus becomes dislodged and blocks the blood supply to the lungs, causing pulmonary emboli. Such blockage may cause shortness of breath, respiratory failure, or death. Therefore, preventing the formation of DVTs in at-risk patients is imperative.

Various approaches, including compression stockings, IPC, calf muscle electrical stimulation, and anticoagulant medications, reduce the risk of DVT formation. The 2018 update of the Cochrane Collaboration systematic review and meta-analysis evaluating the efficacy of graded compression stockings for DVT prevention, which included 20 studies, mostly in postoperative patients, found that graded compression stockings reduced the overall risk of DVT formation and may also reduce the risk of pulmonary embolus (PE).[4] Although most studies used thigh-length stockings, given that a 2012 systematic review comparing knee-length with thigh-length compression stockings for DVT prevention found insufficient evidence to recommend one over the other, the length of the compression stocking probably does not affect efficacy, and shorter stocking are easier to put on.[30] Evidence also supports that IPC applied to the foot and calf (Fig. 21.6) reduces the incidence of DVT formation in hospitalized patients. A 2005 meta-analysis of 15 studies in 2270 surgical patients found that IPC reduced the risk of DVT formation by 60%.[31] Similarly, a 2018 meta-analysis of seven studies (four in English and three in Chinese) on the effects of IPC on DVT prevention in people with stroke found that IPC was associated with a 50% reduction in risk of DVT formation compared with no IPC, but IPC also increased adverse events such as sleep disturbance, skin breakdown, and risk of falls, resulting overall in minimal, if any, improvement in quality-adjusted survival.[32] An area of considerable interest is whether IPC and medications are more effective alone or together for the prevention of DVT and PE. Anticoagulation medications are clearly effective in reducing the risk of DVT formation, but they come with an increased risk of hemorrhage, making compression appealing. A 2016 Cochrane Collaboration review on this topic found that adding medication to IPC reduced the rate of DVT formation but not the rate of PE and also increased the rate of bleeding (from 0.1% to 1.5%). Adding IPC to medication

reduced the rate of PE but did not alter the rate of DVT or bleeding.[33] Based on these findings, the authors support combining IPC with medications in hospitalized patients with trauma or undergoing surgery who are at risk of developing DVT or PE.

Long air flights are also associated with DVT formation, probably because prolonged sitting and reduced external air pressure can impair lower extremity circulation. The 2006 and 2016 Cochrane database systematic reviews discussed earlier in this chapter that found the wearing of compression stockings for flights of at least 5 to 7 hours to be associated with less edema formation also found that wearing compression stockings was associated with a substantial reduction in asymptomatic DVT formation.[1,6]

Compression is thought to reduce DVT formation primarily by improving venous blood flow, thus reducing venous stasis and the opportunity for thrombus formation.[1,34] Intermittent compression may also inhibit tissue factor pathways that initiate blood coagulation or may degrade thrombi by enhancing fibrinolysis.[35–38]

VENOUS STASIS ULCERS

A **venous stasis ulcer** is an area of tissue breakdown and necrosis that occurs in areas of impaired venous circulation (see Fig. 21.5). The exact mechanism by which poor venous circulation causes ulcers is still uncertain. It is thought that increased venous pressure and deep venous reflux lead to the leakage of white blood cells and matrix metalloproteinases, resulting in local inflammation and delayed migration and proliferation of cells required for healing.[39–41]

Compression is the gold-standard, first-line approach for treating and preventing the recurrence of venous stasis ulcers.[42] Compression can improve venous circulation, which may reduce the adverse effects of poor venous flow, diminish the risk of vascular ulcer formation, and facilitate healing of previously formed ulcers.[43,44]

Compression has been recommended for promoting leg ulcer healing[45] since the time of Hippocrates (400 BCE), and the most recent Cochrane Collaboration systematic review of studies on compression for venous leg ulcers, published in 2012, also concluded, based on 48 studies, that compression increases the rate of healing of venous stasis ulcers compared with no compression.[43] Compression may facilitate healing by improving venous circulation, reducing venous pooling and reflux, improving tissue oxygenation, altering white cell adhesion, and reducing edema. Multilayered compression (two or four layer) is more effective for healing venous ulcers than single-layer compression, with systems including elastic components being most effective.[43] Consistently wearing compression stockings also reduces the likelihood of venous ulcer recurrence.[44] Venous ulcers have been found to recur more often in patients who do not wear compression stockings consistently.[46] IPC may be used to treat venous stasis ulcers that do not heal using other methods, and at least in the short term, patient compliance may be higher with this than with other methods of compression.[47] A recent meta-analysis also found that adding exercise, such as heel raises and walking, to compression therapy accelerates healing and is associated with a higher incidence of healing compared with compression therapy alone.[48]

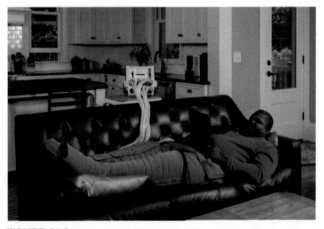

FIGURE 21.6 Use of intermittent pneumatic compression to prevent deep vein thrombosis (DVT) formation in a bedridden patient. (Courtesy Tactile Medical, Minneapolis, MN.)

Compression therapy is the cornerstone of treatment for venous stasis ulcers. Multilayered compression is more effective than single-layer compression, and adding exercise to compression provides additional benefit.

Although compression is recommended for the treatment of venous ulcers, compression is generally contraindicated with arterial insufficiency because compression of the arteries may further impair arterial flow, aggravating the condition. However, surprisingly, compression has been found to sometimes facilitate the healing of arterial insufficiency ulcers. A meta-analysis found that some studies demonstrated improved wound healing with IPC in patients with severe peripheral artery disease who were not candidates for surgery.[49] It is possible that compression helped these patients by reducing chronic edema that places pressure on the arterial vessels. However, because of the risk of further impairment of arterial flow with compression, compression should not be used on most patients with peripheral artery disease.

RESIDUAL LIMB SHAPING AFTER AMPUTATION

Residual limb reduction and shaping are required to prepare for functional weight bearing on a prosthetic device. The residual limb must be shaped so that the prosthesis maintains its position and alignment and promotes weight bearing on appropriate structures. Excessive pressure on unprotected bony prominences should be avoided to promote comfort and function and to limit the risk of tissue breakdown (Fig. 21.7).[50]

Both static and intermittent compression are used for limb shaping, although intermittent compression can reduce the residual limb in approximately half the time required by other techniques,[51] and a temporary prosthesis may achieve ideal stump shaping even more quickly than compression bandaging or pneumatic compression.[52] When intermittent compression is used for limb shaping, it is applied in conjunction with an elastic bandage. Compression reduces residual limb size because it controls postsurgical edema and prevents stretching of the soft tissues by accumulated fluids.

CONTROL OF HYPERTROPHIC SCARRING

Hypertrophic scarring, which is excessive scarring within the boundaries of the original site of skin injury, is a common complication of deep burns and other extensive skin and soft tissue injuries. Normal skin is pliable, is esthetically pleasing, and has clearly identifiable layers, whereas hypertrophic scars are not pliable, have a raised and ridged appearance, and do not have clearly identifiable skin layers (Fig. 21.8). The risk of hypertrophic scarring is increased with delayed healing, a deep wound, repeated trauma, infection, or the presence of a foreign body and in individuals with a genetic predisposition. Hypertrophic scarring is most common around the sternum, upper back, and shoulders. **Keloid**s are also a form of excessive scarring, but in contrast to hypertrophic scars that stay within the boundaries of the initial injury, keloids extend beyond the boundaries of the original site of skin injury. The risk of keloids after injury is largely genetically determined. Hypertrophic scars and keloids result in poor cosmesis and the development of contractures that may restrict ROM and function.

Although many approaches, including surgery, pharmaceuticals, passive stretch with positioning, massage, and silicone gel, are used to control the formation of hypertrophic scars, compression is the standard, first-line approach.[53,54] Based on a

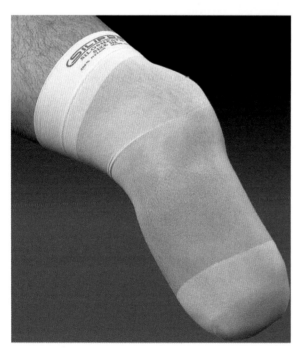

FIGURE 21.7 Compression for residual limb shaping. (Courtesy Silipos, Niagara Falls, NY.)

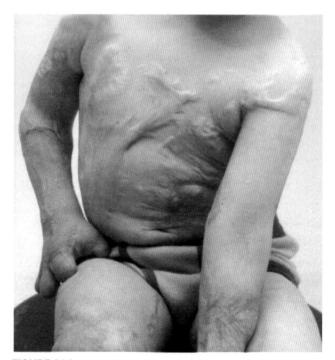

FIGURE 21.8 Hypertrophic scarring. (From Cameron MH, Monroe LG: *Physical rehabilitation: evidence-based examination, evaluation, and intervention,* St Louis, 2007, Saunders.)

systematic review of 28 articles, compression for at least 23 h/day for 12 months, with 20 to 30 mm Hg of pressure, is recommended to decrease scar height and erythema for wounds at risk for hypertrophic scarring.[55] Many mechanisms have been proposed to explain the effects of compression on hypertrophic scarring. Compression may directly shape the scar tissue by acting as a mold for the growth of new tissue. It also decreases the formation of local edema and improves collagen orientation. Compression may also improve the extracellular matrix organization in hypertrophic scars and may increase collagenase activity as a result of increased skin temperature or increased release of prostaglandin E_2.[56,57] Alternatively, compression may control scar formation by inducing local tissue hypoxia[58] or by altering the release and activity of matrix metalloproteinases thought to be involved in wound healing.[59] Compression has been shown to induce apoptosis (cell death) and to regulate cytokine release in hypertrophic scars, thus reducing the hyperproliferation that underlies excessive scarring.[60]

When compression is applied to control hypertrophic scar formation, treatment is generally initiated once the new epithelium has formed and is continued for 12 months or longer until the scar has reached maturity and is no longer growing. Compression can be applied with elastic bandages, self-adherent wraps, tubular elastic cotton supports, or custom-fit elastic garments. With any of these, the compression pressure is maintained at approximately 20 to 30 mm Hg. It is recommended that the compression device be worn 23 to 24 h/day to achieve maximum benefit.[55] Compression garments should be replaced every 2 to 3 months so that the level of compression force is maintained. Overall, 60% of patients with hypertrophic scarring treated with compression show 80% to 100% improvement.[61] Common complications of this treatment include skin irritation, constriction of circulation, and restricted joint motion.

◎ Clinical Pearl

To control hypertrophic scar formation, compression producing 20 to 30 mm Hg of force should be worn for 23 to 24 h/day for 12 months or longer.

Compression may also be used to try to manage keloids, but keloids tend to be less responsive to treatment than hypertrophic scars.[61,62] Because an individual's risk of keloid formation may be known from previous injury, people who have developed keloids in the past are generally advised to avoid nonessential or cosmetic surgery.

Contraindications and Precautions for External Compression

Few contraindications apply to all compression devices; however, when compression is used to treat edema or impaired circulation, the underlying cause of these problems should be addressed before compression therapy is initiated. Compression therapy will be ineffective and contraindicated in cases where edema is caused by blockage of the circulation or if there is active infection or malignancy in the affected extremity. When peripheral edema is caused by cardiovascular disease, such as congestive heart failure (CHF) or cardiomyopathy, one must ensure that the increased fluid load that could be placed

on the heart by the shifting of fluid from the periphery in response to treatment with compression will not be detrimental to the patient. In such cases, the patient's physician should always be consulted before compression therapy is begun.

All forms of compression are contraindicated in patients with symptomatic heart failure (because of the risk of system overload) and in patients with a thrombus (because of the risk of dislodgment) and may not be appropriate if an arterial revascularization has been performed on the involved limb. In addition, the clinician must evaluate for the presence and severity of arterial insufficiency before compressing a limb. This is most often determined by calculating the **ankle-brachial index (ABI)**. If the ABI is less than 0.6, all forms of static compression are contraindicated. If the ABI is over 0.8, standard or full compression (30 to 40 mm Hg) may be used. When the ABI is between 0.5 and 0.8, the compression pressure should be reduced to between 23 mm Hg and 27 mm Hg. If the patient also has neuropathy, careful monitoring is necessary because they may fail to recognize symptoms of ischemia, such as pain, numbness, or tingling.

Particular care should be taken when applying and removing compression bandages and garments to avoid trauma to healing tissue or fragile skin. Details of contraindications and precautions for the use of compression pumps are provided next.

CONTRAINDICATIONS FOR INTERMITTENT OR SEQUENTIAL COMPRESSION PUMPS

✱ CONTRAINDICATIONS

for Intermittent or Sequential Compression Pumps

- Symptomatic heart failure or pulmonary edema
- Recent or acute DVT, thrombophlebitis, or pulmonary embolism
- Obstructed lymphatic or venous return
- Severe peripheral arterial disease
- Acute local skin infection (e.g., cellulitis)
- Significant hypoproteinemia (protein levels <2 g/dL)
- Acute trauma or fracture
- Arterial revascularization

Symptomatic Heart Failure or Pulmonary Edema

Although edema of the dependent parts of the body is a common consequence of CHF, compression pumps should only be used to treat edema of this origin if the increased stress on the failing heart from the shift of fluid from the peripheral to the central circulation is deemed safe. CHF results from a decrease in the ability or efficiency of cardiac muscle contraction and subsequent decreased cardiac output. This increases venous pressure and sodium and water retention, which cause edema. Peripheral edema caused by CHF is usually of the bilateral lower extremities and is symmetrical. Treating CHF requires decreasing the load on the heart using a variety of medications. Compression increases the cardiac load by increasing the amount of fluid in the veins. Thus, compression tends to aggravate the underlying condition and can result in worsening edema and potentially other more serious side effects, such as pulmonary edema. However, with appropriate medical management and guidance, compression may be safely used to remove edema accumulated over time from the lower extremities, and this edema reduction can be maintained with daily use of below-knee compression socks.

Pulmonary edema occurs with prolonged or severe CHF. Pulmonary edema is the result of elevated lung capillary pressure causing fluid to leave the circulation and accumulate in alveolar air spaces in the lungs. Compression is contraindicated when pulmonary edema is present because compression increases the fluid load of the vascular system and pressure in the lung capillaries, potentially aggravating this serious medical condition.

> **■ Ask the Patient**
> - "Do you have any heart or lung problems?"
> - "Do you have difficulty breathing?"
> - "Are you taking any medications for your heart or blood pressure?"
> - "Do you have swelling in both legs?"
>
> **■ Assess**
> - Check for the presence of bilateral edema.

Compression should not be used to treat edema until the clinician has ascertained that this is safe with a patient with CHF and that they do not have pulmonary edema.

Recent or Acute Deep Venous Thrombosis, Thrombophlebitis, or Pulmonary Embolism

Although compression is recommended for DVT prevention, intermittent compression should not be used when the patient is known to have a DVT, thrombophlebitis, or a pulmonary embolus because the thrombus may become dislodged or the embolus may travel. This can occur because of direct mechanical agitation of the clot by compression or because of increased circulation produced by compression. If a thrombus or embolus becomes dislodged, it may travel in the bloodstream to a distant site and lodge in a location where it impairs blood flow to an organ sufficiently enough to cause organ damage, severe morbidity, or even death. For example, an embolus in the pulmonary arteries produces approximately a 30% mortality rate, whereas an embolus that lodges in the arteries supplying the brain may cause stroke or death. Compression can help prevent the formation of DVTs, but it should not be used when it is thought that a thrombus may already be present.

> **■ Ask the Patient**
> - "Do you have pain in your calves?"
> - "How long have you not been walking?"
>
> **■ Assess**
> - Check for Homans sign (discomfort in the calf on forced dorsiflexion of the foot), a sign of thrombosis in the leg.

Further evaluation by a physician should be requested if the clinician suspects that there may be a thrombus in the deep veins of the leg. The use of compression should be delayed until the patient has been cleared for the presence of thromboses or thrombophlebitis in the area to be treated.

Obstructed Lymphatic or Venous Return

Although compression is recommended for the treatment of edema resulting from lymphatic or venous insufficiency, compression is contraindicated when lymphatic or venous return is completely obstructed because increasing the fluid load of the vessels in such cases cannot reduce the edema until the obstruction has been removed. Lymphatic or venous return may be obstructed by a thrombus, radiation damage to the lymph nodes, an inguinal or abdominal tumor, or other masses. With partial obstruction of the vessels or complete occlusion of only a few of the vessels, treatment with compression may enhance the functioning of intact collateral vessels.

> **■ Ask the Patient**
> - "Do you know why you have swelling in your legs/ arms?"
> - "Is something obstructing your circulation?"

If there is complete lymphatic or venous obstruction, compression should not be used. Such obstruction may need to be treated surgically. When there is partial obstruction, compression may be used in conjunction with careful monitoring of the patient's response to the treatment to ensure that the treatment is helping to resolve the edema, rather than just shifting the fluid to a more proximal area of the affected limb.

Severe Peripheral Artery Disease

Compression should not be used in patients with severe peripheral artery disease because it can aggravate this condition by closing down diseased arteries, further impairing circulation in the area.

> **■ Ask the Patient**
> - "Do you get pain in your calves when walking?"
> - If an ulcer is present: "Have you had problems with your arteries, for example, heart bypass surgery or bypass surgery in your legs?"

Pain in the calves while walking can be the result of intermittent claudication, a sign of peripheral artery disease. A history of bypass surgeries suggests the presence of arterial disease in other areas.

> **■ Assess**
> - If an ulcer is present, try to determine whether it is the result of arterial insufficiency. Ulcers caused by arterial insufficiency are usually small and round, with definite borders, and painful. They occur most often on the interdigital spaces between the toes or on the lateral malleolus.
> - Request that an ABI be obtained. This is generally performed by vascular services and is a measure of the ratio of systolic blood pressure in the lower extremity to systolic blood pressure in the upper extremity. Compression should not be applied if the ABI is less than 0.6, indicating that blood pressure at the ankle is less than 60% of that in the upper extremity. If the ABI is over 0.8, standard or full compression (30 to 40 mm Hg) may be used. When the ABI is between 0.5 and 0.8, the compression pressure should be reduced to between 23 mm Hg and 27 mm Hg.

Acute Local Skin Infection

A local skin infection is likely to be aggravated by the application of compression because the sleeves and skin coverings used increase the moisture and temperature of the area, encouraging the growth of microorganisms. If a chronic skin infection is present, single-use sleeves that avoid cross-contamination from one patient to another or reinfection of the same patient may be used to apply intermittent compression.

■ **Ask the Patient**
• "Do you have any skin infections in the area to be treated?"

■ **Assess**
• Inspect the skin for rashes, redness, or skin breakdown, indicating the possible presence of infection.

Significant Hypoproteinemia

Although peripheral edema is a common symptom of severe hypoproteinemia, when the serum protein level is less than 2 g/dL, resulting edema should not be treated with compression because returning fluid to the vessels will further lower the serum protein concentration, potentially causing severe adverse consequences, including cardiac and immunological dysfunction. Severe hypoproteinemia can occur because of inadequate food intake, increased nutrient losses, or increased nutrient requirements resulting from an underlying disease.

■ **Ask the Patient**
• "Have you recently lost weight?"
• "Have you changed your diet?"
• "Do you have any other disease?"

■ **Assess**
• Check the laboratory values section of the patient's chart for the serum protein level.

The use of compression should be delayed until the patient's serum protein level is greater than 2 g/dL.

Acute Trauma or Fracture

Intermittent compression is contraindicated immediately after acute trauma because compression may cause excessive motion at the site of trauma, increasing bleeding, aggravating the acute inflammation, or destabilizing an acute fracture.[63] Such effects can further damage the site of injury and can impair healing. Intermittent compression should be used for treating posttraumatic edema only after the initial acute inflammatory phase has passed, bleeding has stopped, and the area is mechanically stable. Static compression, as provided by stockings or wraps, may be used immediately after acute trauma to prevent edema and reduce bleeding. Directly after an injury, static compression is frequently applied in conjunction with rest, ice, and elevation to optimize the control of pain, edema, and inflammation.

◎ **Clinical Pearl**

Immediately after acute trauma, static compression, often in conjunction with rest, ice, and elevation, can be applied to prevent edema and reduce bleeding. Do not apply intermittent compression immediately after acute trauma because this can aggravate bleeding or destabilize the site.

■ **Ask the Patient**
• "When did your injury happen?"
• "Do you know if a bone was broken?"

Arterial Revascularization

Intermittent compression is contraindicated after arterial revascularization surgery because of the risk of occluding arterial vessels and preventing blood from reaching the extremities, leading to ischemia. If the patient has had recent arterial revascularization, elevation of the extremity and exercise may be used to decrease edema.

■ **Ask the Patient**
• "Have you had surgery on your arteries?"

■ **Assess**
• Look for scars that would indicate vascular surgery, especially on the legs.

PRECAUTIONS FOR INTERMITTENT OR SEQUENTIAL COMPRESSION PUMPS

✱ **PRECAUTIONS**

for Intermittent or Sequential Compression Pumps

• Impaired sensation or mentation
• Uncontrolled hypertension
• Cancer
• Superficial peripheral nerves

Impaired Sensation or Mentation

Compression should be applied with caution to patients with impaired sensation or mentation because such patients may be unable to recognize or communicate when pressure is excessive or painful.

■ **Ask the Patient**
• "Do you have normal feeling in this area?"

■ **Assess**
• Sensation in the area
• Alertness and orientation

Compression garments or low levels of intermittent compression may be used if the patient has impaired sensation or mentation; however, such patients must be carefully monitored for adverse effects such as skin irritation or aggravated edema caused by constriction of garments in tight areas.

Uncontrolled Hypertension

Compression should be applied with caution to patients with uncontrolled hypertension because compression can further elevate blood pressure by increasing the vascular fluid load. Blood pressure should be monitored frequently while treating these patients, and treatment should be stopped if their blood pressure increases above the safe level determined by their physician.

> ■ **Ask the Patient**
> • "Do you have high blood pressure? If so, is it well controlled with medication?"
>
> ■ **Assess**
> • Resting blood pressure

The clinician should check with the patient's physician for guidelines on blood pressure limits.

Cancer

Compression can increase circulation, which may disturb or dislodge metastatic tissue, promoting metastasis, or may improve tissue nutrition, promoting tumor growth. Although no reports have described metastasis or accelerated tumor growth caused by the use of compression, it is generally recommended that compression not be applied where a tumor is present or when it is thought that an increase in circulation may cause a tumor to move or grow more rapidly. However, compression is frequently used to control lymphedema that results from the treatment of breast cancer with mastectomy or radiation and may even be used directly after surgery to prevent lymphedema formation. Experts in this field vary in their opinions regarding the safety of this treatment and the precautions to be applied.[64–66] Although some experts do not consider the presence or history of malignancy to contraindicate the use of compression, others recommend avoiding the use of compression in areas close to the malignancy, and still others recommend not applying this type of intervention until the patient has been cancer-free for 5 years. In general, most experts agree that the use of compression need not be restricted during the time that patients are receiving chemotherapy, hormone therapy, or biological response modifiers for treatment of their cancer.

> ■ **Ask the Patient**
> • If edema results from the treatment of breast cancer: "Are you receiving chemotherapy, hormone therapy, or biological response modifiers for treatment of your cancer?"
>
> ■ **Assess**
> • Determine how recently the cancer diagnosis was made.

If the cause of edema is unknown and the patient has signs of cancer such as recent unexplained changes in body weight or constant pain that does not change, treatment with compression should be deferred until a follow-up evaluation that can rule out malignancy has been performed by a physician.

Superficial Peripheral Nerves

Peroneal nerve palsy has been documented after the application of intermittent sequential compression.[67,68] Significant weight loss resulting in loss of fat and muscle mass around the peroneal nerves may predispose these nerves to injury from compression devices. When compression is applied over an area where there is a superficial nerve, particularly in a patient with significant weight loss, the clinician should monitor closely for symptoms of nerve compression, including distal changes in, or loss of, sensation or strength.

Adverse Effects of External Compression

The potentially adverse effects of compression generally relate to aggravating a condition that is causing edema or is impairing circulation if excessive pressure is used. When edema is the result of heart, kidney, or liver failure or circulatory obstruction, compression may aggravate the underlying condition. Also, if too much pressure is used, the compression device may cause soft tissue injury or act as a tourniquet, impairing arterial circulation and causing ischemia and edema or compression of peripheral nerves.[63,67–69] If ischemia is prolonged, impaired healing or tissue death can occur. When compression is effective in reducing edema in an extremity, it is recommended that if this fluid accumulates at the proximal end of the extremity or where the extremity attaches to the trunk, it should be mobilized using massage. To minimize the probability of adverse circulatory effects from treatment with compression, it is recommended that the patient always be monitored closely for undesired changes in blood pressure or edema, particularly with the first application of the treatment or with changes in treatment parameters.

Application Techniques

Compression can be applied in several ways, depending on the patient's clinical presentation and the treatment goals.[26] Static compression can be applied with bandages or garments, whereas intermittent compression can be applied with electrical pneumatic pumps.

COMPRESSION BANDAGING

Compression bandaging, also known as *compression wrapping*, is used in patients with lymphedema to decrease limb volume. Compression bandages should be worn for 23 to 24 hours/day. Compression bandages work by applying resting or working pressure or a combination of the two. **Resting pressure** is exerted by elastic when it is put on stretch. An elastic bandage exerts this pressure whether the patient is moving or immobile. **Working pressure** is produced by active muscles pushing against an inelastic bandage (Fig. 21.9) and is produced only when the patient is moving and contracting the muscles. Compression bandages come in varying degrees of extensibility and may be applied as a single layer or in multiple layers. Types of compression bandages include long-stretch, short-stretch, multilayered, and semi-rigid bandages.

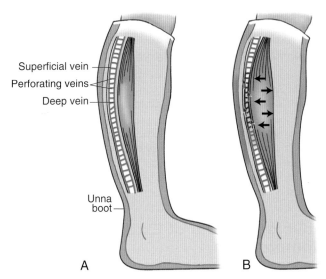

FIGURE 21.9 Development of working pressure. (A) Muscle relaxed. (B) Calf muscle contracting and pressing against Unna boot to compress the veins.

A **long-stretch bandage** (also known as *high-stretch bandage*) can extend by 100% to 200%. These bandages provide the greatest resting pressure because they exert the greatest restoring force. When stretched, a long-stretch bandage typically applies approximately 60 to 70 mm Hg pressure. These highly elastic bandages provide little to no working pressure because they stretch rather than resist when the muscles expand. Long-stretch bandages are most effective for applying compression to immobile patients or limbs. Examples of long-stretch bandages include Ace wraps and Tubigrip (ConvaTec, Skillman, NJ). In general, it is recommended that if high-stretch bandages, such as a new Ace wrap, are used to control edema, they should be applied with only moderate tension to avoid excessive resting pressure because without activity, the high resting pressure provided by this type of bandage may impair circulation.

A **short-stretch bandage** (also known as *low-stretch bandage*) has low elasticity, with 30% to 90% extension. These bandages produce a low resting pressure but cause resistance and high working pressure during muscle activity. Because low-stretch bandages provide a degree of both resting and working pressures, they can be somewhat effective during activity or at rest. For an inelastic bandage to produce working pressure, the patient must have a functional calf muscle and a functional gait pattern. Short-stretch bandages are most useful during active movement when the activity of the muscles results in high working pressure; generally, they do not control edema effectively or improve circulation in a flaccid or inactive limb. Patients wearing short-stretch lower extremity bandages are encouraged to walk, and those wearing short-stretch upper extremity bandages are encouraged to use their wrapped limb as much as possible throughout the day. Examples of short-stretch bandages are Comprilan (Smith & Nephew/Beiersdorf, London, UK) and Artico (Activa Healthcare, Burton-upon-Trent, UK).

Multilayered bandage systems use a combination of inelastic and elastic layers to apply moderate to high resting pressure through the use of two, three, or four layers of different

bandages (Fig. 21.10). For example, one type of multilayered bandage system (Profore; Smith & Nephew) provides approximately 40 mm Hg of resting pressure at the ankle, graduating to 17 mm Hg at the knee.[70] The layers of bandages provide protection and absorption, as well as compression. This type of bandage system is most commonly used for the treatment and prevention of venous leg ulcers and can maintain high compression for up to 1 week after application. A 2012 systematic review of 48 trials concluded that multicomponent

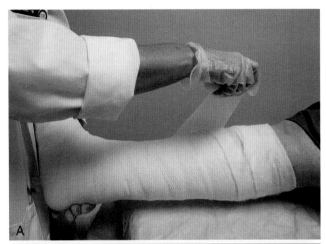

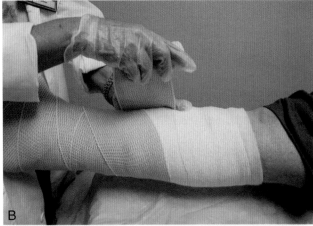

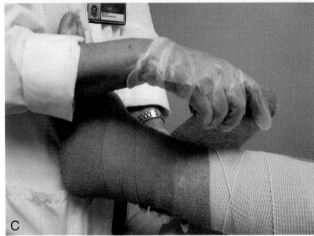

FIGURE 21.10 Application of a four-layer compression bandage. (From Cameron MH, Monroe LG: *Physical rehabilitation: evidence-based examination, evaluation, and intervention*, St Louis, 2007, Saunders.)

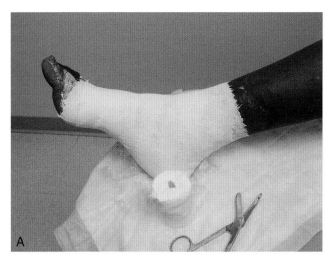 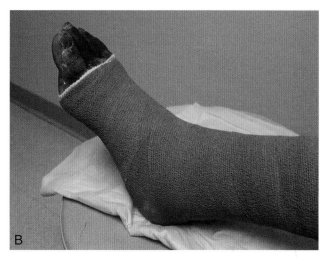

FIGURE 21.11 Unna boot. (From Cameron MH, Monroe LG: *Physical rehabilitation: evidence-based examination, evaluation, and intervention,* St Louis, 2007, Saunders.)

bandaging is more effective than single-component compression in the treatment of venous leg ulcers and that including an elastic component is more effective than using mainly inelastic constituents.[43] Examples of multilayered bandages include Profore and Dyna-Flex.

A semi-rigid bandage formed of zinc oxide–impregnated gauze is commonly used to exert working pressure. When this type of bandage is applied to the lower extremity, it is known as an **Unna boot** (Fig. 21.11). This bandage is typically used to treat venous stasis ulcers. Zinc oxide–impregnated gauze bandages become soft when wet to allow molding around the involved limb and then harden as they dry to form a semi-rigid boot. The boot is left on the patient for 1 to 2 weeks and is then removed and replaced. An Unna boot provides a sustained compression force of 35 to 40 mm Hg.

Compression bandages are generally applied by wrapping them around the limb in a figure-eight manner, starting distally and progressing proximally. Circular, circumferential, and spiral wrappings are generally not recommended because these configurations can result in uneven pressure and thus uneven control of edema. The bandage should be applied tightly enough to apply moderate, comfortable compression without impairing circulation. To avoid the compression bandage slipping on the skin, cohesive gauze or foam bandages are often applied under the compression bandages directly against the patient's skin. Soft cotton may be used as an underwrapping to absorb sweat and to help distribute pressure more evenly.

For all types of bandages, it is recommended that compression have a pressure gradient, being greatest distally and gradually decreasing proximally. This is generally produced by keeping consistent equal tension in the bandage all the way up. This is because, according to Laplace's law (pressure = tension/radius), if tension is constant and the radius of the limb increases, as it generally does moving proximally, pressure will decrease. To maintain consistency of pressure around anatomical indentations, such as the ankles, pieces of foam or cotton cut to size should be placed in these indentations before the bandage is applied (Fig. 21.12).

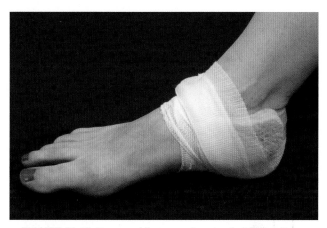

FIGURE 21.12 Foam padding around anatomical indentations.

◎ Clinical Pearl

For all types of compression bandages, compression should be greatest distally and gradually decrease proximally.

COMPRESSION GARMENTS

Compression garments provide various degrees of compression and are available in custom-fit sizes for all areas of the body and in standard off-the-shelf sizes for the limbs. Compression garments are generally made of washable Lycra spandex and nylon and have moderate elasticity to provide a combination of moderate resting and working pressures. Inelastic or low-stretch garments, which provide more working pressure, are not made because they are too difficult to put on and take off; however, low-stretch Velcro closure static-compression garments that are easier to use are available.

APPLICATION TECHNIQUE 21.1   COMPRESSION BANDAGE

Equipment Required

- Cohesive gauze, foam, or cotton underbandage
- Bandages of appropriate elasticity
- Cotton or foam for padding

Procedure

1. Remove clothing and jewelry from the area to be treated.
2. Inspect the skin in the area.
3. Apply foam or cotton padding around anatomical indentations.
4. Dress and cover any wound according to the treatment regimen being used for that wound.
5. Apply a cohesive gauze, foam, or cotton under the bandage to protect the skin from the compression bandage and to minimize slipping of the compression bandage. Start distally and progress proximally.
6. Apply the compression bandage, starting distally and progressing proximally. When applying a bandage to the lower extremity, first apply it around the ankle to fix the bandage in place, then wrap the foot, and then bandage the leg and thigh. Wrapping around the foot should be from medial to lateral when on the dorsum of the foot.[71] When applying a bandage to the upper extremity, first apply it to the wrist to fix it in place, then wrap the hand, and then bandage the forearm and arm. For all areas, slightly more tension should be applied distally than proximally, and the bandage should be applied in a figure-eight manner (Fig. 21.13).

Advantages

- Inexpensive
- Quick to apply once skill is mastered
- Readily available
- Extremity can be used during treatment
- Safe for acute conditions

- The frequent rewrapping of bandages ensures optimal compression throughout the limb as the limb shape and size change during the initial weeks of treatment.

Disadvantages

- Requires moderate skill, flexibility, and level of cognition to apply
- Compression not readily quantifiable or replicable
- Bulky and unattractive
- Inelastic bandages do not control edema in flaccid limb.

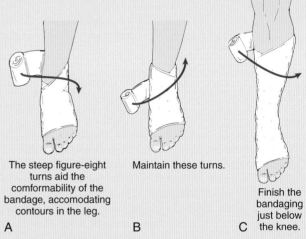

The steep figure-eight turns aid the comformability of the bandage, accomodating contours in the leg.   Maintain these turns.   Finish the bandaging just below the knee.

A   B   C

FIGURE 21.13 Elastic compression wrap of the foot, ankle, and leg. Note the figure-eight wrap at the ankle. (Redrawn from Morrison M, Moffat C: *A colour guide to the assessment and management of leg ulcers,* ed 2, London, 1994, Mosby.)

Off-the-shelf stockings, known as **antiembolism stockings,** provide a low compression force of approximately 16 to 18 mm Hg and are used to prevent DVT formation in bedridden patients (Fig. 21.14). These stockings are not intended to provide sufficient compression to prevent DVT formation or alter circulation when the lower extremities are in a dependent position. These stockings should fit snugly but comfortably around the lower extremities, and they should be worn by the patient 24 hours a day except when bathing. Knee-high and thigh-high antiembolism stockings have been found to be similarly efficient in reducing venous stasis, and knee-high stockings are more comfortable to wear and wrinkle less than thigh-high stockings.[71]

Custom-fit and off-the-shelf compression garments that provide sufficient compression to control edema and counteract the effects of gravity on circulation in active patients, or to modify scar formation after burns, are available in different thicknesses and with different degrees of pretensioning to provide pressure ranging from 10 to 80 mm Hg (Fig. 21.15). A pressure of 20 to 30 mm Hg is generally appropriate to control the formation of scar tissue or upper extremity lymphedema, whereas 30 to 40 mm Hg pressure will control lower extremity edema in most ambulatory patients.[72]

Some garments provide a pressure gradient so that compression is greatest distally and decreases proximally. Although

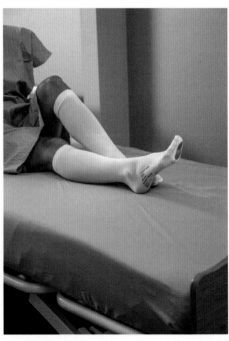

FIGURE 21.14 Antiembolism stockings. (Courtesy Cardinal Health, Dublin, OH.)

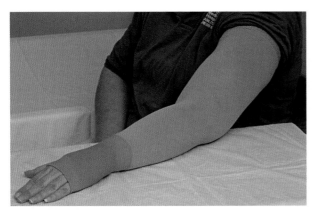

FIGURE 21.15 Upper extremity compression garment. (From Fairchild SL: *Principles and techniques of patient care,* ed 5, St Louis, 2013, Saunders.)

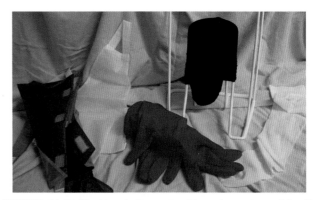

FIGURE 21.16 Stocking butler and rubber gloves to assist with donning compression stockings. (From Cameron MH, Monroe LG: *Physical rehabilitation: evidence-based examination, evaluation, and intervention,* St Louis, 2007, Saunders.)

off-the-shelf stockings can improve venous circulation and control edema in most patients, custom-fit garments may be necessary in severe conditions or when an individual's limb contours do not match off-the-shelf sizing. Custom-fit garments may include options such as zippers and reinforced padded areas to improve ease of use and fit and are effective in normalizing venous flow in many cases in which off-the-shelf garments are ineffective.[73] For sizing to be appropriate, both custom-fit and off-the-shelf compression garments should be fitted when edema is minimal. This is generally done first thing in the morning or after treatment with an intermittent compression pump. Garments are available for both upper and lower extremities, as well as for the trunk and head (see Fig. 21.15). They are also available in a number of colors.

Compression garments are sometimes difficult for patients to put on and take off, especially for patients with poor vision, manual dexterity, coordination, or balance and for patients

who are weak or cannot reach their feet.[74] This can affect adherence to compression therapy. Assistive devices, such as the stocking butler and rubber gloves, can assist with donning compression stockings, but many people still have difficulty wearing compression devices as recommended (Fig. 21.16). A patient's belief that wearing stockings is worthwhile and that the stockings are comfortable to wear may be the greatest determinants of adherence.[75] It is recommended that compression garments be replaced approximately every 6 months because they lose compression force over time.[44] Machine washing preserves pressure delivery better than hand washing.

Clinical Pearl

Compression garments lose compression force over time and should therefore be replaced about every 6 months.

APPLICATION TECHNIQUE 21.2   COMPRESSION GARMENT

Compression garments should be applied by gathering them up, placing them on the distal area first, and then gradually unfolding them proximally. Because higher-compression garments have greater pretensioning, some patients have difficulty putting them on. Specific devices have been developed to assist with this, or the patient may wear two sets of lower-compression garments to provide a total compression equal to the sum of the two. For example, the patient could wear two pairs of 20 mm Hg compression stockings instead of one pair of 40 mm Hg stockings to achieve the same effect.

When used to control edema, compression garments are usually used to maintain edema control after bandaging has successfully achieved edema reduction. When used for this purpose, the garment is usually only worn during the day, donning it in the morning and doffing it before sleep. When compression garments are used for scar control, they need to be worn every day for at least 23 h/day and removed only while bathing. In general, with proper care, these garments last about 6 months, after which time they lose their elasticity and no longer exert the appropriate amount of pressure.

Advantages

- Compression quantifiable (unlike bandaging)
- Extremity can be used during treatment (unlike IPC)

- Less expensive than intermittent compression devices for short-term use
- Thin and attractive, available in various colors
- Safe for acute condition
- Can be used 24 h/day
- Preferred over compression bandages by patients

Disadvantages

- When used alone, may not reverse edema that is already present
- More expensive than most bandages
- Need to be fitted appropriately
- Require strength, flexibility, and dexterity to put on
- Hot, particularly in warm weather
- Expensive for long-term use because they need to be replaced at least every 6 months, and patient requires at least two identical garments so that one is available when the other is being laundered

Garments need to be replaced if there is a significant change in limb size, which may occur with changes in edema or in body weight. For the compression device to be effective and to avoid the expense of purchasing many sets of garments, it is recommended that compression garments be ordered only once compression bandaging has achieved a stable limb size.

Successful treatment in the long-term management of lymphedema requires successful fitting of a compression garment and the individual's ability to safely don and doff the garment. Goals to address donning and doffing the garment should include the following:

1. Patient will independently don and doff compression garment with (or without) use of assistive device as needed.
2. Caregiver will independently don and doff compression garment with (or without) use of assistive device as needed.

A sample SOAP note for a therapy session in donning and doffing a compression garment follows:

S: Pt reports difficulty with donning and doffing compression garment.

O: Focus of treatment on donning and doffing compression garment for long-term management of lymphedema in R UE. Pt instructed in proper method for donning and doffing compression garment. Pt performed three trials of donning and doffing compression garment. She initially required minimal assistance; however, with repeated trials, she was able to don and doff the compression garment independently. Education was provided on the wear and care schedule of stocking.

A: Pt demonstrates ability to independently don and doff compression garment for R UE. She verbalizes understanding of wear and care schedule.

P: Follow up next treatment session to ensure adherence to recommended wearing schedule and continued independence with donning and doffing of compression garment for R UE.

Velcro Closure Garments

Readily removable and adjustable compression garments that fasten with Velcro straps are also available (Fig. 21.17). Although these can improve patient acceptance, ease of removal can also decrease adherence. These garments provide inelastic compression similar to an Unna boot, but the patient can adjust the amount of compression during daily activities. With optimal use, companies claim that these devices provide 30 to 40 mm Hg gradient compression.[73] Because the Velcro bands are nonstretch, the amount of compression does not decrease with the age of the device.

INTERMITTENT PNEUMATIC COMPRESSION PUMP

IPC pumps are used to provide the force for intermittent compression. The pump is attached via a hose to a chambered sleeve placed around the involved limb (Fig. 21.18). Methods of application differ slightly among pumps, and specific instructions for the application of intermittent compression are provided with all pumps. General instructions for applying most pumps are given in Application Technique 21.4. Although intermittent compression is suitable for home use, the patient should always begin the course of therapy under clinician supervision.

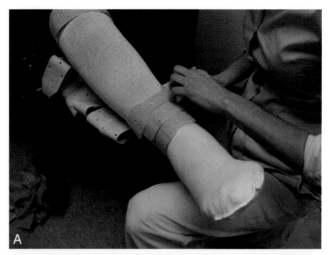
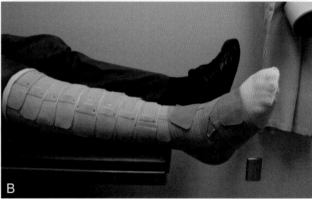

FIGURE 21.17 Velcro closure compression device. (From Cameron MH, Monroe LG: *Physical rehabilitation: evidence-based examination, evaluation, and intervention,* St Louis, 2007, Saunders.)

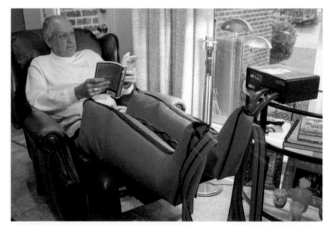

FIGURE 21.18 Intermittent pneumatic compression being applied for treatment of lymphedema. (Courtesy Vasocare, Baton Rouge, LA.)

Once edema has been satisfactorily reduced with the pump, the clinician should determine whether control will be maintained with continued use of the pump or if better results would be obtained with a compression garment or bandage. In general, because a compression pump is used for only a number of hours each day, the patient should use a static compression device between treatments with the pump to

APPLICATION TECHNIQUE 21.3

VELCRO CLOSURE COMPRESSION GARMENTS

Equipment Required

- Stockinette
- Velcro closure device

Procedure

1. Remove clothing and jewelry from the area to be treated.
2. Inspect skin for infection and wounds.
3. Dress and cover any wound according to the treatment regimen being used for that wound.
4. Apply stockinette.
5. Apply Velcro closure garment and close it, starting at the foot and working upward toward the knee.

Advantages

- Easier for patient to apply than other compression garments providing comparable compression
- Does not lose effectiveness with use or washing
- More adjustable to limb shape or volume changes than standard garments
- Can adjust the tightness of the garment depending on activity

Disadvantages

- Easy to remove, with decreased effectiveness if patient removes garment
- Loosening Velcro straps reduces compression to levels that may be insufficient for controlling edema

---

maintain the reversal of edema produced by the pump. In patients with chronic venous insufficiency and resulting edema and leg ulcers, adding intermittent compression to the use of compression stockings or bandages may accelerate wound healing, but it is unclear if intermittent compression can be used instead of compression bandages or stockings.[5,76] Similarly, IPC can help control lymphedema but is likely not a substitute for bandages or garments. Intermittent compression generally is not used to decrease the formation of scar tissue because compression is required at all times for this effect.

Parameters for Intermittent Pneumatic Compression Pumping

Inflation and Deflation Times. Inflation time is the period during which the compression sleeve is being inflated or is at the maximal inflation pressure; deflation time is the period during which the compression sleeve is being deflated or is fully deflated. For the treatment of edema or venous stasis ulcers or for DVT prevention, the inflation time is generally between 80 and 100 seconds, and the deflation time is generally between 25 and 50 seconds to allow for venous refilling after compression. No difference in volume reduction was found in patients with upper extremity lymphedema between 90-second inflation/90-second deflation compared with 45-second inflation/15-second deflation.[77] For residual limb volume reduction, these periods are generally shorter, with inflation time between 40 and 60 seconds and deflation time between 10 and 15 seconds. Usually, pressure is applied in approximately a 3:1 ratio of inflation to deflation time; it is then adjusted if necessary according to the patient's tolerance and response.

Inflation Pressure. Inflation pressure, which is the maximum pressure during inflation time, is measured in millimeters of mercury (mm Hg). Most units can deliver between 30 and 120 mm Hg of inflation pressure. When a single-chamber sleeve is used to provide intermittent compression, the chamber inflates to the maximum pressure and then deflates. When a multichamber sleeve is used to provide sequential compression, the distal segment inflates first to the maximum pressure, and then, as it deflates, the more proximal

segments inflate sequentially, generally to a slightly lower pressure. Some recommend that inflation pressure should not exceed diastolic blood pressure in the belief that higher pressures may impair arterial circulation; however, because the tissues of the body protect arterial vessels from collapse, higher pressures may be used if this is necessary to achieve the desired clinical outcome and does not cause pain, although close patient supervision is recommended when higher pressures are used. For all indications, inflation pressure is generally between 30 and 80 mm Hg and frequently is just below the patient's diastolic blood pressure. Because venous pressure is usually lower in the upper extremities than in the lower extremities, the lower end of the pressure range, 30 to 60 mm Hg, is generally used for the upper extremities, and the higher end of the range, 40 to 80 mm Hg, is generally used for the lower extremities. Lower pressures are generally recommended for residual limb reduction and shaping and to treat posttraumatic edema rather than the problems caused by venous insufficiency.

The ideal amount of pressure for the treatment of edema resulting from venous or lymphatic insufficiency is controversial. Clinical practice guidelines and systematic reviews on treatment of lymphedema indicate that lower pressures, 30 to 60 mm Hg, are safer and may still be effective for this condition,[78–80] but one study found that adding IPC at 120 mm Hg to manual lymphatic drainage and multilayer bandaging was significantly more effective for controlling lower extremity edema than adding IPC at 60 mm Hg or not adding IPC at all.[24] This may be in part because the pressure achieved in the tissue fluid is lower than in the compression chambers of an IPC device.[81] Treatment with inflation pressures below 30 mm Hg is not likely to affect circulation or tissue formation and therefore is not recommended for any condition.

Total Treatment Time. Total treatment time recommendations vary from 20 minutes to 4 hours per treatment, with treatment frequency ranging from three times per week to four times per day. For most applications, treatments of 2 to 3 hours once or twice a day are recommended. The frequency and duration of treatment should be the minimum necessary to maintain good edema control or satisfactory progress toward the goals of treatment (Table 21.1).

TABLE 21.1	Recommended Parameters for Application of Intermittent Compression		
Problem	Inflation/Deflation Time in Seconds (ratio)	Inflation Pressure (mm Hg)	Treatment Time
Edema due to venous insufficiency, DVT prevention, venous stasis ulcer	80–100/25–50 (3:1)	30–60 UE; 40–80 LE	2–3 hours
Lymphedema	80–100/25–50 (3:1)	30–60 UE; 40–80 LE	20–60 minutes, 1–2×/day
Residual limb reduction	40–60/10–15 (4:1)	30–60 UE; 40–80 LE	2–3 hours

DVT, Deep venous thrombosis; *LE,* lower extremity; *UE,* upper extremity.

APPLICATION TECHNIQUE 21.4

Equipment Required

- Intermittent pneumatic compression unit
- Inflatable sleeves for upper and lower extremities
- Stockinette
- Blood pressure cuff
- Stethoscope
- Tape measure

Procedure

1. Determine that compression is not contraindicated for the patient or the condition. Be certain to check for signs of DVT, including calf pain or tenderness associated with swelling and take the patient's history or check the chart for CHF, pulmonary edema, or other contraindications that may be the cause of the edema.
2. Remove jewelry and clothing from the treatment area, and inspect the skin. Cover any open areas with gauze or an appropriate dressing.
3. Place the patient in a comfortable position, with the affected limb elevated. Limb elevation reduces the pain and edema caused by venous insufficiency if applied soon after these symptoms develop, as elevation allows gravity to accelerate the flow of blood in the veins toward the heart. With chronic venous insufficiency or lymphatic dysfunction, elevating the limbs is generally less effective in reducing edema because the fluid is trapped within fibrotic tissue and cannot return as readily to the venous or lymphatic capillaries, from where it can flow back to the central circulation.

INTERMITTENT PNEUMATIC COMPRESSION PUMP

4. Measure and record the patient's blood pressure.
5. Measure and record the limb circumference at a number of places with reference to bony landmarks, or take volumetric measurements by displacement of water from a graduated cylinder.
6. Place a stocking or stockinette over the area to be treated and smooth out all the wrinkles (Fig. 21.19).
7. Apply the sleeve from the unit (Fig. 21.20). Reusable sleeves made of washable Neoprene and nylon are generally used, although single-use vinyl sleeves are also available when there is concern about cross-contamination. The Neoprene and nylon sleeves can be machine washed in warm water and air dried or dried at low heat in a dryer. The sleeves provide intermittent or sequential compression, depending on their design. Single-chamber sleeves provide intermittent compression only, and sleeves composed of a series of overlapping chambers can inflate sequentially, starting distally and progressing proximally, to produce a milking effect on the extremity. As noted, sequential compression has been shown to result in more complete emptying of the deep veins, better control of lymphedema, and greater increase in fibrinolytic activity than single-chamber, intermittent compression and is therefore

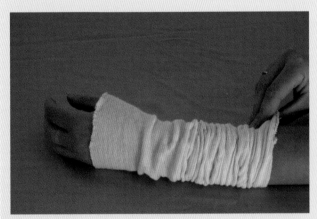

FIGURE 21.19 Application of stockinette before application of compression sleeve.

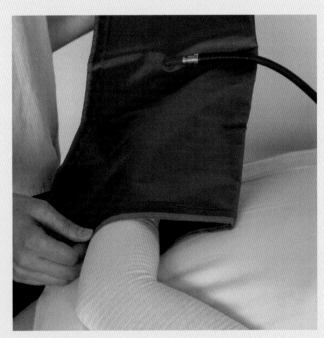

FIGURE 21.20 Application of compression sleeve.

APPLICATION TECHNIQUE 21.4—*cont'd*

preferred for most applications.[82–84]Single-chamber and multichamber sleeves are available in a variety of lengths and widths for treatment of upper or lower extremities of various sizes. When a compression pump is used for the treatment of edema, it is recommended that the sleeve be long enough to cover the entire involved limb so that fluid does not accumulate in areas of the limb proximal to the end of the sleeve. When a compression pump is used for the prevention of DVT formation, calf-high or thigh-high sleeves can be used because both have been found to be effective for this application.

8. Attach the hose(s) from the pneumatic compression pump to the sleeve. Pumps vary in size and complexity from small home units intended for the treatment of one extremity to larger clinical units that can be used to treat multiple extremities at different settings all at one time (Fig. 21.21).

9. Set the appropriate compression parameters, including inflation and deflation times, inflation pressure, and total treatment time. Because few research data are presently available to guide the precise selection of any of these parameters, the parameters used clinically are based on an understanding of the pathology being treated and measures of the patient's blood pressure and comfort, as well as the observed efficacy of treatment in the individual patient. Most protocols use an inflation pressure slightly below the patient's diastolic blood pressure, although higher pressures can be used, and all units come with treatment guidelines based on their design and manufacture. A 2019 systematic review provides guidance for parameter selection for IPC use in patients with lymphedema.[80] The parameters listed in Table 21.1 cover the ranges from this review for lymphedema and the ranges suggested by most pump manufacturers for other indications.

10. Provide the patient with a means to call you during the treatment. Measure and record the patient's blood pressure during treatment, and discontinue treatment if the systolic or diastolic pressure exceeds the limits set for the patient by the physician.

11. When the treatment is complete, turn off the unit, disconnect the tubing, and remove the sleeve and the stockinette.

12. Remeasure and record limb volume in the same manner as in step 5.

13. Reinspect the patient's skin.

14. Remeasure and document the patient's blood pressure.

15. Apply a compression garment or bandage to maintain the reduction in edema between treatments and after discontinuing the use of a compression pump. Maximum reduction of edema is usually achieved by using the pump for 3 to 4 weeks.

Advantages

- Actively moves fluids and therefore may be more effective than static devices, particularly for a flaccid limb
- Compression quantifiable
- Can provide sequential compression
- Requires less finger and hand dexterity to apply than compression bandages or garments
- Can be used to reverse and control edema
- Use can be supervised in a patient who is noncompliant with static compression

Disadvantages

- Used only for limited times during the day and therefore not appropriate for modification of scar formation
- Generally requires a static compression device to be used between treatments
- Expensive to purchase unit or to pay for regular treatments in a clinic
- Requires moderate comfort using machinery to apply
- Requires electricity
- The extremity cannot be used during treatment.
- The patient cannot move about during treatment.
- The pumping motion of the device may aggravate an acute condition.

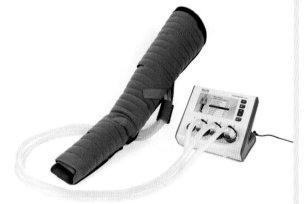
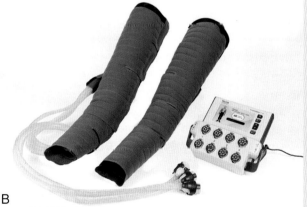

A   B

FIGURE 21.21 Intermittent compression units. (Courtesy Tactile Medical, Minneapolis, MN.)

Documentation

When applying external compression, document the following:
- Type of compression device
- Area of the body being treated
- Inflation and deflation times
- Compression or inflation pressure
- Total treatment time
- Patient's response to the treatment

Documentation is typically written in the SOAP format. The following examples summarize only the modality component of treatment and are not intended to represent a comprehensive plan of care.

EXAMPLES

When applying a compression bandage to the left ankle after an acute sprain, document the following:

S: Pt reports L ankle swelling that increases in the PM.
O: Ankle girth R 9 inches, L 10½ inches, 3 days ago, before placement of elastic bandage.
Today, L ankle girth 10 inches.
Treatment: Replaced elastic bandage to L ankle and leg, figure-eight, and instructed Pt in bandage application.
A: Pt responding to treatment, with reduced edema 3 days after injury.
P: Continue high-stretch elastic bandage to L ankle and leg. Pt to keep LE elevated.

When applying IPC to the right arm to treat lymphedema, document the following:

S: Pt reports decreasing R UE edema in the past 2 weeks and is now able to use a key with her R hand.
O: Pretreatment arm volume to elbow: R 530 cc, L 410 cc.
BP pretreatment: 135/80 mm Hg; during and immediately after treatment: 140/85 mm Hg. No overall change in pretreatment blood pressure during 2-week course of treatment.
Treatment: IPC R UE, 80 s/30 s, 50 mm Hg, 2 h twice daily. After 1 treatment: R 500 cc; after 2 weeks of treatment: R 450 cc.
A: Pt tolerating treatment well, with decreased edema, increased R hand function, and no change in BP over 2 weeks.
P: Continue IPC R UE, 80 s/30 s, 50 mm Hg, 2 h twice daily. When R UE volume stabilizes, consider fitting for compression garment.

When applying compression hose to prevent DVT formation, document the following:

S: Pt not oriented; bedridden.
O: Negative Homans sign. No other signs of DVT formation.
Treatment: Compression hose both LEs, approximately 20 mm Hg compression.
A: Bedridden Pt at risk for DVT.
P: Pt to wear compression hose 23 h/day while in bed. Instruct other caregivers in compression hose program.

CLINICAL CASE STUDIES

The following case studies summarize the concepts of compression discussed in this chapter. Based on the scenarios presented, an evaluation of the clinical findings and goals of treatment are proposed. These are followed by a discussion of the factors to be considered in selecting compression as the indicated intervention and in selection of the ideal compression device and treatment parameters to promote progress toward the goals of treatment.

CASE STUDY 21.1

Chronic Lymphedema
Examination
History

FR is a 40-year-old right-handed female carpenter. FR reports that 8 years ago, she had a right mastectomy with 16 lymph nodes removed as part of her treatment for breast cancer. She was treated with chemotherapy and radiation therapy at that time and has had no recurrence of the malignancy. FR has been advised by her physician to reduce the use of her right arm and to elevate it when possible to control the swelling. At her request, she has been referred to therapy for further management of her lymphedema.

FR has chronic lymphedema of her right upper extremity and complains of pain and swelling in this extremity that worsens with use but is moderately alleviated by elevation and avoiding use of the extremity. She rates her pain severity as 4 to 8/10. She first noticed the swelling 2 or 3 years ago, but at that time it occurred only after extensive use of her upper extremity at work; the swelling was mild and resolved with a night's rest. Over the last year, the swelling has worsened. Now, it never resolves fully and is easily aggravated by even light activity at work or by yard work, and she has reduced her work hours by 50%.

Systems Review

FR appears well overall. She is alert and cooperative with testing. She reports that her pain severity today is 5/10 after doing light chores around the house this morning. She reports "minimal" weakness and ROM restrictions in right upper extremity. She does not report swelling.

Tests and Measures

The objective examination reveals moderate pitting edema of the right arm and forearm, with circumferential measurements of 7 inches at the right wrist compared with 6 inches at the left wrist, 11 inches at the right elbow compared with 9½ inches at the left elbow, and 14 inches at the right midbiceps compared with 11 inches at the same level on the left. The swelling also causes moderate restriction of elbow, wrist, hand, and finger ROM. Passive elbow ROM was measured as 130 degrees flexion and –10 degrees extension on the right compared with 145 degrees flexion and full extension on the left. The skin of the patient's right upper extremity appears thin, flaky, and red, and her blood pressure is 120/80 mm Hg. All other tests, including shoulder ROM and upper extremity sensation, are within normal limits.

CLINICAL CASE STUDIES—cont'd

Based on the patient's history, is the lymphatic system in her right upper extremity blocked? What parts of the history lead you to this conclusion? Is malignancy a concern when compression is considered as an intervention for this patient?

Evaluation and Goals

ICF Level	Current Status	Goals
Body structure and function	Increased girth and loss of motion of right UE	Control and reduce edema until measurement of right arm girth equals left arm girth Restore ROM so that right UE ROM becomes equal to left UE ROM within 3 months
Activity	Reduced tolerance for using and lifting with right arm	Able to use right UE for all daily activities and to lift 40 lb
Participation	Reduced work hours by 50%	Improve work hours to 100% of normal over next 3 months

ICF, International Classification for Functioning, Disability and Health; *ROM,* range of motion; *UE,* upper extremity.

◆ FIND THE EVIDENCE

PICO Terms	Natural Language Example	Sample PubMed Search
P (Population)	Patients with symptoms due to chronic lymphedema	("Lymphedema" [MeSH] OR "Lymphedema" [text word])
I (Intervention)	Compression therapy	AND ("Compression Bandages" [MeSH] OR "compression therapy" [text word]
C (Comparison)	No compression therapy	
O (Outcome)	Reduction of pain and swelling; increased ROM	AND ("pain reduction" [text word] OR "Range of Motion, Articular" [MeSH] OR "ROM" [text word])
		AND ("Humans" [MeSH] AND English [lang])

Key Studies or Reviews

1. Fu MR, Deng J, Armer JM: Putting evidence into practice: cancer-related lymphedema. *Clin J Oncol Nurs* 18(Suppl):68–79, 2014.

   This systematic review evaluated 75 selected articles from 2009 to 2014 and supported compression bandages

and compression garments, as well as complete decongestive therapy, with the highest level of evidence for best clinical practice.

2. Tan K, Argáez C: *Intermittent pneumatic compression devices for the management of lymphedema: a review of clinical effectiveness and guidelines* [Internet], Ottawa (ON), 2017, Canadian Agency for Drugs and Technologies in Health, CADTH Rapid Response Reports.

   This extensive and thorough research report concludes that although IPC may not provide any additional benefits when used in combination with routine management of lymphedema, current guidelines recommend short-term use of IPC in combination with other approaches to lymphedema management.

Prognosis

Although the recommendations of experts in the field vary for the treatment of lymphedema, most agree that some form of compression is indicated. Compression can provide working or resting pressure to control fluid flow out of the venous circulation and into the lymphatic circulation and can promote the movement of fluid through the lymphatic vessels. Some experts recommend the use of special massage techniques in conjunction with compression to promote lymphatic flow, particularly in proximal areas such as the axilla and the trunk, to aid or divert flow in areas where lymphatic function is compromised and where most compression devices are not effective. Without such additional treatment, compression alone may allow fluid proximal to the compression device to accumulate, particularly if proximal lymphatic function is impaired.

Although the use of compression generally is not recommended in the presence of active malignancy, because this patient has had no recurrence of her disease after more than 5 years, most experts agree that compression may be used. Although the lymphatic circulation in this patient is clearly impaired, the fact that the severity of her edema varies, resolving to some extent with rest and elevation, indicates that the lymphatic circulation in the right upper extremity is not completely blocked, and therefore compression is not contraindicated.

Intervention

Initially, an IPC can be used to apply compression. This form of compression is likely to produce the quickest and most effective reversal of edema because it provides both compression and the milking action of sequential distal-to-proximal compression. To control the formation of edema between treatments with the pneumatic device, an inelastic bandage was applied during the day to provide a high working pressure. When the reduction of edema plateaus, which usually takes 2 to 3 weeks, pumping can be gradually discontinued. The patient should continue to use the bandages when working or exercising her upper extremity. If the patient is not adherent to long-term use of bandages or cannot perform her job duties while bandaged, a compression garment may be

Continued

used. However, because this type of garment is made of a moderately elastic material that develops limited working pressure, it may not be as effective as an inelastic bandage in maintaining edema control during exercise or other heavy upper extremity activity. The patient should not be measured for fitting of a compression garment at the initiation of treatment because a garment fitted at that time will soon be too big if pumping or bandaging reverses any edema. Measurement for fitting of the garment should be performed when limb volume stabilizes.

Optimal treatment parameters at the initiation of treatment, when the sequential IPC pump is being used, are 80 to 100 seconds of inflation and 25 to 35 seconds of deflation, with a maximum inflation pressure of 30 to 60 mm Hg, potentially increasing up to 120 mm Hg if needed. The lowest inflation pressure that achieves reduction of edema should be used to minimize the risk of collapsing the superficial lymphatic or venous vessels. For most patients, treatment with the pump for 45 to 60 minutes once or twice per day is sufficient. All parameters may be adjusted within these ranges to achieve optimal edema control without pain and with the least disruption of the patient's regular activities. Compression bandages or garments should be worn at all times, except for bathing, when the pump is not being used.

Appropriate use of massage, exercise, and activity modification should be considered, in addition to treatment with compression, to achieve the optimal outcome for this patient. The patient's blood pressure should be monitored before, during, and after use of the compression pump. If her blood pressure gets too high, the pressure and, if necessary, the duration, of pumping should be reduced. During pumping, the patient's upper extremity should be elevated above the level of her heart. This is most readily achieved if she lies supine and places her arm on a pillow.

Documentation

S: Pt reports swelling and pain, severity 4 to 8/10, in R UE that worsens with use and at the end of the day.

O: Pretreatment: Moderate pitting edema R arm and forearm. R wrist circumference 7 inches, R midbiceps 14 inches, L wrist circumference 6 inches, L midbiceps 11 inches. Passive ROM R elbow 130 degrees flexion, –10 degrees extension.

Treatment: IPC to R UE 80 s inflation, 25 s deflation for total treatment time 60 minutes.

Posttreatment: Minimal edema R arm and forearm. R wrist circumference 6½ inches, R midbiceps 12 inches. Passive ROM R elbow 140 degrees flexion, –5 degrees extension.

A: Good response to compression with IPC, with reduced edema, increased functional ROM, decreased pain.

P: Instruct Pt on home use of IPC device 1 h once daily. Instruct Pt on application of bandages or compression garment to R UE after IPC. Follow-up 1 week for reassessment.

CASE STUDY 21.2

Venous Stasis Ulcer
Examination
History

JU is a 65-year-old man with a full-thickness venous stasis ulcer on his distal medial left leg. He reports that the ulcer is minimally painful at 1/10 on the pain scale but requires frequent dressing changes because a large amount of fluid leaks from it. The ulcer has been present for 4 to 6 months and is gradually getting larger. The only treatment being provided for the ulcer is gauze dressing application, which the patient changes two or three times a day when he notices seepage.

This wound has significantly affected JU's activities. He stopped attending biweekly bingo games and weekly church services 4 months ago because he found that prolonged sitting made his left leg swell and hurt and because he was embarrassed by his weeping ulcer. He has decreased his physical activity at home, spending most of the day sitting indoors in his recliner with his legs up, rather than gardening for 2 hours when the weather permitted. He reports that his ankle is often uncomfortable to move and that swelling worsens when he is upright for longer than an hour.

JU had coronary artery bypass surgery 2 years ago, at which time the left saphenous vein was removed to be used for the graft. He is currently taking medication to control hypertension.

Systems Review

JU is a well-appearing man. He is alert, cooperative, and eager to return to the activities that contributed to his quality of life. He has no atrophy or self-reported weakness, ROM restrictions, or sensory changes in either upper or lower extremities.

Tests and Measures

JU has a shallow, flat ulcer with a red base fully covered with granulation tissue, approximately 5 cm × 10 cm in area on the distal medial left leg, with darkening of intact skin around the ulcer. Edema of the left foot, ankle, and leg is noted. Ankle girth, measured at the medial malleolus, is 9 inches on the right and 10½ inches on the left. No signs of edema are noted in the right lower extremity. Ankle ROM is +10 degrees of dorsiflexion to 60 degrees plantar flexion on the right and 0 degrees of dorsiflexion to 50 degrees of plantar flexion on the left. The patient's blood pressure is 140/100 mm Hg.

Why does this patient have a venous stasis ulcer? What other aspect of the patient's examination is a matter of concern? What would you tell this patient about the lifetime use of compression? What measurement needs to be taken before compression is applied to this patient?

Evaluation and Goals

ICF Level	Current Status	Goals
Body function and structure	Enlarging left LE venous stasis ulcer	Heal the ulcer
	Increased girth left lower distal extremity	Reduce edema so that left ankle girth matches right ankle girth and prevent ulcer recurrence
	Restricted left ankle ROM	Increase left ankle ROM to match right ankle ROM
Activity	Sitting with LE dependent and walking limited to 60 min	Sitting with LE dependent and walking tolerated for up to 2 h
Participation	Decreased gardening, bingo, and church attendance	Return to prior level of gardening, bingo, and church attendance within 2 months

ICF, International Classification for Functioning, Disability and Health; *LE,* lower extremity; *ROM,* range of motion.

◆ FIND THE EVIDENCE

PICO Terms	Natural Language Example	Sample PubMed Search
P (Population)	Patients with symptoms due to venous stasis ulcer	("Varicose Ulcer/Therapy" [MeSH] OR "venous stasis ulcer" [text word])
I (Intervention)	Compression therapy	AND ("Compression Bandages" [MeSH] OR "compression therapy" [text word])
C (Comparison)	No compression therapy	
O (Outcome)	Reduction of pain and swelling; increased quality of life	AND "Wound Healing/ Physiology" [MeSH] AND ("humans" [MeSH] AND English [lang])

Key Studies or Reviews

1. Chapman S: Venous leg ulcers: an evidence review. *Br J Community Nurs* 22(Suppl 9):S6–S9, 2017.
   This evidence-based review concludes that compression therapy with bandages or stockings promotes healing of venous leg ulcers by aiding venous return and is the first-line treatment for venous leg ulcers.
2. Jull A, Slark J, Parsons J: Prescribed exercise with compression vs compression alone in treating patients with venous leg ulcers: a systematic review and meta-analysis. *JAMA Dermatol* 154(11):1304–1311, 2018.

This systematic review with meta-analysis, which included five trials with a total of 190 participants, found that adding exercises to compression therapy was associated with increased venous leg ulcer healing, with the combination of progressive resistance exercise with prescribed physical activity being most effective.

Prognosis

JU presents with loss of skin and subcutaneous tissue integrity, requiring him to change wound dressings frequently and placing him at risk for local infection and possible sepsis. His ulcer and edema of the distal lower extremity are probably a result of poor venous circulation. Compression is an indicated intervention because it can improve venous circulation to facilitate wound healing and edema control. Specialized dressings that are more absorbent and less adherent than gauze should be used to reduce the frequency of dressing changes and thus reduce the potential for wound trauma and inconvenience to the patient. Contraindications for the use of compression, including arterial insufficiency, heart failure, and DVT, should be ruled out before initiating treatment with compression. The patient's history of cardiac bypass surgery suggests the possibility of arterial insufficiency in the lower extremities, although the presence of edema and the conformation of the leg ulcer indicate that it is probably a result of venous, rather than arterial, insufficiency. To rule out arterial insufficiency, an ABI should be obtained, and compression should be applied only if this is above 0.8. The presence of unilateral rather than bilateral edema indicates that this patient's edema is probably not a result of cardiac failure. Assessment for Homans sign should be performed to rule out a DVT before treatment with compression is initiated.

Intervention

Initially, JU was treated with intermittent compression applied with a sequential pneumatic pump twice a week, with static compression with a two-layer bandage system between pumping sessions. The pump was used to reduce the edema through the milking action associated with sequential distal-to-proximal intermittent compression, and edema control was maintained by the continuous compression of the compression bandage system boot. Recommended treatment parameters for the sequential IPC pump to promote circulation and control edema are 80 to 100 seconds of inflation and 25 to 35 seconds of deflation, with a maximum inflation pressure of 30 to 60 mm Hg and treatment duration of 2 to 3 hours. Adjustments should be made within these ranges to achieve optimal edema control without pain and with the least disruption of the patient's regular activities. The Unna boot should be worn at all times between intermittent compression treatments. If the compression bandage is not tolerated, compression stockings providing 30 to 40 mm Hg of pressure or a Velcro closure device may be worn between pumping treatments. Although stockings are easier to remove and reapply than the compression bandage system, a Velcro closure

Continued

CLINICAL CASE STUDIES—*cont'd*

device is likely to be a better choice for this patient because of the risk of damaging the skin when donning and doffing stockings. The patient's blood pressure should be monitored before, during, and after using the compression pump. If his blood pressure increases, the force and, if necessary, the duration of pumping should be reduced. An appropriate dressing should be placed on the ulcer site before the compression sleeve, bandage, or stocking is applied. A single-use sleeve should be used for pumping, or an occlusive barrier should be placed over the ulcer during pumping, to avoid cross-contamination.

It is essential that the patient continue to wear a compression stocking after the ulcer has healed because his circulatory compromise puts him at high risk for recurrence of edema and tissue breakdown in this extremity. In addition, JU should perform progressive resistive exercises of his lower extremities, engage in aerobic physical activity, and have gait training to ensure a functional gait pattern with active use of his plantar flexors to optimize his wound healing.

Documentation

S: Pt reports a nonhealing ulcer present for 4 to 6 months on his L medial lower extremity and increased edema of his L LE.

O: Pretreatment: 5 cm × 10 cm shallow ulcer on the distal medial L leg, with darkening of intact skin around the ulcer. L ankle girth measured at the medial malleolus is 10½" and R ankle girth is 9". L ankle ROM 0 to 50 degrees, R ankle ROM +10 to 60 degrees.

Treatment: IPC to L leg at 80 s inflation and 35 s deflation, and maximum inflation pressure of 50 mm Hg × 2 h. Leg presses, 2 × 10, 30 lb, and stationary cycling × 5 minutes. Pt instructed to perform these daily at home.

Posttreatment: Ulcer unchanged in size after one treatment. L ankle girth 10 inches.

A: Good response to treatment. No adverse effects.

P: Continue twice-weekly treatments with intermittent sequential pneumatic compression at 80 s inflation and 35 s deflation, and maximum inflation pressure of 50 mm Hg for 2 h. Pt should perform exercises and wear two-layer compression bandage between intermittent compression treatments and may switch to compression hose when ulcer begins to heal. Reassess each time patient comes for intermittent compression treatment and Unna boot application.

Chapter Review

1. Compression applies an inwardly directed force to the tissues, increasing extravascular pressure and venous and lymphatic circulation.
2. External compression can be used to control edema, prevent the formation of DVT, facilitate venous stasis ulcer healing, and shape residual limbs after amputation.
3. Compression devices include compression bandages, compression garments, Velcro closure devices, and pneumatic pumps. Bandages and garments provide static compression and can be worn throughout the day, whereas pneumatic pumps provide intermittent compression for limited periods of time.
4. The choice of compression device depends on the problem being treated and the ability of the patient to comply with the treatment.
5. The use of compression is contraindicated in patients with heart failure, pulmonary edema, DVT, thrombophlebitis, pulmonary embolism, obstructed lymphatic or venous return, peripheral artery disease, skin infection, hypoproteinemia, and trauma. Caution should be used in patients with impaired sensation or mentation, uncontrolled hypertension, or cancer and in the application of compression over superficial peripheral nerves.

Glossary

Ankle-brachial index (ABI): Ratio of systolic blood pressure at the ankle to systolic blood pressure in the upper arm (brachium). An ABI lower than 1, indicating lower blood pressure at the ankle than in the arm, suggests reduced distal lower extremity blood flow as a result of peripheral artery disease.

Antiembolism stockings: Knee-high or thigh-high stockings that provide low compression force to prevent DVT formation.

Compression: The application of a mechanical force that increases external pressure on a body part to reduce swelling, improve circulation, or modify scar tissue formation.

Deep venous thrombosis (DVT): Blood clot in a deep vein.

Edema: Swelling caused by increased fluid in the interstitial spaces of the body.

Hydrostatic pressure: Pressure exerted by a fluid, for example, in the blood vessels. It is determined by the force of the heart and gravity and contributes to movement of fluid into or out of blood vessels and lymphatics.

Hypertrophic scarring: Excessive scarring with a raised and ridged appearance that does not extend beyond the boundaries of the original site of skin injury. This type of scar has poor flexibility and can result in contractures and poor cosmesis.

Intermittent pneumatic compression (IPC): Pressure that is alternately applied and released by a pneumatic compression pump.

Keloid: Excessive scarring that extends beyond the boundaries of the original site of skin injury.

Long-stretch bandage: An elastic bandage that can extend by 100% to 200% and provides high resting pressure; also called a *high-stretch bandage*.

Lymphatic fluid (lymph): Fluid rich in protein, water, and macrophages that is removed from the interstitial space by the lymphatic system and is returned to the venous system.

Lymphatic system: A system of vessels and nodes designed to carry excess fluid from the interstitial space to the venous system and to filter the fluid, removing bacteria and other foreign particles.

Lymphedema: Swelling caused by excess lymphatic fluid in the interstitial space.

Oncotic pressure: Pressure determined by the concentration of proteins inside and outside blood vessels that contributes to movement of fluid into or out of blood vessels and lymphatics.

Phlebitis: Inflammation of the veins; the most common cause of venous insufficiency.

Resting pressure: Pressure exerted by elastic when put on stretch.

Short-stretch bandage: A bandage with low elasticity and 30% to 90% extension that provides a low resting pressure but a high working pressure during muscle activity; also called a *low-stretch bandage*.

Static compression: Steady application of pressure.

Unna boot: A semi-rigid bandage made of zinc oxide–impregnated gauze that is applied to the lower extremity to exert pressure.

Venous insufficiency: Decreased ability of the veins to return blood to the heart.

Venous stasis ulcer: An area of tissue breakdown and necrosis that occurs as a result of impaired venous return.

Working pressure: Pressure produced by active muscles pushing against an inelastic bandage.

References

1. Clarke MJ, Broderick C, Hopewell S, et al. Compression stockings for preventing deep vein thrombosis in airline passengers. *Cochrane Database Syst Rev* 2016(9):CD004002, 2016. doi:10.1002/14651858. CD004002.pub3.
2. Rohner-Spengler M, Frotzler A, Honigmann P, et al. Effective treatment of posttraumatic and postoperative edema in patients with ankle and hindfoot fractures: a randomized controlled trial comparing multilayer compression therapy and intermittent impulse compression with the standard treatment with ice. *J Bone Joint Surg Am* 96(15):1263–1271, 2014.
3. Heiss R, Hotfiel T, Kellermann M, et al. Effect of compression garments on the development of edema and soreness in delayed-onset muscle soreness (DOMS). *J Sports Sci Med* 17(3):392–401, 2018.
4. Sachdeva A, Dalton M, Lees T: Graduated compression stockings for prevention of deep vein thrombosis. *Cochrane Database Syst Rev* 2018(11):CD001484, 2018. doi:10.1002/14651858.CD001484. pub4.
5. Nelson EA, Hillman A, Thomas K: Intermittent pneumatic compression for treating venous leg ulcers. *Cochrane Database Syst Rev* 2014(5):CD001899, 2014. doi:10.1002/14651858.CD001899.pub4.
6. Clarke M, Hopewell S, Juszczak E, et al. Compression stockings for preventing deep vein thrombosis in airline passengers. *Cochrane Database Syst Rev* 2006(2):CD004002, 2006.
7. Olsen JHH, Öberg S, Rosenberg J: The effect of compression stocking on leg edema and discomfort during a 3-hour flight: a randomized controlled trial. *Eur J Intern Med* 62:54–57, 2019. doi:10.1016/j. ejim.2019.01.013.
8. Smyth RM, Aflaifel N, Bamigboye AA: Interventions for varicose veins and leg oedema in pregnancy. *Cochrane Database Syst Rev* 2015(10): CD001066, 2015.
9. Barrett KE, Barman SM, Brooks HL, et al. *Ganong's review of medical physiology*, ed 26, New York, NY, 2019, McGraw Hill Education.
10. Grada AA, Phillips TJ: Lymphedema: pathophysiology and clinical manifestations. *J Am Acad Dermatol* 77(6):1009–1020, 2017. doi:10.1016/j.jaad.2017.03.022.
11. Leung EY, Tirlapur SA, Meads C: The management of secondary lower limb lymphoedema in cancer patients: a systematic review. *Palliat Med* 29:112–119, 2015.
12. Biglia N, Zanfagnin V, Daniele A, et al. Lower body lymphedema in patients with gynecologic cancer. *Anticancer Res* 37(8):4005–4015, 2017.
13. Poage E, Singer M, Armer J, et al. Demystifying lymphedema: development of the lymphedema putting evidence into practice card. *Clin J Oncol Nurs* 12:951–964, 2008.
14. King M, Deveaux A, White H, et al. Compression garments versus compression bandaging in decongestive lymphatic therapy for breast cancer-related lymphedema: a randomized controlled trial. *Support Care Cancer* 20:1031–1036, 2012.
15. Ochalek K, Gradalski T, Partsch H: Preventing early postoperative arm swelling and lymphedema manifestation by compression sleeves after axillary lymph node interventions in breast cancer patients: a randomized controlled trial. *J Pain Symptom Manage* 54(3):346–354, 2017. doi:10.1016/j.jpainsymman.2017.04.014.
16. Ochalek K, Partsch H, Gradalski T, et al. Do compression sleeves reduce the incidence of arm lymphedema and improve quality of life? Two-year results from a prospective randomized trial in breast cancer survivors. *Lymphat Res Biol* 17(1):70–77, 2019. doi:10.1089/lrb.2018.0006.
17. Zasadzka E, Trzmiel T, Kleczewska M, et al. Comparison of the effectiveness of complex decongestive therapy and compression bandaging as a method of treatment of lymphedema in the elderly. *Clin Interv Aging* 13:929–934, 2018. doi:10.2147/CIA.S159380.
18. Thomaz JP, Dias TDSM, de Rezende LF: Effect of taping as treatment to reduce breast cancer lymphedema: literature review. *J Vasc Bras* 17(2):136–140, 2018. doi:10.1590/1677-5449.007217.
19. Pajero Otero V, García Delgado E, Martín Cortijo C, et al. Kinesio taping versus compression garments for treating breast cancer-related lymphedema: a randomized, cross-over, controlled trial. *Clin Rehabil* 33(12):1887–1897, 2019. doi:10.1177/0269215519874107.
20. Ergin G, Şahinoğlu E, Karadibak D, et al. Effectiveness of Kinesio taping on anastomotic regions in patients with breast cancer-related lymphedema: a randomized controlled pilot study. *Lymphat Res Biol*, 2019. doi:10.1089/lrb.2019.0003. Aug 1[Epub ahead of print].
21. Tran K, Argáez C: *Intermittent pneumatic compression devices for the management of lymphedema: a review of clinical effectiveness and guidelines [Internet]*, Ottawa (ON), 2017, Canadian Agency for Drugs and Technologies in Health, CADTH Rapid Response Reports.
22. Sanal-Toprak C, Ozsoy-Unubolo T, Bahar-Ozdemir Y, et al. The efficacy of intermittent pneumatic compression as a substitute for manual lymphatic drainage in complete decongestive therapy in the treatment of breast cancer related lymphedema. *Lymphology* 52(2):82–91, 2019.
23. Feldman JL, Stout NL, Wanchai A, et al. Intermittent pneumatic compression therapy: a systematic review. *Lymphology* 45:13–25, 2012.
24. Taradaj J, Rosińczuk J, Dymarek R, et al. Comparison of efficacy of the intermittent pneumatic compression with a high- and low-pressure application in reducing the lower limbs phlebolymphedema. *Ther Clin Risk Manag* 11:1545–1554, 2015.
25. Desai SS, Shao M, Vascular Outcomes Collaborative: Superior clinical, quality of life, functional, and health economic outcomes with pneumatic compression therapy for lymphedema. *Ann Vasc Surg* (19):30774–30779, 2019. doi:10.1016/j.avsg.2019.08.091. pii: S0890-5096.
26. Xiong Y, Tao X: Compression garments for medical therapy and sports. *Polymers (Basel)* 10(6), 2018. doi:10.3390/polym10060663. pii: E663.
27. Zaleska M, Olszewski WL, Cakala M, et al. Intermittent pneumatic compression enhances formation of edema tissue fluid channels in lymphedema of lower limbs. *Lymphat Res Biol* 13:146–153, 2015.
28. Heit JA: The epidemiology of venous thromboembolism in the community: implications for prevention and management. *J Thromb Thrombolysis* 21:23–29, 2006.
29. Heit JA, O'Fallon WM, Petterson TM, et al. Relative impact of risk factors for deep vein thrombosis and pulmonary embolism: a population-based study. *Arch Intern Med* 162:1245–1248, 2002.
30. Sajid MS, Desai M, Morris RW, et al. Knee length versus thigh length graduated compression stockings for prevention of deep vein thrombosis in postoperative surgical patients. *Cochrane Database Syst Rev* 2012(5):CD007162, 2012.
31. Urbankova J, Quiroz R, Kucher N, et al. Intermittent pneumatic compression and deep vein thrombosis prevention: a meta-analysis in postoperative patients. *Thromb Haemost* 94:1181–1185, 2005.
32. Zhang D, Li F, Li X, et al. Effect of intermittent pneumatic compression on preventing deep vein thrombosis among stroke patients: a systematic review and meta-analysis. *Worldviews Evid Based Nurs* 15(3):189–196, 2018. doi:10.1111/wvn.12288.

33. Kakkos SK, Caprini JA, Geroulakos G, et al. Combined intermittent pneumatic leg compression and pharmacological prophylaxis for prevention of venous thromboembolism. *Cochrane Database Syst Rev*, 2016(9):CD005258, 2016. doi:10.1002/14651858.CD005258.pub3.

34. CLOTS (Clots in Legs or sTockings after Stroke) Trials Collaboration, Dennis M, Sandercock P, et al: Effectiveness of intermittent pneumatic compression in reduction of risk of deep vein thrombosis in patients who have had a stroke (CLOTS 3): a multicentre randomised controlled trial. *Lancet* 382:516–524, 2013.

35. Malone MD, Cisek PL, Comerota Jr AJ, et al. High-pressure, rapid-inflation pneumatic compression improves venous hemodynamics in healthy volunteers and patients who are post-thrombotic. *J Vasc Surg* 29(4):593–599, 1999.

36. Comerota AJ, Chouhan V, Harada RN, et al. The fibrinolytic effects of intermittent pneumatic compression: mechanism of enhanced fibrinolysis. *Ann Surg* 226(3):306–313, 1997. discussion 313–314.

37. Kohro S, Yamakage M, Sato K, et al. Intermittent pneumatic foot compression can activate blood fibrinolysis without changes in blood coagulability and platelet activation. *Acta Anaesthesiol Scand* 49(5):660–664, 2005.

38. Chouhan VD, Comerota AJ, Sun L, et al. Inhibition of tissue factor pathway during intermittent pneumatic compression: a possible mechanism for antithrombotic effect. *Arterioscler Thromb Vasc Biol* 19:2812–2817, 1999.

39. Thomas PR, Nash GB, Dormandy JA: White cell accumulation in dependent legs of patients with venous hypertension (a possible mechanism for trophic changes in the skin). *Br Med J (Clin Res Ed)* 296:1693–1695, 1998.

40. Herouy Y, Trefzer D, Zimpfer U, et al. Matrix metalloproteinases and venous leg ulceration. *Eur J Dermatol* 10:173–180, 2000.

41. Corrow K, Callas PW, Zhar R, et al. Pressure elevation slows the fibroblast response to wound healing. *J Vasc Surg* 42(3):546–551, 2005.

42. Evidently Cochrane: Venous leg ulcers. https://www.evidentlycochrane.net/venous-leg-ulcers-evidence/. (Accessed October 27, 2019).

43. O'Meara S, Cullum N, Nelson EA, et al. Compression for venous leg ulcers. *Cochrane Database Syst Rev* 2012(11):CD000265, 2012.

44. Nelson EA, Bell-Syer SE: Compression for preventing recurrence of venous ulcers. *Cochrane Database Syst Rev* 2014(9):CD002303, 2014.

45. Felty CL, Rooke TW: Compression therapy for chronic venous insufficiency. *Semin Vasc Surg* 18:36–40, 2005.

46. Mayberry JC, Moneta GL, Taylor Jr LM, et al. Fifteen-year results of ambulatory compression therapy for chronic venous ulcers. *Surgery* 109:575–581, 1991.

47. White JV, Ryjewski C: Chronic venous insufficiency. *Perspect Vasc Surg Endovasc Ther* 17:319–327, 2005.

48. Jull A, Slark J, Parsons J: Prescribed exercise with compression vs compression alone in treating patients with venous leg ulcers. A systematic review and meta-analysis. *JAMA Dermatol* 154(11):1304–1311, 2018. doi:10.1001/jamadermatol.2018.3281. PMCID: PMC6248128. PMID: 30285080.

49. Labropoulos N, Wierks C, Suffoletto B: Intermittent pneumatic compression for the treatment of lower extremity arterial disease: a systematic review. *Vasc Med* 7:141–148, 2002.

50. Johannesson A, Larsson GU, Ramstrand N, et al. Outcomes of a standardized surgical and rehabilitation program in transtibial amputation for peripheral vascular disease: a prospective cohort study. *Am J Phys Med Rehabil* 89:293–303, 2010.

51. Ibegbuna V, Delis KT, Nicolaides AN, et al. Effect of elastic compression stockings on venous hemodynamics during walking. *J Vasc Surg* 37:420–425, 2003.

52. Alsancak S, Kose SK, Altinkaynak H: Effect of elastic bandaging and prosthesis on the decrease in stump volume. *Acta Orthop Traumatol Turc* 45:14–22, 2011.

53. Staley MJ, Richard RL: Use of pressure to treat hypertrophic burn scars. *Adv Wound Care* 10:44–46, 1997.

54. Kant SB, Ferdinandus PI, den Kerckhove EV, et al. A new treatment for reliable functional and esthetic outcome after local facial flap reconstruction: a transparent polycarbonate facial mask with silicone sheeting. *J Plast Surg* 40(5):407–416, 2017. doi:10.1007/s00238-017-1306-y.

55. Sharp PA, Pan B, Yakuboff KP, et al. Development of a best evidence statement for the use of pressure therapy for management of hypertrophic scarring. *J Burn Care Res* 37:255–264, 2016.

56. Lee RC, Capelli-Schellpfeffer M, Astumian RD: A review of thermoregulation of tissue repair and remodeling, Abstract, Society for Physical Regulation in Biology and Medicine, 15th annual meeting, 1995, Washington, DC.

57. Larson DL, Abston S, Evans EB, et al. Techniques for decreasing scar formation and contractures in the burned patient. *J Trauma* 11:807–823, 1971.

58. Ward RS: Pressure therapy for the control of hypertrophic scar formation after burn injury: a history and review. *J Burn Care Rehabil* 12:257–262, 1991.

59. Reno F, Sabbatini M, Stella M, et al. Effect of in vitro mechanical compression on Epilysin (matrix metalloproteinase-28) expression in hypertrophic scars. *Wound Repair Regen* 13:255–261, 2005.

60. Costa AM, Peyrol S, Porto LC, et al. Mechanical forces induce scar remodeling: study in non-pressure-treated versus pressure-treated hypertrophic scars. *Am J Pathol* 155:1671–1679, 1999.

61. Berman B, Maderal A, Raphael B: Keloids and hypertrophic scars: pathophysiology, classification, and treatment. *Dermatol Surg* 43(Suppl 1):S3–S18, 2017. doi:10.1097/DSS.0000000000000819.

62. Sadawi-Konefka R, Watson D: Nonsurgical treatment of keloids and hypterophic scars. *Facial Plast Surg* 35(3):260–266, 2019.

63. Datta I, Ball CG, Rudmik L, et al. Complications related to deep venous thrombosis prophylaxis in trauma: a systematic review of the literature. *J Trauma Manag Outcomes* 4(1), 2010.

64. Brennan MJ, DePompolo RW, Garden FH: Focused review: post-mastectomy lymphedema. *Arch Phys Med Rehabil* 77:S74–S80, 1996.

65. Renò F, Sabbatini M, Lombardi F, et al. In vitro mechanical compression induces apoptosis and regulates cytokines release in hypertrophic scars. *Wound Repair Regen* 11:331–336, 2003.

66. Swedborg I: Effects of treatment with an elastic sleeve and intermittent pneumatic compression in post-mastectomy patients with lymphoedema of the arm. *Scand J Rehabil Med* 26:35–41, 1984.

67. Wright RC, Yacoubian SV: Sequential compression device may cause peroneal nerve palsy. *Orthopedics* 33:444, 2010.

68. McGrory BJ, Burke DW: Peroneal nerve palsy following intermittent sequential pneumatic compression. *Orthopedics* 23:1103–1105, 2000.

69. Rhee SY, Lee SY, HR Jeon: Radial nerve injury caused by compression garment for lymphedema: a case report. *PM R* 11(4):436–439, 2019. doi:10.1016/j.pmrj.2018.09.039.

70. Smith & Nephew: Profore. http://wound.smith-nephew.com/no/Product.asp?NodeId=857. (Accessed August 16, 2006).

71. Hiatt WR: Contemporary treatment of venous lower limb ulcers. *Angiology* 43:852–855, 1992.

72. Partsch H, Damstra RJ, Mosti G: Dose finding for an optimal compression pressure to reduce chronic edema of the extremities. *Int Angiol* 30:527–533, 2011.

73. *The at-a-glance guide to vascular stockings*, Charlotte, NC, 1991, Jobst.

74. Balcombe L, Miller C, McGuiness W: Approaches to the application and removal of compression therapy: a literature review. *Br J Community Nurs* 22(Suppl 10):S6–S14, 2017. doi:10.12968/bjcn.2017.22.Sup10.S6.

75. Jull AB, Mitchell N, Arroll J, et al. Factors influencing concordance with compression stockings after venous leg ulcer healing. *J Wound Care* 13:90–92, 2004.

76. Alpagut U, Dayioglu E: Importance and advantages of intermittent external pneumatic compression therapy in venous stasis ulceration. *Angiology* 56:19–23, 2005.

77. Pilch U, Wozniewski M, Szuba A: Influence of compression cycle time and number of sleeve chambers on upper extremity lymphedema volume reduction during intermittent pneumatic compression. *Lymphology* 42:26–35, 2009.

78. *Lymphoedema Framework: Best practice for the management of lymphoedema, international consensus,* London, 2006, MEP Ltd.

79. Harris SR, Hugi MR, Olivotto IA, et al. Clinical practice guidelines for the care and treatment of breast cancer: lymphedema. *Can Med Assoc J* 164:191–199, 2001.

80. Phillips JJ, Gordon SJ: Intermittent pneumatic compression dosage for adults and children with lymphedema: a systematic review. *Lymphat Res Biol* 17(1):2–18, 2019. doi:10.1089/lrb.2018.0034.

81. Olszewski WL, Jain P, Ambujam G, et al. Tissue fluid pressure and flow during pneumatic compression in lymphedema of lower limbs. *Lymphat Res Biol* 9:77–83, 2011.

82. Pidala MJ, Donovan DL, Kepley RF: A prospective study on intermittent pneumatic compression in the prevention of deep vein thrombosis in patients undergoing total hip or total knee replacement. *Surgery* 175:47–51, 1992.

83. Pekanmaki K, Kolari PJ, Kirstala U: Intermittent pneumatic compression treatment for post-thrombotic leg ulcers. *Clin Exp Dermatol* 12:350–353, 1987.

84. Fife CE, Davey S, Maus EA, et al. A randomized controlled trial comparing two types of pneumatic compression for breast cancer-related lymphedema treatment in the home. *Support Care Cancer* 20:3279–3286, 2012.

Appendix

Units of Measure

Ampere (A): Electrical current; 1 ampere = 1 coulomb per second.

Bar: Pressure; 1 bar = 100,000 pascal, which is slightly less than the average pressure at sea level or roughly the atmospheric pressure on Earth at an altitude of 111 m at 15°C.

Calorie (C): Energy; 1 calorie = energy required to increase the temperature of 1 g of water by 1°C.

Coulomb (C): Electrical charge.

Gauss (G): Magnetic field strength.

Hertz (Hz): Frequency; 1 hertz = 1 cycle per second.

Joule (J): Energy; 1 J = 1W × 1 second.

Ohm (Ω): Electrical resistance; 1 Ω = 1 volt/1 amp.

Pulses per second (pps): Frequency when the events are not cycles.

Volt (V): Electrical potential difference.

Watt (W): Power; 1 W = 1 J/sec.

Watt per centimeter squared (W/cm^2): Intensity.

PREFIXES FOR UNITS

Pico (p): 10^{-12}
Nano (n): 10^{-9}
Micro (μ): 10^{-6}
Milli (m): 10^{-3}
Kilo (K): 10^{3}
Mega (M): 10^{6}
Giga (G): 10^{9}

Commonly Used Abbreviations and Acronyms

AC: Alternating current
ATP: Adenosine triphosphate
BNR: Beam nonuniformity ratio
CNS: Central nervous system
CT: Computed tomography
CVA: Cardiovascular accident (stroke)
DC: Direct current
DOMS: Delayed-onset muscle soreness
DVT: Deep venous thrombosis
ELF: Extremely low frequency (waves)
EMG: Electromyography
ERA: Effective radiating area
ES: Electrical stimulation
ESWT: Extracorporeal shock wave therapy
FES: Functional electrical stimulation
He-Ne: Helium-neon (laser)
HP: Hot pack
HVPC: High-volt pulsed current
ICIDH: International Classification of Impairments, Disabilities, and Handicaps
IP: Ice pack
IR: Infrared
L: Left
LD: Laser diode
LE: Lower extremity
LED: Light-emitting diode
LLLT: Low-level laser therapy
MED: Minimal erythemal dose (for ultraviolet [UV] treatment)
MRI: Magnetic resonance imaging
MVIC: Maximum voluntary isometric contraction
MWD: Microwave diathermy
NDT: Neurodevelopmental training
NMES: Neuromuscular electrical stimulation
OA: Osteoarthritis
PAD: Peripheral artery disease
PC: Pulsed current
PEMF: Pulsed electromagnetic field
PSWD: Pulsed shortwave diathermy
PUVA: Psoralen with ultraviolet A
R: Right
RA: Rheumatoid arthritis
RCT: Randomized controlled trial
RICE: Rest, ice, compression, elevation
ROM: Range of motion
RPW: Radial pressure wave
SLD: Supraluminous diode
SNS: Sympathetic nervous system
SWD: Shortwave diathermy
SWT: Nonthermal shortwave therapy
TENS: Transcutaneous electrical nerve stimulation
UE: Upper extremity
US: Ultrasound
UV: Ultraviolet
#: Pounds

Index

Page numbers followed by "*f*" indicate figures, "*t*" indicate tables, and "*b*" indicate boxes.